T0231053

THE THORAX

Second Edition,
Revised and Expanded
(in three parts)

PART A: PHYSIOLOGY

LUNG BIOLOGY IN HEALTH AND DISEASE

Executive Editor

Claude Lenfant

Director, National Heart, Lung and Blood Institute
National Institutes of Health
Bethesda, Maryland

ADDITIONAL VOLUMES IN PREPARATION

The opinions expressed in these volumes do not necessarily represent the views of the National Institutes of Health.

THE THORAX

Second Edition,
Revised and Expanded
(in three parts)

PART A: PHYSIOLOGY

Edited by

Charis Roussos
National and Kapodistrian
University of Athens Medical School
Athens, Greece

McGill University
Montreal, Quebec, Canada

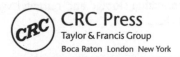

CRC Press
Taylor & Francis Group
Boca Raton London New York

CRC Press is an imprint of the
Taylor & Francis Group, an **informa** business

Library of Congress Cataloging-in-Publication Data

The thorax / edited by Charis Roussos. — 2nd ed., rev. and expanded.
    p.   cm. — (Lung biology in health and disease ; v. 85)
    Contents: pt. A. Physiology — pt. B. Applied physiology — pt. C. Disease.
    ISBN 0-8247-9504-0 (pt. A : alk. paper). — ISBN 0-8247-9600-4 (pt. B : alk. paper).
— ISBN 0-8247-9601-2 (pt. C : alk. paper).
    1. Chest—Diseases. 2. Chest—Muscles. 3. Chest—Physiology. I. Roussos, Charis.
II. Series.
    [DNLM: 1. Thoracic Diseases. 2. Thorax. 3. Respiration.   W1 LU62 v.85 1995 /
WF 970T4877 1995]
RC941.T48   1995
617.5'4—dc20
DNLM/DLC
for Library of Congress   95-32396
                                                                      CIP

The publisher offers discounts on this book when ordered in bulk quantities. For more information, write to Special Sales/Professional Marketing at the address below.

Marcel Dekker, Inc.
270 Madison Avenue, New York, New York 10016

To Ludwig A. Engel,
an example of scientific excellence;
a superb teacher;
an unending source of creativity in research;
a model of strength;
a prototype of dedication and courage;
and our friend.

INTRODUCTION

Although Galen is credited with recognizing that the thorax played some role in moving air in and out of the lungs, it was much later that the function of the thorax was established:

> The lungs do not move naturally of their own motion, but they follow the motion of the thorax and the diaphragm. The lungs are not expanded because they are filled with air, but they are filled with the air because they are expanded.

> *Franciscus Sylvius de la Boe*
> *Opera Medica—1681*

Later physiologists such as the French N. P. Adelon described the thorax as a "cavity situated below the neck but above the abdomen, which contains the heart and the lungs and acts with regard to the latter as a bellows to fill them with air" (Physiologie de l'homme—1831).

It is noteworthy that not until the post-World War II era did a significant research focus on the thorax develop. This occurred essentially because of the compelling need to learn about the mechanics of breathing. Yet, in 1951, Wallace O. Fenn concluded in a review article titled "Mechanics of Respiration" that "At best an outline of the mechanical problems of breathing has been stretched and some possible methods of attack have been suggested for future addition to our knowledge of the subject" (Am. J. Med. 1951; 10).

Exactly 10 years ago Volume 29 of this series of monographs appeared. Charis Roussos and Peter T. Macklem were the editors and its title was *The Thorax*. In the Foreword, E. J. Moran Campbell wrote: "The bibliographies in this book attest to the growth of interest (in the mechanics of breathing) in the last quarter century." The book was in two parts and it included 47 chapters. The average number of references per chapter numbered 50.

This new volume, edited by Charis Roussos, clearly attests to the work that has been done since the first edition. It includes 91 chapters contributed by over 100 authors, and the references number in the thousands. One could say that this three-part book is an encyclopedia of the thorax.

No one, of course, questions that life is inherently tied to the respiratory function that brings oxygen to the tissues. "In some animals air reaches the lung by buccal deglutition that literally pushes it into the lungs as food reaches the stomach. However, in humans, it is because of the action of the thorax that air alternatively enters and exits the lung" (Adelon). In this volume, all the mechanisms of this action in health and disease are described and analyzed in great detail. The editor and the authors have accomplished an extraordinary amount of work to complete this truly landmark book. I am greatly appreciative that they gave me the opportunity to include it in the "Lung Biology in Health and Disease" series.

Claude Lenfant, M.D.

FOREWORD

The second edition of *The Thorax* is a remarkable achievement. I cannot think of an aspect of the respiratory muscles that is not covered. History, anatomy, kinematics, statics, dynamics, energetics, biochemistry, cell and molecular biology, pharmacology, psychophysics, imaging, morphology, patient symptoms, and physical signs are all dealt with—and more. This eclectic approach reflects the current fad in biological research to break a system down into its components, whether they be molecules, forces, strains, vectors, or sensations. The spectacular successes of molecular biology and genetics indicate without a shadow of reservation how successful modern science has been.

Yet reductionism in science, in spite of its successes, has always conflicted with the science that deals with how all the component parts work when they are integrated into a single functioning unit. How the whole works, rather than how each component functions in isolation, also plays a prominent part in *The Thorax*. Indeed, this volume presents a nice balance between reductionist and integrative approaches.

Such a balance is tricky these days. So much of science is molecular that integrative approaches are getting short shrift. Yet understanding of what molecules do in isolation is unlikely to impart understanding (let alone wisdom) of how diseases make human beings sick. Although this book has retained a nice balance, it seems that many of us have been completely seduced by the appeal of molecular science.

Academic clinical department heads appear to have caved into science funding policy so that nowadays a requirement for a full-time position in a subspecialty division is usually expertise in molecular and/or cellular biology.

This is hardly ideal for the teaching and practice of medicine. The science of medicine is above all a study of how molecules and cells within the body function as integrated units; of how disorders can be explained and understood, not as dysfunctions of single molecules or cells but as abnormalities of the *interactions* between many molecules and many cells. *The Thorax* provides state-of-the-art information on interactions and, because it does so, will provide invaluable information to a generation of doctors and scientists who have not been taught how to integrate the individual components of cells, organs, or whole organisms and who, without that knowledge, cannot understand function.

Although the modern physician may have difficulty in coping with the function and dysfunction of whole organisms, it seems likely that the next scientific revolution will be precisely in this area. How complex systems which are never in equilibrium function can now be studied rigorously. Complexity has already given remarkable new insights into Darwinian evolution. The idea that survival of the fittest is limited to systems that can adapt meaningfully means that systems in equilibrium are destined to become extinct because they lack the mechanism for adaptation. Similarly, chaotic systems cannot adapt meaningfully. Thus only systems that function at the edge of order and chaos can survive. Evolution means that all that is living in our universe—ourselves, flora, fauna, and indeed all biological systems—are systems that are neither in equilibrium nor chaotic, but that teeter on the brink between the two.

Teetering on the brink suggests that complex systems may become too ordered or too chaotic. If survival depends on remaining at the border between equilibrium and chaos, then disease is a situation that pushes us into one camp or the other. What determines whether a system is in equilibrium, is chaotic, or functions normally? The answer to this question is profoundly important for the practice of medicine.

Feed-forward systems are important for adaptation; the number of interactions between the nodes of a system is an important determinant of whether the system is chaotic or not; negative feedback loops are essential for homeostasis; sensitivity to initial conditions may determine if a particular environmental insult causes disease or not. These are the parameters that need to be critically examined to determine if a biological system is becoming abnormal because it is approaching equilibrium or because it is becoming chaotic.

The study of complexity is certain to bring remarkable new insights into the mechanisms of disease and new therapeutic interventions. I predict that it will have a profound effect on the practice of medicine—at least as great as the great scientific revolution produced by molecular biology. Nowhere is this more likely to be true than in respiration. The ventilatory mechanisms controlling acid–base balance, oxygen delivery, and CO_2 elimination and which involve complex interactions between receptors, spinal, brainstem, and cortical neural controllers and pathways, respiratory muscles, lungs, and chest wall is obviously a complex system functioning close to, but not in, equilibrium, capable of beneficial adaptations to changing environmental conditions. Thus, understanding of chaotic, complex, and equilibrated systems of respiration is likely to lead to the next major advances in understanding the thorax and the diseases that plague it.

Because it provides an excellent balance between integrative and cellular/molecular approaches, the present volume is well positioned to be an important stepping stone to the newest biology. It gives the basis for understanding respiratory complexity. It should be an essential building block in the construction of the bridge between present-day understanding of disease and the exciting new approaches that students of complexity will bring.

Peter T. Macklem

PREFACE TO THE SECOND EDITION

This first edition of *The Thorax*, published about 10 years ago, was confined to two volumes. Since then, the literature relating to the chest wall has expanded quite rapidly, as indicated by the enormous increase in the size of the reference sections at the end of each chapter. Hence, the second edition consists of three volumes and contains almost double the number of pages of the first edition.

The goal of *The Thorax*, Second Edition, is to provide a comprehensive, authoritative, and contemporary discussion of the physiology (Part A) and pathophysiology (Part B) of the chest wall as well as an overview of the diagnostic and therapeutic modalities (Part C). It also identifies those areas of the field that need further research and investigation. This book will be an invaluable aid to clinical investigators by providing answers to basic questions and helping them gain a better understanding of clinical problems, areas of controversy, and lacunae of knowledge. Hopefully, this will stimulate further research efforts.

The Thorax, Second Edition, was completed with the help of over 125 authors. As in the first edition, contributors were selected based on their knowledge of and expertise in their respective fields. Thus, whether clinicians or scientists, they are at the forefront of their disciplines, and are undoubtedly in the best position to analyze and summarize information and debate controversial issues. The geographical diversity of contributors is striking—Argentina, Australia, Belgium, Canada, England, Finland, France, Greece, Italy, Sweden, and the United States—and reflects the international interest in advancing our knowledge of the function and dysfunction of the chest wall. I believe that these contributors have given the book a lively flavor, making it very up to date and comprehensive, while putting the future of the field in both realistic and exciting perspective.

The first volume, Part A, updates information on the striated muscles and briefly and lucidly relates it to the respiratory muscles. Thus, Chapters 1–12 lead smoothly to the complex subsequent chapters on mechanics and energetics (Chapters 13–25) and control (Chapters 26–34) of respiratory muscles. The second volume, Part B, deals extensively with the methods of measurement of chest wall function. It points out to researchers areas that need further investigation and illustrates to clinicians the pitfalls and limitations of each method (Chapters 35–44). This volume also discusses the relation between the chest wall and commonplace activities or conditions such as speech, dyspnea, exercise, diving, and anesthesia, to mention a few (Chapters 45–60). Thus the significant role that the thorax plays in various physiological and pathological conditions is explained. The third volume, Part C, focuses on disease states. Chapters 61–65 deal with the methods of diagnosis by which to establish the normality or dysfunction of the chest wall. These chapters try to offer as much practical information to the clinician as possible. Chapters 66–76 describe the pathophysiology of the respiratory muscles and the chest wall as a whole in various clinical conditions. Finally, Chapters 77–91 describe the therapeutic approaches necessary to improve the function of the ventilatory pump in various disease states. Some overlap between the chapters was encouraged which allowed for an uninterrupted flow of thoughts and helped to achieve the detailed coverage of the topics.

This book would have been impossible to produce without the help of all the distinguished authors to whom I am profoundly indebted, not only for their contributions but for their support when I began my new position at the University of Athens Medical School. During this interesting period of creativity, they helped mature my thinking through animated discussions. I am grateful to Miss M. Titcomb for her excellent secretarial assistance and cooperation, and I thank my colleagues at Evangelismos Hospital of Athens for creating an environment that, despite the sometimes insurmountable administrative difficulties, has been conducive to scholarly work. Finally, I am most grateful to my family—Alexandra, Konstantinos, and Katerina—for their forbearance during these interesting years, for sharing my excitement, and for supporting me during periods of fatigue.

Charis Roussos

PREFACE TO THE FIRST EDITION

It is only somewhat belatedly that chest physicians have begun to focus their attention on the chest wall. Physiologists have continued their interest since at least the time of Hippocrates, but physicians have mostly avoided the role of the chest wall except when it was obviously involved in diseases such as flail chest, kyphoscoliosis, or neuromuscular disorders.

However, just as hypertension can lead to congestive heart failure, the chest wall can also malfunction due to disorders that are external to it. Lung disease can put such a load on the chest wall muscles and low cardiac output states can sufficiently impair their supply, that they may fail to develop the respiratory pressure swings required for normal alveolar ventilation. It is this growing awareness that is leading chest physicians to become more interested in the chest wall aspect of respiratory disease. Furthermore, chest wall disorders offer new possibilities for treatment, even though the external disorders cannot be effectively reversed. Indeed, a substantial number of chest physicians think that the most crippling aspects of respiratory disease, namely, shortness of breath and hypercapnic respiratory failure, arise from disordered chest wall function and not from the lung.

Thus this book attempts to gather the essence of this timely topic: the function and dysfunction of the chest wall. It is meant to provide a comprehensive view of the physiology and pathophysiology of the chest wall with an overview of the various therapeutic modalities presently available. In its own right, this book is not simply a resumé of current information, but contains several chapters of original scientific contribution. Our aim is not only to describe the burgeoning wealth of information which has accumulated, but also to emphasize what remains unsolved, thereby stimulating further research in this domain.

We are also attempting, as implied by the title, to restore the original meaning of the word "thorax." Most chest physicians equate "thorax" with rib cage. As one of us points out, this is not in accord with its original meaning in ancient Greek. At that time, "thorax" meant "chest wall" and this is how we use the term in this book. We hope our readers will also restore the original meaning to the word "thorax."

During the period needed to produce this book, the infusion of new knowledge continued unabated and new concepts evolved, rendering this work an editorial challenge, but also, we hope, a gratifying scientific contribution.

Charis Roussos
Peter T. Macklem

PROLOGUE
THE THORAX THROUGH
HISTORY INTO MEDICINE

The *Gould Medical Dictionary* defines the term "thorax" as

> The chest. The portion of the trunk above the diaphragm and below the neck. The framework of bones and soft tissues bounded by the diaphragm below: the ribs and the sternum in the front; the ribs and the thoracic portion of the vertebral column behind; above, by the structures in the lower part of the neck; and containing the heart enclosed in pericardium, the lungs invested by the pleura and mediastinal structures.

Clearly, in this definition, the thorax is equivalent to the chest that is also defined in Gould as "the earliest form of container for storing clothes, documents, valuables and other possessions."

It is obvious from the above description that, in the English medical literature, the concept of the term thorax is that of a container along with its contents, i.e., a chest. The Greek word thorax, though, did not always have this meaning. Its conceptual transformation as it passed from Greek into English exemplifies some interesting problems in the history of medicine: for one, how common words are transformed into medical terms, and also how knowledge is transferred from one language to another.

As French (1978) points out in his scholarly review "The Thorax in History," early scholars encountered many difficulties in the transmission of anatomical knowledge from one language to another. The original language presented a technical term which was made clear by the descriptive content, but no corresponding term of sufficient accuracy existed in the language receiving the word. The scholars then had to invent an analogous term which reflected at the same time their understanding of the function of the organ. This problem, as it relates to the history of medicine, is illustrated by the various translations of the term thorax into many different languages—like *clibanus* (oven), a term denoting the rigidity of the thorax as a heat-containing structure holding the heat-producing heart (from a Latin translation of Galen's work, *On the Usefulness of Parts*) or like chest (container) in English.

It is my intention, in this historical search, to credit to the term thorax its original meaning, thus to justify its usage in the title of the present monograph. I will try to trace the word from its earliest beginnings, even before it entered the Greek language, and follow it in its long journey through many centuries of Greek history and cultural evolution. At the crossroads of culture and medicine, I will follow the word as it became a medical term, up to the point where it acquired its present meaning. The search for these roots is aided by the memories of this journey to be found in the nonmedical usage of the word thorax in modern Greek language.

Etymologically, thorax is a word probably of Sanskritic origin and it entered the Greek language very early. It is believed to be derived from the words *dharaka*, *dhara*, *dharahma*, which mean receptacle or vessel and also holding, supporting, life-bearing, containing, maintaining, and protecting. In its transition into the Greek language, thorax retained protection as its primary meaning. Thus, thorax came to signify a wall-like device placed externally around vulnerable parts of the body, of a ship or a city for the purpose of their fortification and therefore protection (Herodotus, Book I).

The use of the word thorax to mean the protective wall of the life-supporting organs of the body, that is, the heart, lungs, and intestines, dates back at least as far as the epic poems of Homer, written in the 8th century B.C. Homer wrote in the *Iliad* about a war between the Trojans and the Greeks which allegedly took place in 1180 B.C. In his vivid descriptions, he referred to the thorax, meaning a leather or copper cover which protected the chest of soldiers. Thorax meant corset, ciurass, breastplate to the Homeric Greeks.

As Greek culture became more sophisticated and advanced and blacksmiths improved and expanded their skills, we find descriptions of more elaborate thoraces. Unlike those of the Homeric Greeks, these later thoraces did not stop at the waistline but covered the whole trunk. Alcaeus, a lyric poet of the 7th century B.C., referred to thoraces using the descriptive adjectives of "complex and elaborate." In another poem he referred to the price of the thorax, implying that the thorax was no longer the simple copper or leather armor of the soldier, but a piece of equipment that reflected the wealth and status of its bearer. There are abundant descriptions of thoraces as armor by other ancient Greek authors too. Herodotus talked about laminated and squamous (scale-bearing) thoraces (Herodotus, Books II and IX), and Pausanias of a thorax consisting of a coat of mail or chain mail.

The 5th century witnessed significant progress and evolution in the Greek culture. It ushered in the classical period of ancient Greece and saw giants of philosophy, art, and science. The Ionian philosophy, based on observation, reached a peak and man started to observe and study his own body very carefully. This meant that he needed new words to name the new concepts and the parts of the body according to their function. Around this time the meaning of thorax undergoes a two-step transformation.

In the first phase, the armor—the thorax—which had until now protected the internal organs from the anterior like a wall, becomes incorporated into the new knowledge of the body structure and function. In this process it moves into the interior and gives its name to the anatomy of the very body structures it used to cover, thus becoming the chest wall. The change in the meaning of the word is reflected in one of the plays of Aristophanes, one of the wittiest Greek writers, who used the word thorax in a pun. In his play *Wasps*, he described a duel and commented on the strength of the "thorax" of the winner. When one of the listeners remarked that fighters were not allowed to wear "thoraces" in this type of a duel, the narrator explained that "thorax" meant the chest wall of the fighter, not his breastplate.

In the second phase we witness a further transformation of the term. As the medical interest during this period gravitates toward the internal organs, the anatomical thorax is losing its exclusive meaning as a wall and by generalization it comes to signify both the wall and the cavity enclosed by this wall. In other words, the conceptualization of the structure termed "thorax" is shifting toward that of a chest. The limits, though, of this chest remain ambiguous, as the meaning of thorax as armor remains vivid in the memory of Greek scientists and philosophers.

Each author defines the boundaries of the thorax according to the shield wall he is referring to (it is interesting to note that the same ambiguity about the precise demarcation of the boundaries of the chest wall is to be found among scientists even to the present day). Evidence of this new evolution of the meaning of the word thorax is to be found in both the writings of Plato, who used the word with its colloquial meaning, and the scientific works of Hippocrates and Aristotle.

Plato in *Timaeus* described the hierarchy of the functions of the human body and related them to the hierarchy of values of human life. In his description of the body, he mentioned that the "cavity of the Thorax" is divided into the upper part over the diaphragm, which contains the heart, and the lower part below the diaphragm, which contains the intestines.

The official entrance of the term into medicine came with Hippocrates, the Father of Medicine. For him the boundaries of the bodily thorax coincided with those of the armor thorax. In his book *The Art*, he describes the thorax as the cavity in which the liver is covered, that is, the trunk.

Aristotle was one of the most germinal minds of antiquity and he became the founder of the scientific thinking of the Western world. It is interesting to note the ambiguity that exists in his writings vis-à-vis the definition of thorax. In his work *Problems*, he differentiates between thorax and abdomen as he refers to the three regions of the body, that is, the head, the thorax (chest), and the stomach. In his *History of Animals*, in the same chapter, he uses the term thorax interchangeably to define both the chest and the trunk. So we first read that the thorax (chest) has a back and a front . . . next after the thorax in front is the belly, and further down he says that the penis is situated externally at the base of the thorax (trunk). In *Parts of Animals*, the thorax is described as extending from the head to the "residual vent."

Medicine as the science we know today started with Galen, the famous Greek physician, the founder of experimental physiology. Using vivisections and dissections as the Egyptians had done centuries before him, he gained a fine knowledge of anatomy and physiology. Galen was a rigorous scientist and, as he was forced to make up medical terminology from common words, he was very careful to define his new terms precisely. An example of this is the definition of thorax. In his *The Usefulness of Parts* we read "all that cavity bounded by the ribs on both sides, extending to the sternum and the diaphragm in front and curving down to the spine in the rear is customarily called Thorax by the physician." It is worth noting how similar this definition is to the one in the *Gould Medical Dictionary*.

Thorax has never become exclusively a medical term in the Greek language, thus it never lost its primary meaning of fortified protective wall. Through the centuries we find the term thorax used figuratively to mean armor or breastplate in the Hellenic Greek of the New Testament. In Paul, we read about the thorax (breastplate) of love and faith. In the contemporary common Greek language thorax means fortified wall [hence the medical term *pneumothorax*, meaning a wall of air around the lungs] and the verb "thorakizo" or "to install a thorax" means to apply external fortification around ships, cars, etc. in the form of armor.

We have now reached the modern era and we find the term thorax once more at the crossroads of history and medicine, at least in the conscience of a Greek scientist, the editor of the present monograph. As it was pointed out in the present search, thorax has maintained the meaning of a protective fortified wall for 30 centuries of Greek culture and history. In medicine the term thorax gradually lost its original meaning when the concept of the chest wall as a vital organ failed to be recognized, thus rendering its symbol "the thorax" void of meaning. Currently, though, we observe new developments in respiratory physiology and medicine with the chest wall becoming the subject of rigorous scientific research. History and medicine thus have met, as "thorax," the old symbol of the fortified wall, is acquiring substance again. Medicine is restoring to the chest wall its appropriate significance. The editor is attempting to do so by giving the title *The Thorax* to the present monograph, the subject matter of which is precisely the chest wall, restoring thus the original meaning to this ancient term.

References

Alcaeus 15, *Codicus Atheneaus*, 1123.560, 11.374, 4.136.
Aristophanes, *Wasps*, 1194.
Aristotle, *History of Animals*, Book I, 493a, 10 and 493a, 25.
Aristotle, *Parts of Animals*, Book IV, 686b, 5.
Aristotle, *Problems*, Book XXXIII, 962a, 35.
French, R. K. (1978). The thorax in history. *Thorax* 33.
Galen, *On the Usefulness of Parts*, Book VI, 300.
Blakiston's Gould Medical Dictionary.
Herodotus, Book I, 181.
Herodotus, Book II, 182.
Herodotus, Book IX, 22.
Hippocrates, *The Art*, Book X, 10.
Homer, *Iliad*, 4.133, 5.99, 11.234, 15.529.
Paul, *Ephesians* 6.14.
Pausanias, Book I, 21.6.
Plato, *Timaeus*, 69.E.

Charis Roussos

CONTRIBUTORS TO PART A: PHYSIOLOGY

Emilio Agostoni, M.D. Professor and Chairman, First Institute of Human Physiology, University of Milan, Milan, Italy

David G. Allen, M.D. Ph.D., Professor, Department of Physiology, University of Sydney, Sydney, New South Wales, Australia

A. Anzueto Case Western Reserve University and Metrohealth Medical Center, Cleveland, Ohio

Robert B. Banzett, Ph.D. Associate Professor, Department of Environmental Health, Harvard School of Public Health; and Department of Medicine, Harvard Medical School, Boston, Massachusetts

Susan V. Brooks, Ph.D. Research Fellow, Institute of Gerontology, University of Michigan, Ann Arbor, Michigan

Shirley H. Bryant, Ph.D. Professor, Department of Pharmacology and Cell Biophysics, University of Cincinnati College of Medicine, Cincinnati, Ohio

xxi

Alain S. Comtois, Ph.D. FRSQ Scholar, Adjunct Professor, Centre de Recherche Louis-Charles Sinard, University of Montreal, Hôpital Notre-Dame, Montreal, Quebec, Canada

Edgardo D'Angelo, M.D. Professor of Physiology, First Institute of Human Physiology, University of Milan, Milan, Italy

J. Andrew Daubenspeck, Ph.D. Professor, Department of Physiology, Dartmouth Medical School, Lebanon, New Hampshire

Paul W. Davenport, Ph.D. Professor, Department of Physiological Sciences, University of Florida, Gainesville, Florida

Jean-Philippe Derenne Professor, Department of Pneumology and Intensive Care, Groupe Hospitalier Pitié-Salpêtrière, Paris, France

André De Troyer, M.D., Ph.D. Professor of Medicine, Chest Service, Erasme University Hospital, and Director, Laboratory of Cardiorespiratory Physiology, Brussels School of Medicine, Brussels, Belgium

Thomas E. Dick, Ph.D. Associate Professor, Division of Pulmonary and Critical Care, Department of Medicine, Case Western Reserve University, Cleveland, Ohio

Norman H. Edelman, M.D. Dean and Professor of Medicine, University of Medicine and Dentistry of New Jersey, Robert Wood Johnson Medical School, New Brunswick, New Jersey

Richard H. T. Edwards, Ph.D., F.R.C.P. Professor, Department of Medicine, University of Liverpool, Liverpool, England

Alexandre Fabiato, M.D., Ph.D. Professor, Department of Physiology, Medical College of Virginia, Virginia Commonwealth University, Richmond, Virginia

John A. Faulkner, Ph.D. Professor of Physiology, Institute of Gerontology, University of Michigan, Ann Arbor, Michigan

Robert S. Fitzgerald, Litt. B., S.T.B., M.A., S.T.M., Ph.D. Professor, Departments of Environmental Health Sciences, Physiology, and Medicine, The Johns Hopkins Medical Institutions, Baltimore, Maryland

John T. Hackett, Ph.D. Professor, Department of Molecular Physiology and Biological Physics, University of Virginia Health Sciences Center, Charlottesville, Virginia

David A. Hood, B.P.H.E., M.Sc., Ph.D. Associate Professor, Department of Physical Education, York University, North York, Ontario, Canada

Sandra Howell, Ph.D. Associate Professor, Departments of Biokinesiology and Biomedical Engineering, University of Southern California, Los Angeles, California

Sabah N. A. Hussain, M.D., Ph.D. Associate Professor, Department of Medicine, McGill University, Montreal, Quebec, Canada

C. David Ianuzzo, Ph.D. Professor of Biology and Physical Education, York University, North York, Ontario, Canada

Yves Jammes Professor of Physiology and Chairman, Laboratoire de Physiopathologie Respiratoire, Faculty of Medicine, Institut Jean Roche, Marseille, France

David A. Jones, B.Sc., Ph.D. Professor; Head, School of Sport and Exercise Sciences, The University of Birmingham, Birmingham, England

Steven G. Kelsen, M.D. Professor of Medicine and Physiology, Director of Research, Division of Pulmonary and Critical Care Medicine, Temple University School of Medicine, Philadelphia, Pennsylvania

Jan Lännergren, M.D., Ph.D. Associate Professor, Division of Physiology II, Department of Physiology and Pharmacology, Karolinska Institute, Stockholm, Sweden

Ann M. Leevers, M.Sc., Ph.D. Assistant Professor, Department of Anatomy and Cell Biology, Queen's University, Kingston, Ontario, Canada

Stephen H. Loring, M.D. Scientific Director of Respiratory Therapy, Department of Anesthesia and Critical Care, Beth Israel Hospital; and Associate Professor of Anesthesia, Harvard Medical School, Boston, Massachusetts

Peter T. Macklem, O.C., M.D., F.R.S.(C). Scientific Director, Respiratory Health Network of Centres of Excellence; Professor of Medicine, McGill University, Montreal, Quebec, Canada

Jere Mead, M.D. Cecil K. and Philip Drinker Professor of Environmental Physiology, Emeritus, Respiratory Biology Program, Department of Environmental Science and Physiology, Harvard School of Public Health, Boston, Massachusetts

Joseph Milic-Emili, C.M., M.D., F.R.S.C. Professor of Physiology; Director, Meakins-Christie Laboratories, Department of Medicine, McGill University, Montreal, Quebec, Canada

Jacopo P. Mortola, M.D. Professor, Department of Physiology, McGill University, Montreal, Quebec, Canada

Dennis Gordon Osmond, B.Sc., M.B., Ch.B., D.Sc. Robert Redford Professor of Anatomy and Chair, Department of Anatomy and Cell Biology, McGill University, Montreal, Quebec, Canada

W. Robert Revelette, M.D., Ph.D. Resident and Associate Professor (Adjunct), Departments of Pediatrics and Physiology, University of Kentucky, Lexington, Kentucky

Jeremy David Road, B.Sc., M.D., F.R.C.P.(C) Associate Professor, Department of Medicine, University of British Columbia, Vancouver, British Columbia, Canada

Dudley F. Rochester, M.D. Professor Emeritus, Pulmonary and Critical Care Division, Department of Medicine, University of Virginia Health Sciences Center, Charlottesville, Virginia

Charis Roussos, M.D., M.Sc., Ph.D., M.R.S., F.R.C.P.(C) Professor of Medicine, Critical Care Department and Thoracic Unit, National and Kapodistrian University of Athens Medical School, Athens, Greece; and Professor of Medicine, McGill University, Montreal, Quebec, Canada

Anthony T. Scardella, M.D. Associate Professor, Department of Medicine, University of Medicine and Dentistry of New Jersey, Robert Wood Johnson Medical School, New Brunswick, New Jersey

Gary C. Sieck, Ph.D. Professor of Physiology and Molecular Neuroscience, Departments of Anesthesiology and Physiology and Biophysics, Mayo Medical School and Mayo Foundation, Rochester, Minnesota

Jeffrey C. Smith, Ph.D. Associate Professor, Department of Physiological Sciences, University of California, Los Angeles, California

Nicholas Sperelakis, Ph.D. The Joseph Eichberg Professor of Physiology and Biophysics, Department of Molecular and Cellular Physiology, University of Cincinnati College of Medicine, Cincinnati, Ohio

Gerald S. Supinski, M.D. Associate Professor, Case Western Reserve University and Division of Pulmonary and Critical Care Medicine, Metrohealth Medical Center, Cleveland, Ohio

Janusz B. Suszkiw, Ph.D. Professor, Department of Molecular and Cellular Physiology, University of Cincinnati College of Medicine, Cincinnati, Ohio

Erik van Lunteren, M.D. Associate Professor, Pulmonary and Critical Care Medicine, Case Western Reserve University, Cleveland, Ohio

Nina K. Vøllestad, Ph.D. Senior Research Scientist, Department of Physiology, National Institute of Occupational Health, Oslo, Norway

Michael E. Ward, M.D., Ph.D. Assistant Professor, Critical Care Division, Department of Medicine, McGill University, Montreal, Quebec, Canada

Håkan Westerblad, M.D., Ph.D. Associate Professor, Division of Physiology II, Department of Physiology and Pharmacology, Karolinska Institute, Stockholm, Sweden

William A. Whitelaw Professor, Department of Medicine, University of Calgary, Calgary, Alberta, Canada

Spyros Zakynthinos, M.D. Assistant Professor, Critical Care Department, Evangelismos Hospital, Athens, Greece

CONTENTS OF PART A: PHYSIOLOGY

PART I PROPERTIES OF STRIATED AND RESPIRATORY MUSCLES

A cumulative index appears in Part C.

CONTENTS OF PART B: APPLIED PHYSIOLOGY

CONTENTS OF PART C: DISEASE

THE THORAX

*Second Edition,
Revised and Expanded
(in three parts)*

PART A: PHYSIOLOGY

Part I

PROPERTIES OF STRIATED AND RESPIRATORY MUSCLES

1

Skeletal Muscle Physiology
Structure, Biomechanics, and Biochemistry

DAVID A. JONES

School of Sport and Exercise Sciences
The University of Birmingham
Birmingham, England

I. Introduction

Although respiratory muscles, and especially the diaphragm, are sometimes spoken of as being distinct from skeletal muscle, this is a false impression. As far as is known, the biochemistry and physiology of the respiratory muscles are the same as any skeletal muscle, and the only distinguishing features are possibly their anatomy and patterns of use. Consequently, the following review describes the basic structure, physiology, and biochemistry of a variety of human and animal muscles, few of which are specifically respiratory muscles.

Skeletal muscle is one of the tissues in which the molecular basis of function is best understood, and an appreciation of the size and shape of the key molecules and the way they are arranged in the muscle fiber is an important prerequisite for understanding the physiology. This chapter ends with a discussion of the way in which energy is provided to the locomotor skeletal muscle during a marathon; at first sight, this may seem to have little relevance to respiratory muscle. However, it should be remembered that together with the heart, the respiratory muscles are continually active throughout life, with bursts of high activity from time to time when we cough, sing, or exercise. As such, the provision of energy for this demanding schedule is of the greatest importance.

II. The Contractile Apparatus

Deliberate movement is one of the features that separates animal from plant life and, clearly, the contractile proteins play an important role in this process.

Nevertheless, contractile proteins, especially actin, are found in all types of cells, being responsible for protoplasmic streaming and the movement of intracellular organelles. Actin is a protein of great antiquity and is highly conserved in the sense that actins from animal and plant cells are functionally and immunologically very similar. Skeletal and cardiac muscle are unusual, not so much for possessing actin and myosin, but for their particularly high content (about 80% of the total protein) and for having these two proteins arranged in a highly ordered array within the cell, permitting the controlled generation of force and movement.

A. Actin

Actin is a globular protein (G-actin), with a relative molecular mass (M_r) of 42,000, that polymerizes into what appears to be double-helical strands (F-actin) (see Cohen and Vibert, 1987, for a general review). The polymerization of actin involves splitting ATP and the binding of ADP. About 90% of the ADP in muscle is bound to actin.

Tropomyosin and the three troponin subunits, TnC, TnT, and TnI, form the other constituents of the thin filaments (Fig. 1). The tropomyosin extends over seven actin subunits and blocks the myosin-binding sites until caused to move by calcium binding to troponin C.

The actin filaments join at one end to form the Z-line structure. At the Z line the actin filaments are in a square array, with each thin filament in one-half sarcomere being linked to four other filaments in the next half sarcomere. The protein α-actinin forms the connections between the actin filaments (Franzini-Armstrong, 1973).

In fast muscles, the linkage is quite simple, giving a thin Z line, whereas in slow fibers, there may be several connections between the two sets of thin filaments, giving a thicker Z line.

B. Myosin

Myosin molecules consist of two identical chains, each with an M_r of approximately 200,000, together with four light chains each of about 20,000 M_r (Fig. 2; see Knight

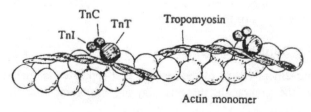

Figure 1   Part of an actin filament together with tropomyosin and the troponin subunits.

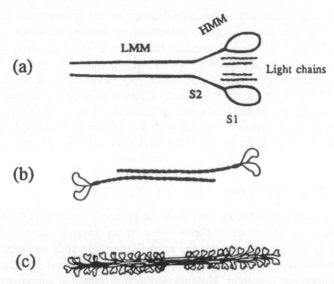

Figure 2 Myosin structure and assembly into thick filaments. (a) Schematic arrangement of myosin subunits; (b, c) the basic double-headed myosin units aggregating to form a thick filament.

and Trinick, 1987, for a general review). In mollusk muscle, the myosin light chains have a clear regulatory role, binding calcium and controlling the activity of myosin. Mammalian light chains can substitute for mollusk light chains, demonstrating that they have functional potential, but no unequivocal role for these proteins has yet been found in mammalian muscle. The composition of the light chains differs between fast and slow muscles.

The myosin molecule can be split enzymatically into various fragments. The globular head, or S1 fragment, contains the enzymic activity and is the portion that can combine with actin. The S2 portion is a flexible region of the molecule, whereas the tail (light meromyosin; LMM) combines with other tails, binding the myosin molecules together to form the *thick filaments*. Thick filaments consist of approximately 300 molecules arranged so that the myosin heads are pointing in one direction, at one end of the filament, and in the opposite direction, at the other end. Consequently, there is a region in the center of each filament where there are only tails and no projecting heads, constituting about 10% of the total length. The thick filaments are very uniform in length throughout the animal kingdom (Offer, 1987).

The thick myosin filaments are arranged so that the thin actin filaments, attached to the Z lines, can slide between. The unit from Z line-to-Z line is known as a sarcomere and, in mammalian muscle held at a resting length in the body, is between 2 and 2.5 μm long. Each thick filament is surrounded by six thin filaments. At the Z lines the thin filaments are held in a square array, whereas in the overlap region they are forced into a hexagonal array by the arrangement of the thick filaments. The thin filaments must, therefore, be somewhat flexible and, in the I-band region where there is no overlap, they have a no regular array (Fig. 3; see Squire et al., 1987, for a general review of the myofibril structure).

The nomenclature of the various bands in a sarcomere is shown in Figure 3. The A and I bands are so called because of their birefringent properties under the light microscope, the I band being *i*sotropic and the A band *a*nisotropic. The area in the A band where there is no overlap with thin filaments is known as the H zone, in the center of which is the region of the thick filaments bare of projecting myosin heads.

C. Structural Proteins

There are a variety of proteins for which the probable function is to maintain the architecture of the sarcomere. Proteins in the M line keep the myosin filaments in the correct spatial arrangement for the actin filaments to slide between them. The thick filaments have a banded appearance, which is enhanced by staining with a specific antibody to C protein. The function of this protein is unknown, but it may be involved in the aggregation of the myosin monomers and regulation of thick filament length.

Titin is an extremely long protein molecule (about 1 μm) that links the myosin filaments to the Z line. The value of such a connection is to keep the A band located in the center of the sarcomere at times when the sarcomere is stretched to lengths at which there is little or no overlap of the thick and thin filaments. Nebulin is another very large protein found associated with actin near the Z line, but the function of which is not known.

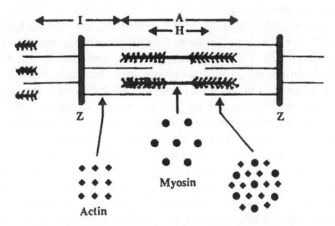

Figure 3   The arrangement of thick and thin filaments to form a sarcomere. Below: cross sections of the sarcomere.

α-Actinin forms part of the Z-line structure, binding the actin filaments together, and *desmin* links the Z lines of adjacent myofibrils, serving to keep the Z lines in register. *Spectrin* and *dystrophin* are proteins that probably have a structural role in the surface membrane of the muscle fiber, the latter being of great current interest because its absence gives rise to the muscular dystrophies.

D. The Myofibril

Bundles of 100–400 thick filaments form *myofibrils* that are separated from one another by sarcoplasmic reticulum, T tubules (see later), and sometimes mitochondria. Myofibrils vary in size, but average about 1 μm in diameter and make up about 80% of the volume of a muscle fiber. The numbers of myofibrils vary with the size of the muscle fiber and can be as few as 50 in a developing fetal muscle fiber, but about 2000 myofibrils in an adult muscle fiber.

E. Sarcoplasmic Reticulum

Each myofibril is enveloped in a complex membranous bag, the interior of which is quite separate from the cytoplasm of the fiber (Fig. 4). The membrane system is known as the sarcoplasmic reticulum and acts as a store for the uptake and release of calcium (Peachey, 1965). The portions near the T tubules are known as the terminal cisternae. In fast muscle fibers the sarcoplasmic reticulum may surround each myofibril, but in slower fibers the membrane system is less well developed (Eisenberg, 1983).

F. T-Tubular System

The plasma membrane of the muscle fiber invaginates to form a complex tubular system, which forms a branching network running across the whole fiber and contacting every myofibril.

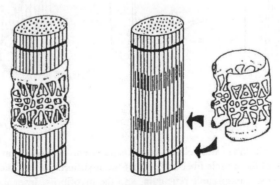

Figure 4 The sarcoplasmic reticulum envelops a myofibril.

In mammalian muscle, the invaginations of the surface membrane occur twice in every sarcomere, approximately at the level of the junction of the A and I bands (Fig. 5).

Where the T tubules meet the sarcoplasmic reticulum the two membranes are closely applied, and electron-dense "feet" have been described linking the two sets of membranes.

In electron micrograph sections, the T tubules are often seen cut in cross section with a potion of the sarcoplasmic reticulum on either side: this is known as a *triad*. When associated with sarcoplasmic reticulum in a triad, the T tubule is flattened, otherwise it tends to be circular in cross section. The lumen of a T tubule is continuous with the extracellular space, but is separated from the interior of the sarcoplasmic reticulum, even though the two membrane systems are in close approximation.

III.   Muscle Organization

Each muscle fiber is bounded by its sarcolemma. The innermost portion of the sarcolemma is the plasma membrane, which is the true boundary of the cell. Outside the plasma membrane is the basement membrane, which is not a membrane in the usually accepted sense of the word in that it does not have a lipid bilayer structure, but is composed of a loose glycoprotein and collagen network. It is freely permeable

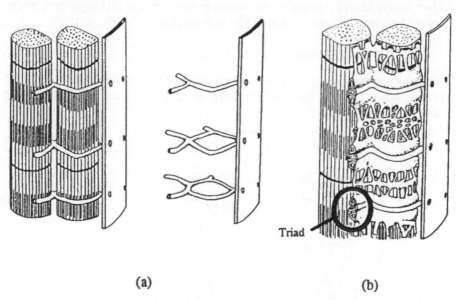

(a)   (b)

Figure 5   (a) The T tubules in relation to the sarcomere. T tubules invaginate from the surface membrane of the muscle fiber and contact the myofibrils at the junction of the A and I band. (b) T tubules, sarcoplasmic reticulum, and the myofibrils. Inset shows the structure of a triad.

and may surround more than one fiber. Following muscle fiber damage, the basement membrane forms a framework within which regeneration occurs.

Adult muscle fibers vary considerably in size and length among various muscles in the body and among persons of different sex, build, and age. Fiber length varies greatly, from a few millimeters in the ciliary muscles of the eye to 10 cm or more in the sartorius, a long, straplike muscle in the inner thigh.

At the ends of a muscle fiber, the outer membranes become irregular and indented to form a close link with the connective tissue. The connective tissue elements all come together to form the tendons, which join the muscle to the bony skeleton.

Between the muscle fibers are fibroblasts that secrete collagen fibers to form a thin connective tissue matrix, the endomysium. Groups of 10–100 muscle fibers are surrounded by a thicker layer of connective tissue, the perimysium, to form fascicles (Fig. 6). Fibroblasts, and their major product collagen, play an important role for maintaining the structure of a muscle, and they may help maintain the environment within which the contractile muscle fiber can function.

Small blood vessels and motor axons traverse the perimysial spaces to make connections with the muscle fibers. Muscle spindles are also found enclosed in connective tissue envelopes in the perimysium. Each muscle is covered by a thick outer connective tissue layer, the epimysium.

IV. Size of Adult Muscle

The number of fibers in each human muscle is probably set by 24 weeks of gestation. In the rat, fiber numbers do not change during life, whereas the mean fiber cross-

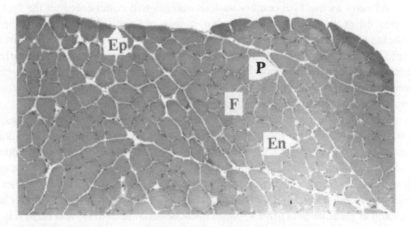

Figure 6 Transverse section through a portion of mouse skeletal muscle. Light microscope; section stained with hematoxylin and eosin. F, fascicle; En, endomysium; P, perimysium; Ep, epimysium.

sectional area increases nearly tenfold from the newborn to adult animal (Rowe and Goldspink, 1969). There are considerable practical and ethical problems involved in making measurements of fiber size and number in children and adults, but the limited data available suggest that there is an increase in size, without a change in fiber numbers (hypertrophy without hyperplasia) as the muscles grow in size and strength. Adult muscle fiber cross-sectional areas are reached shortly after puberty. In an adult man, about 40–45% of the body weight is muscle, and this figure is slightly lower in females. The mean cross-sectional area of fibers in a biopsy from the quadriceps muscle in a normal man is about 3500–7500 μm^2 and, in normal women, 2000–5000 μm^2.

V.   The Motor Unit

In a mature muscle, one motoneuron will, through its axonal branches, supply several fibers scattered throughout the muscle. In a healthy muscle, the innervation is almost entirely random, and adjacent fibers are most likely to be supplied by branches from different motoneurons. All the muscle fibers supplied by one motoneuron form a *motor unit*. Within a single muscle, there is a range of motor unit size, the number and type of fibers in each depending on the function of the motoneuron. The large, high-threshold motoneurons support large motor units, whereas the small low-threshold motoneurons support small units.

The number of fibers constituting a motor unit varies from muscle to muscle and may be as few as ten fibers in a small hand muscle, to several thousand in a large muscle such as the quadriceps. The number of fibers depends not only on the size of the muscle, but also on its function. The finer the control of movement required, the smaller will be the size of the motor units.

As early as the 17th century various authors had commented on the fact that muscles differ in their appearance, but it was not until 1873, that the French physician and physiologist Ranvier recognized that skeletal muscles differ not only in color, some being dark red, others almost white, but that they also have different contractile properties. For example, the soleus muscle at the back of the lower leg is red in appearance and is slow, whereas the extensor digitorum longus, a white muscle at the front of the leg, contracts and relaxes rapidly.

Various histochemical stains are used to identify different fiber types, the most commonly used are the myosin ATPase, with preincubation at either alkaline or acid pH; a marker of mitochondrial activity, such as NADH tetrazolium reductase or succinic dehydrogenase; and a marker of glycolytic activity, with myophosphorylase being the most commonly measured activity. Three main types of fiber can be distinguished. Type I (slow, oxidative) have a low myosin ATPase activity when measured at alkaline pH (pH 9.4), high mitochondrial activities, and relatively low glycolytic enzyme activities. The type II fibers (fast, glycolytic) stain darkly with the myosin ATPase at pH 9.4 and have high levels of glycolytic enzymes, but lower mitochondrial contents, than the type I fibers (Fig. 7). The type II fibers are

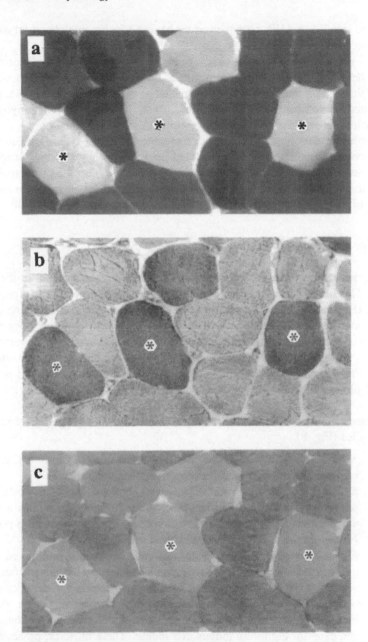

Figure 7 Histochemical stains: Serial sections of human quadriceps muscle stained for (a) myosin ATPase, pH 9.4; (b) mitochondrial enzyme activity (NADH tetrazolium reductase); (c) glycolytic enzyme activity (phosphorylase). Note the same three type I fibers marked (*) in each section.

subdivided into IIA and IIB, with the former having a higher mitochondrial enzyme content and being more fatigue-resistant.

The soleus muscle in mice and rats is composed almost entirely of type I fibers, whereas the extensor digitorum longus consists mainly of type IIA and IIB fibers. This is true of these two muscles in most mammals, but other skeletal muscles contain mixtures of fiber types (Johnson et al., 1973). The high content of myoglobin and cytochrome c in the slow muscle accounts for their red color.

The broad classification of muscle fibers into three fiber types is adequate for most purposes when considering normal and pathological physiology, but modern investigations show that there are a complex set of genes controlling the expression of the characteristic proteins and, especially with the fast fibers, there can be variable amounts of mixed gene expression in single fibers (Pette and Staron, 1990).

VI. Contractile Properties

Fast muscles rapidly develop force and also relax more rapidly than do the slow muscles. The fast extensor digitorum longus muscle, when stimulated at a frequency of 10–20 Hz, reacts quickly enough for the tension to fall back to the baseline before the next impulse, but in the slower soleus muscle, the next impulse comes before relaxation is complete, and the contraction is superimposed on the tension remaining from the previous stimulus. In this way the individual twitches are said to *summate* or *fuse*. When stimulated at a sufficiently high frequency the muscle will produce a smooth plateau of force. The frequency required to achieve this plateau is known as the *fusion frequency*, and this frequency is higher for the fast muscles.

There are several features that distinguish the contractile properties of fast and slow muscles (Fig. 8).

1. *The shape of the twitch*: The twitch of a fast muscle has an earlier peak of force and more rapid relaxation than a slow muscle.
2. *Relaxation from an isometric tetanus*: Figure 8 shows the relaxation phase from a tetanus. The last half of the curve approximates a single exponential, and a useful measure of speed is the half-time of this portion.
3. *Fusion frequency*: This is higher in fast muscles.
4. *Fatigability*: Muscles vary widely in their response to prolonged activity, with the fast muscles, and especially the type IIB fibers, fatiguing very rapidly. As first recorded by Ranvier, there is a clear connection between the appearance and contractile properties of certain skeletal muscles, such as the red and white muscles of a chicken, or the soleus and extensor digitorum longus in a mouse. These muscles, however, are somewhat unusual in consisting preponderantly of one fiber type, whereas most skeletal muscles are a mixture of different types. It is important to know whether the different fiber types within a single muscle also have differing contractile properties.

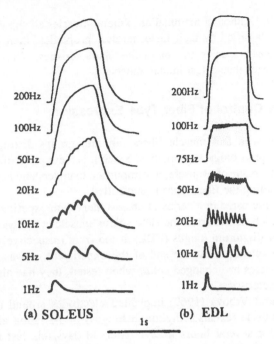

Figure 8 Force generated during a 500-ms tetanus at different frequencies (isolated muscles, 25°C): (a) mouse soleus; (b) mouse extensor digitorum longus (EDL).

A. The Relation Between Histochemistry and Contractile Properties

Sophisticated techniques have been developed that allow the histochemical and physiological properties of individual motor units to be characterized (Burke et al., 1971; Kugelberg, 1973).

By stimulating a single axon, or a single motoneuron, all the fibers in one motor unit can be made to contract simultaneously and, by using sensitive force-recording techniques, the contractile characteristics of this motor unit can be determined. The maximum tetanic force generated by the motor unit gives an indication of the number of fibers of which it is composed. The fibers belonging to a motor unit can be identified in histochemical sections if the motor unit is fatigued by repeated stimulation to deplete the fibers of that one unit of glycogen.

On the basis of size, speed, and fatigability, motor units fall between two extremes, large, fast, and fatigable, or small, slow, and fatigue-resistant.

When examining their histochemical properties, the large units tend to be made up of type IIB fibers, whereas the small, slow units are predominately composed of type I fibers. Type IIA motor units span a range of size and fatigue resistance that is reflected in the broad spectrum of their mitochondrial enzymatic activities (Fig. 9). Although mammalian skeletal muscles all show similar varieties of fibers when classified by their histochemical properties, there are considerable differences between species in contractile characteristics. Thus, a slow mouse muscle is still faster than a fast human muscle.

VII. The Control of Fiber Type Expression

So far we have seen that muscle fibers fall into groups distinguished by their biochemical and physiological properties. Since it is these properties that determine the use that can be made of a muscle, it is important to understand how the expression of genes determining the fiber types is controlled.

The first clue came in a series of cross-innervation experiments by Buller et al. (1960) in which nerves from the slow soleus muscle at the back of the leg and the fast extensor digitorum longus (EDL) at the front (respectively, red and white muscles) were exchanged. At the end of the experiment, it was noticed that the reinnervated muscles had changed color; when tested, they had also changed their contractile characteristics.

Salmons and Vrbova (1969) implanted electrodes around the motor nerve serving a fast muscle (extensor digitorum longus) in the rabbit and stimulated at low frequency for several hours a day. After 30 days this fast muscle came to resemble the slow soleus muscle in its appearance and contractile characteristics.

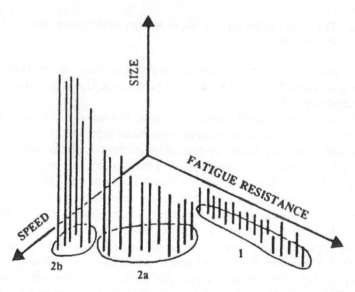

Figure 9 Contractile properties of motor units. The size, speed, and fatigue resistance of different types of motor units, as defined by their histochemical properties.

The same workers later demonstrated that the presence of the nerve itself is not required, since, if conduction along the nerve is blocked and the muscle is stimulated directly, the change from fast to slow characteristics still occurs. These experiments indicate that it is the pattern of activity imposed on the muscle, rather than trophic substances coming from the nerve, that regulates the expression of genes coding for proteins responsible for the slow contractile properties.

The major changes seen after chronic stimulation include an increase in capillary density, proliferation of mitochondria, decrease in sarcoplasmic reticulum, and the expression of different troponin and myosin isoenzymes, which occur with different time courses (Pette and Vrbova, 1992).

Increased capillary density and mitochondrial content, which are among the first changes to be seen in response to prolonged activity, will predominantly affect the fatigability of the muscle. Changes in the sarcoplasmic reticulum and contractile proteins, which require more activity, influence the speed of the muscle. Although there has been a great deal of work on stimulated animal muscle, there are relatively few investigations of the effects of prolonged stimulation on human muscle. The studies that have been undertaken show that changes in fatigability can be produced, but that the stimulation has probably never been sufficient to alter the myosin isoenzyme expression, thus converting the type II fibers to type I (Rutherford and Jones, 1988).

Many top endurance athletes have over 80% type I fibers in their leg muscles (Fig. 10; Saltin and Gollnick, 1983), and there is considerable debate over whether

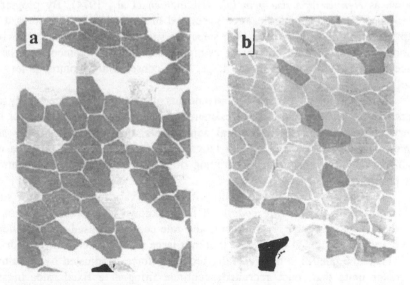

Figure 10 Fiber type composition of the quadriceps in athletes: (a) high jumper; (b) quality marathon runner. Myosin ATPase, pH 9.4; the type II fibers stain dark.

they were born this way or have achieved the fiber type disproportion as a result of their prolonged training. Human stimulation studies have continued for only a few months, whereas most endurance athletes have been training intensively for many years by the time they reach the highest levels of performance. On the other hand, it is well known that attributes, such as maximum aerobic exercise capacity (V_{O_2} max) and sprinting ability that are determined, at least in part, by the fiber type composition, have strong genetic predispositions.

VIII. Motor Unit Recruitment

Motor units vary in their size and contractile characteristics, and these differences reflect different patterns of use during normal activity.

The low-threshold units prove to be small, slow, motor units, whereas those recruited at higher thresholds are larger, fast units (Yemm, 1977), and there appears to be an ordered recruitment of motor units, with small, slow motor units being recruited during low-force contractions, whereas the fast units are active only during high-force contractions. Henneman and co-workers found that, in the cat, small, slow motor units were supplied by small, easily excitable motoneurons, whereas larger units were innervated by motoneurons that had higher thresholds for excitation. Henneman suggested that this difference might be the basis for the modulation of force, with units being recruited in order of size. This has become known as *Henneman's size principle* (Henneman et al., 1974). By progressive recruitment of motor units the force generated in a muscle can be increased in a stepwise fashion. At low forces, the steps are small (small motor units) giving a smooth increase in force; however, at higher forces, the increments are larger, since the recruited motor units are larger and, consequently, control is less precise.

This recruitment pattern has advantages in that the most frequently used units are small, slow, and fatigue-resistant, and can provide fine control for most everyday activities, such as postural adjustments, that require relatively small forces. The large, fast, and rapidly fatigable units are used only for occasional high-force contractions, such as sprinting or jumping, for which fine control is not necessary.

An alternative way of modulating force is to vary the frequency of stimulation; this is known as *rate coding*. It is not known to what extent these two methods of varying force, recruitment, and rate coding are used during a normal voluntary contraction. It is possible that in a large muscle, such as the quadriceps for which fine control is not generally required, force is adjusted by recruitment of motor units that, once recruited, continue firing at a fixed rate. In small muscles, such as those of the hand for which fine control is essential, rate coding may be more important.

IX. Mechanism of Force Generation

A. Length–Tension Relation of Skeletal Muscle

The total force produced by a muscle consists of two components: the *passive tension*, which is due to stretching the connective tissue elements of the muscle and, possibly, the structural proteins of the muscle fiber, such as titin. The *active tension* is superimposed on the passive tension when the muscle is stimulated. In the discussion that follows we are concerned only with the active tension, the passive component being subtracted from the total force.

The main feature of the length–tension relation is that force declines on either side of an optimum length and, by extrapolating the line to longer lengths, a value can be predicted at which no tension would be generated.

If force is generated by the interaction of actin and myosin, this should vary according to the degree of overlap of these two sets of filaments. By knowing the lengths of the filaments, it is possible to predict the length–tension relation and the sarcomere length at which no force would be developed. While taking care to keep the sarcomere lengths constant by length-clamping segments of the muscle fiber, Gordon et al. (1966) found a close fit between the actual and predicted force (Fig. 11). These results constitute one of the foundations of the sliding filament theory, demonstrating that force is generated by the interaction of the overlapping portions of actin and myosin filaments.

Unless great care is taken to keep sarcomere lengths constant, a significant discrepancy is observed between the actual and predicted values for the right-hand descending limb of the length–tension curve. Force is still developed at sarcomere lengths at which no filament overlap would be expected. The reason for the difference between observed and predicted results lies in the phenomenon generally known as "creep." Close examination of the single-fiber preparations used in this type of work shows that the sarcomere spacing is not uniform along the length of a fiber, the sarcomeres at the ends of the fiber being shorter than those in the middle, so that the whole fiber generates more force than would be expected from the length of most sarcomeres.

B. The Nature of the Interaction Between Thick and Thin Filaments

It has long been known that, if an active muscle is rapidly shortened by as little as 1% of its total length, the force generated drops, momentarily, to near zero before redeveloping (e.g., Gasser and Hill, 1924). If the actin and myosin filaments had formed into some kind of long spring when the muscle was activated, the force would be expected to decrease roughly in proportion to the change in its overall length (i.e., about 1%), not the value close to 100% that is found. This important observation suggests that force is generated by components that are very short, compared with the length of a sarcomere, so that a change of 1% of the sarcomere

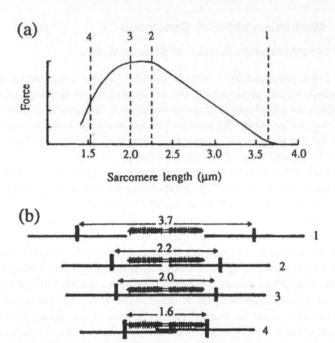

Figure 11 Isometric force at different sarcomere lengths. (a) Force generated; (b) arrangement of filaments at different lengths. At lengths less than 2.0 μm, thin filaments begin to overlap and, at still shorter lengths, the thick filaments come into contact with the Z lines. Values are for frog muscle. Mammalian thin filaments are slightly longer so the corresponding sarcomere lengths are 1–4.0 μm, 2–2.5 μm, 3–2.4 μm, and 4–1.6 μm. (Redrawn from Gordon et al., 1969.)

length is sufficient to take all the stretch out of them, and this fits well with the notion that force is generated by numerous myosin cross-bridges that are each active over a small distance.

The force produced by a muscle is proportional to the cross-sectional area of the muscle, rather than to its length.

By working outward from the central Z line of a muscle fiber, it can be seen that the forces exerted by each half-sarcomere on the adjacent Z line are opposed to one another and so do not summate along the length of the fiber. During an isometric contraction, the intermediate sarcomeres serve to form a rigid connection between the two ends of the muscle (Fig. 12).

Although isometric force is independent of length, this is not true for the speed of shortening. At the onset of contraction, all sarcomeres in a muscle fiber will begin to shorten more or less at the same time and at the same velocity. If the muscle were only one sarcomere long and shortened from 3 to 2 μm in 0.1 s then the velocity of shortening of the two ends would be 10 μm/s, but for a muscle

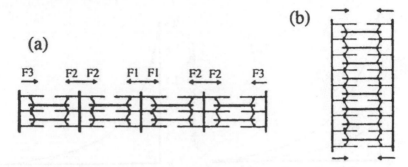

Figure 12 Force generated by sarcomeres in series and in parallel. (a) Sarcomeres in series: The forces F1 and F2 are opposed, leaving only F3 to exert force at the ends of the muscle. (b) The same number of actin and myosin filaments arranged in parallel to give four times the isometric force of (a).

2.5-cm long, containing about 10,000 sarcomeres in series, the velocity of shortening would be 10 cm/s. To compare speed of shortening in muscles of different lengths, the velocity is often expressed as muscle lengths per second, as sarcomere lengths per second, or even half-sarcomere lengths per second.

Power is the product of force and velocity. Since force is proportional to the cross-sectional area of a muscle, and velocity to the length, it follows that power is proportional to the product of these: namely, volume. Thus, a short, fat muscle will generate a high force, but have a low maximum velocity of shortening, whereas a long, thin muscle of the same volume will produce little force, but shorten rapidly. However, they will have the same power output. Maximum power is usually obtained at about one-third V_{max} so that, although the maximum power may be the same in the two muscles, the velocity at which this occurs will be different.

C. Force–Velocity Characteristics

The length–tension characteristics of skeletal muscle, together with the rapid-release experiments, established in broad terms the type of structure required to explain force generation. Further information about the nature of the myosin–actin interaction has been obtained by consideration of the force–velocity characteristics of muscle.

As the velocity of shortening increases, so the force sustained by the muscle rapidly diminishes, eventually reaching a velocity at which force can no longer be sustained at all; this is the maximum velocity of unloaded shortening (V_{max}; Fig. 13). The relation between force and velocity has been described mathematically in a number of ways, but the most widely used is the so-called characteristic equation of A. V. Hill (1938):

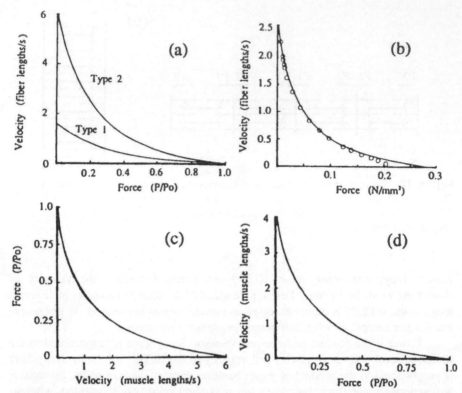

Figure 13 Force–velocity relation for different muscle preparations. (a) Human type I and type II fibers estimated from preparations of isolated human muscle obtained at surgery; 37°C. (b) Frog anterior tibialis, 2.7°C, single fiber with measurements made by length clamping. Hill's equation fitted to data less than 80% P_0, note the deviation at high forces. (c) Rat medial gastrocnemius, 26°C, using isokinetic releases. (d) Human elbow flexors, values estimated from measurements made in situ. (From Wilkie, 1950.)

$$(P + a)V = b(P_0 - P)$$

where P_0 is the isometric force, and P is the force sustained by the muscle when shortening at a velocity V. This is the equation of a hyperbola in which the axes have been moved by the constants a and b. The equation is a valuable way of describing the characteristics of a muscle and estimating V_{max} when this cannot be measured easily, but the equation is an empirical description of the experimental data and does not embody any hypothesis about the way in which force is generated.

During an isometric contraction, there is no movement, no external work is done by the muscle, and all the energy liberated appears in the form of heat. During shortening, heat is still produced, but the muscle also performs work, which is the product of the force and distance moved. It was first observed by Fenn (1923) that during shortening the total energy liberated, in the form of heat plus work, is greater than that occurring during an isometric contraction (Fenn effect). Any explanation of the mechanics of force generation must be able to account, not only for the observed force–velocity characteristics, but also the way in which energy liberation increases with shortening.

D. A. F. Huxley's 1957 Model

In this model, the myosin-binding site oscillates backward and forward and, when it attaches to an actin-binding site, exerts a force pulling the binding site toward the central equilibrium position. To produce movement in one direction, it is necessary to specify that the attachment will occur only when the myosin-binding is on one site of the equilibrium position; the force generated being proportional to the displacement x (Fig. 14a). Cross-bridges that are carried beyond the central position will generate force opposing the movement; to keep this opposing force to a minimum, it is necessary that there should be a rapid dissociation, once the cross-bridge moves into regions for which the value of x is negative; the rate constants for attachment (f) and detachment (g) are postulated to vary with displacement as shown in Figure 14b. The rate constant for detachment at negative values of x is assigned a high and constant value (g_2). With a judicious choice of values for the rate constants, the theory can provide a very good fit to experimental data and demonstrates the reasons why force decreases so rapidly as velocity increases. In the isometric state, all attached cross-bridges are within the region bounded by $x = 0$ and $x = h$. With sliding of the filaments past one another, fewer cross-bridges are attached near the position h, and some will have been carried into the region beyond the equilibrium position, so that the bridges are compressed and

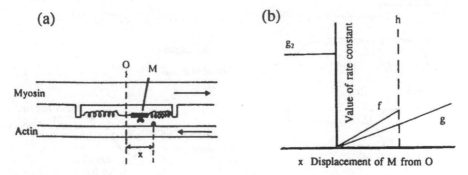

Figure 14 Mechanical model forming the basis of Huxley's 1957 theory. (a) The myosin-binding sites M oscillates about the equilibrium position O and can bind to the actin only for positive values of x. (b) Rate constants for attachment (f) and detachment (g) of myosin to actin: h is the maximum displacement of the myosin head at which binding can occur. For negative values of x, f is zero, and g has a high and constant value (g_2).

oppose movement. The net effect of fewer bridges generating force and some opposing motion is for the force to fall off rapidly as the velocity of shortening increases. At high velocities, a large proportion of cross-bridges will be carried beyond the equilibrium position and, when the opposing force from the cross-bridges in compression equals the force generated by the cross-bridges in the region $0 - h$, the net result is no force production by the muscle. The velocity at which this occurs is the maximum velocity of shortening. For a general review of cross-bridge kinetics and muscle energetics, see Irving (1987) and Woledge and associates (1985).

Huxley's 1957 theory of cross-bridge action does not explain the behavior of muscle subjected to rapid changes in length. If a muscle is rapidly shortened, the force initially falls, and then shows a very rapid recovery (Fig. 15). This rapid phase is followed by a slower return of force to the isometric value. The explanation proposed by Huxley and Simmons (1970) is that the rapid phase of force recovery is due to rotation of the myosin heads of the unloaded bridges, thereby restretching the compliant S2 component.

The slow phase of force recovery, from T_2 to full isometric force, is ascribed to detachment and reattachment of cross-bridges, so that the conditions of the isometric contraction are reestablished.

The size of the various transients differs with the extent of the rapid release. For small releases, the size of the drop from isometric force to T_1 (T_1 curve) is almost linearly related to the size of the release, which is consistent with the transition being due to the S2 portion of the myosin molecule acting as a compliance

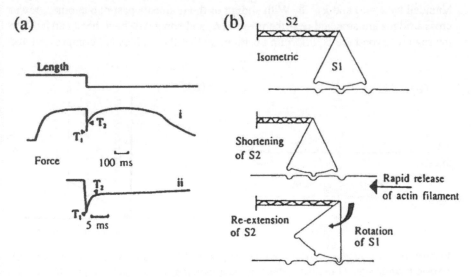

Figure 15   Force transients during rapid release. (a) Force response shown on a slow (i) and fast (ii) time base. (b) Shortening of S2 during rapid release is compensated by the rapid rotation of the myosin head portion, producing the T_1–T_2 recovery.

that obeys Hook's law. The T_1-T_2 transition (T_2 curve) shows a plateau for small releases that is thought to correspond to the range of movement over which rotation of the myosin head can fully take up the slack in the S2 portion (see Fig. 15). For longer releases, the rotation can only partially compensate for the change in length of the S2 portion and so T_2 is less than the isometric force.

E. ATP Splitting During Activity

The basic Huxley 1957 model explains the force–velocity characteristics for skeletal muscle, and it also gives an explanation of the Fenn effect: if one ATP is hydrolyzed with every cross-bridge dissociation, the rate at which heat and work are produced will depend on the rate of cross-bridge turnover. In the isometric state, the rate constant for cross-bridge detachment is relatively low, but in the region beyond the equilibrium position, g_2 is high and, therefore, turnover and liberation of energy will be high. As the velocity of shortening increases, so the number of cross-bridges carried into an orientation for which detachment is rapid, also increases, accounting for the increase in production of heat plus work.

F. Force During Muscle Stretch

Although muscle activity is usually thought of in terms of shortening, there are almost as many occasions, such as when walking down stairs or lowering weights, when the active muscle is stretched.

The maximum forces that can be produced during this type of movement are considerably greater than the isometric force and vary with the velocity of stretch. With increasing velocity, the force reaches a plateau of about 1.8 times the isometric force. The increased force can be explained in terms of Huxley's model, in that during a stretch, the attached cross-bridges are pulled so that $x > h$, stretching the compliant portion of the cross-bridge more than occurs during isometric contractions.

The overall shape of the curve, shown in Figure 16, with force increasing with stretch and decreasing with shortening, has important consequences for the stability of sarcomeres acting in series. If one sarcomere is stronger than the next, it might be imagined that the stronger would pull out and extend the weaker. Such disruption does happen to some extent since stretching active muscle is associated with structural damage of a type that is not seen as a result of other types of muscular exercise. However, this damage is minimized because, when the sarcomeres begin to move, the force generated by the stronger will fall as it shortens (moving down the right-hand portion of the curve), whereas the force of the weaker sarcomere will increase as it is stretched (moving up the left-hand side of Fig. 16).

G. ATP Splitting During Stretching

Heat production falls to low values when muscle is stretched, a fact first noticed by Fenn (1923). More recently, Curtin and Davies (1973) showed that ATP splitting

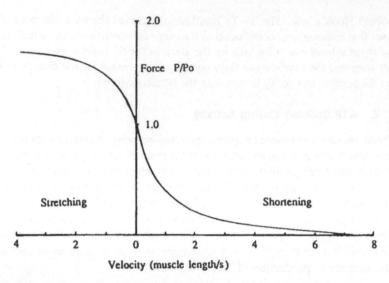

Figure 16 Force of mouse soleus muscle during stretch and shortening; 26°C.

was likewise very low during stretching, and exercise that involves a substantial element of "negative work," such as walking down hill or trying to resist the movement of the pedals on an electrically driven cycle, have a very low oxygen cost (Bigland-Ritchie and Woods, 1976). The implication of this finding is that, when cross-bridges are stretched into the region at which $x > h$, the detachment does not require the binding of ATP, and the linkage is forcibly disrupted.

X. Biochemistry of Force Generation

Force and movement are the result of the cyclic attachment and detachment of myosin bridges in the thick filaments with binding sites on the thin actin filaments (Fig. 17). The attachment of actin and myosin (i) is a reversible process that will give stiffness to the muscle (i.e., it will resist if stretched), but does not itself generate force. The release of phosphate from the actomyosin complex (ii) is thought to initiate the changes that result in force generation (rotation of the S1 head in this model). Toward the end of the rotation phase, ADP is released (iii), and the actomysin complex can then bind ATP (iv). Having done so the actin and myosin dissociate with the ATP bound to myosin (v). The bound ATP is then hydrolyzed and the products remain bound to the protein (vi); this last process is thought to activate the S1 unit, making it ready to bind to actin again. Skinned fiber preparations can be used to investigate the mechanical correlates of the enzymic steps (e.g., Cooke and Pate, 1985). Adding phosphate to contracting, skinned fibers decreases

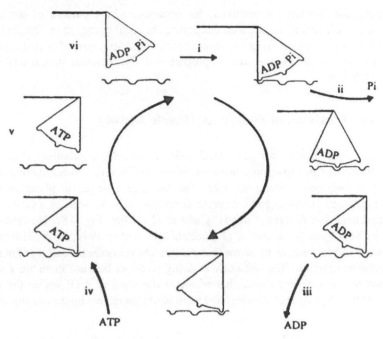

Figure 17 Stages in the cross-bridge cycle. Force is generated between steps ii and iii.

the force generated. This is thought to be a result of slowing the rate of release of phosphate (ii), leading to an accumulation of cross-bridges in the state preceding the development of force. Consequently, there will be a lower proportion of cross-bridges in the high-force state. The rate of unloaded shortening is determined by the rate of cross-bridge detachment in the region beyond the useful range of movement of the cross-bridge head (g_2, −ve values of x). The detachment is thought to correspond to reaction iv involving the binding of ATP and reaction v, the dissociation step. Phosphate does not influence the rate of reaction vi and, therefore, does not affect the force–velocity characteristics. On the other hand, ADP will inhibit reaction iii, the release of ADP, and will thus reduce the proportion of cross-bridges that reach the stage at which they can dissociate. This leads to an accumulation of cross-bridges in a force-generating state. For an isometric contraction, increased ADP causes a higher force, but during shortening, a larger proportion of cross-bridges will be carried into a position where they oppose movement, leading to a reduction in force at a given velocity and in Vmax, the maximum velocity of shortening.

Mechanical experiments with whole muscles, single fibers, and with fragments of fibers have led to a situation for which clear mechanical models of the working cross-bridge have been developed. There is considerable interest in understanding the molecular mechanism involved; for instance, which portion of the myosin molecule is responsible for the transduction of chemical energy to mechanical work? Recent advances determining the three-dimensional structure of myosin S1 point the way ahead in linking mechanical properties to the chemical structure (Rayment et al., 1993a,b).

XI. Provision of Energy for Muscle Activity

Although ATP plays such a central role in muscle metabolism, this is not immediately obvious from measurements of metabolite levels in contracting muscle. During a sustained contraction, there can be large changes in phosphocreatine, breaking down to creatine and inorganic phosphate, together with increases in lactate and hydrogen ion (decrease in pH; Cady et al., 1989; Fig. 18). However, ATP changes very little in the course of a contraction, and in 1949, A. V. Hill issued a challenge to biochemists to prove that ATP is the immediate source of energy for muscular contraction. The difficulty in doing so arises because there are a number of reactions, some very rapid, that maintain the level of ATP within the muscle fiber. ADP is rapidly rephosphorylated from phosphocreatine by the enzyme creatine

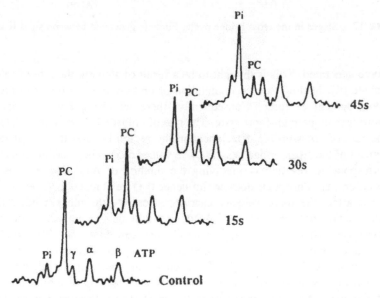

Figure 18 NMR spectroscopy used to measure phosphorus metabolites in human muscle (first dorsal interosseous). Averaged spectra from a fully rested muscle (Control) and from a muscle after 15, 30, and 45 s of maximum voluntary contraction. Note the progressive decrease in phosphocreatine (PC) and increase in inorganic phosphate (Pi) peaks. The α, β, and γ peaks of ATP remain constant.

kinase, which is abundant in muscle, and the equilibrium of the reaction is well over to the side of ATP formation, so that the ATP level remains virtually constant until the phosphocreatine has become almost exhausted. It was not until Cain and Davies (1962) used dinitrofluorobenzene to inhibit creatine kinase that unequivocal evidence of ATP involvement in contraction was first demonstrated. Glycolysis and oxidative metabolism also act to restore levels of ATP, but these processes can be blocked with the inhibitors iodoacetate and cyanide, respectively.

A. Short-Term, High-Intensity Exercise

In many muscles, the generation of high forces leads to high pressures within the muscle that have the effect of cutting off the blood supply and, since human skeletal muscle has relatively small amounts of myoglobin, the muscle must function anaerobically. Figure 18 shows the changes in muscle metabolites during a sustained contraction and illustrates the importance of phosphocreatine and glycolysis in maintaining the ATP content of the cell. Over the course of a 45-s contraction, about half the total energy comes from the splitting of phosphocreatine and half from glycolysis. The final intracellular pH of about 6.5 represents the limit of acidosis seen in human muscle as a result of physical activity.

B. Longer-Term Activity

The provision of energy for any exercise lasting more than a minute or so is limited by the supply of oxygen to the tissue, the availability of fuels for oxidation, and the mitochondrial content. An increase in muscle mitochondrial enzyme content is a well-known result of endurance training, with activities of many mitochondrial enzymes increasing two- to threefold. Muscle biopsies from highly trained endurance athletes show an abundance of mitochondria, often accumulating just beneath the sarcolemma.

The high capillary density and the myoglobin and mitochondrial content of the trained muscle have obvious advantages for endurance exercise and can occur as the result of adaptation to prolonged endurance training in muscles of any fiber composition. The thigh muscles of top-class marathon runners are generally composed preponderantly (about 70%) of type I, slow-oxidative fibers that have a high-oxidative capacity even in the untrained state.

XII. Supply of Oxygen

The supply of oxygen to the tissues may be divided into three areas of interest: ventilation and gas exchange at the lungs, the cardiac output and peripheral circulation, which determines the amount of oxygen delivered to the tissue and, lastly, diffusion into the cells and the capacity of the tissue to utilize oxygen. The first two are dealt with in other chapters; thus, this account will be limited to the potential of the muscle itself.

Factors that improve diffusion of oxygen from capillary to the muscle fiber mitochondria are the size of the muscle fibers and their myoglobin content. Endurance-trained athletes tend to have muscles that are somewhat smaller than the average, because their muscle fibers are smaller in cross section. The advantage of this is that diffusion distances for oxygen are reduced. Patterns of artificial electrical stimulation of muscles in humans and animals, leading to an improvement in fatigue resistance, also result in reduction in muscle force, probably because the muscle fibers become smaller. The myoglobin content of slow fibers is higher than in fast fibers and functions to facilitate oxygen diffusion from the capillary into the fibers. The rate of diffusion is approximately doubled by the presence of myoglobin. Myoglobin content of muscle probably increases with endurance training, but there is little information on this topic.

A. Supply of Fuel

The two major fuels used by muscle are carbohydrate, in the form of glucose or glycosyl units, and free fatty acids. Oxidation of amino acids makes only a minor contribution to the provision of energy during exercise. The carbohydrate and fatty acids either arrive at the muscle in the blood, having been released from liver or adipose tissue, or are obtained from intracellular stores of glycogen and triglyceride within the muscle fiber.

B. Energy Reserves and Rates of Utilization

The central dilemma concerning the selection of fuel for muscular exercise is that there is a choice to be made between the *size* of the reserves and the *rate* at which the energy can be obtained from these stores. In general, the larger the store (i.e., greater endurance) the lower the power output that can be sustained.

The muscle content of ATP, phosphocreatine, and the energy available from glycolysis, is sufficient to sustain activity at a power output equivalent to 80% Vo_2max for about 60 s. Liver glycogen and glucose in the circulation can sustain this level of effort for about 20 min, and oxidation of muscle glycogen stores can further sustain the exercise for about 1 h. Although there may be massive stores of triglyceride in the body, there is a limit to the rate at which this fuel can be used. Oxidation of body fat could theoretically support a high level of activity for over 4000 min, but in practice, nobody can sustain this level for more than a few hours (Newsholme, 1987). Untrained subjects can sustain 80% V_{O_2}max for only about 30 min, whereas a highly motivated, trained athlete can sustain this level for the duration of a marathon (about 3 h). The maximum rate of energy production from the oxidation of fat is about 50% that from the oxidation of carbohydrate. If a subject chooses to exercise at less than 50% Vo_2max, then the work can be sustained by oxidation of fatty acids for very long periods, provided that feet, ankles, and knees survive; this is the strategy that "ultradistance" athletes are forced to adopt for their 100-mile and 6-day races.

XIII. Strategies for Improving Performance in Endurance Exercise

In running a marathon, a compromise must be made between the rate at which energy can be liberated and the size of the store being used. It is possible to sustain a high-power output using muscle glycogen, but those reserves are sufficient for only 1–1.5 h exercise. When muscle glycogen is depleted, there is no alternative but to oxidize fat, which can support power output at about only half that provided by carbohydrates. The time at which the muscle glycogen stores are used up and the body has only fat as a substrate is known as "hitting the wall" and leads to a rapid decline in running speed. In this context, there are two ways in which performance in endurance events can be improved.

A. Increasing Muscle Glycogen Stores

One way of improving endurance of exercise at high levels of oxygen uptake is to increase the muscle glycogen content by the carbohydrate-loading techniques now commonly used by endurance runners. Bergstrom and colleagues (1966, 1967) first noted this effect during an investigation of the rate of glycogen resynthesis after fatiguing exercise. The subjects exercised one leg to exhaustion; the other leg acted as a control. After having depleted the test leg of glycogen, muscle levels were restored after 1 day. However, the surprising finding was that on the second and third days after exercise the muscle glycogen was one and half to twice as high as in the control muscles.

Glycogen levels in muscle can be raised by simply feeding a high-carbohydrate diet, without any exercise, and there have been various suggestions that the loading may be enhanced by taking a low-carbohydrate diet for a week before the race, followed by a high-carbohydrate diet 24–48 h before the exercise. The optimum combination of exercise and diet has not been fully evaluated, but there is no doubt that muscle glycogen stores can be significantly elevated with beneficial effects for running speed and endurance.

B. Increased Utilization of Fats

The maximum rate of energy production from fat oxidation is such as to limit the power output to 50% VO_2max. If fat oxidation is fully utilized, a power output of 80% VO_2max could be achieved if the glycogen stores were to provide the remaining 30%. The limited glycogen store is then used only to "top up" the energy requirement and, consequently, is used up at about a third of the rate that would be required if glycogen were the only source of energy.

If it were possible to consume fatty acids at a maximum and constant rate from the start of exercise, a high and constant power output could be maintained for a longer time in contrast to the abrupt loss of performance seen if the two fuels are used sequentially.

Fatty acid oxidation is largely controlled by the availability of substrate. Fatty acid oxidation appears to spare carbohydrate by two mechanisms; directly reducing glucose uptake by the tissue and decreasing glycolysis as a consequence of the accumulation of citrate which inhibits phosphofructokinase.

In normal, untrained subjects fatty acids are mobilized and make a significant contribution to the energy requirements only after an hour or so of exercise at a time when glycogen stores are becoming depleted. In contrast, elite endurance athletes have high levels of fat oxidation, with sparing of carbohydrate, during exercise. The utilization of fat also begins earlier in the exercise. Trained cyclists working at the same percentage VO_2 max as untrained subjects were found to have lower plasma lactate and higher plasma free fatty acids than untrained controls (Bloom et al., 1976) indicating a greater use of fats and a shift away from carbohydrate utilization.

XIV. Summary

An appreciation of skeletal muscle function requires an understanding of the structure of the tissue at the molecular and cellular levels, together with its neurological control and special biochemical properties: what applies to skeletal muscle, in general, also applies to the respiratory muscles in particular. Advances in understanding respiratory muscle function in health and disease have come about as a result of modifying and applying the techniques of conventional muscle physiology to the respiratory muscles and this will undoubtedly lead to advances in the future. Conversely, the energy and interest generated by clinical problems often provides the stimulus for fundamental advances and this may well prove to be the case with muscle physiology especially in the areas of muscle control, fatigue, and training.

References

Bergström, J., and Hultman, E. (1966). Muscle glycogen synthesis after exercise: An enhancing factor localized to muscle cells in man. *Nature* 210: 309–310.

Bergström, J., Hermansen, L., Hultman, E., and Saltin, B. (1967). Diet, muscle glycogen and physical performance. *Acta Physiol. Scand.* 71: 140–150.

Bigland-Ritchie, B., and Woods, J. R. (1976). Integrated EMG and O_2 uptake during positive and negative work. *J. Physiol.* 260: 267–277.

Bloom, S. R., Johnson, R. H., Park, D. M., Rennie, M. J., and Sulaiman, W. R. (1976).

Differences in the metabolic and hormonal response to exercise between racing cyclists and untrained individuals. *J. Physiol.* 258: 1–18.

Buller, A. J., Eccles, J. C., and Eccles, R. M. (1960). Interactions between motor neurones and muscles in respect of the characteristic speeds of their responses. *J. Physiol.* 150: 417–439.

Burke, R. E., Levine, D. M., Zajac, F. E., Tsairis, P., and Engel, W. K. (1971). Mammalian motor units: Physiological–histochemical correlation in three types in cat gastrocnemius. *Science* 174: 709–712.

Cady, E. B., Jones, D. A., Lynn, J., and Newham, D. J. (1989). Changes in force and intracellular metabolites during fatigue of human skeletal muscle. *J. Physiol.* 418: 311–325.

Cain, D. F., and Davies, R. E. (1962). Breakdown of adenosine triphosphate during a single contraction of working muscle. *Biochem. Biophys. Res. Commun.* 8: 361–366.

Cohen, C., and Vibert, P. J. (1987). Actin filament: images and models. In *Fibrous Protein Structure*. Edited by J. M. Squire and P. J. Vibert. London, Academic Press, pp. 284–306.

Cooke, R., and Pate, E. (1985). The effects of ADP and phosphate on the contraction of muscle fibres. *Biophys. J.* 48: 789–798.

Curtin, N. A., and Davies, R. E. (1973). Chemical and mechanical change during stretching of activated frog skeletal muscle. *Symp. Quant. Biol.* 27: 619–626.

Eisenberg, B. R. (1983). Quantitative ultrastructure of mammalian skeletal muscle. In *Handbook of Physiology*, Section 10, Skeletal Muscle. Edited by L. D. Peachey, R. H. Adrian, and S. R. Geiger. Bethesda, MD, American Physiological Society, pp. 73–112.

Fenn, W. O. (1923). A quantitative comparison between the energy liberated and the work performed by the isolated sartorius muscle of the frog. *J. Physiol.* 58: 175–203.

Franzini-Armstrong, C. (1973). The structure of a simple Z line. *J. Cell Biol.* 58: 630–642.

Gasser, H. S., and Hill, A. V. (1924). The dynamics of muscular contraction. *Proc. R. Soc. B* 96: 398–437.

Gordon, A. M., Huxley, A. F., and Julian, F. J. (1966). The variation in isometric tension with sarcomere length in vertebrate muscle fibres. *J. Physiol.* 184: 170–192.

Henneman, E., Clamann, H. P., Gillies, J. D., and Skinner, R. D. (1974). Rank order of motoneurons within a pool, law of combination. *J. Neurophysiol.* 37: 1338–1349.

Hill, A. V. (1938). The heat of shortening and the dynamic constants of muscle. *Proc. R. Soc. B* 126: 136–195.

Huxley, A. F. (1957). Muscle structure and theories of contraction. *Prog. Biophys. Biophys. Chem.* 7: 255–318.

Huxley, A. F., and Simmons, R. M. (1971). Proposed mechanism of force generation in striated muscle. *Nature* 233:533–538.

Irving, M. (1987). Muscle mechanics and probes of the crossbridge cycle. In *Fibrous Protein Structure*. Edited by J. M. Squire and P. J. Vibert. London, Academic Press, pp. 495–528.

Johnson, M. A., Polgar, J., Weightman, D., and Appleton, D. (1973). Data on the distribution of fibre types in 36 human muscles. An autopsy study. *J. Neurol. Sci.* 18: 111–129.

Knight, P., and Trinick, J. (1987). The myosin molecule. In *Fibrous Protein Structure*. Edited by J. M. Squire and P. J. Vibert. London, Academic Press, pp. 247–281.

Kugelberg, E. (1973). Histochemical composition, contraction speed and fatigability of rat soleus motor units. *J. Neurol. Sci.* 20: 177–198.

Newsholme, E. A. (1987). Application of metabolic logic to the questions of causes of fatigue in marathon races. In *Exercise: Benefits, Limits and Adaptations*. Edited by D. Macleod et al. London, E. & F. N. Spon,Ltd, pp. 181–198.

Offer, G. (1987). Myosin filaments. In *Fibrous Protein Structure*. Edited by J. M. Squire and P. J. Vilbert. London, Academic Press, pp. 307–356.

Peachey, L. D. (1965). The sarcoplasmic reticulum and transverse tubules of the frog's sartorius. *J. Cell Biol.* 25(Suppl. 3): 209–231.

Pette, D., and Staron, R. S. (1990). Cellular and molecular diversities of mammalian skeletal muscle fibres. *Rev. Physiol. Biochem. Pharmacol.* 116: 1–76.

Pette, D., and Vrbova, G. (1992). Adaptation of mammalian skeletal muscle fibres to chronic electrical stimulation. *Rev. Physiol. Biochem. Pharmacol.* 120: 116–202.

Rayment, I., Rypniewski, W. R., Schmidt-Base, K., et al. (1993a). Three dimensional structure of myosin subfragment-1: A molecular motor. *Science* 261: 50–58.

Rayment, I., Holden, H. M., Whittaker, M., et al. (1993b). Structure of the actin–myosin complex and its implications for muscle contraction. *Science* 261: 58–65.

Rowe, R. W. D., and Goldspink, G. (1969). Muscle fibre growth in five different muscles in both sexes of mice: I, normal mice. *J. Anat.* 104: 519–530.

Rutherford, O. M., and Jones, D. A. (1988). Contractile properties and fatiguability of the human adductor pollicis and first dorsal interosseous: A comparison of the effects of two chronic stimulation patterns. *J. Neurol. Sci.* 85: 319–331.

Salmons, S., and Vrbova, G. (1969). The influence of activity on some contractile characteristics of mammalian fast and slow muscles. *J. Physiol.* 201: 535–549.

Saltin, B., and Gollnick, P. D. (1983). Skeletal muscle adaptability: Significance for metabolism and performance. In *Handbook of Physiology*, Section 10, Skeletal Muscle. Edited by L. D. Peachey, R. H. Adrian, and S. R. Geiger. Bethesda, MD, American Physiological Society, pp. 555–631.

Squire, J. M., Luther, P. K., and Trinick, J. (1987). Muscle myofibril architecture. In *Fibrous Protein Structure*. Edited by J. M. Squire and P. J. Vibert. London, Academic Press, pp. 423–450.

Wilkie, D. R. (1950). The relation between force and velocity in human muscle. *J. Physiol.* 110: 249–280.

Woledge, R. C., Curtin, N. A., and Homsher, E. (1985). Energetic aspects of muscle contraction. *Monogr. Physiol. Soc.* No. 41. London, Academic Press.

Yemm, R. (1977). The orderly recruitment of motor units of the masseter and temporal muscles during voluntary isometric contractions in man. *J. Physiol.* 265: 163–174.

2

Electrophysiology and Excitation–Contraction Coupling in Skeletal Muscle

NICHOLAS SPERELAKIS

University of Cincinnati
  College of Medicine
Cincinnati, Ohio

ALEXANDRE FABIATO

Medical College of Virginia
Virginia Commonwealth University
Richmond, Virginia

I. Introduction

The purpose of this chapter is to provide a concise review of the electrophysiology of skeletal muscle fibers and the mechanism of the coupling of contraction to membrane excitation. It is not intended to provide extensive documentation of the statements made and views presented, because the chapter would become unwieldy and too lengthy for the page limitations imposed. Therefore, references are limited to key articles and reviews.

The electrophysiology of muscle is important to an understanding of the factors that control the contraction force of the respiratory muscles, including the fatigue process. It is also crucial to an understanding of the effects, both therapeutic and deleterious, of various drugs. Finally, several disease processes affect the electrophysiological properties of the cell membrane, and the pathological disorders can be explained by the membrane changes. Therefore, it is imperative that the nature of and basis of membrane excitability be understood.

The chapter begins with a discussion of the properties of the resting membrane and ionic basis of the resting potential. This will be followed by a discussion of excitation and conduction of the action potential, and by the process of excitation–contraction coupling. Alterations in membrane properties in some diseases are given in the following chapter.

II. Cell Membrane Structure and Fluidity

The resting potential and the action potential are the direct result of the special properties of the cell membrane, including selective ionic permeability, ion pumping, and ion exchange. The cell membrane is composed of a bimolecular leaflet of phospholipid molecules, with embedded protein. Protein molecules float in the lipid bilayer, some proteins extending into only the inner or outer leaflet of the membrane, and other proteins spanning the entire membrane (Fig. 1). The proteins that span the membrane include the voltage-dependent ionic channels, ion-pumping enzymes, and receptors. The proteins that may insert into half the membrane thickness include some membrane-associated enzymes. The nonpolar hydrophobic ends of the phospholipid molecules project toward the center of the membrane, and the polar hydrophilic ends point toward the edges of the membrane bordering on the water phases; this is their thermodynamically favorable orientation (see Fig. 1). Each phospholipid head group occupies about 60 Å.

The lipid bilayer is about 70-Å thick, and the phospholipid molecules are about 35 Å in length. The membrane-specific capacitance (C_m) is about 1 $\mu F/cm^2$. The capacitance arises because of the lipid bilayer, the lipid acting as a good dielectric (dielectric constant of 3–5) that separates the two conductive plates (the water phases on each side of the membrane contain ions). Experimental measurement of C_m allows the calculation of membrane thickness (δ) (see Sperelakis, 1979). The voltage gradient across the cell membrane at rest (90 mV/70 $\times$ 10^{-8} cm) is about 129,000 V/cm, thus illustrating the effective dielectric properties of the

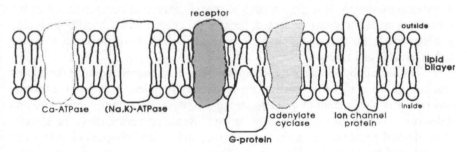

Figure 1   Diagrammatic illustration of cell membrane substructure showing the lipid bilayer with proteins floating in the bilayer. Nonpolar hydrophobic tail ends of the phospholipid molecules project toward the middle of the membrane and polar hydrophilic heads border on the water phase at each side of the membrane. Lipid bilayer is about 70 Å thick. The cholesterol molecules are not shown. Large protein molecules protrude through entire membrane thickness or are inserted into one leaflet only, as illustrated. These proteins include various enzymes associated with the cell membrane as well as membrane ionic channels. The membrane has fluidity, so that the protein and lipid molecules can move around in the plane of the membrane. (Adapted from Singer and Nicolson, 1972.)

biological membrane. Artificial lipid bilayer membranes have a high capacitance, similar to the biological membrane, but have a very high resistance, about 10^3–10^6 times that of the cell membrane. This fact suggests that the relatively high conductance (reciprocal of the resistance) of the cell membrane is due to the membrane-spanning proteins floating in the lipid bilayer. Some of these proteins subserve the ionic conductances for Na^+, K^+, Ca^{2+}, and Cl^- ions in the resting membrane and the gated, voltage-sensitive conductance pathways (channels) that open during excitation. This molecular arrangement of the membrane makes the cell membrane a parallel resistance–capacitance (RC) network.

The proteins floating in the lipid bilayer can move laterally from one area of the membrane to another, unless anchored in place by a special anchoring protein (e.g., *anchorin*). For example, the fast Na^+ channels are anchored in the nodes of Ranvier. The fluidity of the membrane (reciprocal of the microviscosity) can be measured by the use of fluorescent probe molecules that insert into and lodge at different levels of the lipid bilayer (e.g., in the middle), and it is a measure of the ability of the protein molecules to move laterally in the plane of the membrane. A high cholesterol content tends to lower the fluidity of the membrane, whereas a high degree of unsaturation or branching of the phospholipid tails tends to increase the fluidity; chain length also affects fluidity. The polar portion of the planar cholesterol molecule lodges in the hydrophilic part of the membrane, and the nonpolar portion wedges in between the fatty acid tails, thereby restricting their motion and lowering fluidity. Phospholipids with unsaturated and branched-chain fatty acids cannot be packed as tightly because of steric hindrance caused by their greater rigidity; hence, such phospholipids increase membrane fluidity. Low temperature decreases fluidity. Calcium and magnesium ions may diminish the electrostatic charge repulsion between the phospholipid head groups, allowing the bilayer molecules to pack more tightly, thereby reducing fluidity.

Local anesthetics affect membrane fluidity also. The hydrophobic portion of the molecule interposes between the lipid molecules and separates them, thus reducing the van der Waals forces of interaction between adjacent acyl chain tails, and so increasing membrane fluidity. The local anesthetics produce a nonselective depression of most ionic conductances of the resting and excited membrane, and depress the activity of certain membrane-associated enzymes [e.g., the (Na^+, K^+)-ATPase]. The lipid matrix influences the function of membrane proteins, including the (Na^+, K^+)-APTase (for refs., see Sperelakis, 1979).

Changes in membrane fluidity occur during muscle development and in certain muscular diseases. For example, membrane fluidity increases in myotonic dystrophy (Appel and Roses, 1976). Animals given diazocholesterol for several weeks to interfere with cholesterol synthesis develop myotonia (Sha'afi et al., 1975). In chickens with genetic muscular dystrophy, the cholesterol/phospholipid ratio is increased, and membrane fluidity is decreased (Sha'afi et al., 1975).

III. Ionic Basis of the Resting Potential

A. Ion Distributions

The transmembrane resting potential (E_m) of skeletal muscle fibers is about -80 mV in mammals and about -90 mV in amphibians. The ionic composition of the extracellular fluid bathing the muscle fibers is similar to that of the blood plasma. It is high in Na^+ (about 145 mM) and Cl^- (about 125 mM), but low in K^+ (about 4.5 mM). The free-Ca^{2+} concentration is about 1.8 mM. In contrast, the intracellular fluid has a low concentration of Na^+ (about 15 mM or less) and Cl (about 6 mM), but a high concentration of K^+ (about 150 mM) (Fig. 2). The free intracellular Ca^{2+} concentration ($[Ca]_i$) is about 10^{-7} M, but during contraction it rises to 10^{-5} or 10^{-4} M. The total intracellular Ca^{2+} is much higher (about 2 mM/kg), but most of this is bound to molecules, such as proteins, or is sequestered into compartments, such as the sarcoplasmic reticulum. Most of the intracellular K^+ is free, and it has a diffusion coefficient only slightly less than K^+ in free solution (for refs., see Sperelakis, 1979). Thus, under normal conditions, the skeletal muscle fiber maintains its internal ion concentrations markedly different from those in the medium bathing the cells, and it is these ion concentration differences that underlie the resting E_m and excitability.

B. Sodium–Potassium Pump

The intracellular ion concentrations are maintained differently from those in the extracellular fluid by active ion-transport mechanisms that expend metabolic energy to push specific ions against their concentration or electrochemical gradients. These ion pumps are located in the cell membrane at the cell surface (see Fig. 2) and probably also in the transverse (T) tubular membrane. The major ion pump is the Na–K-linked pump, which pumps three Na^+ ions out of the cell against its electrochemical gradient, while simultaneously pumping two K^+ ions in against its electrochemical gradient. The coupling with K^+ pumping is obligatory, since in zero $[K]_o$ the Na^+ can no longer be pumped out. The coupling ratio for the amount of Na^+ pumped out to K^+ pumped in is usually 3:2. If the ratio were 3:3, the pump would be electrically neutral or nonelectrogenic; a potential difference (PD) across the membrane would not be directly produced because the pump would pull in one positive charge (K^+) for every positive charge (Na^+) it pushed out. With a ratio of 3:2, the pump is electrogenic and directly produces a PD that causes the membrane potential (E_m) to be greater (more negative) than it would be otherwise [on the basis of the ion concentration gradients and relative permeabilities or net diffusion potential (E_{diff}) alone]. Under normal steady-state conditions, the contribution of the Na^+ electrogenic pump potential (V_{ep}) to E_m in skeletal muscle fibers is only a few millivolts in frog muscle, but is about 16 mV in mammalian muscle.

The driving mechanism for the Na–K pump is the membrane (Na^+,K^+)-ATPase that requires both Na^+ and K^+ ions for activation. This enzyme requires

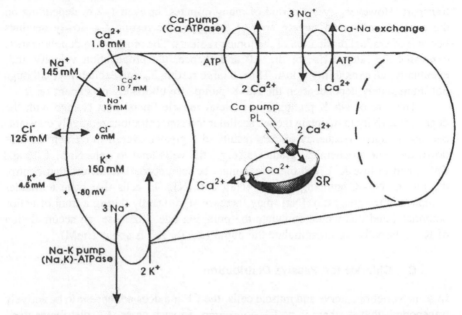

Figure 2 Intracellular and extracellular ion distributions in vertebrate skeletal muscle fibers. Also shown are the polarity and magnitude of the resting potential. Arrows indicate direction of the net electrochemical gradient. The Na^+–K^+ pump and Ca^{2+}–Na^+ exchange carrier are located in the cell surface membrane. A Ca-ATPase and a Ca^{2+} pump, similar to that in the sarcoplasmic reticulum (SR), are located in the cell membrane. Phospholamban (PL) is depicted close to the Ca^{2+} pump of the sarcoplasmic reticulum and serves to regulate pump activity.

Mg^{2+} for activity, and it is inhibited by Ca^{2+}. Thus, ATP, Mg^{2+}, and Na^+ are required at the inner surface of the membrane, and K^+ is required on the outer surface. A phosphorylated intermediate of the (Na^+,K^+)-ATPase occurs in the transport cycle, its phosphorylation being Na^+-dependent and its dephosphorylation being (K^+-dependent) (for refs., see Sperelakis, 1979). The enzyme–pump usually drives three Na^+ ions out and two K^+ ions in for each ATP molecule hydrolyzed. The (Na^+,K^+)-ATPase is specifically inhibited by the cardiac glycosides acting on the outer surface. The enzyme–pump is also inhibited by sulfhydryl reagents (such as *N*-ethylmaleimide, mercurial diuretics, and ethacrynic acid), indicating that the SH groups are crucial for activity.

Blockade of the Na–K pump by ouabain in frog muscle produces a relatively small immediate depolarization of about 2–6 mV, representing the contribution of V_{ep} to E_m. The amount of rapid depolarization in mammalian muscle is greater, about 16 mV. Excitability and the generation of an action potential (AP) are only slightly affected at short times, since excitability is independent of active ion transport. However, over a period of many minutes, or even 1–2 h, depending on the ratio of volume to surface area of the fiber, the resting E_m slowly declines because of gradual dissipation of the ionic gradients. The progressive depolarization depresses the rate of rise of the AP and, hence, the propagation velocity and, eventually, all excitability is lost. Thus, a large resting E_m and excitability, although not immediately dependent on the Na–K pump, are ultimately dependent on it.

The rate of Na–K pumping in skeletal muscle fibers must change with the degree of activity to maintain the intracellular ion concentrations relatively constant, because a higher frequency of APs results in a greater overall movement of ions down their electrochemical gradients (e.g., the cells tend to gain Na^+, Cl^-, and Ca^{2+}, and to lose K^+), and these ions must be repumped. The factors that control the rate of Na–K pumping include $[Na]_i$ and $[K]_o$. In cells that have a smaller volume/surface area ratio, $[Na]_i$ may increase significantly during a train of action potentials, and this would stimulate the pumping rate. Likewise, an accumulation of K^+ externally would stimulate the pump (K_m for K^+ is about 2 mM).

C. Chloride Ion Passive Distribution

In some vertebrate nerve and muscle cells, the Cl^- ion does not appear to be actively transported; that is, there is no Cl^- ion pump. In such cases, Cl^- distributes itself passively (no energy used) in accordance with E_m; E_{Cl} becomes equal to E_m if the cell is at rest. In amphibian and mammalian skeletal muscle fibers also, Cl^- seems to follow passive distribution, because $[Cl]_i$ is at (or slightly above) the value predicted by the Nernst equation from the resting E_m (for refs., see Sperelakis, 1979). When passively distributed, $[Cl]_i$ is low because the negative potential inside the cell (the resting E_m) expels the negatively charged Cl^- ion until the Cl^- distribution is at equilibrium with E_m). Hence, for a resting E_m of –80 mV, and taking $[Cl]_o$ to be 125 mM, $[Cl]_i$ would be 6.1 mM (E_m = +61 mV log $[Cl]_i/[Cl]_o$ (see Fig. 2). However, during the AP, the inside of the cell goes in a positive direction, and net Cl^- influx (outward I_{Cl}) will occur, thereby increasing $[Cl]_i$. The magnitude of the Cl^- influx depends on the Cl^- conductance (g_{Cl}) of the membrane $[I_{Cl}, = g_{Cl}(E - E_{Cl})]$. Thus, the average level of $[Cl]_i$ in working skeletal muscles should depend on the frequency and duration of the APs, that is, on the mean E_m averaged over many AP cycles.

D. Calcium Ion Distribution

For the positively charged Ca^{2+} ion, there must be some mechanism for removing Ca^{2+} from the myoplasm; otherwise the muscle fibers would continue to gain Ca^{2+} until there was no electrochemical gradient for its net influx. (This would occur until the free $[Ca]_i$ in the myoplasm was even greater than that outside (2 mM), because of the negative potential inside the cell.) Therefore, there must be one or more Ca^{2+} pumps operating. The sarcoplasmic reticulum (SR) membrane contains a Ca^{2+}-activated ATPase that actively pumps Ca^{2+} from the myoplasm into the SR lumen at the expense of ATP, and is capable of pumping down the Ca^{2+} to a concentration of less than 10^{-7} M. This sequestration of Ca^{2+} by the SR is essential for muscle relaxation. (The mitochondria also can actively take up Ca^{2+} to about the same degree as the SR, but this Ca^{2+} pool does not play an important role in normal excitation–contraction-coupling processes.) However, the resting Ca^{2+} influx and extra Ca^{2+} influx that enters with each AP (see following section) must be returned to the interstitial fluid. Two mechanisms have been proposed (see Fig. 2) for this (for refs., see Sperelakis, 1979) (1) a Ca–Na exchange occurs across the cell membrane, and (2) a Ca–ATPase, similar to that in the SR, is present in the sarcolemma.

E. Calcium–Sodium Exchange

The Ca–Na exchange reaction exchanges one internal Ca^{2+} ion for the three external Na^+ ions by a membrane carrier molecule (for refs., see Sperelakis, 1979; see Fig. 2). This reaction is facilitated by ATP, but ATP is not hydrolyzed. Instead, the energy for the pumping of Ca^{2+} against its large electrochemical gradient comes from the Na^+ electrochemical gradient. That is, the uphill transport of Ca^{2+} is coupled to the downhill movement of Na^+. Therefore, the energy required for this Ca^{2+} movement is effectively derived from the (Na^+,K^+)-ATPase. Thus, the Na–K pump, which uses ATP to maintain the Na^+ electrochemical gradient, indirectly helps to maintain the Ca^{2+} electrochemical gradient. Hence, the inward Na^+ leak is greater than it would be otherwise. The energy cost (ΔG_{Ca}, in J/mol) for pumping out Ca^{2+} ion is directly proportional to its electrochemical gradient, namely, $\Delta G_{Ca} = zF(E_m - E_{Ca})$. The energy available from the Na^+ distribution is directly proportional to its electrochemical gradient [$\Delta G_{Na} = zF(E_m - E_{Na})$]. Depending on the exact values of $[Na]_i$ and $[Ca]_i$ during rest, the energetics would be adequate for an Na^+/Ca^{+2} exchange ratio of 3:1. An exchange ratio of 3:1 would produce a small depolarization owing to the net inward Na–Ca exchange current. The exchange reaction depends on the relative concentrations of Ca^{2+} and Na^+ on each side of the membrane and on the relative affinities of their binding sites. Because of this Ca–Na exchange reaction, whenever the cell gains Na^+ it will also gain Ca^{2+}, because the exchange reaction becomes slowed (e.g., the Na^+ electrochemical gradient is reduced). In addition, when an elevated $[Na]_i$ occurs, some of the exchange carriers will exchange the ions in reverse (internal Na^+ for external Ca^{2+}) and will thus increase Ca^{2+} influx. The net effect of both mechanisms is to elevate $[Ca]_i$. The Ca–Na exchange process is involved in the positive inotropic action of cardiac glycosides in the heart.

   Reversal of the Ca–Na exchange can also occur during the AP depolarization because of the favorable energetics; the reversal potential (E_{rev}) is at about –80 mV (for $E_{Ca} = 130$ mV, $E_{Na} = 60$ mV, and a coupling ratio of 3:1). The relationship is as follows:

$$E_{rev} = E_{Na/Ca} = 3 E_{Na} - 2E_{Ca}$$

Thus, a Ca^{2+} influx (and net outward current) can occur during the AP by this mechanism. This Ca_o-Na_i exchange is also electrogenic (hyperpolarizing). It has been proposed that this mechanism is important in cardiac excitation–contraction coupling (Mullins, 1979).

F. Equilibrium Potentials

For each ionic species distributed unequally across the cell membrane, an equilibrium potential (E_i) or battery can be calculated for that ion from the Nernst equation (for 37°C): $E_i = -61$ mV/z [log (C_i/C_o)], where C_i is the internal concentration of the ion, C_o is the extracellular concentration, and z is the valance (with sign) (Fig. 3). The Nernst equation gives the PD (electrical force) that would exactly oppose the concentration gradient (diffusion force). Only a very small charge separation (Q, in coulombs) is required to build up a very large PD ($E_m = Q/C_m$). For the ion distributions given previously, the approximate equilibrium potentials are $E_{Na} = +60$ mV, $E_{Ca} = +129$ mV, $E_K = -94$ mV, and $E_{Cl} = -80$ mV (see Fig. 3). The sign gives the direction of the concentration gradient, with the side of higher concentration being negative for positive ions (cations) and positive for negative ions (anions). Any ion for which the equilibrium potential is different from the resting E_m (–80 mV) is off equilibrium and, therefore, must effectively be pumped at the expense of energy. In the muscle fiber, only Cl^- appears to be at or near equilibrium, whereas Na^+, Ca^{2+}, K^+, and H^+ are effectively actively transported. A more detailed discussion of concentration cells and diffusion is given by Sperelakis (1979).

G. Electrochemical Driving Forces and Membrane Ionic Currents

The electrochemical driving force for each species of ion is the algebraic difference between its equilibrium potential, E_i, and membrane potential, E_m (Fig. 4). The total driving force is the sum of two forces: an electrical force (e.g., the negative potential in the cell tends to pull in positively charged ions) and a diffusion force (based on the concentration gradient). Thus, in a resting cell, the driving force for Na^+ is: $E_m - E_{Na} = -80$ mV – (+60 mV) = –140 mV. The negative sign means that the driving force is directed to bring about net movement of Na^+ inward. The driving force for Ca^{2+} is: $E_m - E_{Ca} = -80$ mV – (+129 mV) = –209 mV. The driving force for K^+ is: $E_m - E_K = 80$ mV – (–94 mV) = +14 mV; hence, the driving force for K^+ is small and directed outward (see Fig. 4). The driving force for Cl^- is zero for a cell at rest (assuming passive distribution): $E_m - E_{Cl} = -80$ mV – (–80 mV) = 0). However, during the AP, when E_m is changing, the driving force for Cl^- is not zero, and there is a net driving force for inward Cl^- movement

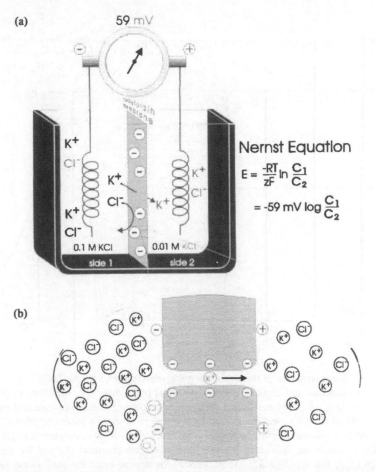

(a)

59 mV

Nernst Equation

$$E = \frac{-RT}{zF} \ln \frac{C_1}{C_2}$$

$$= -59 \text{ mV} \log \frac{C_1}{C_2}$$

K⁺
Cl⁻
K⁺
Cl⁻
K⁺
Cl⁻
0.1 M KCl

K⁺
Cl⁻
K⁺
0.01 M KCl

side 1   side 2

(b)

Figure 3 Development of a potential across the membrane of a concentration cell. (a) In a two-compartment system, a diffusion potential develops across the artificial membrane containing negatively charged pores. The membrane is impermeable to Cl⁻, but permeable to cations such as K⁺. The concentration gradient for K⁺ causes a potential to be generated, the side of higher K⁺ concentration becoming negative (see text for elaboration of the Nernst equation). (b) Expanded diagram of a water-filled pore in the membrane, showing the permeability to K⁺, but lack of penetration of Cl⁻. The potential difference is generated by the charge separation, a slight excess of K⁺ being held close to the right-hand surface of the membrane; a slight excess of Cl⁻ is clustered close to the left-hand surface.

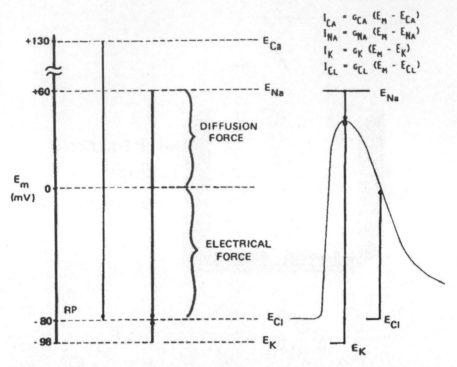

Figure 4 Representation of the electrochemical driving forces for Na^+, Ca^{2+}, K^+, and Cl^- at rest (left diagram) and during the action potential (right diagram). Equilibrium potentials for each ion (e.g., E_{Na}) are positioned vertically according to their magnitude and sign; they were calculated from the Nernst equation for a given set of extracellular and intracellular ion concentrations. Measured resting potential is assumed to be −80 mV. Electrochemical-driving force for an ion is the difference between its equilibrium potential (E_i) and the membrane potential (E_m), that is, ($E_i − E_m$). Thus, at rest, the driving force for Na^+ is the difference between E_{Na} and the resting E_m; if E_{Na} is +60 mV and resting E_m is −80 mV, the driving force is 140 mV. The driving force is then the algebraic sum of the diffusion force and the electrical force, and is represented by the length of the arrows in the diagram. Driving force for Ca^{2+} (about 210 mV) is even greater than that for Na^+, whereas that for K^+ is much less (about 18 mV). Direction of the arrows indicates the direction of the net electrochemical driving force; namely, the direction for K^+ is outward, whereas that for Na^+ and Ca^{2+} is inward. If Cl^- is passively distributed, then its distribution across the cell membrane can be determined only by the net membrane potential; for a cell remaining a long time at rest, E_{Cl} = E_m, and there is no net driving force. The driving forces change during the action potential, as depicted. The equations for the different ionic currents are given in the upper right-hand portion of the figure. (Adapted from Sperelakis, 1979.)

(outward Cl^- current). Similarly, the driving force of K^+ outward movement increases during the AP, whereas those for Na^+ and Ca^{2+} decrease (see Fig. 4).

The net current for each ionic species (I_i) is equal to its driving force times its conductance (g_i, reciprocal of the resistance) through the membrane. This is essentially Ohm's law, $I = V/R$, modified for the fact that in an electrolytic system the total force driving net movement of a charged particle must take into account both the electrical force and the concentration (or chemical) force. Thus, for the four ions, the net current can be expressed as (see Fig. 4):

$$I_{Na} = g_{Na} (E_m - E_{Na})$$
$$I_{Ca} = g_{Ca} (E_m - E_{Ca})$$
$$I_K = g_K (E_m - E_K)$$
$$I_{Cl} = g_{Cl} (E_m - E_{Cl})$$

In a resting cell, Cl^- and Ca^{2+} can be neglected, and the Na^+ current (inward) must be equal and opposite to the K^+ current (outward) to maintain a steady resting potential: $I_K = -I_{Na}$. Thus, although in the resting membrane, the driving force for Na^+ is much greater than that for K^+, g_K is proportionally larger than g_{Na}, so the currents are equal. Hence, there is a continual leak of Na^+ inward and K^+ outward even in a resting cell, and the system would eventually run down if active pumping were blocked. Since the ratio of the Na^+/K^+ driving forces (-140 mV/$+14$ mV) is 10, the ratio of conductances (g_{Na}/g_K) should be about 1:10. The fact that g_K is much greater than g_{Na} accounts for the resting potential being close to E_K and away from E_{Na}.

G. Determination of Resting Potential

For given ion distributions (which normally remain nearly constant under the usual steady-state conditions), the resting potential (actually E_{diff}, which is the net diffusion potential, i.e., exclusive of the electrogenic pump potential contribution) is determined by the relative membrane conductance (g) or permeability (P) for Na^+ and K^+ ions. That is, the resting potential (of about -80 mV) is close to E_K (about -94 mV) because $g_K >> g_{Na}$ or $P_K >> P_{Na}$. From circuit analysis (using Ohm's law and Kirchhoff's law), one can prove that this is true. Therefore, E_m will always be closer to the battery (equilibrium potential) having the lowest resistance (highest conductance) in series with it (Fig. 5). In the resting membrane, this battery is E_K, whereas in the excited membrane it is E_{Na}, because there is a large increase in g_{Na} during the AP. Any ion that is passively distributed cannot determine the resting E_m; instead, the resting E_m determines the distribution of that ion. Therefore, Cl^- drops out of the consideration for skeletal muscle fibers because it seems to be passively distributed. However, transient net movement of Cl^- across the membrane does influence E_m. For example, washout of Cl^- from the cell (in Cl^--free solution) produces a transient depolarization and spontaneous APs and twitches, followed by return to the normal resting potential

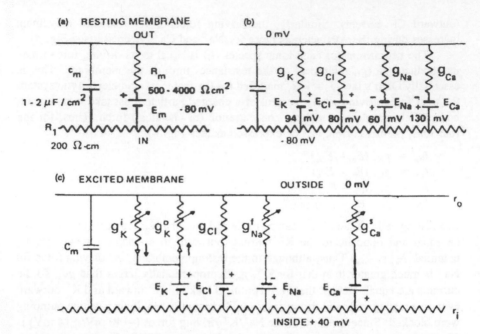

Figure 5 Electrical equivalent circuits for a skeletal muscle fiber cell membrane at rest (a,b) and during excitation (c). (a) Membrane as a parallel resistance capacitance circuit, the membrane resistance (R_m) being in parallel with the membrane capacitance (C_m). Resting potential (E_m) is represented by an 80-mV battery in series with the membrane resistance, the negative pole facing inward. (b) Membrane resistance is divided into four component parts, one for each of the four major ions of importance: K^+, Cl^-, Na^+, and Ca^{2+}. Resistances for these ions (R_K, R_{Cl}, R_{Na}, and R_{Ca}) are parallel to one another, and represent totally separate and independent pathways for permeation of each ion through the resting membrane. These ion resistances are depicted as their reciprocals, namely, ion conductances (g_K, g_{Cl}, g_{Na}, and g_{Ca}). Equilibrium potential, for each ion (e.g., E_K), determined solely by the ion distribution in the steady state and calculated from the Nernst equation, is shown in series with the conductance path for that ion. Resting potential of –80 mV is determined by the equilibrium potentials and by the relative conductances. (c) Equivalent circuit is further expanded to illustrate that for the voltage-dependent conductances. There are at least two separate K^+-conductance pathways (labeled here g_K^o and g_K^i). In series with the K^+ conductances are rectifiers pointing in the direction of least resistance to current flow. Thus g_K^o allows K^+ flux to occur more readily in the outward direction (so-called outward-directed rectification), whereas g_K^i allows K^+ flux to occur more readily in the inward direction (inward-directed rectification). There is one Na^+ conductance pathway, the kinetically fast Na^+ conductance (g_{Na}^f). In addition, there is a kinetically slow pathway that allows Ca^{2+} to pass through. Arrows drawn through the resistors indicate that the conductances are variable, depending on membrane potential and time. (Adapted from Sperelakis, 1979.)

and quiescence when Cl^- is all washed out. Reintroduction of Cl^- produces a transient hyperpolarization, followed by return to the normal resting potential when Cl^- is reequilibrated. The g_{Cl} is relatively high in skeletal muscle fibers. Because of its relatively low concentration, coupled with its relatively low resting conductance, the Ca^{2+} distribution has only a relatively small effect on the resting E_m, and so it can be ignored. Therefore, a simplified version of the Goldman–Hodgkin–Katz *constant-field equation* can be given (for 37°C):

$$E_m = -61 \text{ mV } \ln \frac{[K]_i + P_{Na}/P_K [Na]_i}{[K]_o + P_{Na}/P_K [No]}$$

This equation shows that for a given ion distribution, the resting E_m is determined by the P_{Na}/P_K ratio (the relative permeability of the membrane to Na^+ and K^+). There is a direct proportionality between P_K and g_K and between P_{Na} and g_{Na} at a constant E_m and concentrations (for a discussion of this, see Sperelakis, 1979). For skeletal muscle fibers, the P_{Na}/P_K ratio is about 0.04.

Inspection of the constant-field equation shows that the numerator of the log term will be dominated by the $[K]_i$ term [since (P_{Na}/P_K) $[Na]_i$ will be very small], whereas the denominator will be affected by both the $[K]_o$, and (P_{Na}/P_K) $[Na]_o$ terms. This relationship thus accounts for the deviation of the E_m versus log $[K]_o$ curve from a straight line (having a slope of 61 mV/decade) in normal Ringer solution. When $[K]_o$ is elevated ($[Na]_o$ reduced by an equimolar amount), the denominator becomes more and more dominated by the $[K]_o$ term and less and less by $(P_{Na}/P_K)[Na]_o$. Therefore, in bathing solutions of high K^+, the constant-field equation approaches the simple Nernst equation for K^+, and E_m approaches E_K. As $[K]_o$ is raised, E_K becomes correspondingly reduced, since $[K]_i$ stays relatively constant; therefore, the membrane becomes more and more depolarized (Fig. 6).

An alternative method of approximating the resting potential is by the *chord-conductance equation*:

$$E_m = \frac{g_K}{g_K + g_{Na}} E_K + \frac{g_{Na}}{g_K + g_{Na}} E_{Na}$$

This equation can be derived from Ohm's law and circuit analysis for the condition when net current is zero (see Sperelakis, 1979). The chord-conductance equation again illustrates the important fact that the ratio g_K/g_{Na} determines the resting potential. When $g_K \gg g_{Na}$, then E_m is close to E_K; conversely, when $g_{Na} \gg g_K$ (as during the spike AP), E_m shifts close to E_{Na}.

When $[K]_o$ is lowered below the physiological level (e.g., to 0.1 mM), a depolarization strangely occurs, as shown in Figure 6. This depolarization could be explained by several factors: (1) inhibition of the electrogenic Na^+ pump (V_{ep}), (2) a decrease in P_K (and, therefore, g_K), and (3) a decrease in g_K (but not P_K) owing to the concentration effect.

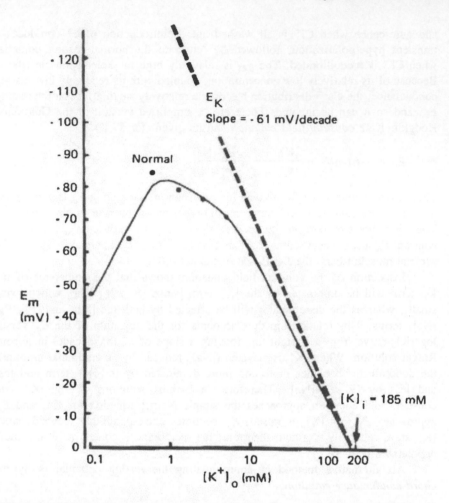

Figure 6 The mean resting membrane potential (E_m) of normal mouse skeletal muscle (extensor digitorum longus, EDL) plotted as a function of the extracellular K^+ concentration ($[K]_o$) on a logarithmic scale. The straight line drawn through the data points for 20 mM $[K]_o$ and above (fitted by method of least squares) has a slope of 50 mV/decade. Extrapolation of this line to zero potential gives the intracellular K^+ concentration ($[K]_i$) of 185 mM. The dashed line gives the calculated E_K values (slope of 61 mV/decade). Note the "foldover" of the E_m curve at $[K]_o$ levels below 1 mM, presumably owing to inhibition of the electrogenic pump potential (V_{ep}) and to a decrease in P_K and g_K at low $[K]_o$ levels. (From Sellin and Sperelakis, 1978.)

Inhibition of the Na–K pump will gradually run down the ion concentration gradients. The cells lose K^+ and gain Na^+; therefore, E_K and E_{Na} become smaller. The cells thus become depolarized (even if the relative permeabilities are unaffected), which causes them to gain Cl^- and, therefore, also water (cells swell). In summary, in the presence of ouabain (short-term exposure only) to inhibit V_{ep}, the resting E_m or net diffusion potential E_{diff} is determined by the ion concentration gradients for K^+ and Na^+ and by the relative permeability for K^+ and Na^+ (Fig. 7). When the Na–K pump is operating, there is normally a small additional contribution of V_{ep} to the resting E_m of about 6–16 mV in mammalian skeletal muscle. Thus, the contribution of V_{ep} to the resting E_m is relatively small. V_{ep} is actually greater than E_{diff}, since V_{ep} and E_{diff} must be in parallel with one another, such that inhibition of V_{ep} allows E_{diff} to be expressed (see Fig. 7).

H. Surface Charge

The cell membrane has fixed negative charges on its outer and inner surfaces (Fig. 8). These charges are due to acidic phospholipids in the bilayer and to charged protein molecules embedded in the lipid bilayer. Because of their acid isoelectric point, the proteins possess a net negative charge at a pH near 7.0. The charge difference between the outer surface of the cell membrane and the bathing solution is known as the *zeta potential*, and is responsible for the passive electrophoretic movement of dead cells in an applied electric field. The surface charge affects the true potential difference (PD) across the membrane. At each surface, the fixed negative charge produces an electric field that extends a short distance into the solution, and causes each surface of the membrane to be a few millivolts more negative than the extracellular and intracellular solutions (see Fig. 8). This surface potential declines exponentially with a length constant of a few angstrom units, depending on the ionic strength of the solution. The magnitude of the surface potential depends on the density of the charges. The number of charges is also affected by the pH.

The membrane potential measured by an intracellular microelectrode (E_M) is the potential of the outer solution (ψ_o) minus the potential of the inner solution (ψ_i): $E_m = \psi_o - \psi_i$ (see Fig. 8a). The true PD directly across the membrane (E_m'), however, is that including the surface charges, and is the PD controlling the ionic conductances of the membrane. E_m' equals E_m only when the surface charges at the two surfaces are equal. If the outer surface charge is decreased by extra binding of cations, such as Ca^{2+}, then the membrane becomes slightly hyperpolarized ($E_m' > E_m$), although this is not measurable by an intracellular microelectrode (see Fig. 8b). Conversely, if the inner surface charge were decreased, then the membrane would become slightly depolarized ($E_m' < E_m$). Because the membrane conductances are controlled by E_m' (and not by E_m), changes in the surface charges by drugs, ionic strength, or pH can lead to apparent shifts in the threshold potential and inactivation potential (e.g., shift in E_m vs h_∞ curve).

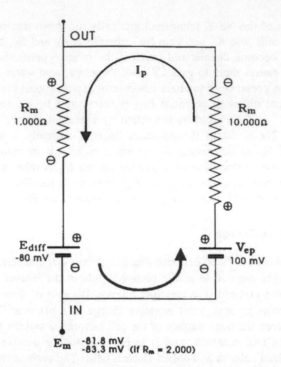

Figure 7 Hypothetical electrical equivalent circuit for the electrogenic Na^+ pump. Model consists of a pump pathway in parallel with the membrane resistance (R_m) pathway and the membrane capacitance (C_m) pathway. This model conforms to the evidence that the pump is independent of short-range membrane excitability and that the pump and channel proteins are embedded in the lipid bilayer as parallel elements. The net diffusion potential [(E_{diff}), determined by the ion equilibrium potentials and relative permeabilities] of –80 mV is depicted in series with R_m. The pump leg is assumed to consist of a battery in series with a fixed resistor [pump resistance (R_p)] that does not change with changes in R_m, the value of which is tenfold higher than R_m. The pump battery is charged up to some voltage [electrogenic pump potential (V_{ep}) of –100 mV, for example] by a pump current generator. The net electrogenic pump current is developed by the pumping in only two K^+ for every three Na^+ pumped out. For the values given in the figure (R_m = 1000 Ω, E_{diff} = –80 mV, R_p = 10,000 Ω; V_{ep} = –100 mV), the measured membrane potential (E_m) can be calculated by circuit analysis to be –81.8 mV; that is, the direct electrogenic pump potential contribution to the resting potential is –1.8 mV. If R_m were raised to 2000 Ω (e.g., by placing the membrane in Cl^--free solution, or by adding Ba^{2+} ion to decrease P_K, or both), then the calculated E_m would be –83.3 mV, thus coming closer to V_{ep} (–100 mV). (Adapted from Sperelakis, 1979.)

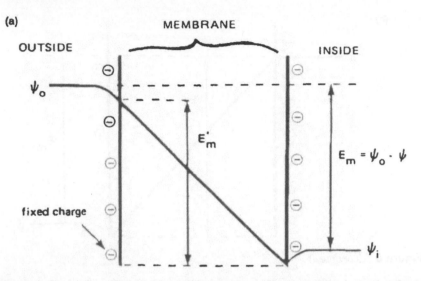

Figure 8   Potential profile across the cell membrane. (a) Because of fixed negative charges (at pH 7.4) at outer and inner surfaces of the membrane, there is a negative potential (indicated as downward) that extends from the edge of the membrane into the solutions on both sides of the membrane. This surface potential falls off exponentially with distance into the solution. Magnitude of the surface potential is a function of the charge density. ψ_o is the electrical potential of the outside solution, ψ_i is that of the inside solution, and membrane potential (E_m) is the potential difference ($\psi_o - \psi_i$). E_m is determined by the diffusion potentials and relative conductances. The potential profile through the membrane is shown as linear (the constant field assumption), although this need not be true. If the outer surface potential is equal to that at the inner surface, then the true transmembrane potential (E_m') is equal to the microelectrode-measured membrane potential (E_m). (b) If the outer surface potential is different from the inner potential (in this example, done by elevating the extracellular Ca^{2+} concentration to bind Ca^{2+} to more of the negative charges), then E_m' is greater than the measured E_m. Diminution of the inner surface charge decreases E_m'. The membrane ion channels are controlled by E_m'. (Adapted from Sperelakis, 1979.)

IV. Automaticity

To maintain a steady resting potential, the outward K^+ current must be equal and opposite to the inward Na^+ current (plus Ca^{2+}). If the inward current exceeds the outward current, then the membrane will depolarize along a certain time course (i.e., slope of the pacemaker potential), depending on the excess (or net) inward current. The inward leak of Na^+ and Ca^{2+} currents is often called the background inward current. For the inward current to exceed the outward current (i.e., for a net inward current), either the inward current can be increased, or outward current I_K can be decreased. Both of these mechanisms are used. For example, if a time-dependent decrease in g_K occurs following an action potential, then I_K decreases

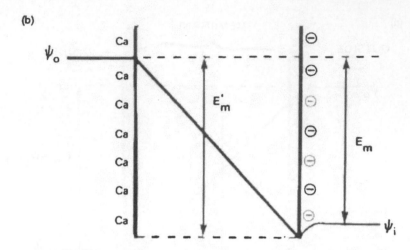

Figure 8   (*continued*)

and the membrane depolarizes (g_{Na}/g_K) progressively increases). Conversely, if an agent increases the resting g_K, then the outward I_K is increased, the membrane hyperpolarizes, and the slope of the pacemaker potential decreases, thus reducing the frequency of firing. Some agents may increase the background inward current and decrease the outward current, thereby increasing the slope of the pacemaker potential by both mechanisms.

A prerequisite for automaticity is that the fibers must have a relatively low Cl^- conductance (g_{Cl}) (Cole, 1968). A high g_{Cl} acts to clamp E_m, making it difficult for a pacemaker potential to be developed. For example, addition of Ba^{2+} (0.5 mM) to frog sartorius muscle fibers, which have a high P_{Cl}/P_K ratio of about 4.0, has very little immediate effect. However, when the fibers are first equilibrated in Cl-free solution to reduce g_{Cl} to zero, Ba^{2+} produces a prompt depolarization, an increase in R_m, and automaticity (Sperelakis et al., 1967). A spontaneous firing of skeletal muscle APs, known as *myotonia*, can occur in fibers with an abnormally low g_{Cl} or P_{Cl} (see Chap. 3).

During the time course of the linear (ramp) pacemaker potential (V_p), membrane resistance (R_m) increases progressively owing to a decrease in g_K (Sperelakis and Lehmkuhl, 1964). There is a progressive turnoff of the g_K increase (delayed rectification) that was responsible for the rapid repolarizing phase of the action potential. The decreasing g_K produces the spontaneous depolarization. Thus, in the presence of a steady inward background current, depolarization of automatic cells is partly explained by deactivation of the outward K^+ current that was activated during the preceding AP.

All excitable cells are capable of exhibiting automaticity under certain conditions. For example, ventricular myocardial cells exposed to Ba^{2+}, to decrease g_K and depolarize, develop automaticity (Sperelakis and Lehmkuhl, 1966). Ventricular muscle depolarized by the application of current also fires spontaneously during the current pulse (Sperelakis and Lehmkuhl, 1964; Katzung, 1975). That is, when E_m is brought into the voltage region that can develop pacemaker potentials, automaticity occurs. In any pacemaker cell, if the membrane potential is hyperpolarized by a current pulse, the frequency of spontaneous firing is slowed and stopped; thus, automaticity is suppressed at high E_m values (Sperelakis and Lehmkuhl, 1964). Conversely, application of depolarizing current increases the frequency of discharge. The slope of the pacemaker potential is exquisitely sensitive to small changes in E_m. The farther E_m is above E_K (within limits), the greater the degree of automaticity. A low g_K, which also means a relatively lower resting E_m, facilitates automaticity. Elevation of $[K]_o$, which increases g_K, suppresses automaticity, despite depolarization (Sperelakis and Lehmkuhl, 1966).

One characteristic of a pacemaker cell is that accommodation does not occur; the cell fires, no matter how slowly E_m is brought to the threshold potential V_{th}.

V. Effect of Resting Potential on Action Potential

Any agent that affects the resting potential has important repercussions on the AP. Depolarization reduces the rate of rise of the AP and, thereby, also slows its velocity of propagation (Fig. 9). A slow spread of excitation throughout the muscle will interfere with its ability to act efficiently. This effect is progressive as a function of the degree of depolarization. If the muscle fibers are depolarized to about –50 mV, by any means, then the rate of rise goes to zero, and all excitability and contraction are lost.

Hyperpolarization usually produces only a small increase in the rate of rise. Larger hyperpolarizations may actually slow the velocity of propagation, and even cause propagation block, because the critical depolarization required to bring the membrane to its threshold potential is increased.

The explanation for the effect of resting E_m (or takeoff potential) on maximum rate of rise (max dV/dt) of the AP is based on the sigmoidal h_∞ versus E_m curve (see Fig. 9). In Hodgkin–Huxley notation, h is the inactivation variable for the fast Na^+ conductance; it is a probability factor that deals with the open ($h = 1.0$) versus closed ($h = 0$) positions of the inactivation (I) gate of the channel (Fig. 10). The h factor varies as a function of E_m and time (t), and h_∞ is the h value at steady state or infinite time (practically, $t > 20$ ms). At the normal resting potential (–80 mV), h_∞ is 0.9–1.0 and diminishes with depolarization, becoming zero at about –50 mV.

lower activation (threshold) potential of about -35 mV (compared with about -55 mV for the fast Na^+ channels).

The resting potential also affects duration of the AP. With polarizing current, depolarization lengthens the AP, whereas hyperpolarization shortens it. In contrast, when elevated $[K]_o$ is used to depolarize the cells, the AP is usually shortened. One important determinant of the AP duration is the K^+ conductance (g_K). Agents or conditions that increase g_K, such as elevation of $[K]_o$, shorten the duration. In contrast, agents that decrease g_K or slow the activation of g_K, such as Ba^{2+} ion or tetraethylammonium ion (TEA^+), lengthen the AP duration. Because of anomalous rectification (i.e., a decrease in g_K with depolarization and an increase with hyperpolarization), depolarization by current prolongs the AP and hyperpolarization shortens it.

Other factors are also important in determining the AP duration. For example, agents that slow the closing of the I-gates of the fast Na^+ channels, such as veratridine, prolong the AP. The AP also becomes prolonged in Cl^--free solution. At high rates of activity, two factors could contribute toward changes in the membrane potentials: (1) The increase in $[Ca]_i$ (resulting from an increase in $[Na]_i$) produces an increase in g_K (the $g_{K(Ca)}$ channel) (the Meech–Gardos effect; Meech, 1972). (2) The K^+ accumulates outside the cell membrane, thereby increasing g_K and decreasing E_K.

VI. Electrogenesis of the Action Potential

A. General Overview

The action potentials in vertebrate skeletal muscle twitch fibers consist of a spike followed by depolarizing ("negative") afterpotential (Fig. 11). A large, fast inward Na^+ current, passing through fast Na^+ channels, is responsible for electrogenesis of the spike, which rises rapidly (400–700 V/s). Subsequently, a small slow inward Ca^{2+} current, passing through kinetically slow channels, may be involved in excitation–contraction coupling (see later). The skeletal muscle cell membrane has at least two types of voltage-dependent K^+ channels (see Fig. 5). One type allows K^+ ions to pass more readily inward (against the net electrochemical gradient for K^+) than outward: the *inward-going rectifier*. This gated channel is responsible for anomalous rectification (i.e., decrease in g_K with depolarization), and quickly decreases its conductance after depolarization and increases its conductance with repolarization. The second type of K^+ channel is similar to the usual K^+ channel found in other excitable membranes; the *delayed rectifier*. Its conductance turns on more slowly than g_{Na} after depolarization. This channel allows K^+ to pass more readily outward (down the electrochemical gradient for K^+) than inward, and so is also known as the *outward-going rectifier*. The activation of this channel produces the large increase in total g_K that terminates the AP (see Fig. 11).

The AP amplitude is about 120 mV, from a resting potential of -80 mV to a

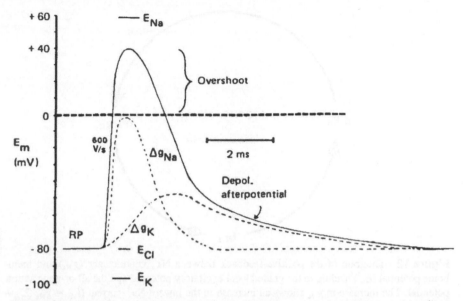

Figure 11 Diagrammatic representation of the relative conductance changes for Na^+ and K^+ during an action potential (AP) in skeletal muscle fibers. The rising phase of the AP is caused by an increase in g_{Na}, which brings the membrane potential (E_m) toward the Na^+ equilibrium potential (E_{Na}). The falling phase the AP is due to the rise in g_K and to the decrease in g_{Na} and to an outward Cl^- current (g_{Cl} constant). The depolarizing afterpotential is explained by the fact that the delayed rectifier K^+ channel is less selective for K^+ (30:1 over Na^+) than is the resting channel (100:1).

peak overshoot potential of about +40 mV (see Fig. 11). The duration of the AP (at 50% repolarization) ranges between 3 and 6 ms, depending on the species and temperature. The threshold potential (V_{th}) for triggering of the fast Na^+ channels is about –55 mV; thus, a critical depolarization of about 25 mV is required to reach V_{th}. The turn-on of the fast g_{Na} (fast I_{Na}) is very rapid (within 0.2 ms), and E_m is brought rapidly toward E_{Na} (see Fig. 11). There is an explosive (positive exponential initially) increase in g_{Na}, caused by a positive-feedback relationship between g_{Na} and E_m (Fig. 12).

From the current versus voltage curves, the maximum inward Na^+ fast current occurs at an E_m of about –20 mV. The current decreases at more depolarized E_m levels because of the diminution in electrochemical-driving force as the membrane is further depolarized, even though the conductance remains high. At the reversal potential (E_{rev}) for the current, the current goes to zero and then reverses direction with greater depolarization.

As E_m depolarizes, it crosses V_{th}, which is about –35 mV, for slow Ca^{2+} channels located in the transverse tubules. Turn-on of the Ca^{2+} conductance (g_{Ca}) and I_{Ca} is slow. The peak I_{Ca} is considerably smaller than the peak I_{Na}.

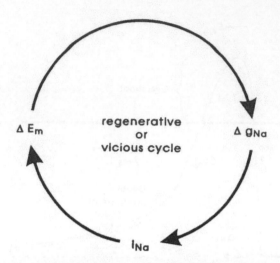

Figure 12 Diagram of the positive-feedback between Na^+ conductance (g_{Na}) and membrane potential (E_m) leading to the graded local excitatory potential and the all-or-none action potential. The increase in g_{Na} allows an increase in the inward Na^+ current [$I_{Na} = g_{Na} (E_m - E_{Na})$], which is depolarizing and so triggers a further increase in g_{Na}. This feedback cycle is enabled by the voltage dependency of the fast Na^+ channels. (Adapted from Hodgkin, 1957.)

B. Fast Sodium Ion Channel Activation

The fast Na^+ channels (and the slow Ca^{2+} channels) have a double-gating mechanism; one gate is the inactivation gate (I-gate), and the second gate is the activation gate (A-gate) (Fig. 13). For a channel to be conducting, both the A-gate and I-gate must be open; if either one is closed, the channel is nonconducting. The A-gate is located somewhere near the middle of the channel; it is not at the outer surface because tetrodotoxin (TTX) does not prevent the movement of this gate, and it is not at the inner surface because proteases do not affect it. The A-gate is closed at the resting E_m and opens rapidly at depolarization (whereas the I-gate is open at the resting E_m and closes slowly at depolarization) (see Fig. 13). In the Hodgkin–Huxley (1952) analysis, the opening of the A-gate requires simultaneous occupation of three negatively charged sites by three positively charged m^+ particles. If m, the activation variable, is the probability of one site being occupied, from m^3 is the probability that all three sites are occupied; therefore, $g_{Na} = \overline{g}_{Na} m^3 h$, where h is the inactivation variable and $\overline{g}_{Na}$ is the maximum conductance.
F13

A gating current (I_g) has been measured that corresponds to the movement of the charged m particles (or rotation of an equivalent dipole). The gating current is very small in intensity and is measured by subtracting the linear capacitative current (to a hyperpolarizing clamp step) from the total capacitative current (linear plus nonlinear) that occurs with a depolarizing clamp step beyond threshold. The outward

I_g leads into the inward I_{Na}. Tetrodotoxim does not block I_g, although it does block I_{Na}. Thus, the gating current is a nonlinear outward capacitative current (not an ionic current) obtained during depolarizing clamps that reflects movement of the A-gate from the closed to the open configuration. The linear capacitative current occurs in the lipid bilayer matrix, whereas the nonlinear capacitative-gating current occurs in the protein channels floating in the lipid matrix.

C. Sodium Ion Inactivation

The fast I_{Na} lasts only for 1–2 ms because of the spontaneous voltage inactivation of the fast Na^+ channels. That is, the fast Na^+ channels inactivate quickly, even if the membrane were to remain depolarized. (In contrast, the slow Ca^{2+} channels inactivate very slowly.) Inactivation is produced in the fast Na^+ channels by the voltage-dependent closing of the inactivation gate (I-gate; see Fig. 13). The I-gate is located near the inner surface of the membrane, as evidenced by the fact that addition of proteolytic enzyme to the inside of a perfused giant axon chops off the I-gate is presumably charged positively to allow it to move with changes in the membrane potential (see Fig. 13). During depolarization, the inside of the membrane becomes positive, and this causes the I-gate to close. At the normal resting potential, the I-gate is open (see Fig. 13).

The voltage dependency of inactivation is given by the h_∞ versus E_m curve (see Fig. 9). The inactivation variable h (probability function), varies between 0 and 1.0, perhaps reflecting occupation of a negatively charged site by a positively charged h particle, and h_∞ is the value of h at infinite time (> 20 ms) or at steady state. When $h = 1.0$, the I-gates of all the fast Na^+ channels are in the open configuration; conversely, when $h = 0$, all the I-gates are closed. Since the Na^+ conductance (g_{Na}) at any time is equal to the maximal value ($\bar{g}_{Na}$) times m^3h, when $h = 0$, $g_{Na} = 0$ and when $h = 1.0$, $gNa = \bar{g}_{Na}$ (if $m = 1.0$). At the normal resting potential, h_∞ is nearly 1.0 and diminishes with depolarization, becoming zero at about -50 mV. Since the maximal rate of rise of the AP (max dV/dt) is directly proportional to the net inward current or I_{Na}, which is directly proportional to g_{Na} [$dV/dt \propto I_{Na}/C_m \ \bar{g}Na \ m^3h \ (E_m - E_{Na})/C_m$], the decrease in h_∞ is the cause of decrease in max dV/dt. At about -50 mV, $h_\infty = 0$, and there is complete inactivation of the fast Na^+ channels. Therefore, depolarization by any means (e.g., elevated $[K]_o$ or applied current pulses) decreases max dV/dt, and excitability disappears at about -50 mV (see Fig. 9).

The slow Ca^{2+} channels behave much the same as the fast Na^+ channels relative to inactivation, with one main difference being the voltage range over which the slow channels inactivate: -45 to -10 mV for the slow channels, compared with -80 to -50 mV for the fast Na^+ channels. Another major difference is that the slow Ca^{2+} conductance inactivates much more slowly than the fast Na^+ conductance; that is, they have a long inactivation time constant (τ_{inact}). (The h variable for the slow channel is referred to as the f variable, and the m variable as the d variable.)

the g_{Na} channels would spontaneously inactivate, and so the g_{Na}/g_K ratio and E_m would slowly be restored to their original resting values.

In skeletal muscle, there is an important third factor involved in repolarization of the AP: the Cl^- current. The Cl^- permeability (P_{Cl}) and conductance (g_{Cl}) are very high in skeletal muscle. In fact, P_{Cl} of the surface membrane is much higher than P_K, the P_{Cl}/P_K ratio being about 3–7. As discussed earlier, the Cl^- ion is passively distributed, or nearly so, and thus cannot determine the resting potential under steady-state conditions. However, net Cl^- movements inward (hyperpolarizing) or outward (depolarizing) do affect E_m transiently until reequilibration occurs. There is no net electrochemical driving force for Cl^- current (I_{Cl}) at the resting potential, since $E_m = E_{Cl}$. However, during the AP depolarization, there is a larger and larger driving force for outward I_{Cl} (i.e., Cl^- influx), since $I_{Cl} = g_{Cl}(E_m - E_{Cl})$ (see Fig. 4). In other words, the large electric field that was keeping Cl^- out (i.e., $[Cl]_i << [Cl]_o$, such that $E_{Cl} = E_m$) is diminishing during the AP, and so Cl ion enters the fiber. This Cl^- entry is hyperpolarizing, and so tends to repolarize the membrane more quickly than would otherwise occur. That is, repolarization of the AP is "sharpened" by the Cl^- mechanism. For this mechanism to occur, there need not be any voltage-dependent gated g_{Cl} channels. All that is necessary is that there be a high g_{Cl}; the higher the g_{Cl}, the greater this effect. The importance of the Cl^- current in repolarization is illustrated by *myotonia* in which an abnormally low P_{Cl} causes repetitive APs to occur (see Chap. 3).

To illustrate some of the foregoing points, if skeletal muscle fibers are placed into Cl^--free Ringer solution (e.g., methanesulfonate substitution), depolarization and spontaneous APs and twitches occur for a few minutes, until most or all of the $[Cl]_i$ is washed out. After equilibration, the resting E_m returns to the original value (ca. −90 mV for frog muscle), clearly indicating that Cl^- does not determine the resting potential, and that net Cl^- efflux produces depolarization. Readdition of Cl^- to the bath produces a rapid, large hyperpolarization (e.g., to −120 mV), owing to net Cl^- influx; the E_m then slowly returns to the original value (−90 mV) as Cl^- reequilibrates (i.e., redistributes itself passively). These same effects would occur in cardiac muscle, smooth muscle, and nerve, but to a lesser extent, because in these tissues P_{Cl} is much lower (e.g., P_{Cl}/P_K ratio is about 0.5 in vascular smooth muscle).

G. Slow Potassium Ion Current

Two types of K^+ delayed rectifier currents occur in skeletal muscle. A slow I_K was first described by Adrian and coworkers (1970a,b) in frog sartorius fibers voltage-clamped at 30°C; the slow component of outward I_K reached a maximum in about 3 s (at −30 mV) and declined with a time constant of about 0.5 s (at −100 mV). In voltage-clamped frog toe muscle, Lynch (1978) observed that, with depolarizing clamps more positive than the threshold of −55 mV for activation of the outward K^+ current (about 5 mS/cm^2), 85% of the fibers had both fast and slow components to the outward I_K. In 7% of the fibers, only the slow component ($Q_{10} = 2.8$) was observed; it had an activation time constant of about 90 ms, and an inactivation time constant of 6.9 s (at 0 mV). The voltage dependence of both K^+ currents were shifted equally in the depolarizing direction by elevated $[Ca]_o$, or $[H]_o$, presumably by altering the net negative outer surface charge of the membrane, thereby "hyperpolarizing" (see foregoing). Acidosis also increased the rate of turn-on of the slow delayed rectifier, so that it became about equal to that of the fast delayed rectifier (pK_a = 5.8). The fast delayed current was relatively selectively blocked by TEA or by a sulfhydryl reagent, whereas the slow delayed current was selectively depressed by a histidine reagent. It was estimated that about 25% of the delayed rectifier channels are in the T-tubular membrane. The functional significance of the slow outward I_K is unknown, although it may be responsible in part for the delayed depolarizing afterpotential (see the following).

VII. Electrogenesis of Afterpotentials

A. Introduction

The AP spike in skeletal muscle fibers is followed by a prominent depolarizing afterpotential (also called a "negative" afterpotential based on the old terminology from external recording; see Fig. 11). In addition to this "early" afterpotential (i.e., emerging from the spike), there is a "late" depolarizing afterpotential that follows a tetanic train of spikes (e.g., ten spikes). The electrogenesis of the early and late afterpotentials is different. The early afterpotential is due to conductance change, whereas the late afterpotential may be due to K^+ accumulation in the T tubules.

B. Early Depolarizing Afterpotentials

The early depolarizing afterpotential of frog skeletal fibers is about 25 mV in amplitude immediately after the spike component, and gradually decays to the resting potential over a period of 10–20 ms. It was shown by Adrian et al. (1970a) to result from the fact that the delayed rectifier K^+ channel that opens during depolarization to terminate the spike is less selective for K^+ (ca. 30:1, K^+/Na^+) than is the K^+ channel in the resting membrane (ca. 100:1 K^+/Na^+). Therefore, from the constant-field equation (see foregoing), one can predict that the membrane should be partly depolarized when the membrane potential is dominated by this K^+ conductance. Thus, the early depolarizing afterpotential seems to be due to the persistence of the slow decay of this less-selective K^+ conductance.

C. Late Depolarizing Afterpotentials

Adrian and Freygang (1962) concluded that the late afterpotential results from accumulation of K^+ ions in the T-tubules. During the AP depolarization and turn-on of the g_K (delayed rectifier), there is a large driving force for K^+ efflux from the myoplasm, coupled with a large K^+ conductance, resulting in a large outward K^+ $[I_K = g_K (E_m - E_K)]$ across all surfaces of the fiber, namely the surface sarcolemma and T-tubule walls. The K^+ efflux at the fiber surface membrane can rapidly diffuse away and mix with the relatively large interstitial fluid (ISF) volume, whereas the K^+ efflux into the T-tubules is trapped in this restricted diffusion space. The resulting high $[K]_{TT}$ decreases E_K across the T-tubule membrane and, thereby, depolarizes this membrane. Because of cable properties, part of this depolarization is transmitted to the surface sarcolemma and is recorded by an intracellular microelectrode. The K^+ accumulation in the T-tubules can be dissipated only relatively slowly by diffusion out of the mouth of the T-tubules and by active pumping back into the myoplasm across the T-tubule wall. Thus, the decay of the late afterpotential will be a function of these two processes.

The amplitude and duration of the late depolarizing afterpotential of frog skeletal muscle fibers is a function of the number of spikes in the train and their frequency. That is, the greater the spike activity, the greater the amplitude and duration of the late afterpotential. If the train consists of 20 spikes at a frequency of 50/s, a typical value for the amplitude of the late afterpotential is about 20 mV. When the diameter of the T-tubules was increased by placing the fibers in a hypertonic solutions, the amplitude of the late afterpotential decreased, as expected, because of the greater dilution of the K^+ ions accumulating in the T-tubule lumen. When the T-tubular system was disrupted and disconnected from the surface membrane by the glycerol osmotic shock method, the late afterpotentials disappeared (whereas the early afterpotentials persisted).

An alternative explanation for the late afterpotential is that proposed by Adrian et al. (1970b), who suggested that it may be due to the slow g_K change described earlier. The equilibrium potential for the slow I_K was −83 mV, and it was found that the sign of the late afterpotential was reversed by depolarizing below −80 mV. Hence, the late afterpotential may arise from the slow relaxation of a component of the K^+ conductance increase, which is less selective for K^+ than the K^+ channels open in resting membrane. That is, in this view, the electrogenesis of the late afterpotential would be similar to that for the early afterpotential described in the previous section, but a different K^+ channel is involved.

D. Hyperpolarizing Afterpotentials

Neurons, pacemaker heart cells, and vascular smooth-muscle cells often exhibit early hyperpolarizing (positive) afterpotentials. These are due to the delayed-rectifier K^+ conductance increase (which terminates the spike) persisting after the spike, thereby bringing E_m closer to E_K. The maximum amplitude of the possible afterpotential is the difference between E_K and the normal resting potential. The time course of this afterpotential is determined by the decay of the K^+ conductance increase.

Some cells, such as nonmyelinated neurons, exhibit late hyperpolarizing afterpotentals following a train of spikes. These afterhyperpolarizations are due to the Na–K pump, because inhibition of the pump by any means (such as ouabain, cold, Li^+) abolishes the afterhyperpolarization. Two mechanisms have been proposed for the afterhyperpolarization: (1) an increased electrogenic Na^+ pump potential (V_{ep}), stimulated by an increase in [Na]$_i$ (since these neurons are small in diameter and, hence, have a large surface area/volume ratio) or by an increase in $[K]_o$ (since these neurons are surrounded by Schwann cells and, hence, there is a narrow intercellular cleft and restricted diffusion space); and (2) an increased E_K caused by K^+ depletion in the intercellular cleft owing to the stimulated Na–K pump overpumping the K^+ back in. It is generally believed that a larger V_{ep} is the most probable mechanism, although it is difficult to distinguish these two possibilities.

E. Importance of Afterpotentials

All afterpotentials, regardless of whether early or late or of their electrogenesis, have physiological importance because they alter excitability and the propagation velocity of the fiber. A depolarizing afterpotential should enhance excitability (lower threshold), and a hyperpolarizing afterpotential should depress excitability to a subsequent AP. This is because the critical depolarization required to reach the threshold potential would be decreased or increased, respectively. A large late depolarizing afterpotential, such as that due to K^+ accumulation in the T-tubules, can, under certain pathological conditions, trigger repetitive APs (see Chap. 3).

The effect of afterpotentials on velocity of propagation involves two opposing factors: (1) the change in critical depolarization required, and (2) the change in maximal rate of rise of the AP (max dV/dt), which is a function of the takeoff potential (h_∞ vs. E_m curve). For example, during a depolarizing afterpotential in skeletal muscle fibers, the critical depolarization required is decreased, but the max dV/dt is decreased. Therefore, which factor dominates will depend on the degree of depolarization and the shape of the h_∞ curve. When frog skeletal fibers are depolarized slightly by elevating $[K]_o$, only a decrease in propagation velocity is observed (Sperelakis et al., 1970).

VIII. Slow Action Potentials

Slow APs are recorded under conditions in which the fast Na^+ current is blocked by Na^+-deficient solution, TTX, or voltage inactivation of the fast Na^+ channels in high $[K]_o$. Under these conditions, the only carrier of inward current available to produce an AP is Ca^{2+} ion. Spontaneously occurring slow APs were first observed by Sperelakis et al. (1967) in frog sartorius fibers equilibrated in Cl⁻-free solution containing TTX to block the fast Na^+ channels. Upon addition of Ba^{2+} ion (e.g., 0.5 mM), which is a potent blocker of K^+ channels and P_K, the fibers became partially depolarized, and spontaneously discharged slowly rising (e.g., 1–10 V/s) overshooting APs of long duration (e.g., several seconds), having a prominent plateau component resembling a cardiac AP in shape. Barium depolarizes rapidly in Cl⁻-free solution, because the voltage-clamping effect of the Cl⁻ distribution (E_{Cl}), caused by the large P_{Cl}, is circumvented. In addition, since Cl⁻-free solution raises the resistance of the cell membrane about sevenfold (Sperelakis et al., 1967), an intracellular microelectrode can better detect the potential changes occurring across the T-tubule wall because of less short-circuiting of the surface membrane.

Subsequently, the slow APs of frog skeletal muscle fibers were further studied using two intracellular microelectrodes, one for applying intracellular current to stimulate the impaled fiber and the other for recording voltage a short distance away in the same fiber (Fig. 14) (Kerr and Sperelakis, 1982). In these experiments, $[K^+]_o$ was elevated to 25 mM to depolarize the fibers to about –45 mV and, thereby, voltage-inactivate the fast Na⁺ channels (rather than using TTX blockade); in addition, $[Na]_o$ was reduced to zero so that there could be no inward fast Na⁺ current, sucrose being used to replace NaCl in the Ringer solution. Application of small hyperpolarizing current pulses during the slow AP indicated that membrane resistance was increased progressively during the plateau component, leading to an abrupt repolarization terminating the AP. The AP responses fatigued with repetitive stimulation. The rate of rise, overshoot, and duration of the slow APs are a function of $[Ca]_o$ (Beaty and Stefani, 1976; Vogel et al., 1978; Kerr and Sperelakis, 1982) (see Fig. 14c,d). For example, the AP duration at 50% amplitude (APD_{50}) was about 8 s when $[Ca]_o$ was 6 mM. The amplitude of the slow AP plotted against log $[Ca]_o$ gave a straight line with a slope of 28 mV/decade, which is close to the theoretical 29 mV/decade (at 21°C) from the Nernst relationship for a situation in which only Ca^{2+} ion carried the inward current. The slow APs were depressed by the Ca-antagonistic and slow channel-blocking drugs, verapamil and bepridil, with a median effective dose (ED_{50}) of about 5×10^{-8} M; complete blockade occurred at 5×10^{-6} M (see Fig. 14e). Elevation of $[Ca]_o$ (e.g., to 5.1 mM), restored large slow APs. The effect of the slow Ca^{2+} channel blockers could be partially reversed by washout of the drugs for 1–3 h.

The slow AP arises from the sarcotubular system of the skeletal muscle fiber [i.e., from the T-tubule or terminal cisternae (TC) of the SR] (Vogel et al., 1978; Kerr and Sperelakis, 1982). The T-tubules were disrupted and disconnected from the surface membrane by the glycerol osmotic shock method (Eisenberg and Gage, 1969). The slow APs continue in the presence of the glycerol (500 mOsm for 45 min), but are lost within a few minutes after washout of the glycerol (see Fig. 14f–h). The normal fast APs are not affected by the glycerol treatment. These results indicate that the slow Ca^{2+} channels giving rise to the slow APs are located primarily in the tubular system. If some slow Ca^{2+} channels also exist in the surface sarcolomma, their density must not be great enough to sustain a regenerative response.

A substantial contraction accompanies the slow APs. For example, Vogel et al. (1978) found that a contractile force of between 20 and 50% of the normal twitch tension accompanies the slow AP. These results suggest that the voltage-dependent, slow Ca^{2+} channels in the tubular system may play a role during excitation–con-

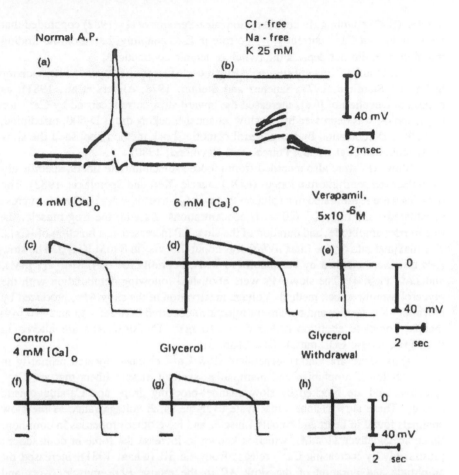

Figure 14 Induction and Ca^{2+}-dependence of slow action potentials (APs) in frog sartorius muscle fibers. (a) Normal fast AP. The resting potential is –85 mV. Depolarizing pulses (50 nA for 5 ms) were applied through an intracellular current microelectrode; potential was recorded with a second microelectrode 2 mm away. The bottom trace represents max dV/dt, the peak excursion of which gives max dV/dt. (b) Fiber equilibrated in the Cl^--free, Na^+-free, high-K^+ (25 mM) solution. The fiber was experimentally hyperpolarized to –85 mV by application of continuous hyperpolarizing current. Application of depolarizing current pulses did not elicit normal (fast) APs. (c–e) The resting potential in Cl^--free, Na^+-free, high-K^+ solution was –45 mV. Increasing $[Ca]_o$ from 2 mM to 4 mM (c) and 6 mM (d) produced an increase in amplitude and duration of the slow AP. A shock artifact occurs during the upstroke. Verapamil (5×10^{-6} M) blocked the slow APs (e). (f–h) Disappearance of slow APs in detubulated fibers. (f) Control slow AP in Cl^--free, Na^+-free, high-K^+ solution; (g) fiber bathed in Cl^--free, Na^+-free, high-K^+ solution containing 550 mM glycerol; (h) within 10 min after abruptly changing bathing solution to a Cl^--free, Na^+-free, high-K^+ solution without glycerol to disrupt the T-tubular system, the slow APs were blocked (only shock artifact visible). The upper horizontal lines in each panel give the zero potential level. (Modified from Kerr and Sperelakis, 1982.)

traction (E–C) coupling. In contrast, Gonzalez-Serratos et al. (1982) concluded that the slow inward Ca^{2+} current plays no role in E–C coupling, based on the finding that diltiazem did not depress the twitch or tetanic contractions.

When the Ca^{2+} inward current in frog muscle was studied by the voltage-clamp technique (Stanfield, 1977; Sanchez and Stefani, 1978; Almers et al., 1981), as expected, elevation of $[Ca]_o$ increased the inward slow current carried by Ca^{2+} ion (I_{Ca}), and I_{Ca} was depressed by the slow–channel-blocking drugs D-600, nifedipine, and Ni^{2+}. Detubulation by the glycerol osmotic shock method abolished the slow I_{Ca} (Nicola-Siri et al., 1980; Potreau and Raymond, 1980).

Slow APs were also recorded from mouse skeletal muscle fibers, specifically from the extensor digitorum longus (EDL) muscle (Kerr and Sperelakis, 1983). The muscles were equilibrated in a solution that was Cl^--free, low Na^+ (10 mM, sucrose substituted), and high K^+ (20 mM) concentrations. As with the frog muscle, the rate of rise, amplitude, and duration of the slow AP increased as a function of $[Ca]_o$. The maximal rate of rise (max dV/dt) was about 0.5 V/s (in 8 mM $[Ca]_o$). The slow APs also were blocked by verapamil (10^{-6} M), bepridil (10^{-6} M), Mn^{2+} (1 mM), and La^{3+} (1 mM). The slow APs were abolished following detubulation with the glycerol osmotic-shock method. Voltage inactivation of the slow APs, produced by elevating $[K]_o$ further and by current injection, occurred between –45 and –10 mV; that is, complete abolition occurred at –10 mV. The slow APs are altered in dystrophic mouse EDL muscle (see Chap. 3).

Thus, there are voltage-dependent slow Ca^{2+} channels located primarily in the T tubules of amphibian and mammalian skeletal muscle fibers that are Ca^{2+} selective, and are blocked by slow channel-blocking drugs and Ca-antagonistic cations. These slow channels inactivate over the same voltage range as the slow channels found in heart and smooth muscle, and have other properties in common. Since acetaldehyde (1 mM), which is known to increase the force of contraction, presumably by increasing Ca^{2+} release from the SR (Khan, 1981), increased the amplitude and duration of the slow AP in the mouse EDL muscle (Kerr and Sperelakis, 1983); this supports the view that the slow Ca^{2+} channels play an important role in E–C coupling. The various conformational states that the Ca^{2+} slow channels undergo during excitation are depicted in Figure 15. These states are similar to those of the fast Na^+ channels (see Fig. 13), except there are only two closed states.

The Ca^{2+} influx into the myoplasm through the voltage-dependent slow channels, as evidenced by the slow APs, may be involved in excitation–contraction coupling. For example, this Ca^{2+} influx could either participate directly in the activation of the myofibrils or trigger the release of more Ca^{2+} from the nearby TC–SR by the Ca^{2+}-trigger–Ca^{2+}-release mechanism (Fabiato, 1981). Estimates of the amount of Ca^{2+} entering through the slow channels are difficult to make because of the number of assumptions required. Although contractions can still be evoked when the inside of the surface membrane is made sufficiently positive (by depolarizing to E_{Ca}) to prevent Ca entry (Miledi et al., 1977), this does not

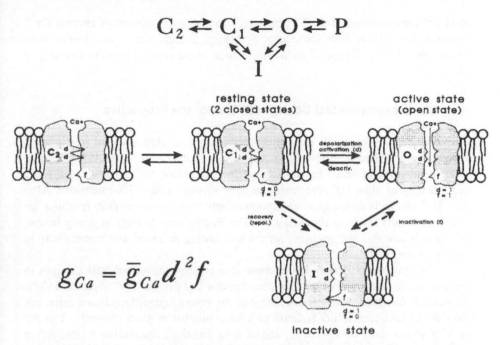

$$C_2 \rightleftarrows C_1 \rightleftarrows O \rightleftarrows P$$

$$g_{Ca} = \bar{g}_{Ca} d^2 f$$

Figure 15 Cartoon model of the four hypothetical states of the slow Ca^{2+} channel. There is evidence for two closed states. As depicted, in the most closed state (C_2), both d gates (or particles) are in the closed configuration. In the least closed state (C_1), one gate is closed and one is open. In the resting closed states (C_2, C_1), the activation gate (A or m) is closed and the inactivation gate (I or h) is open: $d = 0, f = 1$. Depolarization to the threshold activates the channel to the active state, the A-gate opening rapidly and the I-gate still being open: $d = 1, f = 1$. The activated channel spontaneously inactivates to the inactive state owing to closure of the gate: $d = 1, f = 0$. The recovery process upon repolarization returns the channel from the inactive state back to the resting state, thus making the channel again available for reactivation. The Ca^{2+} ion is depicted as being bound to the outer mouth of the channel and poised for entry down its electrochemical gradient when both gates are in the open configuration (active state of channel). The reaction between the resting state and the active state is readily reversible, and there is some evidence of reversibility in the other reactions, as indicated.

exclude a possible role for the Ca^{2+} entry across the T-tubule wall, because it is the ΔE_m across the T-tubule that would affect Ca^{2+} influx at this location. Although the time course of the slow AP recorded under these special experimental conditions is much longer than a twitch contraction, it is not known what the time course of the slow channel activation would be under physiological conditions. It was suggested that the inward Ca^{2+} current may play a role in tetanic contraction, K^+ contracture, or in long-term regulation of contraction, perhaps by increasing the Ca^{2+} concentration in the SR; thereby, increasing the amount of internal Ca^{2+} available for release with subsequent activation (Nicola-Siri et al., 1980). It is known that $[Ca]_{SR}$ increases following tetanic stimulation (Gonzalez-Serratos et al., 1978).

IX. Developmental Changes in Membrane Properties

It appears that most or all excitable membranes pass through similar stages of differentiation during development. For example, young (2- to 3-day-old) embryonic chick heart (tubular heart) has little or no functional fast Na^+ channels, but has a high density of slow Na^+ channels and fires slowly rising TTX-insensitive APs. Fast Na^+ channels then appear and progressively increase in number, reaching the maximal (adult) level on about day 18. The P_{Na}/P_K ratio is high in young hearts, owing to a low P_K, and accounts for the low resting potential and automaticity in nearly all the cells.

Skeletal muscle fibers and neurons also undergo developmental changes in membrane electrical properties (e.g., see Spector and Prives, 1977; Spitzer, 1979). In general, fast Na^+ channels are absent in the young less-differentiated cells, but they do possess excitability because of a large number of slow channels. The AP is TTX-insensitive, slowly rising, and of long duration, resembling a slow AP in cardiac muscle. Later during development, fast Na^+ channels make their first appearance, and both the fast Na^+ channels and slow channels coexist. Tetrodotoxin does not abolish the APs, but reduces max dV/dt, that is, slow APs remain. At a later stage yet, the slow channels in the sarcolemma are lost (or greatly reduced in number), and the fast Na^+ channels progressively increase in density; the APs become fast-rising, of short duration, and completely abolished by TTX. As discussed in Section VIII, some functional slow channels remain in the sarcotubular system.

X. Slow Fibers

One type of skeletal muscle fiber, known as *slow fibers*, subserve tonic functions including posture. They should not be confused with "slow-twitch fibers." The slow fibers do not fire APs, whereas all types of twitch fibers do. The slow fibers are usually smaller in diameter than twitch fibers, and they exhibit a less distinct myofibrillar arrangement. Slow fibers have been found in a number of vertebrate muscles as, for example, in the frog rectus abdominus muscle, frog ileofibularis muscle, and mammalian extraocular muscles. It seems likely that careful searching will reveal some slow fibers in other mammalian muscles.

The slow fibers have multiple innervation, by a series of motor end plates (spaced about 1 mm apart) from a single motoneuron. As with twitch fibers, acetylcholine (ACh) is the synaptic transmitter. The force of contraction of the slow fibers is controlled by graded end-plate potentials (EPPs). That is, an increase in frequency of impulses in the motoneuron produces a larger EPP (by temporal summation), and this, in turn, produces a greater contraction in the vicinity of the end plate. Since the end plates are spaced closely together—at a distance of about 1 length constant—the entire fiber becomes nearly uniformly depolarized, even though there are no propagated APs. Therefore, the entire length of the slow fiber contracts almost uniformly.

The slow fibers do possess T tubules and triadic junctions with the terminal cisternae of the SR (TC-SR). Therefore, the T tubules may act as passive conduits in the slow fibers to bring the depolarization (produced in the surface membrane by the EPP) deep into the fiber interior. If, as discussed in Section XI.E, there is lumen-to-lumen continuity between the TT and TC-SR, then depolarization of the T-tubule by passive cable properties will lead to depolarization of the TC-SR. This, in turn, could bring about the release of Ca^{2+} by activation of voltage-dependent Ca^{2+} slow channels.

Action potentials normally cannot be induced to occur in vertebrate slow fibers in a variety of experimental conditions, including the addition of Ba^{2+} ion. However, denervation of frog slow fibers does allow an AP-generating mechanism to appear (Miledi et al., 1971). In invertebrate slow fibers [e.g., some crustacean skeletal muscles and horseshoe crab (*Limulus*) heart], APs can be induced (Fatt and Ginsborg, 1958). In the neurogenic *Limulus* heart, which normally is activated by summating excitatory postsynaptic potentials, propagating (about 5 cm/s) and overshooting spontaneous APs can be rapidly induced by Ba^{2+} (0.1–10 mM) (Rulon et al., 1971). These slowly rising (ca. 1.0 V/s) APs were resistant to TTX. The voltage-dependent slow channels in *Limulus* heart can pass Ba^{2+}, Sr^{2+}, and Ca^{2+}.

XI. Conduction of the Action Potential

A. Local Circuit Currents

When the end-plate potential (EPP), generated at the neuromuscular junction, reaches threshold for eliciting an AP in the skeletal muscle fiber, an AP is propagated down the muscle fiber in both directions from the end plate. (In some muscle fibers, there is a second end-plate innervated by a motoneuron exciting the spinal cord at another level.) The AP is overshooting (to about +40 mV), and propagates at a constant velocity of about 5 m/s over the surface sarcolemma. Propagation is by means of the local circuit currents that accompany the propagating impulse (Fig. 16). The longitudinal (axial) currents, both inside and outside the fiber, are biphasic: (1) the first phase is most intensive and, if viewed inside the fiber, is in the direction of propagation of the impulse (forward); (2) the second phase is less intensive and is in the backward direction (see Fig. 16).

The radial (transmembrane) currents are triphasic: (1) the first phase is outward across the membrane and is of moderate intensity; (2) the second phase is inward

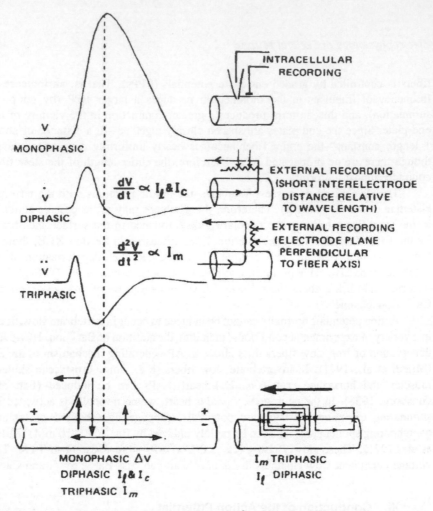

Figure 16 Schematic representation of the first ($\dot{V}$) and second ($\ddot{V}$) time derivatives of the action potential spike and the longitudinal and radial currents associated with the propagating spike. dV/dt ($\dot{V}$) is proportional to the capacitive current ($I_C \rightleftharpoons C_m \cdot dV/dt$) and the longitudinal (axial) current, and is biphasic, having an intense forward phase and a less intense backward phase, as depicted in the diagram at the lower right. d^2V/dt^2 ($\ddot{V}$) is proportional to the radial transmembrane current (I_m), and is triphasic, having a moderately intense initial outward phase, then a very intense inward phase (the "current sink"), followed by a least intense second outward phase, as depicted in the diagram at the lower right. The arrows in the diagram at the lower left also depict the three phases of the membrane current and the two phases of the axial current. dV/dt can be recorded externally by a pair of closely spaced (relative to the spike's wavelength: wl = vel/freq = period · vel = spike dur · vel) electrodes arranged parallel to the fiber axis, as illustrated. d^2V/dt^2 can be recorded by a pair of electrodes arranged perpendicular to the fiber axis, as depicted. The vertical dashed line indicates that when the slope of the spike goes to zero at the peak of the spike, dV/dt is zero; dV/dt is maximum at about the middle of the rising phase of the spike.

and is most intensive (at the current "sink" region); (3) the third phase is outward and is the least intensive (see Fig. 16). The first outward phase corresponds to the passive exponential foot of the AP owing to the passive cable spread of voltage and current. The second inward phase corresponds to the large increase in g_{Na} and fast inward Na^+ current during the later portion of the rising phase and peak of the AP. The third outward phase corresponds to the small increase in g_K and net outward K^+ current and the less steep repolarizing phase of the AP spike.

These currents can be recorded by suitably placed external electrodes: (1) the longitudinal currents by two electrodes (bipolar) placed close together along the length of the fiber; (2) the radial currents by two electrodes placed close together in a plane perpendicular to the fiber axis (see Fig. 16). The former gives a record that approximates the first-time derivative of the intracellularly recorded AP, and the latter electrode arrangement approximates the second-time derivative. The external longitudinal currents must equal the internal axial currents, but they are in the opposite directions. The internal axial currents are confined to the myoplasm, whereas the external longitudinal currents can use the entire ISF space, or *volume conductor* (since "current takes the path of least resistance"). It is this latter fact that allows the electrocardiogram (ECG) to be recorded from the body surface and the electromyogram (EMG) to be recorded from the skin overlying an activated skeletal muscle. The amplitude of the EMG potentials gets larger when more fibers within the muscle are activated (*fiber summation*), owing to summation of the IR voltage drops produced by each fiber activated simultaneously. The frequency of the EMG potentials reflects the frequency and asynchrony of activation of the muscle.

B. Cable Properties

The skeletal muscle fibers, composed of myoblast cells fused end to end and multinucleated, behave as semi-infinite cables. That is, an AP can propagate from one end of the fiber to the other, uniformly and unimpeded. The *space* or *length* constant (λ) of the fiber cable is about 1.5 mm for frog sartorius fibers (Sperelakis et al., 1967) and about 0.75 mm for the rat EDL muscle (Sellin and Sperelakis, 1978). The length constant is the distance over which the potential impressed at one region would decay to $1/e$ ($1/2.717 = 0.37$) or 37% of the initial value. That is, in a cable, voltage (passively) decays exponentially with a certain length constant as given by:

$$V_x = V_o \, e^{-x/\lambda}$$

where V_x is the voltage at the distance x, and V_o is the voltage at the origin ($x = 0$), λ is given by:

$$\lambda = \sqrt{\frac{r_m}{r_i + r_o}} \approx \sqrt{\frac{r_m}{r_i}} = \sqrt{\frac{R_m}{R_i} \frac{a}{2}}$$

where r_m (Ω–cm) is the membrane resistance normalized only for unit length of fiber, r_i (Ω/cm) is the internal longitudinal resistance normalized only for unit length of fiber, R_m (Ω–cm^2) is the membrane resistance normalized for both fiber radius and length, R_i (Ω–cm) is the resistivity of the myoplasm normalized for length and cross-sectional area, and a (cm) is the fiber radius. R_m is often loosely called membrane resistivity or specific resistance, but this is inaccurate because, for true membrane resistivity (ρ_m) there must be correction for membrane thickness δ:

$$\rho_m = R_m/\delta$$
$$(\Omega\text{–cm}) = (\Omega\text{–cm}^2)(\text{cm})$$

The foregoing equation for λ, using R_m and R_i, is an approximation that assumes that r_o (the outside longitudinal resistance) is negligibly small compared with r_i; this would be true for a superficial fiber in a bundle immersed in a large bath. For a derivation of the foregoing equations, and for the interconversions between r_i and R_i, and r_m and R_m, the reader is referred to the chapter by Sperelakis (1979).

Resistance (R) of a material depends on its resistivity (ρ), length (L), and cross-sectional area (A_x):

$$R = \rho \frac{L}{A_x} \qquad \Omega = (\Omega\text{–cm})\ \frac{\text{cm}}{\text{cm}^2}$$

The interconversions for R_m, R_i, and C_m are as follows:

$$R_m = r_m \cdot 2\pi a \quad \Omega\text{–cm}^2 = (\Omega\text{–cm})(\text{cm}) \quad (2\pi a \text{ is the fiber circumference})$$

$$R_i = r_i \cdot \pi a^2 \quad \Omega\text{–cm} = \frac{\Omega}{\text{cm}}\ (\text{cm}^2) \quad (\pi a^2 \text{ is the fiber cross-sectional area})$$

$$C_m = \frac{c_m}{2\pi a} \quad \frac{F}{\text{cm}^2} = \frac{F/\text{cm}}{\text{cm}}$$

Membrane *time constant* (τ_m) is a product of the resistance and capacitance:

$$\tau_m = r\ c = r_m c_m = R_m C_m$$
$$(\text{s}) = \Omega \cdot F$$

The time constant for an exponential charge or discharge of the membrane capacitance is the time required for the voltage to decay to $1/e$ or 37% of the initial voltage or to build up to $1 - 1/e$) or 63% of the final voltage. The appropriate equations are:

$$V_t = V_{max} \cdot e^{-t/\tau} \qquad \text{for decay}$$
$$V_t = V_{max} \cdot (1 - e^{-t/\tau}) \quad \text{for} \quad \text{buildup}$$

where V_t is the potential at any time, t, and V_{max} is the maximum (initial or final) voltage.

The *input resistance* (R_{in}) is the resistance that the current-injecting micro-electrode "looks into," and is defined by the equation:

$$R_{in} = \frac{\Delta V_0}{I_0}$$

where ΔV_0 is the change in potential produced at the site of injection of current of intensity I_0. Input resistance is related to length constant by the following equation:

$$R_{in} = 1/2 \, r_i \quad \lambda = 1/2 \, \sqrt{r_i r_m}$$

Therefore,

$$\Delta V_0 = 1/2 \, r_i \lambda I_0$$

C. Factors That Determine Propagation Velocity

The factors that determine active velocity of propagation (θ_a) include the intensity of the local circuit current, threshold potential, and the passive cable properties: λ and τ_m. As discussed earlier, the greater the rate of rise of the AP, the greater the intensity of the local circuit current, hence, the greater the θ_a. Besides its dependence on the density of the fast Na^+ channels (determinant of the maximum fast Na^+ conductance, g_{Na}), the kinetic properties of the channel gating, and the threshold potential (V_{th}), max dV/dt is determined also by the resting (takeoff) potential (related to the h_∞ vs. E_m curve), as discussed earlier. In addition, since lowered temperature decreases max dV/dt $(Q_{10} \approx 3)$, θ_a is slowed accordingly. R_m also is increased at low temperature, the Q_{10} for R_K in frog sartorius fibers being about 2.8 (ion diffusion in free solution has a Q_{10} of about 1.2) (Sperelakis, 1969).

In a passive cable, such as a nonmyelinated axon or a skeletal muscle fiber, the passive propagation velocity (θ_p) is directly proportional to the length constant [the length constant for sinusoidally varying applied currents (λ_{ac}) is shorter than θ_{dc}, depending on the ac frequency] and inversely proportional to the time constant:

$$\theta_p = \frac{\lambda}{\tau_m} = \sqrt{\frac{R_m}{R_i} \frac{a}{2}} = \frac{\sqrt{a}}{\sqrt{R_m R_i 2 C_m}}$$

Therefore, propagation velocity is directly proportional to the square root of the fiber radius (a), and inversely proportional to membrane capacitance (C_m) and to the square root of R_i and the square root of R_m. For example, the propagation velocity is greater in larger-diameter nerve fibers.

Myelination of neurons is an evolutionary method of reducing C_m (with capacitors in series, the total capacitance decreases); hence, an increase in propagation velocity (myelination increases γ while holding τ_m about the same, since R_m increases about in proportion to the decrease in C_m). In myelinated axons:

$$\theta_p = \frac{\lambda^2}{\tau_m \cdot x} \propto \frac{a}{2 R_i C_m}$$

(where x is a distance term). That is, propagation velocity is proportional to the fiber radius and inversely proportional to C_m.

The membrane current density (I_m) is given by:

$$I_m = \frac{a}{2} \frac{1}{R_i} \frac{1}{\theta^2} \frac{d^2V}{dt^2}$$

$$(\text{amp/cm}^2) = (\text{cm}) \ \frac{1}{\Omega-\text{cm}} \ \frac{1}{\text{cm}^2/\text{s}^2} \ \frac{V}{\text{s}^2}$$

where d^2V/dt^2 is the second-time derivative of the AP. As indicated, membrane current is proportional to d^2V/dt^2, whereas the longitudinal current (I_l) or the capacitive current (I_C) is proportional to dV/dt:

$$I_c = C_m \frac{dV}{dt}$$

D. Conduction into the Sarcotubular System

The experiments of Huxley and Taylor (1958) were the first to provide evidence that there was some structure, located at the level of the Z lines in frog skeletal muscle fibers, that is involved in excitation–contraction coupling. These investigators applied current pulses at different points along the length of the sarcomeres in isolated fibers and found that when the microelectrode tip was opposite the Z line, graded contractions of the two half-sarcomeres occurred. The greater the current, the greater was the inward spread of the contraction. In addition, they discovered that there were sensitive spots located around the perimeter of the fiber at the Z line level; that is, the membrane was not uniformly sensitive. At about the same time, it was discovered by electron microscopists that transverse (T) tubules were located at the level of the Z lines in amphibian skeletal muscle (and at the level of the A–I junctions of the sarcomere in mammalian skeletal muscle). Thus, the T-tubules probably represent the morphological conduit for the findings of Huxley and Taylor.

Diffusion of some substance from the surface membrane into the skeletal muscle fiber interior is much too slow to account for the relatively short latent period of about 1–3 ms between the beginning of the AP and the beginning of contraction. That is, the diameter of the fibers (mean value of about 70 μm in frog sartorius fibers) is much too large for a diffusion mechanism to be responsible. [Diffusion time (for 95% equilibration) increases by the square of the distance, and would require about 2.5 s for a small molecule freely diffusing across a cell radius of 50 μm; estimates for Ca^{2+} diffusion time are considerably longer than this (Podolsky and Costantin, 1964).] Therefore, the T-tubular system serves to bring excitation deep into the fiber interior rapidly and, thereby, to reduce the required diffusion distance to an average value of about 0.7 μm (Sperelakis and Rubio, 1971). Disruption of the T-tubules with their disconnection from the surface membrane by the glycerol osmotic-shock method uncouples contraction from excitation (Eisenberg and Gage, 1969), thus further underscoring the essential role of the T-tubules in excitation–contraction coupling.

Estimates of the length constant of the T tubules (λ_{TT}), assuming the T-tubule membrane has about the same resistivity (R_m) as the surface membrane ($\lambda = \sqrt{R_m/R_i}$ $\sqrt{a/2}$), give values of about 50 μm. The resistivity of the T-tubule membrane is probably higher than that of the surface sarcolemma because of a lower g_{Cl} (Hodgkin and Horowicz, 1959; Adrian and Freygang, 1962; Sperelakis and Schneider, 1968). Therefore, it is possible for the T-tubules to serve as passive conduits to bring the depolarization from the surface membrane (during its AP) into the fiber interior. However, there is evidence that the T-tubules fire APs; that is, they actively propagate impulses inward, and so bring large depolarization deep into the fiber. The evidence for this includes the observation of a threshold for sudden initiation of localized contraction by Costantin and colleagues (1967). The T-tubule AP is sensitive to TTX and is Na^+ dependent, and so seems to be similar in nature to the surface membrane AP. By use of a high-speed cinemicrography to measure sequential activation of the myofibrils in a radial direction, Gonzalez-Serratos (1971) estimated the propagation velocity of the T-tubule AP to be about 10 cm/s. This value is about 50 times slower than propagation down the fiber longitudinally (about 5 m/s).

It has been proposed that fatigue during relatively brief tetanic contractions (i.e., a progressive falloff in the force of contraction) was due to Na^+ depletion in the T-tubule network, particularly in the deeper parts far from the orifice at the fiber surface. Bezanilla et al. (1972) showed that, in fibers preequilibrated in low $[Na]_o$ (e.g., 60 mM), the fatigue occurred more rapidly. It is thought that the Na^+ influx (the inward fast Na^+ current) with each AP in the T-tubule produces a progressive decline in $[Na]_{TT}$, which slows propagation velocity down the T-tubules and eventually leads to loss of excitability when $[Na]_{TT}$ drops below some critical level (e.g., 30 mM). Sodium depletion should occur more rapidly deep in the fiber's T-tubule network because there would be less diffusion of Na^+ in from the mouth of the T-tubule to replenish the Na^+ loss. Active Na–K pumping in the T-tubules may not occur fast enough to keep up with the Na^+ loss into the fiber myoplasm.

There are also voltage-dependent, slow Ca^{2+} channels in the T-tubule membrane, and slow APs that arise from the T-tubule can be recorded under appropriate conditions (Sperelakis et al., 1967; Vogel and Sperelakis, 1978). The evidence for the existence of this type of channel and some of its properties is discussed in Section VIII. The Ca^{2+} influx into the myoplasm through these slow channels could play a role in excitation–contraction coupling.

E. Does the T-Tubule Communicate with the Sarcoplasmic Reticulum Across the Triadic Junction?

The Ca^{2+} for contraction in skeletal muscle is primarily released from the TC-SR (Winegrad, 1968), and there is an internal cycling of Ca^{2+} ion. Changes in $[Ca]_o$ of the bathing solution take a relatively long time (e.g., 30–60 min) before exerting a large effect on the force of contraction in skeletal muscle. In contrast, in cardiac muscle, the effect of lowered $[Ca]_o$ is obvious within a few seconds, indicating that the primary determinant of the force of contraction is the Ca^{2+} influx across the sarcolemma through the slow Ca^{2+} channels. Therefore, in skeletal muscle, excitation propagates actively down the T-tubules and Ca^{2+} is released from the TC-SR, but it is not known how the signal is transferred from the T-tubule to the TC-SR across the triadic junction.

Electron-opaque tracer molecules, such as horseradish peroxidase (HRP; ca. 60 Å diameter), enter into the T-tubules and from there into some of the TC-SR of frog skeletal muscle (Rubio and Sperelakis, 1972; Kulczycky and Mainwood, 1972). Exposure of the fibers to hypertonic solutions facilitated the entry of HRP into the TC-SR, so that under these conditions nearly 100% of the TC-SR became filled. Ruthenium red also stains the SR of skeletal muscle, including the TC and connecting longitudinal elements of the SR (L-SR) (Luft, 1971; Sperelakis et al., 1973). Thus, there may be a functional connection between the SR and the extracellular space (Fig. 17).

It was reported that membranous connections, known as *pillars*, extend between the T-tubule membrane and the TC-SR membrane at the triadic junctions (pillars are also found in cardiac muscle and smooth muscle, between the J-SR and sarcolemma; Forbes and Sperelakis, 1983) and that stimulations of the muscle increased the number of pillars observed by severalfold (Somlyo, 1979; Eisenberg et al., 1979). Eisenberg and Eisenberg (1982) reported that resting fibers had 39 ± 14 pillars per square micron of tubule membrane, and 100 mM K^+-stimulated fibers contained 66 ± 13 pillars per square micron. It was suggested that rapid pillar formation is a normal step in E–C coupling, and that the pillars might be the structures that provide a linking conductance [maximum coupling conductance in Siemens (S; the unit of conductance) of $<10^{-3}$ S/cm^2 and 10^{-14}–10^{-15} S/pillar], which allows ionic current to flow from the T-tubules into the TC-SR to depolarize them (Mathias et al., 1980). If so, there may be lumen-to-lumen continuity between the T-tubules and TC-SR during excitation, allowing the AP in the T-tubules to invade directly into the TC-SR to depolarize and bring about the release of Ca^{2+}.

If the L-SR is electrically isolated from the TC-SR by a substantial resistance (e.g., the zippering between the two SR compartments described in the following), this would account for the relatively low fiber capacitance measured (Mathias et al., 1980). [The region connecting the L-SR with the TC-SR is the intermediate SR (I-SR).] The effect of this would be to remove the very large membrane surface area of the L-SR from the TC-SR and, hence, greatly reduce the capacitance that would be measured (see Fig. 17).

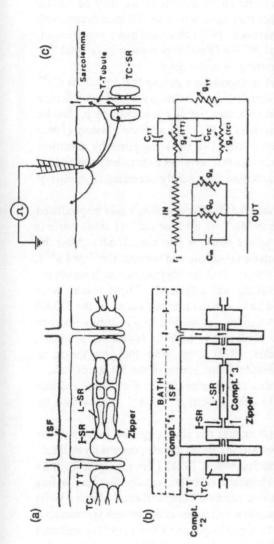

Figure 17 (a) Diagrammatic representation of internal tubular systems of a frog sartorius muscle fiber. Depicted are interstitial space (ISF) between two parallel fibers, the transverse tubules (TT), terminal cisternae (TC) of the sarcoplasmic reticulum (SR), and longitudinal elements of SR (L-SR). TC and L-SR are interconnected, and TT is continuous with ISF, but direct luminal continuity between TT and TC at triadic junctions has not yet been observed. However, indirect evidence, which suggests that TC may be patent with TT, includes entrance of horseradish peroxidase and ruthenium red into TC and swelling of TC in sucrose hypertonic solutions. (b) Block diagram of compartments accessible to [³H]sucrose corresponding to diagram in (a). Compartments are assumed to be in series: compartment 1 being ISF, compartment 2 being TC (and possibly including the TT), and compartment 3 perhaps being L-SR. There appear to be functional connections between TC and TT lumens, perhaps by means of the pillars. There may be some partial diffusion barrier between L-SR and TC, as represented by the "zippers" observed morphologically. The two membranes come close together, forming a restricted diffusion space, in the region of the intermediate SR (I-SR). This region serves to functionally isolate the L-SR from the TC-SR. It is presumed that sucrose penetrates across the sarcolemma, T-tubule membranes, or SR membranes only very slowly, if at all. The ISF compartment connects with the muscle bath. (c) The sarcotubular system (T-tubules and TC-SR) of skeletal muscle fibers represented diagrammatically (upper part of figure) and by one possible electrical equivalent circuit (lower part). As illustrated, the T-tubules and perhaps the TC-SR shunt the cell surface membrane (e.g., when current is injected intracellularly through a microelectrode. C_{TT}, capacitance of T-tubule membrane; C_{TC}, capacitance of the TC-SR membrane; $g_{K(TT)}$, K⁺ conductance of the T-tubule membrane; $g_{K(TC)}$, K⁺ conductance of the TC-SR membrane; g_{tf}, conductance of the lumen of the T- tubule (tubular fluid).

The depolarization of the TC-SR could activate voltage-dependent, Ca^{2+}-selective slow channels. This would allow Ca^{2+} influx into the myoplasm down an electrochemical gradient. The ion concentrations in the SR lumen may be similar to those in the ISF, and a resting potential may exist across the SR membrane, with the lumen side positive. Forbes and Sperelakis (1972) observed that a ouabain-sensitive ATPase activity (presumably (Na^+,K^+)-ATPase) was present in skeletal SR, and so could account for the ion concentrations in the SR.

It has been suggested that the SR is depolarized during the release of Ca^{2+} in E–C coupling. For example, optical signals (e.g., birefringence and fluorescence changes) can be recorded from the SR membranes during contraction (e.g., Baylor and Oetliker, 1975; Bezanilla and Horowicz, 1975). In addition, Natori (1965) demonstrated that propagation of contraction (1–3 m/s) triggered by electrical stimulation can occur in muscle fiber regions that have been denuded (skinned) of their sarcolemma, the propagation of excitation presumably occurring by means of the SR membranes.

Sperelakis et al. (1973) demonstrated that E–C uncoupling could be produced by exposing frog skeletal muscle fibers to Mn^{2+} (1 mM) or La^{3+} (1 mM) while in hypertonic solution (to facilitate entry of the blockers into the TC-SR). After the fibers were returned to normal Ringer solution (isotonic and without Mn^{2+} or La^{3+}), normal fast APs could be elicited, but there were no contractions accompanying them (i.e., a "permanent" E–C uncoupling was produced). These results were interpreted as suggesting that Mn^{2+} and La^{3+} entered into the lumen of the TC-SR and blocked the Ca^{2+} slow channels. A similar exposure of frog sartorius fibers to Mn^{2+}, La^{3+}, or to Ca^{2+}-free solution blocked the caffeine (8–10 mM)-induced contracture as well (Rubio and Sperelakis, 1972). Thus, from these physiological and ultrastructural studies, it was suggested that the lumen of the SR is continuous with that of the T-tubule under conditions of hypertonicity or excitation, and that substances can enter into the TC-SR to exert an effect on Ca^{2+} release into the myoplasm.

Compartmental analysis of skeletal muscle has also suggested that the SR is open to the interstitial fluid (ISF). [In contrast, in cardiac muscle, there is no evidence that the SR is open to the ISF (Rubio and Sperelakis, 1971).] For example, Conway (1957), Harris (1963), and Keynes and Steinhardt (1968) concluded that Na^+ in frog skeletal muscle fibers is distributed in two separate compartments. Harris (1963) suggested that the Na^+, K^+, and Cl^- concentrations in one compartment (presumably the SR) were about equal to those of the ISF, and Rogus and Zierler (1973) concluded that the Na^+ concentration in the SR of rat skeletal muscle (EDL) approximates that of the ISF. The sucrose space and Na^+ space were similar (0.238 ml/g vs. 0.232 mg/g wet weight, respectively), and they found three compartments for ^{24}Na washout: (1) an ISF compartment with a $t_{1/2}$ of 1.4 min, (2) an SR compartment with a $t_{1/2}$ of 7.5 min, and (3) a myoplasmic compartment with a $t_{1/2}$ of 35 min. The volume of the SR compartment was 12.4% of muscle volume (14.3% of fiber volume) and, in hypertonic solution (1.66 times isotonic), the SR volume increased to 16.4% and the washout of the SR compartment was faster ($t_{1/2}$ of 5.3 min). Tasker et al. (1959) also had reported a large sucrose space of 26.5% for frog sartorius fibers.

Birks and Davey (1969) demonstrated that the volume changes of the SR of skeletal muscle in hypertonic (sucrose) and hypotonic solutions were always opposite those occurring within the myoplasmic compartment. They concluded that sucrose must enter into the SR, pulling in water osmotically from the myoplasm, to produce the marked swelling of the SR that occurred in hypertonic solutions. Thus, this is a compelling argument for the SR being open to the ISF. Vinogradova (1968) concluded, from the distribution of nonpenetrating sugars in frog sartorius muscle, that the SR compartment is continuous with the ISF; the insulin space was 19.0% and increased in hypertonic solution and decreased in hypotonic solution and in glycerol-treated fibers.

Sperelakis et al. (1978) found that the total [^{3}H]sucrose space of frog sartorius muscles was 18.0% in isotonic solution and 22.6% in twofold hypertonic solution (Table 1). The relative SR volume (including the small T-tubule volume) was 12.4 and 17.0% of fiber volume, respectively. Half-maximal saturation of [^{3}H]sucrose uptake was achieved in about 8 min. This value for SR volume of frog skeletal muscle

Table 1 Summary of Data with [^{3}H]Sucrose in Washout and Uptake Experiments in Frog Sartorius Muscles[a]

A. Washout experiment (isotonic)			
Compartment no.	$t_{1/2}$ (min)	Rel. vol. (tissue) (%)	Possible identity
1	0.50	7.0	ISF space
2	5.8	9.0	TT and TC-SR
3	60.0	2.0	L-SR
1 + 2 + 3		18.0	SR, TT, and ISF
2 + 3		11.0 (11.8)[c]	SR and TT

B. Uptake experiment			
Tonicity[b]	Rel. vol.$_{ISF}$ (%)	Rel. vol.$_{SR-TT}$[d] (%)	Total sucrose space
1X	6.3	11.6 (12.4)[c]	18.0
2X	6.3	15.9 (17.0)[c]	22.6

[a]Abbreviations: ISF, interstitial fluid; TT, transverse tubular system; TC-SR, terminal cisternae of the sarcoplasmic reticulum; L-SR, longitudinal tubules of the SR.
[b]Twofold hypertonic solution was produced by adding sucrose to Ringer solution.
[c]The numbers in parentheses have been corrected for fiber volume, whereas those without parentheses are for the whole muscle.
[d]The values listed are the average values calculated by two different methods, both of which yielded very similar values.
Source: Data from Sperelakis et al. (1978).

is close to that measured by ultrastructural techniques (Peachey, 1965; Mobley and Eisenberg, 1975). In washout experiments, they observed three exponential components with the following $t_{1/2}$ values and relative tissue volumes: (1) an ISF compartment, 0.50 min and 7.0%; (2) a TC-SR compartment, 5.8 min and 9.0%; and (3) a L-SR compartment, 60 min and 2.0% (see Fig. 17 and Table 1). Evidence that the TC-SR and L-SR may not be freely connected to one another under resting conditions are the observations that (1) the L-SR did not fill with HRP, whereas the TC-SR did (Rubio and Sperelakis, 1972); and (2) there is a "zippering" of the membranes connecting these two components of the SR in mouse and frog skeletal muscle (Howell, 1974; Wallace and Sommer, 1975; Forbes and Sperelakis, 1979).

In ^{45}Ca-washout experiments on frog EDL muscles, Kirby et al. (1975) found three compartments with half-times of 0.26, 1.9, and 22 min, similar to the three sucrose compartments of Sperelakis et al. (1978), except the half-times were about two to threefold shorter. They also suggested that the first compartment was the ISF space, the second compartment was the T-tubule plus the TC-SR, and the third was the L-SR. Also in agreement, Bianchi and Bolton (1974) found a transient increase in ^{45}Ca efflux and a marked loss of muscle Ca^{2+} from frog sartorius muscles exposed to hypertonic solutions (twofold isotonicity using sucrose or NaCl), and suggested that hypertonicity produces transient communication between the TC-SR and the T-tubules, thereby allowing their Ca^{2+} to be lost to the ISF. In addition, it has been reported in a human muscle disease, polymyositis, that the T-tubules were spatially continuous with the SR, as visualized with lanthanum tracer, and that enzymes leak from the TC-SR into the T-tubules and ISF (Chou et al., 1980).

Frog skeletal muscle fibers have an osmotically inactive volume of about 32% when placed into Ringer solution made hypertonic with sucrose or other nonpenetrating solutes; that is, fiber diameter does not shrink to the theoretical value expected if it were a perfect osmometer (Sperelakis and Schneider, 1968; Sperelakis et al., 1970). For example, in twofold hypertonic solution, there should be a decrease in fiber volume to one-half and fiber radius to 0.707 $(1/\sqrt{2})$ of the original value. The observed change is to only 0.81 of the original diameter. Since the SR volume *increases* in hypertonic solution (Huxley et al., 1963; Sperelakis and Schneider, 1968; Birks and Davey, 1969), it is likely that the osmotic inactive volume is due to the SR. The swollen SR would prevent the fiber volume from decreasing to one-half in twofold hypertonic solution, even if the volume of the myoplasm proper were to decrease to one-half. In cardiac muscle, an osmotically inactive volume is not present (Sperelakis and Rubio, 1971), electron-opaque tracers do not enter the SR (Sperelakis et al., 1974), and the SR volume does not increase with hypertonicity (Sperelakis and Rubio, 1971).

F. Electric Field and Current Interactions Between Cell Membrane and Sarcoplasmic Reticulum Membrane

Sperelakis and colleagues (1977) developed an hypothesis for the electrical interaction between two contiguous excitable short cells that did not require low-resistance connections between the cells at the cell junction. The mechanism of the electrical interaction was the electrical field that develops in the narrow junctional cleft between the cells, provided that the prejunctional and postjunctional membranes are ordinary excitable membranes. When the prejunctional membrane fires, the cleft between the cells becomes negative relative to ground (the interstitial fluid surrounding the cells), and this negative cleft potential acts to depolarize the postjunctional membrane by an equal amount, by a patch-clamplike effect and, thereby, bring it to its threshold. The inner surface of the postjunctional membrane remains at nearly constant potential relative to ground, because virtually no local circuit current flows through the postjunctional cell. Thus, intercellular transmission can occur electrically without low-resistance connections between the cells. The key feature of the hypothesis is that the postjunctional membrane is depolarized to threshold by change of its outer surface potential by the electric field that develops in the narrow junctional cleft when the prejunctional membrane fires an AP, coupled with the fact that the membrane conductances are controlled by the transmembrane potential and not by the absolute potentials.

The same principles of electric field interactions may apply whenever two membranes are held in close apposition, such as the SR membrane (junctional or J-SR) forming a junction either with the surface sarcolemma (diad junction) in cardiac muscle and smooth muscle or with the T-tubule invaginations in some myocardial cells and in skeletal muscle (where triad junctions are formed). That is, an AP in the cell membrane should develop a positive cleft potential (opposite of the negative intercellular cleft potential, because the inner surface of the membrane is involved at diads or triads). If the SR has a "resting potential," positive inside the lumen (equivalent to outside of the cell membrane) and negative on the myoplasmic side, then the positive cleft potential would depolarize the SR membrane. This, in turn, could bring about a Ca^{2+} influx into the myoplasm through voltage-dependent Ca^{2+} slow channels and down an electrochemical gradient for Ca^{2+}.

The role of the pillars could be to somehow facilitate the influence of the electric field developed by the T-tubule membrane on the TC-SR membrane. Since pillars should have a high transverse resistance, this would allow a greater influence of the electric field on the postjunctional membrane. In this model there would then be no problem concerning why the large capacitance of the large SR network is not measured in standard experiments in skeletal muscle.

When the diad junction was modeled, it was found that current flow also produced an interaction between the two closely apposed membranes (Sperelakis et al., 1992). It was concluded that any organelle, such as junctional SR, that is physically in very close proximity to the cell membrane will "hear" the electrical activity occurring in the cell membrane. When the contiguous cell membrane fires an AP, current is forced to flow through the J-SR, hyperpolarizing the contiguous J-SR membrane, but depolarizing the opposite (or distal) J-SR membrane, and causing it to fire an AP, which then propagates to the contiguous J-SR membrane.

Even if the J-SR is not an excitable membrane, there would still be a significant potential reflection across the diadic junction. The passive depolarization of the distal J-SR membrane could be sufficient to trigger the opening of Ca^{2+} channels.

XII. Excitation–Contraction Coupling

A. Introduction

Respiratory muscles have not been extensively used for the study of the mechanism of excitation–contraction (E–C) coupling. These muscles, in particular the diaphragm, are mixed muscles composed of fast-twitch type and slow-twitch type fibers (Gunn and Davies, 1971). The fast-twitch fibers have a more developed sarcoplasmic reticulum (SR) than the slow ones. Consequently, the mechanism of E–C coupling may differ quantitatively in these two types of fibers, but is unlikely to be fundamentally different. Yet it must be stressed that the mechanism of E–C coupling is not fully known for any type of skeletal muscle fibers. It is well established that Ca^{2+} is released from the SR between the depolarization of the T-tubules and the development of tension (Ridgway and Ashley, 1967), but the mechanism linking depolarization of the T-tubules and Ca^{2+} release is not established. Several hypotheses have been proposed. Those that are reviewed in this chapter have not been either excluded or definitively established by experimental evidence. Our goal is not to present a complete review of these hypotheses, which can be found elsewhere for both skeletal (Rios and Pizzaro, 1991) and cardiac muscle (Feher and Fabiato, 1990), but to propose some critical insight on topical subjects based on our experience in structural and electrophysiological studies.

B. Ionic Shifts in the Sarcoplasmic Reticulum and Myoplasm During Calcium Release

The membranes of the T-tubule and the SR come in structural apposition at the site of the triadic junction (Franzini-Armstrong, 1971). Tracers of the extracellular space, such as horseradish peroxidase, penetrate into the lumen of the SR (Rubio and Sperelakis, 1972), but a positive peroxidase reaction has also been found in the SR, even in the absence of extrinsic horseradish peroxidase (Forbes et al., 1977). Thus, there is no strong evidence in favor of a continuity of the lumen of the transverse tubules and of the SR. On the contrary, most investigators now think that the lumen of the SR is not in continuity with the extracellular space (Franzini-Armstrong et al., 1978; Neville, 1979).

Electron probe studies (Somlyo et al., 1981) indicate that the Ca^{2+} concentration is much higher in the terminal cisternae of the SR (TC-SR) than in the myoplasm (Table 2). During tetany, the Ca^{2+} release from the SR increases the free Ca^{2+} concentration in the myoplasm and decreases it in the TC-SR. During this Ca^{2+} release, there is also an increase of K^+ and Mg^{2+} concentrations, but the increase in these concentrations is insufficient to compensate for the change of

Table 2 Elemental Concentrations in the Terminal Cisternae and Longitudinal Elements of the Sarcoplasmic Reticulum and the Myoplasm of Frog Skeletal Muscle Under Resting Conditions (Control) and Tetanic Stimulation

Location	Condition	Concentration of element (mM)						
		Na	Mg	P	S	Cl	K	Ca
Terminal cisternae	Control	22	23	161	83	17	215	46
	Tetanus	23	28	161	88	16	235	19
Myoplasm	Control	11	14	85	66	14	128	1.1
	Tetanus	10	12	85	64	14	126	2.0

Source: Data recalculated from Somlyo et al. (1981).

charge caused by the Ca^{2+} release. If there were a potential across the SR membrane, the release of 1 pmol of Ca^{2+} would result in a positive potential of about 100 mV outside the SR, which would prevent the completion of the release of Ca^{2+} if K^+ and Mg^+ were the only counterions. The only major ion that is not accessible to the electron probe analysis is H^+. Thus, it is still possible that H^+ is an additional counterion during Ca^{2+} release (Chiesi and Inesi, 1980), and Ca^{2+} release may still be electrically silent. Autohistoradiographic studies with ^{45}Ca suggest that C^{2+} is released at the level of the terminal cisternae of the SR and, subsequently, is reaccumulated in the longitudinal SR (Winegrad, 1968). Electron probe analysis, however, failed to show either a large increase of Ca^{2+} in the longitudinal SR during the presumed reaccumulation of Ca^{2+}, or a long delay before the return of Ca^{2+} into the terminal cisternae.

C. Calcium-Induced Calcium Ion Release from the Sarcoplasmic Reticulum

The hypothesis of a Ca^{2+}-induced release of Ca^{2+} from the SR is that a small influx of Ca^{2+} across the T-tubule membrane, including at the T-tubule–SR junction into the myoplasm in the vicinity of the SR induces the release of a large amount of Ca^{2+} from the SR (Bianchi and Shanes, 1959; Frank, 1980). This hypothesis has been tested mostly in mechanically skinned fibers, which are single fibers from which the sarcolemma has been removed by microdissection (Natori, 1954). With Natori's preparation, a Ca^{2+}-induced release of Ca^{2+} can indeed be obtained in skeletal muscle fibers, but only under conditions that seemed to exclude any physiological role of the Ca^{2+}-induced release of Ca^{2+} from the SR (Endo, 1977). These conditions include the following: (1) a very high preload of the SR with Ca^{2+} was required; (2) the free Mg^{2+} concentration had to be more than ten times lower than the presumed physiological level; and (3) the increase of free $[Ca]_i$ had to be so large that this would be sufficient to activate the myofilaments directly. Some investigators, however, maintain that such an exclusion of any physiological role of Ca^{2+}-induced release of Ca^{2+} in the E–C coupling of skeletal muscle was premature (Stephenson, 1981).

It is possible that ions other than Ca^{2+} may participate in the trigger mechanism. One possible candidate among these other ions is H^+ (Shoshan et al., 1981).

D. Depolarization-Induced Release of Calcium from the Sarcoplasmic Reticulum

Soon after the morphological description of the SR, Peachey and Porter (1959) suggested the hypothesis of an electrical coupling between T-tubules and TC-SR. This hypothesis has received some enthusiasm, but it has not yet been supported by any compelling data, nor has it been completely rejected.

The question of whether there are changes of potential across the SR membrane is still unresolved. It is not possible to place microelectrodes in the tubules and cisternae of the SR because of their small sizes. Attempts to depolarize SR by externally applied electrical currents (Costantin and Podolsky, 1967) resulted in Ca^{2+} release only through damage of the SR by the thermic effect of the high-intensity current (Endo, 1977). A more satisfactory approach seemed to be provided by the substitution of ions with different permeability to the SR membrane in the solution bathing skinned fibers, to produce an ionically induced depolarization of the SR membrane. These ionic substitution maneuvers indeed appeared to induce a Ca^{2+} release from the SR of skinned fibers, and this has been considered as a possible (Endo, 1977), if not likely (Ebashi, 1976), mechanism for the induction of Ca^{2+} release from the SR. Subsequently, this interpretation has been largely, if not completely, discounted. First, the Ca^{2+} release could be triggered by depolarization of sealed-over T-tubules that remain present in the skinned fibers, as first suggested by Costantin and Podolsky (1967) and confirmed by several other investigators (e.g., Donaldson, 1982). Second, the ionic substitutions could induce Ca^{2+} release by their osmotic effect on the SR, rather than by the depolarization that they might cause (Meissner and McKinley, 1976). Experiments with potential-sensitive dyes have neither eliminated nor supported the possibility of a potential across the SR membrane (Russell et al., 1979a,b). The signals obtained with these dyes could be caused by change of surface-charge distribution on the SR membrane, without the necessary implication of a transmembrane potential change (Russell et al., 1979a,b).

Potential-sensitive dyes have also been used in intact fibers in the hope of detecting the electrical activity of the SR, and one of the components of the optical signals has been tentatively attributed to a depolarization of the SR (see Ebashi, 1976 for a review). Yet more recent results suggest that this component may, in fact, be caused by an event subsequent to the Ca^{2+} release (Suarez-Kurtz and Parker, 1977). The results of measurements of the passive electrical properties, both linear and nonlinear, of intact skeletal muscle do not seem compatible with a simple resistive or capacitive coupling between T-tubules and SR (Mathias et al., 1977). The effective capacitance of resting muscle is much too small to account for an electrical connection between surface membrane and SR, if the specific capacitance of the SR membrane is of the same order of magnitude as that for other excitable membranes. The rate of rise of the depolarization phase of the AP is much too high to be compatible with loading from a predicted large SR capacitance.

Yet for the problem of the coupling between adjacent myocardial cells, models have been developed that are compatible with an electrical coupling, with practically no current flow (Sperelakis and Mann, 1977). Similarly, all the possibilities for a current spread between the transverse tubules and the SR have not yet been explored experimentally, as suggested by the modeling of Mathias et al. (1980), especially if the terminal cisternae were electrically isolated by a high resistance from the longitudinal SR (Sommer et al., 1978). It seems unlike that a high resistance isolates the triadic junction from the myoplasm (Franzini-Armstrong, 1971; Eisenberg et al., 1979).

E. Calcium Release Coupled to Charge Movement in the T-Tubules

Electrophysiological experiments have provided evidence for very low level currents caused by the displacement of charged macromolecules embedded in the surface membrane of skeletal muscle and probably in the T-tubule (Chandler et al., 1976). It is also established that there is a tight control of the contractile activation by the potential imposed experimentally on the sarcolemma and, presumably, on the T-tubules (Costantin and Taylor, 1973).

An electron microscopic description of the triadic junction between T-tubules and the SR is emerging and may provide some basis for the coupling between the movement of charge in the T-tubules and the release of Ca^{2+} from the SR. Two types of structures have been described in this space, which is about 22 nm wide. Foot processes are made of a solid, electron-dense material (Franzini-Armstrong, 1975), and a similarity was observed between the number of charged groups detected electrophysiologically and the number of feet determined by electron microscopy (Schneider and Chandler, 1973). Recent data, however, suggest that the relation may be more complex than one charged molecule attached to one foot process (Schneider, 1981). A different structure is represented by pillars, which are made by a pair of electron-opaque lines bounding an electronlucent interior (Somlyo, 1979). In fact, it is not certain that pillars and foot processes are different structures. The appearance of the structures in the junction between T-tubules and TC-SR varies with the method of staining and fixation (Somlyo, 1979) and with the degree of tilting of the thin section in the electron microscope (Fig. 18). Thus, pillars and foot processes might correspond to the same structure observed under different conditions. A very challenging observation on the possible physiological role of the

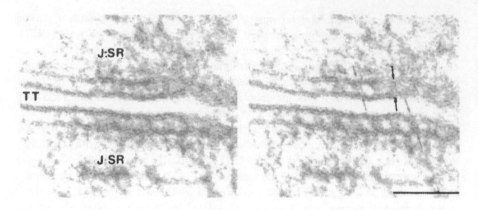

Figure 18 Pillars and junctional foot processes at the triadic junction in mouse skeletal muscle (tibialis anterior). The two cisternae of junctional SR (J-SR) face one another across a transverse tubule (TT). In the junctional gap between the coupling components are located periodically spaced, opaque structures, the junctional processes. The two panels constitute a stereoscopic pair of micrographs (10° angle of convergence). In the right-hand panel, several linear membranelike junctional processes, the "pillars," which extend between the apposed unit membranes, can be detected (arrows). The appearance of such pillars varies substantially according to the degree of tilting of the thin section in the electron microscope, as can be discerned by comparison of profiles between the right and left panels. That is, these two images are identical except for the 10° difference in tilt angle. Scale bar = 0.1 μm. (Micrographs courtesy of Dr. Michael S. Forbes.)

pillars is that the number of these pillars seemed to increase when the surface membrane, and presumably the T-tubules, were depolarized by K^+ ion (Eisenberg and Eisenberg 1982) (Fig. 19).

It is still possible that either of these structures may permit ionic current to flow from the T-tubules to the TC-SR; for instance, according to the hypothesis of Mathias et al. (1980). An alternative possibility has been proposed, however. It consists of considering pillars or foot processes as mechanical links between the charged macromolecules embedded in the T-tubules and openings plugged in the SR membrane. The depolarization-induced movement of charge in the T-tubules would then unplug channels in the SR membrane through which Ca^{2+} would flow into the myoplasm (Fig. 20). This hypothesis is still very weakly supported because of the difficulty of correlation between structure and function. Yet, no data accumulated until now have permitted its elimination (Schneider, 1981; however, see the critical calculations of Oetliker, 1982).

The preceding discussion had been written originally in 1984, and we thought it was still valuable to leave it approximately intact in the new edition of the book. However, since the original writing of this discussion, progress has been made in the description of the triad between the transverse tubule and the SR (Kawamoto et al., 1986; Chadwick et al., 1988; Block et al., 1988; Caswell and Brandt, 1989;

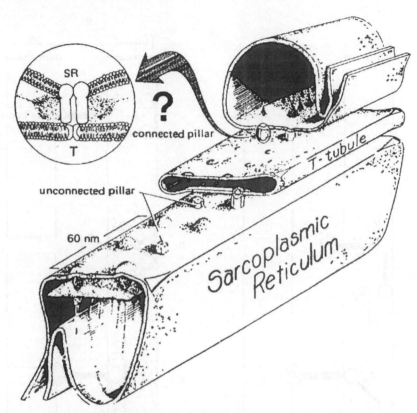

Figure 19 Schematic representation of the pillars between the T-tubules and the TC-SR. The small unlabeled hemispheres represent the foot processes. Connection of the pillars presumably is induced by depolarization of the transverse (T) tubules. The insert indicates one possible hypothesis for the role of the pillars: that they could represent ionic channels for an electrical coupling between the T-tubules and TC-SR. An alternative hypothesis is that the pillars may represent mechanical links between macromolecules embedded in the T-tubule membranes and sites plugged in the SR membrane. (From Eisenberg and Eisenberg, 1982.)

Dulhunty, 1989). The feet are now considered by most investigators to be identical with the pillars and to correspond to the ryanodine receptors, which have been demonstrated to correspond to the sarcoplasmic reticulum Ca^{2+} channels, whereas the periodic structure of the transverse tubules is believed to correspond to the dihydropyridine receptor of these tubules (Block et al., 1988). These structural data and many important electrophysiological findings have given much more strength to the hypothesis that dihydropyridine and ryanodine receptors physically interact (Block et al., 1988), and that this physical interaction is important in excitation–contraction coupling (Caswell and Brandt, 1989), as reviewed by Rios and Pizzaro (1989). This is not true, however, for cardiac muscle, in which any charge movement

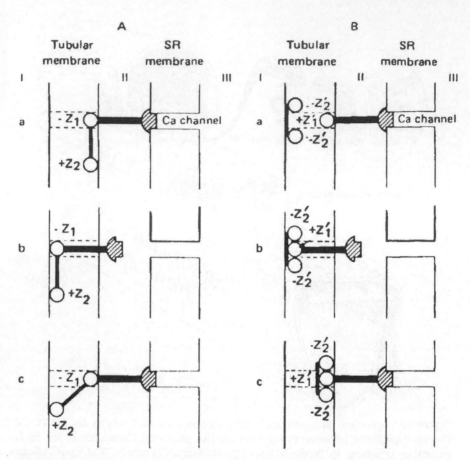

Figure 20   A mechanical hypothesis for Ca^{2+} release from the TC-SR. The diagrams give hypothetical examples of how a charged complex might regulate Ca^{2+} release from the SR. I denotes the lumen of the T-tubules, the space labeled II is continuous with the sarcoplasm, and III indicates the inside of the terminal cisterna of the SR (TC-SR), where Ca^{2+} is thought to be stored. Z denotes the valence of the charged groups. In (A) Z_2 is greater than Z_1, by about 3. In (B) Z_1' is 3; the other charged complex consists of two groups of valence Z_2' connected by a basket which can move Z_1' to the right; $2Z_2' > Z_1'$. Configuration (a) corresponds to the resting state, (b) to the activated state, and (c) to the refractory state. (From Chandler et al., 1976.)

in the transverse tubules seems to play no major role in the triggering of Ca^{2+} release from the SR (Fabiato, 1989).

Considerable progress has also been made through single calcium channel recordings from sarcoplasmic reticulum incorporated into lipid bilayers (Smith et al., 1985, 1986) and from reconstituted ryanodine receptor (Smith et al., 1988), as reviewed by Rios and Pizzaro (1991). This brings the problem of excitation–contraction coupling to a nearly molecular level, but does not yet help in identifying the physiologically relevant mechanism triggering the Ca^{2+} release from the SR of either skeletal (Rios and Pizzaro, 1991) or cardiac muscle (Feher and Fabiato, 1990).

F. Modulation of Calcium Release from the Sarcoplasmic Reticulum

Although the mechanism of induction of Ca^{2+} release from the SR is still unknown, an abundant body of data has been reported concerning the regulation of the amount of Ca^{2+} released from the SR. Ions other than Ca^{2+} modify the amount Ca^{2+} released from the SR (Ebashi, 1976; Endo, 1977). The ionic balance most likely to be perturbed during respiratory diseases is that of H^+ ions. A modification of pH induces a change of both Ca^{2+} release from, and Ca^{2+} accumulation into, the SR, which is variable depending on the level of Ca^{2+} loading in the SR (Fabiato and Fabiato, 1978). A decrease of pH also decreases the sensitivity of the myofilaments to Ca^{2+} as well as the maximum tension developed by the myofilaments (Fabiato and Fabiato, 1978).

Several drugs modify E–C coupling (Ebashi, 1976; Endo, 1977). Some of these drugs, such as dantrolene or caffeine, are used as tools for understanding the mechanism of cardiac E–C coupling (Ebashi, 1976; Endo, 1977).

Finally, data are starting to emerge on the pathophysiological modifications of E–C coupling in muscle diseases. Thus, for instance, the Ca^{2+} release from the SR is depressed in Duchenne muscular dystrophy and in enhanced malignant hyperthermia and myotonia (Wood, 1978; Wood et al., 1978).

Acknowledgments

The authors thank Anthony Sperelakis and Glenn Doerman for drawing the figures, and Rhonda Hentz for typing manuscript.

References

Adrian, R. H., and Freygang, W. H. (1962). The potassium and chloride conductance of frog muscle membrane. *J. Physiol. (Lond.)* 163: 61–103.

Adrian, R. H., Chandler, W. K., and Hodgkin, A. L. (1970a). Voltage clamp experiments in striated muscle fibers. *J. Physiol. (Lond.)* 208: 607–644.

Adrian, R. H., Chandler, W. K., and Hodgkin, A. L. (1970b). Slow changes in potassium permeability in skeletal muscle. *J. Physiol. (Lond.)* 208: 645–668.

Almers, W., Fink, R., and Palade, P. T. (1981). Calcium depletion in frog muscle tubules: The decline of calcium current under maintained depolarization. *J. Physiol. (Lond.)* 312: 177–207.

Appel, S. H., and Roses, A. D. (1976). Membrane biochemical studies in myotonic muscular dystrophy. In *Membranes and Disease*. Edited by L. Bolis, J. F. Hoffman, and A. Leaf. New York, Raven Press, pp. 183–195.

Baylor, S. M., and Oetliker, H. (1975). Birefringence experiments on isolate skeletal muscle fibres suggest a possible signal from the sarcoplasmic reticulum. *Nature* 253: 97–101.

Beaty, G. N., and Stefani, E. (1976). Calcium dependent electrical activity in twitch muscle fibers of the frog. *Proc. R. Soc. Lond. (Biol.)* 194: 141–150.

Bezanilla, F., and Horowicz, P. (1975). Fluorescence intensity changes associated with contractile activation in from muscle stained with Nile Blue A. *J. Physiol. (Lond.)* 246: 709–735.

Bezanilla, F., Caputo, C., Gonzalez-Serratos, H., and Venosa, R. A. (1972). Sodium dependence of the inward spread of activation in isolated twitch muscle fibres of the frog. *J. Physiol. (Lond.)* 223: 507–523.

Bianchi, C. P., and Bolton, T. C. (1974). Effect of hypertonic solutions and glycerol treatment on calcium and magnesium movements of frog skeletal muscle. *J. Pharmacol. Exp. Ther.* 188: 536–552.

Bianchi, C. P., and Shanes, A. M. (1959). Calcium influx in skeletal muscle at rest, during activity, and during potassium contracture. *J. Gen. Physiol* 42: 803–815.

Birks, R. I., and Davey, D. F. (1969). Osmotic responses demonstrating the extracellular character of sarcoplasmic reticulum. *J. Physiol. (Lond.)* 21: 171–188.

Block, B. A., Imagawa, T., Campbell, K. P., and Franzini-Armstrong, C. (1988). Structural evidence for direct interaction between the molecular components of the transverse tubule/sarcoplasmic reticulum junction in skeletal muscle. *J. Cell Biol.* 14: 161–165.

Caswell, A. H., and Brant, N. R. (1989). Does muscle activation occur by direct mechanical coupling of transverse tubules to sarcoplasmic reticulum? *TIBS* 14: 161–165.

Chadwick, C. C., Inui, M., and Fleischer, S. (1988). Identification and purification of a transverse tubule coupling protein which binds to the ryanodine receptor of terminal cisternae at the triad junction in skeletal muscle. *J. Biol. Chem.* 263: 10872–10877.

Chandler, W. K., Rakowski, R. F., and Schneider, M. F. (1976). Effects of glycerol treatment and maintained depolarization on charge movement in skeletal muscle. *J. Physiol. (Lond.)* 254: 285–316.

Chiesi, M., and Inesi, G. (1980). Adenosine 5'-triphosphate dependent fluxes manganese and hydrogen ions in sarcoplasmic reticulum vesicles. *Biochemistry* 19: 2912–2918.

Chou, S. M., Nonaka, I., and Voice, G. F. (1980). Anastomoses of transverse tubules with terminal cisternae in polymyositis. *Arch. Neurol.* 37: 257–266.

Cole, K. S. (1968). *Membranes, Ions and Impulses: A Chapter of Classical Biophysics.* Berkeley, University of California Press.

Constantin, L. L., and Podolsky, R. J. (1967). Depolarization of the internal membrane system in the activation of frog skeletal muscle. *J. Gen. Physiol.* 50: 1101–1124.

Constantin, L. L., and Taylor, S. R. (1973). Graded activation in frog muscle fibers. *J. Gen. Physiol.* 61: 424–443.

Conway, E. J. (1957). Nature and significance of concentration relations of potassium and sodium ions in skeletal muscle. *Physiol. Rev.* 37: 84–132.

DiFrancesco, D. (1981). A new interpretation of the pacemaker current in calf Purkinje fibers. *J. Physiol.* 314: 359–376.

Donaldson, S. K. (1982). Mammalian skinned muscle fibers: Evidence of a ouabain-sensitive component of Cl^--stimulated Ca^{2+} release. *Biophys. J.* 37: 23a.

Dulhunty, A. F. (1989). Feet, bridges and pillars in triad junction of mammalian skeletal muscle: Their possible relationship to calcium buffers in terminal cisternae and T-tubules and to excitation–contraction coupling. *J. Membr. Biol.* 109: 73–83.

Ebashi, S. (1976). Excitation–contraction coupling. *Annu. Rev. Physiol.* 38: 293–313.

Eisenberg, B. R., and Eisenberg, R.-S. (1982). The T-SR junction in contracting single skeletal muscle fibers. *J. Gen. Physiol.* 79: 1–19.

Eisenberg, R. S., and Gage, P. W. (1969). Ionic conductances of the surface and transverse tubular membranes of frog sartorius fibers. *J. Gen. Physiol.* 53: 279–297.

Eisenberg, B. R., Mathias, R. T., and Gilai, A. (1979). Intracellular localization of markers within injected or cut frog muscle fibers. *Am. J. Physiol.* 237: C50–C55.

Endo, M. (1977). Calcium release from the sarcoplasmic reticulum. *Physiol. Rev.* 57: 71–108.

Fabiato, A. (1981). Mechanism of calcium-induced release of calcium from the sarcoplasmic reticulum of skinned cardiac cells studied with potential-sensitive dyes. In *The Mechanism of Gated Calcium Transport Across Biological Membranes*. Edited by S. T. Ohnishi and M. Endo. New York, Academic Press, pp. 237–255.

Fabiato, A. (1989). Appraisal of the physiological relevance of two hypotheses for the mechanism of calcium release from the mammlian cardiac sarcoplasmic reticulum: calcium-induced release versus charge-coupled release. *Mol. Cell. Biochem.* 89: 135–140.

Fabiato, A., and Fabiato, F. (1978). Effects of pH on the myofilaments and the sarcoplasmic reticulum of skinned cells from cardiac and skeletal muscles. *J. Physiol. (Lond.)* 276: 233–255.

Fatt, P., and Ginsborg, B. L. (1958). The ionic requirements for the production of action potentials in crustacean muscle fibers. *J. Physiol. (Lond.)* 142: 516–543.

Feher, J. J., and Fabiato, A. (1990). Cardiac sarcoplasmic reticulum: Calcium uptake and release. In *Calcium and the Heart*. Edited by G. Langer. New York, Raven Press, pp. 200–267.

Ferrier, G. R., and Moe, G. K. (1973). Effect of calcium on acetylstrophanthidin-induced transient depolarizations on canine Purkinje tissue. *Circ. Res.* 33: 508–515.

Forbes, M. S., and Sperelakis, N. (1972). (Na^+,K^+)-ATPase activity in tubular systems of mouse cardiac and skeletal muscles. *Z. Zellforsch.* 134: 1–11.

Forbes, M. S., and Sperelakis, N. (1979). Ruthenium red staining of skeletal and cardiac muscles. *Z. Zellforsch/Cell Tissue Res.* 200: 367–382.

Forbes, M. S., and Sperelakis, N. (1983). Bridging junctional processes in the junctional gap of couplings in striated and smooth muscle cells. *Muscle Nerve* 5: 674–681.

Forbes, M. S., Plantholt, B. A., and Sperelakis, N. (1977). Cytochemical staining procedures selective for sarcotubular systems of muscle: Modifications and applications. *J. Ultrastruct. Res.* 60: 306–327.

Frank, G. B. (1980). The current view of the source of trigger calcium in excitation–contraction coupling in vertebrate skeletal muscle. *Biochem. Pharmacol.* 29: 2399–2406.

Franzini-Armstrong, C. (1971). Studies of the triad. II. Penetration of tracers into the junctional gap. *J. Cell Biol.* 49: 196–203.

Franzini-Armstrong, C. (1975). Membrane particles and transmission at the triad. *Fed. Proc.* 34: 1382–1389.

Franzini-Armstrong, C., Heuser, J. E., Reese, T. S., Somlyo, A. P., and Somlyo, A. V. (1978). T-tubule swelling in hypertonic solutions: A freeze substitution study. *J. Physiol. (Lond.)* 283: 133–140.

Gonzalez-Serratos, H. (1971). Inward spread of activation in vertebrate muscle fibers. *J. Physiol. (Lond.)* 212: 777–799.

Gonzalez-Serratos, H., Somlyo, S. V., McClellan, H., Shuman, H., Borrero, L. and Somlyo, A. P. (1978). Composition of vacuoles and sarcoplasmic reticulum in fatigued muscle: Electron probe analysis. *Proc. Natl. Acad. Sci. USA* 75: 1329–1333.

Gonzalez-Serratos, H., Valle-Aguilera, R., Lathrop, D. A., and del Carmen Garcia, M. (1982). Slow inward calcium currents have no obvious role in muscle excitation–contraction coupling. *Nature* 298: 292–294.

Gunn, H. M., and Davies, A. S. (1971). Histochemical characteristics of muscle fibers in the diaphragm. *Biochem. J.* 125: 108P–109P.

Harris, E. J. (1963). Distribution and movement of muscle choride. *J. Physiol. (Lond.)* 166: 87–109.

Hodgkin, A. L. (1957). *Conduction of the Nervous Impulse*. Springfield, IL, Charles C Thomas.

Hodgkin, A. L., and Horowicz, P. (1959). The influence of potassium and chloride ions on the membrane potential of single muscle fibers. *J. Physiol. (Lond.)* 148: 127–160.

Hodgkin, A. L., and Huxley, A. F. (1952). Currents carried by sodium and potassium ions through the membrane of the giant axon of *Loligo*. *J. Physiol. (Lond.)* 116: 449–472.

Howell, J. N. (1974). Intracellular binding of ruthenium red in frog skeletal muscle. *J. Cell Biol.* 62: 242–247.

Huxley, A. F., and Taylor, R. E. (1958). Local activation of striated muscle fibres. *J. Physiol. (Lond.)* 144: 426–441.

Huxley, H. E., Page, S., and Wilkie, D. R. (1963). Appendix. In M. Dydynsk and D. R. Wilkie.

An electron microscopic study of muscle in hypertonic solutions. *J. Physiol. (Lond.)* 169: 312–329.

Irisawa, H. (1980). Ionic currents underlying spontaneous rhythm of the cardiac primary pacemaker cells. In *The Sinus Node*. Edited by F. I. M Bonke. The Hague, Martinus Nijhoff, pp. 368–375.

Kass, R. S., Lederer, W. J., Tsien, R. W., and Weingart, R. (1978). Role of calcium ions in transient inward currents and aftercontractions induced by strophanidin in cardiac Purkinje fibres. *J. Physiol. (Lond.)* 281: 187–208.

Katzung, B. G. (1975). Effects of extracellular calcium and sodium on depolarization-induced automaticity in guinea-pig papillary muscle. *Circ. Res.* 37:118–127.

Kawamoto, R. M., Brunschwig, J. P., Kyungsook, K., and Caswell, A. H. (1986). Isolation, characterization, and localization of the spanning protein of skeletal muscle triads. *J. Cell Biol.* 103: 1405–1414.

Kerr, L. M., and Sperelakis, N. (1982). Effects of the calcium antagonists verapamil and bepridil (CERM-1978) on Ca^{2+}-dependent slow action potentials in frog skeletal muscle. *J. Pharmacol. Exp. Ther.* 222: 80–86.

Kerr, L. M., and Sperelakis, N. (1983). Membrane alterations in skeletal muscle fibers in dystrophic mouse. *Muscle Nerve* 6: 3–13.

Keynes, R. D., and Steinhardt, R. A. (1968). The components of the sodium efflux in frog muscle. *J. Physiol. (Lond.)* 198: 581–599.

Khan, A. R. (1981). Influence of ethanol and acetaldehyde on electromechanical coupling of skeletal muscle fibres. *Acta Physiol. Scand.* 111: 425–430.

Kirby, A. C., Lindley, B. D., and Picken, J. R. (1975). Calcium content and exchange in frog skeletal muscle. *J. Physiol. (Lond.)* 253: 37–52.

Kulczycky, S., and Mainwood, G. W. (1972). Evidence for a functional connection between the sarcoplasmic reticulum and the extracellular space in frog sartorius muscle. *Can. J. Physiol. Pharmacol.* 50: 87–98.

Lehmkuhl, D., and Sperelakis, N. (1967). Electrical activity of cultured heart cells. In *Factors In Influencing Myocardial Contractility*. Edited by R. D. Tanz, F. Kavaler, and J. Roberts. New York, Academic Press, pp. 245–278.

Luft, J. H. (1971). Ruthenium red and violet. 2. Fine structural localization in animal tissues. *Anat. Rec.* 171: 369–416.

Lynch, C. III. (1978). *Kinetic and biochemical separation of potassium currents in frog striated muscle.* Ph.D. dissertation. New York, University of Rochester.

Mann, J. E., Sperelakis, N., and Ruffner, J. A. (1981). Alterations in sodium channel gate kinetics of the Hodgkin–Huxley equations on an electric field model for interaction between excitable cells. *IEEE Trans. Biomed. Eng.* 28: 655–661.

Mathias, R. T., Eisenberg, R. S., and Valdiosera, R. (1977). Electrical properties of frog skeletal muscle fibers interpreted with a mesh model of the tubular system. *Biophys. J.* 17: 57–93.

Mathias, R. T., Levis, R. A., and Eisenberg, R. S. (1980). Electrical models of excitation–contraction coupling and charge movement in skeletal muscle. *J. Gen. Physiol.* 76: 1–31.

Meech, R. W. (1972). Intracellular calcium injection causes increased potassium conductance in aplysia nerve cells. *Comp. Biochem. Physiol.* 42: 493–499.

Meissner, G., and McKinley, D. (1976). Permeability of sarcoplasmic reticulum membrane. The effect of changed ionic environments on Ca^{2+} release. *J. Membr. Biol.* 30: 79–88.

Miledi, R., Stefani, E., and Steinbach, A. B. (1971). Induction of the action potential mechanism in slow muscle fibres of the frog. *J. Physiol. (Lond.)* 217: 737–754.

Miledi, R., Parker, R. I., and Schalow, G. (1977). Measurement of calcium transients in frog muscle by the use of arseno III. *Proc. R. Soc. Lond. B* 198: 201–210.

Mobley, B. A., and Eisenberg, B. R. (1975). Sizes of components in frog skeletal muscle measured by methods of stereology. *J. Gen. Physiol.* 66: 31–45.

Mullins, L. J. (1979). The generation of electric currents in cardiac fibers by Na/Ca exchange. *Am J. Physiol.* 263: C103–C110.

Natori, R. (1954). The property and contraction process of isolated myofibrils. *Jikeikai Med. J.* 1: 119–126.

Natori, R. (1965). Propagated contractions in isolated sarcolemma-free bundle of myofibrils. *Jikeidai Med. J.* 12: 214–221.

Neville, M. C. (1979). The extracellular compartments of frog skeletal muscle. *J. Physiol. (Lond.)* 288: 45–70.

Nicola-Siri, L., Sanchez, J. A., and Stefani, E. (1980). Effect of glycerol treatment on calcium current of frog skeletal muscle. *J. Physiol. (Lond.)* 305: 87–96.

Oetliker, H. (1982). An appraisal of the evidence for a sarcoplasmic reticulum membrane potential and its relation to calcium release in skeletal muscle. *J. Muscle Res. Cell Motil.* 3: 247–272.

Peachey, L. D. (1965). The sarcoplasmic reticulum and transverse tubules of the frog's sartorius. *J. Cell Biol.* 25: 209–231.

Peachey, L. D., and Porter, K. R. (1959). Intracellular impulse conduction in muscle cells. *Science* 129: 721–722.

Pelleg, A., Vogel, S., Belardinelli, L., and Sperelakis, N. (1980). Overdrive suppression of automaticity in cultured chick myocardial cells. *Am. J. Physiol.* 238: H24–H30.

Podolsky, R. J., and Costantin, L. L. (1964). Regulation by calcium of the traction and relaxation of muscle fibers. *Fed. Proc.* 23: 933–939.

Potreau, D., and Raymond, G. (1980). Calcium-dependent electrical activity and contraction of voltage-clamped frog single muscle fibers. *J. Physiol. (Lond.)* 307: 9–22.

Ridgway, E. B., and Ashley, C. C. (1967). Calcium transients in single muscle fibers. *Biochem. Biophys. Res. Comm.* 29: 229–234.

Rios, E., and Pizarro, G. (1991). Voltage sensor in excitation–contraction coupling in skeletal muscle. *Physiol. Rev.* 71: 849–908.

Rogus, E., and Zierler, K. L. (1973). Sodium and water contents of sarcoplasm and sarcoplasmic reticulum in rat skeletal muscle: Effects of anisotonic media, ouabain, and external sodium. *J. Physiol. (Lond.)* 233: 227–270.

Rubio, R., and Sperelakis, N. (1971). Entrance of colloidal ThO2 tracer into the T-tubules and longitudinal tubules of the guinea pig heart. *Z. Zellforsch.* 116: 20–36.

Rubio, R., and Sperelakis, N. (1972). Penetration of horseradish peroxidase the terminal cisternae of frog skeletal muscle fibers and blockade of caffeine contracture by Ca^{++} depletion. *Z. Zellforsch.* 124: 57–71.

Ruffner, J. A., Sperelakis, N., and Mann, J. E., Jr. (1980). Application of the Hodgkin–Huxley equations to an electric field model for interaction between excitable cells. *J. Theor. Biol.* 87: 129–152.

Rulon, R., Hermsmeyer, K., and Sperelakis, N. (1971). Regenerative action potentials induced in the neurogenic heart of *Limulus polyphemus*. *Comp. Biochem. Physiol.* 39A: 333–335.

Russell, J. T., Beeler, T., and Martonosi, A. (1979a). Optical probe responses on sarcoplasmic reticulum: Oxycarbocyanines. *J. Biol. Chem.* 254: 2040–2046.

Russell, J. T., Beeler, T., and Martonosi, A. (1979b). Optical probe response on sarcoplasmic reticulum merocyanine and oxonol dyes. *J. Biol. Chem.* 254: 2047–2052.

Sanchez, J. A., and Stefani, E. (1978). Inward calcium current in twitch muscle fibers of the frog. *J. Physiol. (Lond.)* 283: 197–209.

Schneider, M. F. (1981). Membrane charge movement and depolarization–contraction coupling. *Annu. Rev. Physiol.* 43: 507–517.

Schneider, M. F., and Chandler, W. K. (1973). Voltage dependent charge movement in skeletal muscle: A possible step in excitation–contraction coupling. *Nature* 242: 244–246.

Sellin, L. C., and Sperelakis, N. (1978). Decreased potassium permeability in dystrophic mouse skeletal muscle. *Exp. Neurol.* 62: 609–617.

Sha'afi, R. I., Rodan, S. B., Hintz, R. L., Fernandez, S. M., and Rodan, G. A. (1975). Abnormalities in microviscosity and ion transport in genetic muscular dystrophy. *Nature* 254: 525–526.

Shoshan, V., MacLennan, D. H., and Wood, D. S. (1981). A proton gradient controls a calcium-release channel in sarcoplasmic reticulum. *Proc. Natl. Acad. Sci. USA* 78: 4828–4832.

Singer, S. J., and Nicolson, G. L. (1972). The fluid mosaic model of the structure of cell membranes. *Science* 175: 720–731.

Smith, J. S., Coronado, R., and Meissner, G. (1985). Sarcoplasmic reticulum contains adenine nucleotide-activated calcium channels. *Nature* 316: 446–449.

Smith, J. S., Coronado, R., and Meissner, G. (1986). Single channel measurements of the calcium release channel from skeletal muscle sarcoplasmic reticulum. Activation by Ca^{2+}, ATP, and modulation by Mg^{2+}. *J. Gen. Physiol.* 88: 537–588.

Smith, J. S., Imagawa, T., Ma, J., Fill, M., Campbell, K. P., and Coronado, R. (1988). Purified ryanodine receptor from rabbit skeletal muscle is the calcium release channel of sarcoplasmic reticulum. *J. Gen. Physiol.* 92: 1–26.

Somlyo, A. V. (1979). Bridging structures spanning the junctional gap at the triad of skeletal muscle. *J. Cell Biol.* 80: 743–750.

Somlyo, A. V., Gonzalez-Serratos, H., Shuman, H., McClellan, G., and Somlyo, A. P. (1981). Calcium release and ionic changes in the sarcoplasmic reticulum of tetanized muscle: An electron-probe study. *J. Cell Biol.* 90: 577–594.

Sommer, J. R., Wallace, N. R., and Hasselbach, W. (1978). The collapse of the sarcoplasmic reticulum in skeletal muscle. *Z. Naturforsch.* 33C: 561–573.

Spector, I., and Prives, J. M. (1977). Development of electrophysiological and biochemical membrane properties during differentiation of embryonic skeletal muscle in culture. *Proc. Natl. Acad. Sci. USA* 74: 5166–5170.

Sperelakis, N. (1967). Electrophysiology of cultured chick heart cells. In *Electrophysiology and Ultrastructure of the Heart*. Edited by T. Sano, V Mizuhira, and K. Matsuda. Tokyo, Bunkodo Co., pp. 81–108.

Sperelakis, N. (1969). Changes in conductance of frog sartorius fibers produced by CO_2, ReO_4, and temperature. *Am. J. Physiol.* 217: 1069–1075.

Sperelakis, N. (1979). Origin of the cardiac resting potential. In *Handbook of Physiology*, The *Cardiovascular System*, Vol. 1, The Heart. Edited by R. Berne and N. Sperelakis. Bethesda, MD, Amican Physiological Society, Chap. 6, pp. 267.

Sperelakis, N. (1980). Changes in membrane electrical properties during development of the heart. In *The Slow Inward Current and Cardiac Arrhythmias*. Edited by D. P. Zipes, J. C. Bailey, and V. Elharrar. The Hague, Martinus Nijhoff, pp. 221–262.

Sperelakis, N. (1982). Electrophysiology of vascular smooth muscle of coronary artery. In *The Coronary Artery*. Edited by S. Kalsner. London, Croom Helm, pp. 118–167.

Sperelakis, N., and Lehmkuhl, D. (1964). Effect of current on transmembrane, potentials in cultured chick heart cells. *J. Gen. Physiol.* 47: 895–927.

Sperelakis, N., and Lehmkuhl, D. (1966). Ionic interconversion of pacemaker and nonpacemaker cultured chick heart cells. *J. Gen. Physiol.* 49: 867–895.

Sperelakis, N., and Mann, J. E., Jr. (1977). Evaluation of electric field change in the cleft between excitable cells. *J. Theor. Biol.* 64: 71–96.

Sperelakis, N., and Rubio, R. (1971). Ultrastructural changes produced by hypertonicity in cat cardiac muscle. *J. Mol. Cell. Cardiol.* 3: 139–156.

Sperelakis, N., and Schneider, M. F. (1968). Membrane ion conductances of frog sartorius fibers as a function of tonicity. *Am. J. Physiol.* 215: 723–729.

Sperelakis, N., Schneider, M. F., and Harris, E. J. (1967). Decreased K^+ conductance produced by Ba^{++} in frog sartorius fibers. *J. Gen. Physiol.* 50: 1565–1583.

Sperelakis, N., Mayer, G., and Macdonald, R. (1970). Velocity of propagation in vertebrate cardiac muscles as functions of tonicity and $[K^+]_0$. *Am. J. Physiol.* 219: 952–963.

Sperelakis, N., Valle, R., Orozco, C., Martinez-Palomo, A., and Rubio, R. (1973). Electromechanical uncoupling of frog skeletal muscle by possible change in sarcoplasmic reticular content. *Am. J. Physiol.* 225: 793–800.

Sperelakis, N., Forbes, M. S., and Rubio, R. (1974). The tubular systems of myocardial cells: Ultrastructure and possible function. In *Recent Advances in Studies on Cardiac Structure and Metabolism*. Edited by N. S. Dhalla and G. Rona. Myocardial Biology, Vol. 4. Baltimore, University Park Press, pp. 163–194.

Sperelakis, N., Shigenobu, K., and Rubio, R. (1978). ^{3}H-sucrose compartments in frog skeletal muscle relative to sarcoplasmic reticulum. *Am J. Physiol.* 234: C181–C190.

Sperelakis, N., Ortiz-Zwazaga, H., Picone, J., and Mann, J. E., Jr., (1992). Voltage interaction between sarcolemma and junctional SR membrane. *J. Math. Comp. Model.* 16: 101–115.

Spitzer, N. C. (1979). Ion channels in development. *Annu. Rev. Neurosci.* 2:363–397.

Stanfield, P. R. (1977). A calcium dependent inward current in frog skeletal muscle fibers. *Pflugers Arch.* 368: 267–270.

Stephenson, E. W. (1981). Activation of fast skeletal muscle: Contributions of studies on skinned fibers. *Am. J. Physiol.* 240: C1–19.

Suarez-Kurtz, G., and Parker, I. (1977). Birefringence signals and calcium transients in skeletal muscle. *Nature* 270: 746–748.

Tasker, P., Simon, S. E., Johnstons, B. M., Shankly, K. H., and Shaw, F. H. (1959). The dimensions of the extracellular space in sartorius muscle. *J. Gen. Physiol.* 43: 39–53.

Vassalle, M. (1970). Electrogenic suppression of automaticity in sheep and dog Purkinje fibers. *Circ. Res.* 27: 361–377.

Vinogradova, N. A. (1968). Distribution of nonpenetrating sugars in the frog's sartorius muscle under hypo- and hypertonic conditions. *Tsitologiia* 10: 831–838.

Vogel, S., and Sperelakis, N. (1978). Valinomycin blockade of myocardial slow channels is reversed by high glucose. *Am. J. Physiol.* 235: H46–H51.

Vogel, S., Harder, D., and Sperelakis, N. (1978). Ca^{++} dependent electrical and mechanical activities in skeletal muscle. *Fed. Proc.* 37: 517.

Wallace, N., and Sommer, J. R. (1975). Fusion of sarcoplasmic reticulum with ruthenium red. *Proc. Electron Microsc. Soc. A.*, 33rd, Las Vegas, pp. 500–501.

Winegrad, S. (1968). Intracellular calcium movements of frog skeletal muscle during recovery from tetanus. *J. Gen. Physiol.* 51: 65–83.

Wood, D. S. (1978). Human skeletal muscle: Analysis of Ca^{2+} regulation in skinned fibers using caffeine. *Exp. Neurol.* 58: 218–230.

Wood, D. S., Sorenson, M. M., Eastwood, A. B., Charash, W. E., and Reuben, J. P. (1978). Duchenne dystrophy: Abnormal generation of tension and Ca^{++} regulation in single skinned fibers. *Neurology* 28: 447–457.

3

Pathophysiology of Skeletal Muscle

SHIRLEY H. BRYANT and NICHOLAS SPERELAKIS

University of Cincinnati College of Medicine
Cincinnati, Ohio

I. Introduction

The purpose of this chapter is to describe and discuss a few selected conditions or diseases of skeletal muscle, to illustrate some of the pathophysiological changes that can occur in muscle function under a variety of conditions. The chapter material has been extensively reorganized and modified from the previous edition. Several new areas have been included that touch on the important advances that have come about through application of molecular biology. The text continues to emphasize the importance of understanding the electrophysiological properties described and discussed in Chapter 2. This is because the changes that occur in hereditary diseases of muscle (such as the myotonias, muscular dystrophies, and the periodic paralyses; and in conditions such as fatigue, denervation, and malignant hyperthermia) affect the electrical properties of the cell membrane. This chapter will also describe the effects of two hormones, insulin and β-adrenergic agonists, on the electrical properties of skeletal muscle fibers. Extensive documentation of many of the statements that are made and views presented cannot be done because of size limitations.

A. Ion Channel Disease in Skeletal Muscle

Many of the important conditions affecting muscle function result from abnormal ion channel function. These ion channel diseases are often due to genetic mutations. Ion channels are involved in many critical cellular processes: from the transmission of impulses in excitable membranes, to linking excitation with contraction. Probably most spontaneous genetic mutations of ion channels or of their regulators may prove to be lethal, but humans and other mammals can survive, at least to reproductive age, and pass on some severe alterations that we recognize as those hereditary diseases for which the target is ion channels. A gene mutation can affect channels in one of the following ways: (1) A defective channel protein is expressed, or its expression is blocked. (2) A nonchannel protein on which channel function depends is expressed, but is defective, or its expression is blocked. Defective and malfunctioning proteins may be expressed as a result of improper coding. However, certain mutations can completely block the expression of a product. Furthermore, it is possible for a defect to occur in a subunit or in a regulator shared by several types of channels. This may offer an explanation of how a single defective gene could lead to malfunction of more that one type of channel. A mutation in the gene for a specific channel can also alter the function of an unrelated channel. This is referred to as a *pleotropic* effect, and the mechanism of such effects is generally unknown. Some of these possibilities are illustrated with our discussion of certain classic muscle syndromes. Knowledge of the molecular details of channel diseases is increasing at an astounding rate as new techniques of molecular genetics are being applied. Therefore, some information is so new that inclusion of details here may be premature.

B. Cloning of Disease Genes

Identification of genes involved in ion channel diseases is currently very labor-intensive. The effort appears to have been worth it, as evidenced by the recent successes of the "candidate gene approach" (see Fontaine, 1993, for further discussion). A scheme of this approach is shown in Figure 1. The circled area represents a new disease locus assigned to a chromosome. The genes located around this locus are analyzed for the several features shown on the right-hand side and compared with features of the diseases shown on the left. The order of comparison of these features must correspond to match the gene with the disease. In like manner, when a new gene is assigned to a chromosome region, the candidate diseases are analyzed in an analogous fashion. At the experimental level two principal search strategies have evolved: (1) functional or expression cloning, and (2) positional cloning. In *expression cloning*, the gene is isolated on the basis of information about the expressed protein product (e.g., its amino acid sequence or antibody reactivity) or about its function (e.g., receptor–ligand reactivity or ion channel characteristics). Complementary DNA libraries are screened using different types of probes, including antibodies and oligonucleotides. The polymerase chain reaction (PCR) is often employed to amplify the cDNA, using oligonucleotides derived from the protein sequence. Functional cloning was used to characterize the CLC-1 chloride channel gene involved in the arrested development of righting response (ADR) myotonic mouse, myotonia congenita (MC), and recessive generalized myotonia (RGM); and the Na^+ channel

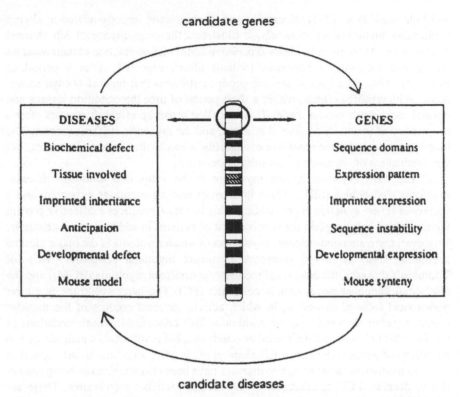

Figure 1   The candidate gene approach to identifying disease genes. (From George et al., 1993.)

mutants causing paramyotonia congenita (PC) and hyperkalemic periodic paralysis (HYPP). In contrast, *positional cloning* is the process of isolating the gene starting from information about its genetic or physical location in the genome. Often, little or nothing may be known about the function of the product. The work involved is enormous, since it relies on the method of chromosomal walking and identification of expressed sequences. Positional cloning is a "brute force" approach, which will probably give way to more efficient methods in time. In spite of these difficulties, 19 important disease genes were identified in this way between 1989 and 1993 (Ballabio, 1993), including myotonic dystrophy (DM) and cystic fibrosis. Some newer strategies combine both expression and positional cloning to identify the genes.

II. Myotonia

A. General Description

Myotonia is a bizarre syndrome seen in several classic hereditary muscle diseases of humans and animals, and occasionally in response to chemicals or disease (Rüdel and Lehmann-Horn, 1985). Because myotonia is usually directly related to altered excitability involving ion channels, it illustrates the consequence of ion channel dysfunction. Myotonic individuals experience additional contraction of their muscles during and following a voluntary (willed) effort, especially after a period of inactivity. This extra contraction can produce stiffness that hinders normal movement. With repeated efforts, within a short period of time the condition lessens and normal movements can be made. This so-called warm-up effect disappears after a new period of inactivity of several minutes, and the myotonic stiffness returns. The biophysical bases for the repetitive excitability is established in most instances, but the mechanism of warm-up is not fully understood.

The most common human myotonia is the autosomal dominant disease, myotonia dystrophica (MD), which is accompanied by muscular dystrophy and a variety of severe systemic abnormalities. This mutation produces a defective protein kinase, which helps explain the involvement of systems in addition to ion channels. However, there are nondystrophic myotonias in which myotonia is the major clinical presenting sign, as in the autosomal dominant myotonia congenita (MC) (or Thomsen's disease), the autosomal recessive generalized myotonia (RGM), and the autosomal dominant paramyotonia congenita (PC). The latter syndrome is a rarer paradoxical form of myotonia, in which activity or local cooling of the muscles *worsens* (rather than reduces) the myotonia. This condition involves mutations of an Na^+ channel gene, unlike the other nondystrophic myotonias, which are due to mutations of genes coding for a Cl^- channel or, in MD, a protein kinase regulator.

In nonhuman myotonias, two diseases have been characterized as being mainly due to decreased Cl^- conductance of the muscle excitable membranes. These are the hereditary myotonia of the goat and the myotonia of the ADR or myotonic mouse. Myotonia has been described in other species, such as the dystrophic chicken. In the latter species, the biophysical basis is not precisely known, although it is definitely not due to decreased Cl^- permeability (Entrikin and Bryant, 1979). The importance of the role of Cl^- current in stabilizing the membrane of skeletal muscle is nicely illustrated by the myotonic goat. Bryant and colleagues (see Bryant, 1979) have shown that there is a genetically determined, abnormally low permeability of Cl^- (P_{Cl}) in a myotonic goat colony (resembling in many respects the human MC (Fig. 2)). The low P_{Cl}, and hence Cl^- conductance (g_{Cl}), produces the characteristic myotonic symptoms, which are chiefly *hyperexcitability*, *repetitive firing* to single stimulations, *after-depolarization*, and *after-discharges* to prolonged depolarizing pulses. These electrical abnormalities prevent the animal or person from relaxing the voluntary muscles in a normal manner. Thus, the myotonic patient has difficulty in relaxing a handshake or starting up the stairs. In myotonia, there is a partial loss of motoneuron control over the skeletal muscles. In the myotonic goat, as expected, membrane resistivity (R_m) is elevated by severalfold, but the resting potential is normal. The repetitive firing causes the diagnostic "dive-bomber" response in the electromyogram (EMG) following needle electrode insertion into the muscle (mechanical stimulation).

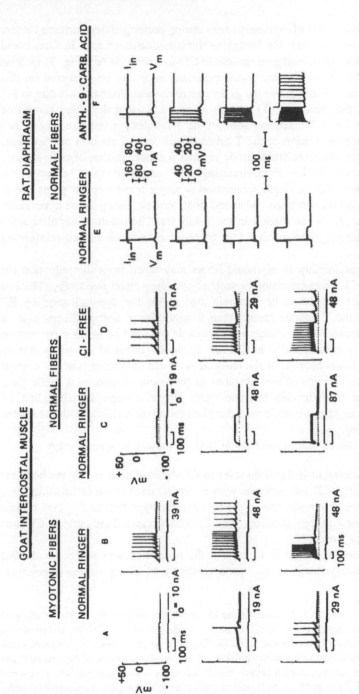

Figure 2 Excitation of normal and myotonic fibers with constant-current pulses recorded with a microelectrode close to the microelectrode passing current. Duration and magnitude of the currents are indicated below (A–D) or above (E–F) the potential traces. (A,B) Intercostal muscle fibers from a myotonic goat in normal Ringer at 37°C. (C,D) Intercostal fibers from a normal goat in normal Ringer at 37°C (C) and in a Cl⁻-free Ringer (sulfate substituted) at 37°C (D). (E,F) Normal rat diaphragm fibers in a normal physiological solution at 30°C (E) and in presence of 5×10^{-5} M anthracene-9-carboxylic acid (F). (A–D, from Adrian and Bryant, 1974; E, F from Furman and Barchi, 1978; modified from Bryant, 1982b).

The repetitive firing of myotonic fibers during prolonged depolarizing current pulses can be predicted from the Hodgkin–Huxley equations[*] and, in fact, could be modeled by placing normal goat muscle in Cl^--free solution (see Fig. 2) (Adrian and Bryant, 1974). However, the afterdepolarization cannot be predicted on this basis. The afterdepolarization (which gives rise to the afterdischarge) is due to K^+ accumulation in the transverse (T) tubules. It was estimated that there should be approximately 0.3 mM K^+ accumulation in the T-tubules per impulse, giving rise to a theoretical depolarization of the T-tubule membrane of about 3 mV/impulse. However, an intracellular microelectrode records a depolarization of only about 1 mV/impulse, because of the "short-circuiting" or "voltage-clamping" effect of the surface membrane. Thus, a single stimulation or single nerve impulse gives rise to multiple muscle action potentials (APs) and contractions, owing to the hyperexcitability and to the K^+ accumulation in the T-tubules. The resultant depolarization gives rise to multiple impulses in a sort of positive-feedback or self-reinforcing arrangement.

The hyperexcitability in myotonic fibers may result from the reduction (or removal) of the Cl^- short-circuiting or voltage-clamping effect due to P_{Cl}. The low g_{Cl} of the surface membrane in myotonia also makes the depolarization by K^+ accumulation in the T tubules greater than it would be in normal fibers, and so reinforces the uncontrolled discharge. As expected from the discussion in the section on mechanisms of repolarization in Chapter 2, repolarization of the AP is slowed in the myotonic fibers because of the reduced or absent contribution of Cl^- current to repolarization. The role of the T-tubules in the myotonic pattern is made clear by the fact that the after-depolarization and after-discharge are abolished by detubulating the myotonic muscle with the glycerol osmotic-shock method (Adrian and Bryant, 1974).

Myotonia can be induced in normal skeletal muscle in several ways:

1. The bathing of isolated muscles in Cl^--free solution is one method (see Fig. 2). In Cl^--free solution with an impermeant anion as substitute, g_{Cl} becomes zero regardless of the fact that the hypothetical P_{Cl} may remain high because, by definition, for a Cl^- conductance there must be Cl^- ions to carry current.
2. A second approach is to expose the normal muscle to chemicals that specifically decrease g_{Cl}, presumably by blocking voltage-dependent,

---

[*]A classic way to view this is that raising the Cl^- resistance reduces the short-circuiting of the parallel LC (inductance–capacitance) membrane equivalent circuit of Cole, and so allows spontaneous oscillations in membrane potential (E_m) to occur at the resonant frequency (for each E_m level). The L component arises because of the peculiar behavior of R_K, namely, the anomalous rectifier pathway, which causes an increase of R_K with depolarization. This tends to keep I_K constant [$I_K = g_K (E_m - E_K)$], and so conferring a large apparent inductive property to the membrane (for further discussion, see Sperelakis, 1979).

gated Cl^- channels or pathways. The aromatic monocarboxylic acids such as (2,4-dichlorophenoxyacetic acid and anthracene-9-carboxylic acid), are such agents (see Fig. 2). At $10^{-5}-10^{-3}$ M, they decrease g_{Cl} within a few minutes and induce myotonia (Bryant, 1979). There are also chiral derivatives of clofibric acid (e.g., 4-chlorophenoxy-2-propionic acid), the enantiomers of which have opposite effects (Conte-Camerino, et al., 1988). One enantiomer (S–) blocks g_{Cl} and induces myotonia, whereas the other (R+) increases g_{Cl} and antagonizes myotonia. Divalent cations, such as Zn^{2+} (ca. 1–5 mM) may also decrease g_{Cl}.

3. Theoretically, acidosis (e.g., pH 6.6–6.1) should exert the same effect as the carboxylic acids because it known that acidosis markedly depresses g_{Cl} in frog skeletal muscle (Hutter and Warner, 1967; Sperelakis, 1969) and mammalian skeletal muscle (Palade and Barchi, 1977). However, myotonia is not seen, and this is most likely due to the depressive action of low pH on the Na^+ channels.

4. Diazacholesterol (and other hypocholesterolemic agents), fed for several weeks to inhibit cholesterol synthesis, induces myotonia. The mechanism of this effect is unknown, but presumably, the decreased cholesterol (and increased desmosterol) content of the cell membrane somehow alters g_{Cl} and possibly Na^+ channels as well. However, very high doses can induce myotonia in hours, well before changes occur in membrane sterols. Clofibrate, another hypercholesterolemic agent, causes myotonia acutely owing to hydrolysis, which produces a carboxylic acid, and chronically by block of cholesterol synthesis (Kwiecinski, 1981; Rüdel and Lehmann-Horn, 1985).

5. Vitamin E deficiency can induce myotonia by an unknown mechanism.

6. Drugs, such as aconitine and veratridine, and some polypeptide toxins, also induce myotonialike symptoms by an Na^+ channel mechanism. Veratridine, for example, acts by holding open the fast Na^+ channels (i.e., by keeping the I-gate from closing), thereby giving rise to prolonged APs with repetitive firing (Sperelakis, 1981). Thus, this mechanism of inducing myotonia is completely independent of the Cl^- mechanism.

7. Colchicine also induces myotonia. This agent disrupts microtubules and blocks fast axoplasmic flow in neurons, and it decreases g_{Cl} (and g_K) in the muscle fibers, presumably by affecting the neurotropic behavior of the neuron on the muscle.

8. Denervation of mammalian skeletal muscle after 2 weeks induces fibrillation of the fibers, but this phenomenon should not to be confused with myotonia. The basis of fibrillation is not hyperexcitability of the membranes, as in myotonia. Fibrillation potentials arise as a type of pacemaker potential from near the denervated end-plate region. Denervation decreases g_{Cl} of mammalian muscle within a few days (but affects only g_K in frog muscle). Thus, denervated mammalian fibers might be expected

to be myotonic. On the contrary, permanently denervated fibers are slightly depolarized, less excitable, and actually resistant to development of myotonia with g_{Cl} blockers (Iyer et al., 1981; Caccia et al., 1975).

9. Phorbol esters can block g_{Cl} and induce myotonia in mammalian (but not frog) skeletal muscle (Bryant and Conte-Camerino, 1991; Tricarico et al., 1991, 1993). Because phorbol esters activate protein kinase C (PKC) through the diacylglycerol pathway, it suggests that PKC is a negative regulator of skeletal muscle g_{Cl} in mammals.

10. Sea anemone toxin, ATX II, can delay inactivation of skeletal muscle sodium channels thereby producing a myotonia similar to that seen in paramyotonia and hyperkalemic periodic paralysis (Cannon and Cory, 1993) (see Sec. V).

In other studies, Bryant and colleagues (Bryant, 1979, 1982a,b; Bryant and DeCoursey, 1980) have reported that there is also an increased inactivation time for the fast Na^+ channels in myotonic goats in addition to the defective g_{Cl}. If so, this would act like veratridine, as discussed earlier. In addition, they suggest that the T-tubular and sarcoplasmic reticulum (SR) membranes, and excitation–contraction coupling, may be affected in myotonic goat muscle. They also suggest that a higher mechanical threshold may protect the myotonic fibers from destructive contractures that might otherwise occur. We will see further that other autosomal dominant skeletal muscle diseases are associated with Na^+ channels having prolonged inactivation.

In the realm of pure nondystrophic myotonia of animals, there is the strain of goats, referred to earlier, that have a hereditary myotonia as an autosomal dominant mutation, and the one that occurs in the arrested development of righting response (ADR) or myotonic mouse as an autosomal recessive mutation. Myotonia reported in most other animal models is contaminated by muscular dystrophy and other systemic complications. In all of these myotonic conditions, the phenomenon is due to abnormalities of the excitable skeletal muscle membranes (sarcolemma and T-tubule membranes), and not to the neuromuscular junction or the nervous system. We know this because true myotonia persists after blocking the neuromuscular junctions with curarelike drugs, or by stimulating the muscle membranes directly immediately after acute denervation to remove control by the motor nerve. Pseudomyotonia (i.e., myotonia blocked by neuromuscular blockers) occurs in some human diseases and in the recessive *dy*-type dystrophic mouse. In the *dy* mouse model the repetitive firing has been attributed to a reverberating circuit set up by electrical interaction between motor fibers that have undergone demyelination at the nerve roots (Rasminsky, 1980).

An impressive sign of myotonia can be seen during a routine electromyographic (EMG) examination of skeletal muscles when recording needle electrodes are inserted into the muscle, and the action potentials (APs) are amplified and played through a loudspeaker. A normal muscle gives slight static when the electrode is gently moved about in the muscle, damaging and depolarizing a few fibers that fire only briefly. In stark contrast, the myotonic fiber with identical treatment produces long runs of repetitive APs that sound musical and are often compared with the sound of a diving propeller-driven airplane (the dive-bomber effect). The sound of the myotonic EMG is a very useful diagnostic sign. The mechanism involved here is that moving the electrode within the muscle mechanically injures individual muscle fibers, causing a steady depolarization at the site of the injury. Normal fibers are stimulated initially to fire only a few APs and then become quiescent. The persistent depolarization causes the Na^+ channels in the depolarized region to inactivate, which prevents further APs. In contrast, the myotonic fibers have a lower threshold, so they can fire with depolarizations too small to seriously inactivate the Na^+ channels. In addition, the potassium currents at the falling phase of each AP resets the membrane potential below threshold, allowing the continued depolarization to produce long trains of repetitive APs.

B. Biophysics of Myotonia

There are many models for generating the normal oscillations or repetitive activity seen in biological systems. In myotonia, however, the repetitive responses are abnormal, but the underlying processes are the same. Among the simplest ideas is the so-called integrate-and-fire model (Glass and Mackey, 1988). In this model (Fig. 3a), a quantity called *activity* starting from a lower threshold increases with time until it reaches an upper firing threshold, at which time an event occurs. The event then causes the activity to relax back to the lower threshold, from which the process can be indefinitely repeated. Providing the functions causing the upward and downward relaxations of activity are fixed, and further if the two thresholds remain constant, a repetitive sequence of events will be generated, from which the frequency can be easily determined. Since the frequency is determined by the speed of the relaxations, in this case, the term *relaxation oscillator* is often applied to such a system. To complete the analogy to the myotonic fiber, *activity* corresponds to the varying membrane potential, and *lower threshold* to the fixed potential from which the membrane potential begins depolarizing after being reset to this value by a preceding AP. The *firing threshold* corresponds to that fixed membrane potential where the AP is triggered. The AP process is not shown in this simplified scheme. The rapid relaxation to lower threshold in a real myotonic fiber is due to the transient turn on of g_K, which brings the membrane potential below firing threshold to the lower threshold and begins the next cycle. The more intense the depolarizing current, the more rapidly the depolarization (activity) reaches the firing threshold; hence, firing frequency increases. The cause of the depolarizing current when no external source is applied can be accounted for by the presence of a small "window" Na^+ current (see Bryant, 1982a) which is effective only when g_{Cl} is low or when Na^+ inactivation is prolonged. Either or both of the latter conditions are seen in different myotonias.

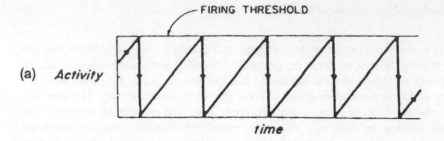

(a) *Activity*

FIRING THRESHOLD

time

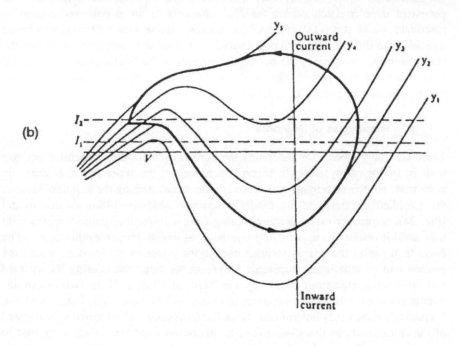

(b)

y_5
Outward current
y_4
y_3
y_2
y_1

I_2
I_1
V

Inward current

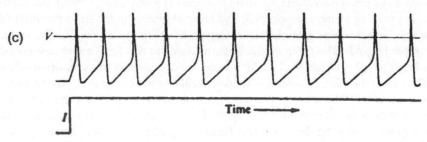

(c) V

Time ⟶

I

Figure 3 Repetitive firing mechanisms. (a) The integrate-and-fire model. (b) The forms of the voltage–current relation frozen at different times in a cell capable of repetitive firing, see text. (c) Membrane potential (V) as a function of time in response to the superthreshold depolarizing current pulse (I_2). The repetitive action potential spikes correspond to the voltage current trajectory (thick line) shown in (b). (a, from Glass and Mackey, 1988; b and c, from Jack et al., 1985.)

Mathematical models have been constructed to simulate myotonia caused either by abnormal Cl^- channels or by abnormal Na^+ channels. A description of the nonlinearity of the membrane is required, and the Hodgkin–Huxley (1952) equations are sufficient for this task. Several workers have modeled repetitive firing in excitable cells using simple modifications of these equations. One important finding from the simulations is the necessity of the T-tubule membrane system for attaining a myotonic afterdischarge comparable with a real fiber. This is true for both Na^+ (Cannon et al., 1993) and low-Cl^- types of myotonia (Adrian and Marshall, 1976). The firing frequency of APs in myotonia increases with depolarization over a limited range, thus resembling a classic relaxation oscillator. One striking difference between simple electrical models of repetitive-firing and real myotonic fiber behavior is that the firing of the myotonic fiber is self-limited and stops after a short time. Simple models without a T-system load fail to turn off (i.e., once started, they fire forever). More complicated models based on the actual physiology of fibers (e.g., including potassium accumulation and diffusion in the T system with each AP) will turn off and duplicate many of the real fiber characteristics.

Figure 3b shows the forms of the voltage–current relation of the skeletal muscle membranes as they would be seen frozen at different times in a cell capable of repetitive firing (see Jack et al., 1983). The curve y_1 is the resting condition. Curves y_2–y_5 progressively represent the voltage–current curves being altered in time by sodium inactivation and potassium activation during depolarization. I_1 is a subthreshold current that only depolarizes the cell, I_2 is a superthreshold depolarizing current that causes V to cycle through the curves y_2–y_5 following the trajectory shown in the thick line in the direction indicated by the arrowheads. The trajectory (also known as a phase portrait, or phase–plane trajectory) is an important analysis tool in the field of nonlinear dynamics. In this particular case the phase plane contains information concerning the stability of the fiber and its tendency to fire repetitively. Figure 3c shows the membrane potential (V) as a function of time showing the repetitive action potential spikes produced in response to the super-threshold depolarizing current pulse (I_2). These potentials correspond to the voltage–current phase–plane trajectory (thick line) shown in 3b. The mechanisms involved in myotonia obviously implicate membrane ionic channels, but it appears that there are differences in membrane mechanisms for the repetitive firing, as well as in the molecular genetics for the myotonic conditions described in the following.

III. Chloride Channel Diseases

A. Which Is the Major Chloride Channel?

The problem of low Cl^- conductance myotonia brings up the question of which is the normal Cl^- channel that is responsible for the stabilizing conductance of mammalian skeletal muscle fibers, and the absence of which produces myotonia. The identity of this channel, called CLC-1 (see Fig. 4) has only recently been clarified in spite of the fact that skeletal muscle g_{Cl} has been studied in such detail for so many years. There are still confusing data relative to its cellular location (surface or T-tubular membrane?), and its small unit conductance (ca. 1 pS) will make a detailed kinetic analysis of single data very difficult.

Many years ago it was thought that g_{Cl} of skeletal muscle was due to an identical "chloride channel" in all vertebrate species. Thus, frog muscle fibers, which are large (up to 130 μm in diameter or greater) and easy to study with microelectrodes, were used to study Cl⁻ conductance. Eventually, it was appreciated that frog and mammalian Cl⁻ channels must be quite different in several properties: (1) denervation blocks mammalian g_{Cl}, but does not affect g_{Cl} in the frog; (2) aromatic carboxylic acids, such as anthracene-9-carboxylic acid (9-AC) block g_{Cl} in mammalian fibers and induce myotonia, but are without either effect in the frog; (3) mammalian channels may reside mainly in the T-tubules, whereas frog channels may largely be on the surface; (4) the kinetics and the voltage dependence of g_{Cl} are different in these species; (5) phorbol esters block mammalian g_{Cl}, but not that of frog (Tricarico et al., 1993), and (6) no Cl⁻ channel has yet been identified that is the same in the frog and mammal. The channels responsible for the main resting conductance in frogs have not yet been identified, but it is clear that they are different from CLC-1.

The discovery of CLC-1 is interesting. Jentsch and his colleagues, after cloning and expressing the principal Cl⁻ channel (called CLC-0) of the *Torpedo* electroplax, turned their attention to the mammalian skeletal muscle. With the knowledge that the electroplax and skeletal muscle are embryologically related, they made polypeptides from short sequences of the *Torpedo* channel and probed a rat skeletal muscle cDNA library. By injecting derived cRNA into xenopus oocytes, they expressed a Cl⁻ current that was blocked by low concentrations of 9-AC and had voltage dependence and kinetic properties similar to what is expected for the main mammalian Cl⁻ channel (Steinmeyer et al., 1991b). They further found that RNA for this protein was almost entirely in adult skeletal muscle (a small amount in brain and kidney) and was not present in immature skeletal muscle. This rat channel was called CLC-1; but they were unable to make single-channel records because, as we now know, the conductance was too low. Meanwhile, Jockusch and colleagues, using a ligand that blocks g_{Cl} and induces myotonia when injected internally, isolated a Cl⁻ channel from the surface membranes (but *not* the T-tubules) of mouse fibers (Weber-Schürholz et al., 1993). Furthermore, they recorded 40-pS single-channel activity by patch-clamping fused ("giant") liposomes containing the channels. There were other confusing results during this period, for which we may now have an explanation. First, careful patch-clamping studies of surface membranes of freshly dissociated rat and mouse fibers by at least two laboratories, report that only 0–2% (of 200–350) clean patches contained Cl⁻ channels (Chua and Betz, 1991; R. Wagner, D. Tricarico, D. Conte-Camerino, and S. H. Bryant, unpublished observations). Possibly all of the Cl⁻ channels are in the T-tubular membrane, as suggested earlier by Dulhunty (1979). Indeed, 40-pS Cl⁻ channels have been reported from T-tubular membrane incorporated into planar bilayers (Hidaka et al., 1993). Future studies with immunological probes to CLC-1 may resolve this problem of the location of the channels. The mystery of the absence of single-channel records from rat rCLC-1 expressed in xenopus oocytes, in mammalian cell lines, or from the surface of mammalian fibers (assuming some surface density) appears to be resolved by the new finding that human hCLC-1 and rat rCLC-1 channels may have open conductances of only 1 pS (range 0.4–1.2 pS). This estimate comes from a most recent study of Jentsch and collaborators in which they examined currents from human and rat CLC-1 that was expressed in the human cell line, HEK-293 (Pusch et al., 1993). Since these single-channel currents were too small to detect within the noise present in the conventional patch clamp, a nonstationary state analysis method using the parabolic mean–variance relation of the macroscopic channel current was employed (for an explanation of this method, see Heineman and Conti, 1992). The method is restricted by some simplifying assumptions and can yield only estimates of the single-channel current (hence, its conductance), the total number of channels in the cell, and the open probability. The channel is voltage-sensitive, with a 50% activation at −100 mV and a gating valence of about one electronic charge. When saturated at positive potentials the currents still show a fluctuation between open and closed states. These new results imply that the many previously reported skeletal muscle chloride channels ranging from 10 to 300 pS are not CLC-1, and possibly not even related to the majority of g_{Cl}.

B. Myotonic Goat

Pursuant to the brief foregoing account, more details are given here. This hereditary myotonia has been known for over a century and has been studied as an animal model of myotonia for over 50 years. The condition is due to an autosomal dominant mutation (Bryant, 1979). The tendency of goats to move quickly when disturbed (*startle reaction*) can lead to a sudden attack of muscular stiffness, causing the animal to lose balance and fall on its side, the goat is unable to get up for several seconds. The goat then gets up a little stiff, but with repeated movements over the next few seconds, the phenomenon of warm-up appears. The lay public refer to these animals as "falling" or "fainting" goats. The gene has been bred into all varieties of goats, and special interest groups have maintained the defect out of curiosity and for the novelty. Physiological studies of the myotonia in these goats helped develop our modern concepts of this phenomenon. When human fibers were more difficult to study, this animal model was very useful, in that it allowed investigators in the 1960s and 1970s to demonstrate that a lack of Cl⁻ permeability of the fibers could account for the repetitive firing of myotonia (Adrian and Bryant, 1974; Rüdel and Lehmann-Horn, 1985). The actual studies were performed on small biopsies of external intercostal muscle. It is presumed that dysfunctional or absent Cl⁻ channels are involved in this disease, but the precise gene defect in the goat has not yet been determined. Identical experiments were performed on human muscle biopsies during this early period, and many, but not all, of the human myotonic fibers had low Cl^- permeability and Cl^- conductance. It became clear eventually that there was more than one type of human myotonia. In some patients, the mechanism of the low Cl^- conductance, similar to that found in the goat, appeared to operate. In many myotonic patients, Cl^- conductance was not greatly affected, in spite of severe myotonia, and we are led to conclude that other mechanisms, most likely involving abnormal Na^+ channels, are the cause.

C. Arrested Development of Righting (Myotonic) Mouse

A mouse that had difficulties in righting when placed on its back was discovered at the Jackson Laboratories (Mehrke et al., 1988). This condition was due to a recessive mutation, and at first was thought to be a neurological condition affecting the righting mechanism and thus received the name of arrested development of righting response or ADR mouse. Later, it became clear that the major problem was myotonia of the skeletal muscles, and thus the term myotonic mouse is also used. The repetitive firing and other defects in excitability were shown to be due to a specific lack of membrane Cl^- conductance, as with the myotonic goat and some myotonic patients. This, in turn, means that Cl^- channels were either not functioning or were absent. Unlike the dominant mutation of the goat, where the heterozygous animals also showed reduced Cl^- conductance, in the mouse, the heterozygous animals had nearly normal Cl^- conductance and behaved normally. This indicates that the normal allele in the heterozygous mouse is capable of coding for and expressing a normal density of Cl^- channels. Jentsch and his colleagues (Steinmeier et al., 1991a,b) have shown that the normal Cl^- channel of mammalian skeletal muscle is the second in their family of Cl^- channels (CLC-0 through CLC-2) called CLC-1, shown diagrammatically in Figure 4. This channel is coded by a single gene, which they argue is the same one affected in the myotonic mouse mutation. Indeed, they showed that the mutation was caused by a transposon (i.e., a nonsense code) inserted into this gene at a region that would otherwise code for an essential part of the channel protein. Actually, the defect is so severe that no mRNA for this channel was detected in the myotonic mouse.

D. Thomsen's Disease (Myotonia Congenita)

An autosomal dominant condition, myotonia congenita, was first recognized in the family of Dr. Thomsen, a Danish physician living in Germany in the 1870s. The condition resembles myotonia in the goat, but when studies were done on muscle biopsies of living descendants of Dr. Thomsen, the investigators did not see the profound lack of Cl^- conductance in these individuals, as reported in the myotonic goat or in patients having RGM. The mechanism of the myotonia in MC may involve a fraction of abnormal Na^+ channels that inactivate too slowly

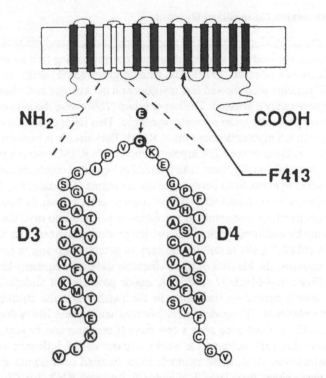

Figure 4 (Top) Model of the CLC-1 mammalian skeletal muscle chloride channel showing 12 membrane-spanning segments and the intracellular COOH-terminus. (Bottom) The domains D3 and D4 are shown enlarged and indicate the location where the glycine (G) is replaced by glutamic acid (E) in myotonia congenita (MC) (or Thomsen's disease); shown also is the position of the conserved phenylalanine, F413, at the end of domain D8 where substitution of cysteine produces recessive generalized myotonia (RGM). (Modified from George et al., 1993.)

(Iaizzo et al., 1991). Sodium ion currents of this type were also noticed in myotonic goat fibers (Bryant and Decoursey, 1980), but their presence was not necessary to account for the myotonia, since computer models showed that the lack of Cl⁻ conductance alone was sufficient (Adrian and Marshall, 1976). Interestingly, it has been reported that the gene coding for CLC-1 (see Fig. 4) is defective in myotonia congenita. It was also suggested that pleotropic action is at work (i.e., the Cl⁻ channel gene influences the expression or function of other proteins including Na^+ channels), thus accounting for the myotonic excitability. It is now clear that dominant MC is distinct from recessive RGM, but both diseases may be result from separate defects in the CLC-1 gene. As shown in Figure 4 (Koch et al., 1992), the defect producing MC is a single-point mutation in which glycine (G) is replaced by glutamic acid (E).

E. Recessive Generalized Myotonia

Professor R. Becker of Germany studied a large population of nondystrophic myotonic patients, and distinguised two separate diseases, corresponding to their dominant or recessive inheritance (Becker, 1973). The smaller group (30%) were the autosomal dominant MC patients who showed less myotonia on the average and whose physiology we have previously discussed. The larger group (70%) were the autosomal recessives, who were generally more severely myotonic. This latter condition was termed recessive generalized myotonia congenita or RGM. This disease in humans somewhat resembles the condition of the ADR myotonic mouse. In RGM there is a reduced Cl^- conductance, but additionally, there is an altered Na^+ channel conductance, and these two ionic channel abnormalities account for the myotonia (Franke et al., 1991).

Investigators have frequently studied muscle cells grown in tissue culture. One popular preparation, consisting of myoblast cells fused into myotubes and then caused to clump by addition of colchicine (which produces microtubular disruption), is called a "myoball." Cells in culture are easy to patch clamp and to record single Cl^- channel currents; the kinetics of these channels have consequently been studied extensively (Blatz and Magleby, 1985). A major problem not understood is why these Cl^- channels appear so frequently in the patch when the cultured cell has minuscule macroscopic Cl^- conductance. Mammalian muscle fibers denervated in vivo lose their Cl^- conductance after a few days (Camerino and Bryant, 1976), so it is predictable that cells cultured for weeks without neural influence would have little Cl^- conductance. Also, these channels from cultured cells do not appear to be the CLC-1 type, since they lack 9-AC sensitivity, and RNA for CLC-1 is not detectable in northern blots. The adult CLC-1 requires innervation of the adult cell for continuous expression, and cells in culture lack such nerve influence.

With the caveat that cultured muscle cells do not contain the adult-type major Cl^- channel, abnormalities have been reported in single Cl^- channel currents from myoballs cultured from biopsies of three RGM patients (Fahlke, et al., 1993). Four differnt types of Cl^- channels were studied, of which two types differed from control channels by having only half of the unitary single-channel conductance. One of these was the channel accounting for most of the conductance of the myoball. Only the unitary conductance was affected, the kinetics of these channels being normal. On the basis of these data, it would appear that a protein regulating more than one channel type may be at fault, rather than mutations of several ion channel genes.

As seen in Figure 4, the mutation producing RGM is a point mutation in which the highly conserved phenylananine (F) at position 413 is replaced by cysteine (C).

IV. Muscular Dystrophies

A. Myotonic Dystrophy (Myotonia Dystrophica)

Myotonic dystrophy (MD) is the most common form of inherited skeletal muscle disease in human adults and the most frequent form where myotonia is present

(Harper, 1989). The disease is clearly a distinct entity from other myotonias. The affected gene is on chromosome 19 and, with one rare exception, the mutation is an unstable trinucleotide, cytosine–thymine–guanine (CTG), repeat in the 3'-untranslated region. The gene product is believed to be a protein having serine–threonine protein kinase activity. The CTG repeat has a copy number varying from 50 to over 2000, and the disease severity increases with the degree of amplification of the repeat. This offers an explanation for the observation that the disease may increase in severity in succeeding generations (Harley et al., 1993). However, the systemic nature of the disease, with life-shortening conditions present in many other organs, makes the myotonia relatively less important to the patient. Also present may be severe muscle dystrophy with weakness. The myotonia is probably associated with presence of some Na^+ channels that have prolonged inactivation, since Cl^- conductance can be normal in these muscles. Only a small fraction of Na^+ channels need to be defective to produce profound effects on membrane excitability. The defective protein kinase would explain the widespread nature of the disease, affecting various physiological systems. Relative to the Na^+ channel dysfunction, this would be another example of pleotropic action by the defective gene, since it not believed that the Na^+ channel gene of skeletal muscle is defective in this disease.

B. Duchenne Muscular Dystrophy

There are several types of nonmyotonic muscular dystrophies, but the type to be discussed here is the human Duchenne muscular dystrophy (DMD). The gene associated with this sex-linked disease (Zubrzyka-Gaarn et al., 1988) is the largest that has been isolated to date (2.3 million base pairs). The disease afflicts 1 in 3500 boys and is the most severe of the dystrophies, causing muscular wasting and death by about age 20. In normal muscle, this gene codes for the product *dystrophin*, which is localized in the sarcolemma of the skeletal muscle cell, where it is a major constituent of the subsarcolemmal cytoskeleton. However, dystrophin is only 0.002% of the total skeletal muscle protein (Blau, 1993). The defective gene in the DMD patient produces a deficiency of dystrophin, with consequent loss of all dystrophin-associated proteins, which renders the DMD fibers susceptible to dysfunction and ultimately to necrosis (Ohlendieck et al., 1993). The Becker muscular dystrophy is also due to defective dystrophin expression, but the level of dystrophin is not as low; consequently, the symptoms are not as severe as with DMD. In general, in the various dystrophies, the muscle fibers progressively degenerate and become necrotic and are replaced by fatty tissue and connective tissue. A theoretical scheme (after Ohlendieck et al., 1993) for the overall mechanism of DMD is given in Table 1.

C. The *mdx* Mouse

Cloning of the DMD gene has had a great impact on the diagnosis of DMD, but treatment continues to be only palliative. There is great interest in developing

Table 1   Scheme of the Mechanism of Muscle Fiber Necrosis in DMD

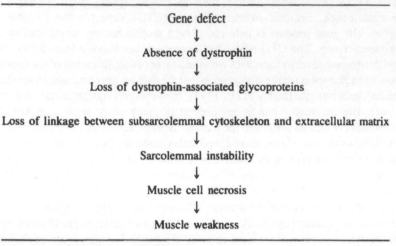

Gene defect

↓

Absence of dystrophin

↓

Loss of dystrophin-associated glycoproteins

↓

Loss of linkage between subsarcolemmal cytoskeleton and extracellular matrix

↓

Sarcolemmal instability

↓

Muscle cell necrosis

↓

Muscle weakness

Source: After Ohlendieck et al. (1993).

gene replacement therapy, and this appears to be a possibility in the near future. An important animal model is the *mdx* mouse, which has an aberrant gene leading to lack of dystrophin production. Although these animals do not show the degree of muscular weakness or impaired movement so obvious in human DMD, they do undergo a severe degeneration of the diaphragm muscle that closely resembles what occurs in human DMD. This is of particular interest because respiratory failure is the principal cause of death in these patients. In a recent study (Cox et al., 1993), a transgenic *mdx* mouse expressing a recombinant gene for dystrophin was able to correct the dystrophic signs in the diaphragm. The level of expression of dystrophin was 50 times normal in the transgenic *mdx* mouse, but this produced no toxic effects.

D.   The *dy* Mouse

For completeness one should mention the autosomal recessive mutant *dy/dy* mouse, which served as a model for Duchenne dystrophy for two decades. Although the pathophysiology seen in the *dy* mouse model is now believed to be different from that of human Duchenne dystrophy, many of the clinical signs in these animals, such as weakness, wasting of muscle tissue, and a multitude of biochemical and morphological alterations, were strikingly similar. For a review of the *dy* dystrophic mouse one should consult Mendell et al. (1979).

V. Periodic Paralyses and Sodium Ion Channel Diseases

A. General Comments

There are various inherited diseases in which periodic bouts of paralysis occur. Some of these conditions are associated with either hyper- or hypokalemia, and myotonia may also be present. For a general review of the periodic paralyses see, Ruff and Gordon, 1986. Recent studies have brought considerable light to understanding many of these conditions, with the discovery that several genetic forms of myotonia and periodic paralysis may be due to failure of a small fraction of the skeletal muscle voltage-gated Na^+ channels to inactivate normally (Rüdel and Lehmann-Horn, 1985). There are multiple subtypes of Na^+ channels in skeletal muscle, based on sensitivity to toxins and to antibodies, and these subtypes may be located preferentially in the T-tubules or surface membrane. Two Na^+ channels, specific to skeletal muscle, known as SkM1 (Trimmer et al., 1989; George et al., 1992) and SkM2 (Kallen et al., 1990), have been cloned and sequenced. Skeletal muscle. Na^+ channels are heterodimers having a 260 kDa α-subunit and a 38 kDa β-subunit (Kraner et al., 1985). Type SkM1 is expressed in both innervated and denervated adult muscle and is blocked by nanomolar concentrations of tetrodotoxin (TTX) and μ-conotoxin. Type SkM2 is TTX-insensitive and is not found in innervated adult mammalian muscle, but appears within hours following denervation, reaching a maximum at 48 h and then decreasing. The type SkM2 is expressed in early development and disappears as type SkM1 increases and becomes the only adult form. Type SkM2 is also seen in vitro in skeletal muscle culture (absence of nerve control) where it is about 30% of the functioning channels, its sequence is essentially the same as the normal TTX-insensitive Na^+ channel of heart (Rogart, et al., 1989). In the following we will discuss first the hypokalemic periodic paralysis, which may have a metabolic basis. We will then combine our discussion of the hyperkalemic periodic paralysis with the related myotonia syndromes. We do this because these latter two conditions appear to be due to different mutations of the *SCN4A* gene (on chromosome 17q) that codes for the SkM1-type Na^+ channel.

B. Hypokalemic Periodic Paralysis

Hypokalemic periodic paralysis (HOPP) is the common form of this group of diseases, and is characterized by a greatly lowered serum K^+ concentration (e.g., to 1.7 mM) during attacks. As the name implies, there are periodic episodes of extreme muscle weakness and flaccid paralysis (e.g., in the limbs). There is hyporeflexia and areflexia as well, and respiration is sometimes difficult. Myotonia may develop transiently as the weakness develops (Resnick and Engel, 1967). The heart is also affected during HOPP attacks, the ECG reflecting the hypokalemic state. There is ST-segment depression, T-wave flattening, and appearance of U waves. Diverse stimuli can trigger attacks, including stress, exercise, cold, insulin, and high-carbohydrate meals (presumably mediated by insulin release). A combination of insulin and glucose is well known to lower serum potassium concentrations by stimulating K^+ uptake into the skeletal muscles. The disease is inherited as an autosomal dominant trait, but strikes males more often, the onset usually occurring in the teens and early 20's. The oral or intravenous administration of K^+ relieves an attack usually within one or a few hours. Acetazolamide, a carbonic anhydrase inhibitor, also is effective in therapy of HOPP, presumably owing to the metabolic acidosis it produces (by promoting the loss of bicarbonate through the kidneys). It is not known how acidosis terminates an attack (bicarbonate infusion antagonizes the acetazolamide, whereas, NH_4Cl potentiates it). This might be related to the fact that acidosis inhibits the (Na^+, K^+)-ATPase and Na–K pump (e.g., Sperelakis and Lee, 1971), and hence K^+ uptake into the muscles.

Single-fiber EMG studies, during an attack induced by insulin plus glucose infusion, showed a decrease in propagation velocity, a lengthening of the AP duration, and a failure of excitability in the muscle fibers (DeGrandis et al., 1978). Depolarization of the skeletal muscle fibers was reported both in vivo (Creutzfeld et al., 1963) and in vitro (Hofmann and Smith, 1970). A reduced amplitude of the miniature end-plate potentials (MEPPs) was also observed (Hofmann and Smith, 1970), but this might be explained, at least partially, by the depolarization [since the amplitude of postsynaptic potentials (PSP) is a function of the difference between the resting potential and the equilibrium potential for the PSP]. Electrical stimulation of the paralyzed muscles is ineffective. Since sensation and nerve conduction appears to be normal, this suggests that the abnormality is limited to the muscles.

As discussed in the section on resting potential in Chapter 2, a low $[K]_o$ (e.g., to 1.0 mM) should hyperpolarize normal skeletal muscle fibers, but a further decrease to 0.3 or 0.1 mM sharply depolarizes. This depolarization is presumably due to two factors: (1) inhibition of the Na–K pump (since the K_m for external K^+ is about 2 mM) and, hence, the reduction or entire removal of the electrogenic pump contribution to the resting potential; (2) a lowered K^+ conductance (g_K) of the membrane, since conductance for an ion is a function of its concentrations outside and inside the cell; in addition, there some evidence that a low $[K]_o$ reduces P_K (Carmeliet et al., 1976), and hence g_K (since g_K is a function of P_K). This second factor would act to increase the g_{Na}/g_K ratio and thereby depolarize, as discussed in the previous chapter. Therefore, normal skeletal muscle should not depolarize at a $[K]_o$ level of 1.5 mM, as seen during attacks on HOPP patients, but should actually hyperpolarize. But if in the HOPP patient there was an alteration in membrane properties such that prominent depolarization occurred at 1.5 mM $[K]_o$, then the symptoms could be explained; for example, if the K_m (Michaelis-Menten constant) for $[K]_o$ the Na–K pump was substantially higher than normal; or if a lowered $[K]_o$ had a more prominent effect on P_K, thereby raising the P_{Na}/P_K ratio. That is, a relatively small shift in the dependence of the Na–K pump or of P_K on $[K]_o$ could produce a large depolarization. Depolarization, in turn, would slow the rate of rise of the APs, slow propagation velocity, and lead to loss of excitability in the muscle fibers, as discussed in Chapter 2. Even though intracellular K^+ ($[K]_i$) should increase somewhat during an attack because of the increased K^+ uptake into the muscles, and although his would tend to hyperpolarize (since E_K is increased for two reasons: a decrease in $[K]_o$ and an increase in $[K]_i$), this effect is outweighed by the changes in the pump and g_K discussed earlier.

It was shown by Eckel and Sperelakis (1963) that, in rats fed a K^+-deficient diet for 2 weeks, the intracellular K^+ concentration in the skeletal muscle fell (fibers gained Na^+, H^+, and basic amino acids) considerably (to 66% of control muscles), but that because of the concomitant decrease in serum K^+ level (to 49% of the control animals), E_K was actually larger (more negative by several millivolts). However, the fibers in the K-deficient muscles were considerably depolarized (to about -55 mV), indicating that there was a decrease in g_K and probably in electrogenic pump activity. More recently, Bond and Gordon (1993) showed that insulin depolarized K^+-depleted fibers in the presence of low $[K^+]$ solutions. This depolarization was blocked by TTX if added before the insulin, but if added after insulin, there was only a partial block of the depolarization. This is interpreted to mean that noninactivating SkM1 channels contribute to the depolarization; however, insulin must alter some other non–TTX-sensitive conductance. In voltage-clamp measurements it appeared that insulin blocked a K^+ conductance, which could account for the resistant depolarization. The presence of altered Na^+ channel inactivation may not be caused by mutant genes in HOPP, but rather, to the dependence of wild-type SkM1 channel kinetics upon $[K^+]$. It will be seen in the HYPP studies (see Sec. V.C) that this dependence of Na^+ channel inactivation on $[K^+]$ is exaggerated in the mutant SkM1 channels. The preceding and other studies support the validity of the K^+-depleted rat as a realistic model for HOPP.

C. Hyperkalemic Periodic Paralysis and Paramyotonia

Hyperkalemic periodic paralysis (HYPP) and paramyotonia (PC) are related because they are due to autosomal dominant mutations of the type SkM1 Na^+ channel, located in the surface and T-tubule membranes of mammalian skeletal muscle fibers. These channels are normally responsible for conducting the skeletal muscle AP throughout the tubular membranes, which is necessary for excitation–contraction coupling. The genetic studies to date have associated HYPP with defects in the α-subunit of the adult SkM1-type Na^+ channel, which is located on chromosome 17q (locus *SCN4A*) (Fontaine et al., 1990). Figure 5a shows the location of frequent PC and HYPP mutations of the a subunit of the Na^+ channel. In Figure 5b the lack of effect on activation and the profound effect on inactivation is clearly seen in mutant constructs having point mutations in these regions (location numbers differ slightly between 5a and 5b owing to species differences). Note in the single channel records, the longer openings and repeated reopenings of the mutant constructs through inactivation of Na^+ channels.

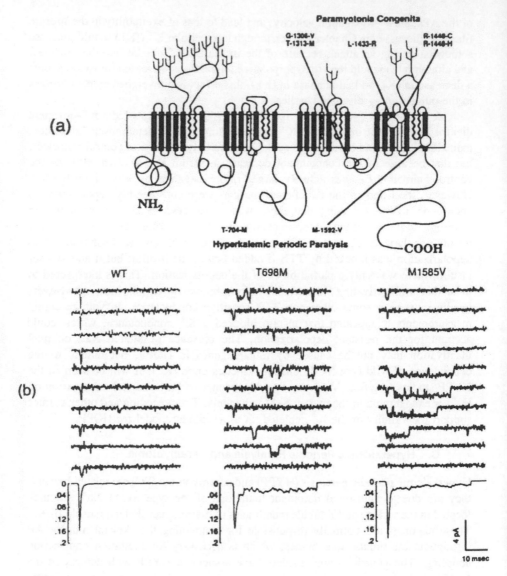

Figure 5 The mutations of the type SkM1 Na$^+$ channel of skeletal muscle cause PC or HYPP, depending on their location (a) Model of the type SkM1 Na$^+$ channel with the COOH-terminus intracellular. Five point mutations producing PC are indicated on the top, and two point mutations producing HYPP are on the bottom. (b) Single-channel records with ensemble averages are shown for the wild type (WT) and two point mutant constructs (*T698M* and *M1585V*) after expressing the cRNA in HEK293t cells. Slight differences in numbered positions occur between top and bottom figures owing to species source. Note the repetitive openings in the mutants that give rise to the noninactivating Na$^+$ current similar to the condition seen in HYPP. [From (a) Ptacek et al., 1991, 1993; (b) Cannon and Strittmatter, 1993.]

Hyperkalemic Periodic Paralysis

Hyperkalemic periodic paralysis (HYPP), like paramyotonia, is also an autosomal dominant mutation in which one sees recurrent episodes of weakness, with small elevations in the serum potassium concentration. In this particular form of the disease, first described by Gamstorp (1956) who called the condition, *adynamia episodica hereditaria*, there is marked depolarization of skeletal muscle fibers during an attack that makes the fiber inexcitable and leads to a flaccid paralysis of the muscle (Creutzfeld et al., 1963). Under voltage-clamp conditions, diseased biopsied fibers produce a noninactivating Na^+ current that can be blocked by TTX and, furthermore, this has been shown to be the mechanism for the depolarization (Lehmann-Horn et al., 1987). In turn, single-channel recordings have shown that the Na^+ channels giving rise to the depolarizing current lack normal inactivation. These channels have prolonged open times and tend to open repetitively (Cannon et al., 1991). This is shown in Figure 5b. The wild SkM1-type channels very rarely show this noninactivating behavior, as do the mutant channels when exposed to low extracellular potassium. However, in high potassium concentrations (around 10 mM compared with a normal of 4–5 mM), a small fraction (5–10%) of the mutant channels do not inactivate, and this produces a constant open probability of between 0.02 and 0.05, yielding a steady depolarizing current large enough to account for the depolarization block (Cannon et al., 1993). As mentioned when discussing the mechanisms of myotonia, delayed inactivation of Na^+ channels can lead to myotonia, and myotonia has been observed in HYPP patients.

An abnormal noninactivating, TTX-sensitive, inward current appeared in muscle fibers of biopsies taken from patients with hyperkalemic periodic paralysis (HYPP) (Lehmann-Horn et al., 1987; Ricker et al., 1989) and paramyotonia congenita (PC) (Lehmann-Horn et al., 1981). These abnormal Na^+ channels (type SkM1 mutants) also displayed sensitivity of the inactivation process to the presence of potassium. The presence of 10 mM extracellular K^+, caused the Na^+ channels from HYPP muscles to enter a noninactivating mode of gating in 5–10% of trials, as evidenced by prolonged open times and persistent reopenings (Cannon et al., 1991). *SCN4A*, located on chromosome 17q, is the genetic locus of the α-subunit of the adult isoform of skeletal muscle Na^+ channels (Fontaine et al., 1990; Ptacek et al., 1991). Both HYPP and PC show autosomal dominant inheritance with tight genetic linkage, with no recombinations to *SCN4A*. Many point mutations have been identified in this locus from families with HYPP (Ptacek et al., 1991) and PC (McClatchey et al., 1992). The HYPP mutations can be made in Na^+ channel cDNA from rat skeletal muscle, and the channels fail to inactivate completely when expressed (Cannon and Strittmatter, 1993). Decreased Na^+ channel inactivation is also found in patch-clamp studies in muscle from patients with MD (Franke et al., 1990), RGM (Franke et al., 1991), and the Schwartz–Jampel syndrome (SJS) (Lehmann-Horn, et al., 1990). As yet, linkages or mutations implicating the *SCN4A* locus have not been demonstrated for MD, RGM, and SJS.

A condition closely resembling HYPP of humans has also been described in mutant quarter horses (Pickar, et al., 1991). These authors suggest that increase in P_{Na}, rather than altered pump activity, is the cause, since in vitro diseased fibers hyperpolarize in response to TTX, whereas normal fibers do not. The disease in the horse is most likely due to mutations in the TTX-sensitive Na^+ channel comparable with those that have been reported for the human HYPP.

There have been two approaches to demonstrate that lack of Na^+ channel inactivation is the possible cause of some forms of myotonia and periodic paralysis. In the first approach, an in vitro model was created in rat muscle exposed to a polypeptide toxin (ATX II) obtained from a sea anemone. The toxin at 10 μM produced a noninactivating open probability at -10 mV of approximately 0.02, similar to what was reported in myotubes from HYPP patients, and myotonia was apparent (Cannon and Corey, 1993). In the second approach, a computer simulation was developed, based on modifications of the Hodgkin–Huxley equations adapted to skeletal muscle fibers. This approach is similar to that discussed for computer simulation of low-g_{Cl} myotonia. The simulated fiber, like the low-chloride model, required a T-tubule compartment to act as a diffusion-limited space in which activity-induced K^+ can accumulate. The computed APs for increasing degrees of incomplete inactivation of Na^+ channels, effectively simulated normal, myotonic, and paralytic muscle. The simulated APs with altered Na^+ inactivation compared favorably with the abnormal APs produced pharmacologically with ATX II (Cannon et al., 1993).

Paramyotonia Congenita

Paramyotonia congenita (PC), an autosomal dominant condition, has also been referred to as paradoxical myotonia because the signs of myotonia increase with use of the skeletal muscles, rather than diminish, and there is an increase in myotonia and a dramatic increase in the response of a muscle to percussion with local cooling. At least in vitro, low-Cl^- conductance myotonias are quite different, since the signs are diminished with cooling below 27°C (Furman and Barchi, 1978). If one replaces the sensitivity to cooling with the worsening of symptoms with elevated serum potassium levels, there is a physiological resemblance between PC and HYPP. Both of these conditions have myotonia with episodic weakness, and the similarities appear to be explained by the findings that both diseases are due to different mutations, but on the same skeletal muscle Na^+ channel gene (Ptacek et al., 1993). Figure 5a diagrams the relation of some of the common mutations that have been identified. The most highly conserved region of the various Na^+ channels, which, as a family, show remarkable homology, are the S4 segments of each domain. This region is commonly believed to function in Na^+ gating and inactivation. These segments contain positively charged arginines and glycines at every third position, with principally neutral amino acids interdigitated between. Figure 5b shows single-channel recordings from cells expressing constructed mutants similar to those shown in Figure 5a. Note the lack of inactivation, as evidenced by repeated openings and longer open times, compared with the wild type (WT). The ensemble averages shown immediately below the single-channel records of the constructs in Figure 5b display the prolonged sodium currents capable of causing depolarization and myotonia.

VI. Malignant Hyperthermia

Malignant hyperthermia (MH) is a rare autosomal dominant condition in humans that predisposes these persons to react to anesthesia with muscle rigidity, hyper-metabolism, and high fever, in which the muscles become highly stimulated metabolically, with a consequent rise in body temperature (MacLennon and Phillips, 1992). A popular form of anesthesia, involving use of halothane in conjunction with a depolarizing neuromuscular blocker, succinylcholine, can trigger MH. If not treated immediately, these patients may die within a few minutes from ventricular fibrillation or within hours to days from neurological or renal complications. Malignant hyperthermia is rare in humans, but is serious enough to be fatal in apparently healthy individuals undergoing anesthesia. In MH, the physiological and biochemical changes that occur are similar to those that occur in normal individuals following severe exercise. There is an increased O_2 consumption and CO_2, production, a high plasma lactate level because of the increased glycolytic rate of the muscles, and respiratory acidosis and metabolic acidosis. The blood glucose and glycerol levels are elevated, but there is a fall in free fatty acids. The blood electrolyte concentrations are also altered, and hyperkalemia occurs. There is an increase in muscle tone, first in the legs and then the arms, sometimes with extreme extensor rigidity. The muscles of the chest wall are also affected, decreasing compliance and making pulmonary ventilation difficult. There is a generalized increase in muscle stiffness, but without convulsions or spasmodic contractions. In some cases, the limbs do not become rigid. Body temperature can rise at the rate of about 0.2°C/min, the major source of heat being the contracted skeletal muscles; thus, the temperature rise is secondary to the elevated muscle metabolism. Cardiac muscle is also involved, and may account for the observed heart failure. Cardiac dysrhythmias also develop during the course of MH. A rise in blood pressure usually occurs, and there is intense peripheral vasoconstriction, which also contributes to the hyperthermia by reducing heat loss. There is reduced blood flow to the rigid (contracted) muscles, which hampers nourishment of the muscles. Near death, cardiac arrest occurs and blood pressure falls, and there is severe hemoconcentration.

Malignant hyperthermia is also be seen in animals, where it is often triggered by heat stress. Pigs susceptible to MH have been recognized for many years (Lucke et al., 1979), and genetic and physiological studies of the MH pigs have hastened our understanding of the comparable condition in human patients. In susceptible pigs given the "halothane test" (4–8% halothane in O_2 for 5 min), the reactor pigs become distressed, have an increased heart rate and respiratory rate, and twitching of the legs occurs (often followed by leg stiffness). Once the MH syndrome is well established, the animals go on to die, even though the halothane administration is stopped. Suxamethonium (succinylcholine) a depolarizing neuromuscular blocking agent, induces violent muscle fasciculations in susceptible pigs that can be stopped by d-tubocurarine.

In both humans and pigs, abnormalities in the peripheral innervation of the skeletal muscles have been reported. In addition, the muscles of susceptible animals exhibit some supercontracted and degenerating and regenerating myofibrils. The main symptoms of MH, such as increased muscle tone, heat production, and glycogenolysis, suggest that $[Ca]_i$ is elevated. There is some evidence that, in susceptible animals, there is an enhanced Ca^{2+} loss from muscle mitochondria in response to hypoxia. The acidosis probably inhibits the Ca-ATPase and may impair the ability of the SR to sequester Ca^{2+}. Acidosis also inhibits (Na^+, K^+)-ATPase and, hence, Na–K pumping (e.g., see Sperelakis and Lee, 1971). The blockade of the myocardial slow (Ca–Na) channels by acidosis (e.g., see Sperelakis, 1981) may contribute to the heart failure during MH.

Some of the features of MH are similar to those of increased activity of sympathetic nervous system and high levels of circulating catecholamines. Pretreatment of animals with phentolamine (an α-adrenergic receptor blocker) prevents the MH response to suxamethonium, even though muscle stimulation is not blocked; propranolol (a β-adrenergic blocker) is not effective here. In addition, infusion of norepinephrine produces a mild hyperthermia, whereas infusion of both norepinephrine and propranolol produces a fatal hyperthermic response. Infusion of phenylephrine (a more selective α-adrenergic agonist) into anesthetized pigs produces a severe hyperthermia. Thus, there is an important relation between α-adrenergic receptor stimulation and heat production. Catecholamine depletion by reserpinization protects susceptible pigs against suxamethonium-induced MH. Adrenalectomy and blockers of postganglionic adrenergic neurons both provide protection against halothane-induced MH. However, it has been suggested that the observed rise in circulating catecholamines in MH could be secondary to the changes in muscle metabolism. On the other hand, the sensitivity to stress suggests that catecholamines may also play a more primary role in MH. The mechanisms by which norepinephrine and epinephrine might stimulate muscle in MH is unknown, although elevation of cyclic-AMP has been found.

The mechanism of MH is the presence of a mutated Ca^{2+} release channel located in the sarcoplasmic reticulum (SR) of skeletal muscle. The specific mutations that account for the dysfunction of this channel are different in humans and pigs. The Ca^{2+} release channel is a key element of the process known as excitation–contraction coupling or simply E–C coupling. This is the chain of events beginning with the muscle AP which invades the T-tubular membrane, causing movement of gating charge in the dihydropyridine (DHP)-sensitive Ca^{2+} channel–voltage sensor, which in turn, activates the Ca^{2+} release channel on the SR to release Ca^{2+} from stores from within the SR to initiate contraction. The exact means by which the voltage sensor of the T-tubular membrane couples with the release channel of SR is not yet fully understood (Rios and Pizarro, 1991). In addition, there are pumps and regulators that accumulate and store the Ca^{2+} for release. These events and a scheme to explain the pathophysiology of a MH attack are depicted in Figures 6 and 7. Shown in Figure 6 is the junctional terminal cisternae of the SR containing the Ca^{2+}-release channels (portrayed as square pyramids) butting up against the T membrane, which contains the tetradic DHP receptors. Within the lumen of the junctional cisternae of the SR are shown calsequestrin, calreticulin, the structural protein HRP, and the two most common glycoproteins, gp53 and gp160. Within the membrane of the junctional SR are shown triadin, phospholamban, and Ca^{2+}-ATPase (or Ca^{2+} pump).

In MH, as first mentioned, there is a paradoxical stimulatory response of the skeletal muscles to certain general anesthetics and to stress; with a consequent rise in body temperature, there is pronounced metabolic stimulation, with high serum lactate, levels acidosis, and hyperkalemia. There is an increase in muscle tone and stiffness, and $[Ca]_i$ is abnormally elevated. Figure 7 suggests the underlying mechanism involved in MH. In the swine model and, in most of the human cases, MH is due to mutations in the gene expressing the sarcoplasmic reticulum calcium release channel, also known as the ryanodine receptor. The mutations then produce a release channel that is more sensitive to opening stimuli and fails to close rapidly, thereby leading to the abnormally high calcium levels that, in turn, lead to the other signs of a MH attack.

The Ca^{2+}-release channel is specifically opened at nanomolar concentrations and blocked at micromolar concentrations by the toxin, ryanodine. Thus, this channel is often referred to as the ryanodine receptor. With use of this high-affinity ligand, the protein was purified and several full-length cDNAs from different species were subsequently cloned. The channel is coded by two different genes: *RYR1* on chromosome 19 codes for the skeletal muscle channel, and *RYR2* on chromosome 1 codes for heart and brain channel. These major isoforms of the ryanodine receptor are the only known cellular-binding sites for the ligand. The protein is a large homotetrameric complex constructed from 565-kDa subunits. The channel region is probably located in the membrane-spanning segments, which are 20% of the subunit from the carboxy-terminus. The remainder of each subunit is cytoplasmic, and the four subunits together form a cytoplasmic structure holding the four extended channels that empty into lateral vestibules. This cytoplasmic region also must contain the sites for coupling to the DHP receptor. Ryanodine-sensitive release channels have been studied in planar bilayer experiments during which they exhibit open conductances greater than 100 pS in 50 mM Ca^{2+}. Ryanodine tends to bind to the channel when it is open. In studies in isolated vesicles, Ca^{2+} and ATP can open the channel, and Mg^{2+} and calmodulin can inhibit the channel. However, the actual physiological control signal is not yet established.

All of the signs of MH, as seen in Figure 7, can be explained by a defect

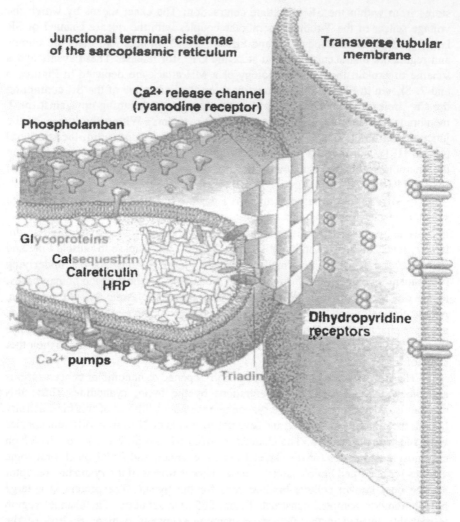

Figure 6 Cartoon showing the arrangement of important proteins in the T-tubule (TT) and sarcoplasmic reticulum (SR) of skeletal muscle as currently conceived. See text for details. (From MacLennan and Phillips, 1992.)

in the regulation of intracellular Ca^{2+}. Sustained Ca^{2+} levels in the fiber would cause contracture; increased glycolytic and anaerobic metabolism, with depletion of ATP, glucose, and oxygen; and overproduction of CO_2, lactic acid, and heat. Other ionic concentrations would also become abnormal. After eliminating possible genetic defects in Ca^{2+} pump protein and other regulators, workers turned their attention to the release channel as having the major abnormality in MH. Some

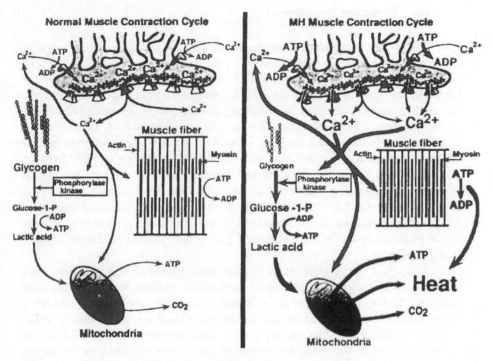

Figure 7 Scheme showing the mechanism of malignant hyperthermia based on abnormality of the Ca^{2+} release channel of the sarcoplasmic reticulum of skeletal muscle. Explanation is discussed in the text. (From MacLennan and Phillips, 1992.)

abnormal cDNA sequences for the Ca-release channel have been described. In pigs the cDNA sequences for *RYR1* between normal and MH pigs predict a single amino acid difference, a cysteine for an arginine. In human studies two mutations of *RYR1* are associated with MH, but some MH patients have no linkage with this gene and, furthermore, mutations of this gene may cause unrelated forms of muscle disease. Human MH may, therefore, involve other gene mutations and interactions.

A specific antagonist for the MH reaction is dantrolene sodium, which is capable of blocking release of intracellular calcium from the SR. The mechanism is not completely established. There is evidence that dantrolene sodium is active at the coupling steps between the T-tubules and the SR, there is also evidence that there is direct block of calcium release from the ryanodine-release channel. Dantrolene is relatively insoluble so a special high-concentration release form is available clinically for use in operating rooms for acute treatment of MH. [For specific references in support of the statements made in this section, the reader is referred to the references cited in the article by MacLennon and Phillips (1992).]

VII. Muscular Dysgenesis

Mice that are homozygous for the autosomal recessive dysgenic gene mutation (*mdg/mdg*) lack excitation–contraction (E–C) coupling and the slow calcium current. These animals, therefore, are incapable of muscular movement and survival. The fetuses do not move in utero and die at birth, presumably from respiratory paralysis. Cultured myotubes that carry the mdg/mdg phenotype can also be produced for experimentation. The physiological problem is related to lack of function of the DHP receptor. In the mutant dysgenic animals there is a fivefold decrease in DHP binding in skeletal muscle, there is a low level of mRNA encoding the DHP receptor, and monoclonal antibodies detect no DPH receptors. On the other hand, cardiac DHP binding in normal, illustrating the fact that the L-type calcium channels (or DHP receptors) are distinctly different in these two tissues. Muscular dysgenesis appears to have been the first documented example of a genetic disease in vertebrates that is produced by a defect in a structural gene coding for an ion channel (Tanabe et al., 1988).

Although a human counterpart has not been reported for this mutation, basic studies with the dysgenic mouse model have helped confirm the role of the DHP receptor as both a voltage sensor and a channel in the T-tubular membrane. A critical experiment was done by Tanabe and co-workers (Tanabe et al., 1988) in which both E–C coupling and slow calcium current were restored in the dysgenic muscle by microinjection of the expression plasmid (pCAC6) carrying cDNA for the missing DHP receptor. The restoration of both voltage sensing and ion channel functions with the single cDNA confirmed the dual role of this protein in the T-tubule. It should be noted, however, that the slow calcium current in skeletal muscle can be blocked without interfering with E–C coupling (Walsh et al., 1986, 1987, 1988), so the function of this current is not understood.

Further experiments (Tanabe et al., 1990) have shown that cardiac L-type channel cDNA expressed in dysgenic skeletal muscle functioned only as an ion channel and do not support E–C coupling. Physiologically this makes sense, since only the calcium currents, hence, ion channel function, are important in the heart. In contrast, the skeletal muscle requires only the voltage sensor function of its DHP receptor to trigger release of calcium from the SR.

VIII. Fatigue

There is considerable interest, particularly clinical, in the mechanisms of muscle fatigue. At first one must distinguish muscle weakness from muscle fatigue. *Muscle weakness* is the inability of an otherwise fresh muscle to generate force, whereas *fatigue* is a phenomenon, caused by the previous activity of the muscle, that results in deterioration of performance (see Bryant et al., 1986). In a fatigued muscle, both force and speed decrease, resulting in a lower-power output. Two basic mechanisms of fatigue will be considered; the *high-frequency* type, in response to continuous high-frequency stimulation; and the *intermittent tetanic* type, from repeated bouts of tetanic stimulation.

In general, fatigue can occur at a number of points in the neuromuscular system. These are illustrated in Figure 8, which depicts the major paths (i–ix) leading to muscle activation and relaxation (Westerblad et al., 1991). Starting with the central voluntary command (i), which is conducted by central conducting axons and synapses, an α-metoneuron is excited, and impulses travel down the motor axon (ii) to the neuromuscular junction (iii), where acetylcholine is released from the nerve terminal to activate the nicotinic receptors on the postjunctional membrane, causing depolarization of the end plate. This depolarization, in turn, activates voltage-dependent Na^+ and K^+ channels, located in the surface membrane (iv) and T-tubular membrane (v), to propagate APs in both directions away from the end plate and to invade the T-tubules (v). The AP in the T-tubule can cause a significant increase in K^+ concentration within the T-tubule lumen because of their relatively small volume. This decreases the K^+ concentration ratio (hence, E_K) across the T-tubular membrane, with a resultant depolarization. As discussed for the myotonia models, this depolarization can accumulate if the AP frequency is more rapid than the time constant of disappearance of this late afterpotential, and this depolarization is important for sustaining repetitive myotonic behavior. This phenomenon can also play a role in promoting fatigue of the high-frequency type because the steady depolarization can increase Na^+ channel inactivation, which decreases Na^+ activation currents which, in turn, decreases AP amplitude and slows conduction velocity.

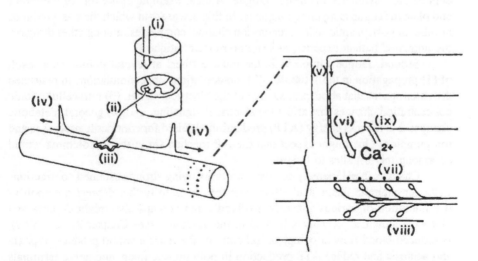

Figure 8 Scheme showing paths leading to muscle activation and relaxation. Explanation given in text. (From Westerblad et al., 1991.)

The tubular AP activates the DHP-sensitive voltage sensors of the T-tubular membrane that are coupled to, and cause Ca^{2+} to be released from, the Ca^{2+}-release channels of the SR (vi) into the myoplasm and on to the troponin C-binding sites (vii). The latter binding by removing tropomyosin from the actin filaments initiates cross-bridge cycling (viii) and force development. After Ca^{2+} release ceases, the continually active ATP-dependent pump (ix) allows reuptake of Ca^{2+} by the SR, lowering Ca^{2+} in the myoplasm, which stops cross-bridge recycling, unloads the troponin C, and allows relaxation. The contraction–relaxation process is also depicted in Figure 7.

Fatigue can occur at the synapses, both in the spinal cord (such as synapses on the anterior horn cells, i.e., motoneurons) and at the neuromuscular junction. Several lines of evidence suggest that the central nervous system, including the motoneurons are not a significant source of fatigue (Merton, 1954). However, in vitro studies can illustrate that the neuromuscular junction can be a site of fatigue by a simple experiment in an isolated nerve–muscle preparation (e.g., frog sciatic nerve–gastrocnemius muscle preparation). If the nerve is stimulated until the muscle shows signs of substantial fatigue, then direct stimulation of the muscle demonstrates that most of the fatigue resided at the neuromuscular junction, because the muscle is able to develop almost its original force of contraction. Therefore, in any whole-animal type study, this factor must be taken into account. Fatigue can also occur at the neuromuscular junction if the readily releasable pool of synaptic transmitter becomes depleted; for example, if the rate of transmitter release is greater than the rate of synthesis for a relatively long period. In addition, since synthesis of acetylcholine (ACh) requires ATP, depression of metabolism by any means will depress ACh synthesis and hasten fatigue. A clear example of the role of the motor end plate in fatigue is myasthenia gravis. In this disease—in which there is a reduced number of postsynaptic ACh receptor–ion channel complexes, among other things— the untreated patient experiences extreme muscle fatigue.

Second, fatigue can occur in the muscle fibers at several points, as a result of (1) propagation in the T-tubules, (2) ion depletions or accumulations in restricted diffusion spaces that affect propagation of the electrical signal, (3) intracellular ionic concentration changes that affect the electrical signaling, and (4) general metabolic changes that depress energy (ATP) production required for contractile processes and ion pumping. One might expect that the AP mechanism in the sarcolemma would be among the last sites to fatigue.

Changes in pH, namely acidosis, accompanying strong sustained contractions with, for example, lactic acid efflux, can feed back to further depress metabolism (by inhibition of various enzymes involved), and perhaps also might depress and block the slow Ca^{2+} channels located in the T-tubules (see Chapter 2, Sec. VIII). A reduced blood flow or complete ischemia of the muscle would produce hypoxia and acidosis and reduce ATP production in both muscle fibers and nerve terminals and, thereby, accelerate fatigue.

Fatigue would occur in the muscle fibers when metabolism is depressed by any means, thereby reducing the ATP available for contraction (e.g., Ca-ATPase activity of the myosin), for ion pumping (e.g., resequestration of Ca^{2+} into the SR), and eventually for other important cell functions, such as protein synthesis. As mentioned in the section of propagation of the AP into the sarcotubular system in Chapter 2, fatigue can occur owing to Na^+ depletion in the T-tubules, with resultant failure of the Na-dependent APs (Bezanilla et al., 1972).

If the ion concentration inside the fiber or outside the fiber (either at fiber surface or in T-tubules) is altered by rapid firing of APs, such that ion-pumping cannot keep up, then this could affect the APs, which would, in turn, affect the developed force of contraction. For example, if $[K]_o$ just outside of the surface membrane were to increase substantially, this $[K^+]_o$ increase would partially depolarize the fibers and, thereby, slow down the velocity of propagation (see Chapter 2, Sec. V). Slowed activation of the fibers might reduce the force of contraction because of the resultant series elasticity and other possible factors.

It has been proposed by Bianchi and Narayan (1982) that some Ca^{2+} from the terminal cisternae of the SR (TC-SR) enters the T-tubules during muscle activation, and could cause muscle fatigue by raising the threshold for coupling of the AP to contraction. The exact mechanism for the latter effect is unclear, but it may be related to charge immobilization of the DHP-sensitive voltage sensors of the T-tubular membrane (Rios et al., 1992). The T-tubules also play a major role in removing the Ca^{2+} that is released from the TC-SR during excitation–contraction (E–C) coupling. Consistent with this view, Howell and Snowdowne (1981) showed that, in single frog skeletal muscle fibers, an elevated $[Ca]_o$, between 5 and 20 mM, rapidly depressed force of contraction to about 60% of the control value (in 1 mM$[Ca]_o$); since they also found that propagation velocity was slowed in high $[Ca]_o$ (to about 50% of the control value at 20 mM$[Ca]_o$), and since AP amplitude and duration were unaffected, they suggested that the depression of contraction resulted from a failure of AP propagation within the T-tubules.

IX. Denervation

Denervation of skeletal muscle produces some interesting changes in the electrical properties of the cell membrane. The changes occur within 2–3 days in mammal (e.g., rat), but more slowly in amphibians (e.g., 2–3 weeks). Thesleff and his colleagues (Redfern et al., 1970; Redfern and Thesleff, 1971) have shown that, in the rat, the fast Na^+ channels are partly replaced by newly synthesized, fast Na^+ channels that are insensitive to TTX, but retain sensitivity to saxitoxin (STX), a poison that is structurally related to TTX, but has two guanidinium groups instead of one. Thus, TTX reduces the maximal rate of rise of the AP (max dV/dt), but does not block excitability. In addition, the max dV/dt is reduced to about 65% of the control (innervated) value, in the absence of TTX.

We can now explain these effects by the development of the SkM2 sodium channel, which is normally inhibited from expression by activity and trophic influences from the nerve. When this new low TTX-affinity denervation channel is studied in planar bilayers, it shows pharmacological sensitivity and electrical properties similar to the normal heart channel (Guo et al., 1987). This "denervation" Na^+ channel is also seen in cultured muscle cells in the absence of nerve influence. Both the heart and denervation channels have been cloned and sequenced, and these two channels differ only slightly, as might be expected (Rogart et al., 1989; Kallen et al., 1990).

Denervation also depolarizes the fibers partially (e.g., to –60 mV). The mechanism of this depolarization is an increase in the P_{Na}/P_K ratio due to a decreased P_K, resulting from the denervation. The cause for the decrease in P_K with denervation is unknown. The low P_K and low resting potential facilitate automaticity of the fibers, and so spontaneous APs are often produced.

In addition to the P_K decrease, P_{Cl} is also decreased in rat muscle (but apparently not in frog muscle). This also acts to raise membrane resistivity (R_m) and to enhance automaticity and spontaneous firing of APs, because, as discussed in Sec. II, the Cl^- distribution (E_{Cl}) and conductance act to "clamp" the membrane potential and to depress excitability. Therefore, a decrease in P_{Cl} should enhance automaticity and excitability; however, this is not true in the denervated mammalian fiber. Possibly the changes in the sodium channels produce lessened excitability and account for this paradox.

It has also been known for a long time that marked changes occur in the ACh: newly synthesized ACh receptors appear in the extrajunctional regions of the fiber (the so-called spreading of ACh receptors, which really is misleading). (The experiments are done by examining the binding of labeled α-bungarotoxin, which binds specifically and tightly to ACh receptors, and by using microelectrode and iontophoresis studies.) The sensitivity to ACh in the extrajunctional regions becomes nearly as great as in the junctional region (original end plate) (e.g., about one-tenth as high), and this can account for some of the supersensitivity to ACh. In cultured skeletal muscle studies, following fusion of the myoblasts end to end to form myotubules, there is sensitivity to ACh along the entire myotube. However, when innervation of the myotubes is allowed to occur in vitro, the ACh receptors are lost in the extrajunctional regions; thus, this process is the reverse of that which occurs after denervation of differentiated muscle. Denervation is also known to stimulate cell proliferation ([3H]thymidine incorporation) in mouse skeletal muscle by 48 h (McGeachie and Allbrook, 1978), and to cause overdevelopment of the sarcotubular system (Pellegrino and Franzini, 1963).

X. Hyperpolarization by Insulin and Isoproterenol

Insulin slowly hyerpolarizes rat and frog skeletal muscle by 4–7 mV over a period of 10–30 min (Zierler, 1959; Moore and Rabovsky, 1979; Flatman and Clausen,

1979). There are four main possibilities by which insulin can hyperpolarize skeletal muscle membrane: (1) an increase in the ratio of K^+ to Na^+ permeability, (i.e., P_{Na}/P_K) (2) a stimulation of Na^+-H_+ exchange, which increases $[Na]_i$; (3) a stimulation of the (Na^+, K^+)-ATPase; and (4) an increased number of (Na^+, K^+)-ATPase sites on the membrane (Li and Sperelakis, 1993a,b).

Since the insulin (100 mg/ml)-induced hyperpolarization is not prevented by ouabain (10^{-5} M), an inhibitor of the (Na^+, K^+)-ATPase (Zierler and Rogus, 1981b), Zierler and Rogus concluded that this insulin effect in rat muscle is not due to stimulation of the electrogenic pump. In contrast, other investigators have proposed that insulin does stimulate the electrogenic pump. For example, Gavryck et al. (1975) reported that insulin (400 mU/ml) stimulates (mean increases of 25%) the (Na^+, K^+)-ATPase activity in a membrane fraction isolated from frog skeletal muscle. Insulin stimulation of the electrogenic pump (hyperpolarizing pump potential, V_p) was proposed for rat soleus muscle (Flatman and Clausen, 1979) and frog sartorius muscle (Moore and Rabovsky, 1979). Zierler (1972) and Zierler and Rogus (1981a) proposed that the hyperpolarization in rat muscle was by decreasing the P_{Na}/P_K ratio, due to a decrease in P_{Na}. In contrast, Moore and Rabovsky (1979) have suggested that the insulin-induced hyperpolarization in frog muscle is due to a reduced $[K]_o$ in a restricted diffusion space, such as the T-tubules, resulting from stimulation of an electrically neutral, Na–K exchange pump.

The recent studies of Li and Sperelakis (1993a,b) support the fourth of the possibilities initially proposed [i.e., there is an increase in the number of (Na^+, K^+)-ATPase or "pump" sites brought about by insulin], and this produces hyperpolarization. The increase in number of sites is proposed to be due to translocation of sites from intracellular storage sites, possibly by stimulation of increased expression of the protein. These data are based on measurements of pump currents (I_p) in skeletal muscle myoballs using the whole-cell, patch-clamp method, and on ouabain-binding studies (Incerpi and Luly, 1989) on muscle, with and without insulin.

β-Adrenergic agonists, such as isoproterenol, also hyperpolarize rat skeletal muscle fibers (Clausen and Flatman, 1977; Flatman and Clausen, 1979; Li and Sperelakis, 1993a). The magnitude of the hyperpolarization produced by 10^{-6} M isoproterenol in rat caudofemoralis muscle within 15 min averaged -8.3 ± 2.2 mV, and this effect was blocked by ouabain (10^{-5} M). Therefore, it was concluded that activation of the β-adrenergic receptor stimulates the electrogenic Na^+ pump and hyperpolarizes. As further evidence, it was shown that isoproterenol also stimulates the Na–K exchange in skeletal muscle (Flatman and Clausen, 1979; Rogus et al., 1977).

In contrast, in frog semitendinosus muscle, Gonzalez-Serratos et al. (1981) reported that epinephrine (10^{-5}–10^{-6} M) did not significantly increase the resting potential (or AP amplitude). However, there was an increase in twitch tension and in maximal rate of force development; this inotropic effect began at 3 min and reached maximum at 8 min. Since, in split fibers, the force developed by caffeine

(25 mM) was considerably greater when cyclic AMP (1×10^{-4} M) was added to the previous loading solution, it was concluded that β-adrenergic agonists, through cyclic AMP elevation, stimulate the Ca^{2+} pump in the SR so that extra Ca^{2+} can be released during subsequent activation.

XI. Summary and Conclusions

This chapter described some selected conditions and diseases affecting skeletal muscle and the effects of two hormones that hyperpolarize skeletal muscle membrane. It was seen that many of the diseases afflicting skeletal muscle are genetically determined and involve mutations of genes coding for Cl^-, Na^+, or Ca^{2+} channels; thus, the new methods of cloning of diseased genes was summarized. Because defective ion channel function is often the basis of skeletal muscle pathology, a knowledge of the electrophysiological discussions in Chapter 2 becomes very useful in understanding the recent developments in this field.

Myotonia is the unstable repetitive excitability that can arise in skeletal muscle membrane when either the normal stabilizing Cl^- channel leak conductance is decreased, or Na^+ channel inactivation is prolonged. Either of these conditions, or the two together, can be present in naturally occurring or drug-induced myotonia. The biophysical basis of myotonia was discussed in terms of the classic relaxation oscillator (i.e., the integrate-and-fire model). Modern dynamic analysis methods utilizing the phase-plane trajectory are becoming useful in understanding membrane instability.

The Cl^- channel diseases of skeletal muscle are all associated with myotonia and occur in both humans and animals. The myotonic goat and the ADR (myotonic) mouse have a greatly reduced g_{Cl}, leading to the myotonia. The human counterpart is the generalized recessive myotonia (RGM), in which g_{Cl} is also reduced sufficiently to explain the myotonia. On the other hand, Thomsen's disease (myotonia congenita or MC) in humans appears to have myotonic excitability, more because of defective Na^+ channel function, in spite of the fact that the mutation occurs on the Cl^- channel gene. This is one of two examples of pleotropic action for which alterations in channels or other protein products occur in response to mutations in an unrelated gene. The other example is the myotonia seen in myotonic dystrophy (MD) in which Na^+ function is affected, but the gene defect codes for an abnormal kinase.

Two important muscular dystrophies were discussed, the autosomal dominant myotonic dystrophy (MD), which is the most common inherited neuromuscular disease (seen in adults), and the rarer, but clinically more severe, sex-linked Duchenne muscular dystrophy (DMD) seen largely in young boys. Myotonic dystrophy is due to mutation (a CTG repeat in the 3'-untranslated region) of the gene that codes for serine–threonine protein kinase. The severity of the disease varies with the repeat number, which correlates with the loss of kinase function.

This accounts for the increased severity in succeeding generations. Multiple organ systems are adversely affected in addition to skeletal muscle. The myotonia in this case is probably due to Na^+ channel dysfunction secondary to the metabolic abnormality. On the other hand, DMD is due to a defect in a very large gene coding for dystrophin, a protein that is necessary for normal cytoskeleton, hence membrane function. The lack of dystrophin leads to instability of the sarcolemma and necrosis and, ultimately, accounts for the muscle weakness and death. Becker's variation of DMD is not as severe because there is some dystrophin produced in this variant. There is no myotonia present in DMD. The *mdx* mouse model for DMD, although it lacks dystrophin, does not show the severe effects seen in humans. In the *mdx* mouse, only dystrophy of the diaphragm is observed. The classic *dy* "dystrophic mouse" is no longer believed to be a model for known human dystrophies.

In hypokalemic periodic paralysis (HOPP), in which there are periodic episodes of muscle weakness and flaccid paralysis, and which can be triggered by a number of stimuli including stress, exercise, cold, and insulin, the serum K^+ becomes abnormally low owing to enhanced uptake into the skeletal muscles. The skeletal muscle fibers become partially depolarized, and there is a decrease in propagation velocity and failure of excitability in some fibers. The reason for the depolarization is not exactly known, since the decrease in $[K]_o$ and increase in $[K]_i$, and resultant greater E_K, should hyperpolarize. Therefore, there must be some alteration in membrane properties, such as a longer inactivation of Na^+ channels owing to the high intracellular K^+. Hyperkalemic periodic paralysis (HYPP) and paramyotonia congenita (PC) are now believed to be due to different mutations on the *S4CNA* gene that codes for the TTX-sensitive Na^+ channel. Two classes of mutations are recognized. The first type causing PC codes for a Na^+ channel in which inactivation is abnormally prolonged in response to intracellular K^+. The second type causing HYPP codes for Na^+ channels in which inactivation is greatly prolonged by decreased temperature. In PC or HYPP it is important to realize that the fraction of Na^+ channels having the slow inactivation is small, usually less that 10%.

Malignant hyperthermia (MH) is a rare autosomal dominant condition that predisposes an individual to a dangerous release of Ca^{2+} from the sarcoplasmic reticulum in response to anesthesia, most commonly triggered by halothane with succinylcholine. The major signs are muscular rigidity, hypermetabolism, and high temperature. A defective calcium release channel expressed by mutations in the *RYR1* gene is the major cause.

Muscular dysgenesis is a genetic mutation in mice in which the main subunit of the dihydropyridine receptor–voltage sensor of the transverse tubular system is not functional, hence, depolarization of the T system by an action potential does not cause calcium release from the sarcoplasmic reticulum. The newborn mouse cannot survive since it lacks E–C coupling. Transfecting the muscle with normal subunit restores function in vitro. This animal model has given experimental support for accepted notions of E–C coupling.

Skeletal muscle fatigue can occur at the synapses in the spinal cord, at the neuromuscular junction, and in the muscle fiber proper. Fatigue to high-frequency stimulation in the muscle fiber can occur because of failure of excitation and propagation in the T-tubules, as, for example, by Na^+ ion depletion in the lumen of the T-tubule. Potassium ion accumulation in the T-tubule and at the outer surface sarcolemma can partially depolarize, and thereby, affect the characteristics of the APs and slow their propagation velocity. A slowed propagation can allow the series elasticity, owing to as yet uncontracted portions of the fibers, to become a significant factor. Intracellular changes in ion concentrations, such as a rise in free $[Ca]_i$, can affect some of the membrane electrical properties. For example, $[Ca]_i$ is known to activate (open) two types of voltage-independent ion channels: one for K^+ $[g_{K(Ca)}]$ and a nonspecific Na–K channel $[g_{Na, K(Ca)}]$; in addition, $[Ca]_i$ has effects on the slow Ca^{2+} channels (g_{si}). Metabolic depression during fatigue, owing to insufficient blood flow and nutrient–metabolite exchange, depresses ATP production required for contraction and for ion pumping. The depressed ion pumping would allow $[Ca]_i$, $[Na]_i$, and $[Cl]_i$ to rise, and $[K]_i$ to fall; the fibers would also gain H_2O and swell. The altered internal and external ion concentrations would affect the resting potentials and APs, including the driving forces for the ionic currents and the ionic conductances. The acidosis accompanying the fatigue could further depress metabolism, block the slow Ca^{2+} channels, depress g_{Cl}, and inhibit the (Na^+, K^+)-ATPase.

Denervation of rat skeletal muscle produces partial depolarization within 48 h, because of decreased P_K and P_{Cl}. Inhibition of the SkM2, TTX-resistant Na^+ channel is released, and these new channels are expressed for about a week, allowing action potentials in the presence of micromolar TTX. In about 2 weeks a pacemaker activity develops that generates repetitive action potentials, in spite of the fact that, at this time, the fiber excitability is actually reduced and myotonia is inhibited. In addition, denervation causes newly synthesized ACh receptors to appear in the extrajunctional regions of the fibers, allowing the fiber to respond to ACh anywhere along its length. The reverse process also occurs. For example, innervation of cultured skeletal myotubes in vitro causes the ACh to be lost in the extrajunctional regions. Denervation also causes overproliferation of the tubules and stimulates cell proliferation.

Insulin slowly hyperpolarizes skeletal muscle, in vivo or in virto, by 4–7 mV over a period of 10–30 min. There is evidence both for and against stimulating the Na–K pump. Other mechanisms include a decrease in P_{Na}, or a reduced $[K]_o$ in the T-tubules, resulting from stimulation of the Na–K pump. There is recent evidence for increased number of pump sites in response to insulin. β-Adrenergic agonists, such as isoproterenol, also hyperpolarize skeletal fibers by about 8 mV. Since ouabain blocks the effect, it is concluded that the hyperpolarization is due to stimulation of the Na–K pump. Epinephrine also increases the twitch tension and elevates cyclic AMP, and it is proposed that Ca^{2+} sequestration in the SR is enhanced, allowing extra Ca^{2+} release during subsequent activation.

References

Adrian, R. H., and Bryant, S. H. (1974). On the repetitive discharge in myotonic muscle fibres. *J. Physiol. (Lond.)* 240:505–515.

Adrian, R. H., and Marshall, M. W. (1976). Action potentials reconstructed in normal and myotonic muscle fibres. *J. Physiol. (Lond.)* 258: 125–143.

Ballabio, A. (1993). The rise and fall of positional cloning? *Nature Genet.* 3: 277–279.

Becker, P. E. (1973). Generalized non-dystrophic myotonia: The dominant (Thomsen) type and the recently identified recessive type. In *New Developments in Electromyography and Clinical Neurophysiology*, Vol. 1. Edited by J. E. Desmedt. Basel, S. Karger, pp. 407–412.

Bezanilla, F., Caputo, C., Gonzalez-Serratos, H., and Venosa, R. A. (1972). Na^+ dependence of the inward spread of activation in isolated twitch muscle fibres of the frog. *J. Physiol. (Lond.)* 223: 507–523.

Bianchi, C. P., and Narayan, S. (1982). Muscle fatigue and the role of transverse tubules. *Science* 215: 295–296.

Blatz, A. L., and Magleby, K. L. (1985). Single chloride-selective channels active at resting membrane potentials in cultured rat skeletal muscle. *Biophys. J.* 47: 119–123.

Blau, H. M. (1993). Muscular dystrophy: Muscling in on gene therapy. *Nature* 364: 673–675.

Bond, E. F., and Gordon, A. M. (1993). Insulin-induced membrane changes in K^+-depleted rat skeletal muscle. *Am. J. Physiol.* 265: C257–C265.

Bryant, S. H. (1979). Myotonia in the goat. *Ann. N. Y. Acad. Sci.* 317: 314–325.

Bryant, S. H. (1982a). Abnormal repetitive impulse production in myotonic muscles. In *Abnormal Nerves and Muscles as Impulse Generators*. Edited by W. Culp and H. Ochoa. New York, Oxford University Press, pp. 702–725.

Bryant, S. H. (1982b). Physical basis of myotonia. In *Disorders of the Motor Unit*. Edited by D. L. Schotland. New York, John Wiley & Sons, pp. 381–389.

Bryant, S. H., and Conte-Camerino, D. (1991). Chloride channel regulation in the skeletal muscle of normal and myotonic goats. *Pflugers Arch.* 417: 605–610.

Bryant, S. H., and DeCoursey, T. E. (1980). Sodium currents in cut skeletal muscle fibres from normal and myotonic goats. *J. Physiol. (Lond.)* 307: 31p–32p.

Bryant, S. H., Edwards, R. H. T., Faulkner, J. A. Hughes, R. L., and Roussos, C. (1986). Respiratory muscle failure: Fatigue or weakness? *Chest* 89: 118–124.

Caccia, M. R., Boiardi, A., Andreuss, I. L., and Cornelio, F. (1975). Nerve supply and experimental myotonia in rats. *J. Neurol. Sci.* 24: 145–150.

Camerino, D., and Bryant, S. H. (1976). Effects of denervation and colchicine treatment on the chloride conductance of rat skeletal muscle fibers. *J. Neurobiol.* 7: 221–228.

Cannon, S. C., and Corey, D. P. (1993). Loss of sodium channel inactivation by anemone toxin (ATX II) mimics the myotonic state in hyperkalemic periodic paralysis. *J. Physiol. (Lond.)* 466: 501–520.

Cannon, S. C., and Strittmatter, S. M. (1993). Functional expression of Na^+ channel mutations identified in families with periodic paralysis. *Neuron* 10: 317–326.

Cannon, S. C., Brown, R. H., and Corey, D. P. (1991). A sodium channel defect in hyperkalemic periodic paralysis: Potassium-induced failure of inactivation. *Neuron* 6: 619–626.

Cannon, S. C., Brown, R. H., Jr., and Corey, D. P. (1993). Theoretical reconstruction of myotonia and paralysis caused by incomplete inactivation of sodium channels. *Biophys. J.* 65: 270–288.

Carmeliet, E. E., Horres, C. C., Lieberman, M., and Vereecke, J. S. (1976). Developmental aspects of potassium flux and permeability of the embryonic chick heart. *J. Physiol. (Lond.)* 254: 673–692.

Chua, M., and Betz, W. J. (1991). Characterization of ion channels on the surface membrane of adult rat skeletal muscle. *Biophys. J.* 59: 1251–1260.

Clausen, T., and Flatman, J. A. (1977). The effect of catecholamines on Na–K transport and membrane potential in rat soleus muscle. *J. Physiol. (Lond.)* 270: 383–414.

Conte-Camerino, D., Mambrini, M., Deluca, A., Tricarico, D., Bryant, S. H., Tortorella, V., and Bettoni, G. (1988). Enantiomers, of clofibric acid analogs have opposite actions on rat skeletal muscle chloride channels. *Pflugers Arch.* 413: 105–107.

Cox, G. A., Cole, N. M., Matsumura, K., Phelps, S. F., Hauschka, S. D., Campbell, K. P., Faulkner, J. A., and Chamberlain, J. S. (1993). Overexpression of dystrophin in transgenic *mdx* mice eliminates dystrophic symptoms without toxicity. *Nature* 364: 725–729.

Creutzfeld, O. D., Abbott, B. C., Fowler, W. M., and Pearson, C. M. (1963). Muscle membrane potentials in episodic adynamia. *Electroenchephalogr. Clin. Neurophysiol.* 15: 508–519.

De Grandis, D., Fiaschi, A., Tomelleri, G., and Orrico, D. (1978). Hypokalemic periodic paralysis. *J. Neurol. Sci.* 37: 107–112.

Dulhunty, A. F. (1979). Distribution of potassium and chloride permeability over the surface and T-tubule membranes of mammalian skeletal muscle. *J. Membr. Biol.* 45: 293–310.

Eckel, R. E., and Sperelakis, N. (1963). Membrane potentials in K-deficient muscle. *Am. J. Physiol.* 205: 307–312.

Entrikin, R. K., and Bryant, S. H. (1979). Suppression of myotonia in dystrophic chicken muscle by phenytoin. *Am. J. Physiol.* 237: C131–C136.

Fahlke, C., Zachar, E., and Rüdel, R. (1993). Cl⁻ channels with reduced single-channel conductance in recessive myotonia congenita. *Neuron* 10: 225–232.

Flatman, J. A., and Clausen, T. (1979). Combined effects of adrenaline and insulin on active electrogenic Na–K transport in rat soleus muscle. *Nature* 281: 580–581.

Fontaine, B. (1993). Periodic paralysis, myotonia congenita and sarcolemmal ion channels: A success of the candidate gene approach. *Neuromusc. Disord.* 3: 101–107.

Fontaine, B., Khurana, T. S., Hoffman, E. P., Bruns, G. A. P., Haines, J. L., Trofatter, J. A., Hanson, M. P., Rich, J., McFarlane, H., Yasek, D. M., Romano, D., Gusella, J. F., and Brown, R. H. (1990). Hyperkalemic periodic paralysis and the adult muscle sodium channel alpha-subunit gene. *Science* 250: 1000–1002.

Franke, C., Hatt, H., Iazzo, P. A., and Lehmann-Horn, F. (1990). Characteristics of Na⁺ channels and Cl⁻ conductance in resealed muscle fibre segments from patients with myotonic dystrophy. *J. Physiol. (Lond.)* 425: 391–405.

Franke, C., Iazzo, P. A., Hatt, H., Spittlemeister, W., Ricker, K., and Lehmann-Horn, F. (1991). Altered Na channel activity and reduced Cl conductance cause hyperexcitability in recessive generalized myotonia (Becker). *Muscle Nerve* 14: 762–770.

Furman, R. E., and Barchi, R. L. (1978). The pathophysiology of myotonia produced by aromatic carboxylic acids. *Ann. Neurol.* 4: 357–365.

Gamstorp, I. (1956). Adynamia episodica hereditaria. *Acta Paediatr. Scand.* [Suppl.] 108: 1–126.

Gavryck, W. A., Moore, R. D., and Thompson, R. C. (1975). Effect of insulin upon membrane-bound (Na + K)-ATPase extracted from frog skeletal muscle. *J. Physiol. (Lond.)* 252: 43–58.

George, A. L., Komisarof, J., Kallen, R. G., and Barchi, R. L. (1992). Primary structure of the adult human skeletal muscle voltage-dependent Na⁺ channel. *Ann. Neurol.* 31: 131–137.

George, A. L., Crackower, M. A., Abdalla, J. A., Hudson, A. J., and Ebers, G. C. (1993). Molecular basis of Thomsen's disease (autosomal dominant myotonia congenita). *Nature Genet.* 3: 305–310.

Glass, L., and Mackey, M. C. (1988): *From Clocks to Chaos*. Princeton, NJ, Princeton University Press.

Gonzalez-Serratos, H., Hill, L. N., and Valle-Aguilera, R. (1981). Effects of catecholamines and cyclic AMP on excitation–contraction coupling in isolated skeletal muscle fibres of the frog. *J. Physiol. (Lond.)* 315: 267–282.

Guo, X., Uehara, A., Ravindran, A., Bryant, S. H., Hall, S., and Moczydlowski, E. (1987). Kinetic basis for insensitivity to tetrodotoxin and saxitoxin in sodium channels of canine heart and denervated rat skeletal muscle. *Biochemistry* 26: 7546–7556.

Harley, H. G., Rundle, S. A., MacMillan, J. C., Myring, J., Brook, J. D., Crow, S., Reardon, W., Fenton, I., Shaw, D. J., and Harper, P. S. (1993). Size of the unstable CTG repeat sequence in relation to phenotype and parental transmission in myotonic dystrophy. *Hum. Genet.* 52: 1164–1174.

Harper, P. S. (1989). *Myotonic Dystrophy*, 2nd ed. London, W. B. Saunders.

Heinemann, S. H., and Conti, F. (1992). Nonstationary noise analysis and application to patch clamp recordings. *Methods Enzymol.* 207: 131–148.

Hidaka, J., Ide, T., Kawasaki, T., Taguchi, T., and Kasai, M. (1993). Characterization of a Cl^- channel from rabbit transverse tubules in the planar lipid bilayer system. *Biochem. Biophys. Res. Commun.* 191: 977–982.

Hodgkin, A. L., and Huxley, A. F. (1952). A quantitative description of membrane current and its application to conduction and excitation in nerve. *J. Physiol. (Lond.)* 117: 500–544.

Hofmann, W. W., and Smith, R. A. (1970). Hypokalemic periodic paralysis studies in vitro. *Brain* 93: 455–474.

Howell, J. N., and Snowdowne, K. W. (1981). Inhibition of tetanus tension elevated extracellular Ca^{2+} concentration. *Am. J. Physiol.* 240: C193–C200.

Hutter, O. F., and Warner, A. E. (1967). The pH sensitivity of the Cl^- conductance of frog skeletal muscle. *J. Physiol. (Lond.)* 189: 403–425.

Iaizzo, P. A., Franke, C., Hatt, H., Spittelmeister, W., Ricker, K., Rüdel, R., and Lehmann-Horn, F. (1991). Altered sodium channel behavior causes myotonia in dominantly inherited myotonia congenita. *Neuromusc. Disord.* 1: 47–53.

Incerpi, S., and Luly, P. (1989). Insulin sensitivity of rat muscle sodium pump. *Membr. Biochem.* 8: 187–196.

Iyer, V. G., Ranish, N. A., and Fenichel, G. M. (1981). Ionic conductance and experimentally induced myotonia. *J. Neurol. Sci.* 49: 159–164.

Jack, J. J. B., Noble, D., and Tsien, R. W. (1983). *Electrical Current Flow in Excitable Cells*, 2nd ed. Oxford, Oxford University Press.

Kallen, R. G., Sheng, Z.-H., Yang, J., Chen, L., Rogart, R. B., and Barchi, R. L. (1990). Primary structure and expression of a sodium channel characteristic of denervated and immature rat skeletal muscle. *Neuron* 4: 233–242.

Koch, M. C., Steinmeyer, K., Lorenz, C., Ricker, K., Wolf, F., Otto, M., Zoll, B., Lehmann-Horn, F., Grzeschik, K.-H., and Jentsch, T. J. (1992). The skeletal muscle Cl^- channel in dominant and recessive human myotonia. *Science* 257: 797–800.

Kraner, S. D., Tanaka, J. C., and Barchi, R. L. (1985). Purification and functional reconstitution of the voltage-sensitive sodium channel from rabbit T-tubular membranes. *J. Biol. Chem.* 25: 6341–6347.

Kwiecinski, H. (1981). Myotonia induced by chemical agents. *Crit. Rev. Toxicol.* 8: 279–310.

Lehmann-Horn, F., Rüdel, R., Dengler, R., Lorkovic, H., Haass, A., and Ricker, K. (1981). Membrane defects in paramyotonia congenita with and without myotonia in a warm environment. *Muscle Nerve* 4: 396–406.

Lehmann-Horn, F., Kuther, G., Ricker, K., Grafe, P., Ballanyi, K., and Rüdel, R. (1987). Adynamia episodica hereditaria with myotonia: A non-inactivating sodium current and the effect of extracellular pH. *Muscle Nerve* 10: 363–374.

Lehmann-Horn, F., Iaizzo, P. A., Franke, C., Hatt, F., and Spaans, F. (1990). Schwartz–Jampel syndrome: Na^+ channel defect causes myotonia. *Muscle Nerve* 13: 528–535.

Li, K.-X., and Sperelakis, N. (1993a). Isoproterenol and insulin-induced hyperpolarization in rat skeletal muscle. *J. Cell. Physiol.* 157: 631–636.

Li, K.-X., and Sperelakis, N. (1993b). Electrogenic Na–K pump in rat skeletal myoball. *J. Cell. Physiol.* 159: 181–186.

Lucke, J. N., Hall, G. M., and Lister, D. (1979). Malignant hyperthermia in the pig and the role of stress. *Ann. N. Y. Acad. Sci.* 317: 326–337.

MacLennan, D. H., and Phillips, M. S. (1992). Malignant hyperthermia. *Science* 256: 789–794.

McClatchey, A. I., Van den Bergh, P., Pericak-Vance, M. A., Raskind, W., Verellen, C., McKenna-Yasek, D., Rao, K., Haines, J. L., Bird, T., Brown, R. H., and Gusella, J. F. (1992). Temperature-sensitive mutations in the III–IV cytoplasmic loop region of the skeletal muscle sodium channel gene in paramyotonia congenita. *Cell* 68: 769–774.

McGeachie, J., and Allbrook, D. (1978). Cell proliferation in skeletal muscle following denervation or tenotomy. A series of autoradiographic studies. *Cell Tissue Res.* 193: 259–267.

Mehrke, G., Brinkmeier, H., and Jockusch, H. (1988). The myotonic mouse mutant ADR: Electrophysiology of the muscle fiber. *Muscle Nerve* 11: 440–446.

Mendell, J. R., Higgins, R., Sahnek, Z., and Cosmos, E. (1979). Relevance of genetic animal models of dystrophy to human muscular dystrophies. *Ann. N. Y. Acad. Sci.* 317: 409–430.

Merton, P. A. (1954). Voluntary strength and fatigue. *J. Physiol. (Lond.)* 123: 553–564.

Moore, R. D., and Rabovsky, J. L. (1979). Mechanism of insulin action on resting membrane potential of frog skeletal muscle. *Am. J. Physiol.* 236: C249–C254.

Ohlendieck, K., Matsumura, K., Ionasescu, V. V., Towbin, J. A., Bosch, E. P., Weinstein, S. L., Sernett, S. W., and Campbell, K. P. (1993). Duchenne muscular dystrophy: Deficiency of dystrophin-associated proteins in the sarcolemma. *Neurology* 43: 795–800.

Palade, P. T., and Barchi, R. L. (1977). On the inhibition of muscle membrane chloride conductance by aromatic carboxylic acids. *J. Gen. Physiol.* 69: 879–896.

Pellegrino, C., and Franzini, C. (1963). An electron microscope study of denervation atrophy in red and white skeletal muscle fibers. *J. Cell Biol.* 17: 327–349.

Pickar, J. G., Spier, S. J., Snyder, J. R., and Carlsen, R. C. (1991). Altered ionic permeability in skeletal muscle from a horse with hyperkalemic periodic paralysis. *Am J. Physiol.* 260: C926–C933.

Ptacek, L. J., George, A. L., Griggs, R. C., Tawil, R., Kallen, R. G., Barchi, R. L., Robertson, M., and Leppert, M. F. (1991). Identification of a mutation in the gene causing hyperkalemic periodic paralysis. *Cell* 67: 1021–1027.

Ptacek, L. J., Gouw, L., Kwiecinski, H., McManis, P., Mendell, J. R., Barohn, R. J., George, A. L., Barchi, R. L., Robertson, M., and Leppert, M. F. (1993). Na^+ channel mutations in paramyotonia congenita and hyperkalemic periodic paralysis. *Ann. Neurol.* 33: 300–307.

Pusch, M., Steinmeyer, K., and Jentsch, T. J. (1993). Low single channel conductance of the major skeletal muscle chloride channel, ClC-1. *Biophys. J.* 66: 149–152.

Rasminsky, M. (1980). Ephaptic transmission between single nerve fibres in the spinal nerve roots of dystrophic mice. *J. Physiol. (Lond).* 305: 151–169.

Redfern, P., and Thesleff, S. (1971). AP generation in denervated rat skeletal muscle. II. The action of tetrodotoxin. *Acta Physiol Scand.* 82: 70–78.

Redfern, P., Lundth, H., and Thesleff, S. (1970). Tetrodotoxin resistant APs in denervated rat skeletal muscle. *Eur. J. Pharmacol.* 11: 263–265.

Resnick, J. S., and Engel, W. K. (1967). Myotonic lid lag in hypokalemic periodic paralysis. *J. Neurol. Neurosurg. Psychiatry* 30: 47–51.

Ricker, K., Camacho, L. M., Grafe, P., Lehmann-Horn, F., and Rüdel, R. (1989). Adynamia episodica hereditaria: What causes the weakness? *Muscle Nerve.* 12: 883–891.

Rios, E., and Pizarro, G. (1991). Voltage sensor of excitation–contraction coupling in skeletal muscle. *Physiol. Rev* 71: 849–908.

Rios, E., Pizarro, G., and Stefani, E. (1992). Charge movement and the nature of signal transduction in skeletal muscle excitation-contraction coupling. *Annu. Rev. Physiol.* 54: 109–133.

Rogart, R. B., Cribbs, L. L., Muglia, L. K., Kephart, D. D., and Kaiser, M. W. (1989). Molecular cloning of a putative tetrodotoxin-resistant rat heart Na^+ channel isoform. *Proc. Natl. Acad. Sci. USA* 86: 8170–8174.

Rogus, E. M., Cheng, L. C., and Zierler, K. (1977). β-Adrenergic effect on Na^+-K^+ transport in rat skeletal muscle. *Biochim. Biophys. Acta* 464: 347–355.

Rüdel, R., and Lehmann-Horn, F. (1985). Membrane changes in cells from myotonia patients. *Physiol. Rev.* 65: 310–356.

Ruff, R. L., and Gordon, A. M. (1986). Disorders of muscles. The periodic paralyses. In *The Physiology of Membrane Disorders*. Edited by T. E. Andreoli, J. F. Hoffmann, D. P. Fanestil, and S. G. Schultz. New York, Plenum Press, pp. 825–839.

Sperelakis, N. (1969). Changes in conductance of frog sartorius fibers produced by CO_2, ReO_4^- and temperature. *Am. J. Physiol.* 217: 1069–1075.

Sperelakis, N. (1979). Origin of the cardiac resting potential. In *Handbook of Physiology, The Cardiovascular System, Vol. 1: The Heart.* Edited by R. M. Berne and N. Sperelakis. Washington, DC, American Physiological Society, pp. 187–267.

Sperelakis, N. (1981). Effects of cardiotoxic agents on the electrical property of myocardial cells. In *Cardiac Toxicology*, Vol. 1. Edited by T. Balazs. Boca Raton, FL, CRC Press, pp. 39–108.

Sperelakis, N., and Lee, E. C. (1971). Characterization of (Na^+-K^+)-ATPase isolated from embryonic chick hearts and cultured chick heart cells. *Biochim. Biophys. Acta* 233: 562–579.

Steinmeyer, K., Klocke, R., Ortland, C., Gronemeier, M., Jockusch, H., Grunder, S., and Jentsch, T. (1991a). Inactivation of muscle chloride channel by transposon insertion in myotonic mice. *Nature* 354: 304–308.

Steinmeyer, K., Ortland, C., and Jentsch, T. (1991b). Primary structure and functional expression of a developmentally regulated skeletal muscle chloride channel. *Nature* 354:301–304.

Tanabe, T., Beam, K. G., Powell, J. A., and Numa, S. (1988). Restoration of excitation–contraction coupling and slow calcium current in dysgenic muscle by dihydropyridine receptor complementary DNA. *Nature* 336: 134–139.

Tanabe, T., Mikami, A., Numa, S., and Beam, K. G. (1990). Cardiac-type excitation–contraction coupling in dysgenic skeletal muscle injected with cardiac dihydropyridine receptor cDNA. *Nature* 344: 451–453.

Tricarico, D., Conte-Camerino, D., Govoni, S., and Bryant, S. H. (1991). Modulation of rat skeletal muscle chloride channels by activators and inhibitors of protein kinase C. *Pflugers Arch.* 418: 500–503.

Tricarico, D., Wagner, R., Bryant, S. H., and Conte, C. D. (1993). Regulation of resting ionic conductances in frog skeletal muscle. *Pflugers Arch.* 423: 189–192.

Trimmer, J. S., Cooperman, S. S., Tomiko, S. A., Zhou, J., Crean, S. M., Boyle, M. B. Kallen, R. G., Sheng, Z., Barchi, R. L., Sigworth, F. J., Goodman, R. H., Agnew, W. S., and Mandel, G. (1989). Primary structure and functional expression of a mammalian skeletal muscle sodium channel. *Neuron* 3: 33–49.

Walsh, K. B., Bryant, S. H., and Schwartz, A. (1984). Diltiazem potentiates mechanical activity in mammalian skeletal muscle. *Biochem. Biophys.* 122: 1091–1096.

Walsh, K. B., Bryant, S. H., and Schwartz, A. (1986). Effect of calcium antagonist drugs on calcium currents in mammalian skeletal muscle fibers. *J. Pharmacol. Exp. Ther.* 236: 403–407.

Walsh, K. B., Bryant, S. H., and Schwartz, A. (1987). Suppression of charge movement by calcium antagonists is not related to calcium channel block. *Pflugers Arch.* 409: 217–219.

Walsh, K. B., Bryant, S. H., and Schwartz, A. (1988). Action of diltiazem on excitation-contraction coupling in bullfrog skeletal muscle fibers. *J. Pharmacol. Exp. Ther.* 245: 531–536.

Weber-Schürholz, S., Wischmeyer, E., Laurien, M., Jockusch, H., Schürholz, T., Landry, D. W., and Al-Awqati, Q. (1993). Indanyloxyacetic acid-sensitive chloride channels from outer membranes of skeletal muscle. *J. Biol. Chem.* 268: 547–551.

Westerblad, H., Lee, J. A., Lannergren, J., and Allen, D. G. (1991). Cellular mechanisms of fatigue in skeletal muscle. *Am. J. Physiol.* 261: C195–C209.

Zierler, K. L. (1959). Effect of insulin on membrane potential and potassium content of rat muscle. *Am. J. Physiol.* 197: 515–523.

Zierler, K. L. (1972). Insulin, ions, and membrane potential. In *Handbook of Physiology*, *Endocrinology*, Vol. 1. Washington, DC, American Physiological Society, pp. 347–368.

Zierler, K., and Rogus, E. (1981a). Insulin does not hyperpolarize rat muscle by means of a ouabain-inhibitable process. *Am. J. Physiol.* 241: C145–C149.

Zierler, K., and Rogus, E. M. (1981b). Rapid hyperpolarization of rat skeletal muscle induced by insulin. *Biochim. Biophys. Acta* 640: 687–692.

Zubrzycka-Gaarn, E. E., Bulman, D. E., Karpati, G., et al. (1988). The Duchenne muscular dystrophy gene product is localized in sarcolemma of human skeletal muscle. *Nature* 333: 466–469.

4

The Neuromuscular Junction

NICHOLAS SPERELAKIS
and JANUSZ B. SUSZKIW

University of Cincinnati
  College of Medicine
Cincinnati, Ohio

JOHN T. HACKETT

University of Virginia
  Health Sciences Center
Charlottesville, Virginia

I. Introduction

A basic problem of cell physiology is the nature of the communication between excitable cells that is mediated by a chemical transmitter substance. The functional contact between nerve cells or nerve and muscle cells that mediates the cell-to-cell communication is termed a *synapse*. The vast majority of synapses in vertebrates operate by means of a chemical synaptic transmitter, but a few synapses have been reported to operate electrically, without a neurotransmitter. Chemical synapses are of two types: excitatory (E–) synapses and inhibitory (I–) synapses. The *excitatory synapses* tend to depolarize the postsynaptic cell to threshold and cause it to fire an action potential, whereas *inhibitory synapses* tend to hyperpolarize the postsynaptic cell and so tend to keep it from firing an action potential. At synapses in the CNS (e.g., on the anterior horn cell of the spinal cord), the excitatory and inhibitory synaptic currents add and subtract (i.e., these are integrating synapses), and the postsynaptic cell fires only when the net depolarizing synaptic current is sufficient to bring the postsynaptic cell to its threshold (Eccles, 1964).

The *neuromuscular junction* between a motor neuron and a skeletal muscle fiber is one example of an excitatory chemical synapse. The properties and functioning of this particular synapse are relatively well known, and these properties apply to other excitatory synapses, at which the analysis of the synaptic transmission

141

process is more difficult. Therefore, the skeletal neuromuscular junction may be viewed as a model excitatory synapse. Acetylcholine (ACh) is the neurotransmitter at this synapse (Katz, 1966).

The term *synapse* refers to the motor nerve terminal (and presynaptic membrane), the intervening synaptic cleft, and the contacted muscle surface (postsynaptic membrane). In the region of innervation, the nerve forms a specialized plate-shaped junction, the end plate, which may range in size from about 20 to 50 μm in diameter. As the nerve terminal approaches the end plate, it loses its myelin sheath and branches extensively. The junction region is covered by Schwann cells and perineural sheath cells. After presenting an overview of the entire synaptic transmission process and listing some of the general properties of the neuromuscular junction, we shall discuss the presynaptic and postsynaptic events in sequence. Finally, the actions of some drugs and toxins at the neuromuscular junction will be reviewed, followed by a discussion of one particular disease of this synapse.

II. Overview of Entire Process

The function of the neuromuscular junction (NMJ) is to transfer excitation from the motor neuron to the skeletal muscle fiber. Because the nerve terminal is very small in diameter and the muscle fiber is very large in diameter, the action potential (AP) cannot simply be transferred from the nerve cell membrane to muscle cell membrane, even if these two membranes were continuous with one another, because of the impedance mismatch explained later. Therefore, the impulse signal is interrupted at the NMJ by an intervening process that utilizes chemical amplifications of the signal. This process involves the fast release of synaptic transmitter molecules— acetylcholine (ACh) in all vertebrate NMJs—from the nerve terminal, triggered by the arrival of the nerve AP at the nerve terminal.

The released ACh molecules diffuse quickly (e.g., ca. 10 μs) over the short distance (approx. 600 Å) between the presynaptic (nerve) and postsynaptic (muscle) membranes, and bombard the postsynaptic membrane (PSM). The ACh molecules randomly bind to specific ACh (nicotinic) receptor sites on the outer surface of the channels of the PSM. The ACh receptor sites are located on the two α-subunits of the channels; both sites must be occupied for the channel to open. The chemically activated receptor gates (opens) the ionic channel, which is nonselective and allows Na^+, Ca^{2+}, and K^+ cations to pass through, but not anions, such as Cl^-. The simultaneous openings of a large number of such channels causes (1) the resistance of the PSM to be lowered and (2) the depolarization of the PSM. Because the adjacent conductile (electrically excitable) membrane is contiguous to the PSM, a local synaptic current flows between the PSM and conductile membrane, such that the conductile membrane also becomes depolarized. When the threshold potential of the conductile membrane is reached, an AP is triggered that propagates down the muscle fiber in both directions from the NMJ. The ACh molecules in the synaptic cleft are rapidly hydrolyzed by a specific acetylcholinesterase (AChE), and the system returns to its resting condition, available for the next nerve impulse to arrive.

Thus, the NMJ normally has a transfer function of 1.0 (i.e., one nerve AP leads to the generation of one muscle AP). If more than one muscle AP is generated per nerve AP, as in myotonia or anti-AChE poisoning, then the system is pathological and malfunctions. If less than one muscle AP is generated per muscle AP, as in severe fatigue, curare poisoning, or myasthenia gravis, again the system is malfunctioning and pathological.

The schematic summary of presynaptic and postsynaptic processes at the vertebrate NMJ is provided in Figure 1.

III. General Properties of Neuromuscular Junction

A. Synaptic Transmitter

Several criteria must be fulfilled before a substance is recognized as a synaptic transmitter. It must be synthesized by the presynaptic neuron and released by electrical stimulation of the presynaptic neuron. Furthermore, microapplication of putative neurotransmitter substance to the postsynaptic membrane should mimic the physiologically evoked response and be similarly modified by drugs. Presently, only about 24 substances fulfill all or most of the criteria for a neurotransmitter function in the nervous system of the entire animal kingdom.

Acetylcholine is the transmitter at all vertebrate skeletal NMJs. As described in the following, ACh is stored in small membrane-delimited vesicles (electron-lucent in electron microscopy) that are about 400–500 Å in diameter, and each contains between 1,500 and 50,000 molecules of ACh. There is a small spontaneous release of packets of ACh (each packet represents the contents of one vesicle) under resting conditions at a rate of about 1–3/s, generating small depolarizing potential changes in the PSM of about 0.4 mV each, called the *miniature end-plate potentials* (MEPPs). During the nerve AP, there is a nearly simultaneous release of about 200–300 vesicles, or *quanta*, that gives rise to a large end-plate potential capable of triggering an AP (Katz, 1966).

B. Impedance Mismatch; Chemical Amplification

As stated in the Introduction, there is an impedance mismatch between the small-diameter nerve fiber, which has a very high output impedence (or resistance), and the muscle fiber, which has a very low input impedence. This means that even if all the local circuit action current from the propagating AP in the nerve fiber could be funneled into the muscle fiber, the amount of depolarization it could produce (e.g., 1 mV) would be much too low to bring the muscle fiber membrane to its threshold potential (about −60 mV) from its resting potential (about −80 mV).

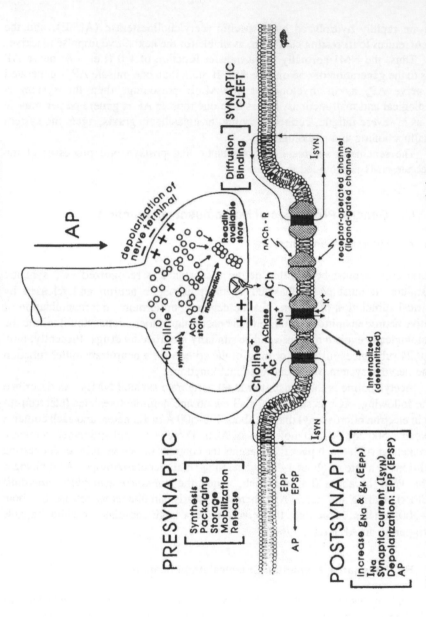

Figure 1 General scheme of the processes involved in neuromuscular transmission.

That is, there is no way that an electrical (low-resistance) synapse could work successfully at the NMJ.

Therefore, the role of the chemical transmitter is to allow sufficient depolarization of the muscle fiber to occur by drawing energy for this depolarization from the muscle fiber itself (from its resting potential or battery storehouse) and not from the nerve fiber. Energy from the nerve fiber is used for the uptake (of precursors), synthesis, storage, and release of the chemical transmitter, but not for direct depolarization of the muscle fiber by current flow. Thus, the synaptic transmitter acts as a *chemical amplifier* that, in effect, opens ion-channel gates in the PSM, allowing synaptic current to flow from one part of the muscle fiber to another, leading to the generation of an AP.

C. Electrical Inexcitability of Postsynaptic Membrane

The post-SM is electrically inexcitable, that is, it cannot fire an AP (even if the muscle fiber is stimulated directly at one end, and propagation of the impulse past the NMJ is allowed to occur). The PSM has little or no voltage-dependent ionic channels, such as fast Na^+ channels and K^+ channels. Instead, the PSM has preponderantly ionic channels that are opened only by the specific synaptic transmitter (ACh) or a close analogue. These are the so-called receptor-operated channels or ligand-gated channels. Binding of ACh to its nicotinic cholinergic receptor, presumably by producing some protein conformational change, opens a gate that allows the ion channel to switch to the conducting or open mode from the nonconducting or closed mode. Two ACh molecules must bind to one channel for activation to occur. The property of the PSM of electrical inexcitability is important functionally because it means that there is no positive-feedback mechanism between membrane potential (E_m) and membrane conductance (g_m), as in the conductile membrane. Therefore, the amount of depolarization of the PSM that is produced is strictly a function of the amount of ACh released. This underlies phenomena such as facilitation and fatigue.

D. Unidirectionality

All chemical synaptic junctions in vertebrates are unidirectional; thus, under physiological conditions there is only one-way traffic. For example, at the skeletal neuromuscular junction, the signal passes from the motor neuron to the muscle fiber. The reason for the unidirectionality is the morphological and biochemical specialization of the presynaptic and postsynaptic regions and membranes. For example, ACh is synthesized and stored in the presynaptic nerve terminal, whereas the nicotinic cholinergic receptors are on the postsynaptic (muscle) membrane. Unidirectionality of chemical synapses is often known as the law of Bell–Magendie.

E. Delay Time

There is a small delay at all chemical synaptic junctions of about 0.2–1.0 ms (i.e., the time lost in the synaptic transmission process). Most of the synaptic delay is due to the neurotransmitter release process. Diffusion across the short synaptic gap of about 1000 Å is very rapid, because the diffusion distance is short; diffusion time (e.g., for 90% equilibration; $t_{90\%}$) varies directly with the square of the diffusion distance (d): $t_{90\%} \propto d^2$. Table 1 illustrates how diffusion time for a small molecule or ion varies with distance. The time required for generation of the postsynaptic potential and action potential is also very brief. The delay time is increased with cooling.

F. Local Graded End-Plate Potential

Activation of the postsynaptic channels allows a Na^+ influx (and K^+ efflux) to occur into the muscle fiber through the PSM. This produces depolarization of the postsynaptic membrane, which is termed the *excitatory postsynaptic potential* (EPSP), or *end-plate potential* (EPP) in the case of the neuromuscular junction.

The EPP is a local potential; that is, it is not actively propagated down muscle fiber. It decays exponentially with distance away from the PSM, in accordance with the length constant of the fiber cable.

The EPP is a graded potential; it is not all-or-none or refractory in nature. Thus, two or more EPPs can summate (in time) to produce a larger EPP. Hence, EPPs have different properties from action potentials (APs), being both graded and localized (nonpropagating).

G. Rapid Inactivation of the Chemical Transmitter

The synaptic transmitter—ACh in the vertebrate NMJ—is rapidly inactivated by the enzyme, AChE, localized in the PMJ (outer surface) and in the synaptic cleft. This enzyme hydrolyzes ACh into choline and acetic acid. Acetylcholinesterase is one

Table 1 Sample Illustration of How Diffusion Time for a Small Molecule or Ion Varies with Diffusion Distance

Diffusion distance (mm)	Diffusion time (90% equilibration) (ms)
0.1	0.01
1.	1.
10.	100.
100.	10,000.

of the fastest-acting enzymes, producing hydrolysis in about 1 μs and having a turnover rate of about 1 million/s. The rapid inactivation of ACh allows the system to rapidly return to the resting or nonactivated state, and so enables the NMJ to monitor and respond to the subsequent motor nerve impulse. That is, the next nerve impulse can produce another EPP which, in turn, can trigger another muscle AP. This system allows high-frequency tetanic contractions of the muscle fibers to be produced.

The NMJ normally works such that for every nerve AP, there is one EPP and one muscle AP. That is, the nerve and muscle are coupled 1:1 in an obligatory fashion. This arrangement enables the nervous system to exercise tight control over the skeletal muscles. In some abnormal states, such as fatigue, or disease states, such as myasthenia gravis, the 1:1 coupling is lost, one nerve AP producing less than one muscle AP. In other conditions, such as myotonia, in which the muscle conductile membrane is abnormal (see Chap. 3, Sec. II), several muscle APs may be triggered by one nerve AP.

When anticholinesterase (anti-AChE) drugs are used to prolong the life of the released ACh, this has profound effects on neuromuscular transmission (discussed later).

H. Facilitation and Fatigue

The NMJ exhibits the properties of both facilitation and fatigue. In *facilitation*, the quantity of synaptic transmitter (ACh) released per nerve impulse is increased on subsequent stimulations, compared with the first stimulation (after a relatively long rest period). That is, more quanta are released per nerve impulse (increased quantal content). This phenomenon is known as *postactivation* (or *posttetanic*) *potentiation* of transmitter release. The system behaves as though more synaptic vesicles (quanta) are mobilized and available for release (e.g., aligned along the active zones of the pre-SM). However, the small gain in $[Na]_i$ and $[Ca]_i$ in the fine (small-diameter, high-surface–area/volume ratio) nerve terminals after repetitive firing may be involved in this phenomenon; in addition, the presence of a hyperpolarizing afterpotential following the AP in the nonmyelinated, fine nerve endings may contribute to the increased transmitter release to subsequent nerve APs, by increasing the electrochemical driving force $(E_m - E_i)$ for Na^+ and Ca^{2+} entry. Facilitation is further discussed in Section IV.F.

In *fatigue* of the neuromuscular junction, the quantity of synaptic transmitter released per nerve impulse is decreased. The reason for this is depletion of synaptic vesicles; that is, ACh is released faster than what can be resynthesized and repackaged into synaptic vesicles. The net effect of this ACh depletion is that the EPPs produced are smaller in amplitude and slower rising, and may fail to depolarize the adjacent conductile membrane to threshold, and so fail to trigger a muscle AP. In such a condition, many of the muscle fibers may fail to become activated at the same time, or at a high enough tetanic frequency, such that the individual exhibits a weakened muscle. In such conditions, temporal summation of two or more EPPs may be required to trigger one muscle AP.

In some cases of muscle fatigue in humans, the fatigue resides primarily in the neuromuscular junction; thus it is a synaptic fatigue, and not a true fatigue of the muscle fibers proper. This can be demonstrated in the laboratory by stimulating the nerve of a nerve–muscle preparation until the muscle fails to contract, and then immediately stimulating the muscle directly and seeing that the muscle is fully capable of contracting forcefully. Since the nerve APs are very resistant to fatigue, the fatigue resides primarily at the NMJ.

I. Sensitivity to Drugs

Chemical synapses, including the NMJ are very sensitive to drugs. In contrast, the nerve fibers and skeletal muscle fibers themselves are more resistant to drug action, as they are more resistant to fatigue. Drugs acting on the neuromuscular junction can act either presynaptically (on the motor nerve terminals) to affect the amount of neurotransmitter released (or synthesized), or postsynaptically (on the PSM) to affect the binding of the neurotransmitter ACh, to its receptor (nicotinic), or to affect the AChE. A more detailed discussion of the various categories of such drugs and how they act is given in Section VI.

IV. Presynaptic Physiology of Motor Nerve Terminals

A. Synaptic Vesicle Cycling

Perhaps the most striking feature of presynaptic terminals is the presence of many vesicular structures within the nerve terminal. The site where exocytosis of the synaptic vesicles occurs in the presynaptic active zone. This region was first defined by Couteaux and Pecot-Dechavassine (1970) as a series of dense bars attached to the internal face of the plasma membrane. The synaptic vesicles are arranged in rows on either side of these bars. One or two rows of large intramembranous particles are found along both margins of each bar (Figs. 2 and 3), which are thought to be calcium channels (Pumplin et al., 1981). If calcium conductance (or permeability) of a stimulated nerve terminal is divided by the number of particles, a value is obtained that is approximately the amount of conductance measured for a single Ca channel. During synaptic activity, synaptic vesicles fuse with the presynaptic membrane and form pits along the rows of large intramembranous particles (see Fig. 3). However, physiological evidence indicates that these are not the only sites from which ACh can be released (Colmeus et al., 1982; Evers et al., 1989).

The life history of presynaptic vesicles has been described by the elegant morphological experiments of Heuser and Reese (1973) (cf., Ceccareli et al., 1973). They showed that, with prolonged repetitive stimulation (10 Hz for 1 min), the number of presynaptic vesicles transiently decreased, but the decreased amount of

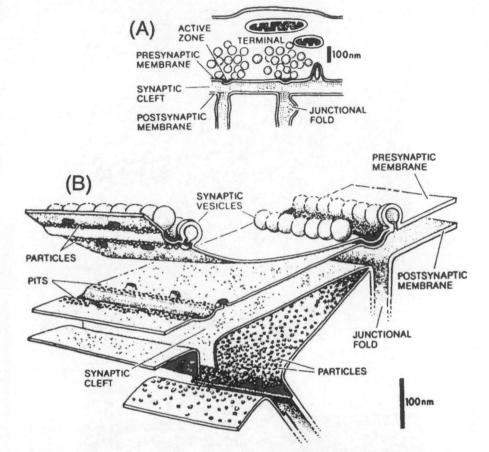

Figure 2 Structure of a neuromuscular junction. (A) Schematic representation of a longitudinal section through a portion of a nerve terminal containing a number of vesicles near an active zone opposite a junctional fold in the postsynaptic membrane. (B) The plasma membranes are split, as they would be by freeze-fracturing, to show the particles and pits in the active zone adjacent to where synaptic vesicles can empty their contents into the synaptic cleft. The particles in the postsynaptic membrane are thought to be acetylcholine receptors. (From Kuffler and Nichols, 1977.)

vesicular membrane was balanced by an increase in the plasma membrane of the nerve terminal. The idea proposed was that the vesicle membrane became incorporated into the plasma membrane. After longer stimulation times (15 min), cisternae were formed within the terminals. Following a period of rest, the cisternae were replaced by synaptic vesicles.

The picture that emerged (Fig. 4) has synaptic vesicles (SVs) fused with the plasma membrane, followed by a membrane conservation mechanism whereby some

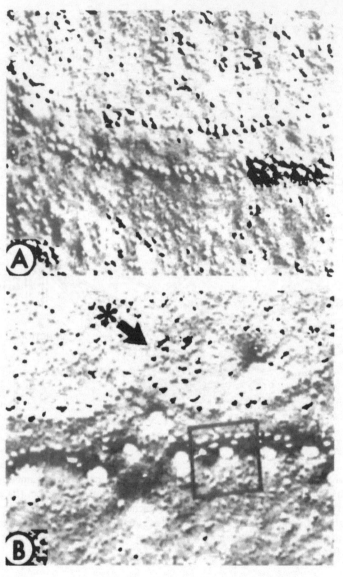

Figure 3 (A) Freeze-fractured replicas of one active zone from a nerve terminal in the "resting" state. Note the ridge bordered by parallel rows of large intramembrane particles. (B) An active zone from a nerve terminal treated like the one in (A), but given one nerve stimulus 5 ms before freezing. As the nerve begins to discharge large numbers of acetylcholine quanta, many membrane perturbations appear along the edges of the active zone. The two areas marked by asterisks are probably vesicles that have collapsed after opening. Note that these areas have a cluster of two or more large intramembrane particles like those found in intact synaptic vesicle membranes. The area in the square represents a characteristic domain of exocytosis. (From Heuser et al., 1979.)

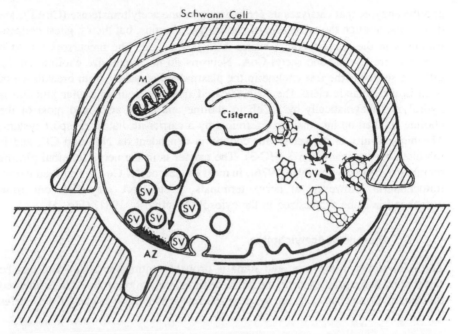

Figure 4 The life history of synaptic vesicles. Arrows indicate the direction of movement of synaptic vesicles. The nerve terminal is depicted as lying in a groove in a muscle surface that has a secondary groove opposite the active zone (AZ). The nerve terminal is covered by a Schwann cell and contains mitochondria (M), synaptic vesicles (SV), coated vesicles (CV), and a cisterna. (From Heuser and Reese, 1973.)

of the terminal membrane was internalized into the cisternae, from which new vesicles could be formed. Support for this conclusion was obtained by using an extracellular electron-opaque tracer, the formation of which was amplified by exogenous horseradish peroxidase (HRP). The reaction product was found first in cisternae and then in the vesicles. To demonstrate that this was a one-way cycle, preparations were washed to remove extracellular tracer, and then stimulated to see if tracer could be found internally; none was found. The mechanism by which vesicles are retrieved may involve the formation (next to the plasma membrane) of weblike membrane to decrease the energy barrier for endocytosis. Coated vesicles (CVs) appear at this stage, and lose their coat when they fuse with the cisternae.

B. Acetylcholine Metabolism

Acetylcholine is the chemical neurotransmitter substance at the NMJ. A prerequisite for a putative neurotransmitter is the demonstration that it be synthesized and stored in the motoneuron in a form that can be released by an action potential. Acetylcholine and the enzyme that catalyzes its formation, choline acetyltransferase (ChAT), are distributed through the cytoplasm of cholinergic neurons, but their highest concentration is in the nerve terminal where ACh is released. The precursors for ACh synthesis are choline and acetyl-CoA. Neurons do not synthesize choline, so the ultimate source is the free choline in the plasma and recycling from breakdown of ACh in the synaptic cleft. The ACh released from the neuromuscular junction is hydrolyzed enzymatically by AChE to choline and acetic acid, and most of the choline is taken up into the nerve terminal by a carrier-mediated transport system. The high affinity of the carrier for choline is dependent on Na^+ and Cl^-, and is inhibited by hemicholinum-3 (HC-3). The carrier is in the nerve terminal plasma membrane (Suszkiw and Pilar, 1976). In most tissues, acetyl-CoA is confined within mitochondria. However, at nerve terminals, acetyl-CoA may leak out from mitochondria or be synthesized in the cytosol (MacIntosh, 1981) (Fig. 5).

C. Storage of Acetylcholine

The ACh stored in the axon and soma is probably entirely unbound and can be released by homogenization. In the nerve endings, only 50% of the ACh is released by osmotic or mechanical lysis, whereas the rest is found in vesicles. The vesicles

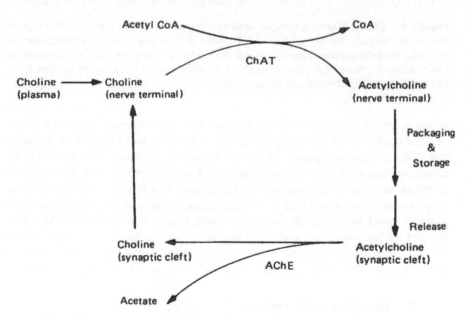

Figure 5 Synthesis, storage, and release of acetylcholine. Arrows indicate various metabolic pathways that interlock in synthesis of acetylcholine. Release of acetylcholine into the synaptic cleft is in quantal form from a vesicle. Choline is taken up from the synaptic cleft by nerve terminals and muscles (Hubbard et al., 1969).

are approximately 40–50 nm in diameter, and contain 1,500–50,000 ACh molecules in a volume of about 2.7×10^{-17} cm^3. There are about 900 vesicles per cubic meter of axon terminal (Steinbach and Stevens, 1976). For chemical analysis and metabolic studies, it is possible to extract a nearly pure population of synaptic vesicles from electromotor nerve terminals of *Torpedo* (electric ray) (Sheridan et al., 1966). The vesicles are considerably larger (ca. 84 nm) than those of mammalian motor nerve terminals, and they each may contain about 300,000 molecules of ACh. Following exhaustive nerve stimulation, the vesicles depleted of ACh become smaller.

Both ATP and ACh are taken up into the synaptic vesicles by a carrier-mediated transport system (Whittaker, 1982). The vesicles have to take up and retain ACh against a large concentration gradient. There are five major proteins in the membrane of the vesicles, four of which have been identified: (1) a (Ca^{2+}, Mg^{2+})-activated ATPase, (2) a form of actin, (3) an ATP carrier, and (4) an acetylcholine carrier. The molar ratio of ACh to ATP in torpedo vesicles is about 1:4–1:5. The role of ATP in the synaptic vesicle is unknown. Perhaps the ATP and protein complexes are counterions for ACh, helping to keep it inside the vesicles. In the sympathetic nerves of vascular smooth muscle, ATP and norepinephrine (NE) are cotransmitters; ATP produces the fast EPSP (or EJP; excitatory junction potential) and NE produces the slow EPSP.

D. Release of Acetylcholine

The *quantal theory* of synaptic transmission says that action potential-evoked postsynaptic potentials are made up of quantal components of the same shape and size as MEPPs. The *vesicular theory*, an extension, of the quantal theory, suggests that the presynaptic vesicles are the storage sites for the multimolecular package or quanto of ACh, and that they are released by exocytosis.

Although ACh can be measured by biochemical and bioassay techniques, these are not sensitive enough to detect the multimolecular package form of ACh released from the nerve terminal. To detect this very small amount of ACh (on the order of 10,000 molecules), electrophysiological techniques have been used (Kuffler and Yoshikami, 1975). These techniques also can resolve the rapid time course of the release process, which can increase 10^5-fold in 1 ms when an action potential invades the nerve terminal. The multimolecular package of ACh was first measured as a small-amplitude depolarization (less than 1 mV) lasting about 10 ms, which was recorded by a microelectrode, the tip of which had penetrated the muscle fiber close to the end-plate region (Fig. 6A–C). These events, the miniature end-plate potentials (MEPPs), occur spontaneously and reflect ACh released from the nerve terminal. They are about 1/100 the size of the end-plate potential evoked by an action potential invading the nerve terminal with a normal external Ca^{2+} ion concentration.

Beside the MEPPs, there are (1) subminiature EPPs (Kriebel and Gross, 1974), which may represent the release of a partially filled vesicle, and (2) giant MEPPs,

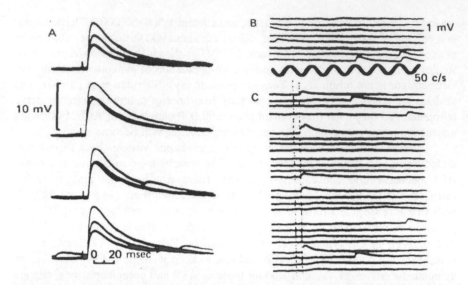

Figure 6 Magnesium ions act to block synaptic transmission. (A) End-plate potentials reduced to subthreshold responses (10 mM MgCl, 1.8 mM CaCl, 10^{-6} M prostigimine). Note the fluctuations in the amplitude of the evoked response (three superimposed traces in each set of records) that is approximately equivalent to the amplitude of spontaneous miniature end-plate potentials. (B,C) Further depression of synaptic transmission (14 mM MgCl, 0.9 mM CaCl). In (B) four spontaneous miniature end-plate potentials were recorded, and in (C) five end-plate potentials were evoked by single nerve impulses. (The first dotted line marks the beginning of the stimulus, and the second, the start of the end-plate potential.) Note that 19 nerve impulses failed to evoke end-plate potentials, and there were four spontaneous end-plate potentials. (From del Castillo and Katz, 1954.)

which may be the result of the fusion of a number of vesicles (Pecot-Dechavassine, 1976). There is also nonquantal release of ACh (molecular leakage or unpackaged), which may be important to the trophic maintenance of muscle by the nerve (Katz and Miledi, 1977; Vyskocil and Illes, 1977). Only the vesicular release is involved in transmission of nerve impulse. Nerve degeneration results in loss of MEPPs (Miledi and Slater, 1966). After the removal of nerve, Schwann cells can take over the release of ACh in an unpackaged form (Dennis and Miledi, 1974).

The evidence for release of multimolecular packages (or quanta) of neurotransmitter comes from recording at only the end-plate region of a minimum-sized postsynaptic potential. Large and small MEPPs may indicate release from sites proximal and distal to the microelectrode. Electrophoretic application of ACh to the postsynaptic membrane does not produce "quantal" potentials, but instead, a graded postsynaptic depolarization proportional to the amount of ACh applied.

The frequency of occurrence of MEPPs is increased with depolarization of the presynaptic terminal (in the presence of Ca^{2+}) or by agents that alter nerve terminal function. Thus, the frequency of MEPPs is related to presynaptic events, whereas a change in amplitude usually reflects altered postsynaptic responsiveness. One exception to this rule is HC-3, which blocks ACh synthesis and thus decreases the size of a quantum. Pharmacological agents that act on the postsynaptic membrane affect MEPP amplitude (e.g., curare).

E. Role of Calcium in Acetylcholine Release by Nerve Terminal Action Potentials (Phasic Release)

A brief summary of the ionic requirements for ACh release is as follows:

1. The release of neurotransmitters and hormones is dependent on the extracellular Ca^{2+} concentration ($[Ca]_o$). The intracellular free Ca^{2+} concentration ($[Ca]_i$) is very low (about $0.1 \mu M$).
2. The entry of Ca^{2+} into activated giant squid nerve terminals has been demonstrated using the bioluminescent protein, aequorin, which emits light when it binds Ca^{2+} (Llinas and Nicholson, 1975).
3. Iontophoretic injection of Ca^{2+} into nerve terminals results in transmitter release (Miledi, 1973). In addition, intracellular injection of Ca^{2+} by means of lipid vesicles (liposomes) containing high internal concentrations of Ca^{2+} evokes ACh release (Rahamimoff et al., 1978). The liposomes transfer their contents through the cell membrane and, thus, increase $[Ca]_i$ inside the nerve terminal.
4. Tetrodotoxin (TTX) and tetraethylammonium (TEA) can block the active Na^+ and K^+ conductances, respectively, that underlie the APs, but they do not block the depolarization-evoked transmitter release. Therefore, by exclusion, Ca^{2+} ions are the species of ion required for phasic ACh release.
5. Blockage of ACh release by the divalent cations, Mg^{2+}, Mn^{2+}, Co^{2+}, Cd^{2+}, occurs only when the cations are on the outside of the nerve terminal (Kharasch et al., 1981). These cations are known to block Ca^{2+} influx.
6. An inward Ca^{2+} current can be measured in voltage-clamped squid nerve terminals (in the presence of TTX and TEA) that is correlated with neurotransmitter release (Fig. 7; Llinas et al., 1981). Presynaptic depolarization to the equilibrium potential for Ca^{2+} (E_{Ca}) blocks inward Ca^{2+} current and subsequent transmitter release, but the tail current following repolarization evokes transmitter release with a briefer synaptic delay (200 μs). The Ca^{2+} current in response to an AP is similar to the tail current because it continues into the falling phase of the AP, when the driving force for Ca^{2+} is increasing.

Similarly, in voltage-clamped presynaptic motor neuron of the skeletal neuromuscular junction, an inward Ca^{2+} current that is sufficient for ACh release

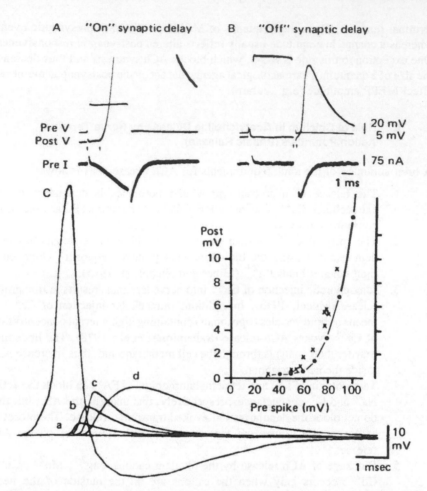

Figure 7 Synaptic transmission during voltage-clamp of presynaptic terminal. (A) A depolarizing command voltage evoked a presynaptic current change that was followed 700 μs later by the postsynaptic response. (B) With a larger command pulse, there is suppression of synaptic transmission that began after the pulse was off (200 μs synaptic delay): Top trace, presynaptic voltage (Pre-V); middle trace, postsynaptic response (Post-V); lower trace, calcium current (Pre-I). (C) Theoretical solution for propagating action potential in the presynaptic terminal and related steps in synaptic transmission: a, calcium ion channel formation; b, calcium current; c, postsynaptic current; d, postsynaptic potential. (From Llinas et al., 1981.)

can be recorded in the presence of TTX and TEA (Fig. 8; Brosius et al., 1990). Depolarization to E_{Ca} abolishes the inward current and synaptic transmission (see Fig. 8C), thus demonstrating that the Ca^{2+} current is necessary for release. Upon repolarization (after the depolarization; see Fig. 8C), there is a transient Ca^{2+} tail current that occurs while the gradient is inward and the channels remain open. The transmission evoked by this tail current has a brief latency, because triggering neurosecretion does not require time to open the Ca^{2+} channels.

F. Cumulative and Persistent Effects of Synaptic Activation

There is a random fluctuation in the amplitude of EPPs evoked by nerve stimulation, which is attributed to the average probability (p) that quanta are released, as well as to the number (n) of available quanta. Thus, the number of quanta released or quantal number (m) is a function of the probability that a quantum is released times the number of quanta available for release: $m = np$.

If the probability of release is reduced, for example, by lowering the $[Ca]_o$, then one observes only a few quantal components of the EPP. Under these conditions and with repetitive stimulation, the EPPs grow in amplitude with each successive stimulus, presumably because the probability (p) increases. This is called *facilitation*. It has been demonstrated at the squid giant synapse (Charlton et al., 1982) that facilitation of synaptic transmission is not related to an increase in Ca^{2+} conductance of the nerve terminal, but is due to the residual buildup of internal Ca^{2+} following electrical activity (Fig. 9). If, in contrast, the $[Ca]_o$ is normal or high, each stimulus releases a large number of transmitter packages, and the store of ACh is depleted. This results in depression of synaptic transmission. A possible physical basis for n is the number of active sites in the nerve terminal (Atwood and Johnston, 1968; Wernig, 1976; Kuno, 1964; Jack et al., 1981; Korn et al., 1982).

G. Proteins Associated with the Molecular Machinery of Quantal Release

Immediately after a presynaptic depolarization, there occurs a brief and highly localized increase in $[Ca]_i$, which results in fusion of synaptic vesicles with the presynaptic plasma membrane. Calcium may act directly on the membrane to cause vesicular fusion, or by interacting with an intermediary agent. Evidence from a broad range of studies indicates that the latter mechanism dominates, and that presynaptic proteins are the most likely targets for Ca^{2+} interaction. Calcium may modulate presynaptic protein function by binding-mediated conformational changes, or by activating a calcium-dependent enzyme. One protein associated with quantal release is synapsin I (Hackett et al., 1990).

Synapsin I (SYN-I) was first isolated from particulate synaptic fractions of brain as an endogenous substrate for cAMP-dependent protein kinase (Johnson et al., 1972; Ueda et al., 1973). It was later found to be an endogenous substrate for

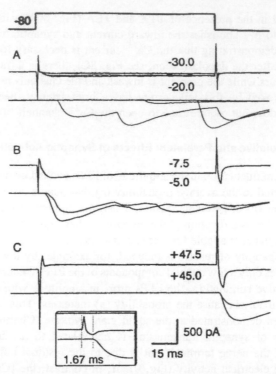

Figure 8 Presynaptic Ca^{2+} current is necessary and sufficient for eliciting quantal release at a nerve–muscle synapse. (A–C) Superimposed traces of presynaptic current (top) and postsynaptic current (bottom) elicited by presynaptic depolarizing commands (voltage protocol illustrated in A). (A) Depolarizing test pulses to –30, –27.5, –25, and –22.5 mV from a holding potential of –80 mV. The corresponding quantal postsynaptic currents were evoked by –27.5 mV and more depolarized values. Larger amplitude test pulses recruited more quantal units. Synaptic transmission occurred throughout the duration of the test pulse, beginning after synaptic delay. The synaptic delay shortened as the test pulses grew in amplitude, although there was considerable variability. (B) Test pulses to –7.5 and –5.0 mV evoked near maximal Ca^{2+} currents. The activation time constant was 3.54 ms. The postsynaptic responses elicited by the tail currents overlapped those stimulated during the test pulses. (C) Large depolarizing command pulses beyond the suppression voltage for evoked release. No transmission is seen in response to the depolarizing pulse. The release evoked by the tail currents is highly synchronized. The amplitudes of the postsynaptic responses fluctuated in a random fashion, indicative of quantal release. (Inset) The mean synaptic delay of eight averaged response pairs was 1.67 ms. (From Brosius et al., 1990.)

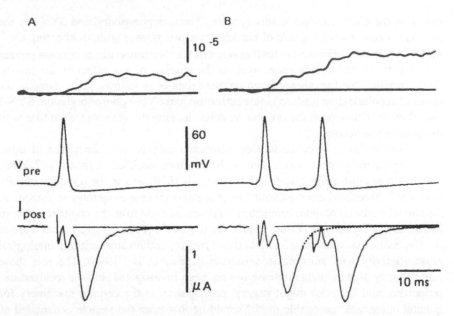

Figure 9 Absorbance changes at 660 nm to single and paired action potentials in terminal filled with arsenazo III. Presynaptic potential was recorded with the dye-injecting electrode, and postsynaptic current (I_{post}) was recorded from a postsynaptic axon under voltage clamp. Absorbance records are averages of responses to 160 stimuli repeated every 45 s, and postsynaptic currents are averages of 16 responses. The dotted line in B shows the postsynaptic current tail traced from A. The second postsynaptic response is 11% larger than the first. (From Charlton et al., 1982.)

a Ca^{2+}-dependent protein kinase found in isolated synaptic fractions (Krueger et al., 1977; Sieghat et al., 1979), and was purified to homogeneity (Ueda and Greengard, 1977). Synapsin I was purified from bovine brain, but has been identified in squid (Llinas et al., 1985) and fish brain (T. Ueda, personal communication); thus it is likely to be of general distribution and importance. Synapsin is phosphorylated at three serine sites: site 1 is phosphorylated by both cAMP-dependent protein kinase and Ca^{2+}–calmodulin-dependent protein kinase II (Hunter et al., 1981; Kennedy and Greengard, 1981). Synapsin I is localized to synaptic vesicles, as shown by immunoferritin labeling (De Camilli et al., 1983). Ferritin-labeled vesicles were found distributed throughout the cytoplasm, but no label was seen on the plasma membrane. This SYN-I localization to neuronal synaptic vesicles suggests that SYN-I is specific to neurons or to the neuronal mode of secretion, since labeling in endocrine secretory cells is not found. Llinas et al. (1985) have shown in physiological experiments that SYN-I might be involved in neurosecretion. The dephosphorylated form of SYN-I, but not the phosphorylated form, inhibits synaptic transmission when introduced into the squid giant synapse. No effect was found on the Ca^{2+} currents at this synapse. Thus, dephosphorylated SYN-I is the only agent now known capable of blocking synaptic release without affecting Ca^{2+} influx. An equally provocative finding was that Ca^{2+}–calmodulin-dependent protein kinase II facilitated transmission, again in the absence of any effect on the inward Ca^{2+} current. One hypothesis based on these data is as follows: Ca^{2+} entry as the result of depolarization leads to kinase activation and SYN-I phosphorylation; SYN-I may then dissociate from the synaptic vesicles, leaving the vesicles free to fuse with the plasma membrane.

Vesicle fusion with the plasma membrane may involve the action of other Ca^{2+}-dependent proteins associated with secretory vesicles. Synexin (47 kDa), isolated from chromaffin granules (Creutz et al., 1978) acts in the presence of 0.01 mM Ca^{2+} (threshold concentration) to promote membrane–membrane fusion. A functionally similar protein, calelectrin, has been isolated from the cholinergic nerve terminals of *Torpedo marmorata* (Sudhof et al., 1985; Walker, 1982). It has a lower relative molecular mass (M_r; 32 kDa) than synexin, and no apparent immunological cross-reactivity with antisynexin antiserum (Creutz et al., 1986). The role these proteins may play in quantal release has not been investigated, but the localization, properties, and behavior might suggest participation in the cellular machinery for quantal release. A reasonable model would be that once the vesicle is denuded of SYN-I, Ca^{2+} in the cytoplasm activates these proteins to promote vesicle fusion and exocytosis.

V. Postsynaptic Physiology of the Neuromuscular Junction

A. Acetylcholine Receptor–Ion Channel Complex

Function and Localization

The ACh receptor (AChR) of the vertebrate skeletal muscle is a channel-forming protein complex the function of which is to increase the permeability of the motor end plate to cations. The ACh molecules released by nerve impulses bind to the receptors and, thereby, open the associated ion channels for 1–2 ms. During this time, roughly 10^4 Na^+ ions flow into the cell, and somewhat fewer K^+ ions flow out through each activated channel. The ensuing depolarization of the end-plate region (end-plate potential; EPP) triggers a regenerative muscle AP and muscle contraction.

The ACh receptors are concentrated at the juxtaneuronal region of the postjunctional folds. The localization of receptors at the crests of postjunctional folds has been demonstrated by electron microscopic autoradiography of motor end plates labeled with α-[^{125}I]-bungarotoxin (α-[^{125}I]BGT), an 8000-Da polypeptide component of snake (Formosan krait) venom, which binds with high affinity and specificity to the ACh receptors (Fig. 10). By employing quantitative autoradiography of α-[^{125}I]BGT-labeled sternomastoid muscles in mice, Fertuck and

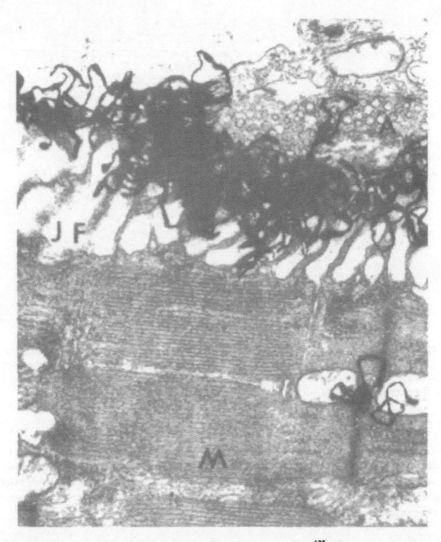

Figure 10 Localization of the acetylcholine receptors with α-[^{125}I]-bungarotoxin. Electron microscope autoradiogram of end-plate from mouse sternomastoid muscle incubated with α-[^{125}I]-bungarotoxin until all neurally evoked muscle contractions were blocked. The autoradiogram is overexposed to dramatize the illustration that the label is not uniformly distributed throughout the postjunctional membrane, but is concentrated near the axonal interface. JF, junctional folds; A, axon; M, muscle. ×21,000. (From Fertuck and Saltpeter, 1976b.)

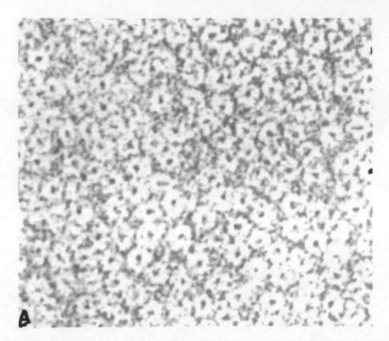

Figure 11 Uranyl acetate-stained AChR membrane sheets from preparations rich in dimeric AChR. In a portion of the membranes, the density packed AChR molecules (A) have been dispersed by excessive base treatment and sonication (B). Circles outline some membranes of the dimeric pairs of AChR in the membrane. (From Kistler et al., 1982.)

Saltpeter (1976a,b) estimated 30,000 ± 8,000 toxin sites per square micron of membrane. Since each receptor contains two toxin-binding sites, the corresponding number of receptors would be about $15,000/\mu m^2$. In contrast, the receptor density at about 7 μm away from the end plate is less than 0.2% of the subsynaptic concentration.

Molecular Structure of Acetylcholine Receptor

The PSM of vertebrate skeletal muscle constitutes less than 0.1% of the total cell membrane. Thus, despite the high density of AChR at the end plate, the amount of receptor protein that can be isolated from muscle is not sufficient for detailed biochemical analyses. Fortunately, large quantities of nicotinic receptor obtained from electric organs of electric eels and electric fish (*Torpedo* and *Electrophorus*) permit detailed characterization of the receptors. Biochemical characteristics of receptors isolated from electric organ and those from vertebrate skeletal muscle appear quite similar (Conti-Tronconi and Raffery, 1982).

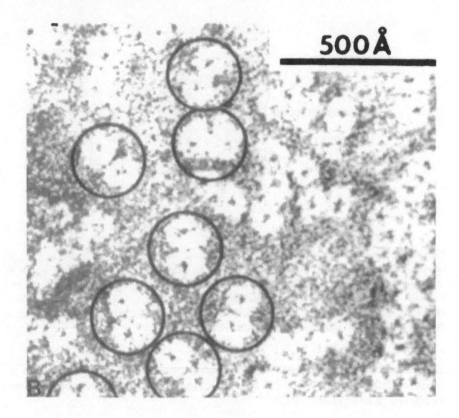

500 Å

The torpedo ACh receptor is a large ($\sim$250 kD, M_r) protein complex composed of two identical α-subunits ($\sim$40 kDa) and three nonidentical subunits: β- 4($\sim$50 kDa), γ- 4($\sim$60 kDa), and δ ($\sim$65 kDa). Each of the two α-subunits contains one ACh-binding site.

Negative staining of receptor-rich membranes with electron-dense dyes, such as uranyl acetate, reveals a pentameric arrangement of the subunits into rosettes. The rosettes are about 85 Å in diameter and enclose a central cavity approximately 25 Å in diameter (Fig. 11). The cavity spans across the entire membrane and represents the receptor channel. Frequently, receptors dimerize through disulfide bond formation between cysteine residue in the δ-subunits (Karlin, 1983). The functional significance of receptor dimerization is unclear, but it may play a role in aggregation and dense packing of receptors at the end plate.

A three-dimensional model of the AChR, determined by X-ray diffraction analyses and multiple electron microscopic imagings, is shown in Figure 12. In the direction normal to the plane of the membrane, the receptor complex is 110 Å long, with all five subunits spanning the membrane. The receptor extends approximately 50 Å on the extracellular side and 20 Å on the cytoplasmic side beyond the borders

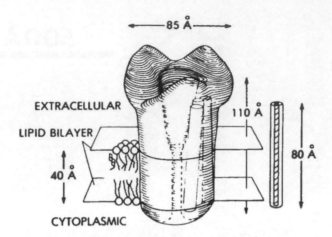

Figure 12 A three-dimensional model for the funnel-shaped AChR molecule in the lipid bilayer. On average, 80-Å-long α-helices indicate an elongated shape of subunits, which are arranged perpendicular to the membrane channel. The protein topography has been inferred from the densities in computer-filtered images of AChR tubular lattices, from side views, and from X-ray diffraction. Note that the funnel-shaped interior portion of the receptor is thought to be the ion channel. (From Kistler et al., 1982.)

of the lipid bilayer. The funnel-shaped channel forms a 25-Å–wide opening to the synaptic cleft and narrows to 7.5 Å at the cytoplasmic side of the postjunctional membrane (Kistler et al., 1982).

Cation-Gating Function of Acetylcholine Receptor

The ACh-gated channels are permeable to cations and exclude anions. Electrophysiological analyses of the permeability properties of end-plate channels in frog muscle indicate that the channel is a water-filled pore through which a variety of monovalent inorganic and organic cations can pass with relative ease. The selectivity among alkali metal ions is weak, with permeability ratios of $Ca^{2+}/Rb^+/K^+/Na^+/Li$ being 1.4:1.3:1.1:1.0:0.9. The channel also allows passage of divalent ions, such as Mg^{2+}, Ca^{2+}, Ba^{2+}, and Sr^{2+}. The estimated Ca/Na permeability ratio (P_{Ca}/P_{Na}) is about 0.2 (Adams et al., 1980).

The postsynaptic channel is gated by the ligand (ACh in this case) and not by voltage. Therefore, the PSM is inexcitable by electrical stimulation (see Sec. III.C).

The ACh-gated channel exists either in closed (nonconducting) or open (conducting) states (Anderson and Stevens, 1973). The binding of two ACh molecules (Dionne et al., 1978) to the receptor induces a conformational transition to the open state. The channel remains open for a few milliseconds and then spontaneously reverts to the closed state. This process may be described by the kinetic scheme below:

$$2ACh + R \rightleftharpoons (ACh)_2R^c \rightleftharpoons (ACh)_2R^o$$

where ACh_nR^c and ACh_nR^o represent the closed conformation and open conformation of the receptor complex. By analogy to enzyme–substrate interactions, the binding step is thought to be very fast. The transition of the AChR to the open conformation is slower, but is fast relative to the conformational transition from the open state back to the closed state. Channel closure probably is the slowest step that determines the mean open time of the channel. The mean channel open time and single-channel conductance have been estimated from statistical analyses of ACh noise (Anderson and Stevens, 1973; Neher and Stevens, 1977) and confirmed by direct measurements of single-channel currents in patch-clamp recordings (Neher and Sakmann, 1976). The best estimates give a single-channel conductance of 20–30 pS (picosiemens), allowing the transfer of approximately 1.5×10^4 univalent cations per millisecond of channel open time. The opening of a single channel produces a depolarization of postsynaptic membrane by about 0.3 μV (at or near the resting potential) (Katz and Miledi, 1972). Therefore, to produce an EPP of 30 mV, there must be nearly simultaneous opening of about 10^5 channels.

Desensitization

Desensitization of nicotinic AChR was first demonstrated electrophysiologically as a decrease in the postsynaptic membrane responsiveness to prolonged application of ACh (Katz and Thesleff, 1957). The phenomenon of desensitization is thought to involve an agonist-induced transition of the receptor to a locked conformation that has high affinity for agonists, but is unable to open the channel. The rates of desensitization depend on ligand concentration, are accelerated by high Ca^{2+}, and occur on the time scale of seconds. Recovery from desensitization occurs over a period of seconds to minutes, and does not appear to depend on the specific agonist agent used to cause the initial conversion to the desensitized state. Desensitization is occasionally caused by a rapid internalization (and possible degradation) of the activated receptors, a type of down-regulation.

Denervation Supersensitivity

Because ACh receptors are normally restricted to end-plate regions, healthy muscles are responsive to ACh only at the end-plates. However, when the motor nerves are severed and the axon terminals degenerate, the whole muscle fiber becomes sensitive to acetylcholine. This response to denervation is associated with the appearance of new extrajunctional ACh receptors, and is termed *denervation supersensitivity* (Axelsson and Thesleff, 1959). The relative densities of junctional and extrajunctional receptors have been estimated by the use of a-[^{125}I]-bungarotoxin. In innervated diaphragm muscles of mouse and rat, the density of receptors at the end plate is of the order of $10^4/\mu m^2$ and less than $50/\mu m^2$ at the extrajunctional sites. Following denervation, the extrajunctional receptors increase to 10^2–$10^3/\mu m^2$ (Hartzell and Fambrough, 1972). Although the precise mechanism by which denervation brings about increased synthesis and incorporation of new receptors into extrajunctional membrane is not known, it is generally thought that trophic factor(s) (possibly including ACh itself) released by the presynaptic nerve terminals regulate the distribution and turnover of receptors in the muscle membrane. The degree of muscle activity also may be an important factor (Thesleff, 1974).

B. Ionic Basis of the End Plate Potential

Postsynaptic Ion Channel

When the synaptic transmitter molecules bind to the postsynaptic receptors, the associated ion channels are opened. That is, these are receptor-operated or ligand-gated channels in which a gate opens when the receptor is occupied. A conformational change in the channel protein could effectively serve to gate the water-filled central pore. The postsynaptic channel at the vertebrate neuromuscular junction is a nonselective (or mixed) channel, allowing many cations, such as Na^+, Ca^{2+}, and K^+, to pass through, but it screens out anions, such as Cl^-, presumably owing to the presence of negative charge in the pore. The fact that cations of greatly different unhydrated (crystal) radii and hydrated radii can pass through about equally well [e.g., the Na^+ conductance (g_{Na}) is about equal to the K^+ conductance (gK)] suggests that the diameter of the pore must be large enough to fit the largest of these cations (Fig. 13). The approximate order of hydrated radii for these ions is: Ca^{2+} (5.2 Å) > Na^+ (3.8 Å) > K^+ (2.5 Å) ≥, Cl^- (2.4 Å).

The ACh receptor–ion channel complexes appear to be packed very tightly (i.e., nearly shoulder to shoulder) in the postsynaptic membrane. It is estimated that there are about 10^4 channels per square micron of membrane area, but only about 10% are activated (10^3 channels open per square micron). The remainder are essentially spare receptors. The conductance per opened channel is about 2.5×10^{-11} ohm^{-1} (or mho or siemens, S; 25 pS/channel). Thus, the total maximal conductance would be 25×10^{-9} S/μm^2 or 2.5 S/cm^2; for an end-plate area of 2500 μm^2, this would give a total conductance of 6.25×10^{-5} S/end plate. Converting to resistance gives a value of 1.6×10^4 ohm or 16 kΩ for the postsynaptic membrane. This value is close to that experimentally measured (see later Figs. 17 and 18). The single-channel conductance of 25 pS/channel corresponds to the inward movement of about 15×10^6 Na^+ ions per second through each channel (assuming a constant driving force of 100 mV). [This is the same as the value of 1.5×10^4 ions per millisecond mentioned in Sec. V.A.] The mean open time for the ACh-activated ion channel is a few milliseconds. The opening and closing rate

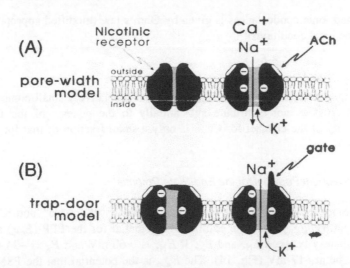

Figure 13 Cartoon model for a receptor–ion channel complex in the postsynaptic membrane at the vertebrate neuromuscular junction. This is a receptor-operated channel. The gate is opened by ACh binding to nicotinic receptor sites on the channel. Gating may be effectively accomplished by a conformational change in the protein molecule. A twitching of the alignment of the five subunits (α_1, α_2, β, γ, and δ) may result in opening the channel. The channel is nonselective, allowing many cations to pass through, including Na^+, Ca^{2+}, and K^+. However, anions, such as Cl^-, cannot pass through, presumably because of fixed negative charges in the wall of the central, water-filled pore of the channel. Two molecules of ACh bound to two receptor sites (on the two α-subunits) are required to open one channel.

constants for the channels are slightly affected by E_m (only about twofold slowing per 100 mV hyperpolarization).

Equilibrium Potentials, Electrochemical Driving Forces, and Ionic Currents

When the postsynaptic channel is in the open state, the cations can pass through down their electrochemical gradients. The net electrochemical driving force for Na^+ ($E_m - E_{Na}$) is in the inward direction, allowing an Na^+ influx, which is depolarizing and tends to bring the membrane potential (E_m) of the SM toward the Na^+ equilibrium potential (E_{Na}). The net driving force for Ca^{2+} ($E_m - E_{Ca}$) is also inward, allowing a Ca^{2+} influx, which is also depolarizing. The net driving force for K^+ ($E_m - E_K$) is outward, allowing a K^+ efflux, which is hyperpolarizing and tends to bring E_m toward E_K. A thorough discussion of equilibrium potentials, electrochemical driving forces, and ionic currents is given in Chapter 2 (also see Sperelakis, 1979).

The relation between the individual ionic currents, electrochemical driving forces, and ionic conductances is given by Ohm's law (modified appropriately for electrochemical conditions):

$$I_{Na} = g_{Na} (E_m - E_{Na})$$
$$I_K = g_K (E_m - E_K)$$

We can ignore the Ca^{2+} current (I_{Ca}) because it is relatively small compared with I_{Na}, and so does not contribute substantially to the genesis of the EPP. The permeability of the channel for Ca^{2+} is only a small fraction of that for Na^+ (see Sec. V.A).

Equilibrium Potential for the End-Plate Potential

Since the opened postsynaptic channel has conductances for Na^+ and K^+ that are about equal (g_{Na}/g_K), then the equilibrium potential for the EPP (E_{epp}) should be about half-way between E_{Na} and E_K. If E_{Na} is +60 mV and E_K is –94 mV, then E_{epp} will be at –17 mV (Fig. 14). The E_{epp} is the potential that the PSM "seeks" when all of the postsynaptic channels are fully activated.

If the PSM is experimentally hyperpolarized or depolarized by application of polarizing current, then the EPP becomes larger and faster-rising when hyperpolarized, or smaller and slower-rising when depolarized. In fact, if the depolarization is to the other side of E_{epp}, then the EPP goes in a hyperpolarizing direction, rather than the usual depolarizing direction. Exactly at E_{epp}, there would be no EPP whatsoever. Therefore, the E_{epp} is often termed the *null point* or the *reversal potential* for the end-plate potential. This behavior is illustrated in Figure 15.

The theoretical value that the membrane potential should reach during maximal activation of the PSM, namely the E_{epp}, may be calculated from the chord-conductance equation:

$$E_{epp} = \frac{g_{Na}}{g_{Na} + g_K} E_{Na} + \frac{g_K}{g_{Na} + g_K} E_K$$

In this simplified form, it was assumed that the contribution of Ca^{2+} is small and can be ignored, so the Ca^{2+} term has been omitted from the equation. If it is assumed that $g_{Na} = g_K$ in the opened postsynaptic channel (actual ratio of g_{Na}/g_K was found to be 1.3), then the value of the E_{epp} is

$$
\begin{aligned}
E_{epp} &= 0.5\, E_{Na} + 0.5\, E_K \\
&= 0.5\, (+60 \text{ mV}) + 0.5\, (-94 \text{ mV}) \\
&= -17 \text{ mV}
\end{aligned}
$$

Any given postsynaptic channel does not carry current simultaneously in two directions (e.g., an inward Na^+ and an outward K^+ current). Near the resting potential (e.g., –80 mV), the electrochemical driving force for Na^+ (inward) is much greater than that for K^+ (outward), so the vast majority of channels carry an inward Na^+ current (depolarizing) initially (Ca^{2+} is ignored). However, as the postsynaptic

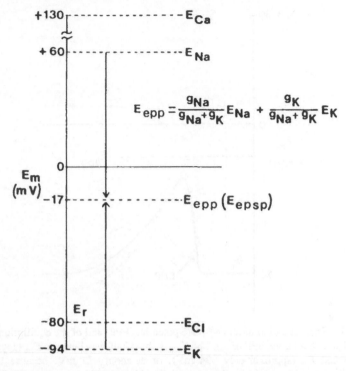

Figure 14 Equilibrium potentials for the four major ions relevant to the generation of synaptic potentials (E_{Na}, E_{Ca}, E_K, and E_{Cl}) and for the end-plate potential (E_{epp}, or excitatory postsynaptic potential, E_{epsp}). The ion channel opened by ACh in the postsynaptic membrane of the vertebrate neuromuscular junction is nonselective for cations (Na^+, K^+, Ca^{2+}), but screens out anions, such as Cl^-. Therefore, since the effect of Ca^{2+} is small and so can be ignored, and since the Na^+ conductance (g_{Na}) of these opened, receptor-operated channels is about equal to the K^+ conductance (g_K), E_{epp} should be about half-way between E_{Na} and E_K, or at about -17 mV, as depicted. This may be calculated from the chord-conductance equation shown.

membrane depolarizes, the driving force for Na^+ becomes less and less, and that for K^+ becomes greater and greater. At the E_{epp}, the two driving forces are equal, and so half the channels would carry an inward Na^+ current and half would carry outward K^+ current (assuming continued activation of the ACh receptors); thus, the net current would be zero, and the membrane potential would not change.

Calculation of End-Plate Potential Amplitude by Circuit Analysis

Using Ohm's law and Kirchhoff's laws, it is possible to calculate the amplitude of the end-plate potential (EPP). The synaptic current (i_{syn}) flows outward through the conductile membrane, producing an I_R drop across the input resistance (R_{in}) of the

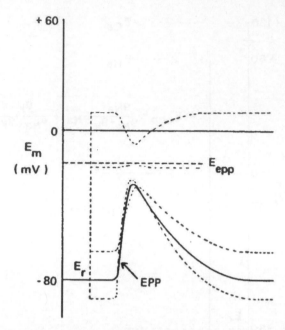

Figure 15 Representation of an end-plate potential (EPP) and of the equilibrium potential or reversal potential for the EPP (E_{epp}). The E_{epp} is about half-way between E_{Na} (approximately +60 mV) and E_K (approximately −94 mV), or at about −17 mV, because the opened postsynaptic channel is about equally conductive to Na$^+$ and K$^+$ ($g_{Na} \simeq g_K$). This E_{epp} value is for a maximally stimulated (by ACh) postsynaptic membrane (i.e., all nicotinic receptors occupied). The EPP is normally initiated from the normal resting potential of the skeletal muscle fiber (approximately −80 mV for mammalian muscle), and tends to approach E_{epp} (solid curve). However, because of the loading-down of the postsynaptic membrane by the adjacent conductile membrane (see circuits in Figs. 17 and 18), the EPP never reaches E_{epp}, but may only reach about −22 mV. If the muscle fiber at the end-plate region is hyperpolarized (by an applied current pulse), the EPP becomes greater in amplitude, as depicted (broken curve). If the muscle fiber is depolarized, the EPP becomes smaller in amplitude, as depicted. If the fiber is depolarized to near the E_{epp} value, the EPP almost entirely disappears (the "null point" or reversal potential). If the fiber is depolarized to the other side of E_{epp}, the EPP inverts in polarity, becoming hyperpolarizing. This illustrates the principle of a reversal potential.

fiber that subtracts from the resting potential (E_r) generated across the conductile membrane (Fig. 16). The i_{syn} flows inward through the postsynaptic membrane, producing an IR drop across its resistance (R_{psm}) that adds to E_{epp} as depicted in Figure 16.

The following equations can be written for the potential difference (PD) across the two legs of the equivalent circuit depicted in Figure 17. The PD across the postsynaptic membrane (E_m', right leg of circuit) and the PD across the adjacent conductile membrane (E_m'', left leg) are

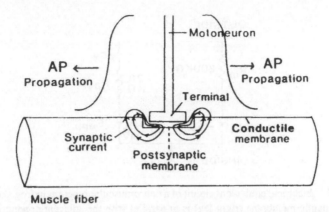

Figure 16 Diagrammatic representation of the neuromuscular junction of vertebrate skeletal muscle, illustrating the close contact between the motor nerve terminal and the postsynaptic membrane of the muscle fiber. Also depicted is the synaptic current (i_{syn}) that flows through the narrow synaptic cleft (≈ 1000 Å), passing inward through the postsynaptic membrane (current sink area) and outward through the adjacent conductile membrane (current source region). Synaptic current produces depolarization in both types of muscle membrane. When the conductile membrane reaches threshold, an action potential is triggered, and propagates in both directions down the muscle fiber toward each end. The end plate is generally located somewhere near the middle region of the longitudinal length of the fiber. The end-plate region occupies about half of the circumferential area of the muscle fiber.

$$E_m' = E_{epp} - i_{syn} R_{psm} \tag{1}$$
$$E_m'' = E_r - i_{syn} R_{in} \tag{2}$$

Since the tops and bottoms of the two legs are connected by relatively low resistances (internal myoplasm and extracellular interstitial fluid), these resistances can be assumed to be zero, as depicted in Figure 17. Therefore, the PD across each leg must be the same, and the following is true:

$$E_m = E_m' = E_m'' \tag{3}$$

To solve Eqs. (1) and (2), the total net synaptic current (i_{syn}) can be calculated from the following relationship (based on Ohm's law):

$$
\begin{aligned}
i_{syn} &= \frac{E_r - E_{epp}}{R_{in} + R_{psm}} \\
&= \frac{(-90 \text{ mV}) - (-15 \text{ mV})}{200 \text{ k}\Omega + 20 \text{ k}\Omega} \\
&= \frac{-75 \text{ mV}}{220 \text{ k}\Omega} \\
&= 0.341 \text{ }\mu\text{A}
\end{aligned}
$$

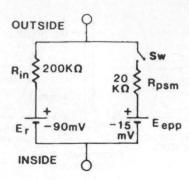

Figure 17 Electrical equivalent circuit of a neuromuscular junction in frog skeletal muscle. The postsynaptic membrane (right leg) is in parallel with the adjacent conductile membrane (left leg of circuit). The input resistance (R_{in}) of the muscle fiber is about 200 kΩ. The resistance of the postsynaptic membrane (R_{psm}), when fully activated by ACh, is about 20 kΩ. Therefore, the membrane potential (E_m) at the neuromuscular junction becomes dominated by the synaptic battery (E_{epp}, equilibrium potential of the end-plate potential) when the synapse is activated (switch, S_w, closed). When the switch is open (psm not activated by ACh), the membrane potential is dominated almost entirely by E_r (resting potential of –90 mV generated across the conductile membrane).

This calculated value for i_{syn} of 0.341 μA is a relatively high value. Assuming the total end-plate area to be 2500 μm² (50 μm × 50 μm), or 2.5×10^{-5} cm² (since 1×10^8 μm²/cm² = 1cm²), this gives a calculated synaptic current density (i_{syn}) of 13.6 mA/cm². This value is even somewhat greater than the current density during the action potential of squid giant nerve fiber.

The calculated value for i_{syn} can now be substituted into Eqs. (1) and (2), and E_m' and E_m'' calculated:

$$E_m' = (-15 \text{ mV}) - (+0.341 \text{ μA}) (20 \text{ kΩ})$$
$$= -15 \text{ mV} - 6.82 \text{ mV}$$
$$= 21.8 \text{ mV}$$
$$E_m'' = (-90 \text{ mV}) - (-0.341 \text{ μA}) (200 \text{ kΩ})$$
$$= -90 \text{ mV} + 68.2 \text{ mV}$$
$$= 21.8 \text{ mV}$$

Therefore, $E_m' = E_m'' = -21.8 \text{ mV} = E_m$.

The current, i_{syn}, flows in opposite directions through the two legs, as depicted in Figure 18, and so has opposite signs. It may be considered as positive in the right leg, because the I_R drop it produces is in such a polarity that it adds to the voltage of E_{epp} [when two batteries are in series (+ – + –), their voltages add]. In the left leg, the current is considered to be negative, because the I_R drop is in such a polarity that it subtracts from the voltage of E_R (the voltages subtract when two batteries in series are back to back: – + + –).

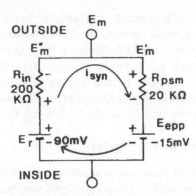

Figure 18 Circuit diagram of the circuit analysis applicable to the generation of the end-plate potential. When the postsynaptic membrane is fully activated by ACh, the membrane potential (E_m) approaches E_{epp}. The synaptic current (i_{syn} flows outward through the conductile membrane (left leg of diagram) and inward through the postsynaptic membrane (right leg of diagram). The synaptic current produces I_R voltage drops across the input resistance (R_{in}) and resistance of the postsynaptic membrane (Rpsm) in opposite polarities, as depicted. These I_R drops subtract from E_r (resting potential of conductile membrane) and add to E_{epp}.

Thus, it is seen that the membrane potential at the peak of the EPP, when the postsynaptic membrane is maximally activated by ACh, is not the theoretical –17 mV (i.e., at E_{epp}), but is about –6.8 mV more negative, namely, –21.8 mV. This difference is caused by the loading-down of the postsynaptic membrane PD by the adjacent conductile membrane. Beginning from a resting potential (E_R) of –90 mV, the total amplitude of the maximal EPP would then be 68.2 mV:

$$\Delta V_{epp} = E_R - E_m$$
$$= (-90 \text{ mV}) - (-21.8 \text{ mV})$$
$$= 68.2 \text{ mV}$$

It becomes evident from Figure 18 and from the circuit analysis presented in the foregoing that the higher the input resistance (R_{in}) of the muscle fiber, the greater is the amplitude of the EPP (ΔV_{epp}), because there is less loading-down of the potential developed across the postsynaptic membrane. Therefore, if membrane-specific resistance (R_m) of the muscle fiber sarcolemma is increased, then ΔV_{epp} becomes greater. Likewise, if the muscle fiber diameter is smaller, R_{in} is greater (since $R_{in} = 1/2 \sqrt{r_m r_i}$), and so ΔV_{epp} would be greater (assuming area of PSM unchanged).

The synaptic current is approximately proportional to the first time-derivative of the EPP; that is, the greatest intensity of synaptic current occurs during the rising phase (depolarizing) of the EPP. (However, the synaptic current does not reverse in direction during the repolarizing phase of the EPP.) The synaptic current rapidly diminishes in intensity and decays to a very low level. Repolarization of the EPP is essentially passive, and occurs after the cause for the depolarization has been removed; namely, the ACh-operated postsynaptic ion channels have reclosed, thereby shutting off the synaptic current. The EPP-repolarizing phase is exponential (after the brief initial portion), and follows the resistance–capacitance (RC) time constant (τ_{rm}) of the muscle cell membrane: about 20 ms for frog sartorius muscle fibers and 1.5 ms for rat EDL muscle (Sellin and Sperelakis, 1978). When membrane-specific resistance (R_m) is altered (e.g., in muscular dystrophy, the τ_m and EPP repolarization change accordingly (Sellin and Sperelakis, 1978).

C. Genesis of the Muscle Impulse

The EPP is generated in the postsynaptic membrane of the muscle fiber, which is an electrically inexcitable membrane. The postsynaptic membrane is chemically excited only by the specific neurotransmitter (and closely related analogues). The EPP is a depolarizing potential. Because of the cable behavior of the muscle fiber, with a length constant (λ) of about 1.0 mm, the EPP causes a depolarization to occur in the conductile membrane (electrically excitable) adjacent to the postsynaptic membrane (see Fig. 16). If this conductile membrane is depolarized to or beyond its threshold potential (V_{th}), it fires an AP. That is, the depolarizing* synaptic current flows inward through the postsynaptic membrane (current *sink* region) and outward through the adjacent conductile membrane (current *source* region), as depicted in Figure 16.

When recording intracellularly near the end-plate region, the EPP is buried or largely masked by the AP that it triggers, but is evident as a step on the rising phase of the AP. The APs that are recorded several millimeters away from the end-plate region are smoothly rising, without any evidence of the EPP, because of the spatial decay of the local EPP caused by the cable properties of the fibers ($\lambda \simeq 1$ mm). If the muscle AP were to be blocked by some means, then the entire EPP would be seen.

Since the neuromuscular junction is usually located somewhere near the middle region of the long muscle fiber, two APs are simultaneously propagated down the fiber, one toward each end. The APs are all-or-none, and propagate at a constant velocity of about 3 m/s. The electrogenesis of skeletal muscle APs and their propagation are discussed in Chapter 2.

In a fraction of the skeletal muscle fibers in a given muscle, there may be two NMJs (motor end plates), each spaced at a distance of about 40% of the fiber length from each end of the fiber, and each arising from a different motoneuron, and usually from different levels of the spinal cord. This arrangement is termed *overlap of motor units*, meaning that a given muscle fiber may be part of two different motor units. (A motor unit consists of one motoneuron and all of the muscle fibers that it innervates.) The origin of the motoneurons from adjacent levels of the

---

*Note that in an excited membrane (e.g., chemically activated postsynaptic membrane or voltage-activated conductile membrane during the peak of an AP), inward current is depolarizing, whereas in a passive (resting) membrane, outward current is depolarizing (and inward current is hyperpolarizing).

spinal cord (e.g., L-3 and L-4) may subserve a small degree of protective function in the event that injury occurs at one level of the spinal cord.

D. Tetanic Contractions

Contractions of skeletal muscles do not occur as twitches (i.e., the brief contractile response to a single muscle AP), but rather, as short or prolonged tetanic contractions. For complete (fused) tetanic contractions, the frequency of muscle APs is between 30 and 60/s, depending on the muscle type. The force of tetanic contraction in a given fiber is severalfold greater than the twitch force, because of the series elastic problem (see Chap. 1). Under physiological conditions, the force of contraction of a given muscle is regulated by (1) increasing the *number of motor units* activated (fiber summation) and (2) increasing the *frequency* of firing of each motor unit (more complete tetanic contraction of each fiber). In addition, the stronger contractions preferentially employ the larger motor units (Henneman's size principle).

E. Slow Fibers

Some skeletal muscle fibers, namely, the true slow fibers, do not fire action potentials under physiological conditions, as do the twitch fibers, in the foregoing described. Instead, the contraction of such fibers is controlled by graded EPPs; the greater the amplitude of the EPP, the greater the force of contraction. The EPPs add by temporal summation. The resting potential of the slow fibers is relatively low, about –60 mV, compared with the values of –80 mV (mammalian) or –90 mV (amphibian) found in the twitch fibers. Each slow fiber has a series of motor end plates distributed along the entire length of the fiber, and spaced about 1 mm apart. All of these end plates are innervated by the same motor neuron. Because the length constant (λ) of the muscle fiber is about 1 mm (i.e., about the interval between neighboring motor end plates), the membrane potential change (depolarization) produced by the summated EPPs is relatively uniform along the entire length of the muscle fiber. Therefore, the contraction produced is relatively uniform along the length of the fiber. Slow fibers are generally found in higher proportion in the postural–tonic skeletal muscles. The slow fibers are smaller in diameter than the twitch fibers, and the myofibrillar organization is less distinct in histological sections.

VI. Actions of Drugs and Toxins

A. Presynaptic Actions

Blockade of Precursor Uptake and Deficiency of Transmitter Synthesis

Hemicholinium-3 (HC-3), a potent competitive inhibitor of the high-affinity choline transport system, effectively prevents synthesis of ACh, which depends on the supply of choline from extracellular medium. During repetitive stimulation in the presence of HC-3, the transmitter store is depleted and MEPP size is smaller; presumably, because synaptic vesicles are unable to replenish their normal content of ACh. This is the only instance known in which an agent reduces quantal size by a presynaptic mechanism. Hyperactive cholinergic neurons may be selectively depressed by this compound. The molecular structure of hemicholinium-3 is given in Figure 19.

Disruption of Transmitter Packaging

α-Latrotoxin, a major polypeptide component of black-widow spider venom, causes massive transmitter exocytosis and depletion of synaptic vesicles from nerve terminals, as revealed by electron microscopy. Synaptic transmission fails in the presence of the toxin. This toxin is not specific to cholinergic terminals.

Uncoupling Secretion From Nerve Terminal Depolarization

Botulinus toxins produced by several strains of *Clostridium botulinum* are responsible for the symptoms associated with food poisoning. The *C. botulinum* neurotoxin is one of the most potent neuroparalytic agents known, with the median lethal dose (LD_{50}) in humans estimated at the submicrogram range. The action of this toxin is essentially irreversible and is exerted following internalization of the molecule or its subunit into the nerve terminal. The block of transmitter release appears to occur at some step of Ca^{2+}-mediated synaptic vesicle exocytosis. Botulinus neurotoxin is specific for cholinergic nerve endings.

Tetanus toxin (*C. tetani*) enters motoneurons at their terminals in muscle—presumably binding to di- and trisialogangliosides—and is transported in retrograde fashion to the cell bodies. The mechanism of action may be to either increase the excitability of motoneurons at postsynaptic sites, or to decrease the release of inhibitory neurotransmitters. The latter requires that the toxin pass across the synaptic cleft and enter the presynaptic nerve terminals. The toxin affects only the inhibitory synapses that are blocked by strychnine, an agent that antagonizes amino acid-mediated inhibitory synaptic events.

Calcium Antagonistic Drugs

Organic calcium antagonist drugs, such as verapamil, D-600, and dihydropyridine derivatives, are not effective blockers of presynaptic Ca^{2+} channels. Verapamil or D-600, at concentrations (10^{-6}–10^{-7} M) that block Ca^{2+} currents in cardiac and vascular smooth muscles (see Sperelakis, 1981), are without effect on evoked release of ACh at vertebrate neuromuscular junctions, or on voltage-dependent influx of Ca^{2+} in isolated nerve endings (synaptosomes) (Gotg'lif and Magazanik, 1977; Nachshen and Blaustein, 1979). Although the calcium antagonistic drugs have little or no effect on the voltage- and time-dependent Ca^{2+} channels in the presynaptic

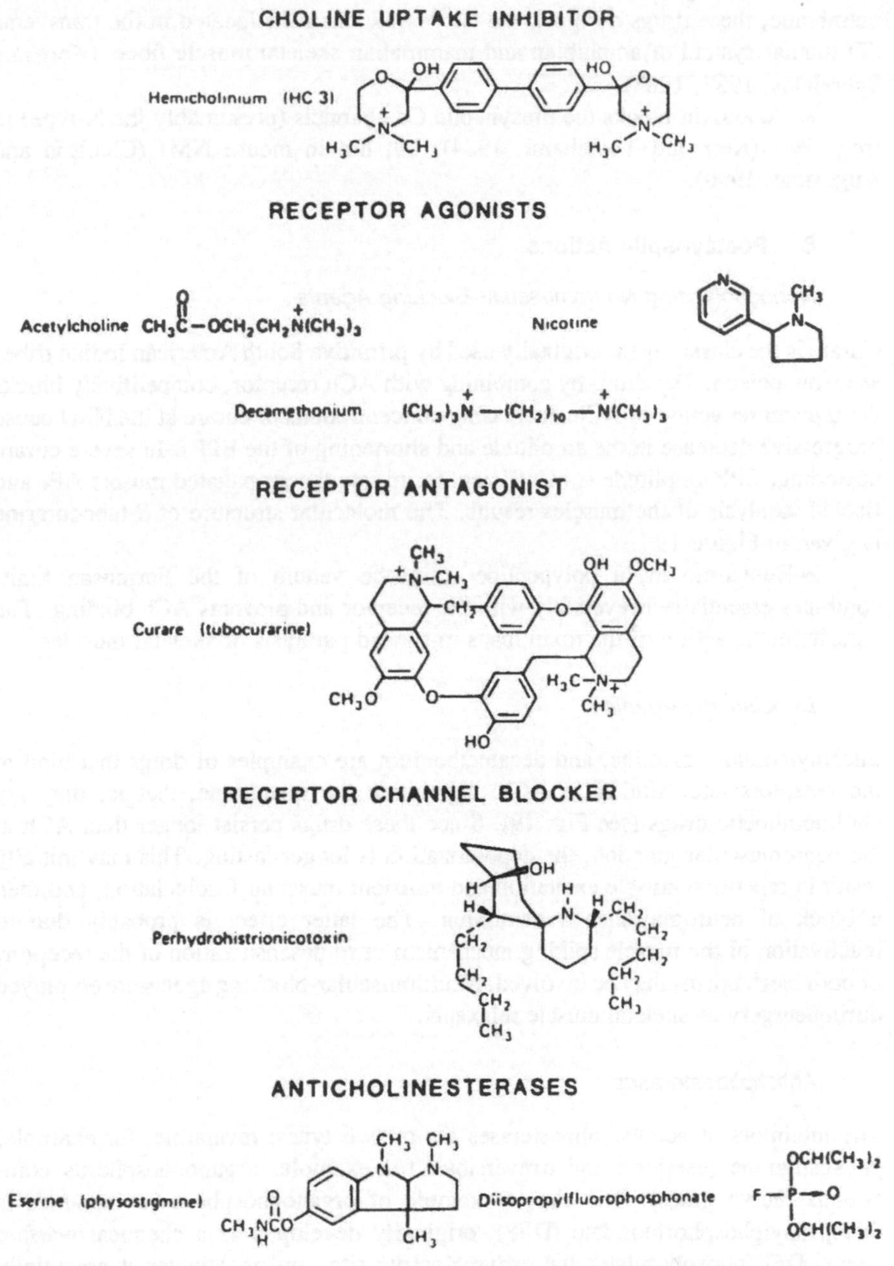

CHOLINE UPTAKE INHIBITOR

Hemicholinium (HC 3)

RECEPTOR AGONISTS

Acetylcholine $CH_3\overset{O}{\underset{}{C}}-OCH_2CH_2\overset{+}{N}(CH_3)_3$

Nicotine

Decamethonium $(CH_3)_3\overset{+}{N}-(CH_2)_{10}-\overset{+}{N}(CH_3)_3$

RECEPTOR ANTAGONIST

Curare (tubocurarine)

RECEPTOR CHANNEL BLOCKER

Perhydrohistrionicotoxin

ANTICHOLINESTERASES

Eserine (physostigmine)

Diisopropylfluorophosphonate

Figure 19 Chemical structures of some drugs active at the neuromuscular junction.

membrane, these drugs do block the Ca^{2+} slow channels located in the transverse (T) tubular system of amphibian and mammalian skeletal muscle fibers (Kerr and Sperelakis, 1982, 1983).

ω-Conotoxin blocks the presynaptic Ca channels (presumably the N-type) in frog NMJ (Kerr and Yoshihami, 1984), but not in mouse NMJ (Charlton and Augustine, 1990).

B. Postsynaptic Actions

Nondepolarizing Neuromuscular-Blocking Agents

Curare is the classic agent originally used by primitive South American Indian tribes as arrow poison. The drug, by combining with ACh receptor, competitively blocks the transmitter action of ACh. Increasing concentrations of curare at the NMJ cause progressive decrease in the amplitude and shortening of the EPPs. In severe curare poisoning, EPP amplitude is insufficient to initiate the propagated muscle AP, and flaccid paralysis of the muscles results. The molecular structure of d-tubocurarine is given in Figure 19.

α-Bungarotoxin, a polypeptide from the venom of the Formosan krait, combines essentially irreversibly with the receptor and prevents ACh binding. The curarimimetic action of the toxin leads to flaccid paralysis of skeletal muscles.

Depolarizing Agents

Succinylcholine, nicotine, and decamethonium are examples of drugs that bind to the receptors and, similar to ACh, depolarize the membrane; that is, they are cholinomimetic drugs (see Fig. 19). Since these drugs persist longer than ACh at the neuromuscular junction, the depolarization is longer-lasting. This may initially result in repetitive muscle excitation and transient muscular fasciculation, and then a block of neuromuscular transmission. The latter effect is probably due to inactivation of the muscle spiking mechanism or to desensitization of the receptor, or both mechanisms may be involved. Neuromuscular-blocking agents are employed during surgery as skeletal muscle relaxants.

Anticholinesterases

The inhibitors of acetylcholinesterases are of two types: reversible, for example, physostigmine (eserine); and irreversible, for example, organophosphorus compounds (nerve gases). The classic example of organophosphorus compounds is diisopropylphosphofluoridate (DFP), originally developed as a chemical warfare agent. DFP phosphorylates the enzyme-active site, and inactivates it essentially irreversibly, since dephosphorylation occurs extremely slowly ($t_{1/2}$ several weeks). The reversible agents are generally compounds that carbamylate the enzyme's active site. Decarbamylation of the enzyme is slow (several minutes), and the enzyme is effectively inhibited against ACh only as long as the inhibitor is present. The result of AChE inhibition is a buildup of ACh concentration in the synaptic cleft. This allows multiple interactions of ACh with the receptors and leads to a longer-lasting depolarization of the end plate. As with the depolarizing neuromuscular blockers, this may initially give rise to repetitive excitation, which is then followed by flaccid paralysis of muscle. The molecular structures of two anti-AChEs are given in Figure 19.

Receptor Channel Blockers

In addition to drugs that interact with ACh-binding sites, various antagonists may interfere with cationic ionophore of the receptors. Examples of this type of action are provided by histrionicotoxin (HTX; an alkaloid from the skin of the Colombian frog *Dendrobates histrionicus*) and phencyclidine (PCP; a hallucinogen) (Eldefrawi, 1979). The molecular structure of a perhydro derivative of HTX is given in Figure 19. Other drugs that modify the end-plate currents by interacting either with the receptor channel or with its microenvironment include the antimalarial drug quinacrine, local anesthetics procaine and lidocaine, the antiviral and antiparkinsonian drug amantadine, and the antispasmodic drug adiphenine (Albuquerque et al., 1980). There is also some evidence that some anti-AChEs also act on the receptor channel, in addition to their action on the enzyme (Albuquerque et al., 1980).

VII. Diseases of the Neuromuscular Junction: Myasthenia Gravis

Myasthenia gravis (MG) is a disorder caused by autoimmune response to ACh receptors, which leads to a reduction in the number of functional receptors and destruction of postsynaptic membrane and, thereby, impairs neuromuscular transmission (reviewed by Drachman, 1981). The characteristic feature of the disease is muscle weakness, especially affecting cranial muscles and limb muscles. There is a tendency for the weakness to vary in severity over a time period (day to day), with remissions and exacerbations evident over longer periods.

Before 1970, the defect in the myasthenic neuromuscular junctions was thought to be of presynaptic origin. This concept was based on the report of Elmquist et al. (1964) that the miniature end-plate potentials recorded from human intercostal muscle were greatly reduced in myasthenia. Since there was no apparent reduction in the responsiveness of the postjunctional membrane, it appeared that a reduction in the amounts of acetylcholine released underlay the impairment of neuromuscular transmission. However, Albuquerque et al. (1976) repeated the intercoastal muscle studies and found a decreased postjunctional responsiveness in myasthenic muscle. The latter electrophysiological studies substantiated the earlier autoradiographic work of Fambrough et al. (1973), who demonstrated a decreased number of α-[^{125}I]-bungarotoxin-binding sites (AChR) in human myasthenic end-plates.

The clue to the autoimmune nature of the disease was provided by the observation of Patrick and Lindstrom (1973) that rabbits injected with an AChR, purified from electric eel for the purpose of obtaining anti-AChR antibodies, developed typical myasthenic symptoms. This serendipitous discovery soon led to the demonstration of receptor antibody titers in myasthenic sera. The role of the antibody in the pathogenesis of MG and experimental autoimmune MG (EAMG, induced by injection of purified receptors) was confirmed by the demonstration that injection of IgG from myasthenic patients into mice caused a reduction in the number of functional receptors and a reduced amplitude of EPPs (Toyka et al., 1977).

The mechanism for the reduction of ACh receptors in MG and EAMG appears to involve an increase in rate of receptor turnover. This is thought to result from cross-linkage of receptors by antibody, with consequent stimulation of endocytosis and degradation of receptors (Appel et al., 1977). Additionally, the characteristic alterations of postsynaptic morphology, which indicate a destruction of the postjunctional membrane, are probably due to membrane complement-mediated focal lysis after binding of antireceptor antibodies activating complement (Engel et al., 1979).

The myasthenic symptoms are improved by anticholinesterases, such as physostigmine, which, as discussed in the preceding sections, elevate ACh concentration and prolong its action at the synaptic cleft. In some patients, administration of anticholinesterase produces a striking, albeit temporary, relief from myasthenic symptoms. For more prolonged treatments, thymectomy, steroids, immunosupportive drugs, and plasmaphoresis have been employed.

References

Adams, D. J., Dwyer, T. M., and Hille, B. (1980). The permeability of endplate channels to monovalent and divalent cations. *J. Gen. Physiol.* 75: 493–510.

Albuquerque, E. X., Rash, J. E., Mayer, R. F., and Satterfield, J. R. (1976). An electrophysiological and morphological study of the neuromuscular junction in patients with myasthenia gravis. *Exp. Neurol.* 51: 536–563.

Albuquerque, E. X., Adler, M., Spinak, C. E., and Aquayo, L. (1980). Mechanism of nicotinic channel activation and blockade. *Ann. N. Y. Acad. Sci.* 358: 204–238.

Anderson, C. R., and Stevens, C. F. (1973). Voltage clamp analysis of acetylcholine produced endplate current fluctuations at frog neuromuscular junction. *J. Physiol. (Lond.)* 235: 655–691.

Appel, S. H., Anwyl, R., McAdams, M. W., and Elias, S. (1977). Accelerated degradation of acetylcholine receptor from cultured rat myotubes with myasthenia gravis sera and globulins. *Proc. Natl. Acad. Sci. USA* 74: 2130–2134.

Atwood, H. L., and Johnston, H. S. (1968). Neuromuscular synapses of a crab motor axon. *J. Exp. Zool.* 167: 457–470.

Axelsson, J., and Thesleff, S. (1959). A study of supersensitivity in denervated mammalian skeletal muscle. *J. Physiol. (Lond.)* 149: 178–193.

Brosius, D. C., Hackett, J. T., and Tuttle, J. B. (1990). Presynaptic calcium currents evoking quantal transmission from avian ciliary ganglion neurons. *Synapse* 5: 313–323.

Ceccareli, B., Hurlbut, W. P., and Mauro, A. (1973). Turnover of transmitter and synaptic vesicles at the frog neuromuscular junctions. *J. Cell. Biol.* 51: 499–524.

Charlton, M. P., and Augustine, G. J. (1990). Classification of presynaptic calcium channels at the squid giant synapse: Neither T-, L-, nor N-type. *Brain Res.* 525: 133–139.

Charlton, M. P., Smith, S. J., and Zucker, R. S. (1982). Role of presynaptic calcium ions and channels in synaptic facilitation and depression at the squid giant synapse. *J. Physiol. (Lond.)* 323: 173–193.

Colmeus, C., Gomez, S. Molgo, J., and Thesleff, S. (1982). Discrepancies between spontaneous and evoked synaptic potentials at normal, regenerating and botulinum toxin poisoned mammalian neuromuscular junctions. *Proc. R. Soc. Lond. B.* 215: 63–74.

Conti-Tronconi, B. M., and Raffery, M. A. (1982). The nicotonic cholinergic receptor: Correlation of molecular structure with functional properties. *Annu. Rev. Biochem.* 51: 491–530.

Couteaux, R., and Pecot-Dechavassine, M. (1970). Vesicules synaptiques et poches au niveau des zones actives de la jonction neuromusculaire. *C. R. Seances Acad. Sci. D.* 271: 2346–2349.

Creutz, C. E., Pazoles, C. J., and Pollard, H. B. (1978). Identification and purification of an adrenal medullary protein (synexin) that causes calcium-dependent aggregation of isolated chromaffin granules. *J. Biol. Chem.* 253: 2858–2866.

Creutz, C. E., Zaks, W. J., Hamnan, H. C., and Martin, W. H. (1986). The roles of Ca^{2+}-dependent, membrane binding proteins in the regulation and mechanism of exocytosis. In *Cell Fusion*. Edited by A. Sowers. New York, Plenum Press.

De Camilli, P., Harris, S. M., Huttner, W. B., and Greengard, P. (1983). Synapsin I (protein I), a nerve terminal-specific phosphoprotein: II. Its specific association with synaptic vesicles demonstrated by immunocytochemistry in agrarose-embedded synaptosomes. *J. Cell Biol.* 96: 1355–1373.

del Castillo, T., and Katz, B. (1954). Quantal components of the endplate potential. *J. Physiol.* 124: 560–593.

Dennis, M. J., and Miledi, R. (1974). Electrically induced release of acetylcholine from denervated Schwann cells. *J. Physiol. (Lond.)* 237: 431–452.

Dionne, V. E., Steinbach, J. N., and Stevens, C. F. (1978). An analysis of the dose–response relationship at voltage-clamped frog neuromuscular junctions. *J. Physiol. (Lond.)* 281: 421–444.

Drachman, D. (1981). The biology of myasthenia gravis. *Annu. Rev. Neurosci.* 4: 195–225.

Eccles, J. C. (1964). *The Physiology of Synapses*. New York, Academic Press, 1964.

Eldefrawi, M. E. (1979). Interactions of drugs with the nicotinic acetylcholine receptor. In *Membrane Mechanisms of Drugs and Abuse*. Edited by C. W. Sharp and L. G. Abood. New York, Alan R. Liss, pp. 63–71.

Elmquist, D., Hofmann, W. W., Kugelberg, J., and Quastel, D. M. J. (1964). An electrophysiological investigation of neuromuscular transmission in myasthenia gravis. *J. Physiol. (Lond.)* 174: 417–434.

Engel, A., Satrashi, K., Lambert, E., and Howard, F. (1979). The ultrastructural localization of the acetylcholine receptor, immunoglobulin G, and the third and ninth complement components at the motor endplate and implications for the pathogenesis of myasthenia gravis. *Excerpta Medica Int. Congr. Ser.* 455: 111–122.

Evers, J., Laser, M., Sun, Y.-A., Xie, Z.-P., and Poo, M.-M. (1989). Studies of nerve–muscle interactions in xenopus cell culture: Analysis of early synaptic currents. *J. Neurosci.* 9: 1523–1539.

Fambrough, D. M., Drachman, D. B., and Satyamurti, S. (1973). Neuromuscular junction in myasthenia gravis: Decreased acetylcholine receptors. *Science* 183: 293–295.

Fertuck, H. C., and Saltpeter, M. M. (1976a). Localization of acetylcholine receptor by ^{125}I-labeled α-bungarotoxin binding at mouse motor endplates. *Proc. Natl. Acad. Sci USA* 71: 1376–1378.

Fertuck, H. C., and Saltpeter, M. M. (1976b). Quantitation of junctional and extrajunctional acetylcholine receptors by electron microscope autoradiography after ^{125}I-α-bungarotoxin binding at mouse neuromuscular junctions. *J. Cell Biol.* 69: 144–158.

Gotg'lif, L. M., and Magazanik, L. G. (1977). Effect of substances blocking calcium channels (verapamil, D-600, manganese ions) on transmitter release from motor nerve endings in frog muscle. *Neirofiziologiia (Kiev)* 9: 320–325.

Hackett, J. T., Cochran, S. C., Greengard, L. J., Brosius, D. C., and Ueda, T. (1990). Synapsin I injected presynaptically into the goldfish Mauthner axon reduces quantal synaptic transmission. *J. Neurophysiol.* 63: 701–706.

Hartzell, H. C., and Fambrough, D. M. (1972). Acetylcholine receptors. Distribution and extrajunctional density in rat diaphragm after denervation correlated with acetylcholine sensitivity. *J. Gen. Physiol.* 60: 248–262.

Heuser, J. E., and Reese, T. S. (1973). Evidence for recycling of synaptic vesicle membrane during transmitter release at the frog neuromuscular junction. *J. Cell Biol.* 57: 315–344.

Heuser, J. E., Reese, T. S., Dennis, M. J., Jan, Y., Jan, L., and Evans, L. (1979). Synaptic vesicle exocytosis captured by quick freezing and correlated with quantal transmitter release. *J. Cell Biol.* 81: 275–300.

Hubbard, J. I., Llinas, R., and Quastel, D. M. J. (1969). *Electrophysiological Analysis of Synaptic Transmission.* London, Edward Arnold Publishers.

Hutter, W. B., DeGennano, L. J., and Greengard, P. (1981). Differential phosphorylation of multiple sites in purified protein I by cyclic AMP-dependent protein kinases. *J. Biol. Chem.* 256: 1482–1488.

Jack, J. J. B., Redman, S. J., and Wong, K. (1981). The components of synaptic potentials evoked in cat spinal motoneurons by impulses in single group Ia afferents. *J. Physiol. (Lond.)* 321: 65–96.

Johnson, E. M., Ueda, T., Maeno, H., and Greengard, P. (1972). Adenosine $3',5',$-monophosphate-dependent phophorylation of a specific protein in synaptic membrane fractions form rat cerebrum. *J. Biol. Chem.* 247: 5650–5652.

Karlin, A. (1983). The anatomy of a receptor. *Neurosci. Commen.* 1: 111–123.

Katz, B. (1966). *Nerve, Muscle, and Synapse.* New York, McGraw-Hill, pp. 1–193.

Katz, B., and Miledi, R. (1972). The statistical nature of the acetylcholine potential and its molecular components. *J. Physiol. (Lond.)* 224: 665–699.

Katz, B., and Miledi, R. (1977). Transmitter leakage from motor nerve endings. *Proc. R. Soc. Lond. B.* 196: 59–72.

Katz, B., and Thesleff, S. (1957). A study of the "desensitization" produced by acetylcholine at the motor endplate. *J. Physiol. (Lond.)* 138: 63–80.

Kennedy, M. B., and Greengard, P. (1981). Two calcium/calmodulin-dependent protein kinases, which are highly concentrated in brain, phosphorylated protein I at distinct sites. *Proc. Natl. Acad. Sci. USA* 78: 1293–1297.

Kerr, L. M., and Sperelakis, N. (1982). Effects of the calcium antagonists verapamil and bepridil (CERM-1978) on Ca^{2+}-dependent slow action potentials frog skeletal muscle. *J. Pharmacol. Exp. Ther.* 222: 80–86.

Kerr, L. M., and Sperelakis, N. (1983). Ca^{2+}-dependent slow action potentials in normal and dystrophic mouse skeletal muscle. *Am. J. Physiol.* 245: C415–C422.

Kerr, L. M., and Yoshikami, D. (1984). A venom peptide with a novel presynaptic blocking action. *Nature* 308: 282–284.

Kharasch, E. D., Mellow, A. M., and Silinsky, E. M. (1981). Intracellular magnesium does not antagonize calcium-dependent acetylcholine secretion. *J. Physiol. (Lond.)* 314: 255–263.

Kistler, J., Stroud, R. M., Klymkowsky, M. W., LaLancette, R. A., and Fairclough, R. H. (1982). Structure and function of an acetylcholine receptor. *Biophys. J.* 37: 371–383.

Korn, H., Triller, A., Mallet, A., and Faber, D. S. (1982). Transmission at a central inhibitory synapse. II. Quantal description of release, with a physical correlate for binomial *n*. *J. Neurophysiol.* 48: 679–707.

Krueger, B. K., Forn, J., and Greengard, P. (1977). Depolarization-induced phosphorylation of specific proteins, mediated by calcium ion influx, in rat brain synaptosomes. *J. Biol. Chem.* 252: 2764–2773.

Kriebel, M. E., and Gross, C. E. (1974). Multimodal distribution of frog miniature and endplate potentials in adult, denervated, and tadpole leg muscle. *J. Gen. Physiol.* 64: 85–103.

Kuffler, S. W., and Nichols, C. (1977). *From Neutron to Brain.* Sunderland, MA, Sinaur Associates.

Kuffler, S. W., and Yoshikami, D. (1975). The number of transmitter molecules in a quantum: An estimate from iontophoretic application of acetylcholine at the neuromuscular synapse. *J. Physiol. (Lond.)* 251: 465–482.

Kuno, M. (1964). Quantal components of excitatory synaptic potentials in spinal motoneurons. *J. Physiol. (Lond.)* 175: 81–99.

Llinas, R., and Nicholson, C. (1975). Calcium role in depolarization–secretion coupling: An aequorin study in squid giant synapse. *Proc. Natl. Acad. Sci. USA* 72: 187–190.

Llinas, R., Steinberg, I. Z., and Walton, K. (1981). Presynaptic calcium currents in squid giant synapse. *Biophys. J.* 33: 289–322.

Llinas, R., McGuinness, T. L., Leonard, C. S., Sugimori, M., and Greengard, P. (1985). Intraterminal injection of synapsin I or calcium/calmodulin-dependent protein kinase II alters neurotransmitter release at the squid giant synapse. *Proc. Natl. Acad. Sci. USA* 82: 3035–3039.

MacIntosh, F. C. (1981). Acetylcholine. In *Basic Neurochemistry.* Edited by G. S. Siegel, R. W. Albers, B. W. Agranoff, and R. Katzman. Boston, Little, Brown & Co., pp. 183–204.

Miledi, R. (1973). Transmitter release induced by injection of calcium ions into nerve terminals. *Proc. R. Soc. Lond. B.* 183: 421–425.

Miledi, R., and Slater, C. R. (1966). The action of calcium on neuronal synapses in the squid. *J. Physiol. (Lond.)* 184: 473–498.

Nachshen, D. A., and Blaustein, M. P. (1979). The effects of some organic "calcium antagonists" on calcium influx in presynaptic nerve terminals. *Mol. Pharmacol.* 16: 579–586.

Neher, E., and Sakmann, B. (1976). Single-channel currents recorded from membrane of denervated frog muscle fibers. *Nature* 260: 799–802.

Neher, E., and Stevens, C. F. (1977). Coductance fluctuations and ionic pores in membranes. *Annu. Rev. Biophys. Bioeng.* 6: 365–381.

Patrick, J., and Lindstrom, J. (1973). Autoimmune response to acetylcholine receptor. *Science* 180: 871–872.

Pecot-Dechavassine, M. (1976). Action of vinblastine on the spontaneous release of acetylcholine at the frog neuromuscular junction. *J. Physiol. (Lond.)* 261: 31–48.

Pumplin, D. W., Reese, T. S., and Llinas, R. (1981). Are the presynaptic membrane particles the calcium channels? *Proc. Natl. Acad. Sci. USA* 78: 7210–7213.

Rahamimoff, R., Meiri, H., Erulkar, S. D., and Barenholz, Y. (1978). Changes in transmitter release induced by ion-containing liposomes. *Proc. Natl. Acad. Sci. USA* 75: 5214–5216.

Sellin, L. C., and Sperelakis, N. (1978). Decreased potassium permeability in dystrophic mouse skeletal muscle. *Exp. Neurol.* 62: 605–617.

Sheridan, M. V., Whittaker, V. P., and Israel, M. (1966). The subcellular fractionation of the electric organ of *Torpedo. Z. Zellforsch. Mikrosk. Anat.* 74: 291.

Sieghat, W., Fom, J., and Greengard, P. (1979) Ca^{2+} and cyclic AMP regulated phosphorylation of same two membrane-associated proteins specific to nervous tissue. *Proc. Natl. Acad. Sci. USA* 76:2475–2479.

Sperelakis, N. (1979). Origin of the cardiac resting potential. In *Handbook of Physiology, The Cardiovascular System,* Vol. 1: The Heart. Edited by R. M. Berne and N. Sperelakis. Washington, DC, American Physiological Society, pp. 187–267.

Sperelakis, N. (1981). Effects of cardiotoxic agents on the electrical properties of myocardial cells. In *Cardiac Toxicology,* Vol. 1. Edited by T. Balazs. Boca Raton, FL, CRC Press, pp. 39–108.

Steinbach, J. H., and Stevens, C. F. (1976). Neuromuscular transmission. In *Frog Neurobiology.* Edited by R. Llinas and W. Precht. New York, Springer-Verlag, pp. 33–92.

Sudhof, T. C., Walker, J. H., and Fritsche, U. (1985). Characterization of calelectrin, a Ca^{2+}-binding protein isolated from the electric organ of *Torpedo marmorata. J. Neurochem.* 44: 1302–1307.

Suszkiw, J. B., and Pilar, G. (1976). Selective localization of a high affinity choline uptake system and its role in ACh formation in cholinergic nerve terminals. *J. Neurochem.* 26: 1133–1138.

Thesleff, S. (1974). Physiological effects of denervation of muscle. *Ann. N.Y. Acad. Sci.* 228: 89–109.

Toyka, K. V., Drachman, D. B., Griffin, D. E., Pestronk, A., Winkelstein, Y. A. Fischbeck, K. H., and Kao, I. (1977). Myasthenia gravis: Study of humoral immune mechanisms by passive transfer to mice. *N. Engl. J. Med.* 269: 125–131.

Ueda, T., Maeno, H., and Greengard, P. (1973). Regulation of endogenous phosphorylation of specific proteins in synaptic membrane fractions from rat brain by adenosine $3',5',$-monophosphate. *J. Biol. Chem.* 248: 8295–8305.

Ueda, T., and Greengard, P. (1977). Adenosine $3':5',$-monophosphate-regulated phosphoprotein system of neuronal membranes. I. Solubilization, purification, and some properties of an endogenous phosphoprotein. *J. Biol. Chem.* 252: 5155–5163.

Vyskocil, F., and Illes, P. (1977). Nonquantal release of transmitter at mouse neuromuscular junction and its dependence on the activity of (Na^+-K^+)-ATPase. *Pflugers Arch.* 370: 295–297.

Walker, J. H. (1982). Isolation from cholinergic synapses of a protein that binds to membranes in a calcium-dependent manner. *J. Neurochem.* 39: 815–823.

Wernig, A. (1976). Localization of active sites in the neuromuscular junction of the frog. *Brain Res.* 118: 63–72.

Whittaker, V. P. (1982). Biophysical and biochemical studies of isolated cholinergic vesicles from *Torpedo marmorata*. *Fed. Proc.* 41: 2759–2764.

5

Structure and Function of the Respiratory Muscles

RICHARD H. T. EDWARDS

University of Liverpool
Liverpool, England

JOHN A. FAULKNER

University of Michigan
Ann Arbor, Michigan

I. Introduction

The diaphragm and accessory (external and internal intercostals, abdominal, scalenes, and sternomastoid) muscles of respiration are embryologically, morphologically, and functionally skeletal muscles. These respiratory muscles are the only skeletal muscles that contract with a regular rhythm throughout the life span. During walking or running, skeletal muscles of the arms and legs contract rhythmically as the muscles of respiration do during breathing, but when the walking or running ceases, breathing continues. In this way, continuous rhythmic activity of the respiratory muscles is analogous to the activity of the heart.

The diaphragm and accessory muscles are also unique in their resting position (Fenn, 1963). The resting position of the respiratory muscles is dictated by the elastic recoil forces of the lung and the effect of gravity on the ribs and on the contents of the thorax and the abdomen. The resting position of the diaphragm muscle and the accessory muscles of respiration (Rochester, 1992) are in dynamic equilibrium as a result of these several forces. The point of equilibrium may change as a result of posture; neural input to the respiratory muscles; or a state of disease in the lungs, tissues of the chest wall, muscles of respiration, or respiratory passages. The accessory muscles, because of their attachments and architecture, are less likely to be affected than the diaphragm muscle. The resting position of the respiratory muscles has a significant effect on their functional capacities. Skeletal muscles in the arms and legs have no such unique dynamic equilibrium in their resting position. Compared with skeletal muscle fibers, fibers in respiratory muscles have a higher oxidative capacity, higher capillary density, higher maximum blood flow, and greater resistance to fatigue. These structural and functional properties of respiratory muscles differ from those of limb muscles, presumably because of the frequency of their use (see Chap. 9). In spite of these quantitative differences, the muscles of respiration are skeletal muscles, and they have the basic anatomical, physiological, and biochemical characteristics of skeletal muscles.

II. Structural Properties of Respiratory Muscles

The structural characteristics of the fibers in the diaphragm and in the accessory muscles of respiration can be described in terms of the proportions of the different types of fibers present, the morphological characteristics of the fibers, and the motor unit organization.

A. Classification of Fibers

Muscles were described initially as red or white, based on gross differences in color that result from myoglobin content (Needham, 1926). This terminology was later applied to skeletal muscle fibers (Gauthier and Padykula, 1966). Since the classification "red" included fibers with low and high activities for myofibrillar ATPase, the term "intermediate" was used for fast-red fibers (Table 1). More recent classification systems have designated single fibers as type I, type IIA, and type IIB, based on myofibrillar ATPase activity, measured histochemically at different pHs (Brooke and Kaiser, 1970), or slow-oxidative, fast-oxidative–glycolytic, and fast-glycolytic according to histochemical myofibrillar ATPase activity and succinic acid dehydrogenase (SDH) activity (Peter et al., 1972). Motor units have been

Table 1 The Different Terms Applied to the Three Types of Mammalian Skeletal Muscle Fibers

Ref.	Classification		
Brooke and Kaiser, 1970	Type I	Type IIA	Type IIB
Burke et al., 1973	Slow	Fast–fatigue-resistant	Fast-fatigable
Peter et al., 1972	Slow-oxidative	Fast-oxidative–glycolytic	Fast-glycolytic
Needham, 1926	Red	Intermediate	White

Note: Initially, the designation "red" included type I and type IIA fibers based on their redness caused by high myoglobin concentration. The classification "intermediate" was added much later to bring the red–white classification in line with the other classification systems.

classified as slow (S), fast–fatigue-resistant (FR), and fast-fatigable (FF) on the basis of the contraction time, the "sag" during unfused tension, and the fatigability, as measured by the proportion of initial force remaining after 2 min of repeated isometric contractions (Burke et al., 1973; Fig. 1). This functional classification of motor units appears valid for the hind limb muscles of rats (Côté and Faulkner, 1986) and cats (Burke et al., 1973); the diaphragm muscle of cats (Sieck, 1988); the medial gastrocnemius muscle of humans (Garnett et al., 1978); and with modifications the thenar muscles of humans (Bigland-Ritchie et al., 1992).

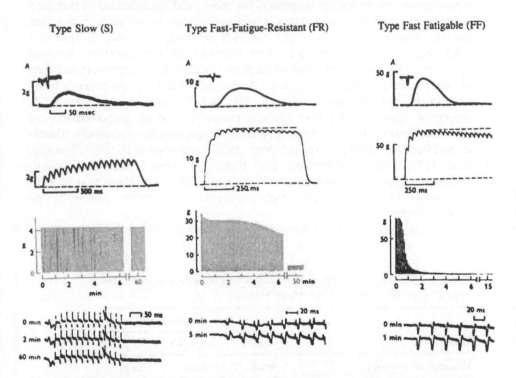

Figure 1 The contractile properties of single motor units from a gastrocnemius muscle of a cat. Isometric contractile properties of type S, type FR, and type FF motor units are shown for a twitch contraction; an infused tetanic contraction (50–40 Hz); and a graph of tension development during stimulation at a firing frequency of 70/s, each tetanic contraction lasting 200 ms and repeated every 1 s throughout the duration of time shown on the abscissa of the graph. Time to peak twitch tension and half-relaxation time are longest for type S, shortest for type FF, and intermediate for type FR. Type FR and FF motor units show "sag," whereas type S do not. No loss of tension is observed for type S motor units, a rapid loss of tension occurs for type FF motor units, and for type FR motor units tension is lost gradually over a period of 50 min. Under most circumstances, type S are equivalent to type I, type FR to type IIA, and type FF to type IIB, but there are exceptions (see text). (Modified from Burke et al., 1973.)

   Under most conditions, each method provides a similar general scheme of classification for single fibers or for fibers within a given motor unit (see Table 1). The three major fiber types have characteristic histochemical, biochemical, and physiological properties (Table 2), but circumstances exist wherein the histochemical assays give erroneous predictions of the true functional properties of fibers (Gollnick and Hodgson, 1986). Several investigators have postulated the presence of more than three fiber types in mammalian skeletal muscles (Edjtehadi and Lewis, 1979; Romanul, 1974). From data obtained by both biochemical assays and measurements of contractile properties, the most valid interpretation is that each property on which the classification is based constitutes a continuum, rather than discrete divisions among fiber types (Gollnick and Hodgson, 1986). In spite of a valid rationale for a continuum for each characteristic, conceptual and practical advantages exist for the utilization of the three fiber types. Throughout this chapter we will use the classification of type I, IIA, and IIB when the classification is based on histochemical analyses and type S, FR, and FF when based on contractile properties. Each of these fiber types is present in varying proportions in the intercostal, abdominal, sternomastoid, and diaphragm muscles of mammals (Gauthier and Padykula, 1966; Davies and Gunn, 1972; Lieberman et al., 1973; Faulkner et al., 1979; McCully and Faulkner, 1983; Sieck et al., 1983; Metzger et al., 1985), including humans (Lieberman et al., 1973; Keens et al., 1978; Hards et al., 1990). Presumably, the same three fiber types are present in the scalene muscle, but no data are available.

   Gauthier and Padykula (1966) noted that, although the diaphragm muscle has

Table 2 Summary of the Relative Characteristics Generally Associated with Type I, Type IIA, and Type IIB Motor Units

Characteristics	Type of motor unit		
	Type I	Type IIA	Type IIB
Motoneuron diameter	Small	Medium	Large
Fibers per motor unit	Few	Intermediate	Many
Myoglobin concentration	High	High	Low
Mitochondrial density	High	High	Low
Oxidative phosphorylation potential	High	High	Low
Glycolytic potential	Low	High	High
Myosin ATPase activity	Low	High	High
Ca^{2+} uptake	Slow	Fast	Fast
Maximum blood flow	High	High	Low
Recruitment frequency	Often	Occasional	Seldom
Rate of development of force	Slow	Fast	Fast
Force development per motor unit	Low	Moderate	High
Resistance to fatigue	High	High	Low

a similar function in all species, there are striking differences in the frequency and "speed" of contraction. They concluded that red fibers are preponderant in the diaphragms of small mammals with high metabolic rates and high respiratory frequencies, whereas white fibers are preponderant in the diaphragms of large species with low metabolic activities and low respiratory frequencies. The classification of red fibers includes both type I and type IIA fibers, both with a high-oxidative capacity. The white fibers are all of type IIB.

The proportions of the different fiber types in the diaphragm muscles of small mammals, body masses 5–100 g, are similar. A 40-g mouse and a 100-g hamster each has a diaphragm muscle composed exclusively of type IIA fibers. In contrast, although 100% of the fibers in the diaphragm muscle of 5- to 20-kg dogs are highly oxidative, approximately 40% of the fibers are type I and the remainder are type IIA. Between these two species are various medium-sized mammals, ranging in weight from 400-g rats to 15-kg monkeys. In spite of a fivefold difference in respiratory frequencies of these mammals, the composition of the diaphragm of each of them is approximately 40% type I, 30% type IIA, and 30% type IIB fibers. The interpretation is that, within a given species, the classification type I, IIA, and IIB signifies the same relative differences among fibers for a wide variety of structural and functional characteristics (Table 3). In contrast, between species, fibers classified as the same fiber type show major differences in structure and function.

In large (500-kg) mammals (oxen, cows, and horses), 80% of the fibers in the diaphragm are type I (Gauthier and Padykuka, 1966). Of the type II fibers, approximately half are type IIA and half type IIB. Specific groupings in the proportions of fiber types are observed in the diaphragm muscles of animals across large ranges in body mass, metabolic rate, and respiratory frequencies. The percentage of highly oxidative fibers remains above 60% for all mammalian species (Faulkner et al., 1979).

Table 3 Contractile Properties of Muscles[a] of the Limbs and of Respiration

Muscle	TPT (ms)	1/2 RT (ms)	V_o (L_o/s)	P_o (N/cm^2)	P_t/P_o
EDL ($N = 8$)	19 ± 1	18 ± 1	14.2 ± 1.3	28.5 ± 1.1	0.16 ± 0.03
Soleus ($N = 7$)	92 ± 7	122 ± 11	5.7 ± 0.3	26.9 ± 1.3	0.24 ± 0.03
Diaphragm ($N = 4$)	30 ± 1	38 ± 2	9.3 ± 0.8	27.8 ± 1.6	0.36 ± 0.03
Intercostals ($N = 13$)	26 ± 1	24 ± 2			0.20 ± 0.02

[a]Muscles were obtained from adult cats (body weights 2.5–4.8 kg).
Note TPT, = time to peak twitch tension; 1/2 RT, half relaxation time from peak twitch tension; V_o, maximum velocity of shortening; P_o, maximum isometric tetanic tension; P_t/P_o, twitch tension/tetanic tension ratio, EDL, extensor digitorum logus muscle.
Source: ELD, Faulkner et al., 1980; soleus, Murphy and Beardsley, 1992; diaphragm, McCully and Faulkner, 1983; intercostals, Anderson and Sears, 1964.

In the diaphragm, the histochemical representation of fiber types appears to provide an accurate representation of the functional properties. The 100% type II fibers in the diaphragms of very small mammals represent fast-twitch fibers (unpublished data, University of Michigan). Similarly, in the diaphragm of the rat, single permeabilized fibers demonstrate almost 100% consistency between the classification of type I and II fibers histochemically and that of slow and fast fibers based on maximum velocity of unloaded shortening (V_{max}) (Eddinger and Moss, 1987). The high respiratory frequencies of the very small rodents require high velocities of shortening and, consequently, sustained high-power outputs, thus the high percentage of fast fibers (Brooks and Faulkner, 1991). The requirements for sustained power and respiratory frequency are much less for medium- and larger-sized animals. As a result, medium-sized animals have as few as 60% type II fibers and the very large have 20% (Gauthier and Padykula, 1966).

During the first week after birth, developmental changes occur in the histochemistry, biochemistry, and contractile properties of limb muscles (Drachman and Johnston, 1973). The slow soleus muscles of rats develop a higher proportion of type I fibers and the speed of contraction slows (Close, 1964). The fast muscles do not change as dramatically with age, but tend to have a slightly slower contractile response at maturity compared with the values at birth (Close, 1964). The exact mechanism of the change is complicated because of differences between fetal, neonatal, and adult myosin isoforms (Hoh and Yeoh, 1979). The different myosin isoforms cause differences in the pH stability of the myofibrillar ATPase, demonstrated histochemically, that may lead to errors in the classification of fibers (Gollnick and Hodgson, 1986).

Following birth, the percentage of type I fibers in the diaphragm of humans increases rapidly from preterm infants up to children 1 year of age. Diaphragm muscles of adult humans are composed of 55 ± 5% type I fibers, 21 ± 6% type IIA fibers, and 24 ± 3% type IIB fibers (Lieberman et al., 1973). The percentage of type I fibers then remains constant at 55–60% throughout adult life. Muscle fiber diameters are greater in men than in women. In the diaphragm muscle, there is no evidence of the type II fiber atrophy so often observed in the limb muscles of elderly, sedentary, persons (Aniansson et al., 1981).

When the composition of the diaphragm muscle of humans has stabilized, samples obtained from the same subject indicate the percentage composition of the intercostal muscles to be 63 ± 2.7% type I fibers, about 10% greater than the diaphragm muscle (Keens et al. 1978). No significant differences were observed between the internal and external intercostal muscles at any age. The intercostal muscles achieve stability in fiber composition during the first few weeks, which is much earlier than the diaphragm muscle.

Although the percentage composition of type I fibers of the intercostal muscles was higher than the diaphragm muscle, the diaphragm muscle shows higher activity for oxidative enzymes (Keens et al. 1978). The abdominal muscles are much more variable in composition than the other muscles of respiration; the range is 40–70%

type II fibers (unpublished data). The oxidative capacity of the abdominal muscles also fluctuates widely.

B. Fiber Isoform Composition

As in skeletal muscles in the limbs, the fibers in the diaphragm and other muscles of respiration are composed of different isoforms of contractile, regulatory, metabolic, and structural proteins. The major differences in the properties of slow and fast fibers are associated with the myosin ATPase activity, which is determined by the myosin isoforms (Staron and Pette, 1986; Pette and Vrbova, 1992). In adult muscle fibers, myosin heavy chain genes express three fast isoforms: MHC-IIa, MHC-IIb, and MHC-IId, and one slow MHC isoform (Pette and Vrbova, 1992; Staron and Pette, 1986). Furthermore, myosin light chain genes express three fast and two slow isoforms (Gauthier and Lowey, 1979).

Compared with myosin obtained from slow fibers, myosin from fast fibers has a higher ATPase activity (Barany, 1967), decreased ATPase stability under acid or alkaline conditions (Barany et al., 1965), differences in the electrophoretic pattern for light chains (Sarkar et al., 1971; Lowey and Risby, 1971) and heavy chains (Pette and Vrbova, 1992). The V_{max}, in particular, correlates significantly with calcium-activated myosin ATPase (Barany, 1967), but the underlying determinant of V_{max} appears to be the myosin heavy chains (Reiser et al., 1985), with modulation by the myosin light chains (Sweeney et al., 1986).

The histochemical analysis of fiber types depends on myofibrillar ATPase activity and, consequently, on the isoforms of myosin, particularly those of the myosin heavy chain (Billeter et al., 1981). In spite of the dependence of fiber classification on the isoforms of myosin, other proteins display different isoforms. Fast and slow isoforms of troponin and tropomyosin have been described (Greaser, et al., 1988), but their functions are less well characterized.

Within a given muscle fiber, the genes for the various proteins tend to express either fast or slow isoforms. Consequently, the histochemical classification (Brooke and Kaiser, 1970; Peter et al., 1972) and the functional classification (Burke et al., 1973) are usually in good agreement. In addition to the expression of fast, rather than slow, isoforms of MHCs, compared with type I fibers, type II fibers show a faster calcium transport ATPase (Heilmann and Pette, 1979) and a higher total uptake and initial rate of uptake of calcium by sarcoplasmic reticulum (Heilmann and Pette, 1979). Structural differences include a more complex neuromuscular junction in type II than in type I fibers. Although homogeneity of gene expression within a given muscle fiber is usually observed, variations do occur particularly during transitions (see Chaps. 9 and 11).

C. Morphological Characteristics of Fibers

The fibers of the diaphragm and accessory muscles of respiration are arranged in fascicles separated by connective tissue. The peripheral portion of the diaphragm is composed of a continuous flat band of fibers (Fig. 2). The different embryological

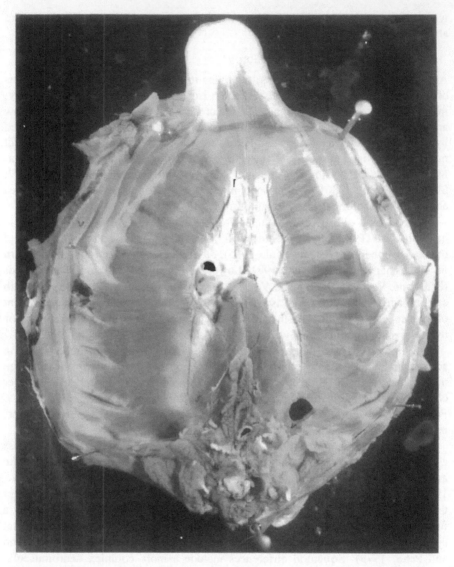

Figure 2 The abdominal surface of the diaphragm of a rat shows the central tendon and the attachments of sheets of fibers to specific ribs. Note the differences in fiber lengths and fiber orientations in different parts of the muscle.

origins of crural, compared with the costal, part of the diaphragm and the differences in function have led to the concept of the diaphragm as being composed of two muscles (de Troyer et al., 1981). The one muscle acts in series and the other in parallel with the rib cage. This concept is developed in detail by de Troyer and Loring (see Chap. 19, Section II.). On the basis of their origin, fibers of the diaphragm are grouped into sternal, costal, and lumbar portions. The sternal fibers have their origin in the xyphoid process and extend to the central tendon. The costal portions also join the central tendon and form the right and left domes of the diaphragm. The right and left crura originate in the lumbocostal spine. The crura pass on either side of the aorta and the esophagus to join the central tendon. The fibers in each crus are parallel (see Fig. 2). The fiber lengths vary considerably in different portions of the diaphragm (Rochester, 1992). The longest fibers are in portions of the crura and in the costal region. Fibers in other portions of the diaphragm may be as much as 50% shorter.

The ultrastructural characteristics of fibers from the diaphragm support the histochemical evidence of many fibers with subsarcolemmal aggregations of mitochondria. The small mammals, such as mice, have considerably more mito-chondria under the sarcolemma and throughout the fiber than do rabbits and other larger species (Leak, 1979). In the diaphragm muscle, each of the three types of fibers tend to have a higher mitochondrial density than the same type of fiber located in a limb muscle. In any given species, more high-oxidative fibers are observed in the diaphragm muscle than in limb muscles. For humans, 80% of the diaphragm muscle is composed of oxidative fibers (i.e., types I and IIA), whereas limb muscles of untrained men vary from 36 to 46% (Gollnick et al. 1972). These differences between the diaphragm muscle and limb muscles result in the diaphragm muscle having a volume density of mitochondria per unit volume of muscle fibers twofold greater than limb muscles (Hoppeler et al., 1981). These characteristics of the diaphragm muscle result in a high capacity to oxidize various substrates and a high resistance to fatigue (Edwards, 1979; Faulkner and Brooks, 1992). Although fewer data are available on the accessory muscles of respiration, data on proportions of fiber types suggest that the intercostal muscles have characteristics similar to the diaphragm muscle. The abdominal, scalenes, and sternomastoid muscles are not as tightly coupled to the respiratory process, and considerable variability in oxidative capacity is observed with differences attributable to both age (see Chap. 10) and physical activity (see Chap. 9).

The histochemical and ultrastructural composition of the respiratory muscles appear to have evolved for multiple functions (Faulkner et al., 1993). The high percentage of oxidative fibers in these muscles, regardless of the species, provides a large number of fatigue-resistant motor units composed of type I and type IIA fibers to sustain respiration at rest. The moderately high percentage of fast type IIA fibers provides an increased power and increased respiratory rate during exercise, and the relatively small proportion of type IIB fibers permit high-power outputs necessary for sneezing and coughing. The presence of exclusively type IIA fibers in the diaphragm muscles of mice and hamsters supports the extremely high respiratory frequencies, even at rest, with over 100 breaths per minute (Gauthier and Padykula, 1966).

D. Motor Unit Organization

Just as in limb muscles (Kugelberg and Edstrom, 1968; Burke et al., 1973), skeletal muscle fibers within a given motor unit (Krnjevic and Miledi, 1957) are broadly dispersed throughout a region of the diaphragm muscle. The dispersion is both horizontally across the surface of the diaphragm and vertically, with fibers at different depths. In cats, the average maximum isometric tetanic force (maximum force) of type II motor units in the diaphragm is 110 mN (Sieck, 1988) compared with 600 mN for those in the medial gastrocnemius muscle (Burke et al., 1973). This indicates that the average size of the fast motor units in the diaphragm is about one-sixth that of units in the medial gastrocnemius muscle. The slow units are small in both muscles, with a range in maximum forces of 30–60 mN. Thus, although the organization and dispersion of fibers within motor units in the diaphragm do not appear to be different from those of limb muscles (Kugelberg and Edstrom, 1968), the area over which fibers are dispersed is smaller (Krnjevic and Miledi, 1957; Sieck, 1988).

In the cat diaphragm, the concentration of motor units innervated by specific nerve roots in a given region of the diaphragm provides evidence for somatotopic organization of motor units (Sieck, 1988). Motor units innervated by C-5 ventral root are found only in the sternocostal and ventral crural regions of the diaphragm, whereas units innervated by C-6 are observed in the dorsal costal and dorsal crural regions. Recruitment of motor units in the diaphragm appears to follow the general principles of the "Henneman size principle" as do other muscles in most circumstances (Henneman and Olson, 1965). For the diaphragm muscle, recruitment by the size principle is modulated, to some degree, by the respiratory rhythm (Sieck, 1988). For the thenar muscles of humans, motor units reach 50% of maximum force at a stimulation frequency between 8 and 10 Hz and maximum force occurs at 30 Hz (Bigland-Ritchie et al., 1992). The narrow range of frequencies involved, coupled with the relatively high forces required during shortening (Brooks and Faulkner, 1991), leaves little room for modulation of force by rate coding.

III. Functional Properties of Respiratory Muscles

Motor units in all skeletal muscles, including those involved in respiration, may be recruited during three different types of contractions: isometric, shortening, or lengthening. A contraction of each of the fibers in a motor unit occurs when a single, or under physiological conditions, multiple action potentials are transmitted across the neuromuscular junction. The action potentials spread across the membrane, through the T-tubule system, and all the myofrils within the activated fiber contract. If the muscle is held at optimum length for force development (L_o), the single action potential will produce an isometric twitch in the activated fibers. Multiple action potentials at a frequency of 10 Hz, or higher, result in a summation of force. If the frequency of stimulation is gradually increased, force plateaus at maximum force. The achievement of maximum force indicates full-activation of a fiber, motor unit, or muscle.

Under any given set of circumstances, when activated by action potentials, muscle fibers actually "attempt" to shorten. Whether the activated fibers remain at the same length, shorten, or lengthen depends on the relative force developed by the activated fibers and the load placed on the muscle. If the force developed by the fibers in a muscle is the same as the load, or a muscle contracts against a fixed load, a fixed length, or isometric, contraction results. If the the force developed by the muscle is greater than the load, a shortening contraction occurs, and if development of a force is less than the load, a lengthening contraction is produced. Forces developed are greatest during lengthening, intermediate during isometric, and least during shortening contractions (Fig. 3). The same number of cross-bridges are strongly bound during each type of contraction (Lombardi and Piazzesi, 1990). Consequently, the differences in force development during the three types of contractions appear to result from variations in the strain on individual cross-bridges.

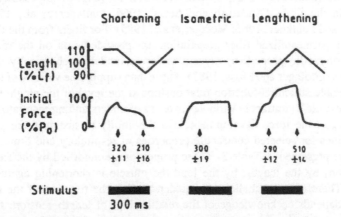

Figure 3 Representative recordings of length (upper traces) and force (lower traces) for shortening, isometric, and lengthening contractions. For each trace the muscle was stimulated for 300 ms at 150 Hz. Isometric contractions (center panel) were initiated at L_o, and muscle length was held constant. Shortening (left panel) and lengthening (right panel) contractions were initiated at 110% of L_f and 90% of L_f, respectively. After 100 ms of stimulation, muscle length was shortened or lengthened by 20% of L_f at a velocity of 1 L_f/s. Power output is the average force developed by the muscle during the shortening contraction times, the velocity of shortening. During a lengthening contraction, external work must be done on the muscle to lengthen it; therefore, power is absorbed. (Modified from McCully and Faulkner, 1985.)

The contractile properties of muscles during isometric, shortening, or lengthening contractions may be assessed in vivo, in situ, or in vitro. Although in vivo tests of muscle function are useful clinically (Edwards et al., 1977b), accurate measurements of contractile properties of the respiratory muscles are difficult. The difficulty arises from the inaccessibility of the muscles of respiration and the complexity of their architecture, including their origins and insertions. To measure contractile properties of respiratory muscles directly, Kim et al., (1976) developed an in situ whole-muscle preparation of the diaphragm muscle of dogs, and Andersen and Sears (1964), an in situ bundle preparation of intercostal muscles in cats. Sieck (1988) has contributed an in situ preparation for investigations of the motor units in the diaphragm muscle of cats.

Ritchie (1954) reported the first data obtained in vitro on the contractile properties of small bundles of fibers from the rat diaphragm muscle. Faulkner et al. (1982) subsequently developed a technique for measuring the contractile properties of small bundles of fiber segments. This technique permits measurements of contractile properties of small segments obtained by open biopsy from muscles with long fibers, such as the human diaphragm. The unique anatomical resting position of the diaphragm, and to a lesser extent, the accessory muscles of respiration, exerts no clear modulating effect on the contractile properties of these muscles. The contraction, relaxation and shortening properties of the respiratory muscles are qualitatively and quantitatively within the range of other skeletal muscles located in the limbs (Andersen and Sears, 1964; Faulkner et al., 1979, 1982; McCully and Faulkner, 1983; Metzger et al., 1985). For fibers from the diaphragm, the single permeabilized fiber preparation has provided data on the relationships among contractile properties, myosin isoforms, and histochemically determined fiber types (Eddinger and Moss, 1987). These data support the validity of the concept of predictable structure–function relationships at the level of the single fiber.

The critical contractile variables in terms of understanding respiratory function are the V_{max}, the force development, and the ability to sustain force and power. Mean values for selected contractile properties of respiratory and limb muscles of the cat are presented in Table 3. These properties are modified by the frequency of stimulation, by the length, by the load the muscle is shortening against, and by fatigue. Therefore, the challenge of understanding the function of the respiratory muscles depends on knowledge of the relationships of length–tension, frequency–force, force–velocity, frequency–power, and frequency–fatigability (see Figs. 4–9).

A. Length–Force Relationships

Muscle fibers produce substantially less force at shorter or longer lengths than at optimal length (Gordon et al., 1966; Fig. 4). McCully and Faulkner (1983) measured the length–force relation of bundles of fiber segments from diaphragm muscles of five mammalian species. The fiber length was adjusted to L_o and stimulation duration was 400 ms. Under these circumstances, no difference is observed between the

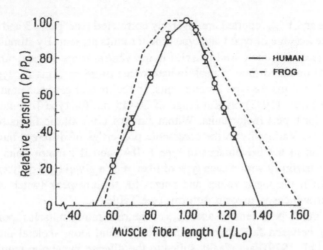

Figure 4 The length–tension relationships for a single frog skeletal muscle fiber (dotted line) and a small bundle of cut fibers from a human diaphragm (solid line). (Modified from Gordon et al., 1966.)

length–active force curves of diaphragm muscles and muscles from the limbs. Similarly, data on bundles of fiber segments from the diaphragm and intercostal muscles of humans are not significantly different from the classic length–force relationship (see Fig. 10), except for the lack of the clear inflection point at 80% of L_0 observed for the single fibers from amphibian muscles (Gordon et al., 1966). The smoothed length–active force curve is obtained when data are collected on bundles of fiber segments (McCully and Faulkner, 1983), or whole limb muscles (Rack and Westbury, 1969). The passive force developed by bundles of fiber segments from the diaphragm muscles of the different species was extremely low. Significant passive forces were not encountered until the length exceeded 115% of L_0 (see Fig. 4).

The amount of shortening that occurs during a contraction is a function of the initial length of the fibers, the angle of pennation, the afterload, and the duration of the contraction. The initial length for most shortening contractions is usually between 100 and 115% of L_0, and shortening occurs to about 75% of L_0 (McCully and Faulkner, 1983). Contractions through more than 25% of fiber length are unusual.

B. Time-Dependent Characteristics of the Twitch

The time-dependent characteristics of the twitch, time to peak twitch force, and half-relaxation time are functions of the kinetics of the release and uptake of calcium by the sarcoplasmic reticulum (SR) (Heilman and Pette, 1979) and of the myosin ATPase activity (Barany, 1967). The characteristics of a twitch are measured at L_0 with a current flow that provides maximum twitch force. In a stable muscle that is not undergoing developmental or experimental changes, the values for time to peak twitch force and V_{max} reported are inversely correlated (see Table 3 and Fig. 5) and represent the average of type I and type II motor units present. By stimulating single motor nerves of the intercostal muscles in the ventral roots of cats, Andersen and Sears (1964) obtained time to peak twitch forces of 25 ± 2 ms for type II motor units and 47 ± 2 ms for type I motor units. In the medial gastrocnemius muscle of cats, Burke et al. (1973) cited a range of 20–55 ms for type II motor units and 58–110 ms for type I motor units. Within a motor unit, all the fibers have similar characteristics. Variability in the contractile properties of different muscles result from variation in the percentages of type I, IIA, and IIB motor units, as well as from some variability within each type of fiber. For a given type of fiber (i.e., type I, IIA, or IIB), the mean values and ranges for time to peak twitch tension vary owing to differences in myosin isoforms (see Table 3).

The time to peak tension and V_{max} of the respiratory muscles, poised as they are halfway between fast skeletal muscle fibers and slow skeletal muscle fibers (Faulkner et al. 1979), are ideally suited to the diverse metabolic requirements of the respiratory muscles for sustained nonfatiguing contractions of type I and IIA fibers and the high-power output of type IIB fibers that cannot be sustained.

C. Frequency–Force Relationships

The frequency–force relationship is presented normally with muscles at L_o (Fig. 6A). With fibers at L_o, the force developed by a skeletal muscle is a function of

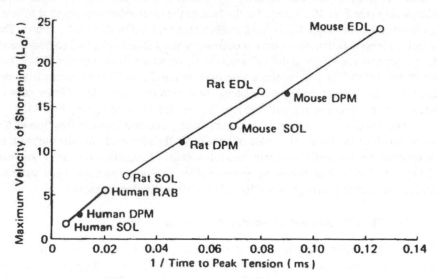

Figure 5 The maximal velocity of shortening expressed as a function of the reciprocal of the time to peak twitch tension of type I slow-twitch soleus (SOL), and of type II fast-twitch extensor digitorum longus (EDL), and the mixed diaphragm (DPM) muscles of mice, rats, and humans. (Modified from Faulkner et al., 1979.)

the frequency of stimulation. The frequency–force relationship results from the summation of twitch force during repeated stimulation. Slow muscles will show summation at lower frequencies of stimulation than fast muscles and, accordingly, higher relative force at a given frequency of submaximum stimulation (see Fig. 6A); consequently, compared with fast muscles, the maximum force development of slow muscles will occur at a lower stimulation frequency.

The effect of fiber length on the frequency–force relationship is complex. The complexity is aggravated by uncontrolled variations in the amount of shortening during the presumably "isometric" contraction as a function of both initial length and frequency of stimulation. Consequently, the effect on force development of lengths shorter than the L_o is of greater magnitude at low frequencies of stimulation than at high frequency (Rack and Westbury, 1969; see Fig. 6B).

The frequency–force relationship is useful in comparisons of force development by different muscles (Fig. 7A) and for the evaluation of high- and low-frequency fatigue by the same muscle (Laroche et al., 1989; see Fig. 7B).

The isometric force developed by a skeletal muscle is a function of the average of the forces developed by the cross-bridges in a strongly bound state present in the total fiber cross section. Consequently, the maximum force can be normalized by the total fiber cross-sectional area (CSA). The total fiber CSA can be obtained from the equation:

$$CSA \ (cm^2) = \frac{Muscle \ mass \ (g)}{Fiber \ length \ (cm) \times muscle \ density}$$

Note: CSA = total fiber cross-sectional area and muscle density = 1.06 g/cc. Muscle density is measured in mass (g) per unit volume of tissue (cc). A "ml" is a measure of the volume of a fluid.

For control muscles, motor units, or single fibers, regardless of fiber type, normalization of the maximum force by total fiber CSA gives a value of ~280 kN/m^2 for the maximum specific force (Brooks and Faulkner, 1988; Close, 1972; Murphy and Beardsley, 1974; Faulkner et al., 1980, 1982; see Table 3).

D. Force–Velocity Relationship

The V_{max} is a linear function of the calcium-activated myosin ATPase activity (Barany, 1967). The relationship between V_{max} and myosin ATPase is valid for muscles from different species, different muscles within the same species, and for single fibers from a given muscle. The myosin ATPase activity is determined primarily by the expression of either slow or fast myosin heavy chains (Reiser et al., 1985), with modulation by the presence of different isoforms of slow and fast myosin light chains (Sweeney et al., 1986). This accounts for a V_{max} for the diaphragm muscle intermediate between the V_{max} of the classic slow soleus and fast EDL muscles (see Table 3 and Fig. 5). In human muscle, the normalized V_{max} (L_f/s) for a number of limb and trunk muscles, measured at 35°C, range from 2 to 6 L_f/s (Faulkner et al., 1986, 1991).

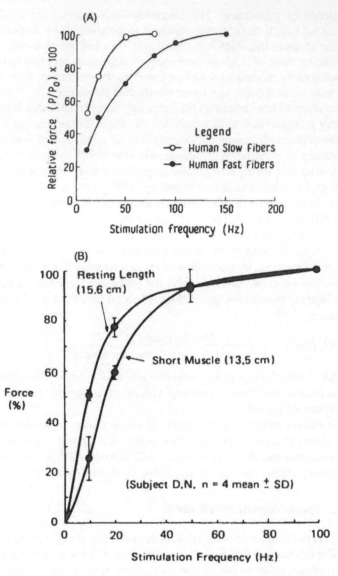

Figure 6 Frequency–force curves for (A) bundles of slow- and fast-fiber segments of muscles from humans; (B) the sternomastoid muscle in a normal subject at optimum length for force development (L_o) and at 87% of L_o. Note the shift to the right of the curve at a shorter length despite the fact that muscle is not fatigued. (A: From Faulkner, 1983.)

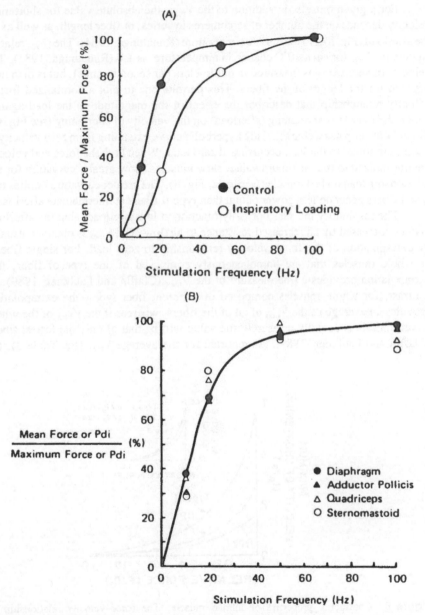

Figure 7 Frequency–force curves for (A) the sternomastoid muscle of a normal subject after a fatiguing respiratory maneuver induced by inspiratory loading. Note the significant loss of force at low frequencies of stimulation. (B) The diaphragm, adductor pollicis, quadriceps, and sternomastoid muscles in normal subjects. Mean values shown. [From Moxham et al. (A) 1981; (B) 1980.]

For a given muscle, in addition to the V_{max}, the absolute value for shortening velocity depends on the number of sarcomeres in series, or fiber length, as well as on the afterload (Fig. 8) and the muscle temperature (Ranatunga, 1984). The Q_{10}, relative change in V_{max} for each 10°C change in temperature, is 1.8 (Ranatunga, 1984). The velocity of shortening is measured in millimeters per second (mm/s), but is then normalized for the length of the fibers. This permits one to plot a normalized force–velocity relationship that describes the effect of the magnitude of the load against which the muscle is shortening (afterload) on the velocity of shortening (see Fig. 8). The relationship has a characteristic hyperbolic curve extending from zero velocity at maximum force, to the V_{max} occurring at zero load. When both the force and velocity are normalized to the maximum value, slow muscles show greater curvature for the relationship than do fast muscles (see inset, Fig. 8). The greater curvature implies that type I fibers generate less power output than type II fibers at intermediate afterloads.

The respiratory muscles normally function at low afterloads, but the afterload may be increased by an increased resistance to airflow. The V_{max} is obtained usually by extrapolation of the force–velocity relationship to zero load. For single fibers, or whole muscles that are homogeneously composed of one type of fiber, this extrapolation provides a true measure of the V_{max} (Claflin and Faulkner, 1989). In contrast, for whole muscles composed of different fiber types, the extrapolation provides an average of the V_{max} of all of the fibers, whereas if the V_{max} of the whole mixed muscle is actually measured, the value will be that of only the fastest fibers (Claflin and Faulkner, 1989). As reported for the average V_{max} (see Table 3), the

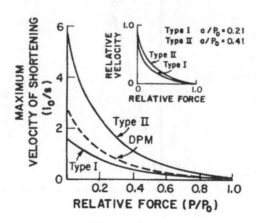

Figure 8 Contractile properties of human muscle. The force–velocity relationship of bundles of type I and type II fibers from limb muscles and for bundles of fibers from the diaphragm (DPM) muscle. The bundles from the diaphragm muscle contained both type I and type II fibers. The inset shows the force–velocity curves for type I and type II fibers, with the abscissa normalized for P_o and the ordinate normalized for V_o. This clarifies the greater curvature of the relationship for type I fibers.

normalized force–velocity relationship of bundles of fiber segments from the diaphragm muscle is intermediate between those of slow (type I) and fast (type II) skeletal muscles (see Fig. 5).

E. Frequency–Power Relationship

The production of airflow into the lungs requires power output by the muscles of respiration; consequently, the ability to develop and sustain power is the most important characteristic of respiratory muscle function. Power may be calculated as the product of the values for velocity and force associated with the force–velocity relationship (see Fig. 8). Under these circumstances, instantaneous peak power occurs at approximately one-third of maximum force and one-third of V_{max}. The most meaningful comparisons are possible when maximum power is measured during a single isovelocity, shortening contraction (Brooks et al., 1990; Fig. 9). The optimum velocity of shortening for the development of power is determined empirically for a given muscle (Fig. 10A). The value (mm/s), always ~30% of the V_{max}, multiplied by the integrated area under the curve for force (mN) equals the power (mW).

As with the frequency–isometric force relationship (see Figs. 6 and 7), the frequency–shortening force (see Fig. 10B) and frequency–power (see Fig. 10C) relationships show a similar dependency of force and power on the frequency of stimulation. The relationships ultimately plateau at maximum values for shortening force and power (see Fig. 10B,C). Similar to force, which is normalized per unit of total fiber CSA, the power, a product of force times velocity, is normalized by muscle mass (Brooks et al., 1990). Under circumstances of a single contraction, fast muscles of mice generate 275 W/kg and slow muscles 75 W/kg (Brooks et al., 1990). During a single maximum voluntary contraction, the biceps muscle of an adult man generates 226 W/kg.

Power decreases rapidly from the value produced during a single contraction to the power sustained during repeated contractions (Fig. 11). The decrease in sustained, compared with maximum, power results from the introduction of a duty cycle that is less than 1.0 and the loss of shortening force (Brooks and Faulkner, 1991). Even for exhaustive exercise of a few minutes duration, the sustained power is reduced to 30% of the maximum power during a single contraction. The energy cost of ventilation at rest has been estimated to be 5% of the resting metabolic rate. This would calculate to a sustained power output of 2 W/kg for the diaphragm muscle, which seems excessively high.

F. Respiratory Muscle Function and Fatigue

Failure to sustain force or power output is one of the defining characteristics of fatigue (Macklem, 1990), but fatigue also includes a deterioration in the capacity to generate maximum force or power output with continued or repeated submaximum

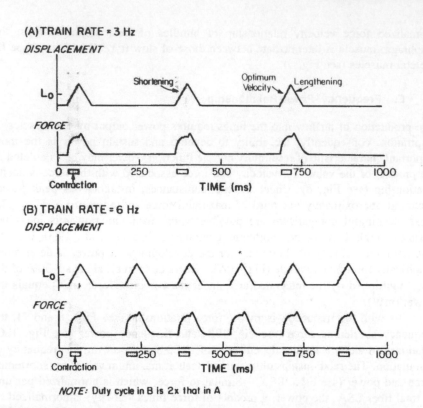

Figure 9 Drawings of examples of experimental records of repeated shortening contractions at two different train rates in identical time scales. Repeated contractions at a train rate of (A) three contractions per second and (B) at six contractions per second. Upper traces in both A and B show displacements of lever during shortening and lengthening of muscle. Displacement of muscle occurs around optimum muscle length (L_o). Lower traces show forces developed by muscle. Stimulation duration is designed by stippled bars during shortening ramp. (Modified from Faulkner et al., 1990.)

activity (Faulkner and Brooks, 1992). In the latter context, fatigue is an ongoing process. For the respiratory muscles, power is approximately equal to pressure (mm Hg) times airflow (ml/s). A failure to sustain power, or to generate maximum power, may reflect a loss in the ability to develop force, velocity, or both (Metzger and Moss, 1987). The metabolic requirements of ventilation on the muscles of respiration, even during heavy exercise, are low relative to the metabolic requirements of a maximum voluntary ventilation test (Vollestad et al., 1988). Consequently, the impaired development of maximum force, power, or both, is not only an important manifestation of diaphragmatic fatigue, but the defining character of fatigue of the respiratory muscles (Macklem, 1990).

    Important distinctions can be made between the central and peripheral

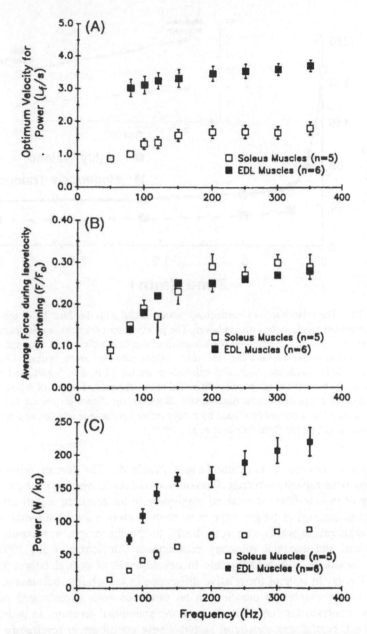

Figure 10 The relationships between frequency of stimulation and (A) optimum velocity for the development of power; (B) the average force developed during the isovelocity shortening contraction; and (C) the normalized power (W/kg) during a single contraction. The data were collected on in situ muscle preparations of slow soleus and fast extensor digitorum longus muscles of mice. Muscle temperature was 35°C.

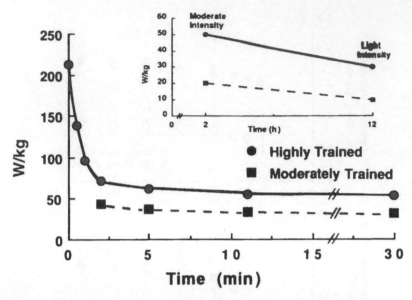

Figure 11 The relationship of normalized power output with the duration of the physical activity in minutes and, in the inset, in hours. The power is for cycling on a stationary bicycle ergometer. The power is normalized per kilogram of active muscle on the assumption that 7 kg of muscle is active in each leg (see text). (Data modified from Wilkie, 1960.) The designations light, moderate, high, and exhaustive are for 12 h, 2 h, 5 min, and <5 min. The data are in reasonable agreement with actual measurements of power of whole muscles during single and repeated contractions in situ. Note the significant difference in the effect of time on the relative power developed by highly trained endurance athletes and moderately trained adults. (Modified from Faulkner et al., 1992.)

mechanisms involved in muscular fatigue (Table 4). The former represents an alteration in the capacity to recruit all possible motor units, whereas the latter reflects a failure of muscle fibers to respond maximally in the presence of full activation. Central mechanisms of fatigue have been studied using a sensitive twitch interpolation technique in which electrical shocks to the diaphragm were made during submaximal and maximal voluntary contractions (McKenzie et al., 1992). The human diaphragm is less susceptible to development of central fatigue than the elbow flexors. In spite of the relative difference in fatigability, substantial central fatigue of the diaphragm muscle can be produced with a prolonged series of expulsive contractions that markedly raise the abdominal pressure. In pathological states, both central and peripheral factors likely contribute to respiratory muscle fatigue (Moxham, 1992). Whether respiratory fatigue occurs spontaneously, or whether built-in compensatory mechanisms intervene and delay the onset of fatigue has not been resolved. Muscles may fail to generate sufficient force as the result of being inadequately driven by their motor innervation, as during a failure of

Table 4 Physiological Classification of Fatigue

Type fatigue	Possible definition	Mechanism
Central	Force or heat generated by voluntary effort less than that by electrical stimulation	Failure to sustain recruitment or decreased frequency of stimulation of motor units
Peripheral	Same force loss or heat generation with voluntary and stimulated contractions	
High-frequency fatigue	Selective loss of force at high-stimulation frequencies	Impaired neuromuscular transmission or propagation of muscle action potential
Low-frequency fatigue	Selective loss of force at low-stimulation frequencies	Impaired excitation–contraction coupling or direct impairment of force development by cross-bridges

Source: Based on Edwards (1979).

motivation in voluntary muscular contractions, or possibly, a failure of central respiratory drive, as the result of depressant drugs or CO_2 narcosis. In spite of the possibilities, fatigue arising because of a decreased central respiratory drive is not a likely factor in most cases of impaired respiratory function (Bigland-Ritchie et al., 1978).

When central fatigue is excluded, two forms of muscle fatigue can be demonstrated following electrical stimulation (see Table 4). High-frequency fatigue occurs after brief periods of stimulation at a frequency of 60–80 Hz. The loss in force is most pronounced at high frequencies and may be almost normal at lower frequencies (Edwards et al., 1977a; Sandercock et al., 1985). Under these circumstances, the mechanism responsible for the fatigue is impaired neuromuscular transmission or impaired muscle action potential propagation along the sarcolemmal membrane. Recovery from high-frequency fatigue is rapid, occurring within, at the most, a few minutes. Patients with myasthenia gravis and myotonia congenita demonstrate high-frequency fatigue (Edwards, 1980), and the phenomenon has been studied experimentally in normal subjects (Jones et al., 1979).

Low-frequency fatigue is much more common, particularly in terms of normal respiratory muscle function. Low-frequency fatigue develops slowly, with a long, sustained contraction, or with contractions repeated over a long period. Low-frequency fatigue is evidenced by a greater loss of force at lower stimulation frequencies of 10 to 40 Hz, than at higher frequencies of 100 Hz (Jones et al., 1979; Sandercock et al., 1985). Low-frequency fatigue results from an increased concentration of inorganic phosphate (Hibberd et al., 1985), an increased hydrogen ion concentration (Metzger and Moss, 1987), or some combination of these factors (Faulkner and

Brooks, 1992). Impaired excitation–contraction coupling may occur secondary to impaired propagation of action potentials, or the increased concentration of inorganic phosphate, hydrogen ions, or both (Westerblad et al., 1991). After several hours of repeated contractions, low-frequency fatigue may reflect a depletion of muscle glycogen stores and low blood glucose concentrations (Goll-nick et al., 1972).

Low-frequency fatigue of the sternomastoid muscle can be produced by inspiratory loading sufficient to generate 70% of the maximum inspiratory mouth pressure with each breath or by sustained isocapnic maximum voluntary ventilation (see Fig. 7B). In each case, the frequency–force characteristics of the muscle, determined 10 min after the end of the fatiguing exercise, separates the low- (Edwards et al., 1977a) from high-frequency fatigue (Jones et al., 1979; Edwards, 1981). Figure 12 shows the slow time course of recovery of low-frequency fatigue of the sternomastoid muscle (Moxham et al., 1980).

The studies of low-frequency stimulation are of significance because stimulation frequencies in the 10- to 40-Hz range produce the normal contractions of the diaphragm muscle at rest and likely even during light physical activities (Bigland-Ritchie et al., 1992). In the presence of low-frequency fatigue, an increased

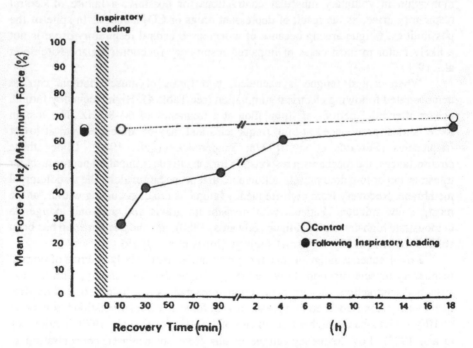

Figure 12   Time course of recovery of low-frequency fatigue in the sternomastoid muscle. (From Moxham et al., 1980.)

neuromuscular drive is expected (Mador and Acevedo, 1991). The increased neuromuscular drive is necessary to maintain a constant ventilation through the recruitment of more motor units, an increased firing frequency of each unit, or a combination of the two (Edwards, 1979; Moxham et al, 1981). Support for this interpretation is provided by the increase in the smooth, rectified electromyogram from a sternomastoid muscle exhibiting low-frequency fatigue compared with that of a fresh muscle, even though the absolute force is unchanged (Moxham et al., 1980).

Fatigue resistance and oxidative capacity are the characteristics that separate type I and IIA fibers from the highly fatiguable glycolysis-dependent type IIB fibers (Burke et al., 1973; Peter et al., 1972). Consequently, the observation of an inverse correlation between the development of low-frequency fatigue and the proportion of the oxidative muscle fibers (Kugelberg and Lindegren, 1979) is hardly surprising. Since immobilization of a muscle results in a decreased oxidative capacity and atrophy of muscle fibers (see Chap. 9), prolonged artificial ventilation would likely cause fibers in the ventilatory muscles to regress toward more fatigue-susceptible, glycolytic-dependent muscle fiber types. Such fiber types appear to characterize the neonatal diaphragm (Keens and Ianuzzo, 1979) and may account for some of the respiratory problems of the neonate.

In view of the importance of breathing for life, a matter of strategic significance is to determine the likelihood of weaning a patient successfully from an artificial ventilator after a prolonged period of artificial ventilation. Practical and reliable tests of the effects of activity on the respiratory muscles are the maximum relaxation rate following a brief tetanic stimulation of the sternomastoid muscle (Mak et al., 1991); or, even more practical for the diaphragm muscle, the "sniff" test (Moxham, 1992). The sniff tests requires either a brief voluntary inspiratory maneuver, with recording of the mouth pressure, or a temporary increase in resistance to inspiratory flow in intubated patients, with the measurement, albeit indirectly, of the relaxation rate of the respiratory muscles. With physical activity, especially in the presence of resistance to inspiratory flow, relaxation rate slows. The slowing of the rate of relaxation, although a valuable indication of metabolic changes in muscle (Wiles and Edwards, 1982), is not a synonym for fatigue (Edwards, 1992). For example, late in recovery from physical activity that causes low-frequency fatigue, the relaxation rate may recover to its prefatigue value, even though fatigue may persist. Slowing of relaxation, although not a linear function of force loss (Vollestad et al., 1988), may be a useful precursor of fatigue (Roussos and Macklem, 1977; Macklem, 1990). For intubated patients in the process of being weaned from a ventilator, changes in the relaxation rate might provide the needed prediction of the likelihood of success (Moxham, 1992).

Electrically stimulated isometric contractions of hand and limb muscles of humans have been useful in dissecting out what appear to be the components of respiratory muscle fatigue (Bigland-Ritchie et al., 1992; Edwards et al., 1977a; Jones, 1981), but differences exist. During respiratory muscle activity, the phasic recruitment of motor units postpones the development of fatigue that would occur if the same absolute force, or pressure, were to be generated as a single bout of static exercise. Furthermore, the shortening of the respiratory muscles would appear to result in a greater loss of force than occurs during isometric contractions, since in muscle strips of the canine diaphragm in situ, the decrement in force was greater during isovelocity shortening than during isometric contractions (Ameredes and Clanton, 1990).

IV. Respiratory Muscle Function in Humans

The diverse activities of the diaphragm, intercostal, abdominal, and sternomastoid muscles result in the range and variety of ventilatory maneuvers. The mechanism by which the muscles of respiration act on the volume of the thorax to achieve various ventilatory maneuvers is through contractions at varied power outputs (force $\times$ distance $\times$ time^{-1}). Ventilatory maneuvers thus involve contractions that vary in force development, distance shortened, and velocity of shortening. These intrinsic characteristics of skeletal muscle fibers are functions of the type of myosin present in fibers, the fiber length, and the fiber cross-sectional area.

Because in vivo respiratory muscles are inaccessible for the measurement of force directly, force development is measured indirectly as the differences in the transdiaphragmatic pressure (P_{di}) (Derenne et al., 1978). The transformation of muscle force to pressure may be estimated for the diaphragm muscle from the LaPlace relationship, but this is complicated by changes in the curvature of the muscle. Although other muscles of inspiration contribute to the P_{di}, the mechanism by which they do so is unknown. For the respiratory muscles, force developed and the length shortened cannot be measured, but the external work performed is estimated correctly by the area under the pressure–volume curve.

The overall strength developed by the respiratory muscles is estimated from measurements of the maximum inspiratory or expiratory pressures. These measurements have been extremely useful in describing normal function and in clinical evaluations. The forces developed by the respiratory muscle displace the chest wall and inflate the lung (Knowles et al., 1967). The chest wall includes the diaphragm, the rib cage with its musculature, and the abdomen with its musculature. Contraction of the diaphragm muscle forces the viscera downward and pushes the abdomen outward. The extent to which the contraction lifts and expands the ribs depends on the resistance of the abdomen to displacement and, thus, the increase in abdominal pressure (Derenne et al., 1978). The external intercostal muscles expand the rib cage. The abdominal muscles usually function during expiration, but their contraction during inspiration will increase abdominal pressure and, consequently, rib expansion (Grimby et al., 1976).

During quiet breathing, there is controversy over the interaction of the diaphragm muscle (Grimby et al., 1976) and the accessory muscles of respiration

(Delhez, 1974). The consensus is that, although the diaphragm muscle is involved consistently and has the most motor units active, parts of the internal intercostals (the interchondrals), the external intercostals, and frequently the scalene and sternomastoid muscles are also active (Derenne et al., 1978). Increases in minute ventilation are accompanied by progressive recruitment of motor units in each of the muscles of respiration. The exact pattern of recruitment varies with differences in the stimuli that cause the hyperpnea (Derenne et al., 1978).

Electrical and magnetic techniques have been developed to stimulate the phrenic nerve to facilitate the study of the contractile properties of the diaphragm (McKenzie et al., 1992; Alex et al., 1992; Bigland-Ritchie et al., 1992). From the early studies (Sant' Ambrogio and Saibene, 1970; Mognoni et al., 1968) to the present, nerve stimulation has been used for noninvasive studies of the diaphragm (Moxham et al., 1981; Aubier et al., 1981) and sternomastoid muscles (Moxham et al., 1980). In addition, the contractile properties of the intrinsic muscles of of the hand have been measured during voluntary contractions and in response to electrical stimulation, and the data then used to interpret the function of the respiratory muscles (Bigland-Ritchie et al., 1992; Edwards et al., 1977b). With these techniques, frequency–force curves were recorded similar to those obtained on isolated bundles of muscles (Moxham et al., 1980). In practice, the attachment of the force transducer to the mastoid process is uncomfortable, and a more useful method for studies of patients is to apply the force transducer to the sternal attachment of the sternomastoid (Edwards et al., 1980).

The recording of P_{di} in response to electrical stimulation of the right phrenic nerve allows a myogram to be obtained from the diaphragm similar to that obtained on the adductor policis muscle. The frequency–force curve for the respiratory muscles is similar to those of other human skeletal muscles (see Fig. 7A). The characteristics of normal respiratory muscles of humans, as with those of small mammals, are those of a muscle intermediate between slow and fast that possesses the qualities of energy economy and resistance to fatigue. The higher resistance to fatigue of the diaphragm and accessory muscles of respiration than of most limb muscles results from the relatively high values for oxidative capacity and maximum blood flow of the respiratory muscles (Bellemare and Grassino, 1982; Gandevia and McKenzie, 1988). Force–velocity characteristics may possibly be a factor for airflow limitation (Agostoni and Fenn, 1960), but only if there is no limiting airway collapse. Adjustments to internal loading appear to influence diaphragm contraction according to known force–length and force–velocity characteristics (Pengelly et al., 1971).

The traditional length–force curve describes the characteristics of the muscle under conditions of maximal activation. Compared with maximally stimulated contractions, when a muscle is stimulated at low frequencies, muscles at shorter lengths show a disproportionate reduction in the force generated (Rack and Westbury, 1969; Edwards, 1979). A similar result was found for a human sternomastoid muscle measured in vivo when the muscle length was reduced by 15% (see Fig. 6B). This disproportionate reduction in the force generated at low-stimulation frequencies and short muscle lengths is in the same direction, and could compound the changes seen if the muscle develops low-frequency fatigue (see Table 4).

The preponderance of highly oxidative fibers allows the diaphragm muscle to perform at high percentages of maximum voluntary ventilation for long periods. Some of the variability in the sustained maximum voluntary ventilation (MVV), curves (Zocche et al., 1960; Tenney and Reese, 1968; Freedman, 1970; Lieberman et al., 1973) may result from differences in the experimental protocols, but a substantial part of the differences likely reflects real differences owing to either hereditary influences or to the state of training of the individuals tested. Endurance athletes demonstrate a fourfold greated endurance time at 80% of MVV than nonathletes and nonathletes show an improvement in short-term MVV following a 5-week training program (Martin and Stager, 1981; see also Chap. 9).

V. Summary

The structural and functional properties of the diaphragm intercostal, abdominal, and sternomastoid muscles are well suited to the unique functional requirements of respiration. The diaphragm muscle, with a high-oxidative capacity, a high, maximum skeletal muscle blood flow, and a velocity of shortening intermediate between that of fast and slow muscles, is highly resistant to fatigue. In spite of these characteristics, the diaphragm can be fatigued by breathing against a high resistance or by a high duty/rest ratio and a high cycle rate. The causes of muscle fatigue are numerous and closely interrelated (Edwards, 1983). The factors underlying diaphragmatic fatigue do not appear to be different from those well studied in fatigue of muscles in the limbs and in the intrinsic muscles of the hand.

Acknowledgments

The authors would like to thank Drs. Susan Brooks-Herzog, Henry Gibson, T. Helliwell, and Veronica Toescu, as well as Miss Gail Gibson and Mrs. Gabriele Wiernert for their assistance in the preparation of the revised manuscript. Support for the research and editorial effort for the preparation of the manuscript was provided by a Program Project grant from the National Institute of Dental Research DE-07687; the Welcome Trust; the Muscular Dystrophy Group of Great Britain and Northern Ireland; and I. C. I. Pharmaceuticals.

References

Agostoni, E., and Fenn, W. O. (1960). Velocity of muscle shortening as a limiting factor in respiratory air flow. *J. Appl. Physiol.* 15: 349–353.
Alex, C. G., Jubran, A., Goldstone, J., and Tobin, M. J. (1992). Noninvasive measurement of

force–frequency curves to guide a phrenic nerve pacing program [Abstract]. *Am. Thorac. Soc.*

Ameredes, B. T., and Clanton, T. L. (1990). Increased fatigue of isovelocity vs. isometric contractions of canine diaphragm. *J. Appl. Physiol.* 69: 740–746.

Andersen, P., and Sears, T. A. (1964). The mechanical properties and innervation of fast and slow motor units in the intercostal muscles of the cat. *J. Physiol. (Lond.)* 173: 114–129.

Aniansson, A., Grimby, G., Hedberg, M., and Krotkiewski, M. (1981). Muscle morphology, enzyme activity and muscle strength in elderly men and women. *Clin. Physiol.* 1: 73–86.

Aubier, M., de Troyer, A., Sampson, M., Macklem, P. T., and Roussos, C. (1981). Aminophylline improves diaphragm contractility. *N. Engl. J. Med.* 305: 249–252.

Barany, M. (1967). ATPase activity of myosin correlated with speed of muscle shortening. *J. Gen. Physiol.* 50: 197–216.

Barany, M., Barany, K., Reckard, T., and Volpe, A., (1965). Myosin of fast and slow muscles of the rabbit. *Arch. Bicohem. Biophys.* 109: 185–191.

Bellemare, F., and Grassino, A. (1982). A effect of pressure and timing of contraction on human diaphragm fatigue. *J. Appl. Physiol.* 53: 1190–1195.

Bigland-Ritchie, B., Jones, D. A., Hosking, G. P., and Edwards, R. H. T. (1978). Central and peripheral fatigue in sustained maximum voluntary contractions of human quadriceps muscle. *Clin. Sci. Mol. Med.* 54: 609–614.

Bigland-Ritchie, B., Thomas, C. K., and Rice, C. L. (1992). Contractile properties of human motor units in relation to diaphragm fatigue. In *Breathlessness*. The Campbell Symposium, Edited by N. L. Jones and K. J. Killian. Boehringer Ingelheim, Ontario, pp. 34–42.

Billeter, R., Heizmann, C. W., Howald, H., and Jenny E. (1981). Analysis of myosin light and heavy chain types in single human muscle fibers. *J. Biochem.* 116: 389–395.

Brooks, S. V., and Faulkner J. A. (1988). Contractile properties of skeletal muscles from young, adult, and aged mice. *J. Physiol. (Lond.)* 404: 71–82.

Brooks, S. V., and Faulkner, J. A. (1991). Forces and powers of slow and fast skeletal muscles in mice during repeated contractions. *J. Physiol. (Lond.)* 436: 701–710.

Brooke, M. H., and Kaiser, K. K. (1970). Muscle fiber types: How many and what kind. *Arch. Neurol.* 23: 369–379.

Brooks, S. V., Faulkner, J. A., and McCubbrey, D. A. (1990). Power outputs of slow and fast skeletal muscles of mice. *J. Appl. Physiol.* 68: 1282–1285.

Burke, R. E., Levine, D. N., Tsairis, P., and Zajac, F. E. III. (1973). Physiological types and histochemical profiles in motor units of the cat gastrocnemius. *J. Physiol. (Lond.)* 234: 723–748.

Claflin, D. R., and Faulkner, J. A. (1989). The force–velocity relationship at high shortening velocities in the soleus muscle of the rat. *J. Physiol. (Lond.)* 411: 627–637.

Close, K. (1964). Dynamic properties of fast and slow skeletal muscles of the rat during development. *J. Physiol. (Lond.)* 173: 74–95.

Close, R. I. (1972). Dynamic properties of mammalian skeletal muscles. *Physiol. Rev.* 52: 129–197.

Côté, C., and Faulkner, J. A. (1986). Characteristics of motor units in muscles of rats grafted with nerves intact. *Am. J. Physiol.* 250: C828–C833.

Davies, A. S., and Gunn, H. M. (1972). Histochemical fibre types in the mammalian diaphragm. *J. Anat.* 112: 41–60.

de Troyer, A., Sampson, M., Sigrist, S., and Macklem, P. T. (1981). The diaphragm: Two muscles. *Science* 213: 237–238.

Delhez, L. (1974). *Contribution Electromyographique a l Etude de la Mecanique et du Controle Nerveux des Mouvements Respiratoires de l'Homme*. Liege, Vailant Carmanne, p. 380.

Derenne, Macklem, P. T., and Roussos, C. (1978). The respiratory muscles: Mechanics, control and pathophysiology. *Am. Rev. Respir. Dis.* Part I 118: 119–113. Part II 118: 373–390.

Drachman, D. B., and Johnston, D. M. 1973). Development of a mammalian fast muscle: Dynamic and biochemical properties correlated. *J. Physiol.* 234: 29–42.

Eddinger, T. J., and Moss, R. L. (1987). Mechanical properties of skinned single fibers of identified types from rat diaphragm. *Am. J. Physiol.* 253: C210–C218.

Edjtehadi, G. D., and Lewis, D. M. (1979). Histochemical reactions of fibres in a fast twitch muscle of the cat. *J. Physiol.* 287: 439–453.

Edwards, R. H. T. (1979). The diaphragm as a muscle: Mechanisms underlying fatigue. *Am. Rev. Respir. Dis.* 119: 81–84.

Edwards, R. H. T. (1980). Studies of muscular performance in normal and dystrophic subjects. *Br. Med. Bull.* 36: 159–164.

Edwards, R. H. T. (1981). Human muscle function and fatigue. In *Human Muscle Fatigue*: *Physiological Mechanisms*. Ciba Foundation Symposium No. 82. London, Pitman Medical.

Edwards, R. H. T. (1983). Biochemical bases of fatigue in exercise performance: Catastrophe theory of muscular fatigue. In *Proceedings of the Fifth International Symposium on the Biochemistry of Exercise*. Edited by H. G. Knuttgen, J. A. Vogel, and J. Poortmans. Champaign, IL, Human Kinetics Publishers.

Edwards, R. H. T. (1992). Respiratory muscle impairment. In *Breathlessness*. The Campbell Symposium, Edited by N. L. Jones and K. J. Killian. Ontario, Boehringer Ingelheim, pp. 43–44.

Edwards, R. H. T., Hill, D. K., Jones, D. A., and Merton, P. A. (1977a). Fatigue of long duration in human skeletal muscle after exercise. *J. Physiol.* 272: 769–778.

Edwards, R. H. T., Young, A., Hosking, G. P., and Jones, D. A. (1977b). Human skeletal muscle function: Description of tests and normal values. *Clin. Sci. Mol. Med.* 52: 283–290.

Edwards, R. H. T., Moxham, J., Newham, D., and Wiles, C. M. (1980). Alternative techniques for recording the frequency:force curve of the sternomastoid muscle in man. *J. Physiol.* 305: 83–84P.

Faulkner, J. A., and Brooks, S. V. (1992). Fatigability of mouse muscles during constant length, shortening, and lengthening contractions: Interactions between fiber types and duty cycles. In *Neuromuscular Fatigue*. Edited by T. Sargeant and D. Kernell, Amsterdam, Elsevier Publishers.

Faulkner, J. A., Maxwell, L. C., Ruff, G. L., and White, T. P. (1979). The diaphragm as a muscle. Contractile properties. *Am. Rev. Respir. Dis.* 119: 89–92.

Faulkner, J. A., Jones, D. A., Round, J. M., and Edwards, R. H. T. (1980). Dynamics of energetic processes in human muscle. In *Exercise Bioenergetics and Gas Exchange*. Edited by P. Ceretelli and G. J. Whipp. Amsterdam, Elsevier North Holland, pp. 81–90.

Faulkner, J. A., Claflin, D. R., McCully, K. K., and Jones, D. A. (1982). Contractile properties of bundles of fiber segments from skeletal muscles. *Am. J. Physiol.* 243: C66–C73.

Faulkner, J. A., Claflin, D. R., and McCully, K. K. (1986). Power output of fast and slow fibers from human skeletal muscles. In *Human Power Output*. Edited by N. L. Jones, N. McCartney, and J. McComas. Champaign, IL, Human Kinetics Publishers, pp. 81–91.

Faulkner, J. A., Zerba, E., and Brooks, S. V. (1990). Muscle temperature of mammals: Cooling impairs most functional properties. *Am. J. Physiol.* 259: R259–R265.

Faulkner, J. A., Claflin, D. R., Brooks, S. V., and Burton H. W. (1991). Power output of fiber segments from human latissimus dorsi muscles: Implications for cardiac assist devices. In *Proceedings of the International Symposium on Basic and Applied Myology*: Perspectives for the 90's. Edited by U. Carraro. Padova, Italy, Unipress, Chap. 2, p. 31.

Faulkner, J. A., Green, H., and White, T. P. (1993). Skeletal muscle responses to acute and adaptations to chronic physical activity. In *Physical Activity, Fitness and Health*. Edited by C. Bouchard, R. Shephard, and T. Stephens. Champaign IL, Human Kinetics Publishers.

Fenn, W. O. (1963). A comparison of respiratory and skeletal muscles. In *Perspectives in Biology*. Edited by C. F. Cori, V. G. Foglia, L. F. Leloir, and S. Ochoa. New York, Elsevier, pp. 294–300.

Freedman, S. (1970). Sustained maximum voluntary ventilation. *Respir. Physiol.* 8: 230–244.

Gandevia, S. C., and McKenzie, D. K. (1988). Human diaphragmatic endurance during different maximal respiratory efforts. *J. Physiol.* (*Lond.*) 395: 625–638.

Garnett, R. A. F., O'Donovan, M. J., Stephens, J. A., and Taylor, A. (1978). Motor unit organization of human medial gastrocnemius. *J. Physiol.* (*Lond.*) 287: 33–43.

Gauthier, G. F., and Lowey, S. (1979). Distribution of myosin isoenzymes among skeletal muscle fiber types. *J. Cell Biol.* 81: 10–25.

Gauthier, G. F., and Padykula, H. A. (1966). Cytological studies of fiber types in skeletal muscle. A comparative study of the mammalian diaphragm. *J. Cell Biol.* 28: 333–354.

Gollnick, P. D., and Hodgson, D. R. (1986). The identification of fiber types in skeletal muscle: A continual dilemma. In *Exercise and Sport Science Reviews*. Edited by K. B. Pandolf. New York, Macmillan, pp. 81–103.

Gollnick, P. D., Armstrong, R. B., Saubert, C. W. IV, Piehl, K., and Saltin, B. (1972). Enzyme activity and fiber composition in skeletal muscle of untrained and trained men. *J. Appl. Physiol.* 33: 312–319.

Gordon, A. M., Huxley, A. F., and Julian, F. J. (1966). The variation in isometric tension with sarcomere length in vertebrate muscle fibres. *J. Physiol. (Lond.)* 184: 170–192.

Greaser, M. L., Moss, R. L., and Reiser P. J. (1988). Variations in contractile properties of rabbit single muscle fibres in relation to troponin T isoforms and myosin light chains. *J. Physiol. (Lond.)* 406: 85–98.

Grimby, G., Goldman, M., and Mead, J. (1976). Respiratory muscle action inferred from rib cage and abdominal V–P partitioning. *J. Appl. Physiol.* 41: 739.

Hards, J. M., Reid, W. D., Pardy, R. L., and Pare, P. D. (1990). Respiratory muscle fiber morphometry. Correlation with pulmonary function and nutrition. *Chest* 97: 1037–1044.

Heilmann, C., and Pette, D. (1979). Molecular transformations in sarcoplasmic reticulum of fast-twitch muscle by electrostimulation. *Eur. J. Biochem.* 93: 437–446.

Henneman, E., and Olson, C. B. (1965). Relations between structure and function in the design of skeletal muscles. *J. Neurophysiol.* 28: 599–620.

Hibbert, M. G., Danzig, J. A., Trentham, D. R., and Goldman, Y. E. (1985). Phosphate release and force generation in skeletal muscle fibers. *Science* 228: 1317–1319.

Hoh, J. F. Y., and Yeoh, G. P. S. (1979). Rabbit skeletal myosin isoenzymes from fetal, fast-twitch and slow twitch muscles. *Nature* 280: 321–323.

Hoppeler, H., Mathieu, O., Weibel, E. R., Krauer, R., Lindstedt, S. L., and Taylor, C. R. (1981). Design of the mammalian respiratory system. VIII. Capillaries in skeletal muscles. *Respir. Physiol.* 44: 129–150.

Jones, D. A. (1981). Muscle fatigue due to change beyond the neuromuscular function. In *Human Muscle Fatigue: Physiological Mechanisms*. Edited by R. Porter and J. Whelan. Ciba Foundation Symposium No. 81. London, Pitman Medical.

Jones, D. A., Bigland-Ritchie, B., and Edwards, R. H. T. (1979). Excitation frequency and muscle fatigue: Mechanical responses during voluntary and stimulated contractions. *Exp. Neurol.* 64: 401–413.

Keens, T. G., and Ianuzzo, C. D. (1979). Development of fatigue-constant muscle fibers in human ventilatory muscles. *Am. Rev. Respir. Dis.* 119: 139–141.

Keens, T. G., Bryan, A. C., Levison, H., and Ianuzzo, C. D. (1978). Developmental pattern of muscle fiber types in human ventilatory muscles. *Am. J. Physiol.* 44: 909–913.

Kim, M. J., Druz, W. S., Danon, J., Machnach, W., and Sharp, J. T. (1976). Mechanics of the canine diaphragm. *J. Appl. Physiol.* 41: 369–382.

Knowles, J. H., Hong, S. K., and Rahn, H. (1967). Possible errors using esophageal ballon in determining the pressure volume characteristics of the lung and thorax cage. *J. Appl. Physiol.* 22: 407.

Krnjevic, K., and Miledi, R. (1957). Motor units in the rat diaphragm. *J. Physiol.* 140: 427–439.

Kugelberg, E., and Edstrom, L. (1968). Differential histochemical effects of muscle contractions on phosphorylase and glycogen in various types of fibers: Relation to fatigue. *J. Neurol. Neurosurg. Psychiatry* 31: 415–423.

Kugelberg, E., and Lindegren, B. (1979). Transmission and contraction fatigue of rat motor units in relation to succinate dehydrogenase activity of motor unit fibres. *J. Physiol.* 288: 285–300.

Laroche, C. M., Moxham, J., and Green, M. (1989). Respiratory muscle weakness and fatigue. *Q. J. Med.* 71: 373–397.

Leak, L. V. (1979). Gross and ultrastructural morphological features of the diaphragm. *Am. Rev. Respir. Dis.* 119: 3–21.

Lieberman, D. A., Faulkner, J. A., Craig, A. B., Jr., and Maxwell, L. C. (1973). Performance and histochemical composition of guinea pig and human diaphragm. *J. Appl. Physiol.* 34: 233–237.

Lombardi, V., and Piazzesi, G. (1990). The contractile response during steady lengthening of stimulated frog muscle fibres. *J. Physiol. (Lond.)* 431: 141–171.

Lowey, S., and Risby, D. (1971). Light chains from fast and slow muscle myosins. *Nature* 234: 81–85.

Macklem, P. T. (1990). The importance of defining respiratory muscle fatigue. *Am. Rev. Respir. Dis.* 142: 274.

Mador, M. J., and Acevedo, F. A. (1991). Effect of respiratory muscle fatigue on breathing pattern during incremental exercise. *Am. Rev. Respir. Dis.* 143: 462–468.

Mak, V. H. F., Chapman, F., James, C., and Spiro, S. G. (1991). Sternomastoid muscle twitch maximum relaxation rate: Prolonged slowing with fatigue and post-tetanic acceleration. *Clin Sci.* 81: 669–676.

Martin, B. J., and Stager, J. M. (1981). Ventilatory endurance in athletes and non-athletes. *Med. Sci. Sports Exerc.* 13: 21–26.

McCully, K. K., and Faulkner, J. A. (1983). Length–tension relationship of mammalian diaphragm muscles. *J. Appl. Physiol.* 54: 1681–1686.

McCully, K. K., and Faulkner, J. A. (1985). Injury to skeletal muscle fibers of mice following lengthening contractions. *J. Appl. Physiol.* 59: 119–126.

McKenzie, D. K., Bigland-Ritchie, B., Gorman, R. B., and Gandevia, S. C. (1992). Central and peripheral fatigue of human diaphragm and limb muscles assessed by twitch interpolation. *J. Physiol.* 454: 643–656.

Metzger J. M., and Moss, R. L. (1987). Greater hydrogen ion-induced depression of tension and velocity in skinned single fibres of rat fast than slow muscles. *J. Physiol. (Lond.)* 393: 727–742.

Metzger, J. M., Scheidt, K. B., and Fitts, R. H. (1985). Histochemical and physiological characteristics of the rat diaphragm. *J. Appl. Physiol.* 58: 1085–1091.

Mognoni, P., Saibene, G., Sant'Ambrogio, G., and Agostoni, E. (1968). Dynamics of the maximal contraction of the respiratory muscles. *Respir. Physiol.* 4: 193–202.

Moxham, J. (1992). Respiratory muscle fatigue: Central, peripheral or both. In *Breathlessness*. The Campbell Symposium. Edited by N. L. Jones and K. J. Killian. Ontario, Boehringer Ingelheim, pp. 45–51.

Moxham, J., Wiles, C. M., Newham, D., and Edwards. R. H. T. (1980). Sternomastoid function and fatigue in man. *Clin. Sci.* 59: 433–468.

Moxham, J., Morris, A. J. R., Spiro, S. G., Edwards, R. H. T., and Green, M. (1981). Contractile properties and fatigue of the diaphragm in man. *Thorax* 36: 154–168.

Murphy, R. A., and Beardsley, A. C. (1974). Mechanical properties of the cat soleus muscle in situ. *Am. J. Physiol.* 227: 1008–1013.

Needham, D. M. (1926). Red and white muscle. *Physiol. Rev.* 6: 1.

Pengelly, L. D., Alderson, A. M., and Milic-Emili, J. (1971). Mechanics of the diaphragm. *J. Appl. Physiol.* 30: 797–805.

Peter, J. B., Barnard, R. J., Edgerton, V. R., Gillespie, C. A., and Stempel, K. E. (1972). Metabolic profiles of three fiber types of skeletal muscle in guinea pigs and rabbits. *Biochemistry* 11: 2627–2633.

Pette, D., and Vrbova, G. (1992). Adaptation of mammalian skeletal muscle fibers in chronic electrical stimulation. *Rev. Physiol. Biochem. Pharmacol.* 120: 116–202.

Rack, P. M. H., and Westbury, D. R. (1969). The effects of length and stimulus rate on tension in the isometric cat soleus muscle. *J. Physiol.* 204: 443–460.

Ranatunga, K. W. (1984). The force–velocity relation of rat fast- and slow-twitch muscles examined at different temperatures. *J. Physiol. (Lond.)* 351: 517–529.

Reiser, P. J., Moss, R. L., Giulian, G. G., and Greaser, M. L. (1985). Shortening velocity in single fibers from adult rabbit soleus muscles is correlated with myosin heavy chain composition. *J. Biol. Chem.* 260: 9077–9080.

Ritchie, J. M. (1954). The relation between force and velocity of shortening in rat muscle. *J. Physiol. (Lond.)* 123: 633–639.

Rochester, D. (1992). Respiratory muscles: Structure, size and adaptive capacity. In *Breathlessness*. The Campbell Symposium. Edited by N. L. Jones and K. J. Killian. Ontario, Boehringer Ingelheim, pp. 1–12.

Romanul, F. C. A. (1974). Enzymes in muscle. *Arch. Neurol.* 11: 355–368.

Roussos, C., and Macklem, P. T. (1977). Diaphragmatic fatigue in man. *J. Appl. Physiol.* 43: 189–197.

Sandercock, T. G., Faulkner, J. A., Albers, J. W., and Abbrecht, P. H. (1985). Single motor unit and fiber action potentials during fatigue. *J. Appl. Physiol.* 58: 1073–1079.

Sant'Ambrogio, G., and Saibene, F. (1970). Contractile properties of the diaphragm in some mammals. *Respir. Physiol.* 10: 349–357.

Sarkar, S., Sreter, F. A., and Gergely, J. (1971). Light chains of myosins from white, red, and cardiac muscles. *Proc. Natl. Acad. Sci. USA* 68: 946–950.

Sears, T. A. (1964). The fibre-calibre spectra of sensory and motor fibres in the intercostal nerves of the cat. *J. Physiol.* 172: 150–161.

Sieck, G. C. (1988). Diaphragm muscle: Structural and functional organization. *Clin. Chest Med.* 9: 195–210.

Sieck, G. C., Roy, R. R., Powell, P., Blanco, C., Edgerton, V. R., and Harper, R. M. (1983). Muscle fiber type distribution and architecture of the cat diaphragm. *J. Appl. Physiol. Respir. Environ. Exerc. Physiol.* 55: 1386–1392.

Staron, R. S., and Pette, D. (1986). Correlation between myofibrillar ATPase activity and myosin heavy chain composition in rabbit muscle fibers. Histochemistry 86: 19–23.

Sweeney, H. L., Kusmerick, M. J., Mabuchi, J., Gergely, J., and Streter, F. A. (1986). Velocity of shortening and myosin isozymes in two types of rabbit fast-twitch muscle fibers. *Am. J. Physiol.* 259: C431–C434.

Tenney, S. M., and Reese, R. E. (1968). The ability to sustain great breathing efforts. *Respir. Physiol.* 5: 187–201.

Vollestad, N. K., Sejersted, O. M., Bahr, R., and Bigland-Ritchie, B. (1988). Motor drive and metabolic responses during repeated sub-maximal contractions in man. *J. Appl. Physiol.* 63: 1–7.

Westerblad, H., Lee, J. A., Lännergren, J., and Allen, D. G. (1991). Cellular mechanisms of fatigue in skeletal muscle. *Am. J. Physiol.* 261: C195–C209.

Wiles, C. M., and Edwards, R. H. T. (1982). The effect of temperature ischaemia and contractile activity on the relaxation rate of human muscle. *Clin. Physiol.* 2: 485–497.

Zocche G. P., Fritts, H. W., and Cournand, A. (1960). Fraction of maximum breathing capacity available for prolonged hyperventilation. *J. Appl. Physiol.* 15: 1073–1074.

6

Fatigue of Striated Muscles
Metabolic Aspects

HÅKAN WESTERBLAD and
JAN LÄNNERGREN

Karolinska Institute
Stockholm, Sweden

DAVID G. ALLEN

University of Sydney
Sydney, New South Wales, Australia

I. Introduction

The performance of skeletal muscles is limited by the development of *fatigue* (i.e., a decline in performance with time of activity, manifested as reduced force, diminished contractile speed, and slower relaxation). The combination of reduced force and lower shortening velocity results in reduced mechanical power output, which is of great functional importance during most types of physical activity. Fatigue is caused mainly by intramuscular factors: thus, neither the central nervous system (CNS), the motor nerve, nor the neuromuscular junction set a significant limit for muscle performance (for review see Bigland-Ritchie and Woods, 1984). In this chapter we will deal with metabolic alterations within the muscle fibres that may be important for the reduced performance in fatigue. We will deal mainly with effects on isometric force production, because this is where most experimental data is available and the causal relations probably best understood; toward the end we will very briefly discuss known metabolic influences on shortening speed and relaxation rate. We will primarily consider fatigue produced by brief maximal contractions, repeated at short intervals, leading to severe fatigue within a few minutes. This type of intermittent maximal activity is known to cause large chemical changes and, therefore, is a good model for studies of the role of metabolic factors in the development of fatigue. Metabolic factors may also be involved in fatigue with other types of activity: for example, fatigue developing during long-lasting, submaximal work is associated with glycogen depletion, but this is beyond the scope of this review.

Recent studies have shown that force decline in fatigue is due to both direct impairment of cross-bridge function and to changes in intracellular activation. Three principal fatigue mechanisms can now be identified (Westerblad and Allen, 1991): (1) reduction of the maximum tension (i.e., the tension at saturating Ca^{2+} levels), (2) reduced myofibrillar Ca^{2+} sensitivity, and (3) reduced Ca^{2+} levels during tetanic contractions. Some metabolic factor(s) may be implicated in all these three mechanisms, or they may be related to different metabolic alterations—such putative relations will be discussed in detail later in the chapter.

II. Metabolic Changes in Fatiguing Muscles

In general, metabolic changes may cause fatigue either through a reduction of high-energy compounds (e.g., phosphocreatine and ATP) or through an accumulation of breakdown products. Figure 1 illustrates some important metabolic changes that occur during fatiguing stimulation. Important changes are the following: a breakdown of phosphocreatine, with a concomitant formation of inorganic phosphate (P_i); a formation of lactate, which usually is accompanied by an accumulation of hydrogen ions and, thus, reduced intracellular pH (pH_i).

Adenosine triphosphate (ATP) is the immediate energy source for energy-requiring processes, such as cross-bridge cycling and ion pumping, and a significant reduction of the myoplasmic ATP concentration would affect cell function. Generally, reported reductions of ATP in fatigue are small (from about 6 to 5 mM; for review see Vøllestad and Sejersted, 1988) and, if representative, would be unlikely to affect cell function. However, there are several studies in which considerably larger reductions (up to about 50%) have been found (Hultman et al., 1986; Harris et al., 1987; Söderlund and Hultman, 1990; Nagesser et al., 1992), and these may influence some cellular processes. Local concentrations, at sites where ATP turnover is particularly high, may well be lower than the cell average (discussed later).

Among all the breakdown products of energy metabolism P_i and hydrogen ions have the greatest effect on the contractile apparatus (Godt and Nosek, 1989): an increased concentration of these ions results in both a reduced maximum tension production and a reduced myofibrillar Ca^{2+} sensitivity.

III. Relation of Fatigue Resistance to Metabolic Capacity

As discussed in the foregoing, there are metabolic changes in fatigue that can reduce the contractile performance. Thus, it appears likely that metabolic factors are involved in the development of fatigue. If this is so, there should be a correlation

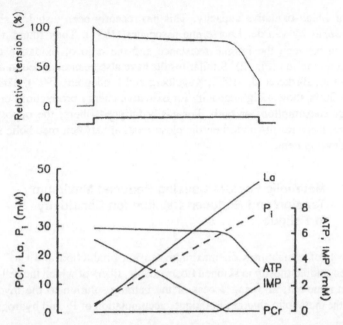

Figure 1 Characteristic pattern of tension decline (upper panel) and metabolic changes (lower panel) during fatigue produced by repeated tetanic stimulation. The tension trace is the envelope of the peak force of a large number of tetanic contractions. The period of fatiguing stimulation is indicated below the tension record; the duration of this period depends on the fiber's fatigue resistance and the pattern of stimulation (i.e., duration of tetani vs. rest period between contractions). Metabolic changes described by full lines are replotted from data in Nagesser et al., (1992) obtained from easily fatigued fibers of *Xenopus*. The metabolites are lactate (La), ATP, inosine monophosphate (IMP), and phosphocreatine (PCr). The change of inorganic phosphate (P_i; dashed line) was calculated from the changes of PCr and ATP. Easily fatigued fibers of *Xenopus* have a very low oxidative capacity and, therefore, during a period of increased energy consumption, they depend on the breakdown of high-energy phosphates (PCr and ATP) and anaerobic glycolysis. The latter process results in an accumulation of lactate ions and an acidosis of up to 0.8 pH-units (Westerblad and Lännergren, 1988). Note that ATP does not start to decline until the store of PCr is almost fully depleted. This pattern can be predicted if the Lohmann reaction (PCr + ADP $\Longleftrightarrow$ Cr + ATP) and the myokinase reaction (2ADP $\Longleftrightarrow$ ATP + AMP) remain at equilibrium during fatiguing stimulation. Note also that the final rapid tension reduction coincides with the decline of ATP.

between a fiber's metabolic profile and fatigue resistance. More specifically, for fatigue resistance, the increased energy demand during contraction should be met without significant depletion of energy stores (phosphocreatine and ATP) and without a large accumulation of lactate and hydrogen ions. Accordingly, a fatigue-resistant fiber should consume as little energy as possible to meet the task and have a high-oxidative capacity. This has recently been tested in single fibers from *Xenopus* by van der Laarse and associates (1991). They found a very good correlation between the fatigue resistance and the ratio of oxidative capacity to energy consumption (Fig. 2). Similar results have also been obtained in mammalian muscle (e.g., Burke et al., 1973; Kugelberg and Lindegren, 1979). Thus, fatigue-resistant fibers show a high capacity for oxidative energy production, or a low rate of energy consumption, or both. For easily fatigued fibers, the opposite is true. Therefore, these results underline the close relation between metabolic factors and fatigue development.

IV. Metabolic Factors Causing Reduced Maximum Tension and Reduced Calcium Ion Sensitivity in Fatigue

The effects of metabolites on maximum tension production and Ca^{2+} sensitivity have been studied mostly in skinned fibers; that is, fibers of which the cell membrane has been removed, allowing access of the bathing solution to the myofilaments. Among the metabolic changes in fatigue, accumulation of P_i and hydrogen ions has

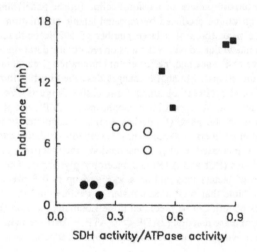

Figure 2 An illustration of the good correlation between endurance, on one hand, and the ratio of oxidative capacity to energy consumption, on the other. The endurance was, in this case, defined as the time taken for tension to decline to 75% of the control. The activity of a mitochondrial enzyme, succinate dehydrogenase (SDH), was used to assess the oxidative capacity, and the myofibrillar ATPase activity was used as a measure of energy consumption. Data were obtained from three types of muscle fibers from *Xenopus*: easily fatigued (●), fatigue-resistant (○), and very fatigue-resistant (■). (Data replotted from van der Laarse et al., 1991.)

a marked effect on maximum tension and myofibrillar Ca^{2+} sensitivity (e.g., Godt and Nosek, 1989).

In skinned fibers, there is a logarithmic relation between the P_i concentration and both maximum tension and Ca^{2+} sensitivity (Millar and Homsher, 1990). This means that small changes of the low P_i at rest have a much larger effect on tension and Ca^{2+} sensitivity than similar changes at the higher P_i in fatigue. This is important to keep in mind when comparing studies on skinned fibers, for which the control medium usually has no P_i added, which gives a P_i concentration of about 0.7 mM (from contamination), and intact fibers, for which the resting P_i concentration is about 3 mM (for recent review see Westerblad et al., 1991). A typical change of the P_i in fatigue of intact fibers would be from 3 to about 30 mM (see Fig. 1; also see Westerblad et al., 1991), which corresponds to about 30% decrease of the maximum tension in skinned fibers (Cooke and Pate, 1985; Millar and Homsher, 1990).

One way to quantify changes in Ca^{2+} sensitivity is to use the Ca_{50} [i.e., the intracellular Ca^{2+} concentration ($[Ca^{2+}]_i$) that gives half maximum tension]. The expected P_i increase in fatigue (see foregoing) results in a 1.7 times increase of Ca_{50} in skinned fibers (Millar and Homsher, 1990). The effect of P_i accumulation on maximum tension and Ca^{2+} sensitivity has not yet been studied in intact fibers.

The accumulation of hydrogen ions in fatigue causes a typical pH_i decline from about 7.0 to 6.5 (Kushmerick and Meyer, 1985; Renaud et al., 1986; Juel, 1988a; Westerblad and Lännergren, 1988; Cady et al., 1989b). In some situations, fatigue may occur without any significant pH_i decline (Le Rumeur et al., 1989; Westerblad and Allen, 1992a). In skinned fibers, a 0.5 pH-unit acidosis causes approximately a 25% reduction of the maximum tension and a doubling of Ca_{50} (Donaldson and Hermansen, 1978; Fabiato and Fabiato, 1978; Godt and Nosek, 1989; Metzger and Moss, 1990) in intact fibers. A similar acidosis reduces the maximum tension by about 15% and increases Ca_{50} by about 50% (Westerblad and Allen, 1992a; Westerblad and Allen, 1993a).

There is evidence suggesting that acidosis and P_i accumulation act synergistically on reducing maximum tension. This appears to be the situation in mammalian fast, but not slow, muscle, and has led to the suggestion that diprotonated P_i is the species that causes the tension reduction in fast muscle (Nosek et al., 1990).

A detailed knowledge of the changes of both maximum tension and Ca^{2+} sensitivity that occur in fatigue in intact fibers is available only for fibers from a mouse muscle (Lännergren and Westerblad, 1991; Westerblad and Allen, 1991; Westerblad and Allen, 1993b), and these changes are illustrated in Figure 3; some quantitatively similar results have been obtained in frog fibers (Edman and Lou, 1990; Lee et al., 1991). These mouse fibers display a 20% reduction of maximum tension and a slightly larger increase of Ca_{50} in fatigue. Under normal conditions isolated mouse fibers fatigue without any significant acidosis (Westerblad and Allen, 1992a); hence, the reduction of maximum tension and Ca^{2+} sensitivity observed would be ascribed to an accumulation of P_i. The foregoing values compare with a 30% reduction of maximum

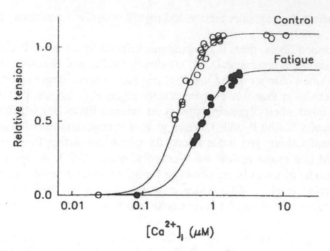

Figure 3 The relation between tetanic tension and $[Ca^{2+}]_i$ obtained in control (O) and during late fatigue (●) in a single mouse muscle fiber. In fatigue, there is both a marked reduction of the stable tension at high $[Ca^{2+}]_i$ (i.e., reduced maximum tension) and a marked rightward shift of the data points (i.e., reduced Ca^{2+} sensitivity). (Data replotted from Westerblad and Allen, 1991.)

tension and a 1.7-fold increase of Ca_{50} in skinned fibers exposed to the expected change of P_i in fatigue (Cooke and Pate, 1985; Millar and Homsher, 1990). Consequently, considering the large methodological differences, there is a reasonable agreement between results from fatigue in intact fibers and results from skinned fibers bathed in a solution similar to the intracellular milieu in fatigue.

Single mouse fibers are fatigued without acidosis because they have an effective extrusion of hydrogen ions by the lactate transporter (Westerblad and Allen, 1992a); that is, a carrier-mediated cotransport of lactate ions and hydrogen ion equivalents (Juel, 1988a; Mason and Thomas, 1988). In the single-fiber experiments, the perfusate was continuously renewed, which allows the lactate transporter to work at a high rate and, consequently, there was no significant acidosis. On the other hand, when fatigue is produced in intact muscle, there will be an accumulation of lactate ions in the extracellular space that will inhibit the lactate transporter. To mimic the situation in whole muscle, single mouse fibers have been fatigued in the presence of the lactate transport inhibitor cinnamate (Westerblad and Allen, 1992a). With cinnamate present, fatigue occurred more rapidly and the fibers showed an acidosis of 0.4 pH units, thus similar to the acidosis frequently observed in fatigued intact muscle. The reduction of the maximum tension was tested in one fiber exposed to cinnamate during fatiguing stimulation, and it was reduced by about 40% (the Ca^{2+} sensitivity was not tested). Accordingly, there was an additional 20% reduction of maximum tension when compared with fatigue under normal conditions, and this extra component can be ascribed to acidosis.

V. Metabolic Factors Causing Reduced Tetanic Calcium Ion Levels in Fatigue

In a classic study, Eberstein and Sandow (1963) showed that the tension produced by fatigued fibers increased substantially when the fibers were exposed to caffeine, or were rapidly depolarized with high K^+ concentrations. Both these maneuvers cause Ca^{2+} release from the sarcoplasmic reticulum (SR) without employing the normal activation pathway. The results of Eberstein and Sandow strongly suggest that excitation–contraction failure is important in fatigue, and similar results have been obtained in many studies thereafter (e.g., Grabowski et al., 1972; Nassar-Gentina et al., 1981; Lännergren and Westerblad, 1991). The role of excitation–contraction failure in fatigue was examined further in a study by Allen and colleagues (1989). They used the photoprotein aequorin to measure $[Ca^{2+}]_i$ during fatiguing stimulation of single xenopus fibers and found a marked reduction of tetanic $[Ca^{2+}]_i$ in fatigue (Fig. 4). Reduced tetanic $[Ca^{2+}]_i$ in fatigue has since been observed with fluorescent indicators (fura-2 and indo-1) in single fibers from *Xenopus* (Lee et al., 1991) and mouse (Westerblad and Allen, 1991; Westerblad and Allen, 1993b), and in whole frog sartorius muscle (Baker et al., 1993). The reduction of tetanic $[Ca^{2+}]_i$ generally occurs late during fatiguing stimulation; initially, there is typically an increase of tetanic $[Ca^{2+}]_i$ (see Fig. 4). The decrease in $[Ca^{2+}]_i$ coincides with a marked decline in tetanic tension, both in easily fatigued and more fatigue-resistant fibers, although the $[Ca^{2+}]_i$ decline occurs after a much longer stimulation period in the latter. This suggests that there is a metabolic factor involved in the reduction of tetanic $[Ca^{2+}]_i$.

In principle, the reduced tetanic $[Ca^{2+}]_i$ in fatigue can be due to a reduced Ca^{2+} release from the SR, or to increased myoplasmic Ca^{2+} buffering. Metabolic changes that occur in fatigue would tend to reduce, rather than increase, Ca^{2+} binding to the main myoplasmic Ca^{2+}-binding sites: H^+ competes with Ca^{2+} for the low-affinity binding sites on troponin C (Blanchard et al., 1984); there is a cooperativity between tension production and Ca^{2+} binding to troponin (Bremel and Weber, 1972; Brandt et al., 1982) and, since an increased P_i concentration reduces the tension, it may also reduce the Ca^{2+} binding to troponin. Thus, the myoplasmic Ca^{2+} buffering would, if anything, fall during fatiguing stimulation; therefore, it can safely be concluded that the declining tetanic $[Ca^{2+}]_i$ reflects reduced SR Ca^{2+} release.

Imaging of $[Ca^{2+}]_i$ has shown the reduction of Ca^{2+} release in fatigue produced by repeated tetany to be homogeneous in fibers from *Xenopus* (Westerblad et al., 1990) and mouse (Duty and Allen, 1994). However, when xenopus fibers were fatigued by continuous high-frequency stimulation, there were gradients, so that the central part of the fibers had a lower $[Ca^{2+}]_i$ (Westerblad et al., 1990). A probable explanation for this latter finding is that K^+ ions accumulate in the T-tubular system during the prolonged stimulation, which results in impaired action potential propagation into the T-system.

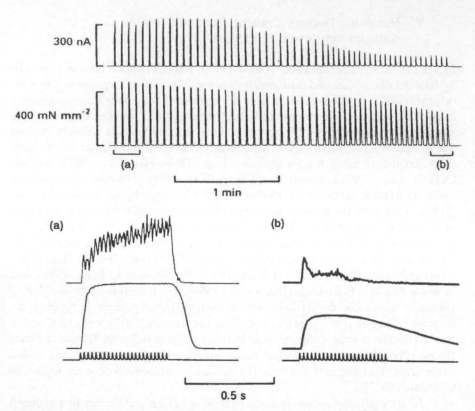

Figure 4 The tension reduction in fatigue is accompanied by declining tetanic $[Ca^{2+}]_i$. Records obtained from an easily fatigued fiber from *Xenopus*. The upper panel illustrates changes in $[Ca^{2+}]_i$ during a period of fatiguing stimulation; $[Ca^{2+}]_i$ was measured with the photoprotein aequorin, the light emission of which is monotonically related to $[Ca^{2+}]_i$. The lower panel shows a continuous tension record. The panels labeled (a) and (b) are averaged records of aequorin light and tension obtained from four tetani at the beginning and the end of the fatigue run, respectively. These panels clearly illustrate the reduced tetanic $[Ca^{2+}]_i$ in fatigue. (Adapted from Allen et al., 1989.)

The lack of $[Ca^{2+}]_i$ gradients in xenopus and mouse fibers fatigued by repeated tetani indicates that the myofibrils are equally well activated across the fiber. However, in frog (*Rana* spp.) fibers, the central part of the fibers appears to be less activated in this type of fatigue, as judged from the appearance of wavy myofibrils (Garcia et al., 1991). Thus, there appears to be a difference between different frog species in this. Gonzalez-Sserratos et al. (1978) have shown swelling and vacuole formation of the T-tubular system in fatigued fibers of *Rana* spp., and Garcia et al. (1991) suggest that this might explain the impaired activation of central myofibrils that they observe. A formation of vacuoles has been demonstrated also in fibers of *Xenopus*, but only during the recovery phase (Lännergren et al., 1990), and this is not associated with any gradients of $[Ca^{2+}]_i$ (Westerblad et al., 1990). Accordingly, vacuole formation, as such, does not necessarily lead to inhomogeneous activation. The smaller cross-sectional area of mammalian fibers, such as those of the mouse, would, all else being similar, simplify diffusion of K^+ out of the T tubules; consequently, impaired action potential propagation would be less likely to occur in these fibers. In the following, we will focus on metabolic correlates for a homogeneous decline of tetanic $[Ca^{2+}]_i$.

An increase of the myoplasmic free Mg^{2+} concentration ($[Mg^{2+}]_i$) may provide a link between metabolism and declining tetanic $[Ca^{2+}]_i$, and this has recently been investigated in mouse fibers (Westerblad and Allen, 1992b) and xenopus fibers (Westerblad and Allen, 1992c). The idea is that breakdown of ATP will result in an increase of $[Mg^{2+}]_i$, and a moderate increase of $[Mg^{2+}]$ can impair SR Ca^{2+} release from skinned fibers with intact T-tubules (Lamb and Stephenson, 1991). During fatiguing stimulation, $[Mg^{2+}]_i$ initially remained essentially constant and, then, started to increase rapidly toward the end of the stimulation period. Thus, $[Mg^{2+}]_i$ followed a time course similar to that of the decline of tetanic $[Ca^{2+}]_i$, which may suggest a causal relation. However, when Mg^{2+} was directly injected into mouse fibers, a much higher $[Mg^{2+}]_i$ was required to give the same tension reduction as in fatigue (Westerblad and Allen, 1992b). The reduction of tetanic $[Ca^{2+}]_i$, then cannot simply be explained by elevated $[Mg^{2+}]_i$, although it is possible that Mg^{2+}-induced inhibition of SR Ca^{2+} release is amplified in fatigue because of other changes, such as a reduction of the myoplasmic ATP concentration ($[ATP]_i$).

Westerblad and Allen (1992b) used modeling to translate the observed increase of $[Mg^{2+}]_i$ to changes of $[ATP]_i$. They found a very good correlation between the reductions of $[ATP]_i$ and $[Ca^{2+}]_i$. There are several mechanisms by which declining $[ATP]_i$ may reduce SR Ca^{2+} release: (1) reduced capacity of the Na–K pumps in the sarcolemma, (2) opening of ATP-sensitive K^+ channels, (3) impaired inositol triphosphate (IP_3) metabolism, (4) direct effect of ATP on SR Ca^{2+} channels, (5) impaired SR Ca^{2+} pumping.

1. A reduction of $[ATP]_i$ will affect membrane-bound, ATP-driven Na–K pumps. A possible scenario involving impaired Na–K pumping in fatigue is as follows. Inhibition of the Na–K pumps causes a membrane depolarization. This results in partial inactivation of voltage-sensitive Na^+ channels, reduced amplitude of action potentials, and finally, impaired voltage activation of Ca^{2+} release. Juel (1988b) studied the role of Na–K pumps by comparing fatigue under control conditions and in the presence of terbutaline, a β_2-adrenoceptor agonist that stimulates Na–K pumping. The results showed that fatigue occurred somewhat more slowly in the presence of terbutaline, and this was accompanied by a less marked depolarization and smaller changes of the intracellular concentration of K^+ and Na^+. A contribution of limited Na–K pumping to fatigue has been suggested by

results from other studies as well (see Vøllestad and Sejersted, 1988); hence, this mechanism is a likely candidate for the reduction of tetanic $[Ca^{2+}]_i$.

2. There are K^+ channels in the sarcolemma that are held close by ATP (K_{ATP} channels) and increase their opening when $[ATP]_i$ falls (Noma, 1983). The K_{ATP} channels are present at high density (Spruce et al., 1985), which means that even a small increase of their opening probability may result in a significant increase of the K^+ permeability (cf. the situation during myocardial ischemia; Nichols et al., 1991). However, $[ATP]_i$ has to be severely reduced to markedly open these channels: half-maximal inhibition occurs at an ATP concentration of 0.14 mM (Spruce et al., 1987) which is markedly lower than the $[ATP]_i$ measured in fatigue (see foregoing). Nevertheless, opening of K_{ATP} channels may contribute to fatigue because acidosis markedly reduces the inhibitory effect of ATP on these channels (Davies, 1990; Standen et al., 1992).

A marked increase of the K^+ permeability would accelerate K^+ loss from muscle fibers, especially from single-fiber preparations, for which the extracellular fluid is continuously renewed. In this situation, no extracellular K^+ accumulation will occur, which may otherwise counteract K^+ extrusion either directly or indirectly by activation of the Na–K pumps. An intracellular loss of K^+ will reduce the K^+ equilibrium potential, which results in a membrane depolarization, inactivation of Na^+ channels, reduced amplitude of action potentials, and eventually reduced SR Ca^{2+} release, as discussed earlier for Na–K pumps. Thus, the opening of K_{ATP} channels provides a likely explanation for the reduced tetanic $[Ca^{2+}]_i$ in fatigue. Their role in fatigue can be tested, since there are drugs that both open and close these channels.

3. In smooth muscle, it is well established that IP_3 has a central role in the coupling between membrane excitation and contraction. In skeletal muscle the physiological importance of IP_3 is less clear: there are experimental data suggesting that IP_3 has a role similar to that in smooth muscle, whereas many other studies have failed to show any physiological importance of IP_3 (for brief review see Jaimovich, 1991). If IP_3 is involved in the excitation–contraction coupling of skeletal muscle, this provides a possible link to energy metabolism, since IP_3 turnover requires ATP (see Donaldson, 1986).

4. The function of the SR Ca^{2+} channels is impaired at very low [ATP] (Smith et al., 1985). However, both ADP and AMP can replace ATP in maintaining opening probability and, therefore, a marked reduction of the total concentration of adenine nucleotides is required to impair Ca^{2+} release. This mechanism is then unlikely to operate in fatigue, at least in its simplest form. There is a possibility that inosine monophosphate (IMP), which is formed by deamination of adenine compounds in fatigue (Sahlin et al., 1978; see also Fig. 1), may directly inhibit the SR Ca^{2+} channels.

5. As $[ATP]_i$ declines the rate and amount of Ca^{2+} pumped into the SR will decline (see e.g., Dawson et al., 1980) and, presumably, this would cause a reduction of the Ca^{2+} release. In accordance with this, there is a marked increase

of the resting $[Ca^{2+}]_i$ in fatigue (Lee et al., 1991; Westerblad and Allen, 1991). This mechanism will work only if a large proportion of the Ca^{2+} ions that are no longer taken up by the SR disappear from the myoplasm; for example, by leaving the cell or by accumulating in some intracellular organelle; a pure redistribution of Ca^{2+} from the SR to the myoplasm will not reduce the amount of Ca^{2+} available for activation of the myofilaments.

The fact that a marked tension increase can be produced in fatigue if the normal activation pathway is bypassed by application of caffeine or high K^+ concentration indicates that the SR is not depleted of Ca^{2+} in fatigue. Moreover, the Ca^{2+} content of the SR in fatigue has been measured with electron microprobe technique and was not reduced (Gonzalez-Serratos et al., 1978); however, some methodological problems with this study should lead to caution (see Westerblad et al., 1991). Thus, although it is not altogether proved, it appears unlikely that reduced SR Ca^{2+} content owing to impaired pumping is an important factor for the reduced tetanic $[Ca^{2+}]_i$ in fatigue.

Han et al. (1992) recently demonstrated a microcompartmentalized system for ATP production and consumption in the triads of skeletal muscle; that is, in the narrow space between the T tubules and the terminal cisternae of the SR. These authors concluded that the ATP pool in the triad may well be out of equilibrium with the major myoplasmic ATP pool owing to a rapid utilization, combined with limited diffusion. This means that the metabolic changes that occur in the triads during fatigue may be quantitatively different from those measured from the whole cell. Thus, although the changes in $[ATP]_i$ and $[Mg^{2+}]_i$ measured from the whole cell appear to be too small to affect the SR Ca^{2+} release channels, these changes may be larger at the triads, affecting Ca^{2+} release.

VI. Causes of Reduced Shortening Velocity and Slowed Relaxation

Apart from diminished force, there is generally reduced shortening speed and slowed relaxation in fatigue, but these parameters have been less studied. The shortening speed can be markedly reduced in fatigue (Edman and Mattiazzi, 1981; de Haan et al., 1989; Lännergren and Westerblad, 1989). This reduction will mainly reflect altered cross-bridge kinetics, and several metabolic factors are known to slow cross-bridges: acidosis (Edman and Mattiazzi, 1981; Metzger and Moss, 1987; Cooke et al., 1988); reduced $[ATP]_i$ (Cooke and Bialek, 1979; Ferenczi et al., 1984); increased myoplasmic ADP concentration ($[ADP]_i$; Cooke and Pate, 1985). Accumulation of P_i, which has a large effect on maximum tension and on myofibrillar Ca^{2+} sensitivity, does not, however, significantly reduce the maximum shortening velocity (Cooke and Pate, 1985; Cooke et al., 1988).

An acidosis of 0.5 pH-units reduces the maximum shortening speed by about 10% (Metzger and Moss, 1987; Cooke et al., 1988). If taken individually, both the changes of $[ATP]_i$ and $[ADP]_i$ that are supposed to occur in fatigue are too small to substantially affect the shortening velocity (Cooke and Bialek, 1979; Ferenczi et al., 1984, Cooke et al., 1988). However, since the PCr concentration is very low in severe fatigue (see foregoing), ATP regeneration is inhibited, and this has a significant effect on the shortening speed (e.g., Cooke and Bialek, 1979). Thus, the slowed shortening in fatigue may be explained by the combined effect of acidosis and impaired ATP regeneration.

The speed of relaxation of skeletal muscle depends on both Ca^{2+} and cross-bridge-related factors; the relative importance of Ca^{2+} versus cross-bridges for the slowing of relaxation in fatigue is not yet clear. If we first consider Ca^{2+}-related factors separately, the speed of relaxation will depend on the rate of $[Ca^{2+}]_i$ decline at the end of a tetanus and the myofibrillar Ca^{2+} sensitivity. In this context, a slowed rate of $[Ca^{2+}]_i$ decline may be counteracted by a reduced Ca^{2+} sensitivity; that is, if the Ca^{2+} sensitivity is low, $[Ca^{2+}]_i$ needs to fall less to reach a level at which cross-bridge detachment overtakes attachment. For example, acidosis is known to inhibit the SR Ca^{2+} pumps (MacLennan, 1970), which will tend to slow relaxation, but this will, to some extent, be compensated by an acidity-induced reduction of Ca^{2+} sensitivity.

Besides pH_i another example of a metabolic change in fatigue that may affect relaxation by Ca^{2+}-related mechanisms is the accumulation of P_i. An increased P_i concentration reduces the myofibrillar Ca^{2+} sensitivity, which should speed up relaxation. However, a P_i accumulation may also reduce the rate of Ca^{2+} uptake by the SR, which would tend to slow relaxation. The mechanism for this slowed uptake would be a reduction of the affinity for ATP hydrolysis that occurs as a consequence of reduced $[ATP]_i$ or increased concentration of the products of its hydrolysis (ADP and P_i) (see Dawson et al., 1980). This also means that a reduction of $[ATP]_i$ or an increase of $[ADP]_i$ can slow relaxation by reducing the rate of SR Ca^{2+} uptake.

Metabolic factors that can affect the relaxation speed by cross-bridge kinetics would be the same as those suggested to slow the shortening velocity (see foregoing). However, it is not immediately evident how slowed cross-bridge detachment during relaxation correlates with reduced shortening velocity.

The slowing of relaxation in fatigue appears to involve one pH-related mechanism and one mechanism that is not related to pH (Cady et al., 1989a; Westerblad and Allen, 1992a). The pH-related mechanism will, as discussed earlier, act both on Ca^{2+} handling and on cross-bridge kinetics.

VII. Conclusions

The tension reduction in fatigue can be ascribed to three factors: reduced maximum tension (i.e., tension at saturating $[Ca^{2+}]_i$), reduced myofibrillar Ca^{2+} sensitivity, and reduced SR Ca^{2+} release. The reduction of maximum tension and Ca^{2+} sensitivity is most likely caused by the combined effect of increased P_i concentration and acidosis. The cause of reduced Ca^{2+} release is less clear, but we speculate that it may be related to declining $[ATP]_i$. Fatigue generally involves reduced shortening speed and reduced relaxation rate. Acidosis slows both shortening and relaxation, but the reduction of these in fatigue appears to involve some other mechanism(s) as well.

References

Allen, D. G., Lee, J. A., and Westerblad, H. (1989). Intracellular calcium and tension in isolated single muscle fibres from *Xenopus*. *J. Physiol.* 415: 433–458.

Baker, A. J., Longuemare, M., Brandes, R., and Weiner, M. W. (1993). Intracellular tetanic calcium signals are reduced in fatigue of whole skeletal muscle. *Am. J. Physiol.* 264: C577–C582.

Bigland-Ritchie, B., and Woods, J. J. (1984). Changes in muscle contractile properties and neural control during human muscular fatigue. *Muscle Nerve* 7: 691–699.

Blanchard, E. M., Pan, B. S., and Solaro, R. J. (1984). The effect of acidic pH on the ATPase activity and troponin Ca^{2+} binding of rabbit skeletal myofilaments. *J. Biol. Chem.* 259: 3181–3186.

Brandt, P. W., Cox, R. N., Kawai, M., and Robinson, T. (1982). Regulation of tension in skinned muscle fibers. Effect of cross-bridge kinetics on apparent Ca^{2+} sensitivity. *J. Gen. Physiol.* 79: 997–1016.

Bremel, R. D., and Weber, A. (1972). Cooperation within actin filament in vertebrate skeletal muscle. *Nature* 238: 97–101.

Burke, R. E., Levine, D. N., Tsairis, P., and Zajac, F. E. (1973). Physiological types and histochemical profiles in motor units of the cat gastrocnemius. *J. Physiol.* 234: 723–748.

Cady, E. B., Elshove, H., Jones, D. A., and Moll, A. (1989a). The metabolic causes of slow relaxation in fatigued human skeletal muscle. *J. Physiol.* 418: 327–337.

Cady, E. B., Jones, D. A., Lynn, J., and Newham, D. J. (1989b). Changes in force and intracellular metabolites during fatigue of human skeletal muscle. *J. Physiol.* 418: 311–325.

Cooke, R., and Bialek, W. (1979). Contraction of glycerinated muscle fibers as a function of ATP concentration. *Biophys. J.* 28: 241–258.

Cooke, R., Franks, K., Luciani, G. B., and Pate, E. (1988). The inhibition of rabbit skeletal muscle contraction by hydrogen ion and phosphate. *J. Physiol.* 395: 77–97.

Cooke, R., and Pate, E. (1985). The effect of ADP and phosphate on the contraction of muscle fibers. *Biophys. J.* 48: 789–798.

Davies, N. W. (1990). Modulation of ATP-sensitive K^+ channels in skeletal muscle by intracellular protons. *Nature* 343: 375–377.

Dawson, M. J., Gadian, D. G., and Wilkie, D. R. (1980). Mechanical relaxation rate and metabolism studied in fatiguing muscle by phosphorus nuclear magnetic resonance. *J. Physiol.* 299: 465–484.

de Haan, A., Lodder, M. A. N., and Sargeant, A. J. (1989). Age related effects of fatigue and recovery from fatigue in rat medial gastrocnemius muscle. *Q. J. Exp. Physiol.* 74: 715–726.

Donaldson, S. K. (1986). Mammalian muscle fiber types: Comparison of excitation–contraction mechanisms. *Acta Physiol. Scand.* [*Suppl.*] 556: 157–166.

Donaldson, S. K. B., and Hermansen, L. (1978). Differential, direct effects of H^+ on Ca^{2+}-activated force of skinned fibers from the soleus, cardiac and adductor magnus muscles of rabbits. *Pflugers Arch.* 376: 55–65.

Duty, S., and Allen, D. G. (1994). The distribution of intracellular calcium concentration in isolated single fibres of mouse skeletal muscle during fatiguing stimulation. Pflügers Arch. 427: 102–109.

Eberstein, A., and Sandow, A. (1963). Fatigue mechanisms in muscle fibres. In *The Effect of Use and Disuse on Neuromuscular Functions.* Edited by E. Gutman and P. Hnik. Amsterdam, Elsevier, pp. 515–526.

Edman, K. A. P., and Lou, F. (1990). Changes in force and stiffness induced by fatigue and intracellular acidification in frog muscle fibres. *J. Physiol.* 424: 133–149.

Edman, K. A. P., and Mattiazzi, A. R. (1981). Effects of fatigue and altered pH on isometric force and velocity of shortening at zero load in frog muscle fibres. *J. Muscle Res. Cell Motil.* 2: 321–334.

Fabiato, A., and Fabiato, F. (1978). Effects of pH on the myofilaments and the sarcoplasmic reticulum of skinned cells from cardaic and skeletal muscles. *J. Physiol.* 276: 233–255.

Ferenczi, M. A., Goldman, Y. E., and Simmons, R. M. (1984). The dependence of force and shortening velocity on substrate concentration in skinned muscle fibres from *Rana temporaria. J. Physiol.* 350: 519–543.

Garcia, M. D. C., Gonzalez-Serratos, H., Morgan, J. P., Cynthia, L., Perreault, C. L., and Rozycka, M. (1991). Differential activation of myofibrils during fatigue in phasic skeletal muscle cells. *J. Muscle Res. Cell Motil.* 12: 412–424.

Godt, R. E., and Nosek, T. M. (1989). Changes of intracellular milieu with fatigue or hypoxia depress contraction of skinned rabbit skeletal and cardiac muscle. *J. Physiol.* 412: 155–180.

Gonzalez-Serratos, H., Somlyo, A. V., McClellan, G., Shuman, H., Borrero, L. M., and Somlyo, A. P. (1978). Composition of vacuoles and sarcoplasmic reticulum in fatigued muscle: Electron probe analysis. *Proc. Natl. Acad. Sci. USA* 75: 1329–1333.

Grabowski, W., Lobsiger, E. A., and Lüttgau, H. C. (1972). The effect of repetitive stimulation at low frequencies upon the electrical and mechanical activity of single muscle fibres. *Pflugers Arch.* 334: 222–239.

Han, J.-W., Thieleczek, R., Varsányi, M., and Heilmeyer, M. G. (1992). Compartmentalized ATP synthesis in skeletal muscle. *Biochemistry* 31: 377–384.

Harris, R. C., Marlin, D. J., and Snow, D. H. (1987). Metabolic responses to maximal exercise of 800 and 2,000 m in the thoroughbred horse. *J. Appl. Physiol.* 63: 12–19.

Hultman, E., Spriet, L. L., and Söderlund, K. (1986). Biochemistry of muscle fatigue. *Biomed. Biochem. Acta* 45: S97–S106.

Jaimovich, E. (1991). Chemical transmission at the triad: $InsP_3$? *J. Muscle Res. Cell Motil.* 12: 316–320.

Juel, C. (1988a). Intracellular pH recovery and lactate efflux in mouse soleus muscles stimulated in vitro: The involvement of sodium/proton exchange and a lactate carrier. *Acta Physiol. Scand.* 132: 363–371.

Juel, C. (1988b). The effect of β_2-adrenoceptor activation on ion-shifts and fatigue in mouse soleus muscles stimulated in vitro. *Acta Physiol. Scand.* 134: 209–216.

Kugelberg, E., and Lindegren, B. (1979). Transmission and contraction fatigue of rat motor units in relation to succinate dehydrogenase activity of motor unit fibres. *J. Physiol.* 288: 285–300.

Kushmerick, M. J., and Meyer, R. A. (1985). Chemical changes in rat leg muscle by phosphorus nuclear magnetic resonance. *Am. J. Physiol.* 248: C542–C549.

Lamb, G. D., and Stephenson, D. G. (1991). Effect of Mg^{2+} on the control of Ca^{2+} release in skeletal muscle fibres of the toad. *J. Physiol.* 434: 507–528.

Lännergren, J., and Westerblad, H. (1989). Maximum tension and force–velocity properties of fatigued, single *Xenopus* muscle fibres studied by caffeine and high K^+. *J. Physiol.* 409: 473–490.

Lännergren, J., and Westerblad, H. (1991). Force decline due to fatigue and intracellular acidification in isolated fibres from mouse skeletal muscle. *J. Physiol.* 434: 307–322.

Lännergren, J., and Westerblad, H., and Flock, B. (1990). Transient appearance of vacuoles in fatigued *Xenopus* muscle fibres. *Acta Physiol. Scand.* 140: 437–445.

Lee, J. A., Westerblad, H., and Allen, D. G. (1991). Changes in tetanic and resting $[Ca^{2+}]_i$ during fatigue and recovery of single muscle fibres from *Xenopus laevis. J. Physiol.* 433: 307–326.

Le Rumeur, E., Le Moyec, L., Chagneau, F., Levasseur, M., Toulouse, P., Le Bars, R., and de Certaines, J. (1989). Phosphocreatine and pH recovery without restoration of mechanical function during prolonged activity of rat gastrocnemius muscle: An in vivo ^{31}P NMR study. *Arch. Int. Physiol. Biochem.* 97: 381–388.

MacLennan, D. H. (1970). Purification and properties of an adenosine triphosphate from sarcoplasmic reticulum. *J. Biol. Chem.* 245: 4508–4518.

Mason, M. J., and Thomas, R. C. (1988). A microelectrode study of the mechanisms of L-lactate entry into and release from frog sartorius muscle. *J. Physiol.* 400: 459–479.

Metzger, J. M., and Moss, R. L. (1987). Greater hydrogen ion induced depression of tension and velocity in skinned single fibres of rat fast than slow muscles. *J. Physiol.* 393: 727–742.

Metzger, J. M., and Moss, R. L. (1990). pH modulation of the kinetics of a Ca^{2+}-sensitive cross-bridge state transition in mammalian single skeletal muscle fibres. *J. Physiol.* 428: 751–764.

Millar, N. C., and Homsher, E. (1990). The effect of phosphate and calcium on force generation in glycerinated rabbit skeletal muscle fibers. *J. Biol. Chem.* 265: 20234–20240.

Nagesser, A. S., van der Laarse, W. J., and Elzinga, G. (1992). Metabolic changes with fatigue in different types of single muscle fibres of *Xenopus laevis*. *J. Physiol.* 448: 511–523.

Nassar-Gentina, V., Passonneau, J. V., and Rapoport, S. I. (1981). Fatigue and metabolism of frog muscle fibers during stimulation and in response to caffeine. *Am. J. Physiol.* 241: C160–C166.

Nichols, C. G., Ripoll, C., and Lederer, W. J. (1991). ATP-sensitive potassium channel modulation of the guinea pig ventricular action potential and contraction. *Circ. Res.* 68: 280–287.

Noma, A. (1983). ATP-regulated K^+ channels in cardiac muscle. *Nature* 305: 147–148.

Nosek, T. M., Leal-Cardoso, J. H., McLaughlin, M., and Godt, R. E. (1990). Inhibitory influence of phosphate and arsenate on contraction of skinned skeletal and cardiac muscle. *Am. J. Physiol.* 259: C933–C939.

Renaud, J. M., Allard, Y., and Mainwood, G. W. (1986). Is the change in intracellular pH during fatigue large enough to be the main cause of fatigue? *Can. J. Physiol. Pharmacol.* 64: 764–767.

Sahlin, K., Palmskog, G., and Hultman, E. (1978). Adenine nucleotide and IMP contents of the quadriceps muscle in man after exercise. *Pflugers Arch.* 374: 193–198.

Smith, J. S., Coronado, R., and Meissner, G. (1985). Sarcoplasmic reticulum contains adenine nucleotide-activated calcium channels. *Nature* 316: 446–449.

Söderlund, K., and Hultman, E. (1990). ATP content in single fibres from human skeletal muscle after electrical stimulation and during recovery. *Acta Physiol. Scand.* 139: 459–466.

Spruce, A. E., Standen, N. B., and Stanfield, P. R. (1985). Voltage-dependent, ATP-sensitive potassium channels of skeletal muscle membrane. *Nature* 316: 736–738.

Spruce, A. E., Standen, N. B., and Stanfield, P. R. (1987). Studies of the unitary properties of adenosine-5'-triphosphate-regulated potassium channels of frog skeletal muscle. *J. Physiol.* 382: 213–236.

Standen, N. B., Pettit, A. I., Davies, N. W., and Stanfield, P. R. (1992). Activation of ATP-dependent K^+ currents in intact skeletal muscle fibres by reduced intracellular pH. *Proc. R. Soc. Lond. B* 247: 195–198.

van der Laarse, W. J., Lännergren, J., and Diegenbach, P. C. (1991). Resistance to fatigue of single muscle fibres from *Xenopus* related to succinate dehydrogenase and myofibrillar ATPase activities. *Exp. Physiol.* 76: 589–596.

Vøllestad, N. K., and Sejersted, O. M. (1988). Biochemical correlates of fatigue. *Eur. J. Appl. Physiol.* 57: 336–347.

Westerblad, H., and Allen D. G. (1991). Changes of myoplasmic calcium concentration during fatigue in single mouse muscle fibers. *J. Gen. Physiol.* 98: 615–635.

Westerblad, H., and Allen, D. G. (1992a). Changes of intracellular pH due to repetitive stimulation of single fibres from mouse skeletal muscle. *J. Physiol.* 449: 49–71.

Westerblad, H., and Allen, D. G. (1992b). Myoplasmic free Mg^{2+} concentration during repetitive stimulation of single fibres from mouse skeletal muscle. *J. Physiol.* 453: 413–434.

Westerblad, H., and Allen, D. G. (1992c). Myoplasmic Mg^{2+} concentration in *Xenopus* muscle fibres at rest, during fatigue and during metabolic blockade. *Exp. Physiol.* 77: 733–740.

Westerblad, H., and Allen, D. G. (1993a). The influence of intracellular pH on contraction, relaxation and $[Ca^{2+}]$; in intact single fibres from mouse muscle, *J. Physiol.* 466: 611–628.

Westerblad, H., and Allen, D. G. (1993b). The contribution of $[Ca^{2+}]_i$ to the slowing of relaxation in fatigued single fibres from mouse skeletal muscle. *J. Physiol.* 468: 729–740.

Westerblad, H., and Lännergren, J. (1988). The relation between force and intracellular pH in fatigued, single *Xenopus* muscle fibres. *Acta Physiol. Scand.* 133: 83–89.

Westerblad, H., Lee, J. A., Lamb, A. G., Bolsover, S. R., and Allen, D. G. (1990). Spatial gradients of intracellular calcium in skeletal muscle during fatigue. *Pflugers Arch.* 415: 734–740.

Westerblad, H., Lee, J. A., Lännergren, J., and Allen, D. G. (1991). Cellular mechanisms of fatigue in skeletal muscle. *Am. J. Physiol.* 261: C195–C209.

7

Changes in Activation, Contractile Speed, and Electrolyte Balance During Fatigue of Sustained and Repeated Contractions

NINA K. VØLLESTAD

National Institute of Occupational Health
Oslo, Norway

I. Introduction

It is well known that muscle strength declines during exercise. This is evident from the continuous fall in force output during sustained maximal voluntary or tetanically stimulated contractions (Fig. 1a) (Merton, 1954; Jones et al., 1979; Hultman and Sjöholm, 1983). During submaximal voluntary exercise a decrease in muscle strength is not necessarily reflected in the performance. Instead, force loss can be determined from test contractions elicited at given intervals during the exercise (see Fig. 1b). Here *fatigue* is defined as any reduction in the force-generating capacity of the muscle, as assessed by the force elicited when the muscle is maximally activated. The schematic example in Figure 1b shows that the muscle strength, tested periodically by brief maximal voluntary contractions (MVCs), starts to decline from the onset of exercise. Moreover, at the time when the MVC force falls below the target force level, subjects can no longer generate the required force. The definition used in many studies, that fatigue occurs when there is "an inability to maintain the required or expected force" (Edwards, 1981), ignores the continuous fall in maximum muscle contractile strength that occurs before this point. Instead, we describe the condition when a subject is no longer able to maintain the target force as *exhaustion*, with fatigue accruing from exercise onset (see Fig. 1b). Therefore, we prefer to define fatigue as "a reduction in the force-generating

235

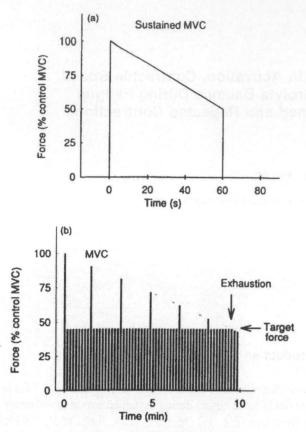

Figure 1 Schematic representation of fatigue protocols with (a) sustained MVC and (b) repeated contractions at 45% of the control MVC. Fatigue was defined as the reduction in the MVC force,

capacity" regardless of the task required (Vøllestad and Sejersted, 1988; Vøllestad et al., 1988). With this definition, we can quantify fatigue from the fall in MVC force or in the force response to electrically stimulated tetanic contractions. The latter definition of fatigue will, therefore, be used here to present novel information concerning changes in mechanical properties and activation processes, which challenges some of the generally accepted facts about events underlying fatigue.

As illustrated in Figure 2, voluntary force generation results from a sequence of events. These events can be divided into seven key processes, each of which is a potential limiting factor for force. The first process (*1*) comprises all central factors influencing activation of the motoneurons. Motivational factors as well as integration of sensory information are included. The next relevant process is the signal transfer in the neuromuscular junction (*2*). In this synapse, acetylcholine released from the

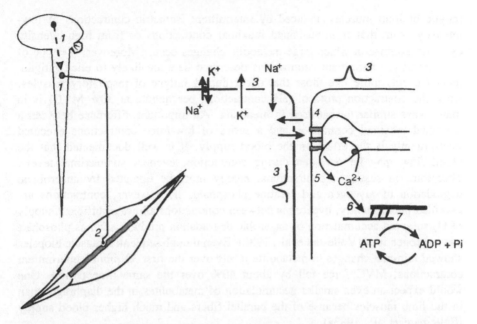

Figure 2 Schematic drawing of events in voluntary activation that may be limiting for force generation. *1*. All central factors influencing activation of motoneurons. *2*. Synaptic signal transfer at the motor end plate. *3*. Propagation of the action potentials along the sarcolemma and the T tubules. *4*. Transfer of signal from depolarization of T-tubular membrane to the SR. *5*. Opening of Ca^{2+} channels in SR. *6*. Binding of Ca^{2+} to troponin. *7*. Interaction of actin and myosin in cross-bridges.

motoneurons will bind transiently to the postsynaptical receptor, and action potentials are generated when sufficient end-plate potentials are summated. Adequate propagation of the action potentials along the sarcolemma and the T tubules depends on the fluxes of Na^+ and K^+ through channels in the membrane (*3*). In addition, activation of the Na–K pumps is required to reestablish the ionic difference between the intra- and extracellular compartments. When the action potentials are propagated, molecules in the membrane of T tubules and sarcoplasmic reticulum (SR) will interact (*4*), and Ca^{2+} channels in SR will open. Because of the electrochemical gradient between SR and cytosol, a Ca^{2+} flux into the cytosol will occur (*5*). The elevated cytosolic Ca^{2+} concentration, in turn, will bind to troponin C (*6*), and subsequently, myosin molecules attach to actin and cross-bridges are formed (*7*). The relevance for fatigue of these seven key processes will differ with the varying degree of metabolic, ionic, and electrical changes seen when different fatigue protocols are used.

In recent years, it has become clear that the changes accompanying fatigue differ, depending on the type of exercise involved. Thus, it is relevant to compare fatigue of limb muscles, induced by intermittent isometric contractions of low-intensity, with that from sustained maximal contractions or from high-intensity dynamic exercise in which large metabolic changes occur. Moreover, the type of low-intensity, intermittent contractions described here are likely to elicit fatigue-related events more like those that occur during fatigue of respiratory muscles, since the contraction protocol (six contractions per minute at 30% MVC) is in many ways similar to that used in breathing. An important difference between a sustained maximal contraction and a series of low-force contractions executed intermittently is the effect on the blood supply. It is well documented that the blood flow may be occluded during contraction, even at submaximal levels. Therefore, in sustained contractions, energy must be liberated by anaerobical degradation of glycogen and creatine phosphate. If, however, contractions are executed intermittently, hyperemia between contractions allows a sufficient supply of O_2 to avoid accumulation of anaerobic degradation products such as phosphate and hydrogen ions (Vøllestad et al., 1988). Even though sequential muscle biopsies showed minimal changes in metabolite levels over the first 30 min of intermittent contractions, MVC force fell by about 40% over the same time period. One would expect an even smaller accumulation of metabolites in the diaphragm than in the limb muscles because of the parallel fibers and much higher blood supply (Bellemare et al., 1983a).

Fatigue is often studied in relation to changes in contractile properties of twitch, MVC, or tetanic responses measured before, during, and after fatiguing voluntary or stimulated contractions. But it is important to point out that normal voluntary activity seldom involves either sustained maximal efforts or single twitches, since the motoneuron firing rates are mainly in the range (10–20 Hz) that results in partial summation of force. This should be kept in mind when interpretations are made concerning fatigue from voluntary contractions.

II. Force Loss: Central and Peripheral Factors

When a maximal voluntary contraction of the adductor pollicis, biceps brachii, or quadriceps muscles is sustained, the MVC force as well as that in response to tetanic stimulation (e.g., at 80 Hz) fall gradually to about 50% of control in approximately 1 min (Jones et al., 1979; Bigland-Ritchie et al., 1986a). These changes recover to preexercise levels within 5–10 min of aerobic rest (Bigland-Ritchie et al., 1986a). When the same values are measured during repeated submaximal contractions, the MVC and tetanic forces both start to decline gradually and in parallel from the onset of exercise (Fig. 3). The rate of force decline, however, is much slower than in an MVC and depends on the contraction intensity, frequency, and duty cycle (Bigland-Ritchie et al., 1986b; Vøllestad et al., 1988). For example, during repeated 6-s contractions of the quadriceps muscles at 30 or 50% MVC (0.6 duty cycle), tetanic force (50 Hz) and MVC force fell in parallel, reaching about 60% of control

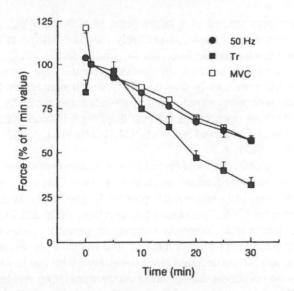

Figure 3 Changes in force responses of MVC, 50-Hz stimulation and single shocks (twitch) during repeated 30% MVC contractions (6-s on, 4-s off) with the quadriceps muscles. *N* = 5.

levels after about 30 and 6 min, respectively (Bigland-Ritchie et al., 1986b, Vøllestad et al., 1988).

For many years, it has been discussed whether fatigue is due to processes in the central nervous system (CNS) or in the muscles themselves. In 1954, Merton reported that the adductor pollicis muscle could be maximally activated during fatigue from ischemic maximal contractions, since there was no additional force generated when a single electrical shock was given during the voluntary contractions. Hence, he concluded that there was no central fatigue. This issue, however, has been reexamined in more recent experiments, in which the same twitch interpolation technique was used, but with an increased sensitivity (McKenzie et al., 1992). These studies showed that attempted maximal voluntary contractions generated 95–100% of the true maximal tetanic force in the diaphragm and the elbow flexor muscles at rest. When maximal contractions were repeated 30 times, the voluntary activation was reduced to 86% of maximum for the limb muscles, but no significant change was observed for the diaphragm. Hence, a small fraction of the fatigue developed during repeated MVCs can be ascribed to factors in the CNS.

An important question is whether the central fatigue develops gradually over time during a fatiguing submaximal exercise. In experiments carried out by several research groups, a repetitive isometric contraction protocol has been used, with contractions lasting 6 s, separated by a 4-s rest. When the quadriceps and the soleus muscles were studied at a target force of 50% of MVC, the MVC was halved over about 4 and 35 min, respectively (Bigland-Ritchie et al., 1986b). In the quadriceps muscle, tetanic force fell in parallel to the MVC and, hence, no central fatigue could be detected. In contrast with this, the tetanic force in the soleus muscle fell more slowly than the MVC, and it was concluded that factors in the CNS and within the muscle itself contributed about equally to the fatigue. Repeated submaximal contractions with the diaphragm induces a degree of central fatigue similar to that observed for soleus (McKenzie et al., 1992; Bellemare and Bigland-Ritchie, 1987).

The different contribution of central factors in fatigue of soleus and quadriceps might be related to the difference in endurance time. One may argue that, with more prolonged exercise, a larger fraction of the fatigue can be ascribed to reduced motor drive from the CNS. To examine this question, we let healthy subjects carry out the same intermittent isometric contraction protocol using the quadriceps muscles, but this time with a target force of 30% MVC. With this target force, the endurance time was 30 min or longer (i.e., comparable with that in which substantial central fatigue was observed during soleus contractions). Our results showed again that the MVC and tetanic forces fell in parallel and, hence, the CNS remained capable of maximally (or nearly maximally) activating the quadriceps muscles over a long time period.

Taken together, these observations show that the degree of central fatigue depends on the muscle being exercised and the contraction protocol. Furthermore, in all muscles studied, it is clear that at least a large fraction of the decline in force-generating capacity can be ascribed to mechanisms within the muscle itself.

It has been a question for many years of to what extent neuromuscular transmission failure contribute to the decline in force-generation capacity during voluntary contraction. In 1954, Merton observed that the amplitude of the muscle compound action potential (M-wave) resulting from a single stimulus applied to the motor nerve remained virtually unchanged during a sustained MVC. This observation suggested that the entire cause of the fatigue was located distally to the excitation of the sarcolemma. At about the same time, however, Næss and Storm-Mathisen (1955) recorded a decline in the amplitude of the M-wave; hence, they concluded that neuromuscular transmission may become a limiting factor for force generation during fatigue. Both these opinions have gained support from studies conducted over the last 30 years. Several research groups have repeatedly found that, in voluntary contraction, the amplitude of the M-wave decrease with fatigue (Bigland-Ritchie et al., 1982; Thomas et al., 1989; Fuglevand et al., 1993; Milner-Brown and Miller, 1986), and this change occurs in parallel with an increasing duration. Therefore, the area remains virtually unchanged by contractile activity. The disparity in opinion of the importance of neuromuscular transmission for fatigue, is based on the interpretation of these results. Thomas and co-workers (1989) suggest that the decline in amplitude and the increase in duration are caused by dispersion of a wider range in conduction velocities of the motor units. They base their interpretation on the view that the efficiency of neuromuscular transmission can be assessed only from the changes in area of the M-wave. Fuglevand and co-workers (1993), on the other hand, argue against this view, because in a sustained contraction at high force the conduction velocity of the faster and most fatiguable motor units would probably be more affected than the fatigue-resistant units. Hence, they suggest that from changes in conduction velocity alone, one would expect the dispersion to decrease, rather than increase. Therefore, they argue that the increased duration of the M-wave is caused by a less efficient signal transfer in the neuromuscular junction.

None of these opinions, however, take into account the observations of decreased amplitude and increased duration of action potentials recorded in single muscle fibers during fatigue using direct stimulation in vitro (Lännergren and Westerblad, 1987). Signal transfer in the neuromuscular junction cannot explain the action potential changes under these circumstances. Rather, it is likely that the increase in extracellular K^+ concentration is an important mechanism for these changes in action potential, as pointed out by Jones (1981). Studies of the M-wave properties, therefore, cannot give conclusive answers to the question of whether neuromuscular transmission failure occurs during fatigue from voluntary contraction. Further studies, with other methodological approaches, are needed to clarify this issue.

During fatigue from voluntary contractions, the force from a single electrical shock (twitch) or from low-frequency stimulation (e.g., 10 Hz) falls faster than the MVC and tetanic forces, reaching about 20% of control value after repeated submaximal isometric contractions as shown in Fig 3. (Bigland-Ritchie et al., 1986b). The same difference is seen during, and for many hours following, fatigue induced by repeated tetanic contractions (Edwards et al., 1977). The disproportional larger decline in the twitch or the low-frequency stimulated response, compared with tetanic stimulation, is often called low-frequency fatigue. As early as 1977, Edwards and co-workers (1977) proposed that this type of fatigue is caused by reduced Ca^{2+} release. More recent studies support this conclusion (Westerblad et al., 1991), although it has not yet been demonstrated directly.

An important factor connected to fatigue is the recovery of the force-generating capacity to preexercise levels. The MVC force recovers within 5–10 min after a sustained MVC (e.g., Bigland-Ritchie et al., 1986a). When fatigue is induced using repeated submaximal contractions, recovery rates are much slower. As illustrated in Figure 4, only about half the reduction in tetanic force was normalized within the first 30 min of postexercise recovery (I. Sejersted and N. K. Vøllestad, unpublished results). The recovery rate was almost the same after repeated contractions at 30, 45, and 60% MVC, suggesting that endurance times (45, 15, and 5 min, respectively) were unrelated to recovery rates.

III. Contractile Speed

Slowing of the contractile properties of the muscle is often considered as an integral part of fatigue (Westerblad et al., 1991). Contractile speed is most often determined

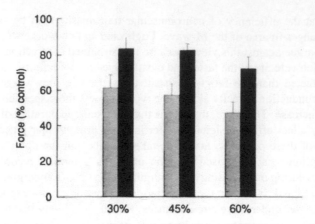

Figure 4   Postexercise recovery of the force response to 50-Hz stimulation of the quadriceps muscle. Hatched bars represent data at exhaustion and solid bars after 30-min recovery. Fatigue was induced by repeated isometric contractions (6 s on, 4 s off) at 30, 45, or 60% of MVC. Mean and SE values for seven subjects. (Courtesy of I. Sejersted.)

by contraction (CT) and half relaxation ($RT_{0.5}$) times, as shown in Figure 5, or their corresponding maximum contraction (MCR) and relaxation (MRR) rates. Several studies of either electrically stimulated contractions or sustained voluntary contractions have shown a 50–100% increase in half relaxation time (Hultman and Sjöholm, 1983; Bergström and Hultman, 1986; Wiles and Edwards, 1982; Bigland-Ritchie et al., 1983b). In all these studies, fatigue was studied under ischemic conditions, resulting in large metabolic changes, and the exercise duration is limited to a few minutes or less. The slowing of contractile speed is then often ascribed to low pH, fall in ATP, increase in inorganic phosphate (P_i), or increase in ADP (Westerblad et al., 1991). By using a more prolonged exercise model, Saltin and coworkers (personal communication) observed a 40% elongation of $RT_{0.5}$ during dynamic knee extension carried out for an hour. Over the first 30 min of postexercise rest, contractile speed recovered to almost preexercise values. These changes could not be ascribed to low pH, since only minor changes in pH were seen. An earlier study demonstrating substantial slowing of muscle in subjects with myophosphorylase deficiency (produced no H^+ from glycolysis) supports that factors other than low pH must be involved in slowing of relaxation (Cady et al., 1989). Saltin and coworkers determined the rate of Ca^{2+} uptake into the sarcoplasmic reticulum (SR) and found a close inverse relation with the changes in $RT_{0.5}$. Their observations indicate that, under these conditions, removal of Ca^{2+} limits relaxation speed. Since the reduced Ca^{2+} uptake into SR and the slowing of contractile speed are thought to be of metabolic origin, it might be hypothesized that fatigue in the absence of changed metabolite levels would not be associated with contractile slowing.

In recent experiments we examined this hypothesis by using repeated isometric

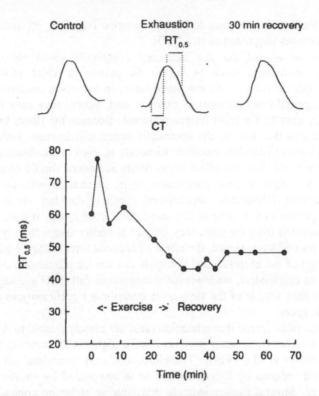

Figure 5 Changes in twitch characteristics during repeated 30% MVC contractions (6 s on, 4 s off) with the quadriceps muscles. Upper tracings show twitches from one subject before exercise (control), at exhaustion, and after 30-min recovery. Contraction time (CT) is measured as the time from 10 to 90% of the peak force. Half-relaxation time ($RT_{0.5}$) is determined as the time from peak force to 50% of the peak force. Lower panel shows changes in twitch $RT_{0.5}$ in one subject during and following the fatiguing exercise. (Courtesy of I. Sejersted.)

voluntary contractions (6-s contractions and 4-s rest) with a target force of 30% of the control MVC. Earlier experiments revealed that for at least 30 min of this type of exercise, only small changes were seen in glycogen, creatine phosphate, and lactate concentrations, and ATP levels remained unchanged (Vøllestad et al., 1988). Twitches elicited from the relaxed muscle between target force contractions showed an *increased* contractile speed as exercise progressed (see Fig. 5) (Sejersted et al., 1993). Twitch contraction time (CT) fell by 19% over the first 5 min of exercise and, thereafter, remained almost unchanged. Twitch half relaxation time, on the other hand, increased only the first minute, before a continuous fall was observed, reaching 71% of control after 30 min. Studies in progress indicate that the increased twitch contractile speed induced by this type of contraction remained almost unchanged for the first 30 min following exercise (see Fig. 5), indicating slow recovery processes (Sejersted et al., 1993).

It may be argued that the increased contractile speed observed in our submaximal contractions could be due to the pattern in which motor units are recruited as fatigue accrues. As discussed later, in low-force contractions, type I fibers are recruited from the start of exercise and, hence, they may fatigue first, although they may be the most fatigue-resistant. Because the fibers first recruited are probably also the slowest, the contractile speed will increase with time when all fiber types are activated by electrical stimulation, even in the absence of changes at the cellular level. But any effect of recruitment pattern should change CT and $RT_{0.5}$ equally, whereas these parameters seem to change with quite different temporal patterns (Vøllestad, unpublished results). Another argument against recruitment pattern as the cause of increased contractile speed, is that, since type I fibers are activated from the start, they fatigue at earlier stages than type II fibers, which are recruited later. Hence, the effect of reduced force in type I will be largest in the first part of the exercise, and diminish as exercise progresses. As illustrated in Figure 5 for one subject, we observed a continuous fall in $RT_{0.5}$, suggesting that factors other than fatigue of the slow units contribute significantly to the increase in contractile speed.

It is generally agreed that relaxation rates are closely related to ATP turnover rates in the muscles [i.e., faster muscles have a higher ATP turnover (Edwards et al., 1975a; Wiles et al., 1979)]. Therefore, one may speculate that changes in relaxation rate induced by fatigue should be accompanied by similar changes in ATP turnover. Several studies indicate that, during ischemic contractions when contractile speed slows, ATP turnover is also reduced (Edwards et al., 1975a, b). It has recently been demonstrated that the energetic cost of contraction *increases* gradually during the repeated submaximal isometric quadriceps contractions in which contractile speed also increases (Vøllestad et al., 1990; Vøllestad and Saugen, 1992). Hence, during fatigue, relaxation rate also seems to be closely coupled to the ATP turnover of the muscle.

IV. Muscle Excitation Rates

When the muscle is stimulated at frequencies that result in submaximal unfused tetanic force, the extent of force summation between successive stimuli is largely determined by its contractile speed. In the unfatigued state, a slow muscle, such as the soleus, generates 50% of its maximum force when excited at a lower rate than a faster muscle (e.g., biceps brachii or adductor pollicis). Thus, when a muscle slows, one may expect the force–frequency curve to be shifted to the left, and a given force may be achieved by a lower excitation frequency. This is consistent with the observation by Bigland-Ritchie and co-workers (1983b) that, following a 60-s MVC, the mean force as well as the degree of fusion increased in response to

7- to 10-Hz stimulation, despite a 50% drop in maximal force. Thus, the eventual outcome in terms of force is uncertain, depending on the balance between force loss and contractile speed changes, which determine whether the force–frequency relation shifts to the left (slowing) or to the right during fatigue. On the other hand, a rightward shift of the force–frequency curve will occur when the muscle becomes faster, and fatigue will enhance this effect. Higher excitation rates are thus needed to maintain force. Indeed, fatigue-induced shifts to both the left and right were about equally evident in force–frequency relations of individual human thenar motor units measured before and after the Burke fatigue test was applied (Thomas et al., 1991).

These observations raise the question: To what extent does the central nervous system change the pattern of muscle excitation to match the contractile speed during fatigue, and thereby optimize force? The excitation rate declines quite rapidly during a sustained maximal contraction (Bigland-Ritchie et al., 1983a). The excitation rates recover rapidly during nonischemic recovery, whereas continued depressed excitation is seen when the muscle blood flow remains occluded following exercise (Bigland-Ritchie et al., 1986a). These data suggest that motor unit-firing rates are regulated to optimize force during a maximal contraction.

We have recently found that the twitches become faster during fatigue from submaximal contractions (see Fig. 5). Recordings from individual muscle fibers with intramuscular flexible electrodes during 30% MVC contractions revealed a firing rate of almost 13 Hz in the unfatigued (control) state. When these submaximal contractions, each held for 6 s with 4 s rest between, were repeated continuously for 30 min, a fall in firing rate (to about 11 Hz) was seen over the first 1–5 min, followed by a gradual increase reaching about 16 Hz (Fig. 6) (Bigland-Ritchie et al., 1986c). The temporal changes in half-relaxation rates and firing rates during target force contractions were closely related, suggesting that CNS motoneuron excitation pattern matches the changes in contractile speed. With excitation rates between 11 and 16 Hz, force is at the steep part of the force–frequency relation and the tetanic responses are unfused (Edwards et al., 1977; Thomas et al., 1991; Bigland-Ritchie et al., 1983b). Hence, when contractile speed increases, as in these experiments, the fatigue-induced decrease in half-relaxation times must reduce twitch summation. This, together with the overall reduction in maximal force, appears to be partly compensated by faster excitation rates as well as by motor unit recruitment. Hence, a maintained target force can be achieved.

During fatigue from prolonged submaximal exercise, force or power output can be maintained by increasing muscle activation by exciting more motor units (recruitment), in addition to increasing the firing rate to those already active (rate coding). Glycogen depletion patterns, examined during low-intensity bicycle exercise ($\sim 40\% V_{O_{2max}}$) show that almost solely type I fibers were recruited initially (Vøllestad and Blom, 1985). At higher intensities, an increasing number of type II fibers were active from the beginning. Studies of exhaustive bicycle exercise at

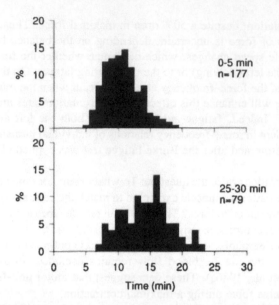

Figure 6 Histograms of motor unit excitation rates in the first 5 min and between 25–30 min of repeated 30% MVC contractions (6 s on, 4 s off) with the quadriceps muscles. (Data from Bigland-Ritchie et al., 1986c.)

75% of Vo_{2max}, showed that type I fibers and type IIA fibers (the most oxidative fast-twitch fibers) were recruited from the beginning (Vøllestad et al., 1984). At later stages, type IIAB and IIB fibers (the least oxidative fibers) were also activated. Hence, all fibers of the vastus lateralis muscle were engaged before exhaustion, and the recruitment pattern followed the sequence I+IIA → IIAB → IIB. The same recruitment pattern was also seen more recently during fatigue from repeated submaximal isometric contractions (Bigland-Ritchie et al., 1986c).

Surface electromyography (EMG) is often used to study the changes in muscle activation, since the integrated rectified EMG amplitude is an integrated measure of the number of action potentials and the area of each. The EMG amplitude of human muscle relates curvilinearly to force in the unfatigued state (Woods and Bigland-Ritchie, 1984). It is not possible to distinguish between the effect of recruitment and firing rate when EMG is used alone. However, in combination with other information, these data may throw some light on the mechanisms involved. In our recent experiments of repeated submaximal contractions, we found that the integrated EMG signal increased almost fourfold, whereas the firing rate increased by only about 25% (Bigland-Ritchie et al., 1986c). Since the changes in the action potential area are small during such prolonged activity, this discrepancy indicated a substantial recruitment. This conclusion was also supported by the glycogen-depletion patterns. Hence, to maintain a constant submaximal target force over a protracted time, increased muscle activity was achieved by recruitment as well as by rate coding.

Another parameter often used when studying muscle fatigue is the shift in the EMG power spectrum toward lower values (Bigland-Ritchie et al., 1981, 1983a; Moxham et al., 1982). This shift occurs during prolonged exercise, as well as during maximal contractions. The underlying causes for the shift in power spectrum are still unresolved. Some studies suggest that a lowered conduction velocity in the muscle fibers is the most important factor (Lindström et al., 1970). Others, in which changes in conduction velocity were assessed from muscle compound action potentials, indicate that this can explain only a fraction of the spectral shift (Moritani et al., 1986; Bigland-Ritchie et al., 1981; Krogh-Lund and Jørgensen, 1992). In one study of repeated submaximal contractions, the power spectrum remained virtually unchanged, both during exercise and in the subsequent 30-min recovery period (Moxham et al., 1982). In these experiments, low-frequency fatigue developed during exercise and remained low during recovery; whereas tetanic force recovered within 10 min. Hence, a normal power spectrum was seen with low tetanic force, together with low-frequency fatigue, and also when tetanic force had recovered. Since the causes of the shifts in EMG power spectrum and its relation to fatigue are poorly understood, one should be careful about using this variable as a measure of fatigue.

V. Electrolyte Shift

Over the last decade, several investigators have focused on the potential effect of altered K^+ balance on muscle function, and they have tried to relate fatigue to shifts in K^+, both intracellularly and extracellularly (Medbø and Sejersted, 1990; Hnik et al., 1972; Vyskocil et al., 1983; Vøllestad et al., 1991; Sjøgaard, 1990; Clausen and Everts, 1991). Interstitial K^+ concentrations were measured directly in only a few of these studies. These indicate that K^+ values between 10 and 15 mM can be reached during 30-s voluntary maximal ischemic contractions, compared with resting values of 4–5 mM (Vyskocil et al., 1983). During maximal treadmill running for 1–4 min, venous effluent blood K^+ concentration reaches about 8 mM at the point of exhaustion and recovers to values below preexercise levels within 1 min of recovery (Medbø and Sejersted, 1990; Vøllestad et al., 1994). With these high K^+ levels, attenuation of the action potential amplitudes can be expected. Moreover, in vitro experiments show that both the resting membrane potential and the amplitude of the action potentials are important for an adequate release of Ca^{2+} from the sarcoplasmic reticulum (SR) (Vergara et al., 1978). Repeated tetanic stimulation of isolated xenopus muscles may induce a 70-mV reduction in the action potential amplitude and a two- to threefold increase in the duration (Lännergren and Westerblad, 1986, 1987). These changes have been attributed to elevated extracellular K^+ concentrations, since similar changes in the action potential amplitude have been observed in unfatigued fibers when extracellular K^+ concentration was raised to 10–15 mM (Lännergren and Westerblad, 1986; Jones, 1981). Thus, an increase in extracellular $[K^+]$ could contribute to the reduction in force-generating capacity in sustained high-force contractions, even though these are not normally associated with a fall in the muscle compound action potential. The rapid increase in the recovery period subsequent to this type of exercise is compatible with a restoration of preexercise interstitial K^+ levels that occur within a minute or less (Medbø and Sejersted, 1990; Vøllestad et al., 1994).

Further support for the possible role of extracellular K^+ for muscular function has come from studies of isolated muscle preparations. During prolonged stimulation at high frequency (80 Hz), intermittent failure to generate action potentials has been shown (Clamann and Robinson, 1985). In these conditions, one may expect extracellular K^+ concentration to rise substantially, especially in the T tubules, and indirect evidence suggests that blockade at T-tubular conduction may develop. By monitoring the intracellular Ca^{2+} concentration in the muscle fibers from *Xenopus* and mouse during stimulation, Westerblad and co-workers (1990) showed that 100-Hz stimulation initially results in homogenous high Ca^{2+} levels in the cells. However, as stimulation continued, the Ca^{2+} concentration in the center of the fibers declined, whereas that near the surface remained high. When they reduced the excitation frequency to 20 Hz, normal homogenous Ca^{2+} distribution was rapidly achieved, together with an augmented force response. These studies suggest that, even when propagation over the muscle fiber surface is unimpaired, failure may occur within the T tubules during high-frequency stimulation.

An important question is whether these changes are relevant during fatigue from normal voluntary contraction, since human motor unit firing rates during maintained contractions are generally below 30 Hz (Bellemare et al., 1983b), and often falling by about 10 Hz over a 60-s sustained MVC contraction (Bigland-Ritchie et al., 1983a). Hence, even with maximal activation, the firing rates are well below the level at which propagation failure would be expected. Furthermore, Thomas and co-workers (1989) showed that, when a sustained MVC was held for up to 5 min, the amplitude of the compound action potential remained unaltered in tibialis anterior, and fell only during the first 2 min (by only 19%) in the much smaller first dorsal interosseus muscle (Fig. 7). These temporal responses differed markedly from the continuous decline in maximal force.

During bicycle exercise at intensities below Vo_{2max}, plasma K^+ increases less than during intense exercise, and a different temporal pattern is seen. At the onset of exercise at 60–85% Vo_{2max}, the extracellular K^+ concentration increases rapidly by about 1–2 mM (Sahlin and Broberg, 1989; Sjøgaard et al., 1985; Vøllestad et al., 1994), but as exercise continues, plasma K^+ concentration either levels off or may even decline. In spite of this, some studies show a continuous net release of K^+ throughout this type of exercise (Sahlin and Broberg, 1989; Sjøgaard et al., 1985), whereas we were unable to detect significant differences between arterial and venous blood after 10 min at 60 and 85% Vo_{2max} (Vøllestad et al., 1994). The

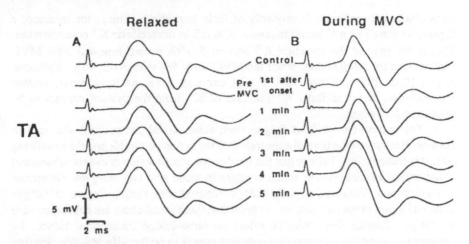

Figure 7 Evoked M waves recorded from a human tibialis anterior muscle before and during a sustained MVC. (From Thomas et al., 1989.)

reason for this discrepancy remains unclear. During prolonged repeated or sustained low-force isometric contractions, there is general agreement that K^+ is continuously lost from the active muscle (Vøllestad et al., 1991; Sjøgaard, 1990). Hence, during submaximal exercise, extracellular K^+ concentrations increase only moderately, but a continuous loss of K^+ from the muscle has been demonstrated.

With submaximal exercise protocols, the rise in extracellular K^+ levels are too low to affect the force-generating capacity noticeably (Sjøgaard, 1990; Vøllestad et al., 1991). However, since the K^+ concentration in the T tubules of human muscle has not yet been measured successfully, one might argue that transient accumulation of K^+ could occur in this compartment during contraction. Diffusion of K^+ is a rapid process, and a homogeneous concentration in the extracellular fluid would be expected within the first second after termination of excitation. Thus, one should expect a rapid recovery of the force-generating capacity within less than a minute if T-tubular accumulation of K^+ is a major determinant for fatigue. In fact, after fatigue from repeated isometric contractions at 30, 45, and 60% MVC, the force from maximal voluntary contractions and from tetanic stimulation recovered only partly over the first 30 min of rest (see Fig. 4; I. Sejersted and N. K. Vøllestad, unpublished results). A large fraction of the near 50% fall in MVC force in this kind of exercise protocol, therefore, must be ascribed to other factors. The accumulation of K^+ ions is probably of even less importance for fatigue in the diaphragm owing to its higher capillarization compared with limb muscles.

The long-lasting release of K^+ from the exercising muscle during repeated submaximal contractions, could result in a gradual depolarization, even though extracellular K^+ is almost unchanged (Byström and Sjøgaard, 1991). This fall in intracellular concentration is probably of little importance, since, for instance, a depolarization of 18 mV would require a 50% fall in intracellular K^+ concentration. This is far beyond the muscular K^+ loss of 5–10% during repeated 30% MVC contractions for 30–100 min, when the MVC force fell with about 40% (Vøllestad et al., 1988, 1991). Hence, during brief exercise at submaximal levels, neither accumulation of extracellular K^+ nor loss of K^+ from the cytosol appears to be important for fatigue.

The mechanisms behind fatigue from submaximal contractions still remain unclear. Because of the normal appearance of the action potentials and the low-firing rate, it is reasonable to believe that the mechanisms must reside in events subsequent to membrane excitation. The minor changes in lactic acid and inorganic phosphate concentrations (Vøllestad et al., 1988), compared with similar degree of fatigue induced by other types of exercise, suggest that these metabolites are not responsible for fatigue through their potential effect on cross-bridge interaction. Hence, by elimination, excitation–contraction coupling seems to be the affected step. Further studies are needed to reveal the true mechanisms.

VI. General Conclusion

Muscle fatigue of voluntary contractions may be accompanied by changes in muscle activation, changes in contractile speed, and in electrolyte shifts, all of which can influence force output. For any given reduction in force-generating capacity, there are both quantitative and qualitative differences in these changes, depending on the type and intensity of exercise. During sustained high-force contractions, or intense dynamic exercise, large metabolic changes occur, and the muscle becomes slower.

In contrast, during repeated submaximal isometric contractions, only negligible accumulation of H^+ and inorganic phosphate occurs, and these metabolites cannot contribute much to fatigue. There is also no reason to believe that the loss of K^+ ions from cytosol, or the elevation in interstitial K^+ concentration, is large enough to cause the 50% decline in maximal force reported for repetitive submaximal exercise (Vøllestad et al., 1988, 1991). With this type of exercise, muscle contractile speed is not reduced. Instead, twitch contraction and half-relaxation times gradually get shorter. The available information indicates that optimization of force by the adjustment of motoneuron-firing patterns to match the contractile speed, is one common response, irrespective of fatigue protocol.

Acknowledgments

I thank Brenda Bigland-Ritchie for her important contributions in preparation of this paper. I also thank Jostein Hallén and Eirik Saugen for stimulating discussions and their comments to previous versions of the paper. Ingrid Sejersted has kindly allowed me to use some of her data. I also thank The Royal Norwegian Council for Scientific and Industrial Research for financial support to my own recent studies included in the review.

References

Bellemare, F., and Bigland-Ritchie, B. (1987). Central components of diaphragmatic fatigue assessed from bilateral phrenic nerve stimulation. *J. Appl. Physiol.* 62: 1307.

Bellemare, F., Wight, D., Lavigne, C. M., and Grassino, A. (1983a). Effect of tension and timing on the blood flow of the diaphragm. *J. Appl. Physiol.* 54: 1597.

Bellemare, F., Woods, J. J., Johansson, R., and Bigland-Ritchie, B. (1983b). Motor-unit discharge rates in maximal voluntary contractions of three human muscles. *J. Neurophysiol.* 50: 1380.

Bergström, M., and Hultman, E. (1986). Relaxation time during intermittent isometric contraction in subjects with different capacity for oxidative work. *Acta Physiol. Scand.* 127: 107.

Bigland-Ritchie, B., Donavan, E. F., and Roussos, C. S. (1981). Conduction velocity and EMG power spectrum changes in fatigue of sustained maximal efforts. *Am. J. Physiol.* 51: 1300.

Bigland-Ritchie, B., Kukulka, C. G., Lippold, O. C. J., and Woods, J. J. (1982). The absence of neuromuscular transmission failure in sustained maximal voluntary contractions. *J. Physiol. (Lond.)* 330: 265.

Bigland-Ritchie, B., Johansson, R., Lippold, O. C. J., Smith, S., and Woods, J. J. (1983a). Changes in motoneurone firing rates during sustained maximal contractions. *J. Physiol. (Lond.)* 340: 335.

Bigland-Ritchie, B., Johansson, R., Lippold, O. C. J., and Woods, J. J. (1983b). Contractile speed and EMG changes during fatigue of sustained maximal voluntary contractions. *J. Neurophysiol.* 50: 313.

Bigland-Ritchie, B., Dawson, N. J., Johansson, R. S., and Lippold, O. C. J. (1986a). Reflex origin for the slowing of motoneurone firing rates in fatigue of human voluntary contractions. *J. Physiol. (Lond.)* 379: 451.

Bigland-Ritchie, B., Furbush, F., and Woods, J. J. (1986b). Fatigue of intermittent submaximal voluntary contractions: Central and peripheral factors. *J. Appl. Physiol.* 61: 421.

Bigland-Ritchie, B., Cafarelli, E., and Vøllestad, N. K. (1986c). Fatigue of submaximal static contractions. *Acta Physiol. Scand.* 128: 137.

Byström, S., and Sjøgaard, G. (1991). Potassium homeostasis during and following exhaustive submaximal static handgrip contractions. *Acta Physiol. Scand.* 142: 59.

Cady, E. B., Elshove, H., Jones, D. A., and Moll, A. (1989). The metabolic causes of slow relaxation in fatigued human skeletal muscle. *J. Physiol. (Lond.)* 418: 327.

Clamann, H. P., and Robinson, A. J. (1985). A comparison of electromyographic and mechanical fatigue properties in motor units of the cat hindlimb. *Brain Res.* 327: 203.

Clausen, T., and Everts, M. E. (1991). K^+-induced inhibition of contractile force in rat skeletal muscle: Role of active Na^+-K^+ transport. *Am. J. Physiol.* 261: C799.

Edwards, R. H. T. (1981). *Human Muscle Fatigue: Physiological Mechanisms.* Edited by R. Porter and J. Whelan. London, Pitman Medical, p. 1.

Edwards, R. H. T., Hill, D. H., and Jones, D. A. (1975a). Metabolic changes associated with the slowing of relaxation in fatigued mouse muscle. *J. Physiol. (Lond.)* 251: 287.

Edwards, R. H. T., Hill, D. K., and Jones, D. A. (1975b). Heat production and chemical changes during isometric contractions of the human quadriceps muscle. *J. Physiol. (Lond.)* 251: 303.

Edwards, R. H. T., Hill, D. K., Jones, D. A., and Merton, P. A. (1977). Fatigue of long duration in human skeletal muscle after exercise. *J. Physiol. (Lond.)* 272: 769.

Fuglevand, A. J., Zackowski, K. M., Huey, K. A., and Enoka, R. M. (1993). Impairment of neuromuscular propagation during human fatiguing contractions at submaximal forces. *J. Physiol.* 460: 549.

Hnik, P., Vyskocil, F., Kriz, N., and Holas, M. (1972). Work-induced increase of extracellular potassium concentration in muscle measured by ion-specific electrodes. *Brain Res.* 40: 559.

Hultman, E., and Sjöholm, H. (1983). Electromyogram, force and relaxation time during and after continuous electrical stimulation of human skeletal muscle in situ. *J. Physiol. (Lond.)* 339: 33.

Jones, D. A. (1981). *Human Muscle Fatigue: Physiological Mechanisms.* Edited by R. Porter and J. Whelan. London, Pitman Medical, p. 178.

Jones, D. A., Bigland-Ritchie, B., and Edwards, R. H. T. (1979). Excitation frequency and muscle fatigue: Mechanical responses during voluntary and stimulated contractions. *Exp. Neurol.* 64: 401.

Krogh-Lund, C., and Jørgensen, K. (1992). Modification of myo-electric power spectrum in fatigue from 15% maximal voluntary contraction of human elbow flexor muscles, to limit of endurance: Reflection of conduction velocity variation and/or centrally mediated mechanisms? *Eur. J. Appl. Physiol.* 64: 359.

Lännergren, J., and Westerblad, H. (1986). Force and membrane potential during and after fatiguing, continuous high-frequency stimulation of single xenopus muscle fibres. *Acta Physiol. Scand.* 128: 359.

Lännergren, J., and Westerblad, H. (1987). Action potential fatigue in single skeletal muscle fibres of *Xenopus. Acta Physiol. Scand.* 129: 311.

Lindström, L., Magnusson, R., and Petersén, I. (1970). Muscular fatigue and action potential conduction velocity changes studied with frequency analysis of EMG signals. *Electromyography* 4: 341.

McKenzie, D. K., Bigland-Ritchie, B., Gorman, R. B., and Gandevia, S. C. (1992). Central and peripheral fatigue of human diaphragm and limb muscles assessed by twitch interpolation. *J. Physiol. (Lond.)* 454: 643.

Medbø, J. I., and Sejersted, O. M. (1990). Plasma potassium changes with high intensity exercise. *J. Physiol. (Lond.)* 421: 105.

Merton, P. A. (1954). Voluntary strength and fatigue. *J. Physiol. (Lond.)* 123: 553.

Milner-Brown, H. S., and Miller, R. G. (1986). Muscle membrane excitation and impulse propagation velocity are reduced during muscle fatigue. *Muscle Nerve* 367.

Moritani, T., Muro, M., and Nagata, A. (1986). Intramuscular and surface electromyogram changes during muscle fatigue. *J. Appl. Physiol.* 60: 1179.

Moxham, J., Edwards, R. H. T., Aubier, M., De Troyer, A., Farkas, G., Macklem, P. T., and Roussos, C. (1982). Changes in EMG power spectrum (high-to-low ratio) with force fatigue in humans. *J. Appl. Physiol.* 53: 1094.

Naess, K., and Storm-Mathisen, A. (1955). Fatigue of sustained tetanic contractions. *Acta Physiol. Scand.* 34: 351.

Sahlin, K., and Broberg, S. (1989). Release of K^+ from muscle during prolonged dynamic exercise. *Acta Physiol. Scand.* 136: 293.

Sejersted, I., Saugen, E., and Vøllestad, N. K. (1993). Muscle fatigue is associated with increased contractile speed during repeated submaximal isometric contractions. *Acta Physiol. Scand.* 149: 35A.

Sjøgaard, G. (1990). Exercise-induced muscle fatigue: Significance of potassium, *Acta Physiol. Scand.* [Suppl.]593: 1.

Sjøgaard, G., Adams, R. P., and Saltin, B. (1985). Water and ion shifts in skeletal muscle of humans with intense dynamic knee extension. *Am. J. Physiol.* 248: R190.

Thomas, C. K., Woods, J. J., and Bigland-Ritchie, B. (1989). Impulse propagation and muscle activation in long maximal voluntary contractions. *J. Appl. Physiol.* 67: 1835.

Thomas, C. K., Bigland-Ritchie, B., and Johansson, R. S. (1991). Force–frequency relationships of human thenar motor units. *J. Neurophysiol.* 65: 1509.

Vergara, J., Bezanilla, F., and Salzberg, B. M. (1978). Nile blue fluorescence signals from cut single muscle fibers under voltage or current clamp conditions. *J. Gen. Physiol.* 72: 775.

Vyskocil, F., Hnik, P., Rehfeldt, H., Vejsada, R., and Ujec, E. (1983). The measurement of

K_e^+ concentration changes in human muscles during volitional contractions. *Pflugers Arch.* 399: 235.

Vøllestad, N. K., and Blom, P. C. S. (1985). Effect of varying exercise intensity on glycogen depletion in human muscle fibres. *Acta Physiol. Scand.* 125: 395.

Vøllestad, N. K., and Saugen, E. (1992). *Current Problems in Neuromuscular Fatigue.* Edited by A. J. Sargeant and D. Kernell. Amsterdam, KNAW.

Vøllestad, N. K., and Sejersted, O. M. (1988). Biochemical correlates of fatigue. A brief review. *Eur. J. Appl. Physiol.* 57: 336.

Vøllestad, N. K., Vaage, O., and Hermansen, L. (1984). Muscle glycogen depletion patterns in type I and subgroups of type II fibres during prolonged severe exercise in man. *Acta Physiol. Scand.* 122: 433.

Vøllestad, N. K., Sejersted, O. M., Bahr, R., Woods, J. J., and Bigland-Ritchie, B. (1988). Motor drive and metabolic responses during repeated submaximal contractions in man. *J. Appl. Physiol.* 64: 1421.

Vøllestad, N. K., Wesche, J., and Sejersted, O. M. (1990). Gradual increase in leg oxygen uptake during repeated submaximal contractions in humans. *J. Appl. Physiol.* 68: 1150.

Vøllestad, N. K., Wesche, J., and Sejersted, O. M. (1991). Potassium balance of muscle and blood during and after repeated isometric contractions in man. *J. Physiol. (Lond.)* 438: 202P.

Vøllestad, N. K., Hallén, J., and Sejersted, O. M. (1994). Effect of exercise intensity on potassium balance in muscle and blood of man. *J. Physiol. (Lond.)* (in press).

Westerblad, H., Lee, J. A., Lamb, A. G., Bolsover, S. R., and Allen, D. G. (1990). Spatial gradients of intracellular calcium in skeletal muscle during fatigue. *Pflugers Arch.* 415: 734.

Westerblad, H., Lee, J. A., Lännergren, J., and Allen, D. G. (1991). Cellular mechanisms of fatigue in skeletal muscle. *Am. J. Physiol.* 261: C195.

Wiles, C. M., and Edwards, R. H. T. (1982). The effect of temperature, ischemia and contractile activity on the relaxation rate of human muscle. *Clin. Physiol.* p. 485.

Wiles, C. M., Young, A., Jones, D., and Edwards, R. H. T. (1979). Relaxation rate of constituent muscle-fibre types in human quadriceps. *Clin. Sci.* 56: 47.

Woods, J. J., Bigland-Ritchie, B. (1984). Linear and non-linear surface EMG/force relationships in human muscles. *Am. J. Phys. Med.* 62: 287.

8

Effects of Acid–Base Balance on Striated Muscles and the Diaphragm

SANDRA HOWELL

University of Southern California
Los Angeles, California

ROBERT S. FITZGERALD

The Johns Hopkins Medical Institutions
Baltimore, Maryland

I. Striated Muscles and Acid–Base Balance

As early as 1807, Berzelius speculated about the relation between lactic acid production and the extent of exercise (Lehman, 1850). Since then, the interaction between changes in acid–base balance and the mechanical output of working muscles has been widely explored. Exercise studies in humans have established a strong relation between increased blood lactate and a decline in the capacity to do exhaustive work (Bang, 1936; Asmussen et al., 1948; Karlsson et al., 1975). Moreover, investigations testing the effects of pharmacologically induced acidosis on human muscular performance have demonstrated a negative effect on endurance (Dennig et al., 1931; Jones et al., 1977). Finally, experiments during which isolated muscle fibers were exposed to an acidotic environment have revealed decreased tension development, suggesting that the site of action for acidosis is on the muscle itself (Fabiato and Fabiato, 1978). In contrast, alkalosis temporarily augments contractility as well as endurance of striated muscle (Creese, 1950; Jones et al., 1977).

It is unclear if the positive effect of alkalosis on physical performance is clinically relevant. However, acidosis has been so convincingly associated with the inability to sustain a given workload that it is generally considered to be consequential in the development of skeletal muscle fatigue (Dawson et al., 1978;

Hermansen, 1981; Sahlin, 1986; March et al., 1991). Lactate ions themselves are not known to have any adverse effect on energy metabolism, nor on the contractile process. At physiological pH, lactate is completely dissociated and H^+ accumulates in an amount equivalent to lactate. Thus, it is the unbuffered H^+ concentration [H^+] inside and outside the muscle fiber that appears to reduce contractility. Recent studies exploring cellular mechanisms of fatigue confirm that increased intracellular [H^+] may contribute to a decline in performance during intense work; however, there is surprisingly little direct evidence that intracellular acidosis plays a major role in skeletal muscle fatigue (Westerblad and Lännergren, 1988; Cady et al., 1989; Edman and Lou, 1990; Weiner et al., 1990; Spriet, 1991). In fact, muscle fatigue is known to occur in the absence of acidosis when central neural mechanisms predominate (Bigland-Ritchie and Woods, 1984) or when long-lasting impaired excitation–contraction coupling prevails (Jones, 1981).

Accordingly, acidosis can alter contractility of striated muscle, quite apart from the effects of exhaustive exercise (Fabiato and Fabiato, 1978). There are many sources of acidosis in the body that can potentially affect physical performance. An important example of this was serendipitously reported in the late 1970s, when it was shown that those patients with chronic airways obstruction who were hypercapnic had reduced ventilatory responses to CO_2, compared with patients with similar airways disease, but who were eucapnic (Altose et al., 1977; Matthews and Howell, 1976; Rochester, 1979). These studies not only demonstrated a correlation between respiratory acidosis and a compromised ability to respond to a respiratory stimulus, but they also represented data correlating respiratory acidosis with decreased inspiratory muscle function. About the same time, other investigators were predicting an important role for diaphragm dysfunction in hypercapnic ventilatory failure (Roussos and Macklem, 1979; Roussos, 1979). These revelations sparked the imagination of researchers who, in the last decade, have turned the study of respiratory muscle function into a special area of pulmonary medicine. Diaphragm dysfunction has been established as a clinical entity, and its role in ventilatory failure is now acknowledged. Moreover, investigation of the interaction between acid–base disorders and the diaphragm has improved the understanding of the pathophysiology of diaphragm dysfunction.

II. The Diaphragm and Acid–Base Balance

The first study revealing the effects of acid–base changes on the diaphragm was conducted in 1950 by Creese, who studied the rat diaphragm, under the assumption that his findings were representative of all striated muscles. Since that time, it has been suggested that the diaphragm is not a typical striated muscle, but has some unique characteristics that are similar to cardiac muscle. Not only do the heart and diaphragm contract continuously throughout life, but studies have shown that the diaphragm, like the heart, depends on the influx of extracellular calcium for activation of the contractile apparatus (Aubier et al., 1985; Viires et al., 1988). Transsarcolemmal calcium does not participate in activation of other skeletal muscles (Sanchez and Stefani, 1978). For these reasons, it is possible that the diaphragm belongs in a functional category that falls between skeletal and cardiac muscle. The myocardium is believed to be far more pH-sensitive than limb skeletal muscle (Fabiato and Fabiato, 1978). This is partly related to the observation that acidosis inhibits the myocardial slow calcium current across the sarcolemma (Vogel and Sperelakis, 1977). Therefore, the reliance of the contracting diaphragm on a transsarcolemmal calcium current may cause it to be more pH-sensitive than other skeletal muscles. This has important implications for the role of diaphragm dysfunction in hypercapnic ventilatory failure.

Fitzgerald et al. (1984) conducted the first comprehensive investigation of the effects of abnormal acid–base balance on contractility of the rat diaphragm in vitro. They simulated classic acid–base disorders by changing the Pco_2 or bicarbonate concentration of the incubation medium. Figure 1a shows that, following a 15-min exposure to respiratory acidosis, diaphragm peak twitch tension was significantly reduced. Figure 1b reveals a similar effect after exposure to metabolic acidosis. When respiratory acidosis was compensated by an increase in bicarbonate, peak twitch tension was again reduced to a small, but significant, degree (see Fig. 1c). The largest decrease in twitch tension was observed during exposure to compensated metabolic acidosis, when a respiratory alkalosis was superimposed on a reduced bicarbonate concentration (see Fig. 1d). This result was surprising because respiratory alkalosis, alone, was observed to potentiate twitch tension in their study.

Investigations designed to study acid–base disorders in an intact physiological model were conducted by Howell et al. (1985a,b), using an in vivo canine diaphragm preparation. Respiratory acidosis was induced in dogs by adding increased CO_2 to the inspired air, and metabolic acidosis was simulated by slow infusion of a weak acid solution. Bilateral phrenicotomy was performed to prevent the diaphragm from contracting (and possibly becoming fatigued) in response to the induced acidotic states. All animals were then mechanically ventilated. Transdiaphragmatic pressure (Pdi) was measured at low and high frequencies of phrenic stimulation, and frequency–Pdi curves were constructed. Figure 2 reveals that, following a 2-h exposure to respiratory or metabolic acidosis, respectively, a moderate, but significant, reduction in Pdi was observed at all frequencies of phrenic stimulation. Figure 2b further shows that compensation of metabolic acidosis with a respiratory alkalosis produced a second marked decrease in Pdi at all stimulation frequencies. This rather dramatic demonstration in an intact animal preparation corroborated the findings in isolated diaphragm by Fitzgerald and co-workers (1984).

Realizing the importance of measuring the effects of acid–base balance on contracting diaphragm, Schnader et al. (1985) studied spontaneously ventilating dogs. Different levels of arterial Pco_2 were induced, including hypocapnia, normocapnia, and hypercapnia, with mean $Paco_2$ values ranging from 17 to 113 torr. Frequency–Pdi curves were constructed while the animals ventilated sponta-

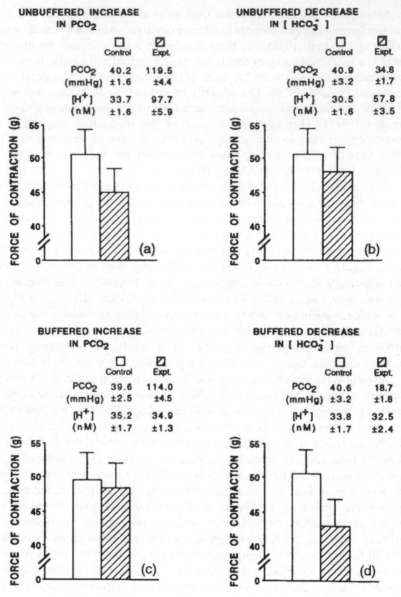

Figure 1 The effect of various forms of acid–base imbalance on the peak twitch force of in vitro rat hemidiaphragm in response to field stimulation. Values above each histogram (mean ± SE; $n = 10$) are the P_{CO_2} (mm Hg) and H^+ (nM). P_{O_2} in the bath was always greater than 400 mm Hg for all experiments. The force of contraction was significantly reduced in all four forms of acid–base imbalance by 11, 5, 3, and 15% in (a), (b), (c), and (d), respectively. (From Fitzgerald, 1984.)

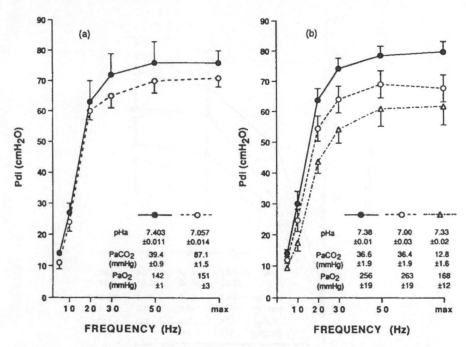

Figure 2 The effect of acid–base imbalance on performance of in vivo canine diaphragm in response to phrenic stimulation at low and high frequencies. (a) Respiratory acidosis (*n* = 6): solid circle, control; open circle, respiratory acidosis. (b) Uncompensated and compensated metabolic acidosis (*n* = 11): solid circle, control; open circle, metabolic acidosis; open triangle, compensated metabolic acidosis. Blood gas values are mean ± SE. In (a) and (b), experimental values of transdiaphragmatic pressure (Pdi) (mean ± SE) at each frequency are significantly less than the control values. Moreover, in (b) the values of Pdi during compensated metabolic acidosis are significantly less than metabolic acidosis. (From Howell, 1985a,b.)

neously in response to each acid–base challenge. Possible development of diaphragm fatigue was averted by resting the animals with mechanical ventilation between challenges. The results showed that, although hypocapnia produced no effect, hypercapnia significantly and rapidly depressed spontaneous contractions of the diaphragm (after 15-min exposures compared with 2 h in the resting diaphragm). Moreover, the effect was more severe than in resting muscle and was dose-dependent. Figure 3 demonstrates that hypercapnic increments progressively decreased the frequency–Pdi curve in the spontaneously breathing animal. Juan and associates (1984) also reported a dose-dependent decrease in Pdi in human subjects breathing increased concentrations of carbon dioxide.

Schnader et al. (1988) further explored the difference between the effects of fatigue and acidosis on the diaphragm. This study would help describe, for example,

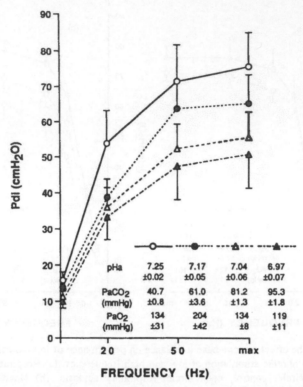

Figure 3 Relation between frequency of phrenic stimulation and transdiaphragmatic pressure (Pdi) at increments of Paco$_2$ in the spontaneously breathing dog. Values of Pdi (mean ± SE; n = 6) at values of Paco$_2$ greater than normocapnia (40.7 ± 0.8 mm Hg) are significantly lower and different from each other at all frequencies except 1 Hz. (From Schnader, 1985.)

the patient with chronic airways obstruction whose diaphragm performs fatiguing work against increased airway resistance, with subsequent carbon dioxide retention. With the in vivo, spontaneously ventilating, canine model, they induced diaphragm fatigue with intermittent phrenic stimulation under hypocapnic, normocapnic, and hypercapnic conditions. Frequency–Pdi characteristics were measured before and after development of fatigue at different Paco$_2$ values. The results of this study and previous findings (Howell and Roussos, 1984; Howell et al., 1985a; Schnader et al., 1985) allow the following characterization of the effects of hypercapnic depression versus fatigue on the diaphragm: (1) The negative inotropic effect of acute hypercapnia on resting and contracting diaphragm function is reversible after restoration of normocapnia or hypocapnia. In contrast, fatigue following repeated intense contractions is a long-lasting phenomenon that was first described by Edwards (1978). (2) Hypercapnia reduces Pdi proportionally at all frequencies of stimulation, whereas fatigue produces more profound effects on Pdi at low frequencies. Hypocapnia has no effect on the frequency–Pdi curve. (3) Development of diaphragm fatigue in hypercapnic animals does not increase the magnitude of fatigue, but greatly reduces endurance. Juan et al. (1984) also demonstrated that respiratory acidosis significantly reduces the ability of the human diaphragm to sustain a given workload over time. As a matter of interest, Esau (1989) has shown that the combination of hypercapnia and hypoxia together produce a greater detrimental effect than either alone and make the diaphragm more susceptible to fatigue. (4) The recovery rate of diaphragm fatigue, induced under acidotic conditions, is enhanced by restoring normocapnia or hypocapnia. (5) Peak twitch tension is reduced by hypercapnia, whereas fatigue reduces twitch tension and increases twitch contraction and relaxation times.

Therefore, it was concluded that the effects of fatigue and hypercapnia on the diaphragm represent different pathophysiological processes, each capable of impairing diaphragm strength, whereas interaction of the two conditions markedly reduces endurance.

III. Factors Influencing Effects of Acid–Base Imbalance on Muscle

A. Fiber Type Composition

The adult human diaphragm is composed of 55% slow-twitch fibers (type I), with the remainder being approximately equally distributed between fast-twitch fatigable (type IIB) and fast-twitch fatigue-resistant (type IIA) (Lieberman et al., 1973). Contractility of slow-twitch fibers is relatively resistant to changes in the pH environment compared with fast-twitch and cardiac fibers (Donaldson and Hermansen, 1978). This may explain the less potent or absent effects of acidosis on some skeletal muscles that have larger populations of slow-twitch fibers. However, with the composition of the diaphragm being nearly 50% fast-twitch fibers, the effects of acidosis on contractility, as described in the foregoing, are not surprising.

B. Intracellular pH

The effects of acid–base balance on striated muscle function, including the diaphragm, are largely mediated by changes in intracellular pH $(pH)_i$. Many studies characterizing how $(pH)_i$ changes in response to altered extracellular pH have been reported (reviewed by Roos and Boron, 1981). Fitzgerald et al. (1988a,b) conducted experiments to clarify the effects of different acid–base environments on resting rat diaphragm. With ^{31}P-nuclear magnetic resonance (NMR) spectroscopy they observed changes in $(pH)_i$ and high-energy phosphates in the diaphragm during exposure to the acid–base imbalances. During respiratory acidosis, $(pH)_i$ rapidly fell from 7.0 to 6.88. The effect of metabolic acidosis on muscle pH was similar. Compensated metabolic acidosis did not cause pH_i to be different from control, but in fact, $(pH)_i$ became slightly alkalotic. Studies in muscles performing fatiguing work have shown that $(pH)_i$ falls to about 6.4 at exhaustion (Hermansen and Osnes, 1972). We are unaware of studies measuring $(pH)_i$ at a time when acid–base disorders have been superimposed on submaximal or maximal muscular work.

C. Energy Metabolism

An increased H^+ concentration inhibits the activity of phosphorylase and phospho-fructokinase (PFK), the key enzymes regulating glycogenolysis and glycolysis, respectively (Ui, 1966; Chasiotis et al., 1983). In vitro experiments reveal that PFK is almost completely inactive at pH 6.9 (Trivedi and Danforth, 1966). However, in situ and in vivo experiments have demonstrated that significant PFK activity is maintained during intense muscular contractions, despite decreases in $(pH)_i$ to 6.4 (Hultman and Sjoholm, 1983; Meyer et al., 1982) and, thus, glycolysis does not appear to be greatly inhibited. The lack of inhibition may result from a combination of decreased inhibitor (ATP) and increased substrate (fructose-6-phosphate) contents, coupled with increases in the contents of several positive modulators (Graham et al., 1986). In contrast, the PFK step was affected when metabolic and respiratory acidosis was experimentally induced in situ in canine hindlimb muscle (Graham et al., 1986; Hirche et al., 1975). The induced acidosis greatly decreased lactate release in contracting muscle. This phenomenon also has been demonstrated in humans (Jones et al., 1977) and is believed to result from both the inhibition of PFK activity and reduced permeability of the sarcolemma for lactate. Fitzgerald et al. (1988b), with ^{31}P-NMR spectroscopy, reported no loss of high-energy phosphate stores in the resting diaphragm during exposure to respiratory or metabolic acidosis, nor in compensated metabolic acidosis. Meyer et al. (1990) concurred with this finding in studies during which both slow- and fast-twitch muscles from the cat hindlimb were exposed to hypercapnia. They detected no change in phosphocreatine (PCr), but in fact, found an increased PCr level in slow-twitch muscle during acidosis. This does not preclude, however, an effect of hypercapnia on the content of PCr, ATP, or P_i in contracting diaphragm.

Oxidative phosphorylation was rather unaffected by an acidotic extramito-chondrial pH, ranging from 6.5 to 7.0 (Mitchelson and Hird, 1973). However, there is evidence that intracellular alkalosis can inhibit oxidative phosphorylation (Lowenstein and Chance, 1968). This could happen if the efflux of $H+$ from the cell dissipated the electrochemical gradient across the mitochondria, which is the source of free energy for ADP phosphorylation. In addition, alkalosis greatly enhances calcium uptake by the mitochondria, and calcium accumulation is a respiratory-dependent process that can replace oxidative phosphorylation (Lehninger, 1970). These hypotheses might help explain the negative inotropic effects of compensated metabolic acidosis on the in vitro and in vivo diaphragm shown in Figures 1d and

2b, respectively. However, this does not help interpret the temporary potentiating effects of respiratory or metabolic alkalosis on physical performance.

D. Calcium Regulation

Acidosis greatly reduces extracellular Ca^{2+} binding to sarcolemmal phospholipids and inhibits Ca^{2+} entry into muscle cells (Seimiya and Ohki, 1983; Langer, 1985). If bound extracellular Ca^{2+} is associated with the function of Ca^{2+} channels, decreased membrane binding would impair transsarcolemmal Ca^{2+} movement, and this would affect contractility of the diaphragm, as it does in the heart. In fact, Viires et al. (1988) have shown that a Ca^{2+}-free incubation medium very rapidly abolishes contractility of in vitro rat diaphragm, whereas rat limb muscle function is affected at a much slower rate. Fitzgerald et al. (1989) have studied Ca^{2+} metabolism in resting rat diaphragm by a method based on simulation and modeling of long-term $^{45}Ca^{2+}$ efflux data from intact muscle. This method allows estimates of the content of Ca^{2+} in discrete cellular locations. They demonstrated that a brief (20-min) exposure of diaphragm tissue to hypercapnia caused rapid release of extracellular bound Ca^{2+} and reduced the content of one intracellular compartment. Howell (1992), employing the Ca^{2+}-tracer method, exposed noncontracting hamster diaphragm to hypercapnia for 1 h during the loading of $^{45}Ca^{2+}$ into the muscle. She observed a release of extracellular Ca^{2+} and a significant increase in the content of one intracellular compartment (believed to represent the SR terminal cisternae). The same experiment in a contracting diaphragm produced different results. The Ca^{2+} content of all extracellular and intracellular compartments was diminished by hypercapnia in the working muscle (S. Howell, unpublished studies, 1993).

It has been speculated that myoplasmic, free Ca^{2+} is elevated during hypercapnia (Lea and Ashley, 1978), although the absolute amount is believed to be small (Lee et al., 1991). This effect may be related to decreased buffering of Ca^{2+} by pH-sensitive cytoplasmic proteins. The pH sensitivity of the myofibrillar ATPase enzyme complex is well known (Blanchard et al., 1984). Acidosis reduces the myofibrillar ATPase activity by an effect of protons on Ca^{2+}-binding sites on troponin. This is not believed to be a simple competition between H^+ and Ca^{2+} for a single class of binding sites on troponin (Fabiato and Fabiato, 1978). The result is that more free Ca^{2+} is required to generate a given submaximal tension, and H^+ reduces the maximum tension development in the presence of saturating free Ca^{2+}.

Several elements in the process of translocating Ca^{2+} into the sarcoplasmic reticulum (SR) have been reported to be pH-dependent, including Ca^{2+}-ATPase activity, the affinity of Ca^{2+} for its binding site on Ca^{2+}-ATPase, the cooperativity of Ca^{2+} binding to Ca^{2+}-ATPase, and dephosphorylation of Ca^{2+}-ATPase (Nakamaru and Schwartz, 1972; Watanabe et al., 1981; Inesi and Hill, 1983; Pick and Karlish, 1982). Interestingly, the pH optimum for skeletal muscle SR Ca^{2+} uptake is equivalent to mild intracellular acidosis (Fabiato and Fabiato, 1978). Therefore, a moderate acidosis would theoretically enhance loading of Ca^{2+} into skeletal muscle SR. A larger SR Ca^{2+} content should lead to increased Ca^{2+} release, which would compensate for the negative effects of acidosis on the myofilaments and preserve the contractile process, to some extent (Fabiato and Fabiato, 1978). Conversely, a mild intracellular alkalosis induces Ca^{2+} release, or halts loading of Ca^{2+} by the SR, which might explain the temporary potentiating effects of respiratory or metabolic alkalosis on physical performance. Under more severe acidotic conditions such as muscular exertion, where $(pH)_i$ is less than 6.6, H^+ competes with Ca^{2+}-binding sites, resulting in a reduced population of activated enzyme (Inesi and Hill, 1983). The result is decreased Ca^{2+} uptake by the SR, with reduced release (Nakamaru and Schwartz, 1972). Functionally, this leads to reduced tension development and slowing of relaxation (Westerblad and Lannergren, 1991).

IV. Summary

In the early days of investigating the decrease in the force of contraction of striated muscle under conditions of acidosis, excess H^+ concentration was understandably designated as the cause. But where and how the H^+ exercised its effect was not designated. The precise, ultimate explanation of why the different forms of acid–base imbalance produce the decrease in the mechanical performance of the diaphragm remains unclear. Particularly perplexing is the effect of compensated metabolic acidosis. For, in this case, the acid–base conditions produce no excess extracellular H^+ at all in either the resting or the exercising muscle; and in the resting diaphragm, the intracellular pH actually becomes slightly alkalotic over 1 h of exposure. It is possible that, in the muscle exercised under conditions of compensated metabolic acidosis, H^+ accumulates more rapidly and to a greater extent inside muscle fibers because of the lower levels in intracellular bicarbonate.

More unlikely as a source of the decreased performance is the effect of H^+ on energy stores. They seem to remain adequate for continued performance. More likely is the effect of H^+ on Ca^{2+} release or uptake from the sarcoplasmic reticulum, or perhaps the interaction of H^+ and the contractile proteins.

However, the failure in the mechanical performance may not be entirely or even largely due to H^+. For in some muscles made acidotic by fatigue, removal of excess H^+ improves the mechanical performance, but does not entirely restore function to control conditions. There is growing evidence that accumulation of inorganic phosphate plays a role; for example, by inhibiting the breakdown of ATP, or by interacting with the contractile proteins. It would be instructive to monitor the levels of this metabolite during exercise under normal conditions compared with exercise under conditions of acid–base imbalance.

Future research goals include a more precise identification of the locus and mechanism of the effect of H^+ in the diaphragm, with a view to reducing this effect, if possible, in those patients who are beset with whatever form of acidosis. Answers to these questions could greatly improve the quality of life of patients who have problems with pulmonary gas exchange, kidney failure, or other conditions creating acid–base imbalance.

References

Altose, M., McCauley, W., Kelsen, S., and Cherniack, N. (1977). Effects of hypercapnia and inspiratory flow-resistive loading on respiratory activity in chronic airway obstruction. *J. Clin. Invest.* 59: 500–507.

Asmussen, E., von Dobeln, W., and Nielsen, M. (1948). Blood lactate and oxygen debt after exhaustive work at different oxygen tensions. *Acta Physiol. Scand.* 15: 57–62.

Aubier, M., Viires, N., Piquet, J., Murciano, D., Blanchet, F., Marty, C., Gherardi, R., and Pariente, R. (1985). Effects of hypocalcemia on diaphragmatic strength generation. *J. Appl. Physiol.* 58: 2053–2061.

Bang, O. (1936). The lactate content of the blood during and after muscular exercise in man. *Scand. Archiv. Physiol.* [*Suppl.*] 10: 51–82.

Bigland-Ritchie, B., and Woods, J. J. (1984). Changes in muscle contractile properties and neural control during human muscular fatigue. *Muscle Nerve* 7: 691–699.

Blanchard, E. M., Pan, B.-S., and Solaro, J. R. (1984). The effect of acidic pH on the ATPase activity and troponin Ca^{2+} binding of rabbit skeletal myofilaments. *J. Biol. Chem.* 259: 3181–3186.

Cady, E. B., Jones, D. A., Lynn, J., and Newham, D. J. (1989). Changes in force and intracellular metabolites during fatigue of human skeletal muscle. *J. Physiol. (Lond.)* 418: 311–325.

Chasiotis, D., Sahlin, K., and Hultman, E. (1983). Acidotic depression of cyclic AMP accumulation and phosphorylase B to a transformation in skeletal muscle of man. *J. Physiol. (Lond.)* 335: 197–204.

Creese, R. (1950). Bicarbonate ion and striated muscle. *J. Physiol. (Lond.)* 100: 450–457.

Dawson, M. J., Gadian, D. G., and Wilkie, D. R. (1978). Muscular fatigue investigated by phosphorus nuclear magnetic resonance. *Nature* 274: 861–866.

Dennig, H., Talbot, J. H., Edward, H. T., and Dill, D. B. (1931). Effect of acidosis and alkalosis upon capacity for work. *J. Clin. Invest.* 9: 601–613.

Donaldson, S. K., and Hermansen, L. (1978). Differential, direct effects of H^+ on Ca^{2+}-activated force of skinned fibers from the soleus, cardiac and adductor magnus muscles of rabbits. *Pflugers Arch.* 376: 55–65.

Edman, K. A. P., and Lou, F. (1990). Changes in force and stiffness induced by fatigue and intracellular acidification in frog muscle fibres. *J. Physiol. (Lond.)* 424: 133–149.

Edwards, R. H. T. (1978). Physiological analysis of skeletal muscle weakness and fatigue. *Clin. Sci. Mol. Med.* 54: 463–470.

Esau, S. A. (1989). Hypoxic, hypercapnic acidosis decreases tension and increases fatigue in hamster diaphragm muscle in vitro. *Am. Rev. Respir. Dis.* 139: 1410–1417.

Fabiato, A., and Fabiato, F. (1978). Effects of pH on the myofilaments and the sarcoplasmic reticulum of skinned cells from cardiac and skeletal muscles. *J. Physiol.* 276: 233–255.

Fitzgerald, R. S., Hauer, M. C., Bierkamper, G., and Raff, H. (1984). Responses of in vitro rat diaphragm to changes in acid–base environment. *J. Appl. Physiol.* 57: 1202–1210.

Fitzgerald, R. S., Howell, S., and Jacobus, W. E. (1988a). ^{31}P-NMR study of resting in vitro rat diaphragm exposed to hypercapnia. *J. Appl. Physiol.* 65: 2270–2277.

Fitzgerald, R. S., Howell, S., Pike, M. M., and Jacobus, W. E. (1988b). NMR study of rat diaphragm exposed to metabolic and compensated metabolic acidosis. *J. Appl. Physiol.* 65: 2278–2284.

Fitzgerald, R. S., Westcott, D., and Phair, R. (1989). The effect of acidosis on calcium in resting in vitro rat diaphragm. *Am. Rev. Respir. Dis.* 139: A167.

Graham, T. E., Barclay, J. K., and Wilson, B. A. (1986). Skeletal muscle lactate release and glycolytic intermediates during hypercapnia. *J. Appl. Physiol.* 60: 568–575.

Hermansen, L. (1981). Effect of metabolic changes on force generation in skeletal muscle during maximal exercise. In *Human Muscle Fatigue: Physiological Mechanisms*. Edited by R. Porter and J. Whelan. London, Pitman (*Ciba Found. Symp*. 82), pp. 75–88.

Hermansen, L., and Osnes, J. B. (1972). Blood and muscle pH after maximal exercise in man. *J. Appl. Physiol*. 32: 304–308.

Hirche, H. J., Homback, V., Langohr, H. D., Wacker, V., and Busse, J. (1975). Lactic acid permeation rate in working gastrocnemii of dogs during metabolic alkalosis and acidosis. *Pflugers Arch*. 365: 209–222.

Howell, S., and Roussos, C. (1984). Isoproterenol and aminophylline improve contractility of fatigued canine diaphragm. *Am. Rev. Respir. Dis*. 129: 118–124.

Howell, S., Fitzgerald, R. S., and Roussos, C. (1985a). Effects of aminophylline, isoproterenol, and neostigmine on hypercapnic depression of diaphragmatic contractility. *Am. Rev. Respir. Dis*. 132: 241–247.

Howell, S., Fitzgerald, R. S., and Roussos, C. (1985b). Effects of uncompensated and compensated metabolic acidosis on canine diaphragm. *J. Appl. Physiol*. 59: 1376–1382.

Howell, S. (1992). Hypercapnia decreases newborn diaphragm calcium content in contrast with an increase in adult diaphragm. *FASEB J*., 6: 6313.

Hultman, E., and Sjoholm, H. (1983). Energy metabolism and contraction force of human skeletal muscle in situ during electrical stimulation. *J. Physiol*. (*Lond*.) 345: 525–532.

Inesi, G., and Hill, T. L. (1983). Calcium and proton dependence of sarcoplasmic reticulum ATPase. *Biophys. J*. 44: 271–280.

Jones, D. A. (1981). Muscle fatigue beyond the neuromuscular junction. In *Human Muscle Fatigue: Physiological Mechanisms*. Edited by R. Porter and J. Whelan. London, Pitman (*Ciba Found. Symp*. 82) pp. 178–192.

Jones, N. L., Sutton, J. R., Taylor, R., and Toews, C. J. (1977). Effect of pH on cardiorespiratory and metabolic responses to exercise. *J. Appl. Physiol*. 43: 959–964.

Juan, G., Calverley, P., Talamo, C., Schnader, J. Y., and Roussos, C. (1984). Carbon dioxide impairs diaphragm function in man. *N. Engl. J. Med*. 310: 874–879.

Karlsson, J., Bonde-Petersen, F., Henriksson, J., and Knuttgen, H. G. (1975). Effects of previous exercise with arms or legs on metabolism and performance in exhaustive exercise. *J. Appl. Physiol*. 38: 763–767.

Langer, G. A. (1985). The effect of pH on cellular membrane calcium binding and concentration of myocardium. *Circ. Res*. 57: 374–382.

Lea, T. J., and Ashley, C. C. (1978). Increase in free Ca^{2+} in muscle after exposure to CO_2. *Nature* 275: 236–238.

Lee, J. A., Westerblad, H., and Allen, D. (1991). Changes in tetanic and resting $[Ca^{2+}]_i$ during fatigue and recovery of single muscle fibres from *Xenopus laevis*. *J. Physiol*. (*Lond*.) 433: 307–326.

Lehman, C. F. (1850). *Lehrbuch der Physiologischen Chemische*, 2nd ed., London, Cavendish Society.

Lehninger, A. L. (1970). Mitochondrial and calcium ion transport. *Biochem. J*. 119: 129–138.

Lieberman, D. A., Faulkner, J. A., Craig, A. B., and Maxwell, L. C. (1973). Performance and histochemical composition of guinea pig and human diaphragm. *J. Appl. Physiol*. 34: 233–237.

Lowenstein, J. M., and Chance, B. (1968). The effect of hydrogen ions on the control of mitochondrial respiration. *J. Biol. Chem*. 243: 3940–3946.

March, G. D., Paterson, D. H., Thompson, R. T., and Driedger, A. A. (1991). Coincident threshold in intracellular phosphorylation potential and pH during progressive exercise. *J. Appl. Physiol*. 71: 1076–1081.

Matthews, A., and J. Howell. (1976). Assessment of responsiveness to carbon dioxide in patients with chronic airways obstruction by rate of isometric inspiratory pressure development. *Clin. Sci. Mol. Med*. 50: 199–205.

Meyer, R. A., Kushmerick, M. J., and Dillon, P. F. (1982). Intracellular pH changes in contracting fast- and slow-twitch muscles. *Proc. FASEB* 41: 979–984.

Meyer, R. A., Adams, G. R., Fisher, M. J., Dillon, P. F., Krisanda, J. M., Brown, T. R., and

Kushmerick, M. J. (1990). Effect of decreased pH on force and phosphocreatine in mammalian skeletal muscle. *Can. J. Physiol. Pharmacol.* 69: 305–310.

Mitchelson, K. R., and Hird, F. J. R. (1973). Effect of pH and halothane on muscle and liver mitochondria. *Am. J. Physiol.* 225: 1393–1398.

Nakamaru, Y., and Schwartz, A. (1972). The influence of hydrogen ion concentration on calcium binding and release by skeletal muscle sarcoplasmic reticulum. *J. Gen. Physiol.* 59: 22–32.

Pick, J., and Karlish, S. J. D. (1982). Regulation of the conformation transition in the Ca-ATPase from sarcoplasmic reticulum by pH, temperature, and calcium ions. *J. Biol. Chem.* 257: 6120–6126.

Rochester, D., Braun, N., and Arora, N. S. (1979). Respiratory muscle strength in chronic obstructive pulmonary disease. *Am. Rev. Respir. Dis.* 119: 151–154.

Roos, A., and Boron, W. F. (1981). Intracellular pH. *Physiol. Rev.* 61: 296–434.

Roussos, C. (1979). Respiratory muscle fatigue in the hypercapnic patient. *Bull. Eur. Physiopathol. Respir.* 15: 117–123.

Roussos, C., and Macklem, P. T. (1979). Diaphragmatic fatigue in man. *J. Appl. Physiol.* 43: 189–197.

Sahlin, K. (1986). Muscle fatigue and lactic acid accumulation. *Acta Physiol. Scand. [Suppl.]* 556: 83–91.

Sanchez, J. A., and Stefani, E. (1978). Inward calcium current in twitch muscle fibres of the frog. *J. Physiol. (Lond.)* 283: 197–209.

Schnader, J. Y., Juan, G., Howell, S., Fitzgerald, R., and Roussos, C. (1985). Arterial CO_2 partial pressure affects diaphragmatic function. *J. Appl. Physiol.* 58: 823–829.

Schnader, J., Howell, S., Fitzgerald, R. S., and Roussos, C. (1988). Interaction of fatigue and hypercapnia in the canine diaphragm. *J. Appl. Physiol.* 64: 1636–1643.

Seimiya, T., and Ohki, S. (1983). Ionic structure of phospholipid membranes and binding of calcium ions. *Biochim. Biophys. Acta* 298: 546–561.

Spriet, L. L. (1991). Phosphofructokinase activity and acidosis during short-term tetanic contractions. *Can. J. Physiol. Pharmacol.* 69: 298–304.

Trivedi, B., and Danforth, W. H. (1966). Effect of pH on the kinetics of frog muscle phosphofructokinase. *J. Biol. Chem.* 241: 4110–4112.

Ui, M. (1966). A role of phosphofructokinase in pH-dependent regulation of glycolysis. *Biochim. Biophys. Acta* 124: 310–322.

Viires, N., Murciano, D., Seta, J. P., Dureuil, B., Parient, R., and Aubier, M. (1988). Effects of calcium withdrawal on diaphragmatic fiber tension generation. *J. Appl. Physiol.* 64: 26–30.

Vogel, S., and Sperelakis, N. (1977). Blockade of myocardial slow inward current in low pH. *Am. J. Physiol.* 233: C99–C103.

Watanabe, T., Lewis, D., Nakamoto, R., Kurzmack, M., Fronticelli, C., and Inesi, G. (1981). Modulation of calcium binding in sarcoplasmic reticulum ATP. *Biochemistry* 20: 6617–6624.

Weiner, M. W., Moussavi, R. S., Baker, A. J., Boska, M. D., and Miller, R. G. (1990). Constant relationships between force, phosphate concentration, and pH in muscle with differential fatigability. *Neurology* 40: 1888–1893.

Westerblad, H., and Lännergren, J. (1988). The relation between force and intracellular pH in fatigued, single *Xenopus* muscle fibres. *Acta Physiol. Scand.* 133: 83–89.

Westerblad, H., and Lännergren, J. (1991). Slowing of relaxation during fatigue in single mouse muscle fibres. *J. Physiol. (Lond.)* 434: 323–336.

9

Structural and Functional Adaptations
of Skeletal Muscle

JOHN A. FAULKNER

University of Michigan
Ann Arbor, Michigan

I. Introduction

The early concepts of adaptation of an organism to its environment can be traced
to the writings of Robert Malthus and Charles Darwin (Leake, 1964). These early
concepts evolved through the work of Claude Bernard, Walter Cannon, Joseph
Barcroft, and L. J. Henderson, to the current perspectives of C. Ladd Prosser (1964),
Hans Selye (1952), and Peter Hochochka and George Somers (1973). For an
extensive review, see *Adaptation to the Environment*, a volume of the *Handbook
of Physiology*, edited by Bruce Dill and his associates (1964). Leake (1964) defined
adaptation as an alteration in the structure or function of an organism that favors
the survival of the organism in an altered environment. The adaptation of a total
organism to environmental change occurs in molecules, cells, tissues, and organs
(Barbashova, 1964; Hochochka and Somers, 1973). Furthermore, at each level,
multiple mechanisms are available for the control of adaptive responses. Consequently, the adaptation of a total organism is highly complex (Adolph, 1956), and
a hierarchical approach to an understanding of structure–function relationships is
advisable (Fig. 1).

In contrast with the organismic definition of adaptation, a muscle physiologist
uses the term "adaptation" in the absence of any direct evidence of a survival value.
For animals, including humans, adaptations of skeletal muscles may enhance survival

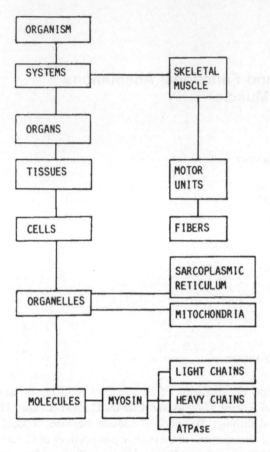

Figure 1 The levels of organization of the total organism at which an adaptive response may occur. Skeletal muscle is presented as an example: architectural changes may occur at the system level and modulation of light or heavy chains at the submolecular level. (From Faulkner, 1983.)

in specific random circumstances, but the adaptations are not directly related to survival. In addition, rather than a response to environmental change, skeletal muscle adaptations occur in responses to some combination of habitual decreases or increases in the frequency, intensity, or duration of contractions of motor units in skeletal muscles (Faulkner et al., 1993). A key concept is that in skeletal muscles, adaptation occurs at the level of single motor units that have undergone a change in the pattern of recruitment or loading beyond the threshold necessary to initiate an adequate stimulus for adaptation (Fig. 2). An *adaptation in skeletal muscle* is defined "as a modification of a morphological, metabolic, or molecular property that alters the functional attributes of fibers in specific motor units" (Faulkner et al., 1993).

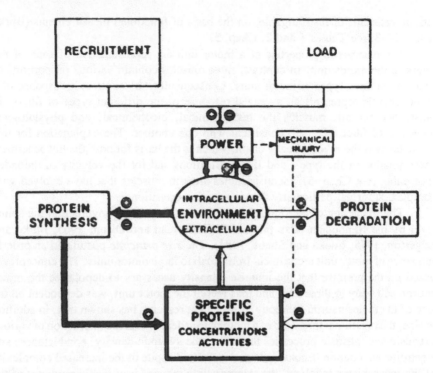

Figure 2 During changes in the level of physical activity the total power developed by a motor unit results from the recruitment of the fibers in motor units and the load against which the fibers contract. If the fibers shorten, power will be developed (+), and if the fibers are lengthened, power will be absorbed (–). Presumably, reduced power, sustained power, or high power result in immediate changes in the cellular environment that then lead to an augmentation or inhibition of gene expression or specific proteases. If sustained, this will lead to altered rates of protein synthesis and degradation, respectively. This, in turn, will lead to changes in the concentrations or activities of specific proteins and thus prolonged, but not permanent, alteration in the cellular environment. These adaptations may increase or decrease the capability of fibers in a motor unit to develop and maintain power. The adaptive responses to some physical activities are known, but the receptors, integrating centers, second messengers, and effectors involved have not been fully identified. Under certain circumstances muscle fibers are injured during sudden contractions and the concentration of myofibrillar proteins is decreased directly. (From Faulkner et al., 1993.)

II. Recruitment of Motor Units

A motor unit consists of an α-motoneuron, its branches, and the muscle fibers innervated by each branch. Motor units are composed of fibers that are more or less homogeneous in fiber type (Nemeth et al., 1981). Consequently, motor units may be classified as type I, IIA, or IIB on the basis of histochemical demonstration of myofibrillar ATPase activity (Brooke and Kaiser, 1970), or as slow, fast fatigue-resistant, or fast-fatigable, on the basis of functional measurements (Burke et al., 1973; see Tables 1 and 2, Chap. 5).

The contractile properties of a motor unit are representative of each of the fibers in the motor unit. In contrast, most muscles contain various proportions of each of the three types of motor units. Consequently, the contractile response of a whole muscle represents an averaged response of the different types of fibers. In most, but not all, muscles the histochemical, biochemical, and physiological measures of fiber types are consistent with one another. The explanation for this consistency is the myosin heavy chain, which is the basis for both the histochemical determination of the type I and II classifications and for the velocity of unloaded shortening (see Chap. 5). Inconsistencies arise in muscles that have evolved with complex isoforms, particularly during adaptive transitions.

The frequency of recruitment of a given motor unit is governed at the spinal level by the Henneman "size principle" (Henneman and Olson, 1965; Burke and Edgerton, 1975; Enoka and Stuart, 1984). The *size principle* postulated an orderly sequence of motor unit recruitment from small to large motor units. The concept was based on the premise that the impulse intensity necessary to depolarize the motor neuron cell body to threshold, and thus recruit the motor unit, was dependent on the size of the motor neuron cell body. Subsequent research has shown that, in addition to size, the functional threshold of a motoneuron depends on the interaction of various extrinsic and intrinsic properties that affect the synaptic density, conductance, and electronic attenuation (Enoka and Stuart, 1984). In spite of the increased complexity of the mechanisms involved, the size principle remains as a viable predictor of the sequence of motor unit recruitment (Enoka and Stuart, 1984). In a relative comparison of motor units, small type I motor units have small motoneurons, are depolarized to threshold by low-impulse intensities, are recruited often, and innervate motor units composed of few fibers. Conversely, large type IIB motor units have large motoneurons, are depolarized to threshold only by high-impulse intensities, are recruited seldom, and innervate large motor units. Type IIA motor units are intermediate between the two extremes in size and frequency of recruitment.

Increases and decreases in habitual recruitment of motor units in limb muscles result from changes in the rates and intensities of the discharge from the motor cortex. At low intensities of discharge only type I motor units are recruited. If discharge from the motor cortex increases, the type I and, possibly, type IIA and type IIB motor units are each recruited more frequently. The rate and intensity of a motor cortical discharge may vary from the impulse intensity required to elicit low-power–high-repetition activities, such as walking or running, to those resulting in maximum voluntary contractions, required for maximum lifts in power training. Similar changes in rates and intensities of discharge may emanate from the respiratory centers and vary the recruitment patterns of the muscles of respiration. In either event, the discharge from the supraspinal level dictates the number of motor units recruited and the stimulus frequency, but the orderly sequence of motor unit recruitment is modulated at the spinal level on the basis of motor unit size.

III. Stimulus for an Adaptive Response

Each individual may be characterized by a habitual level of physical activity in terms of frequency and loading of the skeletal muscles required by the activities (Fig. 3). Adaptations in skeletal muscles arise from decreases and increases in the habitual frequency and loading produced by the voluntary contractions of specific motor units in the muscles of the limbs and trunk. In contrast, decreases and increases in the rate and depth of ventilation are initiated by the changes in the spontaneous contractions of the motor units, the diaphragm, and the accessory muscles of respiration. The adaptive response produced is dependent on the rate of onset and the magnitude of the change (Brooks, 1969; Prosser, 1964). For an adaptive response to occur implies that a stimulus has been detected by a receptor and appropriate signals have been transmitted to an effector (see Fig. 2).

The homogeneity of fibers within a motor unit supports the hypothesis that all fibers within a single motor unit receive the similar adaptive stimuli. With the same protocol of voluntary contractions, different motor units may display very different patterns of recruitment. The intensity of the discharge from the motor cortex or the respiratory center will determine the number of motor units activated during a single contraction (Burke, 1981; Enoka and Stuart, 1984) and, conse-

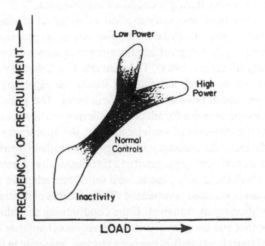

Figure 3 Physical activity is determined by the frequency of recruitment for contractions (ordinate) and the load on the muscle during the contraction (abscissa). Physical activity constitutes a continuum, from the almost complete absence of activity associated with bed rest or immobilization, through the nominal activity levels of sedentary subjects, to high levels observed in physically active subjects. Toward the high end of the continuum, a dichotomy arises as endurance performers increase the frequency of recruitment cycles, without increasing load significantly, whereas strength and power performers increase the load significantly, without much of an increase in frequency.

quently, will determine the mass of muscle involved in the contractions. The specific changes in the habitual pattern of recruitment of a given motor unit that provide the stimulus for an adaptive change are (1) the stimulation frequency (Hz), (2) the duration of the stimulus (ms), (3) the number of contractions per second, (4) the duty cycle (proportion of each second the muscle is contracting), (5) the total duration of the repeated contractions (minutes or hours), (6) the frequency of the bouts of contractions (times per week), and (7) the total duration of the conditioning program (weeks, months, or years). In practical terms, the first four items are grouped into an average "intensity" of physical activity, which can be estimated from velocity of running, cycling, skiing, or swimming.

Under experimental conditions, single contractions of the limb and trunk muscles and of the respiratory muscles can be described in terms of the following: absolute maximum isometric tetanic force (maximum force, newtons; N), maximum specific force (kN/m^2), and submaximum values expressed as a percentage of the value for maximum force; absolute values for maximum power output during shortening and for power input during lengthening (watts; W), power output and input, normalized for the mass of activated muscle fibers (W/kg), and submaximum values expressed as a percentage of maximum power. Similarly, during repeated contractions, sustained force and power can be expressed in absolute, normalized, and relative terms. This provides a potential basis for quantification of the "dose" applied to skeletal muscles during a conditioning program.

In practice, the stimuli necessary to elicit a desired set of adaptive responses in skeletal muscles are organized into a conditioning (training) program. The fundamental principles underlying the design of conditioning programs are "overload," specificity, and reversibility (Faulkner, 1968). The principle of *overload* asserts that for skeletal muscle fibers to increase their structural or functional capability, the capability of the system must be loaded beyond some critical level. The principle of *specificity* maintains that a specific stimulus for adaptation elicits specific structural and functional changes in specific elements of skeletal muscle; the appearance of these changes signals, indeed defines, the adequacy of the prior stimulus (overload). As cellular structures adapt to a conditioning program of a fixed intensity, duration, or frequency, the rate of change will eventually plateau, and no further adaptive change will occur unless the conditioning stimulus is increased. The principle of *reversibility* asserts that the effects of conditioning are transient. If the conditioning stimulus is discontinued, deconditioning occurs and the adaptive changes regress (Faulkner et al., 1972). The process of skeletal muscle adaptation has been studied primarily in terms of responses (i.e., functional changes and their morphological, metabolic, and molecular bases).

IV. Types of Adaptive Responses

The combination of a pattern of motor unit recruitment and the load that produces a power input into the intracellular environment of the fibers of a motor unit is shown in Figure 2. The inputs could be changes in the strain on the contractile and structural proteins; in the rates and magnitudes of flux of ions and other substances across membranes and of substrates through metabolic pathways; in the decreased concentrations of high-energy phosphates; or in the increased concentrations of the end products of metabolism. The exact inputs have not been identified.

The adaptive response may be characterized in terms of its nature, rate, magnitude, and duration. Adaptive responses are regulated by negative feedback. Adaptations of single skeletal muscle fibers can include morphological changes in sarcoplasmic reticulum, fiber length, cross-sectional area (CSA), and isoforms of the contractile and regulatory proteins; and functional changes in force, velocity, and endurance. The adaptation responsible for a structural or functional change may occur at any level of organization of the muscle: the fiber or cell; or the molecules in the contractile, regulatory, structural, or metabolic proteins (see Fig. 1). The nature of some of the responses is known. The CSAs of fibers change when myofibrils in parallel are added or removed, thus changing maximal force or strength (Goldspink, 1970). Length is changed by changing the number of sarcomeres in series (Farkas and Roussos, 1982). A change in fiber length will also change overall velocity of shortening, which may change independently of length changes by variations in myosin isoforms (Pette and Vrbova, 1992). Oxidative capacity (fiber type) is also modified by changing enzyme activities (Holloszy and Booth, 1976); these and other (e.g., vascular) changes are associated with changed endurance (Bradley and Leith, 1978).

The principle of *specificity* states that adaptive changes may be elicited independently by suitable stimuli that require a prescribed pattern of activity for a specific motor unit. An individual motor unit within a muscle is either recruited or not during a contraction of the whole muscle, depending on the overall intensity, duration, and frequency of stimulation; the characteristics of the motoneuron; and the presence or absence of fatigue. The stimuli to different individual motor units within a muscle may be quite different owing to the somatotopic organization of motor units (Sieck et al., 1983). The overall effect is that thresholds for recruitment of individual motor units vary on the basis of the Henneman size principle. Within an individual motor unit, conditioning stimuli can be considered to act more or less in concert on all the muscle fibers. Diverse receptors must reside at multiple sites within fibers, and whether a given adaptive stimulus gives rise to a homogeneous response in each fiber in a motor unit is unknown. Thus, cellular and molecular aspects of conditioning need to be studied at these levels of organization. At the cellular level, four conditioning stimuli have been characterized by identifiable adaptations: endurance conditioning, strength conditioning, stretch conditioning, and deconditioning.

The receptors that receive the adaptive stimuli, the integrating centers, and the effector pathways are unknown. Even with a quantitative assessment of the dose contained in the stimulus for adaptation, the complexity of the interactions between a given dose and the responses of a given muscle is so complex and lacking in stoichiometry that a dose–response approach to the conditioning of skeletal muscles is not feasible (Faulkner et al., 1993).

A. Endurance Conditioning

Endurance conditioning of skeletal muscle fibers is induced by low-power–high-repetition contractions of skeletal muscle fibers. Power is low only relative to its maximum value for a single contraction (see Chap. 5). The 50% drop in maximum power from the value during a single contraction to that during 10 s of repeated contractions results from both the introduction of a duty cycle (the proportion of each second the muscle is contracting) and a decreased average force during the repeated shortening contractions. *High-repetition* implies cyclic activity, wherein the muscle is not continuously active. The timing of activity and rest periods is characterized by the duration of the contraction, the number of contractions per second, and the duty cycle. During dynamic exercise, this rest period involves the recovery and repositioning of a limb, or the diaphragm, for example, for the next stride, or stroke. For persons highly motivated, but with low, moderate, and high levels of conditioning, the highly conditioned are better able to train at a higher percentage of maximum power than those less well trained. For an adaptive response, the intensity must be great enough to satisfy the principle of overload.

Endurance-Conditioning Programs

During endurance conditioning, the number of contractions per minute, the power, and the duration of contractions are designed to stimulate an increased capacity of fibers for sustained effort, without inducing chronic fatigue. *Chronic fatigue* is defined operationally as an impairment in muscle function 24 h after exercise.

Discontinuous or "interval-conditioning" protocols also produce endurance conditioning of muscle fibers. With interval conditioning, the continuity of the duty–rest cycles is broken by longer rest periods. Because this delays the onset of fatigue, interval training permits a higher sustained power, a higher number of contractions per minute, larger duty cycles, or some combination of these variables.

Either continuous or interval protocols for endurance conditioning may involve contractions of large muscle masses, as occurs in running, cycling, swimming, or cross-country skiing. Habitual physical activity of large muscle masses entails large metabolic loads and, indirectly, causes conditioning of some elements of the respiratory and circulatory transport systems. Both respiration and circulation involve the transport processes of bulk flow and diffusion.

When one considers bulk flow of the respiratory and circulatory systems, the focus is on the capacities of the pumps: the heart and the muscles of respiration. The capacities of each of these two pumps can increase in response to overload. Thus, in previously sedentary normal humans, whole-body endurance conditioning is associated with an increase in endurance of inspiratory muscles; their training stimulus presumably is the hyperpnea of muscular exercise (Robinson and Kjeldegaard, 1982). Cellular adaptations in the diaphragm muscles of various rodents have also been shown after endurance conditioning (Farkas and Roussos, 1982; Lieberman et al., 1972; Ianuzzo and Chen, 1979; Supinski and Kelsen, 1982). Fatigue of the respiratory muscles has been demonstrated following a marathon run (Loke et al., 1982), suggesting an overload and, therefore, an adequate training stimulus for the muscles of respiration. A decrease in total respiratory muscle maximum strength (maximum transdiaphragmatic pressure) and endurance (maximum sustained voluntary ventilation) following exhaustive exercise, such as a marathon run, does not imply a loss of power output by the respiratory muscles during the exhaustive exercise when the sustained power output of the diaphragm muscle is significantly less than maximum. During marathon ski races of 160 km (100 miles), the respiratory muscles maintain a minute ventilation of 80–100 L/min for 8–10 h/day without evidence of a diminished power output (Faulkner et al., 1981). A 5-week endurance-conditioning program, which consisted of ventilating to exhaustion three to five times a day, 5 days a week, resulted in a 20% increase in the sustainable ventilatory capacity and a 14% increase in the sustained ventilatory capacity (Leith and Bradley, 1976; Bradley and Leith, 1978). The conclusions are that the respiratory muscles can be trained, and that the stimuli for, and responses to, adaptation are likely the same as for limb muscles.

Adaptation to Endurance Conditioning

The adaptations that result from endurance conditioning increase the capacity of skeletal muscles to sustain force and power. The major adaptations are an increased oxidative capacity and blood flow. The increased oxidative capacity produces a significant transition from type IIB to type IIA fibers, but whether endurance training produces a shift from type II to type I remains controversial (Faulkner et al., 1993).

Muscle Morphology

Single muscle fiber CSA is not increased by endurance conditioning in normal subjects or in rodents. In fact, fibers in the conditioned muscles are often smaller than those in the control muscles (Barnard et al., 1970a; Faulkner et al., 1971; Hermansen and Wachtlova, 1971; Saltin et al., 1968a). The circumstance in which endurance conditioning produces hypertrophy of skeletal muscle fibers is when there has been prior disuse atrophy because of limb immobilization or bed rest (MacDougall et al., 1980).

Oxidative Metabolism and Changes in Fiber Type

Following endurance conditioning, the percentage of fibers classified histochemically as high-oxidative increases in the limb muscles of rats (Barnard et al., 1970a), guinea pigs (Faulkner et al., 1971), and humans (Gollnick et al., 1973a). The same type of change from low-oxidative (type IIB fiber) to high-oxidative (type IIA fiber) is observed in the diaphragm muscle of guinea pigs that were conditioned by 1 h/day of running for 8 weeks (Lieberman et al., 1972).

Reclassification from low- to high-oxidative categories results when enzyme levels reach those used to define high-oxidative groups. The fibers that convert from low-oxidative to high-oxidative are likely to come from among the smallest type IIB motor units, for they are the ones most often recruited in addition to already active type I and type IIA motor units, as the intensity or duration of exercise is increased (Burke and Edgerton, 1975). With repeated protocols of continuous running at submaximum velocities, fibers in the soleus, medial gastrocnemius, and red portion of the vastus lateralis muscles adapt with an increase in the concentration of cytochrome c (Dudley et al., 1982). In contrast, training at high velocities of running are required to produce an increase in the concentration of cytochrome c in fibers in the white portion of the vastus lateralis muscle. Studies that used glycogen depletion to assess the fibers that are active during running have provided evidence that most type IIB fibers are not recruited during activities requiring relatively low-force development (Baldwin et al., 1973). As a consequence, most type IIB fibers show little change in the activity of oxidative enzymes after conditioning at submaximum intensities. The low forces transmitted to the Achilles tendon of cats during running support the view of endurance running as a low-force activity (Walmsley et al., 1978).

Histochemical studies and electron microscopy provide qualitative assessments of adaptations of single fibers. Quantitative measurements of the magnitude of the change in oxidative metabolism are obtained by biochemical assays of whole-muscle homogenates (Baldwin et al., 1972), or of the mitochondrial fraction (Molé et al., 1973). Following a 14-week treadmill-running program, limb muscles of previously sedentary rats undergo a twofold increase in their capacity to oxidize fats and carbohydrates (Baldwin et al., 1972; Dudley et al., 1982; Holloszy, 1967; Molé et al., 1971). The increase in oxidative capacity reflects an increase in a wide variety of mitochondrial enzymes (Holloszy and Booth, 1976) and in total mitochondrial protein (Holloszy, 1967; Morgan et al., 1971). These observations are supported by electron microscopic evidence of increases in the number and size of mitochondria in the skeletal muscles of rats (Gollnick and King, 1969) and humans (Hoppeler et al., 1973; Morgan et al., 1971). The twofold increase in the ability of whole muscle homogenates to oxidize substrates does not reflect a twofold increase in the maximum oxygen uptake of the total organism (Saltin and Gollnick, 1983). When the large muscles' masses are contracting, recruitment of a limited number of motor units and a regional distribution of blood flow reduce the effect of the increase in tissue oxidative capacity. During prolonged physical activity, the enhanced ability to oxidize fatty acids plays a significant role in postponing the onset of metabolic acidosis (Conlee, 1987; Gollnick et al., 1990).

Storage, Synthesis, and Utilization of Glycogen

Although the substrate and enzymes of the glycolytic pathway have not received as much attention as those of the Krebs cycle, some differences attributable to endurance conditioning are known. The endurance in long-term physical activity correlates highly with the glycogen content of skeletal muscle (Bergstrom et al. 1967). Furthermore, compared with unconditioned subjects, conditioned subjects have higher muscle glycogen concentrations (Gollnick et al., 1973b). Both glycogen synthesis and branching enzymes demonstrate increased activity following endurance conditioning (Gollnick et al., 1972, 1973a). Additionally, type IIA fibers, which contribute significantly to the maintenance of a high power output during endurance activity, show a 20% decrease in glycogen phosphorylase activity (Baldwin et al., 1973). Each of these adaptations increases the capacity of skeletal muscle fibers for glycogen storage.

Hexokinase is the only glycolytic enzyme for which activity correlates with the oxidative capacity of skeletal muscle (Baldwin et al., 1973) and for which activity increases with endurance conditioning (Barnard and Peter, 1969; Baldwin et al., 1973). In rats, conditioned by running, the increase in hexokinase activity is greatest (170%) in the portion of the quadriceps composed of type I and IIA fibers, intermediate (50%) in the type I fibers of the soleus muscle, and least (30%) in the portion of the quadriceps composed of type IIB fibers (Baldwin et al., 1973). The remainder of the glycolytic enzymes are highly variable in their response to conditioning (Salmons and Henriksson, 1981; Holloszy and Booth, 1976). Since the capacity for flux through the glycolytic pathway is so much greater than that of oxidative phosphorylation in both unconditioned and conditioned muscles, a rationale for adaptive changes to endurance conditioning in this pathway is difficult to develop. The increase in hexokinase may be either nonspecific or involve other energy fluxes.

In summary, the major adaptations to endurance conditioning enhance glycogen synthesis and glycogen storage. The result is a higher glycogen content in conditioned than in unconditioned muscles. The capacity for energy flux through the glycolytic pathway does not appear to change.

Myosin Isoforms

Skeletal muscles are composed of different proportions of type I, type IIA, and type IIB fibers, or S, FR, and FF (for characteristics, see Chap. 5, Table 1). In rats, the nearly 100% type II-fibered fast extensor digitorium longus (EDL) muscle is almost completely transformed into type I fibers by cross-innervation by a type I-fibered slow soleus nerve (Buller et al., 1960), or by continuous low-frequency (10-Hz) stimulation (Pette and Vrbova, 1992).

Most muscles in larger mammals, including humans, are composed of almost equal proportions of type I and type II fibers. The diaphragm and intercostal muscles of the larger mammals tend to fall into this category (see Chap. 5, Fig. 1). In spite of a mean of approximately 50–50, fluctuations to 80–20 have been observed with a preponderance of either type I (Gollnick et al., 1972) or type II (Tesch, 1988) muscle fibers. Endurance athletes tend to display high proportions of type I fibers, whereas sprinters and power lifters demonstrate high values for type II fibers

(Gollnick et al., 1972; Tesch, 1988). In addition, the high proportions are only observed in the muscles involved specifically in the conditioning program. In spite of these observations, studies of twins indicate a strong genetic influence (Komi and Karlsson, 1979). Furthermore, the cross-sectional studies of athletes do not control for the possibility that athletes who have high proportions of a fiber type gravitate to specific activities that require these attributes.

The dramatic transformations produced by cross-innervation and electrical stimulation have not been observed following endurance-conditioning programs (Faulkner et al., 1993). Experiments on both rats (Green et al., 1984) and humans (Bauman et al., 1987) have been designed to test the hypothesis that endurance training results in a conversion of myosin isoforms from fast to slow. The results have been equivocal. Either no changes in contractile properties were reported (Barnard et al., 1970b), or the changes were small (Green et al., 1984; Bauman et al., 1987). The results are surprising, considering the dramatic difference between the type I fiber composition (80–90%) in the leg muscles of world class marathon runners, compared with the 50% average for control subjects (Gollnick et al., 1972) as well as the demonstrated plasticity of myosin (Pette and Vrbova, 1992). The issue of fiber conversion with endurance conditioning remains unresolved.

Although homogeneity of gene expression within a given muscle fiber is usually observed, variations do occur. The development of antigenic reactions to antibodies of fast and slow myosin has indicated that some skeletal muscle fibers react with antibodies to both fast and slow myosin (Gauthier and Lowey, 1979; Lutz et al., 1979). The interpretation is that these fibers are expressing both fast and slow isoforms of myosin. Such fibers are presumed to be transitional between type IIA and type I. In control muscle of adult animals, the transitional fibers constitute 30% of the total (Lutz et al., 1979). The percentage increases significantly following an experimental intervention. Transitional changes in the myosin heavy chain (MHC) occur in the soleus muscle of rats during development (Reiser et al., 1988).

Contractile Properties

The characteristic contractile properties of fast skeletal muscle fibers undergo a significant conversion to those of slow fibers following cross-innervation of a fast muscle by a slow nerve (Buller et al., 1960) or long-term low-frequency stimulation (Pette and Vrbova, 1992; Salmons and Henriksson, 1981). The low-frequency prolonged stimulation (24 h/day) for several months induces a shift from fast MHC to slow myosin MHC, with a significant slowing of the V_{max} approaching that of the slow soleus muscle (Salmons and Henriksson, 1981). A significant change in V_{max} has not been induced by any endurance-conditioning programs (Faulkner et al., 1993). During development, slow and fast MHC are present in a single fiber (Reiser et al., 1988). Under these circumstances, the V_{max} correlates highly with the proportion of fast MHC present (Reiser et al., 1985). This strong relation of the proportion of fast MHC and V_{max} within single fibers in transition supports the concept of a hierarchical approach to structure–function relationships.

Capillary Density and Muscle Blood Flow

The capillary density and blood flow constitute extrinsic factors within the muscle that impinge on the capability of the fiber to function through the delivery of substrates and oxygen and the removal of end products of metabolism. The capillarity of skeletal muscle can be described quantitatively as capillaries per square millimeter of cross-sectional area, the ratio of the number of capillaries to the number of muscle fibers, or the number of capillaries adjacent to fibers of a given type (Maxwell et al., 1977). There is controversy over whether endurance conditioning induces an increase in the number of capillaries in a skeletal muscle. Studies in both small rodents (Barnard et al., 1970a; Maxwell et al., 1973) and humans (Hermansen and Wachtlova, 1971; Saltin et al., 1968a) showed no change in capillary/muscle fiber ratio or capillaries adjacent to fibers of a given type. In spite of the lack of any change in these variables, an increase in capillaries per square millimeter was observed. The increase in capillaries per square millimeter is associated with a reciprocal decrease in the individual and summed areas of conditioned, compared with nonconditioned, muscle fibers. Other studies have shown an increase in all measures of capillary density following endurance conditioning for guinea pigs (Mai et al., 1970) and for humans (Andersen, 1975; Andersen and Henriksson, 1977; Brodal et al., 1977; Ingjer, 1979). Neither the magnitude of the adaptation nor the significance of an adaptation in capillary density following endurance conditioning has been resolved.

At a given submaximum level of sustained force development, endurance training does not affect the blood flow to the contracting muscles (Armstrong and Laughlin, 1984). The primary effect of endurance training on blood flow is the increase during high-intensity, sustained contractions. In particular, the blood flow to the oxidative portions of the contracting muscles is increased (Armstrong and Laughlin, 1984; Laughlin and Ripperger, 1987). No data are available on the adaptive changes that occur in the blood flow of any of the respiratory muscles with training. Presumably, the control of blood flow and the adaptations to endurance training of the muscles of respiration are comparable with those observed in other skeletal muscles. A possible intervening variable is the very high oxidative capacity and capillary density of the respiratory muscles of untrained animals (see Chap. 5).

At maximum oxygen uptake, a close linear relation is observed between the oxygen consumption and the blood flow of different skeletal muscles in cats, dogs, and humans (Fig. 4). During exhaustive exercise, extraction of oxygen is maximum at approximately 165 ml O_2 per liter of blood flow (Maxwell et al., 1977), and oxygen consumption is entirely dependent on oxygen delivery. Muscles, such as the diaphragm, that have a high capacity to oxidize substrates also have a high capacity for maximum blood flow and, consequently, for oxygen delivery. Since muscles with wide variations in oxidative capacity have quite similar capillary densities (Maxwell et al., 1977, 1980b), capillary density does not appear to be a major determinant of maximum skeletal muscle blood flow. The maximum blood flow and increased flow to specific regions of skeletal muscle appear to depend

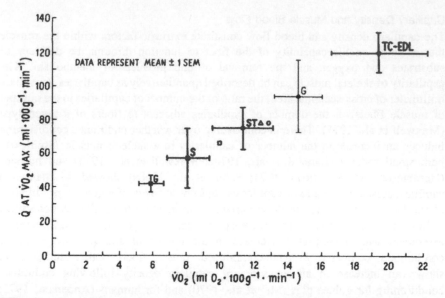

Figure 4 The relation of blood flow (ml · 100 g^{-1} · min^{-1}) and oxygen uptake (ml O$_2$ · 100 g^{-1} · min^{-1}) of selected dog and cat muscles measured at the plateau of oxygen consumption (maximum oxygen uptake). (From Maxwell et al., 1977.)

primarily on the recruitment of existing capillaries through upstream mechanisms of vasodilation and cell-to-cell communication that increase the number of perfused capillaries, the flow through individual capillaries, or both (Segal, 1991). The presence or absence of an increase of capillaries per fiber after endurance conditioning remains controversial.

B. Strength Conditioning

Strength conditioning of skeletal muscle fibers is induced by high-power–low-repetition contractions of skeletal muscle fibers. Power is not only high relative to its maximum value for a single contraction, but may actually be maximum during single lifts (see Chap. 5, Fig. 11). Under these circumstances, adequate time is allowed between lifts for more or less "complete" recovery.

Conditioning Programs

The optimum stimulus for inducing muscle hypertrophy and increasing muscle power appears to be maximum voluntary contractions performed a maximum five to ten times, which is termed a *ten execution maximum* protocol. When resistance can be overcome ten times, a greater resistance is used. The key concept involved is to keep fatigue to a minimum and to maintain force and power. The resistance may involve dynamic (isotonic) free lifts, isokinetic machines, or static (isometric) contractions (Jones et al., 1989). Well-trained lifters will perform two to four sets of five to ten maximum lifts per training session. To recover fully from a strength-conditioning session requires up to 48 h, and sessions are usually performed on alternate days. Although the ten-execution maximum is the most effective protocol, lighter weights of 40–50% of maximum voluntary contraction are advisable during introductory phases to avoid injury to muscles.

Strength-conditioning programs may include static contractions (Jones et al., 1989). The static contraction may be held at a maximum effort or at some percentage of maximum. Protocols can be developed with various combinations of percentage maximum, duty/rest ratio, duty–rest cycle, and duration. The static contraction provides a stimulus similar to that provided by a dynamic lift, at a comparable percentage of maximum effort. There is some evidence that static strength conditioning increases strength only at the specific muscle length or muscle lengths at which static strength was held (Jones et al., 1989). Static strength conditioning appears to be most useful when strength at a specific muscle length limits performance. Strength conditioning should include all of the muscles involved in the specific exercise for which the conditioning is designed. Conditioning should also be carried out through the full range of motion to be used in the exercise. An additional advantage of dynamic lifts, is the inclusion of lengthening contractions at high loads during the lowering of the weights (Jones and Rutherford, 1987).

Leith and Bradley (1976) employed the principles of strength training to design a strength-conditioning program for the muscles of respiration. The program was 5-weeks long with training 5 days a week in the performance of repeated maximum inspiratory and expiratory maneuvers. After strength training, no change was observed in the sustainable ventilatory capacity or the MVV (Bradley and Leith, 1978), which is consistent with data on limb muscles. Whether the respiratory muscles were stronger or more powerful was not determined.

Adaptation to Conditioning

The primary stimuli for an adaptation for strength and power are high-velocity lifts and low-velocity descents with heavy loads. The concept is that the high loads require the recruitment of most of the motor units in the muscle groups, and the high velocity places the major portion of the load on the faster fibers (Fig. 5). Fewer motor units will be recruited during the lowering as the muscles undergo a controlled stretch, but cross-bridges in activated fibers will bear a higher load than during shortening. Therefore, the conditioning stimulus to fibers in these motor units would be even greater than during shortening contraction. The loading of the strained cross-bridges during the lengthening contraction is not velocity-dependent (Lombardi and Piazzesi, 1990). Consequently, the low velocity is advisable to reduce the possibility of contraction-induced injury (McCully and Faulkner, 1985).

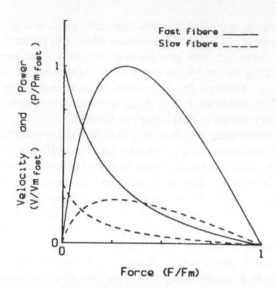

Figure 5   The relation of velocity of shortening and power each plotted against the force or load against which the muscle was shortening. The velocity of shortening was normalized by the velocity of unloaded shortening of the fastest fibers; the power by the maximum power of the fastest fibers; and the force by the maximum isometric tetanic force. Note that maximum power occurs at approximately one-third maximum force and one-third maximum velocity. (From Faulkner et al., 1986.)

Muscle Morphology

The major changes resulting from strength conditioning are in the architecture of the muscle. Following conditioning to heavy-resistance exercise, both type I and type II skeletal muscle fibers increase in cross-sectional area (MacDougall et al., 1980). The significant increase in the type II/type I fiber area ratio indicates a greater involvement of type II fibers in heavy resistive exercise. The increase in single fiber CSA is achieved by increases in the size and number of myofibrils per fiber (Goldspink, 1970). Concurrent with the increase in area, fibers may migrate along fascial planes and increase the angle of attachment relative to the long axis of the muscle (Maxwell et al., 1974).

A major controversy in the response of skeletal muscle to strength conditioning concerns the role of hyperplasia, and the possibilities of fiber splitting, fiber branching, or both (Gonyea and Ericson, 1976; Gollnick et al., 1981). In cat forelimbs conditioned by weight lifting, whole muscle hypertrophy of from 7 to 34% was reported, with an increase of 19% in the total number of fibers in a cross-section area through the belly of the muscle. This is not a definitive method of demonstrating hyperplasia (Maxwell et al., 1974). Gollnick et al. (1981) used ablation of the synergists and exercise to load the soleus, plantaris, and EDL of young rats. The wet mass of the overloaded muscles increased by 29–88% of control values, but when total numbers of individual fibers were counted after nitric acid digestion, no differences were observed between overloaded and control muscles (Gollnick et al., 1981). Furthermore, the frequency of fibers with bifurcations did not change. Compared with the weight-training model for muscle hypertrophy, the ablation model provides a very different set of adaptive stimuli, including differences in intensity, duration, frequency, and variability. Histological evidence purports to show fiber splitting after weight training (Gonyea et al., 1977), whereas as many as 50% of the fibers were branched in dystrophic muscles (Head et a., 1990) and in muscles transplanted in old rats (Blaivas and Carlson, 1991). In the latter two experiments, the fibers are regenerating and the complex patterns of branching likely arise during the growth of new fibers. Although hypertrophy of fibers is the predominant adaptation to strength conditioning, the specific contributions of hyperplasia, fiber splitting, fiber branching, and fiber fusion during muscle enlargement have not been resolved.

Oxidative Metabolism, Capillary Density, and Blood Flow

Programs of high-power–low-frequency contractions designed to increase muscle strength do not increase the oxidative capacity, maximum muscle blood flow, or capillary/muscle fiber ratio (Gollnick et al., 1972; Ianuzzo and Chen, 1979; Vanderhoof et al., 1961). Capillaries per square millimeter may decrease owing to skeletal muscle fiber hypertrophy. The volume density of mitochondria and the mitochondrial volume/myofibrillar volume ratio both decrease following a conditioning program of heavy-resistance exercise (MacDougall et al., 1979).

Contractile Properties

Following strength-conditioning programs, the gains of 30–40% in force development are twofold to threefold greater than the increase in total muscle fiber, or in single muscle fiber CSA (Sale, 1988; Jones et al., 1989). Optimization of recruitment patterns is responsible for at least a part of the early improvements in generation of both strength and power (Sale, 1988). The discrepancy between the structural and functional adaptations are less when participants in conditioning programs are already accustomed to developing maximum strength and power.

Conditioning muscles for the generation of strength and power tend to increase fatigability (Simson and Keys, 1971), possibly through the decrease in mitochondrial protein concentration (MacDougall et al., 1979). In spite of this trend, hypertrophy and fatigability are not immutably linked, since hypertrophied muscles do demonstrate a normal adaptive response to the stimuli of an endurance-conditioning program (Faulkner et al., 1993).

C. Stretch Conditioning

Several different stretch-conditioning models have been developed to investigate the capacity for adaptations increased length of skeletal muscle fibers. The models include the denervated hemidiaphragm (Martin and Sola, 1948), the denervated chicken wing (Feng et al., 1962), ablation of synergistic muscles (Denny-Brown, 1960), shortening of the distal tendon (Schiaffino, 1974), stretched-immobilized ankle flexors (Goldspink, 1977; Laurent and Millward, 1980), spring-loaded extension of the immobilized chicken wing (Holly et al., 1980); stretched myocites in vitro (Vandenburgh et al., 1991a,b); a bite-opening appliance (Maxwell et al., 1981); and hyperinflation of the diaphragm induced by emphysema (Farkas and Roussos, 1982). The conditioning stimulus results from the passive stretch, and in innervated muscles, increased force development owing to the stretch reflex (Laurent and Millward, 1980). An increased protein turnover is associated with the stretch-induced growth. Increases or decreases in the number of sarcomeres in series and, consequently, changes in fiber length, have been observed in several models (Farkas and Roussos, 1982; Holly et al., 1980; Maxwell et al., 1981; Tabary et al., 1972); this appears to be a mechanism to adjust muscle-operating lengths to maintain the optimum length for force development (see Chap. 5).

The ability of skeletal muscles to adjust their lengths appropriately in response to changing operating conditions has profound implications for adaptation of inspiratory muscles to the progressive pulmonary hyperinflation of chronic obstructive lung disease. The adaptation following experimentally induced emphysema in hamsters is an increase in the length of fibers in the diaphragm muscle, proportional to the degree of hyperinflation (Farkas and Roussos, 1982).

D. Deconditioning

The concept of deconditioning presupposes some previous level of muscular activity that can be decreased. If the previous muscular activity involved either an endurance-, strength-, or stretch-conditioning program, after a cessation of the conditioning, the adaptations produced by the conditioning regress back toward the preconditioning values in a matter of weeks or months, depending to some degree on the duration of the conditioning program (Faulkner et al., 1972; Coyle et al., 1984: Larsson, 1985). The conclusion is that the conditioned state requires some maintenance level of increased physical activity (Faulkner et al., 1993).

Because the respiratory muscles are continuously active, they might be proposed as the ideal model for the study of deconditioning. Several factors intervene that result in the respiratory muscles providing less than an ideal model of deconditioning: One, the respiratory muscles of patients who have been on assisted breathing present complications in respiratory function associated with respiratory disease. Second, there are the inherent difficulties of measuring the function of the respiratory muscles of humans accurately (see Chap. 5). Third, the animal models that produce quiescent respiratory muscles employ denervation, and the adaptive responses to denervation are even more complex than other forms of physical inactivity. With denervation, a loss of trophic influences is superimposed on the loss of contractile activity (Guth et al., 1981).

Deconditioning Programs

Deconditioning programs are based on protocols that reduce the recruitment, loading, or both variables, below the habitual level for a muscle, or group of muscles. For humans, bed rest (Saltin et al., 1968b) and space flight (Roy et al., 1991) have been used to reduce the levels of total body physical activity, whereas immobilization of limbs by casting (MacDougall et al., 1980) and unilateral leg suspension (Berg et al., 1991) have been used in animals for recruitment and loading of a group of muscles. For studies of rats, casting (Booth and Kelso, 1973), hind limb suspension (Alford et al., 1987; Musacchia et al., 1990), and space flights (Musacchia et al., 1990) have provided data on different types of deconditioning programs.

Adaptations to Deconditioning

In studies of a return to normal physical activity after a period of high-intensity physical conditioning, the increases in muscle fiber CSA, capacity for oxidative metabolism, muscle blood flow, and in the development of maximum power or the ability to sustain high-power output, each regress back to lower values (Faulkner et al., 1972; Coyle et al., 1984; Larsson, 1985). This supports the concept of the reversibility of adaptive responses. The magnitude of the changes observed in loss of mass, oxidative capacity, and force development of muscle groups deconditioned with the experimental models is no different from that observed after equivalent periods of space flight (Musacchia et al., 1990; Roy et al., 1991). Consequently, the ground-based experiments appear to provide reasonable models for the changes that occur in skeletal muscles during space flight.

Muscle Morphology

In both rats and humans, a significant decrease in muscle mass and in the single muscle fiber CSA results from immobilization (Booth and Kelso, 1973), casting (Sargeant et al., 1977; MacDougall et al., 1980), weightlessness (Mussachia et al., 1990), and edentulation (Maxwell et al., 1980a).

Oxidative Metabolism and Mitochondrial Density

Decreased physical activity of a muscle group results in reductions in oxidative capacity in the muscles of mastication of edentulous monkeys (Maxwell et al., 1980a), in immobilized hind limb muscles of rats (Booth and Kelso, 1973), and in casted limbs of humans (Sargeant et al., 1977; MacDougall et al., 1980). Disuse following almost any surgical intervention results in a decreased oxidative capacity of the muscles involved (Maxwell et al., 1981).

With disuse, a shift occurs from the synthesis of slow to the synthesis of fast myosin (Tsika et al., 1987). A higher proportion of type II fibers is observed after each of the disuse protocols. With immobilization, significant slowing of the contractile response is consistent with the changes in the myosin isoforms (Witzmann et al., 1982).

V. Contraction-Induced Injury

Contraction-induced injury may occur in conditioned, control, or deconditioned skeletal muscles (McCully and Faulkner, 1985; Kasper et al., 1990). Skeletal muscles are more likely to be injured when muscles are stretched during a contraction than when the contraction is either isometric or shortening (Friden et al., 1981; Jones et al., 1986; McCully and Faulkner, 1985; Zerba et al., 1990). The injury produced by muscle contractions is initially focal, but, with repeated contractions, may become more extensive and extend across the total cross section of the fiber. The immediate injury is predominately mechanical, but the secondary aspects, which increase the magnitude of the damage and the deficit in force development, involve oxygen free radicals (Zerba et al., 1990). Injured fiber may display contraction clots, necrosis of some sarcomeres, and eventually, infiltration by phagocytes, with extensive sarcolysis.

Under most circumstances, recovery from contraction-induced injury is complete after a recovery period of several weeks (McCully and Faulkner, 1985). Following sarcolysis of the disrupted cytoplasm, regeneration of injured fibers occurs (Carlson and Faulkner, 1983). Regeneration depends on the presence of a blood supply, either by a surviving vascular bed or by revascularization of the muscle fibers. Phagocytes remove the cellular debris. Satellite cells are activated, and mitotic division results in the formation of myoblasts, myotubes, and eventually muscle fibers. Innervation of fibers is necessary for differentiation into specific fiber types.

The characterization of the prevalence of contraction-induced injury particularly when muscles are stretched during contractions has implications for the design of endurance-conditioning and strength-conditioning programs. Care in the design of programs is of considerable importance when the muscles of the participants have been deconditioned by casting or by long-term bed rest. If these findings are applicable to respiratory muscles, programs designed to wean patients from respirators should be graded for the intensity and duration of the respiratory effort.

VI. Summary

The fibers in skeletal muscle motor units adapt to changes in the frequency of action potentials, the activity–rest cycle, and the pattern in terms of duration of the contraction cycles in a given conditioning session, the number of times per day and per week, and the number of days or weeks. Currently, three patterns of adaptive stimuli have been identified: low-power–high-power–low-repetition stimuli that result in an increased strength; and a stretch stimulus that results primarily in an increased strength. Many of the models used within each of these three conditioning programs vary significantly in their frequency, intensity, duration, and pattern of stimuli, and this may account for some of the controversies that have arisen. The effect of inactivity may be studied during deconditioning programs or by immobilization of limbs. Future research should focus more precisely on the adaptive response to highly prescribed patterns of stimuli.

Acknowledgments

The studies of the adaption of skeletal muscle have been enhanced by long-term collaborations with many colleagues: Bruce M. Carlson, Leo C. Maxwell, Kevin K. McCully, and Timothy P. White. Peter Macpherson provided helpful comments on an earlier draft of the manuscript. Gabriele Wienert and Richard Hinkle provided valuable assistance in the typing and formatting of the manuscript. The research was supported in part by a Program Project grant DE-07687 from the United States Public Health Service, National Institute of Dental Research.

References

Adolph, E. F. (1956). Some general and specific characteristics of physiological adaptations. *Am. J. Physiol.* 184: 18–28.

Alford, E., Roy, R. R., Hodgson, J. A., and Edgerton, V. R. (1987). Electromyography of rat soleus, gastrocnemius, and tibialis anterior during hind limb suspension. *Exp. Neurol.* 96: 635–649.

Andersen, P. (1975). Capillary density in skeletal muscle of man. *Acta Physiol. Scand.* 95: 203–205.

Andersen, P., and Henriksson, J. (1977). Capillary supply of the quadriceps femoris muscle of man: Adaptive response to exercise. *J. Physiol. (Lond.)* 270: 677–690.

Armstrong, R. B., and Laughlin, M. H. (1984). Exercise blood flow patterns within and among rat muscles after training. *Am. J. Physiol.* 246: H59–H68.

Baldwin, K. M., Klinkerfuss, G. H., Terjung, R. L., Molé, P. A., and Holloszy, J. O. (1972). Respiratory capacity of white, red and intermediate muscle: Adaptive response to exercise. *Am. J. Physiol.* 222: 373–378.

Baldwin, K. M., Winder, W. W., Terjung, R. L., and Holloszy, J. O. (1973). Glycolytic enzymes in different types of skeletal muscle: Adaptation to exercise. *Am. J. Physiol.* 255: 962–966.

Barbashova, Z. I. (1964). Cellular level of adaptation. In *Handbook of Physiology*, Section 4. Adaptation to the Environment. Edited by D. B. Dill, E. F. Adolf, and C. G. Wilber. Washington, DC, American Physiological Society, pp. 37–54.

Barnard, R. J., and Peter, J. B. (1969). Effect of training and exhaustion on hexokinase activity of skeletal muscle. *J. Appl. Physiol.* 27: 691–695.

Barnard, R. J., Edgerton, V. R., and Peter, J. B. (1970a). Effect of exercise on skeletal muscle I. Biochemical and histochemical properties. *J. Appl. Physiol.* 28: 762–766.

Barnard, R. J., Edgerton, V. R., and Peter, J. B. (1970b). Effect of exercise on skeletal muscle II. Contractile properties. *J. Appl. Physiol.* 28: 767–770.

Baumann, H., Jaggi, M., Soland, F., Howald, H., and Schaub, M. C. (1987). Exercise training induces transitions of myosin isoform subunits within histochemically typed human muscle fibres. *Pflugers Arch.* 409: 349–360.

Berg, H. E., Dudley, G. A., Häggmark, T., Ohlsén H., and Tesch, P. A. (1991). Effects of lower limb unloading on skeletal muscle mass and function in humans *J. Appl. Physiol.* 70: 1882–1885.

Bergstrom, J., Hermansen, L., Hultman, E., and Saltin, B. (1967). Diet, muscle glycogen and physical performance. *Acta Physiol. Scand.* 71: 140–150.

Blaivas, M., and Carlson, B. M. (1991). Muscle fiber branching—difference between grafts in old and young rats. *Mech. Ageing Dev.* 60: 43–53.

Booth, F. W., and Kelso, J. R. (1973). Effect of hind-limb immobilization on contractile and histochemical properties of skeletal muscle. *Pflugers Arch.* 342: 231–238.

Bradley, E., and Leith D. E. (1978). Ventilatory muscle training and oxygen cost of sustained hyperpnea. *J. Appl. Physiol. Respir. Environ. Exerc. Physiol.* 45: 885–892.

Brodal, P., Ingjer, F., and Hermansen, L. (1977). Capillary supply of skeletal muscle fibers in untrained and endurance-trained men. *Am. J. Physiol.* 232: H705–H712.

Brooke, M. H., and Kaiser, K. K. (1970). Muscle fiber types: How many and what kind. *Arch. Neurol.* 23: 369–379.

Brooks, C. M. (1969). The nature of adaptive reactions and their initiation. In *Physiology and Pathology of Adaptive Mechanisms*. Edited by E. Bajusz. New York, Pergamon Press, pp. 439–451.

Buller, A. J., Eccles, J. C., and Eccles, R. M. (1960). Interactions between motoneuron and muscles in respect of the characteristic speeds of their response. *J. Physiol. (Lond.)* 150: 417–439.

Burke, R. E. (1981). Motor unit recruitment: What are the critical factors? In *Motor Unit Types, Recruitment and Plasticity in Health and Disease*. Edited by J. E. Desmedt. Basel, S. Karger, pp. 61–84.

Burke, R. E., and Edgerton., V. R. (1975). Motor unit properties and selective involvement in movement. In *Exercise and Sports Sciences Reviews*, Vol. 3. New York, Academic Press, pp. 31–81.

Burke, R. E., Levine, D. N., Zajac, F. E. III, Tsairis, P., and Engel, W. K. (1973). Physiological types and histochemical profiles in motor units of the cat gastrocnemius. *J. Physiol. (Lond.)* 234: 723–748.

Carlson, B. M., and Faulkner, J. A. (1983). The regeneration of skeletal muscle fibers following injury. A review. *Med. Sci. Sports Exerc.* 15: 187–198.

Conlee, R. K. (1987). Muscle glycogen and exercise endurance: A twenty-year perspective. In *Exercise Sport Science Review*, Vol. 15. Edited by K. B. Pandolf. New York, Macmillan, pp. 1–28.

Coyle, E. F., Martin, W. M. III, Sinacore, D. R., Joyner, M. J., Hagberg, J. M., and Holloszy, J. O. (1984). Time course of loss of adaptations after stopping prolonged intense endurance training. *J. Appl. Physiol.* 57: 1857–1864.

Denny-Brown, D. E. (1960). Experimental studies pertaining to hypertrophy, regeneration and degeneration. *Res. Publ. Assoc. Res. Nerv. Ment. Dis.* 38: 147–196.

Dill, D. B., Adolph, E. F., and Wilson, C. G., eds. (1964). In *Handbook of Physiology*, Section 4. Adoptation to the Environment. Washington, DC, American Physiological Society, pp. v–1056.

Dudley, G. A., Abraham W. A., and Terjung, R. L. (1982). Influence of exercise intensity and duration on biochemical adaptations in skeletal muscle. *J. Appl. Physiol.* 53: 844–850.

Enoka, R. M., and Stuart, D. G. (1984). Henneman's "size principle": Current issues. *Trends Neurosci.* 7: 226–228.

Farkas, G. A., and Roussos, C. (1982). Adaptability of the hamster diaphragm to exercise and/or emphysema. *J. Appl. Physiol.* 53: 1263–1272.

Faulkner, J. A. (1968). New perspectives in training for maximum performance. JAMA 205: 741–746.

Faulkner, J. A. (1983). The nature of the stimulus for adaptation. In *Frontiers of Exercise Biology*. Edited by K. T. Borer, D. W. Edington, and T. P. White. Champaign, IL: Human Kinetics Publishers, pp. 4–14.

Faulkner, J. A., Maxwell, L. C., Brook, D. A., and Lieberman, D. A. (1971). Adaptation of guinea pig plantaris muscle fibers to endurance training. *Am. J. Physiol.* 221: 291–297.

Faulkner, J. A., Maxwell, L. C., and Lieberman, D. A. (1972). Histochemical characteristics of muscle fibers from trained and detrained guinea pigs. *Am. J. Physiol.* 222: 836–840.

Faulkner, J. A., White, T. P., and Markley, J. M., Jr. (1981). Canadian ski marathon: A natural experiment in hypothermia. In *Exercise in Health and Disease–Balke Symposium*. Edited by F. J. Nagle and H. J. Montoye. Springfield, IL, Charles C Thomas, pp. 184–195.

Faulkner, J. A., Green, H. J., and White, T. P. (1993). Skeletal muscle responses to acute and adaptations to chronic physical activity. In *Physical Activity, Fitness and Health*. Edited by C. Bouchard. Champaign, IL, Human Kinetics Publishers.

Feng, T. P., Jung, H. W., and Wu, W. Y. (1962). The contrasting trophic changes of the anterior and posterior latissimus dorsi of the chick following denervation. *Acta Physiol. Sin.* 25: 304–311.

Friden, J., Sjostrom, M., and Ekblom, B. (1981). A morphological study of delayed muscle soreness. *Experientia* 37: 506–507.

Gauthier, G. F., and Lowey, S. (1979). Distribution of myosin isoenzymes among skeletal muscle fiber types. *J. Cell Biol.* 81: 10–25.

Goldspink, G. (1970). Morphological adaptation due to growth and activity. In *The Physiology and Biochemistry of Muscle as a Food, II.* Edited by E. J. Briskey, R. G. Cassens, and B. B. Marsh. Madison, University of Wisconsin Press, pp. 521–536.

Goldspink, D. F. (1977). The influence of immobilization and stretch on protein turnover of rat skeletal muscle. *J. Physiol. (Lond.)* 264: 267–282.

Gollnick, P. D., and King, D. W. (1969). Effect of exercise and training on mitochondria of rat skeletal muscle. *Am. J. Physiol.* 216: 1502–1509.

Gollnick, P. D., Armstrong, R. B., Saubert, C. W. IV, Piehl, K., and Saltin, B. (1972). Enzyme activity and fiber composition in skeletal muscle of untrained and trained men. *J. Appl. Physiol.* 33: 312–319.

Gollnick, P. D., Armstrong, R. B., Salton, B., Saubert, C. W. IV, Sembrowich, W. L., and Shepherd, R. E. (1973a). Effect of training on enzyme activity and fiber composition of human skeletal muscle. *J. Appl. Physiol.* 34: 107–111.

Gollnick, P. D., Armstrong, R. B., Saubert, C. W. IV, Sembrowich, W. L., Shepherd, R. E., and Saltin, B. (1973b). Glycogen depletion patterns in human skeletal muscle fibers during prolonged work. *Pflugers Arch.* 344: 1–12.

Gollnick, P. D., Timson, B. F., Moore, R. L., and Riedy, M. (1981). Muscular enlargement and number of fibers in skeletal muscles of rats. *J. Appl. Physiol.* 50: 936–943.

Gollnick, P. D., Bertorci, L. A., Kelso, T. B., Witt, E. H., and Hodgson, D. R. (1990). The effect of high intensity exercise on the respiratory capacity of skeletal muscle. Pflugers Arch. 415: 405–413.

Gonyea, W. J., and Ericson, G. C. (1976). An experimental model for the study of exercise-induced skeletal muscle hypertrophy. *J. Appl. Physiol.* 40: 630–633.

Gonyea, W., Ericson, G. C., and Bonde-Petersen, F. (1977). Skeletal muscle fiber splitting induced by weight-lifting exercise in cats. *Acta Physiol. Scand.* 99: 105–109.

Green, H. J., Klug, G. A., Reichmann, H., Seedorf, U., Wiehrer, W., and Pette, D. (1984). Exercise-induced fibre type transition with regard to myosin and sarcoplasmic reticulum in muscles of the rat. *Pflugers Arch.* 400: 432–438.

Guth, L., Kemerer, V. F., Samaras, T. A., Warnick, J. E., and Albuquerque, E. X. (1981). The roles of disuse and loss of neurotrophic function in denervation atrophy of skeletal muscle. *Exp. Neurol.* 73: 20–36.

Head, S. I., Stephenson, D. G., and Williams, D. A. (1990). Properties of enzymatically isolated skeletal fibres from mice with muscular dystrophy. *J. Physiol. (Lond.)* 422: 351–367.

Henneman, E., and Olson, C. B (1965). Relations between structure and function in the design of skeletal muscles. *J. Neurophysiol.* 28: 581.

Hermansen, L., and Wachtlova, M. (1971). Capillary density of skeletal muscle in well-trained and untrained men. *J. Appl. Physiol.* 30: 860–863.

Hochochka, P. W., and Somers, G. N. (1973). *Strategies of Biochemical Adaptation*. Philadelphia, W. B. Saunders, pp. iii–358.

Holloszy, J. O. (1967). Biochemical adaptations in muscle: Effect of exercise on mitochondrial oxygen uptake and respiratory enzyme activity in skeletal muscle. *J. Biol. Chem.* 242: 2278–2282.

Holloszy, J. O., and Booth, F. W. (1976). Biochemical adaptations to endurance exercise in muscle. *Annu. Rev. Physiol.* 38: 273–291.

Holly, R. G., Barnett, G. J., Ashmore, C. R., Taylor, R. G., and Molé, P. A. (1980). Stretch-induced growth in chicken wing muscles: A new model of stretch hypertrophy. *Am. J. Physiol.* 7: C62–C71.

Hoppeler, H., Lüthi, P., Claasen, H., Weibel, E. R., and Howald, H. (1973). The ultrastructure of normal human skeletal muscle. A morphometric analysis of untrained men, women and well-trained orienteers. *Pflugers Arch.* 344: 217–232.

Ianuzzo, C. D., and Chen, V. (1979). Metabolic character of hypertrophied rat muscle. *J. Appl. Physiol.* 46: 738–742.

Ingjer, F. (1979). Effects of endurance training on muscle fibre ATPase activity, capillary supply and mitochondrial content in man. *J. Physiol. (Lond.)* 294: 419–432.

Jones, D. A., and Rutherford, O. M. (1987). Human muscle strength training: The effects of three different regimens and the nature of the resultant changes. *J. Physiol. (Lond.)* 391: 1–11.

Jones, D. A., Newham, D. J., Round, J. M., and Tolfree, S. E. J. (1986). Experimental human muscle damage: morphological changes in relation to other indices of damage. *J. Physiol. (London)* 375: 435–448.

Jones, D. A., Rutherford, O. M., and Parker, D. F. (1989). Physiological changes in skeletal muscle as a result of strength training. *Q. J. Exp. Physiol.* 74: 233–256.

Kasper, C. E., White, T. P., and Maxwell, L. C. (1990). Running during recovery from hindlimb suspension induces transient muscle injury. *J. Appl. Physiol.* 68: 533–539.

Komi, P. V., and Karlsson, J. (1979). Physical performance, skeletal muscle enzyme activities, and fiber types in monozygous twins of both sexes. *Acta Physiol. Scand. [Suppl.]* 462: 1–28.

Larsson, L. (1985). Effects of long-term physical training and detraining on enzyme histochemical and functional skeletal muscle characteristics in man. *Muscle Nerve* 8: 714–722.

Laughlin, M. H., and Ripperger J. (1987). Vascular transport capacity of hindlimb muscles of exercise-trained rats. *J. Appl. Physiol.* 62: 438–443.

Laurent, G. J., and Millward, D. J. (1980). Protein turnover during skeletal muscle hypertrophy. *Fed. Proc.* 39: 42–47.

Leake, C. D. (1964). Perspectives of adaptation: Historical backgrounds. In *Handbook of Physiology*, Section 4. Adaptation to the Environment. Edited by D. B. Dill, E. F. Adolph, and C. G. Wilber. Washington, DC, American Physiological Society, pp. 1–10.

Leith, D. E., and Bradley, M. (1976). Ventilatory muscles strength and endurance training. *J. Appl. Physiol.* 41: 508–516.

Lieberman, D. A., Maxwell, L. C., and Faulkner, J. A. (1972). Adaptation of guinea pig diaphragm muscle to aging and endurance training. *Am. J. Physiol.* 222: 556–561.

Lombardi, V., and Piazzesi, G. (1990). The contractile response during steady lengthening of stimulated frog muscle fibres. *J. Physiol. (Lond.)* 431: 141–171.

Loke, J., Mahler, D. A., and Virgulto, J. A. (1982). Respiratory muscle fatigue after marathon running. *J. Appl. Physiol. Respir. Environ. Exerc. Physiol.* 52: 821–824.

Lutz, H., Weber, H., Billeter, R., and Jenny, E. (1979). Fast and slow myosin within single skeletal muscle fibres of adult rabbits. *Nature* 281: 142–144.

MacDougall, J. D., Sale, D. G., Moroz, J. R., Elder, G. C. B., Sutton, J. R., and Howald, H. (1979). Mitochondrial volume density in human skeletal muscle following heavy resistance training. *Med. Sci. Sports* 11: 164–166.

MacDougall, J. D., Elder, G. C. B., Sale, D. G., Moroz, J. R., and Sutton, J. R. (1980). Effects of strength training and immobilization on human muscle fibers. *Eur. J. Appl. Physiol.* 43: 25–34.

Mai, J. V., Edgerton, V. R., and Barnard, R. J. (1970). Capillarity of red, white and intermediate muscle fibers in trained and untrained guinea pigs. *Experientia* 26: 1222–1223.

Martin, A. W., and Sola, O. M. (1948). The rate of atrophy of rat diaphragm. *Fed. Proc.* 7: 78.

Maxwell, L. C., Faulkner, J. A., and Lieberman, D. A. (1973). Histochemical manifestations of age and endurance training in skeletal muscle fibers. *Am. J. Physiol.* 344: 356–361.

Maxwell, L. C., Faulkner, J. A., and Hyatt, G. J. (1974). Estimation of the number of fibers in guinea pig skeletal muscle. *J. Appl. Physiol.* 37: 259–264.

Maxwell, L. C., Barclay, J. K., Mohrman, D. E., and Faulkner, J. A. (1977). Physiological characteristics of skeletal muscles of dogs and cats. *Am. J. Physiol.* 233: C14–C18.

Maxwell, L. C., McNamara, J. A. Jr., Carlson, D. S., and Faulkner, J. A. (1980a). Histochemistry of fibres of masseter and temporalis muscles of edentulous rhesus monkeys (*Macaca mulatta*). *Arch. Oral Biol.* 25: 87–93.

Maxwell, L. C., White, T. P., and Faulkner, J. A. (1980b). Oxidative capacity, blood flow, and capillarity of skeletal muscles. *Am. J. Physiol.* 49: 627–633.

Maxwell, L. C., Carlson, D. S., McNamara, J. A., and Faulkner, J. A. (1981). Adaptation of the masseter and temporalis muscles following alteration in length, with or without surgical detachment. *Anat. Rec.* 200: 127–137.

McCully, K. K., and Faulkner, J. A. (1985). Injury to skeletal muscle fibers of mice following lengthening contractions. *J. Appl. Physiol.* 59: 119–126.

Molé, P. A., Oscai, L. B., and Holloszy, J. O. (1971). Adaptation of muscle to exercise. Increase in levels of palmityl CoA synthetase, carnitine palmityltransferase and palmityl CoA dehydrogenase and in the capacity to oxidize fatty acids. *J. Clin. Invest.* 50: 2323–2330.

Molé, P. A., Baldwin, K. M., Terjung, R. L., and Holloszy, J. O. (1973). Enzymatic pathways of pyruvate metabolism in skeletal muscle: Adaptations to exercise. *Am. J. Physiol.* 224: 50–54.

Morgan, T. E., Cobb, L. A., Short, F. A., Ross, R., and Gun, D. R. (1971). Effects of long-term exercise on human muscle mitochondria. In *Muscle Metabolism During Exercise*. Edited by B. Pernow and B. Saltin. New York, Plenum Press, pp. 87–95.

Musacchia, X. J., Steffen, R. D., Fell, R. D., and Dombrowski, M. J. (1990). Skeletal muscle response to spaceflight, whole body suspension, and recovery in rats. *J. Appl. Physiol.* 69: 2248–2253.

Nemeth, P. M., Pette, D., and Vrbova, G. (1981). Comparison of enzyme activities among single muscle fibres within defined motor units. *J. Physiol.* (*Lond.*) 331: 489–495.

Pette, D., and Vrbova, G. (1992). Adaptation of mammalian skeletal muscle fibers in chronic electrical stimulation. *Rev. Physiol. Biochem. Pharmacol.* 120: 116–202.

Prosser, C. L. (1964). Perspectives of adaptation: Theoretical aspects. In *Handbook of Physiology*, Section 4. Adaptation to the Environment. Edited by D. B. Dill, E. F. Adolph, and C. G. Wilber. Washington, DC, American Physiological Society, pp. 11–26.

Reiser, P. J., Moss, R. L., Giulian, G. G., and Greaser, M. L. (1985). Shortening velocity in single fibers from adult rabbit soleus muscles is correlated with myosin heavy chain composition. *J. Biol. Chem.* 260: 9077–9080.

Reiser, P. J., Kasper, C. E., Greaser, M. L., and Moss, R. L. (1988). Functional significance of myosin transitions in single fibers of developing soleus muscle. *Am. J. Physiol.* 254: C605–C615.

Robinson, E. P., and J. M. Kjeldgaard. (1982). Improvement in ventilatory muscle function with running. *J. Appl. Physiol. Respir. Environ. Exerc. Physiol.* 52: 1400–1406.

Roy, R. R., Baldwin, K. M., and Edgerton, V. R. (1991). The plasticity of skeletal muscle: Effects of neuromuscular activity. In *Exercise and Sport Sciences Reviews*, Vol. 19. Edited by J. O. Holloszy. Baltimore, Williams & Wilkins, pp. 269–312.

Sale, D. G. (1988). Neural adaptation to resistance training. *Med. Sci. Sports Exerc.* 20: S135–S145.

Salmons, S., and Henriksson, J. (1981). The adaptive response of skeletal muscle to increased use. *Muscle Nerve* 4: 94–105.

Saltin, B., and Gollnick, P. D. (1983). Skeletal muscle adaptability: Significance for metabolism and performance. In *Handbook of Physiology*, Chapter 19. Edited by L. D. Peachey, R. H. Adrian, and S. R. Geiger. Baltimore, Williams & Wilkins, pp. 555–631.

Saltin, B., Blomquist, G., and Mitchell, J. H. (1968a). Response to exercise after bedrest and after training: A longitudinal study of adaptive changes in oxygen transport and body composition. *Circulation* 38(Suppl. 7): 1–78.

Saltin, B., Blomquist, G., Mitchell, J. H., Johnson, R. L. Jr., Wildenthal, K., and Chapman, C. B. (1968b). Response to exercise after bed rest and after training. *Circulation* 38: 1–77.

Sargeant, A. J., Davies, C. T. M., Edwards, R. H. T., Maunder, C., and Young, A. (1977). Functional and structural changes after disuse of human muscle. *Clin. Sci. Mol. Med.* 52: 337–342.

Schiaffino, S. (1974). Hypertrophy of skeletal muscle induced by tendon shortening. *Experientia* 30: 1163–1164.

Segal, S. S. (1991). Microvascular recruitment in hamster striated muscle: Role for conducted vasodilation. *Am. J. Physiol.* 261: H181–H189.

Selye, H. (1952). *The Story of the Adaptation Syndrome Told in the Form of Informal Lectures.* Montreal, Acta.

Sieck, G. C., Roy, R. R., Powell, P., Blanco, C., Edgerton, V. R., and Harper, R. M. (1983). Muscle fiber type distribution and architecture of the cat diaphragm. *J. Appl. Physiol. Respir. Environ. Exerc. Physiol.* 55: 1386–1392.

Simson, E., and Keys, A. (1971). *Physiology of Work Capacity and Fatigue.* Springfield, IL, Charles C. Thomas, pp. 241–284.

Supinski, G. S., and S. G. Kelsen. (1982). Effect of elastase-induced emphysema on the force-generating ability of the diaphragm. *J. Clin. Invest.* 70: 978–988.

Tabary, J. C., Tabary, C., Tardieu, C., and Goldspink, G. (1972). Physiological and structural changes in the cat's soleus muscle due to immobilization at different lengths by plaster casts. *J. Physiol.* 224: 231–244, 1972.

Tesch, P. A. (1988). Skeletal muscle adaptations consequent to long-term heavy resistance exercise. *Med. Sci. Sports Exerc.* 20: S132–S134.

Tsika, R. W., Herrick, R. E., and Baldwin, K. M. (1987). Interaction of compensatory overload and hindlimb suspension on myosin isoform expression. *J. Appl. Physiol.* 62: 2180–2186.

Vandenburgh, H. H., Swasdison, S., and Karlisch, P. (1991a). Computer-aided mechanogenesis of skeletal muscle organs from single cells in vitro. *FASEB J.* 5: 2860–2867.

Vandenburgh, H. H., Karlisch, P., Shansky, J., and Feldstein, R. (1991b). Insulin and IGF-I induce pronounced hypertrophy of skeletal myofibers in tissue culture. *Am. J. Physiol.* 260: C475–C484.

Vanderhoof, E. R., Imig, C. J., and Hines, H. M. (1961). Effect of muscle strength and endurance development on blood flow. *J. Appl. Physiol.* 16: 873–877.

Walmsley, B., Hodgson, J. A., and Burke, R. E. (1978). Forces produced by medial gastrocnemius and soleus muscles during locomotion in freely moving cats. *J. Neurophysiol.* 41: 1203–1216.

Witzmann, F. A., Kim, D. H., and Fitts, R. H. (1982). Recovery time-course in contractile function of fast and slow skeletal muscle following hindlimb immobilization. *J. Appl. Physiol.* 52: 677–682.

Zerba, E., Komorowski, T. E., and Faulkner, J. A. (1990). Free radical injury to skeletal muscles of young, adult, and old mice. *Am. J. Physiol.* 258: C429–C435.

10

Effects of Aging on the Structure and Function of Skeletal Muscle

SUSAN V. BROOKS and JOHN A. FAULKNER

University of Michigan
Ann Arbor, Michigan

I. Introduction

Increasing physical frailty is widely accepted as an inevitable concomitant of old age. Physical frailty describes the summation of the effects of muscle atrophy, declining muscle strength and power, fatigue, and injury (Faulkner et al., 1990). Little is known about specific age-associated changes in either the morphological or functional properties of the respiratory muscles. In spite of the lack of data, a reasonable assumption is that the respiratory muscles display deficits similar to those observed for other skeletal muscles. This chapter will address each of the components of physical frailty and the changes associated with aging. Although most of the data on changes in skeletal muscles with aging are obtained from the upper and lower limb muscles of humans and rodents, data on the respiratory muscles will be presented when available. The implications for the respiratory muscles of the age-related changes observed in limb and trunk skeletal muscles will be discussed.

II. Muscle Atrophy

By 60–70 years of age, the muscle mass of humans decreases by 25–30% (Grimby and Saltin, 1983) and in mice and rats by 10–25% (Gutmann and Carlson, 1976;

Fitts et al., 1984; Larsson and Edström, 1986; Brooks and Faulkner, 1988). Superficially, the decrease in muscle mass that is observed with aging appears to be analogous to the atrophy associated with a decrease in physical activity (for review see Faulkner et al., 1994). With a decrease in physical activity, such as occurs following the casting of a limb or with bed rest, the muscle atrophy results from a decrease in the cross-sectional area (CSA) of individual fibers and no decrease in the total number of fibers. For muscles in young and adult humans, muscle mass is quickly restored when normal activity levels are reestablished (MacDougall et al., 1980).

In contrast, the muscle atrophy that occurs with aging is largely irreversible. Although the decrease in muscle mass may be related to decreased activity levels throughout the lifetime, maintenance of physical activity does not appear to protect skeletal muscles completely from these age-related decrements. Even superbly trained, world class athletes, who at any given age display higher values for maximum and sustained strength and power than untrained individuals, show similar trends and time courses of decline in structural and functional properties (Stones and Kozma, 1980; Schulz and Curnow, 1988). The structural and functional deficits are reflected in decreased performance by these athletes and are typified by the world records for the 200-m sprint and the marathon run by individuals of different ages (Fig. 1). These observations suggest that "real" age-related deficits, which are largely inevitable, occur in the skeletal muscles of animals, including humans.

The muscle atrophy that is observed with aging could be due to loss of muscle fibers, a decrease in individual fiber areas, or some combination of the two. Complete fiber counts in mice and rats indicate that fiber number is highly conserved throughout the lifetime of these rodents, decreasing by at most 5% in old age (White

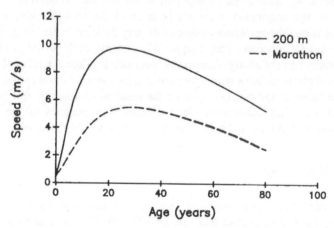

Figure 1 World records for average running speeds of the men's 200-m sprint and marathon (42,195-m) run for men of different ages. (From Moore, 1975.)

et al., 1986; Daw et al., 1988). Some evidence supports the premise that the muscles of humans, unlike those of rodents, lose fibers throughout the life span. In the muscles of humans, of any age, fibers number in the hundreds of thousands. Therefore, direct fiber counts are not feasible. Estimates of fiber number have been made using whole-muscle cross sections from cadavers or indirect measurements of muscle CSA by computed tomography of subjects and mean single-fiber areas from biopsy samples (Grimby and Saltin, 1983). The total number of fibers is estimated by dividing the whole-muscle CSA by the mean single-fiber CSA. The data provided by this technique support the concept that the number of fibers in human muscles decreases continuously throughout the life span (Grimby and Saltin, 1983). The estimates are that a 23% decrease occurs from birth to young adulthood (20–35 years), with a subsequent decrease of 24% in the elderly (70–73 years). In particular, the loss in fiber number early in life is likely to be artifactual, owing to errors in estimation, rather than an actual loss.

Before 60–70 years of age, little change in the single-fiber CSA of any of the three fiber types is observed (Grimby et al., 1982). In spite of this observation, a shift in the proportions of type I and type II muscle fibers cannot be ruled out and may actually contribute to muscle atrophy. Type II fibers tend to be large, whereas, in general, type I fibers are smaller in cross section. An increasing number of type I fibers, with an accompanying decrease in the number of type II fibers, could decrease the total muscle fiber CSA and decrease muscle mass, yet show no differences in the single-fiber CSA of any of the three fiber types.

In age groups older than 70 years, the mean area of type II fibers decrease by about 15% (Grimby et al., 1982) and the percentage of type II fibers decreases by as much as 40% (Larsson, 1983). In fact, elderly bedridden patients often display only two fiber types, type I and type IIB, with complete loss of all type IIA fibers. A clear example of severe type II fiber atrophy is shown in the photomicrograph of a cross section from the vastus lateralis muscle of a 76-year-old woman (Fig. 2A). Type II fiber atrophy has been observed for the abdominal muscles, but not the diaphragm muscles of elderly patients. No data exist on the other accessory muscles of respiration. The decrease in the proportion of type II fibers could be the result of either the conversion of type II fibers to type I fibers, or a direct loss in the total number of type II fibers.

III. Absolute Force

Quetelet (1835) made the original observations of impaired skeletal muscle function with age. During the ensuing 150 years, studies of many different muscles and muscle groups led to the overall conclusion that, between 30 and 80 years of age, muscle strength decreases 30–40% (Fig. 3) (Asmussen, 1980; Larsson et al., 1979; Young et al., 1984, 1985). The decrease in strength correlates well with the decrease in muscle mass. From this equivalency of the decreased strength and decreased

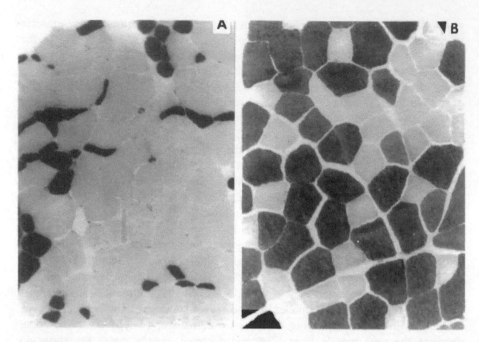

Figure 2 Photomicrographs of myofibrillar ATPase activity (incubated at pH 9.4) of a cross section from the (A) vastus lateralis muscle from a 76-year-old female subject, and (B) rectus abdominis muscle from a 72-year-old male subject. The type II fibers show high myofibrillar ATPase activity.

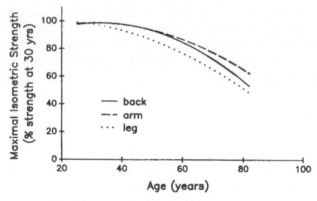

Figure 3 Data from a cross-sectional study of maximum isometric strength of three muscle groups in humans of different ages. Values are expressed as percentages of the strength measured for 30-year-olds. (From Asmussen, 1980.)

mass, Grimby and Saltin (1983) concluded that there was no reason to postulate any intrinsic qualitative changes in skeletal muscle or muscle fibers with aging. This conclusion was based on indirect evidence, and the hypothesis that the loss in strength with aging is fully explained by muscle atrophy is difficult to test rigorously in humans.

The changes in functional properties of skeletal muscles with age may be studied more accurately through measurements of whole skeletal muscles of young, adult, and old rats and mice. Experiments are performed in vitro using supramaximal electrical stimulation. As with humans, a decrease in maximum isometric tetanic force of 20–30% has been reported for muscles of old, compared with adult, mice (Brooks and Faulkner, 1988; Phillips et al., 1991) and rats (Gutmann and Carlson, 1976; Larsson and Edström, 1986; Carlson and Faulkner, 1988). Similar deficits have been observed for both slow and fast muscles (Brooks and Faulkner, 1988; Phillips et al., 1991). Although the deficit in force for the muscles of rodents is less than the deficit in strength reported for elderly humans, the data support the idea that a decrease in maximum force development with age is not unique to humans.

Measurements of maximal voluntary inspiratory and expiratory mouth pressures have been measured on normal adult human subjects (Du Bois and Alcala, 1964; Black and Hyatt, 1969). These measurements provide an indirect measure of the maximum strength of the respiratory muscles, but may be confounded by other effects. Maximum pressures appear to decline for subjects older than 55 years, compared with younger subjects (Black and Hyatt, 1969). The magnitude of the decrease in force exerted by elderly subjects between 75 and 90 years of age was 40–60% and was similar for both men and women (Fig. 4). The respiratory muscles appear to lose at least the same degree of strength as the limb and trunk muscles.

IV. Specific Force

The force-developing capacity of skeletal muscles is proportional to total muscle fiber CSA. Therefore, accurate estimations of the total fiber CSA are necessary to determine the force per unit area or specific force (kN/m^2). An accurate measure of the specific force is essential for the comparison of the intrinsic force-generating capabilities of muscle fibers, muscles, or groups of muscles from individuals of different ages. *Weakness* is the characteristic of a muscle fiber, motor unit, whole muscle, or group of muscles that produces less specific force than expected (Faulkner et al., 1990). Muscles may be relatively small, or atrophied, and still have a normal maximum specific force and, consequently, would not be termed "weak."

Accurate measurements of total muscle fiber CSA in humans are not possible because direct measurements of the muscle mass and the length of fibers cannot be made. Estimates of the total fiber CSA of groups of muscles involved in the contractions depend on indirect measurements by computed tomography, which

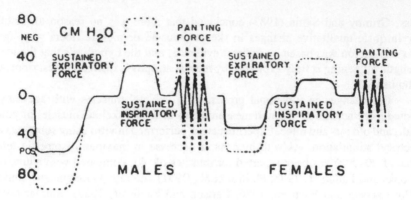

Figure 4 Mean maximal voluntary mouth pressures against a closed tube recorded on moving paper, and showing the diminished force exerted by old subjects (solid line) compared with young subjects (broken line) under identical conditions. (From Du Bois and Alcala, 1964.)

would be accurate for only a completely parallel-fibered muscle. Some estimates of maximum specific strength of humans suggest that atrophy alone does not explain the decrease in voluntary strength with age (Young et al., 1985; Davies et al., 1986; Vandervoort and McComas, 1986; Bruce et al., 1989), and muscles from elderly subjects are, in fact, weaker than those of young subjects. In contrast, others have found no difference in maximum strength normalized for whole-muscle CSA (Frontera et al., 1991). The different results may arise from the architectural complexity of the muscle groups involved.

For isolated whole muscles of rodents, accurate measurements of both muscle mass and fiber length are possible. Therefore, valid estimations of total muscle fiber CSA are possible (see Chap. 5). When the 20–30% decrease in absolute maximum force observed for the muscles of old mice (Brooks and Faulkner, 1988; Phillips et al., 1991) and rats (Gutmann and Carlson, 1976; Fitts et al., 1984; Larsson and Edström, 1986) is normalized for the decrease in total muscle fiber CSA, a deficit of about 20% in maximum specific force remains unexplained by atrophy (Brooks and Faulkner, 1988; Carlson and Faulkner, 1988; Phillips et al., 1991). Muscle weakness does not appear to be limited to the limb muscles. The effect of aging on the contractile properties of isolated diaphragm strips from the hamster has been studied in vitro (Zhang and Kelsen, 1990). Maximum specific force decrease about 20% for diaphragm muscles from 19-month-old hamsters compared with those from 5-month-old animals.

Although the magnitudes of the deficit in maximum specific force observed for muscles from humans and rodents are similar, the mechanisms responsible for the deficit may be quite different. In muscle groups of humans, a change in the complex architecture of muscle with aging could account for some part of the decrease in specific strength (Maughan et al., 1983; Young et al., 1985), but definitive studies have not been possible. In contrast, in single muscles of mice, changes with age in extracellular components are not a major factor and changes in architecture or water content do not occur (Brooks and Faulkner, 1988). Although the concentration of connective tissue in skeletal muscle does increase with age (Alnaqeeb et al., 1984), the magnitude of the increase is not sufficient to affect force development significantly. Consequently, for whole muscles of mammals, the site of the deficit in specific force must be confined to a decrease in the number of cross-bridges per unit area, or to a decrease in the average force developed per cross-bridge (Brooks and Faulkner, 1988; Phillips et al., 1991).

V. Force–Velocity Relationships

In addition to isometric contractions, skeletal muscles may shorten, or be lengthened, during contractions (Faulkner et al., 1994). Following activation, the type of contraction that occurs depends on the interaction between the force developed by the muscle and the load placed on the muscle (see Chap. 5). The force–shortening velocity relationship is hyperbolic, intersecting the force and velocity axes at maximum force and maximum velocity of shortening (V_{max}), respectively. The curvature of the relationship is dependent on the fiber type composition of the muscle, with slow muscles showing greater curvature than fast (Ranatunga, 1984; Faulkner et al., 1986).

The effect of age on the velocity of shortening of human muscles has not been studied extensively (Larsson et al., 1979; Grimby and Saltin, 1983). For the limb muscles of mice and rats, V_{max} of both slow and fast muscles does not appear to change, even in very old animals (Fig. 5) (Fitts et al., 1984; Brooks and Faulkner, 1988; Phillips et al., 1991). In addition, when both force and velocity are normalized to the maximum value, the curvature of the relationships is no different for either slow or fast muscles of old, compared with young, animals. The stability of the entire force–shortening velocity relationship, including V_{max}, with age is consistent with histochemical (Eddinger et al., 1985; Larsson and Edström, 1986; Edström and Larsson, 1987; Florini and Ewton, 1989), and biochemical (Florini and Ewton, 1989) characteristics of slow soleus and fast extensor digitorum longus (EDL) muscles. The data support the hypothesis that, throughout the life span of small rodents, no change occurs in the myosin isoform composition of skeletal muscles composed exclusively of one type of fiber.

Age-associated alterations were observed in the force–velocity relationships of diaphragm strips from hamsters (Zhang and Kelsen, 1990). The V_{max}, as well as the velocity of shortening at given relative afterloads, decreased for the diaphragm strips from the old, compared with the young and adult, animals. These data are consistent with the observation that, compared with younger subjects, the maximum inspiratory and expiratory flow rates decrease by approximately 70% for both male and female subjects 75–90 years of age (Du Bois and Alcala, 1964). A decrease in

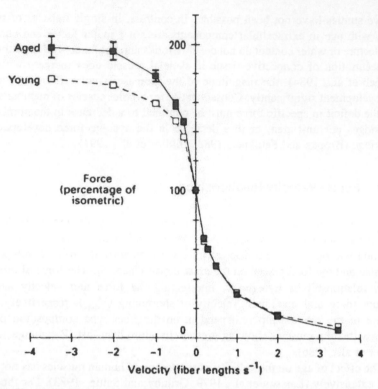

Figure 5 Mean force–velocity relationship during shortening and lengthening (negative velocities) contractions for muscles of young (open squares) and old (filled squares) mice. Velocities are normalized by muscle fiber length, and forces for each aged group ar normalized by the respective maximum isometric forces. Values are means ± SEM. (From Phillips et al., 1991.)

velocity of shortening of the diaphragm muscle with aging may be an indication that, with aging, skeletal muscles that are composed of heterogeneous fiber types do not maintain the same myosin composition.

During lengthening contractions, force increases with velocity to a level approximately two times maximum force (Katz, 1939), but further increases in velocity do not result in higher forces (Katz, 1939; Julian and Morgan, 1979; Edman et al., 1981; Lombardi and Piazzesi, 1990). During lengthening contractions, the number of attached cross-bridges increases by no more than about 10% (Julian and Morgan, 1979; Lombardi and Piazzesi, 1990). Consequently, the predominant factor in the increased active force during lengthening appears to be an increased force developed per cross-bridge, caused by increased cross-bridge strain (Lombardi and Piazzesi, 1990).

Soleus muscles of old mice show significant deficits in specific force during isometric and shortening contractions, but the specific forces developed during lengthening contractions was no different for muscles of old and young mice (Phillips et al., 1991). As a result, when the force–velocity relationships of muscles from young and old mice were normalized by the respective maximum forces, the muscles of old mice developed significantly greater relative forces during lengthening contractions than those of young mice (see Fig. 5). The report that muscle strength of both the knee flexors and extensors in elderly women was much less affected by age during lengthening than shortening contractions is consistent with the observations on mouse muscles (Vandervoort et al., 1990).

The difference in relative force observed during lengthening of muscles of young and old mice most likely is the result of greater average force developed per cross-bridge in the muscles of old mice. The greater average force could be due to a shift in the distribution of cross-bridges between states with different force-generating properties (Phillips et al., 1991). Alternatively, an intrinsic change with age in the compliance of the cross-bridges could lead to greater force developed when the cross-bridges are strained by stretches of the fully activated muscles.

VI. Power Output

Since most everyday tasks, including respiration, require movement, the ability of muscles to generate and sustain power is of great consequence. The power output of a muscle is the product of the velocity of shortening and the average force developed by the muscle. Power output varies parabolically with velocity of shortening (Faulkner et al., 1986). The point along this relationship at which power is maximum, or the optimum velocity for power, occurs at approximately one-third of the maximum velocity of shortening (Hill, 1950; Luff, 1981; Ranatunga, 1984; Faulkner et al., 1986; Brooks et al., 1990). When muscles from young, adult, and old mice were compared at their own optimum velocities for the ability to generate power, the maximum power (watts) developed by muscles of old mice was approximately 30% lower than that of muscles of adult mice (Brooks and Faulkner, 1991). Similar to the age-related deficit in force, about 10% of the deficit in power output could be explained by atrophy, but a 20% deficit in normalized power (W/kg) remained (Brooks and Faulkner, 1991). The primary cause of the deficit in power was the 20% deficit in specific force. The optimum velocity for power increased with age, indicating a more complex mechanism for the decrease in power than the decrease in specific force alone (Brooks and Faulkner, 1991).

VII. Muscle Fatigability

Brooks and Faulkner (1991) have proposed that the fatigability of a muscle is better assessed by the ability of the muscle to sustain force or power, rather than by the decrement in force or power observed over time. The graded exercise test for

physical work capacity has provided a valid measure of the fatigue resistance of the
total organism (Åstrand, 1960) and, similarly, the ability of a muscle to sustain
force or power during repeated contractions provides a valid measure of the fatigue
resistance of a muscle. This type of progressive exercise test initiates contractions
at a low-energy requirement or power and then gradually increases the intensity to
the maximum level that can be sustained. The intensity is increased by increasing
the fraction of the work–rest cycle during which work is done. This duty cycle can
be increased by increasing either the duration of the contractions or the frequency
with which they occur (Brooks and Faulkner, 1991).

 The ability of muscles from young, adult, and old mice to sustain power
during repeated shortening contractions has been measured in situ (Brooks and
Faulkner, 1991). The maximum sustained powers (W/kg) of muscles of adult and
old mice were 55 and 45%, respectively, of the value for muscles from young mice
(Fig. 6). In addition, the muscles of adult and old mice were not able to maintain
the level of duty cycles for repeated contractions achieved by the young mice (see
Fig. 6). Sustained power requires a balance between the rate of energy use and rate
of energy production (Dudley and Fleck, 1984). Both the delivery of oxygen to
muscles through blood flow (Irion et al., 1987) and the capacity for oxidative
metabolism (Farrar et al., 1981; Cartee and Farrar, 1987) provide possible
limitations to the ability of the muscles of adult and old mammals to maintain energy
balance (Dudley and Fleck, 1984). The metabolic limitations appear to arise by 12
months of age in these mice and become increasingly more severe with aging
(Brooks and Faulkner, 1991).

 No data on sustained power of the respiratory muscles in old animals are
available. Isolated diaphragm strips from 19-month-old and 5-month-old hamsters
have been studied in vitro (Zang and Kelsen, 1990). During repeated isometric

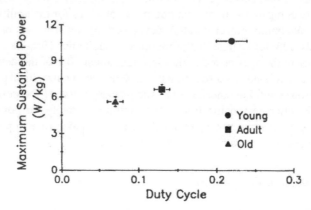

Figure 6 The relationship for young, adult, and old mice between the maximum power
that could be sustained for 30 min and the duty cycle at maximum sustained power. Values
are means ± SEM. (From Faulkner et al., 1990.)

contractions, the diaphragm strips from the old hamsters showed a more rapid decrement in force than those from diaphragm muscles of young hamsters (Zhang and Kelsen, 1990). The conclusion that the fatigability of the diaphragm muscle increases in old compared with younger animals is consistent with the data on limb muscles.

VIII. Contraction-Induced Injury

Skeletal muscles can be injured by their own contractions during everyday activities (see Chap. 9), particularly during lengthening contractions (McCully and Faulkner, 1985). When muscles of young, adult, and old mice were administered the same protocol of lengthening contractions, the amount of injury to muscle fibers in the muscles of old mice was significantly greater than that observed for the muscles of young or adult mice (Fig. 7) (Zerba et al., 1990). In addition, when muscles from young and old mice were injured to the same degree, the muscle fibers in the muscles of old animals recovered less well (see Fig. 7) (Brooks and Faulkner, 1990). Whereas the muscles in young and adult mice recovered fully from contraction-induced injury within a couple of weeks, the muscles of old mice did not recover completely, even after 2 months (Brooks and Faulkner, 1990).

Muscles in old animals also show a decreased regenerative capacity following free whole-muscle transplantation (Carlson and Faulkner, 1988). Under these

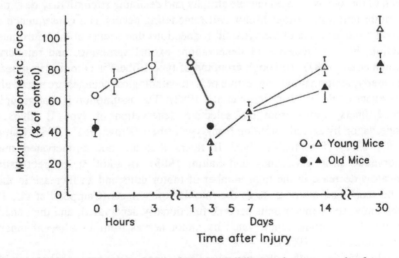

Figure 7 Maximum isometric force of extensor digitorum longus muscles from young (open symbols) and old (filled symbols) mice at selected times after lengthening contractions. Values are expressed as a percentage of the maximum force of the uninjured control muscle. Circles and triangles represent lengthening contraction protocols of different duration. (From Faulkner et al., 1991.)

circumstances, the whole muscle degenerates as a result of the ischemic injury. The recovery of mass and maximum force of grafts following transplantation in young rats was 2.5 times greater than in old rats. Interestingly, the results were the same regardless of the age of the donor. Muscles from young or old rats transplanted into young rats regenerated equally well, whereas muscles from young or old rats transplanted into old rats regenerated equally poorly (Carlson and Faulkner, 1989). Apparently, the inherent regenerative capacity of the muscles in old animals is not decreased, but the host environment is not suitable for successful regeneration. Impaired ability for reinnervation in the old host is a contributing factor to the decrease in muscle regenerative capacity (Carlson and Faulkner, 1992). Other possibilities include impaired, revascularization, hormonal influences, nutrition, disease, or macrophage function.

The prolonged deficits that are observed in the muscles of old mice following degeneration and regeneration resemble those that arise normally in the muscles of old mice. Since various magnitudes of injury are probably occurring throughout the life span of an animal, an increased susceptibility to injury coupled with a decreased ability to recover from injury may well give rise to both muscle atrophy and muscle weakness in old animals.

IX. Motor Unit Remodeling

Much of the age-associated muscle atrophy and declining strength may be explained by motor unit remodeling. Motor unit remodeling occurs as a consequence of the natural turnover cycle of the synaptic connections that occurs at the neuromuscular junction, by the processes of denervation, axonal sprouting, and reinnervation (Brown et al., 1981). Although grouping of type I fibers is common in muscles of the elderly, abnormalities suggestive of histopathological changes are relatively rare (Jennekens et al., 1971; Grimby et al., 1982). The assumption is that grouping of type I fibers results from the selective denervation of type II fibers, with reinnervation by axonal sprouting from type I fibers (Brown et al., 1981; Campbell, et al., 1973). Presumably, type II fibers that are not reinnervated undergo denervation atrophy (Grimby and Saltin, 1983). In addition, indirect estimates indicate a decrease in the total number of motor units and an increase in the size of the remaining motor units in the muscles of humans (Campbell et al., 1973). Apparently, some motor units become functionally denervated, and the denervated muscle fibers become reinnervated by motor nerves from an adjacent innervated unit (Brown et al., 1981).

In muscles with heterogeneous fiber types, data are consistent with the occurrence of similar processes of motor unit remodeling in old rats (Edström and Larsson, 1987; Kanda and Hashizume, 1989). For medial gastrocnemius muscles of 27-month-old rats, the mean maximum force of type II motor units was 70% that of comparable motor units in 12-month-old rats, whereas that of type I motor units was 250% of the adult value (Kanda and Hashizume, 1989). In addition, the total number of motor units in both soleus (Edström and Larsson, 1987) and medial gastrocnemius (Kanda and Hashizume, 1989) muscles of rats decreased by approximately 30%, and the size of the remaining slow motor units increased (Fig. 8). Both the mean number of muscle fibers in a motor unit, as well as the mean total area of the fibers in a motor unit increased (see Fig. 8).

Motor unit remodeling in aging rats appears to occur by selective denervation of type II fibers, with reinnervation by collateral sprouting of nerves from fibers in the type I motor units. An alternative interpretation is that denervation of both type I and type II fibers occurs, but that type I motoneurons are more efficient at reinnervation of muscle fibers (Desypris and Parry, 1990). The greater efficiency might result from faster axonal growth (Lewis et al., 1982) or superiority in establishing permanent connections with muscle fibers (Foehring et al., 1987). Either interpretation is consistent with data from the diaphragm muscles of young, adult, and old rats (Eddinger et al., 1985). Histochemical fiber typing indicates a greater percentage of type I fibers, and a decrease in the percentage of type IIA fibers, in the diaphragm muscles of the old compared with the younger rats (Eddinger et al., 1985).

The concept of selective denervation of fast fibers and reinnervation by sprouting of motor nerves from slow fibers does not contradict the histochemical

(A)　　　　　　　　　(B)

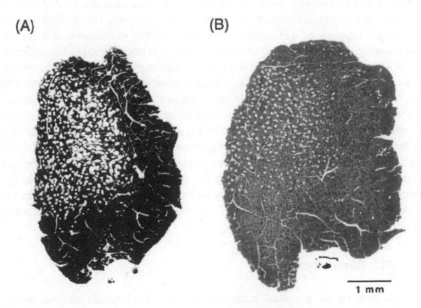

1 mm

Figure 8 Photomicrographs of histochemical preparations of medial gastrocnemius muscles from (A) old and (B) middle-aged rats showing motor unit territories and an enlarged motor unit in the muscle from the old rat. (From Kanda and Hashizume, 1989.)

(Eddinger et al., 1985), biochemical (Florini and Ewton, 1989), or physiological (Brooks and Faulkner, 1988; Phillips et al., 1991) observations that suggest that no changes occur throughout the life span in the myosin composition of the soleus and EDL muscles of rodents. The soleus and EDL muscles of these rodents are very homogeneous in fiber type, and denervation of faster fibers would not produce changes in the proportions of fiber types, the myosin ATPase activity, or the normalized force–shortening velocity relationship that could be identified experimentally. In contrast, most of the muscles in humans, including the respiratory muscles, have approximately equal proportions of slow and fast fibers (Faulkner et al., 1986). With aging, if motor nerves of fast motor units are more likely to degenerate than those of slow motor units, human muscles would show a greater change in fiber type composition, velocity, and power than rodents. The 75% decrease in motor unit number reported for some human muscles (Campbell et al., 1973) compared with the 30% decrease in rat muscles (Edström and Larsson, 1987; Kanda and Hashizume, 1989) suggests that muscles in humans may be more susceptible than those of rodents to the phenomenon of age-related denervation atrophy.

X. Implications for Respiratory Muscles

Although the respiratory muscles are unique skeletal muscles in that they must contract with a regular rhythm throughout the life span, the limited data from diaphragm muscles of old animals indicate that the maintained activity of the respiratory muscles does not spare them from age-related deficits. The deficits that occur with aging in the functional properties of the respiratory muscles do not appear to be of a large enough magnitude to compromise normal respiration. Because of the necessity of respiration, many redundancies and safety factors exist in the respiratory system. In addition, as the limb muscle function declines, one's ability to maintain or initiate a physically active lifestyle during old age would be limited by the periphery. Other age-related changes not related directly to skeletal muscles, such as in chest wall mechanics, increase the effort necessary to maintain normal respiration. As the necessary effort of the respiratory muscles is increasing, the functional capacity of the muscles may be decreasing, placing the older person in a potentially more precarious state, especially when exposed to pathological conditions.

XI. Summary

The phenomena of impaired capacities for the development of maximum and sustained strength and power of muscles of humans appear to begin shortly after the age of 30. The decline progresses slowly, at first, and then more rapidly after aged 65–70. A promising hypothesis for irreversible age-related changes in skeletal muscles is that specific morphological aspects of faster motor nerves result in the preferential degeneration of these nerves and the denervation of the faster muscle fibers (Kanda and Hashizume, 1989). The process of selective denervation, atrophy, and degeneration of motor nerves to muscle fibers in old animals may explain the type II fiber atrophy (Grimby et al., 1982), the loss in the number of fibers (Daw et al., 1988), and the decrease in muscle mass (Grimby and Saltin, 1983; Brooks and Faulkner, 1988). The reinnervation of some denervated fibers by sprouting of motor nerves may account for the clustering of fibers types in muscles of old rodents (Kanda and Hashizume, 1989) and of humans (Grimby and Saltin, 1983), as well as the increase in the size of slow motor units (Kanda and Hashizume, 1989). The process of age-related denervation atrophy may be aggravated by an increased susceptibility of muscles in old animals to contraction-induced injury (Zerba et al., 1990) and by the impaired capacity for regeneration (Carlson and Faulkner, 1988, 1989; Brooks and Faulkner, 1990).

Acknowledgments

Our studies of the effects of aging on skeletal muscle have been enhanced by collaborations with many colleagues: Bruce M. Carlson, Kevin K. McCully, and Eileen Zerba. The research was supported in part by grants from the United States Public Health Service, grant AG06157 from the National Institute on Aging, and grant AG00114 also from the National Institute on Aging, which provided fellowship support to Susan V. Brooks.

Portions of this chapter are excerpts of a review article by Brooks and Faulkner, "Age-associated weakness in skeletal muscles: Underlying mechanisms." *Med. Sci. Sports Exerc.* 26:432–439 (1994). Used with permission.

References

Alnaqeeb, M. A., Al Zaid, N. S., and Goldspink, G. (1984). Connective tissue changes and physical properties of developing and ageing skeletal muscle. *J. Anat.* 139: 677–689.

Asmussen, E. (1980). Aging and exercise. In *Environmental Physiology: Aging, Heat and Altitude*, sec. III. Edited by S. M. Horvath, and M. K. Yousef. New York, Elsevier North-Holland, pp. 419–428.

Åstrand, I. (1960). Aerobic work capacity in men and women with special reference to age. *Acta Physiol. Scand. [Suppl.]* 169: 1–92.

Black, L. F., and Hyatt, R. E. (1969). Maximal respiratory pressures: Normal values and relationship to age and sex. *Am. Rev. Respir. Dis.* 99: 696–702.

Brooks, S. V., and Faulkner, J. A. (1988). Contractile properties of skeletal muscles from young, adult, and aged mice. *J. Physiol. (Lond.)* 404: 71–82.

Brooks, S. V., and Faulkner, J. A. (1990). Contraction-induced injury: Recovery of skeletal muscles in young and old mice. *Am. J. Physiol.* 258: C436–C442.

Brooks, S. V., and Faulkner, J. A. (1991). Maximum and sustained power of extensor digitorum longus muscles from young, adult, and old mice. *J. Gerontol.* 46: B28–B33.

Brooks, S. V., Faulkner, J. A., and McCubbrey, D. A. (1990). Power outputs of slow and fast skeletal muscles of mice. *J. Appl. Physiol.* 68:1282–1285.

Brown, M. C., Holland, R. L., and Hopkins, W. G. (1981). Motor nerve sprouting. *Annu. Rev. Neurosci.* 4:17–42.

Bruce, S. A., Newton, D., and Woledge, R. C. (1989). Effect of age on voluntary force and cross-sectional area of human adductor pollicis muscle. *Q. J. Exp. Physiol.* 74: 359–362.

Campbell, M. J., McComas, A. J., and Petito, F. (1973). Physiological changes in ageing muscles. *J. Neurol. Neurosurg. Psychiatry* 36: 74–182.

Carlson, B. M., and Faulkner, J. A. (1988). Reinnervation of long-term denervated rat muscle freely grafted into an innervated limb. *Exp. Neurol.* 102: 50–56.

Carlson, B. M., and Faulkner, J. A. (1989). Muscle transplantation between young and old rats: Age of host determines recovery. *Am. J. Physiol.* 256: C1262–C1266.

Carlson, B. M., and Faulkner, J. A. (1992). Skeletal muscle regeneration and aging: The influence of innervation. *J. Gerontol.* (submitted).

Cartee, G. D., and Farrar, R. P. (1987). Muscle respiratory capacity and Vo_2 max in identically trained young and old rats. *J. Appl. Physiol.* 63: 257–261.

Davies, C. T. M., Thomas, D. O., and White, M. J. (1986). Mechanical properties of young and elderly human muscle. *Acta Med. Scand.* [*Suppl.*] 711: 219–226.

Daw, C. K., Starnes, J. W., and White, T. P. (1988). Muscle atrophy and hypoplasia with aging: Impact of training and food restriction. *J. Appl. Physiol.* 64: 2428–2432.

Desypris, G., and Parry, D. J. (1990). Relative efficacy of slow and fast α-motoneurons to reinnervate mouse soleus muscle. *Am. J. Physiol.* 258: C62–C70.

Du Bois, A. B., and Alcala, R. (1964). Airway resistance and mechanics of breathing in normal subjects 75 to 90 years of age. In *Aging of the Lung*. Edited by L. Cander and J. H. Moyer. New York, Grune & Stratton, pp. 156–162.

Dudley, G. A., and Fleck, S. J. (1984). Metabolite changes in aged muscle during stimulation. *J. Gerontol.* 39: 183–186.

Eddinger, T. J., Moss, R. L., and Cassens, R. G. (1985). Fiber number and type composition in extensor digitorum longus, soleus, and diaphragm muscles with aging in Fisher 344 rats. *J. Histochem. Cytochem.* 33: 1033–1041.

Edman, K. A. P., Elzinga, G., and Noble, M. I. M. (1981). Critical sarcomere extension required to recruit a decaying component of extra force during stretch in tetanic contractions of frog skeletal muscle fibers. *J. Gen. Physiol.* 78: 365–382.

Edström, L., and Larsson, L. (1987). Effects of age on contractile and enzyme-histochemical properties of fast- and slow-twitch single motor units in the rat. *J. Physiol.* (*Lond.*) 392: 129–145.

Farrar, R. P., Martin, T. P., and Ardies, C. M. (1981). The interaction of aging and endurance exercise upon the mitochondrial function of skeletal muscle. *J. Gerontol.* 36: 642–647.

Faulkner, J. A., Claflin, D. R., and McCully, K. K. (1986). Power output of fast and slow fibers from human skeletal muscles. In *Human Power Output*. Edited by N. L. Jones, M. McCartney, and J. McComas. Champaign, IL, Human Kinetics Publishers, pp. 81–91.

Faulkner, J. A., Brooks, S. V., and Zerba, E. (1990). Skeletal muscle weakness, fatigue, and injury: Inevitable concomitants of aging? *Hermes* 21: 269–280.

Faulkner, J. A., Brooks, S. V., and Zerba, E. (1991). Skeletal muscle weakness and fatigue in old age: Underlying mechanisms. In *Annual Review of Gerontology and Geriatrics*. Edited by V. J. Cristofalo and M. P. Lawton. New York, Springer Publishing, pp. 147–166.

Faulkner, J. A., Green, H. J., and White, T. P. (1994). *Response and Adaptation of Skeletal Muscle to Changes in Physical Activity*. Edited by C. Bouchard, R. J. Shephard and T. Stephens. Champaign, IL, Human Kinetics Publishers, pp. 343–357.

Fitts, R. H., Troup, J. P., Witzmann, F. A., and Holloszy, J. O. (1984). The effect of ageing and exercise on skeletal muscle function. *Mech. Ageing Dev.* 27: 161–172.

Florini, J. R., and Ewton, D. Z. (1989). Skeletal muscle fiber types and myosin ATPase activity do not change with age or growth hormone administration. *J. Gerontol.* 44: B110–B117.

Foehring, R. C., Sypert, G. W., and Munson, J. B. (1987). Motor unit properties following cross-reinnervation of cat lateral gastrocnemius and soleus muscles with medial gastrocnemius nerve. I. Influence of motoneurons on muscle. *J. Neurophysiol.* 57: 1210–1226.

Frontera, W. R., Hughes, V. A., Lutz, K. J., and Evans, W. J. (1991). A cross-sectional study of muscle strength and mass in 45- to 78-yr-old men and women. *J. Appl. Physiol.* 71: 644–650.

Grimby, G., and Saltin, B. (1983). The aging muscle. *Clin. Physiol.* 3: 209–218.

Grimby, G., Danneskiold-Samsoe, B., Hvid, K., and Saltin, B. (1982). Morphology and enzymatic capacity in arm and leg muscles in 78–82 year old men and women. *Acta Physiol. Scand.* 115: 124–134.

Gutmann, E., and Carlson, B. M. (1976). Regeneration and transplantation of muscles in old rats and between young and old rats. *Life Sci.* 18: 109–114.

Hill, A. V. (1950). The dimensions of animals and their muscular dynamics. *R. Inst. Gr. Br. Proc.* 34: 450–471.

Irion, G. L., Vasthare, U. S., and Tuma, R. F. (1987). Age-related change in skeletal muscle blood flow in the rat. *J. Gerontol.* 42: 660–665.

Jennekens, F. G. I., Tomlinson, B. E., and Walton, J. N. (1971). Histochemical aspects of five limb muscles in old age: An autopsy study. *J. Neurol. Sci.* 14: 259–276.

Julian, F. J., and Morgan, D. L. (1979). The effect on tension of non-uniform distribution of length changes applied to frog muscle fibres. *J. Physiol. (Lond.)* 293: 379–392.

Kanda, K., and Hashizume, K. (1989). Changes in properties of the medial gastrocnemius motor units in aging. *J. Neurophysiol.* 61: 737–746.

Katz, B. (1939). The relation between force and speed in muscular contraction. *J. Physiol. (Lond.)* 96: 45–64.

Larsson, L. (1983). Histochemical characteristics of human skeletal muscle during aging. *Acta Physiol. Scand.* 117: 469–471.

Larsson L., and Edström, L. (1986). Effects of age on enzyme-histochemical fibre spectra and contractile properties of fast- and slow-twitch skeletal muscles in the rat. *J. Neurol. Sci.* 76: 69–89.

Larsson, L., Grimby, G., and Karlsson, J. (1979). Muscle strength and speed of movement in relation to age and muscle morphology. *J. Appl. Physiol.* 46: 451–456.

Lewis, D. M., Rowlerson, A., and Webb, S. N. (1982). Motor units and immunohistochemistry of cat soleus muscle after long periods of cross-reinnervation. *J. Physiol. (Lond.)* 325: 403–418.

Lombardi, V., and Piazzesi, G. (1990). The contractile response during steady lengthening of stimulated frog muscle fibres. *J. Physiol. (Lond.)* 431: 141–171.

Luff, A. R. (1981). Dynamic properties of the inferior rectus, extensor digitorum longus, diaphragm and soleus muscles of the mouse. *J. Physiol. (Lond.)* 313: 161–171.

MacDougall, J. D., Elder, G. C. B., Sale, D. G., Moroz, J. R., and Sutton, J. R. (1980). Effects of strength training and immobilization on human muscle fibers. *Eur. J. Appl. Physiol.* 43: 25–34.

Maughan, R. J., Watson, J. S., and Wehr, J. (1983). Strength and cross-sectional area of human skeletal muscle. *J. Physiol. (Lond.)* 338: 37–49.

McCully, K. K., and Faulkner, J. A. (1985). Injury to skeletal muscle fibers of mice following lengthening contractions. *J. Appl. Physiol.* 59: 119–126.

Moore, D. H. II (1975). A study of age group track and field records to relate age and running speed. *Nature* 253: 264–265.

Phillips, S. K., Bruce, S. A., and Woledge, R. C. (1991). In mice, the muscle weakness due to age is absent during stretching. *J. Physiol. (Lond.)* 437: 63–70.

Quetelet, L. A. J. (1835). Sur l'homme et le développement de ses facultés. In *L. Hauman and Cie*, Vol. 2, Paris, Bachelier, Imprimeur-Libraire.

Ranatunga, K. W. (1984). The force–velocity relation of rat fast- and slow-twitch muscles examined at different temperatures. *J. Physiol. (Lond.)* 351: 517–529.

Schulz, R., and Curnow, C. (1988). Peak performance and age among superathletes: Track and field, swimming, baseball, tennis, and golf. *J. Gerontol.* 43: P113–P120.

Stones, M. J., and Kozma, A. (1980). Adult age trends in record running performances. *Exp. Aging Res.* 5: 407–416.

Vandervoort, A. A., and McComas, A. J. (1986). Contractile changes in opposing muscles of the human ankle joint with aging. *J. Appl. Physiol.* 61: 361–367.

Vandervoort, A. A., Kramer, J. F., and Wharram, E. R. (1990). Eccentric knee strength of elderly females. *J. Gerontol.* 45: B125–B128.

White, T. P., Clark, K. I., and Kandarian, S. C. (1986). Mass, fiber number, and cross-sectional area of hindlimb skeletal muscles from C57BL/6 mice at 12 and 28 months of age. *Physiologist* 29: 151.

Young, A., Stokes, M., and Crowe, M. (1984). Size and strength of the quadriceps muscle of old and young women. *Eur. J. Clin. Invest.* 14: 282–287.

Young, A., Stokes, M., and Crowe, M. (1985). The size and strength of the quadriceps muscle of old and young men. *Clin. Physiol.* 5: 145–154.

Zerba, E., Komorowski, T. E., and Faulkner, J. A. (1990). The role of free radicals in skeletal muscle injury in young, adult, and old mice. *Am. J. Physiol.* 258: C429–C435.

Zhang, Y. L., and Kelsen, S. G. (1990). Effects of aging on diaphragm contractile function in golden hamsters. *Am. Rev. Respir. Dis.* 142: 1396–1401.

11

Cellular and Molecular Adaptations of the Respiratory Muscles

C. DAVID IANUZZO and DAVID A. HOOD

York University
North York, Ontario, Canada

The actions of the respiratory muscles are required for life. Like the heart, but in contrast with typical skeletal muscles, they must be continuously active in supporting pulmonary ventilation and must adapt to long-term alteration in respiratory loads. The performance of any skeletal muscle under such conditions is dependent on three main factors: (1) adequate muscle blood flow and oxygen delivery, (2) sufficient mitochondrial content, and (3) economical ATP turnover, determined by the presence of specific myosin and sarcoplasmic reticulum ATPase isoforms (see Holloszy, 1988; Laughlin and Armstrong, 1985; Rall, 1985; Terjung and Hood, 1986, for reviews). The important cellular factors responsible for ATP provision (glycolytic and mitochondrial metabolism) and utilization (calcium cycling and cross-bridge cycling) along with blood flow and O_2 delivery are illustrated in Figure 1. Fortunately, these are not static, immutable components of the muscle cell. Rather, they illustrate a "plasticity" or adaptability, that permits the cell to adjust to changing energy demands over the long term. This occurs in response to regularly performed muscular exercise, usually in the form of endurance training, but also, more dramatically, as induced experimentally with the use of continuous, indirect nerve stimulation. For the respiratory muscles, modifications of blood flow, mitochondrial content, and contractile protein isoforms can also potentially occur during the adaptation to prolonged pathological respiratory load (e.g., emphysema), or in response to specific respiratory muscle training. The adaptations that occur

313

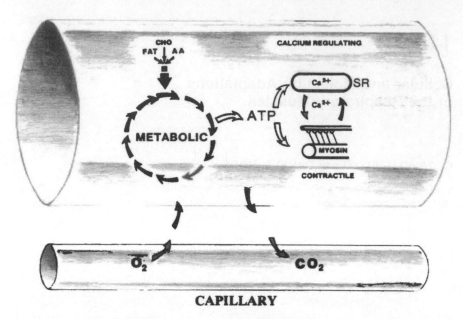

Figure 1 Performance of any skeletal muscle is dependent on the delivery of oxygen, the utilization of oxygen within the mitochondria for the synthesis of ATP, and the utilization of that ATP in the processes of Ca^{2+} handling and actin–myosin interaction for the purposes of force generation and relaxation. As reviewed in the text, adaptations of these factors in response to physiological demand are important for the maintenance of muscle performance and the avoidance of fatigue.

are of physiological benefit in improving the capacity of the muscle for aerobic metabolism and, therefore, prolonging endurance performance under normal, submaximal efforts. This first section will provide an overview of the mitochondrial and blood flow adaptations (ATP provision) in skeletal muscles subject to continual use, with emphasis on the respiratory muscles, and will discuss the metabolic consequences of the adaptations observed. The second and third sections will be devoted to analysis of the ATP-utilizing systems of muscle: Ca^{2+} management in the sarcoplasmic reticulum and the cytosol, and the myofibrillar proteins, which determine the contractile properties of the muscle fiber (see Fig. 1).

I. Metabolic System

A. Skeletal Muscle Fiber Types

Skeletal muscle can be generally classified into two main categories: type I (slow-twitch) and type II (fast-twitch). This histochemical classification system is based on the pH stability and lability of the different slow and fast myosin protein isoforms. From a metabolic standpoint, muscle fibers can be further subclassified as either red or white, depending on the abundance of mitochondria, as well as their blood flow capacities. Thus fibers have been commonly classified as fast-twitch red (FTR) or type II red, fast-twitch white (FTW) or type-II white, and slow-twitch red (STR) or type I red. As outlined in the following, these fiber types respond metabolically in a markedly different way to imposed contractile activity. Any attempt to interpret metabolic findings from a mixed population of these three fiber types is likely to provide misleading results, depending on the relative proportion of each fiber type within the muscle being studied (Terjung and Hood, 1986).

B. Metabolic Responses of Fiber Types During Contractions

Because of the high mitochondrial content and blood flow capacities of red fibers, they are much more reliant on aerobic metabolism for ATP provision than are white fibers. Thus, a given submaximal contractile effort is achieved with a much lower stimulation of glycolytic flux and, therefore, of lactate production. For many years, the metabolic acidosis incurred with lactate production has been associated with muscle fatigue. It occurs largely in white muscle fibers possessing low-oxidative capacities, resulting in rapid fatigue during continued contractions. This is at least partly because of the decreased sensitivity of the contractile proteins to Ca^{2+} in the presence of high H^+ concentrations (Vollestad and Sejersted, 1988). Also evident in white fibers are a greater depletion of high-energy phosphagens (ATP, CP), and an increased production of ammonia, relative to higher oxidative FTR fibers (Dudley and Terjung, 1985). Ammonia, although commonly ignored in metabolic studies of skeletal muscle, is a product of the AMP deaminase reaction, and it has also been associated with fatigue under some conditions, perhaps owing to a central nervous system influence (Mutch and Bannister, 1983). AMP deaminase is activated by the presence of increasing amounts of AMP, as well as by a low pH (Tullson and Terjung, 1990). Both of these conditions are more likely to exist in recruited FTW muscle fibers during exercise.

A contrasting metabolic picture is evident in predominantly STR muscle. In these fibers, AMP deaminase activity is lower and is associated with a different isozyme from that found in fast muscle. This second isozyme is less sensitive to increases in H^+ (Tullson and Terjung, 1990), and since lactate production in STR fibers is much lower than in fast muscle during contractions (Meyer and Terjung, 1979), activation of the enzyme by pH is less likely. Instead, STR muscle fibers (and heart) preferentially metabolize AMP to the dephosphorylated nucleoside, adenosine. This metabolite is exported to the extracellular space, where it exerts a vasodilatory effect. This effect is particularly important for the regulation of blood flow in cardiac muscle (Berne, 1980). In skeletal muscle, the role of adenosine is important, but it is not the sole determinant of metabolically induced increases in blood flow (Poucher et al., 1990).

C. Metabolic Responses of Fiber Types in Respiratory Muscles

In diaphragm muscle of the cat, the proportion of FTR, FTW, and STR fibers is roughly equal (Sieck, 1988). In humans, the relative proportion is approximately 50% STR and 50% fast-twitch. Approximately half of the fast-twitch fibers are red and the other half white (Keens and Ianuzzo, 1979). This resembles the fiber composition of other commonly studied skeletal muscles in the human (e.g., vastus lateralis). Regardless of muscle fiber type differences among species, the metabolic responses observed in a muscle will be a reflection of the weighted average of each fiber type recruited during the period of increased contractile activity. During normal ventilatory behavior, it is the extent of recruitment of each of these different fiber types that appears to be species-specific. In most species, no more than 50% of the motor unit pool will be recruited, even during maximal ventilation (Sieck, 1991). Thus, most ventilation can be accomplished without the use of FTW motor units, these are activated only during maximal expulsive behaviors, such as gagging and sneezing. If the approximately high forces required for ventilation can be attained in the absence of FTW motor unit recruitment, this means that respiratory muscles will largely avoid inordinate increases in lactate and ammonia production, and most energy demands will be met using mitochondrial ATP provision. This emphasizes the importance of adequate mitochondrial synthesis in respiratory muscles during the adaptation to an increased respiratory load, or during development.

Differences in species and the experimental conditions employed have created a controversy over the metabolic response of respiratory muscles to an increased workload. In our estimation, the metabolic response of the respiratory muscles closely resembles that of any other skeletal muscle of similar fiber composition subject to a functional demand. The most important factors that are involved in determining the metabolic behavior of a muscle are (1) the extent and quality of fiber recruitment, (2) the mitochondrial content, and (3) the contractile protein (fast- vs. slow-twitch) isoforms present. That the metabolic behavior of respiratory muscles is similar to the traditional response of other muscles is borne out by a number of studies. For example, during the increased ventilation of prolonged running or swimming, the glycogen and triglyceride contents of diaphragm muscle are reduced, as in other skeletal muscles subject to exercise (Ianuzzo et al., 1987; Górski et al., 1978; Green et al., 1988). This points to the importance of glycogen as a substrate during exercise. Indeed, correlations between the extent of glycogen depletion, lactate accumulation, and diaphragmatic fatigue have been reported (Ferguson et al., 1990).

Losses of ATP, creatine phosphate (CP), and glycogen can also be observed in the diaphragm muscle during inspiratory loading accompanied by hypoperfusion (Lockhat et al., 1988). Under these conditions of increased O_2 demand, accompanied by a deficient O_2 supply, a marked metabolic perturbation in the diaphragm occurs in a fashion similar to other skeletal muscles.

Evidence exists that the diaphragm behaves differently for adenine nucleotide metabolism and lactate production. These metabolites were not detectable in the cannulated phrenic vein of horses during short-term, high-intensity exercise (Manohar and Hassan, 1990). However, it seems unlikely that the intensity of exercise for locomotory skeletal muscles is identical with that for those non-weight-bearing muscles involved in ventilation. Thus, the low lactate and ammonia production evident in the venous effluent of the diaphragm may be due to a lower relative intensity of contractile effort for those fibers, or to a recruitment of predominantly STR and FTR fibers, as described earlier. Stimulation of diaphragm muscle strips in vitro at 20 Hz demonstrated decrements of ATP and increases in IMP and inosine, suggesting that the metabolic capability of the diaphragm to produce IMP and ammonia exists (Massarelli et al., 1989), but that the AMP deaminase reaction is not activated during normal in vivo exercise.

D. Mitochondrial Adaptations in Muscles Responding to Continuous Activity

Wild animals have a greater capacity for prolonged work than their domesticated counterparts. This appears to be related to the darker appearance of the muscles obtained from wild animals which, in turn, is due to the greater capacities for mitochondrial substrate oxidation and blood flow. This adaptation is simply because the muscles of wild animals are recruited more often, and to a greater degree. Historically, endurance training has provided a good model for studying the adaptations of muscle in humans and animals. Convincing changes in the mitochondrial content of muscle were first demonstrated by Holloszy (1967). Since that time, numerous studies have verified that continuous muscle use results in mitochondrial synthesis (or biogenesis). Increases in the size, number, and volume of mitochondria in response to endurance training (Gollnick and King, 1969; Hoppeler, 1986) have been reported. These mitochondria appear to be structurally and functionally normal. Rates of oxidative phosphorylation and electron transport, as well as the activities of enzymes providing reducing equivalents for oxidation, are increased up to twofold, depending on the intensity and duration of the training protocol employed (see Holloszy and Booth, 1976; Saltin and Gollnick, 1983; Terjung and Hood, 1986, for reviews).

The pattern of molecular events underlying these mitochondrial changes remains elusive. To study this, the use of a model that results in a more rapid and extensive mitochondrial biogenesis than found with endurance training would be advantageous. Continued, indirect low-frequency (10-Hz) stimulation of the motor nerve (Salmons and Vrbova, 1969) is a suitable model, since the mitochondrial changes are large (two- to sixfold; Hood et al., 1989; Reichmann et al., 1985) and rapid. With 24 h of continuous stimulation at 10 Hz, a 2.5-fold increase in mitochondrial enzyme activities can be achieved in 5–10 days (Takahashi and Hood, 1993). Thus, mechanisms of mitochondrial biogenesis are more easily studied in the continuous stimulation model.

The adaptive responses of oxidative enzymes within muscle to repeated stimulation are species-specific. The greatest changes are observed in the rabbit, intermediate in the rat and guinea pig, and lowest in the mouse (Simoneau et al., 1990). These differential responses to a standard workload are inversely related to mitochondrial content at the onset of stimulation. Mitochondria are present in skeletal muscle in a variety of shapes and sizes. They exist in two distinct areas of the cell: under the sarcolemma (subsarcolemmal, or SS mitochondria) and between the myofibrils (intermyofibrillar, or IMF mitochondria). Some work has illustrated these as distinct fractions (Ogata and Yamasaki, 1985), whereas other investigators have suggested that mitochondria exist as a continuous reticulumlike structure (Bakeeva et al., 1978; Kirkwood et al., 1986). This may be entirely dependent on the animal species in question. In smaller mammals that possess a higher mitochondrial volume per cell, such as the rat, mitochondria may be a continuous membrane structure. In larger mammals (i.e., horse, humans) in which the cellular mitochondrial volume is lower, individual mitochondria may be found (Kayar et al., 1988). These comparative data are strongly suggestive of a pattern of mitochondrial growth and expansion during adaptation to prolonged muscle use, and confirm the hypothesis that muscle mitochondria are not static structures, but are in a dynamic state of expansion during adaptive increases in mitochondrial volume (Kirkwood et al., 1987).

Evidence also exists that suggests differences in the properties of SS and IMF mitochondria. The SS mitochondria adapt more readily, and to a greater degree, during mitochondrial biogenesis induced by sustained muscle use (Kreiger et al., 1980). The opposite trend occurs during muscle disuse: SS mitochondrial content decreases more than does the IMF mitochondrial content (Desplanches et al., 1990). In cardiac muscle, biochemical studies have indicated that isolated IMF and SS mitochondria possess enzymatic and respiratory properties that distinguish them from one another (Palmer et al., 1985). We have recently confirmed this distinction in skeletal muscle and have found that rates of protein synthesis are higher in IMF than in SS mitochondria (Cogswell et al., submitted). This difference in IMF and SS mitochondria, and their differential behavior during adaptations, may be due to different patterns of mitochondrial biogenesis.

As reviewed in the following, recent work has explored both the underlying cellular mechanisms by which mitochondria are assembled, as well as the physiological consequences of this process.

E. Mitochondrial Gene Expression

The complexity of cellular events involved in the biogenesis of mitochondria is shown in Figure 2. The synthesis of any protein in the muscle cell involves specific gene activation and transcription, export of the resulting mRNA from the nucleus and its stabilization in the cytosol, and translation of the mRNA sequence into protein. The protein is then subject to posttranslational modifications. For example,

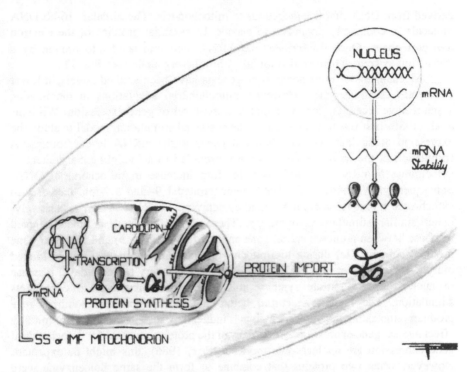

Figure 2 Mitochondrial biogenesis in muscle involves the processes of nuclear gene transcription, mRNA transport to the cytosol where it is stabilized, mRNA translation into protein, and import of the protein into the expanding organelle. A gene expression system endogenous to the mitochondrion performs similar functions (except that import is not necessary) and contributes about 10% of the total mitochondrial protein. Phospholipids, such as cardiolipin, must also be synthesized and incorporated into the organelle membrane system. The pattern of assembly of individual components is not yet firmly established.

most nuclear-encoded mitochondrial proteins are made with a short amino-terminal presequence that is cleaved off once the protein has found its final destination in a mitochondrial compartment. The purpose of this presequence is to recognize receptorlike components found at closely apposed areas of the inner and outer membranes, called contact sites. Penetration of the protein into the mitochondrion at that contact site requires the presence of ATP and a membrane potential. The presequence then serves to "target" the protein to its appropriate location (i.e., matrix, inner or outer membrane) of the mitochondrion. The presequence is finally cleaved by a matrix protease (Attardi and Schatz, 1988).

Approximately 90% of mitochondrial proteins are nuclear-encoded and follow a sequence of events similar to those just described for entry into mitochondria. However, importantly, the remaining 10% of mitochondrial proteins are originally derived from DNA that is endogenous to mitochondria. The circular, 16-kb DNA molecule is compactly organized to encode 13 essential proteins of the electron transport chain. Once transcribed, the mRNAs are translated into protein by a translation system, which is also found within the organelle (see Fig. 2).

Mechanisms of mitochondrial biogenesis have been studied largely in lower eukaryotes, such as yeast. However, mitochondrial adaptations in mammalian systems have recently been investigated at the level of gene expression. Williams et al. (1986) first illustrated the use of the sustained stimulation model to study the expression of nuclear and mitochondrial genes at the mRNA level. Continuous stimulation of the rabbit tibialis anterior muscle led to a fivefold enhancement of cytochrome *b* mRNA, as well as a fourfold increase in mitochondrial DNA. Subsequently, Williams et al. (1987) demonstrated 1.9- and 5.9-fold increases in cytochrome *c* oxidase subunit VIc and cytochrome *b* mRNA levels, respectively, under similar stimulation conditions. These data illustrated an uncoordinated response between a mitochondrial gene product (cytochrome *b*) and a nuclear gene product (subunit VIc) during the mitochondrial biogenesis induced by prolonged muscle use. Annex et al. (1991) have also reported a very rapid (3 days) increase in nuclear-encoded citrate synthase mRNA levels in response to continuous stimulation. The increase occurred before any change in mitochondrial gene products, suggesting that molecular signals induced by sustained muscle use initially affect nuclear gene expression. Since many of the proteins required for mitochondrial gene expression are nuclear gene products (Fox, 1986), this might be expected. However, when two proteins that combine to form the same holoenzyme were examined, a coordinated response was observed. Hood et al. (1989) illustrated increases in cytochrome *c* oxidase subunit VIc mRNA levels in the rat that were coordinated with the level of the mitochondrially encoded subunit III mRNA between 3 and 35 days of continuous stimulation. The increases in mRNA that were observed in these studies could not be accounted for entirely by an increase in transcriptional activity. Thus, some evidence for translational or posttranslational control was found (Hood et al., 1989; Seedorf et al., 1986; Williams et al., 1987). Future work in this area will probably be devoted to investigating whether this posttranslational regulation occurs at the level of holoenzyme mitochondrial protein import, or during assembly.

F. The Pattern of Mitochondrial Assembly

Many studies of endurance training indicate that the resulting mitochondria are normal both functionally and structurally. This suggests that mitochondria are assembled in a coordinated way relative to phospholipid and protein constituents. In support of this, the rate of turnover of mitochondrial inner membrane components of the respiratory chain is approximately equal (5–8 days; Aschenbrenner et al., 1970; Booth and Holloszy, 1977). These components respond in a uniform way (twofold) during the mitochondrial biogenesis induced by endurance training

(Holloszy, 1967). In addition, morphological changes in mitochondrial volume density closely parallel alterations in enzyme activities (Kirkwood et al., 1987; Reichmann et al., 1985).

However, some evidence also exists supporting the stepwise assembly of mitochondria. During development, liver mitochondria exhibit an increase in density during the latter stages of gestation (Aprille, 1984), and the formation of the phospholipid cardiolipin precedes that of cytochrome aa_3 (Hallman and Kankare, 1971). This indicates that the insertion of protein occurs into a preexisting lipid bilayer. This has also been demonstrated in yeast during the transition from an anaerobic to an aerobic environment (Aithal and Tustanoff, 1975). During the process of mitochondrial degradation induced by permanent denervation, the cardiolipin content of muscle decreased significantly by 5 days, and was subsequently followed by declines in the mitochondrial inner membrane enzymes, cytochrome c oxidase and succinate dehydrogenase, by 8–14 days (Wicks and Hood, 1991). Similarly, during mitochondrial biogenesis induced by prolonged stimulation, the time required for the 50% increase in cardiolipin was shorter (4.2 days) than that for succinate dehydrogenase (6.1 days; Takahashi and Hood, 1993). Therefore, these data are supportive of the stepwise accretion and removal of mitochondrial components during organelle turnover, and suggest that initiating events in mitochondrial turnover involve the synthesis or degradation of phospholipids.

G. Respiratory Muscle Adaptations

The oxidative capacity of mammalian diaphragms is directly related to the frequency of breathing across a range of species (Blank et al., 1988). Therefore, it is reasonable to hypothesize that imposed increases in respiratory frequency by regular, endurance exercise will increase the oxidative capacity of the muscle. However, controversy appears to exist concerning the adaptability of the respiratory muscles to endurance training. Lieberman et al. (1972) first indicated that the diaphragm could increase its proportion of red fibers in response to training. Subsequently, Moore and Gollnick (1982) reported small increases (17%) in succinate dehydrogenase (SDH) activity of the diaphragm, but no change in intercostal muscles subjected to up to 26 weeks of endurance training. Ianuzzo et al. (1982) noted training-induced increases of 22–30% in mitochondrial enzymes within the diaphragm. Minimal changes have been reported by Metzger and Fitts (1986), Fregosi et al. (1987), and Green et al. (1989). It may be that the differences reported are due to sampling variability of the various regions of the diaphragm, as well as the intensity and type of endurance training employed. Powers et al. (1990) have recently demonstrated approximately 30% increases in SDH activity of the costal diaphragm of young animals. In older animals, the adaptation within the coastal diaphragm was not found in response to training, but was evident in the intercostal muscles (Powers et al., 1992). These differences are likely due to differential recruitment patterns as a function of age.

In addition, because the respiratory muscles are already continuously active, mitochondrial enzyme activities are even higher than those found in other skeletal muscles that are recruited for posture (i.e., soleus; Moore and Gollnick, 1982), and certainly higher than those muscles that are used only occasionally for ballistic-type movements. Indeed, a training protocol that actively recruits FTR and FTW fibers in locomotory muscles may recruit a different population of fibers within the respiratory muscles. Thus, a greater stimulus for adaptation may be required for the respiratory muscles than that for other skeletal muscles. Furthermore, within the respiratory muscles, a given exercise intensity may impose a stimulus that is adequate for an adaptation to become apparent in one muscle, but not in another.

A stimulus that is more focused on the recruitment of all respiratory muscle fiber types in a prolonged fashion may be more effective in producing an adaptation. Such a situation probably exists in obstructive lung diseases, such as emphysema, in which the load on the respiratory muscles is continuously augmented (Mador, 1991). Experimental models of resistive loading have led to the conclusion that mitochondrial adaptations can occur. Keens et al. (1978) reported significant (30–40%) increases in enzyme activities of the diaphragm and intercostal muscles of the rat in response to tracheal banding. Increases have also been noted in both the crural and costal regions of the diaphragm, and these were associated with improvements in the endurance performance of the muscle, as measured by the maintenance of a higher transdiaphragmatic pressure over a longer period (Akabas et al., 1989). The increases in mitochondrial enzyme activities occurred in both slow-twitch and fast-twitch fibers (Bazzy and Kim, 1992).

Experimentally induced increases in respiratory load can also be accomplished in animals by the administration of elastase. Elastase produces an emphysematous condition, resulting in increases in oxidative enzyme activities (Sieck, 1991). The increases in SDH activity occurred in both type I (slow-twitch) and type II (fast-twitch) fibers. Although this adaptation was not accompanied by increases in capillary density, improvements in fatigue resistance in the emphysematous condition were observed (Lewis et al., 1992).

Thyroid status can also influence diaphragmatic adaptations. Ianuzzo et al. (1984) have reported significant increases (15–30%) in mitochondrial enzyme activities in response to hyperthyroidism. In contrast, hypothyroidism resulted in response to hyperthyroidism. In contrast, hypothyroidism resulted in similar reductions in enzyme activities. These changes were related to 70% differences in minute ventilation between the two groups.

Voluntary, progressive ventilatory muscle training results in an improved maximal voluntary ventilation and performance over a sustained period (Keens et al., 1977). This is particularly evident and beneficial in elderly subjects in whom ventilatory function can be markedly improved (Belman and Gaesser, 1988). Whether, in humans, this is due to an improved oxidative capacity, or to augmented blood flow remains to be determined. Although the maximal blood flow response of ventilatory muscles in response to endurance training has not been measured,

Tamaki (1987) reported increases in capillary/fiber area ratios in trained animals. Individual diaphragm motor unit fatigue resistance has been correlated to both muscle fiber capillarity and mitochondrial enzyme activity (Enad et al., 1989). Thus, it is likely that improvements in endurance performance are related to increases in mitochondrial content, as well as better nutritional perfusion of the active muscles.

H. Respiratory Muscle Adaptations During Development

The development of respiratory muscle fiber composition and functional characteristics is not complete before birth. Despite this, a newborn infant is subject to an obligatory, immediate increase in respiratory work. To avoid muscle fatigue and respiratory failure, rapid adaptive changes in muscle phenotype to the augmented functional demand must occur. Keens et al. (1978) have reported increases in the proportion of type I fibers from approximately 10%, to 25% and 55–65% in the respiratory muscles of premature newborn, full-term newborn, and older (>2-year-old) infants, respectively. This increase in type I fibers results in a muscle that is likely to be more economical in its ATP utilization, accompanied by a high mitochondrial oxidative capacity. The data indicate that the newborn is more susceptible to respiratory muscle fatigue than the older child. Thus, the adaptation observed is important for the transition from a state of high potential of respiratory distress, to one in which the muscles can meet the work demands of ventilation comfortably and with greater fatigue resistance.

However, some species differences appear to exist. In the cat (Sieck et al., 1991) and baboon (Maxwell et al., 1983) fatigue resistance has been noted to be highest at birth, followed by declines as adulthood is approached. In one case (Maxwell et al., 1983), this was correlated with the high oxidative activity of the fibers, whereas in the other (Sieck et al., 1991) a dissociation between oxidative capacity, fiber composition, and fatigue resistance was observed. This observation during development provides an interesting contrast to the typical observation, made in adult animals, that changes in muscle oxidative capacity correlate well with whole-muscle fatigue resistance (Takahashi and Hood, submitted; Sieck, 1991).

I. Physiological Implications of Mitochondrial Biogenesis

The physiological implications of an enhanced mitochondrial content and increased mitochondrial enzymes in muscle are now well established. As illustrated in Figure 3, classic Michealis–Menten kinetics predict that a lower substrate concentration is required to achieve the same biological effect in a tissue with a greater enzyme content (Gollnick and Saltin, 1982; Holloszy et al., 1971). For example, in 1 g of muscle, a lower free ADP (ADP_f) concentration is required to stimulate the same rate of oxygen consumption in trained versus untrained muscle. Since ADP_f is a potent regulator of phosphofructokinase (PFK) and AMP deaminase activities

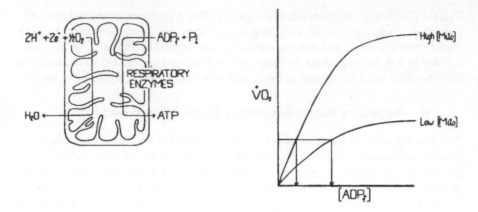

Figure 3 Michealis–Menten plots of reaction rate (Vo_2; oxygen consumed per minute) as a function of its rate-limiting substrate (ADP_f) concentration. High and low [mito] indicate the level of mitochondrial enzymes as a result of mitochondrial biogenesis within muscle responding to a physiological demand, such as endurance training. Note that a given Vo_2 can be achieved with a lower ADP_f concentration in the high mitochondrial content condition.

(Newsholme and Start, 1973; Wheeler and Lowenstein, 1979), the physiological implications of this adaptation include a reduced production of lactate, IMP, and ammonia in the cell (Constable et al., 1987; Dudley et al., 1987). Along with this increase in mitochondrial content is a concomitant increase in enzymatic capacity for fatty acid utilization (Molé et al., 1971). The increase in citrate concentration during free fatty acid metabolism inhibits PFK activity, resulting in diminished glycogen utilization during a given submaximal work bout (Holloszy, 1988). Taken together, these adaptations reduce muscle reliance on limited carbohydrate supplies, limit the production of ammonia and lactate and, therefore, are major reasons for the improved endurance performance that is observed.

J. Blood Flow

Regulation of blood flow in skeletal muscle is mediated by a multiplicity of factors, including metabolic, neural, and myogenic influences. The most important of these appears to be the contribution of neural sympathetic vasoconstrictor tone, competing with the vasodilatory action of local factors (e.g., K^+, adenosine, P_i, and H^+) produced in general proportion to tissue metabolic rate (Laughlin and Armstrong, 1985). The blood flow capacity of skeletal muscle fiber types, similar to the mitochondrial content, is a distinguishing property of each. This suggests that the control of flow differs among fiber types, or that flow is limited by the physical characteristics of the arteriolar networks found within each fiber type.

Differences in the peak blood flow between each fiber type are most easily observed during conditions of high metabolic energy demand, such as muscle contractions. The FTR muscle fibers are endowed with the highest peak blood flow during tetanic contractions ($\sim$300 ml min^{-1} 100 g^{-1}) and locomotory exercise ($\sim$400). The STR fibers have the capacity to increase flow to approximately 200–300 ml min^{-1} 100 g^{-1}, whereas the maximum flows observed in FTW fibers are only approximately 80–100 ml min^{-1} 100 g^{-1}. At rest, blood flows in these fiber types range from 6 to 20 ml min^{-1} 100 g^{-1}, depending on the extent of motor unit recruitment at rest, particularly in STR muscle fibers that are used for postural activities. Thus, 10- to 40-fold increases in flow can be observed during brief contractile activity (Laughlin and Armstrong, 1985; Mackie and Terjung, 1983a). In respiratory muscles, similar increases are found. During exercise, increases of 3- to 12-fold above the flow obtained during quiet breathing are observable (Roussos and Campbell, 1986). Flows of 200–250 ml min^{-1} 100 g^{-1} have been reported for diaphragm muscle during the first minute of moderate exercise in rats (Armstrong and Laughlin, 1984). Similar values have been found at the onset of high-intensity exercise (Laughlin and Armstrong, 1982).

The increase in blood flow in diaphragm muscle during isometric contractions is limited by mechanical impedance above a tension–time index of 20–30% of maximum. At levels above 30%, the pattern of muscle contractions (i.e., the duty cycle) was important in establishing blood flow (Bark et al., 1987). Low duty cycles and high contraction frequencies appear to be important determinants of maximum diaphragmatic blood flow (Buchler et al., 1985).

During resistive inspiratory loading, increases in flow above that seen during spontaneous breathing are also observed (Brancatisano et al., 1991), the magnitude of which has been reported to be as high as 26-fold (Robertson et al., 1977). The extent of the increase also appears to be muscle- and region-specific. During the induction of a progressive increase in the work of breathing by the inhalation of carbon dioxide, blood flow increased most in diaphragm muscle (sixfold) and somewhat less (three- to fivefold) in the intercostal and abdominal muscles (Supinski, 1988). Furthermore, dramatic differences in flow could be seen within the external intercostal muscles. More distal intercostal spaces received markedly less flow than cranial interspaces (Brancatisano et al., 1991). Since flow in skeletal muscle is largely metabolically controlled, these differences within and between muscles are probably a reflection of the degree of motor unit recruitment.

Regularly performed exercise appears to improve the blood flow capacity of those fibers that are poorly perfused to begin with: FTW fibers. Approximately 40–50% increases in blood flow have been noted in this fiber type in response to endurance training, with little change observed in FTR or STR fiber sections (Mackie and Terjung, 1983b). To our knowledge, only one study has reported the effect of training on blood flow to the diaphragm. Armstrong and Laughlin (1984) did not detect an adaptive increase in diaphragm blood flow in response to training. Whether blood flow can be augmented by more specific training of the respiratory muscles in normal individuals, or in patients with respiratory disease, remains to be determined.

II. Contractile System

A. Myosin-Based Muscle Fiber Type and Myosin Heavy Chains

The diaphragm muscle comprised a mixture of fiber types, which express different myosin phenotypes. These phenotypic forms of myosin can be partly differentiated histochemically by their pH-sensitive ATPase activity. With routine histochemical methods, several different myosin-based fiber types have been identified. These are type-I (slow-twitch, red), type-IIA (fast-twitch, red), type-IIB (fast-twitch, white), and type-IC/IIC (neonatal or transitional fiber). With a combination of histochemical, immunohistochemical, and electrophoretic techniques the fiber type classification system can be definitive for the myosin types that exist within individual myofibers. This allows the fiber type classification system to be based on the myosin heavy chain (MHC) phenotype, which reflects the myosin genotype (Table 1). Currently, fibers containing homogeneous myosin phenotypes are classified as types I, IIA, IIB, and IID (same as IIX, see later). Fibers usually contain a single MHC, but at times during development and adaptation, fibers can contain as many as four different myosin types (see Pette and Staron, 1990, for review). Fibers containing heterogeneous isoforms are termed according to the relative amounts of the coexisting myosin types (see Table 1). The use of the type-C classification is the exception and needs to be reconsidered for the terminology to be more meaningful.

The type-IIX fiber, which has only recently been identified (Schiaffino et al., 1986, 1988, 1989), is widely distributed in rat skeletal muscles and comprises a major proportion of the fiber types in the diaphragm. This most recently discovered

Table 1 Adult Fiber Types and Myosin Types

Fiber types	Myosin heavy chain types
Homogeneous phenotypic fibers	
Type I	MHC-I
Type IIA	MHC-IIa
Type IIB	MHC-IIb
Type IID	MHC-IId (same IIx)
Heterogeneous phenotypic fibers	
Type IIAB	MHC-IIa/b
Type IIAD	MHC-IIa/d
Type IIBD	MHC-IIb/d
Type IC	MHC-I/IIa
Type IIC	MHC-IIa/I

MHC-IIx was initially identified by Schiaffino et al. (1986) and later by Bär and Pette (1988), who named it MHC-IId. We have elected to use the IId terminology because it is more in alphabetical sequence with the already identified IIa and IIb MHCs and type-IIC fiber, and goes along with its preponderant presence in the diaphragm, for which the *d* was designated (D. Pette, Univ. Konstanz, personal communication). The adult rat diaphragm contains more fibers with MHC-IId than any of the other rat muscles (Bär and Pette, 1988; Schiaffino et al., 1989).

The IID fibers have not been previously identified and probably unknowingly have been classified as type-IIB, using the pH-based routine histochemical procedures. The identification of this fiber population requires the use of a highly specific myosin antibody (Laframboise et al., 1991) and, furthermore, the IId MHC, which is the basis for this fiber type, cannot be easily separated from the IIb MHC by sodium dodecyl sulfate–polyacrylamide gel electrophoresis (SDS–PAGE) (Laframboise et al., 1991).

The speed of muscular contraction has long been known to correlate with muscle fiber types and myosin ATPase activity (Bárány, 1967). More recently, the maximum velocity of shortening of single fibers was shown to more specifically correlate with the type of myosin heavy chain (Reiser et al., 1985; Sweeney et al., 1986; Eddinger and Moss, 1987). The shortening velocity of fibers containing preponderantly IId MHC has been reported to be intermediate between type IIB and type IIA fibers (Schiaffino et al., 1990). The large percentage of IID fibers in the diaphragm would give it an intermediate, fast, intrinsic-shortening velocity. The physiological meaning derived from these findings is that must be at least four distinct types of highly specialized motor units based on the myosin heavy chain isoform within the diaphragm. This provides the diaphragm with a range of capabilities to generate power and maintain an optimal level of energetic efficiency, with the ultimate purpose of these different myosin-based motor units to provide indefatigable pulmonary ventilation under various normal and pathological conditions.

B. Diaphragm Muscle Development

These four adult MHC isoforms (IIa, IIb, IId, I) are present in the adult rat diaphragm in the proportions of 21, 6, 45, and 28%, respectively (Sugiura et al., 1990). During embryonic development, two other nonadult myosin heavy chain types are also expressed [i.e., embryonic (MHCemb) and neonatal (MHCneo)] (Laframboise et al., 1991). Figure 4 illustrates the MHC expression. By 21 days in utero the diaphragm muscle contained fibers with either MHCemb (100%), MHCemb/neo (90%), and/or MHC-IId (20%). By 4 days postnatal, more than 90% of the fibers contained adult myosin isoforms. At 21 days postnatal, fibers containing only MHC-I comprised 13% of the fibers, which increased to 35% in the fully adult rat diaphragm at 115 days (Laframboise et al., 1991). This is the same percentage of type I fibers reported by us for the rat diaphragm (Keens et al., 1978). The fibers

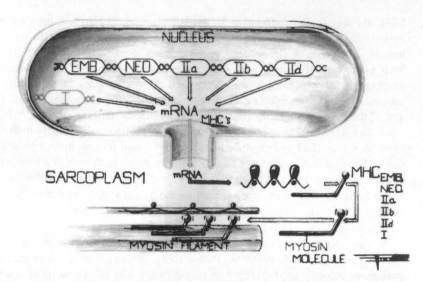

Figure 4   Schematic drawing showing the myosin heavy chain (MHC) genes that are expressed in the embryonic and adult diaphragm. There are a total of six MHCs expressed in the diaphragm. The embryonic (emb) and neonatal (neo) MHCs are expressed during development as well as the MHC-IId. The adult diaphragm contains the four adult MHCs (IIa, IIb, IId, I) in the proportions of 21, 6, 45, and 28%, respectively. (From Sugiura et al., 1990.)

that reacted with the IId antibody declined from 80% at 4 days to 30% at 115 days postnatal, with the remaining fibers containing 31% IIa and 4% IIb MHCs. The sequence and proportion of myosin expression during development reported in the study of Laframboise et al. (1991) are illustrated in Figure 5. In an early attempt to determine diaphragmatic development, we (Keens et al., 1978) used postmortem samples from human diaphragms ranging from 24 weeks gestation to a 59-year-old adult. It was estimated in this study, from routine histochemical studies, that the full complement of type I fibers occurred at approximately 8 months postnatally. In comparison, the expression of MHC-I was optimal at about 60 days in the rat diaphragm (Laframboise et al., 1991). The lack of complete development of the diaphragm at the beginning of postnatal life may make the newborn susceptible to respiratory failure until development of the respiratory muscles is completed.

C.   Factors Involved in Myosin Heavy Chain Expression

Contractile Activity and Anatomical Location

Several possible factors have been suggested to influence the initiation and temporal sequence of myosin expression during development. The contractile activity and

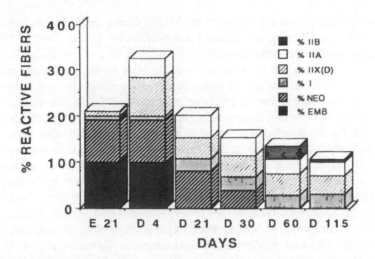

Figure 5 Percentage of muscle fibers that reacted with specific myosin heavy chain antibodies during development of the rat diaphragm from 21 days in utero (E21) to 115–156 days (D 115) postnatal. (Data from LaFramboise et al., 1991.)

the anatomical location in relation to development have been investigated as having possible regulatory influences. Laframboise et al. (1990) compared the developmental expression of the MHC in limb muscles with those in the diaphragm and concluded that neither the contractile activity nor the rostral–caudal position of the diaphragm were factors involved in the temporal elimination of the MHCneo. Kelly et al. (1990) further added that an abrupt change in myosin expression does not occur with the sudden increase in functional challenge that takes place when going from intra- to extrauterine life. The findings from these studies suggest that the developmental expression of myosin is not under the control of inherent contractile activity, respiratory load, or anatomical location.

Thyroid Hormones

Thyroid hormones are also known to have a dramatic effect on switching skeletal muscle fiber types and myosin expression (Ianuzzo et al., 1977), and have been implicated as having a possible influence in the developmental process (Rubinstein et al., 1988). The rate of developmental transition from MHCneo to fast-type MHC is altered by experimental dysthyroidism (Whalen et al., 1985; Russell et al., 1988), which suggests that thyroid hormone is involved in establishing the rate of transition of myosin expression, but is probably not the factor responsible for initiating myosin gene expression during development. The findings of Rubinstein et al. (1988), in which hypo- and hyperthyroidism were combined with innervation and denervation, are consistent with the idea that neither thyroid status nor innervation is the initiating factor of the transitional expression of the MHCs during development, but they do have a role in modulating the temporal and quantitative events. Thyroid hormone was further implicated in the developmental process by a recent study (Brozanski et al., 1991) showing that the attenuation of the time period for the disappearance of MHCneo in the diaphragm of perinatal undernourished rats was caused by a reduced serum triiodothyronine level that was associated with the state of malnutrition. Although thyroid hormones do not appear to be the initiating factor in myosin expression during development, in adult muscle, thyroid hormone does initiate switches in myosin expression in both skeletal and cardiac muscle (Ianuzzo et al., 1977; Hoh et al., 1978; Williams and Ianuzzo, 1988). Chronic experimental dysthyroidism alters the proportions of type I and type II fibers in the diaphragm by twofold, with the hypothroid diaphragm having 45% type I fibers, whereas the hyperthyroid diaphragm had 23% type I fibers (Ianuzzo et al., 1984). It is interesting that when hyperthyroidism was measured against physiological overload, thyroid status was the dominant regulator of myosin expression (Ianuzzo et al., 1991). These findings from experimentally prepared dysthyroid animal models should be helpful for the clinician, since a thyrotoxic myopathy has also been clinically observed in humans (Ayres et al., 1982; Laroche et al., 1988; Martinez et al., 1989; Mier et al., 1989).

Innervation

Innervation has been known to be a prime determinant of myosin types since the classic studies of Buller et al. (1960). The role of innervation in the developmental regulation of myosin expression is still being actively pursued. Innervation of the muscle fiber is required for the complete expression of adult fast myosin to occur, and it is essential for slow myosin expression in regenerating muscles (Ecob-Prince et al., 1986; Cerny and Bandman, 1987). However, in primary myotubes MHC I (slow) is expressed along with MHCemb before innervation, and IIb MHC is expressed in hindlimb muscles denervated at birth (Rubinstein et al., 1988), but the nerve is required for complete expression of I and II MHCs, as well as the repression of the emb and neo MHCs. These findings indicate that the nerve is required for complete expression of both fast and slow myosin, but it does not appear to be necessary for the initiation of expression during development, depending on whether it is a primary or secondary myotube (see Rubinstein et al., 1988; Gunning and Hardeman, 1991, for review).

D. Fiber Type and Myosin Changes in Response to Functional Demand

Electrical Stimulation

Sustained electrical stimulation of fast-twitch muscle is a highly controlled and reproducible experimental procedure, which has been used to determine the temporal transformation of fiber types and expression of myosin types. This approach has led the way in providing insights into the adaptive strategy of the contractile system of muscle fibers that have a continuously imposed physiological overload. In a study by Staron et al. (1987), nearly complete transformation of type II to type I fibers occurred within 60 days following continuous electrical stimulation at a frequency of 10 Hz for 24 h/day (Fig. 6). From this study, it appears that the temporal sequence of the fiber transformation was IIB > IIAB > IIA > IIC > IC > I. The type IID fiber was not identified at the time that this study was being accomplished, so its place in this sequential scheme is not precisely known.

Different Species

The diaphragm muscle of different mammals provides another approach to understanding the strategy of respiratory muscle adaptations to tachypnea, because of the inherent differences in breathing frequencies that are present in nature in different-sized mammals. Diaphragms of different-sized mammals have different proportions of fiber types (Gauthier and Padykula, 1966) and myosin types (Blank et al., 1988), which correlate with the mammals' breathing frequency (Fig. 7). Large mammals, with slow-breathing frequencies, have a greater proportion of slow myosin compared with small mammals with rapid-respiratory rates that have more fast myosin in their diaphragms (Blank et al., 1988). The observed respiratory frequencies of different mammals have been reported to correspond with the calculated optimal-breathing rates (Crosfill and Widdicombe, 1961). An extension of this adaptive hypothesis is that the proportions of type I (slow) and II (fast) fibers have developed to accommodate a particular breathing frequency to provide the optimal contractile and energetic efficiencies for a specific respiratory rate.

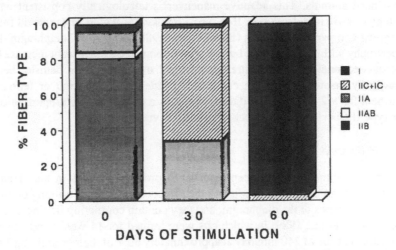

Figure 6 Fiber type transformation in the tibialis anterior of the rabbit during 60 days of continuous electrical stimulation at 10 Hz. (From Staron et al., 1987.)

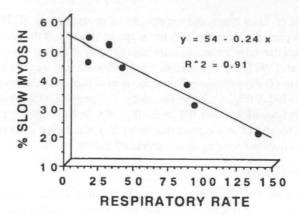

Figure 7 Correlation of breathing frequencies to percentage of slow myosin in the diaphragms of different mammals. (Data taken and estimated from Blank et al., 1988; Sieck et al., 1983; Keens et al., 1978.)

Tracheal Constriction

The initial observation of adaptive fiber type changes in respiratory muscles was from a study using continuous tracheal constriction to produce an increased respiratory load in rapidly growing rats (Keens et al., 1978). Following 5 weeks of tracheal banding, the percentage of type I fibers increased from 35% in the control diaphragms, to 45% in the overloaded diaphragms. These biochemical adaptations were associated with lower breathing frequencies and longer inspiratory times in the banded animals. This adaptive maneuver is teleologically consistent with the strategy of switching from type II to type I myosin, as would be predicted from the foregoing comparative findings (Blank et al., 1988). The costal diaphragm did not hypertrophy with this overload, but the type I fibers had a significant increase (42%) in cross-sectional area. In contrast, prolonged overload of the hamster hemidiaphragm by inactivation of the contralateral side by denervation or tetrodotoxin treatment for a 2-week period did not result in a change in the proportion of type I or type II fiber types (see Sieck, 1991; for review).

Endurance Training

Endurance training has also been reported to produce changes in the diaphragm. These have been only a few studies on the effects of endurance training on the type I and II fiber types of the diaphragm, and they contain conflicting findings. A recent study (Green et al., 1989) in which rats were trained for 14 weeks and achieved a final running time of 240 min/day at approximately 80% of their pretraining VO_{2max}, had an increase of 15% in IIB fibers and a 34% decrease in IIA fibers. No significant change in the percentage type I fibers occurred. In another study, in which weighted rats were swim-trained for 1 h/day, 5 days/week for 4 weeks, a decrease in MHC-IIb from 6.1 to 1.9% was found in the diaphragm of the trained rats, with no significant changes in the other MHCs (i.e., I, IIa, and IId) (Sugiura et al., 1990). The findings of these two studies are obviously conflicting. Even though the type-IIB and IID fibers were not separately classified in the study of Green et al. (1989), the fiber type compared with the myosin heavy chain changes reported in these studies are occurring in opposite directions (i.e., MHC-IIb decreased and type IIB fibers increased). This disagreement may be of only academic concern, since the actual changes were relatively minor (4–6%) and probably would have little physiological consequence to overall respiratory function. However, it does present a problem of how to think about the adaptive strategy of fiber type and myosin changes in the diaphragm in response to the endurance type of respiratory load.

III. Excitation–Contraction Coupling

The events associated with calcium regulation of muscular contraction are central to understanding the adaptive maneuvers of skeletal muscle fibers to altered functional demands, fatigue, and pathological states. The purpose of this section is to present the Ca^{2+}-mediated events that control muscular contraction and relaxation and the adaptive modifications that have been identified to occur in the Ca^{2+} regulatory system with chronically altered functional demands.

A. Sarcolemmal Components

Calcium Channels

The sarcolemma (SL) and transverse tubular system (TTS) contain voltage-sensitive L-type Ca^{2+} channels, which are relatively abundant in skeletal muscle (Fosset et al., 1983). The entry of extracellular Ca^{2+} appears to be important in skeletal muscle, as well as in cardiac muscle, as indicated by the muscles' inability to contract when this Ca^{2+} current is blocked. This suggests that extracellular Ca^{2+} could be involved in the calcium-induced calcium-release (CICR) process (Frank, 1982; Kimura et al., 1987), which is a well-accepted mechanism in cardiac muscle (Fabiato, 1985), but has not been accepted as a primary release mechanism in skeletal muscle (see Rios and Pizarro, 1991, for review).

Sodium–Calcium Exchange

A Na^+–Ca^{2+} exchange electrogenic antiporter has been reported in diaphragm muscle (Yamamoto and Greef, 1981), but with a tenfold smaller maximal capacity than it has in cardiac muscle (Gilbert and Meissner, 1982). The role of this exchanger in skeletal muscle is not yet fully known, but skeletal muscle, like cardiac muscle, needs to finely regulate cytoplasmic Ca^{2+} concentration, which could be partly accomplished using this secondary active transport system. A recent study (Zavecz et al., 1991) has shown that force development of the diaphragm is dependent on $[Ca^{2+}]_o$ and that pharmacological blockade of the Na^+–Ca^{2+} antiport with benzamil dramatically slowed relaxation. These findings suggest that the diaphragm is different from other skeletal muscles in that extracellular $[Ca^{2+}]$ appears to be associated with force development. Furthermore, the diaphragm is affected by cardiac glycosides, which have been reported not to influence force generation in other skeletal muscles (Aubier et al., 1986; Viires et al., 1988). The influence of the Na^+–K^+ pump on the Na^+–Ca^{2+} exchanger allows speculation that the Na^+–Ca^{2+}-exchange capacity in the diaphragm may be higher than that in other skeletal muscles, as is the Na^+–K^+ pump capacity (Ianuzzo and Dabrowski, 1987). The complete understanding of the in vivo functioning of this calcium-regulating antiport system will be necessary for understanding normal diaphragmatic function and probably the etiology of fatigue in certain situations.

The Sarcolemmal Calcium Pump

The SL Ca^{2+} pump is another component of the calcium-regulating system that participates in maintaining low $[Ca^{2+}]_i$, as indicated by its low K_m for Ca^{2+}. This SL Ca^{2+} pump is most abundant in the TTS of skeletal muscle (Brandt et al., 1980) and is a distinctly different pump from the Ca^{2+} pump in the sarcoplasmic reticulum (Schwartzmann, 1989). Little is yet known about its role in skeletal muscle.

B. Sarcoplasmic Reticulum

The sarcoplasmic reticulum (SR) is a canicular organelle that constitutes about 4% of the cellular volume in human skeletal muscle cells (Eisenberg, 1983), depending on the fiber type. This organelle functions primarily to regulate the rapid and fine cytoplasmic Ca^{2+} concentration. It has two morphologically and functionally distinct regions: the terminal cisternae, or the more recent term of junctional SR (jSR), and the longitudinal or the nonjunctional SR (njSR). The jSR interfaces with the TTS and forms a close connection by a pillar or footlike structure (Franzini-Armstrong, 1980). It is at this interface between the jSR and TTS that the initiating signal for intracellular Ca^{2+} release occurs (Fig. 8). Several possible mechanisms for release of Ca^{2+} have been proposed. These possible mechanisms are summarized in the following and are illustrated, in part, in Figure 8. The SR contains a Ca^{2+} pump, which accounts for as much as 90% of the SR protein and has two genotypes in skeletal muscle (i.e., fast and slow cardiac Ca-ATPase) (Brandl et al., 1986). These isoforms have different specific activities and exist in different quantities in fast and slow muscle fibers, which accounts for about a tenfold difference in Ca^{2+}-uptake rates in these fiber types. These two isoforms are under developmental (Brandl et al., 1986) and neural control (Leberer et al., 1986). The SR also contains two

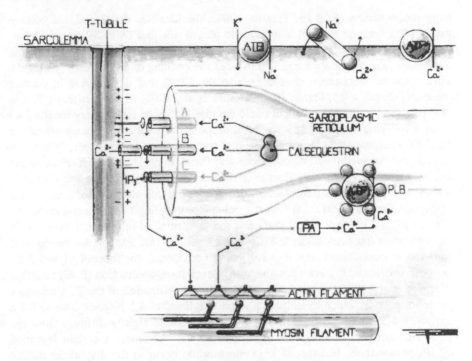

Figure 8 Schematic drawing showing three of the proposed mechanisms that signal calcium release from the sarcoplasmic reticulum (SR). (A). An illustration of the mechanism of direct-coupling of depolarization of the transverse tubular system (TTS) a "plug" that opens the Ca^{2+} channels. (B). An illustration of the mechanism of Ca^{2+}-induced Ca^{2+} release. For this proposed mechanisms Ca^{2+} is released from the TTS into the cytoplasm, which leads to the opening of SR Ca^{2+} channels. (C). An illustration of the proposed mechanism of release caused by inositol 1,4,5-triphosphate (IP_3). Depolarization of the TTS is postulated to activate phospholipase C, which catalyzes the formation of IP_3. IP_3 is assumed to lead to the opening of SR Ca^{2+} channels. Several other mechanisms have also been proposed (see text).

calcium-binding proteins, calsequestrin and high-affinity Ca^{2+}-binding protein. Calsequestrin is the most abundant and is located primarily in the jSR region.

C. Proposed Mechanisms of Intracellular Calcium Release

The depolarization of the SL–TTS is the initial event that precedes the large release of $[Ca^{2+}]_i$ from the SR Ca^{2+}-release channels. The actual signal(s) following the TTS depolarization that leads to the opening of these channels is controversial but is considered to be one of six proposed mechanisms: (1) Depolarization of the TTS has been suggested to induce depolarization of the SR membrane and to cause the opening of voltage sensitive Ca^{2+} channels (Mathias et al., 1980). However, in a more recent review (Ríos and Pizarro, 1991), the idea was developed that voltage gating of the release channel is unlikely to play a role in TTS to SR transmission. (2) It has also been suggested that Ca^{2+} is released from the TTS during the transmembrane potential change that induces the opening of the SR Ca^{2+} channels. This proposed mechanism is analogous to the CICR that is operative in cardiac muscle (Fabiato, 1985; Frank, 1982; Kimura et al., 1987). It appears that CICR is probably not the initial event, but could operate alongside the primary mechanism in an amplifying manner. (3) It has been proposed that sulfhydryl oxidation at the TTS–SR interface could be a mechanism of transmission (Trimm et al., 1986), but this has not received much support (Ríos and Pizarro, 1991). (4) An increase in pH causes contraction of muscle fibers (Shoshan et al., 1981). Thus, a local alkalin-ization was proposed as a mechanism of release, but this also has not found favor (Ríos and Pizarro, 1991). (5) Direct mechanical coupling of a charged molecule with a SR Ca^{2+} channel "plug" that leads to the opening of the channel during TTS depolarization has been suggested (Chandler et al., 1976). Support for mechanical coupling is inconclusive, but it is still being considered. (6) Inositol triphosphate has been implicated to have a possible role in excitation–contraction (E–C) coupling (Vergara et al., 1985; Volpe et al., 1985). The depolarization of the TTS activates phospholipase C, which hydrolyzes phosphotidylinositol 4,5-bisphosphate to form inositol 1,4,5-triphosphate (IP_3). The IP_3 is assumed to rapidly diffuse across the TTS–SR junction to stimulate the opening of SR Ca^{2+} channels. It is then degraded by IP_3 phosphatase. Changes in IP_3 concentration occur in the diaphragm during paced twitching (Nosek et al., 1990). Although the IP_3 system exists in skeletal muscle, opens SR Ca^{2+} channels, and causes Ca^{2+} release and contracture, there are many questions that remain to be answered before the IP_3 system is considered as a primary messenger in E–C coupling (Ríos and Pizarro, 1991). Some of the prime concerns are that this system does not appear to be able to respond in the time frame required to be a messenger capable of rapid signaling of Ca^{2+} release. There are also conflicting findings on whether the concentrations of IP_3 produced are adequate (see Hidalgo and Jaimovich, 1989, for review). Although there are concerns about IP_3 being the primary mechanism (Ogawa and Harafuji, 1989), numerous positive studies suggest the IP_3 system has some function in E–C coupling (Ríos and Pizarro, 1991). It would seem likely that these six proposed mechanisms are not the same in type I and type II fibers because of the heterogeneity of the SR proteins (e.g., Ca^{2+} pump and phospholamban) and membrane protein–lipid composition that exist in different fiber types (Pette and Staron, 1990; Ferguson and Franzini-Armstrong, 1988; Salviati and Volpe, 1988). However, according to Salviati and Volpe (1988) the Ca^2-release mechanisms in fast and slow fibers are homologous, but differ in their sensitivities to Ca^{2+}-modulating drugs.

We (G. Farkas, A. Forer, and C. D. Ianuzzo, unpublished findings) investigated the possibility that IP_3 was involved in force generation and muscle fatigue of the rat diaphragm. Costal diaphragm muscle strips from adult rats were placed in a temperature-controlled (37°C) muscle bath containing either oxygenated

Krebs solution: solution A (NaCl 137 mM, KCl 4 mM, MgCl$_2$ 1 mM, K$_2$HPO$_4$ 1 mM, NaHCO$_3$ 12 mM, CaCl$_2$ 2 mM, glucose 6.5 mM, and *d*-tubocurarine 0.2%); solution B (same as A, but contained 50 mM LiCl and NaCl 87 mM); or solution C (B plus 50 μM *myo*-inositol). Solution A was the control. Solution B inhibited the PI cycle by blocking inositol formation. Solution C bypassed the lithium block by containing inositol. The muscle strips were equilibrated in each of these solutions for 15 min. A force–frequency curve was constructed at frequencies of 5, 10, 20, 35, 50, 70, and 100 Hz (Fig. 9A). The effects of these solutions on diaphragmatic

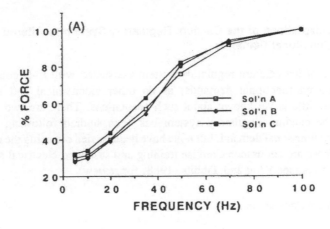

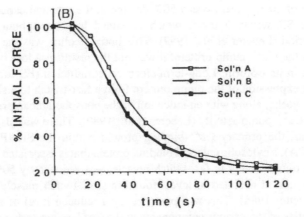

Figure 9 (A) Force–frequency curves of in vitro diaphragm preparations using a control solution (Sol'n A), solution to block the phosphatidyinositol (PI) cycle (Sol'n B), and a solution to bypass the blockade (Sol'n C). For the chemical composition of the solutions see text. (B) These curves show the effects of the three solutions on the fatigue of this in vitro diaphragm preparation. These findings indicate that the PI cycle may not be involved in force generation or in the development of fatigue.

fatigue were determined by direct stimulation with 250-ms, 20-Hz pulses for 120 s (see Fig. 9B). These findings indicate that the possible blockade (solution B) and bypass (solution C) of the IP_3 system did not modify the force–frequency curve or alter fatigability in this in vitro diaphragm preparation.

The definitive mechanisms of primary and secondary Ca^{2+} regulation that are involved in excitation–contraction coupling needs to be resolved by the basic scientists so that the clinical scientists can attempt to determine the role of these mechanism(s) in respiratory failure. This appears to be a fruitful area for respiratory muscle research.

D. Adaptations of the Calcium Regulatory System to Altered Functional Demands

Components of the calcium regulatory system associated with E–C coupling may adapt to altered functional demands, as do other biochemical and subcellular systems, but little is yet known about such adaptations. There are two paradigms in which the calcium regulatory system has been studied following prolonged alterations of functional demand, but none have been carried out using the respiratory muscles. These are endurance exercise training and sustained electrical stimulation of limb muscles (see Klug and Tibbits, 1988, for review).

Electrical Stimulation

When rabbit fast-twitch limb muscles were stimulated with a continuous nerve impulse traffic of 10 Hz, there was a 50% decline in the rate and capacity of Ca^{2+} uptake by the SR within 2 days, which remained low throughout the 28-day stimulation period (Leberer et al., 1987). This initial decline was the result of an inactivation of the Ca^{2+} pump protein: it was not the result of a loss of the protein or of a change in its isoform. Long-term electrical stimulation (ES) does lead to a switch in gene expression of the pump protein from a fast-twitch to a slow, cardiac isoform by 10 weeks, along with an induction of the phospholamban protein, which modulates the Ca^{2+} pump activity (Leberer et al., 1989). There was also a decrease in calsequestrin, the primary Ca^{2+}-binding protein within the SR (Pette, 1984). Parvalbumin (PA), a cytosolic calcium-binding protein that is associated with muscle relaxation and found mainly in fast-twitch muscle, was reduced by 50% following 12 days of ES, and it declined to levels found in slow-twitch muscle by 21 days (Leberer and Pette, 1986). This was preceded by a reduced level of mRNA. The reduced capacities of the various components of the Ca^{2+}-sequestering system were not linearly related to the increase in 50% relaxation time (RT_{50}), but appeared to have a more complex relation. The associated changes in PA and RT_{50} suggested that PA has an important role in relaxation of fast-twitch muscle, whereas, in slow-twitch muscles, Ca^{2+}-uptake capacity appears to be the prime determinant. These biochemical changes result in an increase in the isometric twitch/tetanus ratio, suggested the reduced capacity of this system resulted in an increase in the time of the active state (Klug et al., 1988).

Exercise Training

The reports of the effects of endurance types of exercise training on the Ca^{2+}-sequestering system in muscle have been few and have reported conflicting findings. An increased Ca^{2+}-binding capacity of SR vesicles has been reported, without an increase in the rate of Ca^{2+} uptake (Belcastro et al., 1980). In contrast, endurance training reduced the maximum rate of Ca^{2+} uptake and the K_m for Ca^{2+} (Kim et al., 1981). Klug (G. Klug and colleagues, personal communication) found what appeared to be a significant increase in Ca^{2+}-ATPase activity per milligram of protein in the semipurified SR fraction of the red gastrocnemius and red vastus lateralis of trained rats, but when Ca^{2+}-ATPase was normalized to the total amount of ATPase per sample, the differences were not evident. Klug suggested the initial significant differences were the result of a differential protein contamination of the SR fraction in the trained and control muscles. In another study by Green et al. (1984), in which an exceptionally challenging endurance-training program was imposed on rats, the Ca^{2+} pump protein/30-kDa SR protein concentration ratio declined from 18 to 4. This ratio is consistent with a shift from type IIB to IIA fibers and approaches the ratio found in slow-twitch muscle. There were also significant reductions in the PA concentration in these trained muscles. Although these changes to the Ca^{2+}-sequestering system are not as dramatic as the electrical stimulation changes, the strategy of the adaptive process appears to be similar. There are only a few studies on the effects of exercise training on the Ca^{2+} regulatory system, but these findings are not consistent. There is some evidence from the trends of these studies that begins to provide a basis from which to theoretically discuss the adaptive process that may occur in the respiratory muscles when challenged by a prolonged respiratory overload. The teleologic rationale for adaptations occurring in the calcium regulatory system of the respiratory muscles is to prevent respiratory failure in the processes of excitation–contraction coupling. The review by Luckin et al. (1991) discusses possible locations of conduction and transmission failure.

IV. General Summary

Muscle cells contain three main subcellular systems, which form the underlying basis of their physiological expression: contractile properties, fatigability, and energetic efficiency. These three systems have the inherent property of adapting to persistently altered physiological demands, and their adaptations are dependent on qualitative or quantitative changes in gene expression. The metabolic system has been extensively studied, with the mitochondrion being the central organelle of these adaptations. It is now understood that type II white (FTW) fibers, which have the lowest inherent mitochondrial concentrations, can increase their mitochondrial content from approximately 3% of the cell's volume to 20% by sustained contractile activity. This percentage of cell volume begins to approach that found in cardiac muscle cells. The processes of mitochondrial biogenesis require a symbiotically regulated gene expression occurring between the nuclear and mitochondrial genomes. Newly synthesized mitochondria induced by physiological demand are largely similar in structure and function to those found in the cell before induction of synthesis, although the existence of mitochondrial protein isoforms has not been extensively investigated. Thus, the aerobic metabolic adaptive strategy is to increase the replication of mitochondrial units. Adaptations in the mitochondrial content are associated with commensurate adaptations in the local blood flow capacity. These coadaptations have strong implications for the metabolic response of the muscle cells, since they allow the muscle to rebalance its substrate utilization more toward fatty acid metabolism, thereby conserving the minimal, but necessary, stores of carbohydrates. The functional result of this maneuver is the attenuation of fatigue during long-term submaximal use, which in pulmonary ventilation, would help in the prevention of respiratory failure.

The sarcomere is the basic unit of the contractile system, which comprises numerous sarcomeric proteins that all appear to have polymorhpic forms. The major contractile protein is myosin, which has four known adult myosin heavy chain (MHC) isoforms and two developmental isoforms that are expressed in the diaphragm muscle. These isoforms are sequentially expressed during development, with the adult forms retaining their plasticity of reexpression, which occurs when muscle is challenged by long-term alterations in physiological or pathological demands. The expression of these MHCs are under the controlling influence of at least four factors: myogenic, neural, hormonal, and contractile activity. Continuous contractile activity can result in a complete reexpression from MHC-II to MHC-I, as can many of the other sarcomeric proteins. These MHCs are molecular correlates of contractile velocity and energetic efficiency. They appear to undergo reexpression to provide the most appropriate isoform to accomplish the physiological task. In the diaphragm, prolonged resistive breathing leads to an increase in MHC-I (slow). The adaptive changes in MHC expression that have been observed following daily bouts of pulsed tachypnea resulting from endurance exercise training have been conflicting. Even so, the contractile system in respiratory muscles appears to be adaptable and able to accommodate alterations in functional demand by switching the myosin isoforms, if the level of physiological challenge is adequate.

The processes that regulate the release and uptake of intracellular calcium (i.e., events of excitation–contraction coupling) are essential to the precise regulation and timing of muscular contraction. The actual signal that occurs between the transverse tubular system (TTS) and the sarcoplasmic reticulum (SR) has not yet been identified, but six different transmission mechanisms have been proposed. There are two different isoforms of the SR Ca^{2+} pump in muscle, the quantity and the quality (isoforms) of these pumps can be altered by continuous contractile activity. The calcium-sequestering capacity does adapt to prolonged activity, but the exact adaptive strategy of the calcium regulatory system as a whole is not as well known yet as those of the metabolic and contractile systems.

The general strategy of adaptations of these three subcellular systems to long-term contractile activity is to alter the metabolic capacity, mainly by increasing the mitochondrial content through the coincident expression of the nuclear and mitochondrial genomes. The contractile system adapts to this type of activity by switching protein isoforms to efficiently accommodate the appropriate contractile characteristics. The calcium regulatory system adapts by replicating similar pumping units and also by switching the pump isoform. These subcellular systems appear to maintain a specific ratio of the ATP-utilizing systems (contractile and calcium regulatory) to the ATP-synthesizing system (metabolic). We (Hamilton and Ianuzzo, 1990) have presented this as a capacity quotient (*CQ*).

$$CQ = \frac{1/2 \text{ SR Ca}-\text{pump activity} + 2/3 \text{ contractile ATPase activity}}{\text{Mitochondrial aerobic capacity}}$$

The fractions of 1_3 and 2_3 represent the proportion of the total energetic costs that go to calcium cycling and contractile activity in highly active muscle. Aerobic metabolism is considered to account for almost all ATP synthesis. This *CQ* is different for the various muscle types: cardiac muscle has a $CQ = 5.0 \times 10^{-3}$, whereas type II white (FTW) muscle has a value that is approximately 75-fold greater than heart. When a muscle adapts to endurance types of activity or is transformed by continuous electrical stimulation, it becomes more fatigue-resistant and the value for the CQ approaches that of cardiac muscle, which is the gold standard for indefatigability.

Acknowledgments

The authors wish to thank Ms. Bing Li for helping in the preparation of this manuscript and Mr. Michael Salomon for helping with the library research. Studies of the authors referred to in this manuscript were supported by Canadian NSERC grants and Heart and Stroke Foundation grants.

References

Aithal, H. N., and Tustanoff, E. R. (1975). Assembly of complex III into newly developing mitochondrial membranes. *Can. J. Biochem.* 53: 1278–1281.

Akabas, S. R., Bazzy, A. R., Dimauro, S., and Haddad, G. G. (1989). Metabolic and functional adaptation of the diaphragm to training with resistive loads. *J. Appl. Physiol.* 66: 529–535.

Annex, B. H., Kraus, W. E., Dohm, G. L., and Williams, R. S. (1991). Mitochondrial biogenesis in skeletal muscles: Rapid induction of citrate synthase mRNA by nerve stimulation. *Am. J. Physiol.* 260: C 266–C270.

Aprille, J. R. (1984). Perinatal development of mitochondria in rat liver. In *Mitochondrial Physiology and Pathology*. Edited by G. Fiskum. New York, Van Nostrand Reinhold, pp. 66–99.

Armstrong, R. B., and Laughlin, M. H. (1984). Exercise blood flow patterns within and among rat muscles after training. *Am. J. Physiol.* 246: H59–H68.

Aschenbrenner, B., Druyan, R., Albin, R., and Rabinowitz, M. (1970). Haem *a*, cytochrome *c* and total protein turnover in mitochondria from rat heart and liver. *Biochem. J.* 119: 157–160.

Attardi, G., and Schatz, G. (1988). Biogenesis of mitochondria. *Annu. Rev. Cell Biol.* 4: 289–333.

Aubier, M., Viires, N., Murciano, D., Seta, J.-P., and Pariente, R. (1986). Effects of digoxin on diaphragmatic strength generation. *J. Appl. Physiol.* 61: 1767–1774.

Ayres, J., Rees, J., Clark, T. J. H., and Maisey, M. N. (1982). Thyrotoxicosis and dyspnoea. *Clin. Endocrinol.* 16: 65–71.

Bakeeva, L. E., Chentsov, Y. S., and Skulachev, V. P. (1978). Mitochondrial framework (reticulum mitochondrial) in rat diaphragm muscle. *Biochim. Biophys. Acta* 501: 349–369.

Bär, A., and Pette, D. (1988). Three fast myosin heavy chains in adult rat skeletal muscle. *FEBS Lett.* 235: 153–155.

Bárány, M. (1967). ATPase activity of myosin correlated with speed of muscle shortening. *J. Gen. Physiol.* 50: 197–216.

Bark, H., Supinski, G. S., Lamanna, J. C., and Kelsen, S. G. (1987). Relationship of changes in diaphragmatic muscle blood flow to muscle contractile activity. *J. Appl. Physiol.* 62: 291–299.

Bazzy, A. R., and Kim, Y.-J. (1992). Effect of chronic respiratory load cytochrome oxidase activity in diaphragmatic fibers. *J. Appl. Physiol.* 72: 266–271.

Belcastro, A. N., Wenger, H., Nihei, T., Secord, D., and Bonen, A. (1980). Functional overload of rat fast-twitch skeletal muscle during development. *J. Appl. Physiol.* 49: 583–588.

Belman, M. J., and Gaesser, G. A. (1988). Ventilatory muscle training in the elderly. *J. Appl. Physiol.* 64: 899–905.

Berne, R. M. (1980). The role of adenosine in the regulation of coronary blood flow. *Circ. Res.* 47: 807–813.

Blank, S., Chen, V., and Ianuzzo, C. D. (1988). Biochemical characteristics of mammalian diaphragms. *Respir. Physiol.* 74: 115–126.

Booth, F. W., and Holloszy, J. O. (1977). Cytochrome *c* turnover in rat skeletal muscles. *J. Biol. Chem.* 252: 416–419.

Brancatisano, A., Amis, T. C., Tully, A., and Engel, L. A. (1991). Blood flow distribution within the rib cage muscles. *J. Appl. Physiol.* 70: 2559–2565.

Brandl, C. J., Green, N. M., Korczak, B., and MacLennan, D. H. (1986). Two Ca^{2+} ATPase genes: Homologies and mechanistic implications of deduced amino acid sequences. *Cell* 44: 596–607.

Brandt, N. R., Caswell, A. H., and Brunschwig, J. P. (1980). ATP-energized Ca^{2+} pump in isolated transverse tubules of skeletal muscles. *J. Biol. Chem.* 255: 6290–6298.

Brozanski, B. S., Daood, M. J., LaFramboise, W. A., Watchko, J. F., Foley, T. P., Butler-Browne, G. S. Whalen, R. G., Guthrie, R. D., and Ontell, M. (1991). Effects of perinatal undernutrition on elimination of immature myosin isoforms in the rat diaphragm. *Am. J. Physiol.* 261: L49–L54.

Buchler, B., Magder, S., and Roussos, C. (1985). Effects of contraction frequency and duty cycle on diaphragmatic blood flow. *J. Appl. Physiol.* 58: 265–273.

Buller, A. J., Eccles, J. C., and Eccles, R. M. (1960). Interactions between motoneurons and muscles in respect of the characteristic speeds of their responses. *J. Physiol.* 150: 417–439.

Chandler, W. K., Rakowski, R. F., and Schneider, M. D. (1976). Effects of glycerol treatment and maintained depolarization on charge movement in skeletal muscle. *J. Physiol.* 254: 285–316.

Cogswell, A. M., Stevens, R. J., and Hood, D. A. (1993). Biochemical and functional characteristics of skeletal muscle mitochondria isolated from subsarcolemmal and inter-myofibrillar regions. *Am. J. Physiol.* (Cell Physiol.) 264: C383–C389.

Constable, S. H., Favier, R. J., McLane, J. A., Fell, R. D., Chen, M., and Holloszy, J. O. (1987). Energy metabolism in contracting skeletal muscle: Adaptation to exercise training. *Am. J. Physiol.* 253: C316–C322.

Crosfill, M. L., and Widdicombe, J. G. (1961). Physical characteristics of the chest and lungs and the work of breathing in different mammalian species. *J. Physiol.* 158: 1–14.

Desplanches, G., Kayar, S. R., Sempore, B., Flandrois, R., and Hoppeler, H. (1990). Rat soleus muscle ultrastructure after hindlimb suspension. *J. Appl. Physiol.* 69: 504–508.

Dudley, G. A., and Terjung, R. L. (1985). Influence of acidosis on AMP diaminase activity in contracting fast-twitch muscle. *Am. J. Physiol.* 248: C43–C50.

Dudley, G. A., Tullson, P. C., and Terjung, R. L. (1987). Influence of mitochondrial content on the sensitivity of respiratory control. *J. Biol. Chem.* 262: 9109–9114.

Ecob-Prince, M. S., Jenkison, M., Butler-Browne, G. S., and Whalen, R. G. (1986). Neonatal and adult myosin heavy chain isoforms in an nerve–muscle culture system. *J. Cell Biol.* 103: 995–1005.

Eddinger, T. J., and Moss, R. L. (1987). Mechanical properties of skinned single fibers of identified types from rat diaphragm. *Am. J. Physiol.* 523: C210–C218.

Eisenberg, B. R. (1983). Quantitative ultrastructure of mammalian skeletal muscle. In *Handbook of Physiology*. Section 10. Skeletal Muscle. Edited by L. D. Peachey, R. H. Adrian, and S. R. Geiger. Bethesda, MD, American Physiological Society, pp. 73–112.

Enad, J. G., Fournier, M., and Sieck, G. C. (1989). Oxidative capacity and capillary density of diaphragm motor units. *J. Appl. Physiol.* 67: 620–627.

Fabiato, A. (1985). Calcium-induced release of Ca^{2+} from the cardiac sarcoplasmic reticulum. *Am. J. Physiol.* 245: C1–C14.

Ferguson, D. G., and Franzini-Armstrong, C. (1988). The Ca^{2+} ATPase content of slow and fast twitch fibers of guinea pig. *Muscle Nerve* 11: 561–570.

Ferguson, G. T., Irvin, C. G., and Cherniack, R. M. (1990). Relationship of diaphragm glycogen, lactate, and function to respiratory failure. *Am. Rev. Respir. Dis.* 141: 926–932.

Fosset, M., Jaimovich, E., Delpont, E., and Lazdunski, M. (1983). (^{3}H)Nitrendipine receptors in skeletal muscle. Properties and preferential localization in transverse tubules. *J. Biol. Chem.* 258: 6086–6092.

Fox, T. D. (1986). Nuclear gene products required for translation of specific mitochondrially coded mRNAs in yeast. *Trends Genet.* 2: 97–100.

Frank, G. B. (1982). Roles of intracellular and trigger calcium ions in excitation–contraction coupling in skeletal muscle. *Can. J. Physiol. Pharmacol.* 60: 427–439.

Franzini-Armstrong, C. (1980). Structure of the sarcoplasmic reticulum. *Fed. Proc.* 39: 2403–2409.

Fregosi, R. F., Sanjak, M., and Paulson, D. J. (1987). Endurance training does not affect diaphragm mitochondrial respiration. *Respir. Physiol.* 67: 225–237.

Gauthier, G. F., and Padykula, H. A. (1966). Cytological studies of fiber types in skeletal muscle. A comparative study of the mammalian diaphragm. *J. Cell Biol.* 28: 333–354.

Gilbert, J. R., and Meissner, G. (1982). Sodium–calcium ion exchange in skeletal muscle sarcolemmal vesicles. *J. Membr. Biol.* 69: 77–84.

Gollnick, P. D., and King, D. W. (1969). Effect of exercise and training on mitochondria of rat skeletal muscle. *Am. J. Physiol.* 216: 1502–1509.

Gollnick, P. D., and Saltin, B. (1982). Significance of skeletal muscle oxidative enzyme enhancement with endurance training. *Clin. Physiol.* 2: 1–12.

Górski, J., Namiot, Z., and Giedrojć , J. (1978). Effect of exercise on metabolism of glycogen and triglycerides in the respiratory muscles. *Pflugers Arch.* 377: 251–254.

Green, H. J., Klug, G. A., Reichmann, H., Seedorf, U., Wiehrer, W., and Pette, D. (1984). Exercise-induced fibre type transitions with regard to myosin, parvalbumin, and sarcoplasmic reticulum in muscles of the rat. *Pflugers Arch.* 400: 432–438.

Green, H. J., Ball-Burnett, M. E., Morrissey, M. A., Kile, J., and Abraham, G. C. (1988). Glycogen utilization in rat respiratory muscles during intense running. *Can. J. Physiol. Pharmacol.* 66: 917–923.

Green, H. J., Plyley, M. J., Smith, D. M., and Kile, J. G. (1989). Extreme endurance training and fiber type adaptation in rat diaphragm. *J. Appl. Physiol.* 66: 1914–1920.

Gunning P., and Hardeman, E. (1991). Multiple mechanisms regulate muscle fiber diversity. *FASEB J.* 5: 3064–3070.

Hamilton, N., and Ianuzzo, C. D. (1991). Contractile and calcium regulating capacities of myocardia of different sized mammals scale with resting heart rate. *Mol. Cell. Biochem.* 106: 133–141.

Hallman, M., and Kankare, P. (1971). Cardiolipin and cytochrome aa_3 in intact liver mitochondria of rats. Evidence of successive formation of inner membrane components. *Biochem. Biophys. Res. Commun.* 45: 1004–1010.

Hidalgo, C., and Jaimovich, E. (1989). Inositol trisophosphate and excitation–contraction coupling in skeletal muscle. *J. Bioenerg. Biomembr.* 21: 267–281.

Hoh, J. F., McGraph, P. A., and Hale, P. T. (1978). Electrophoretic analysis of multiple forms of rat cardiac myosin: Effects of hypophysectomy and thyroxine replacement. *J. Mol. Cell. Cardiol.* 10: 1053–1076.

Holloszy, J. O. (1967). Biochemical adaptations in muscle. *J. Biol. Chem.* 242: 2278–2282.

Holloszy, J. O. (1988). Metabolic consequences of endurance exercise training. In *Exercise Nutrition, and Energy Metabolism.* Edited by E. S. Horton, and R. L. Terjung. New York, Macmillan Publishing, pp. 116–131.

Holloszy, J. O., and Booth, F. W. (1976). Biochemical adaptations to endurance exercise in muscle. *Annu. Rev. Physiol.* 38: 273–291.

Holloszy, J. O., Oscai, L. B., Mole, P. A., and Don, I. J. (1971). Biochemical adaptations to endurance exercise in skeletal muscle. *Adv. Exp. Med. Biol.* 11: 51–61.

Hood, D. A., Zak, R., and Pette, D. (1989). Chronic stimulation of rat skeletal muscle induces coordinate increases in mitochondrial and nuclear mRNAs of cytochrome-*c*-oxidase subunits. *Eur. J. Biochem.* 179: 275–280.

Hoppeler, H. (1986). Exercise-induced ultrastructural changes in skeletal muscle. *Int. J. Sports Med.* 7: 187–204.

Ianuzzo, C. D., and Dabrowski, B. (1987). Na^+/K^+-ATPase activity of different types of striated muscles. *Biochem. Med. Metab. Biol.* 37: 31–34.

Ianuzzo, C. D., Patel, P., Chen, V., O'Brien, P., and Willams, C. (1977). Thyroidal trophic influence on skeletal muscle myosin. *Nature* 270: 74–76.

Ianuzzo, C. D., Noble, E. G., Hamilton, N., and Dabrowski, B. (1982). Effects of streptozotocin diabetes, insulin treatment, and training on the diaphragm. *J. Appl. Physiol.* 52: 1471–1475.

Ianuzzo, C. D., Chen, V., O'Brien, P., and Keens, T. G. (1984). Effect of experimental dysthyroidism on the enzymatic character of the diaphragm. *J. Appl. Physiol.* 56: 117–121.

Ianuzzo, C. D., Spalding, M. J., and Williams, H. (1987). Exercise-induced glycogen utilization by the respiratory muscles. *J. Appl. Physiol.* 62: 1405–1409.

Ianuzzo, C. D., Hamilton, N., and Li, B. (1991). Competitive control of myosin expression: Hypertrophy vs. hyperthyroidism. *J. Appl. Physiol.* 70: 2328–2330.

Kayar, S. R., Hoppeler, H., Mermod, L., and Weibel, E. R. (1988). Mitochondrial size and shape in equine skeletal muscle: A three dimentional reconstruction study. *Anat. Rec.* 222: 333–339.

Keens, T. G., and Ianuzzo, C. D. (1979). Development of fatigue-resistant muscle fibers in human ventilatory muscles. *Am. Rev. Respir. Dis.* 119(Suppl.): 139–141.

Keens, T. G., Krastins, I. R. B., Wannamaker, E. M., Levison, H., Crozier, D. H., and Bryan, A. C. (1977). Ventilatory muscle endurance training in normal subjects and patients with cystic fibrosis. *Am. J. Respir. Dis.* 116: 853–860.

Keens, T. G., Bryan, A. C., Levison, H., and Ianuzzo, C. D. (1978a). Developmental pattern of muscle fiber types in human ventilatory muscles. *J. Appl. Physiol.* 44: 909–913.

Keens, T. G., Chen, V., Patel, P., O'Brien, P., Levison, H., and Ianuzzo, C. D. (1978b). Cellular adaptations of the ventilatory muscles to a chronic increased respiratory load. *J. Appl. Physiol.* 44: 905–908.

Kelly, A. M., Rosser, B. W. C., Rubinstein, N. A., and Nemeth, P. M. (1990). Biochemical properties of the diaphragm during development of respiratory function in the rat. In *The Dynamic State of Muscle Fibers*. Edited by D. Pette. New York, Walter de Gruyter, pp. 181–192.

Kim, D. H., Wible, G. S., Witzman, F. A., and Fitts, R. H. (1981). A comparison of sarcoplasmic reticulum function in fast and slow muscle using crude homogenates and isolated vesicles. *Life Sci.* 28: 2761–2677.

Kimura, I., Kimura, M., and Kimura, M. (1987). External Ca^{2+} release in directly stimulated diaphragm muscles of mice. *Jpn. J. Pharmacol.* 44: 510–514.

Kirkwood, S. P., Munn, E. A., and Brooks, G. A. (1986). Mitochondrial reticulum in limb skeletal muscle. *Am. J. Physiol.* 251: C395–C402.

Kirkwood, S. P., Packer, L., and Brooks, G. A. (1987). Effects of endurance training on a mitochondrial reticulum. *Arch. Biochem. Biophys.* 255: 80–88.

Klug, G. A., and Tibbits, G. F. (1988). The effects of activity on calcium-mediated events in striated muscle. *Exerc. Sport Sci. Rev.* 16: 1–59.

Klug, G. A., Leberer, E., Leisner, E., Simoneau, J.-A., and Pette, D. (1988). Relationship between parvalbumin content and the speed of relaxation in chronically stimulated rabbit fast-twitch muscle. *Pflugers Arch.* 411: 126–131.

Kreiger, D. A., Tate, C. A., McMillin-Wood, J., and Booth, F. W. (1980). Populations of rat skeletal muscle mitochondria after exercise and immobilization. *J. Appl. Physiol.* 48: 23–28.

Laframboise, W. A., Daood, M. J., Guthrie, R. D., Butler-Browne, G. S., Whalen, R. G., and Ontell, M. (1990). Myosin isoforms in neonatal rat extensor digitorum logus, diaphragm, and soleus muscle. *Am. J. Physiol.* 259: L116–L122.

Laframboise, W. A., Daood, M. J., Guthrie, R. D., Schiaffino, S., Moretti, P., Brozanski, B., Ontell, M. P., Butler-Browne, G. S., Whalen, R. G., and Ontell, M. (1991). Emergence of the mature myosin phenotype in the rat diaphragm muscle. *Dev. Biol.* 144: 1–15.

Laroche, C. M., Cairns, T., Moxham, J., and Green, M. (1988). Hypothyroidism presenting with respiratory muscle weakness. *Am. Rev. Respir. Dis.* 138: 472–474.

Laughlin, M. H., and Armstrong, R. B. (1982). Muscular blood flow distribution patterns as a function of running speed in rats. *Am. J. Physiol.* 243: H296–H306.

Laughlin, M. H., and Armstrong, R. B. (1985). Muscle blood flow during locomotory exercise. *Exerc. Sport Sci. Rev.* 13: 95–136.

Leberer, E., and Pette, D. (1986). Neural regulation of parvalbumin expression in mammalian skeletal muscle. *Biochem. J.* 235: 67–73.

Leberer, E., Seedorf, U., and Pette, D. (1986). Neural control of gene expression in skeletal muscle. Ca-sequestering proteins in developing and chronically stimulated rabbit skeletal muscles. *Biochem. J.* 239: 295–300.

Leberer, E., Härtner, K.-T., and Pette, D. (1987). Reversible inhibition of sarcoplasmic reticulum Ca-ATPase by altered neuromuscular activity in rabbit fast-twitch muscle. *Eur. J. Biochem.* 162: 555–561.

Leberer, E., Härtner, K.-T., Brandl, C. J., Fujii, J., Tada, M., MacLennan, D., and Pette, D. (1989). Slow/cardiac sarcoplasmic reticulum Ca^{2+}-ATPase and phospholamban mRNAs are expressed in chronically stimulated fast-twitch muscle. *Eur. J. Biochem.* 185: 51–54.

Lewis, M. I., Zhan, W.-Z., and Sieck, G. C. (1992). Adaptations of the diaphragm in emphysema. *J. Appl. Physiol.* 72: 934–943.

Lieberman, D. A., Maxwell, L. C., and Faulkner, J. A. (1972). Adaptation of guinea pig diaphragm muscle to aging and endurance training. *Am. J. Physiol.* 222: 556–560.

Lockhat, D., Roussos, C., and Ianuzzo, C. D. (1988). Metabolite changes in the loaded hypoperfused and failing diaphragm. *J. Appl. Physiol.* 65: 1563–1571.

Luckin, K. A., Biedermann, M. C., Jubrias, S. A., Williams, J. H., and Klug, G. A. (1991). Muscle fatigue: Conduction or mechanical failure? *Biochem. Med. Metab. Biol.* 46: 299–316.

Mackie, B. G., and Terjung, R. L. (1983a). Influence of training on blood flow to different skeletal muscle fiber types. *J. Appl. Physiol.* 55: 1072–1078.

Mackie, B. G., and Terjung, R. L. (1983b). Blood flow to different skeletal muscle fiber types during contraction. *Am. J. Physiol.* 245: H265–H275.

Mador, M. J. (1991). Respiratory muscle fatigue and breathing pattern. *Chest* 100: 1430–1435.

Manohar, M., and Hassan, A. S. (1990). Diaphragm does not produce ammonia or lactate during high-intensity short-term exercise. *Am. J. Physiol.* 259: H1185–H1189.

Martinez, F. J., Bermudez-Gomez, M., and Celli, B. R. (1989). Hypothyroidism. A reversible cause of diaphragmatic dysfunction. *Chest* 96: 1059–1063.

Massarelli, P. S., Green, H. J., Hughson, R. L., and Sharratt, M. T. (1989). Mechanical and metabolic alterations in rat diaphragm during electrical stimulation. *J. Appl. Physiol.* 67: 210–220.

Mathias, R. T., Levis, R. A., and Eisenberg, R. S. (1980). Electrical models of excitation–contraction coupling and charge movement in skeletal muscle. *Biochim. Biophys. Acta* 76: 1–31.

Maxwell, L. C., McCarter, R. J. M., Kuehl, T. J., and Robotham, J. L. (1983). Development of histochemical and functional properties of baboon respiratory muscles. *J. Appl. Physiol.* 54: 551–561.

Metzger, J. M., and Fitts, R. H. (1986). Contractile and biochemical properties of diaphragm: Effects of exercise training and fatigue. *J. Appl. Physiol.* 60: 1752–1758.

Meyer, R. A., and Terjung, R. L. (1979). Differences in ammonia and adenylate metabolism in contracting fast and slow muscle. *Am. J. Physiol.* 6: C111–C118.

Mier, A., Brophy, C., Wass, J. A. H., Besser, G. M., and Green, M. (1989). Reversible respiratory muscle weakness in hyperthyroidism. *Am. Rev. Respir. Dis.* 139: 529–533.

Molé, P. A., Oscai, L. B., and Holloszy, J. O. (1971). Adaptation of muscle to exercise. *J. Clin. Invest.* 50: 2323–2330.

Moore, R. L., and Gollnick, P. D. (1982). Response of ventilatory muscles of the rat to endurance training. *Pflugers Arch.* 392: 268–271.

Mutch, B. J. C., and Bannister, E. W. (1983). Ammonia metabolism in exercise and fatigue: A review. *Med. Sci. Sport Exerc.* 15: 41.

Newsholme, E. A., and Start, C. (1973). in *Regulation in Metabolism.* New York, John Wiley & Sons, pp. 88–137.

Nosek, T. M., Guo, N., Ginsburg, J. M., and Kolbeck, R. (1990). Inositol (1,4,5)-triphosphate (IP3) within diaphragm muscle increases upon depolarization [abstract]. *Biophys. J.* 57: 401a.

Ogata, T., and Yamasaki, Y. (1985). Scanning electron-microscopic studies on the three-dimensional structure of mitochondria in the mammalian and white and intermediate muscle fibers. *Cell Tissue Res.* 241: 251–256.

Ogawa, Y., and Harafuji, H. (1989). Ca-release by phosphoinositides from sarcoplasmic reticulum of frog skeletal muscle. *J. Biochem.* 106: 864–867.

Palmer, J. W., Tandler, B., and Hoppel, C. L. (1985). Biochemical differences between subsarcolemmal and interfibrillar mitochondria from rat cardiac muscle: Effects of procedural manipulations. *Arch. Biochem. Biophys.* 236: 691–702.

Pette, D. (1984). Activity-induced fast to slow transitions in mammalian muscle. *Med. Sci. Sports Exerc.* 16: 517–528.

Pette, D., and Staron, R. S. (1990). Cellular and molecular diversities of mammalian skeletal muscle fibers. *Rev. Physiol. Biochem. Pharmacol.* 116: 2–76.

Poucher, S. M., Nowell, C. G., and Collis, M. G. (1990). The role of adenosine in exercise hyperaemia of the gracilis muscle in anaesthetized cats. *J. Physiol.* 427: 19–29.

Powers, S. K., Lawler, J., Criswell, D., Dodd, S., Grinton, S., Bagby, G., and Silverman, H. (1990). Endurance-training-induced cellular adaptations in respiratory muscles. *J. Appl. Physiol.* 68: 2114–2118.

Powers, S. K., Lawler, J., Criswell, D., Lieu, F.-K., and Martin, D. (1992). Aging and respiratory muscle metabolic plasticity: Effects of endurance training. *J. Appl. Physiol.* 72: 1068–1073.

Rall, J. A. (1985). Energetic aspects of skeletal muscle contraction: Implications of fiber types. *Exerc. Sports Sci. Rev.* 13: 33–74.

Reichmann, H., Hoppeler, H., Mathieu-Costello, O., Von Bergen, F., and Pette, D. (1985). Biochemical and ultrastructural changes of skeletal muscle mitochondria after chronic electrical stimulation in rabbits. *Pfugers Arch.* 404: 109.

Reiser, P. J., Moss, R. L., Giulian, G. G., and Greaser, M. L. (1985). Shortening velocity in single fibers from adult rabbit soleus muscles is correlated with myosin heavy chain composition. *J. Biol. Chem.* 260: 9077–9080.

Ríos, E., and Pizarro, G. (1991). Voltage sensor of excitation–contraction coupling in skeletal muscle. *Physiol. Rev.* 71: 849–898.

Robertson, C. H., Foster, G. H., and Johnson, R. L. (1977). The relationship of respiratory failure to the oxygen consumption of, lactate production by, and distribution of blood flow among respiratory muscles during increasing inspiratory resistance. *J. Clin. Invest.* 59: 31–42.

Roussos, C., and Campbell, E. J. M. (1986). Respiratory muscle energetics. In *Handbook of Physiology*. Section 3. The Respiratory System. Edited by A. P. Fishman, P. T. Macklem, J. Mead, and S. R. Geiger. Bethesda, MD, American Physiological Society, pp. 481–509.

Rubinstein, N. A., Lyons, G. E., and Kelly, A. M. (1988). Hormonal control of myosin heavy chain genes during development of skeletal muscles. In *Plasticity of the Neuromuscular System*. Edited by D. Evered and J. Whelan. New York, John Wiley & Sons, pp. 35–51.

Russell, S. D., Cambon, N., Nadal-Ginard, B., and Whalen, R. G. (1988). Thyroid hormone induces a nerve-independent precocious expression of fast myosin heavy chain mRNA in rat hindlimb skeletal muscle. *J. Biol. Chem.* 263: 6370–7374.

Salmons, S., and Vrbova, G. (1969). The influence of activity on some contractile characteristics of mammalian fast and slow muscles. *J. Physiol.* 201: 535–549.

Saltin, B., and Gollnick, P. D. (1983). Skeletal muscle adaptability: Significance for metabolism and performance. In *Handbook of Physiology: Skeletal Muscle*. Edited by L. D. Peachey. Bethesda, MD, American Physiological Society, pp. 555–631.

Salviati, G., and Volpe, P. (1988). Ca^{2+} release from sarcoplasmic reticulum of skinned fast- and slow-twitch muscle fibers. *Am. J. Physiol.* 254: C459–C465.

Schatzmann, H. J. (1989). The calcium pump of the surface membrane and of the sarcoplasmic reticulum. *Annu. Rev. Physiol.* 51: 473–485.

Schiaffino, S., Saggin, L., Viel, A., Ausoni, S., Sartore, S., and Gorza, L. (1986). Muscle fibre types identified by monoclonal antibodies to myosin heavy chains. In *Biochemical Aspects of Physical Exercise*. Edited by G. Benzi, L. Packer, and N. Siliprandi. Amsterdam, Elsevier, pp. 27–34.

Schiaffino, S., Gorza, L., Sartore, S., Saggin, L., Ausoni, S., Vianello, M., Gundersen, K., and Lomo, T. (1989). Three myosin heavy chain isoforms in type 2 skeletal muscle fibres. *J. Muscle Res. Cell Motil.* 10: 197–205.

Schiaffino, S., Ausoni, S., Gorza, L., Saggin, L., Gundersen, K., and Lomo, T. (1988). Myosin heavy chain isoforms and velocity of shortening of type 2 skeletal muscle fibers. *Acta Physiol. Scand.* 134: 575–576.

Schiaffino, S., Gorza, L., and Ausoni, S. (1990). Muscle fiber types expressing different myosin heavy chain isoforms. Their functional properties and adaptive capacity. In *The Dynamic State of Muscle Fibers*. Edited by D. Pette. New York, Walter de Gruyter, pp. 329–341.

Seedorf, U., Leberer, E., Kirschbaum, B. J., and Pette, D. (1986). Neural control of gene expression in skeletal muscle. *Biochem. J.* 239: 115–120.

Shoshan, V., Maclennan, D. H., and Wood, D. S. (1981). A proton gradient controls a calcium release channel in sarcoplasmic reticulum. *Proc. Natl. Acad. Sci. USA* 78: 4828–4832.

Sieck, G. C. (1988). Diaphragm muscle: Structural and functional organization. *Clin. Chest Med.* 9: 195–210.

Sieck, G. C. (1991). Diaphragm motor units and their response to altered use. *Semin. Respir. Med.* 12: 258–269.

Sieck, G. C., Fournier, M., and Blanco, C. E. (1991). Diaphragm muscle fatigue resistance during postnatal development. *J. Appl. Physiol.* 71: 458–464.

Simoneau, J.-A., Hood, D. A., and Pette, D. (1990). Species-specific responses in enzyme activities of anaerobic and aerobic energy metabolism to increased contractile activity. In *Biochemistry of Exercise VII*. Edited by A. W. Taylor, P. D. Gollnick, H. J. Green, C. D. Ianuzzo, E. G. Noble, G. Metivier, and J. R. Sutton. Champaign, IL, Human Kinetic Books, pp. 95–104.

Staron, R. S., Gohlsch, B., and Pette, D. (1987). Myosin polymorphism in single fibers of chronically stimulated rabbit fast-twitch muscle. *Pflugers Arch.* 408: 444–450.

Sugiura, T., Morimoto, A., Sakata, Y., Watanabe, T., and Murakami, N. (1990). Myosin heavy chain isoform changes in rat diaphragm are induced by endurance training. *Jpn. J. Physiol.* 40: 759–763.

Supinski, G. S. (1988). Respiratory muscle blood flow. *Clin. Chest Med.* 9: 211–223.

Sweeney, H. L., Kushmerick, M. J., Mabuchi, K., Gergely, J., and Sreter, F. A. (1986). Velocity of shortening and myosin isozymes in two types of rabbit fast-twitch muscle fibers. *Am. J. Physiol.* 251: C431–434.

Takahashi, M., and Hood, D. A. (1993). Chronic stimulation-induced changes in cardiolipin, mitochondrial enzymes and performance in rat skeletal muscle. *J. Appl. Physiol.* 74: 934–941.

Tamaki, N. (1987). Effect of endurance training on muscle fiber type composition and capillary supply in rat diaphragm. *Eur. J. Appl. Physiol.* 56: 127–131.

Terjung, R. L., and Hood, D. A. (1986). Biochemical adaptations in skeletal muscle induced by exercise training. In *Nutrition and Aerobic Exercise*. Edited by D. K. Layman. Washington, DC, American Chemical Society, pp. 8–27.

Trimm, J., Soloma, G., and Abramson, J. (1986). Sulfhydryl oxidation induces calcium release from sarcoplasmic reticulum vesicles. *J. Biol. Chem.* 261:16092–16098.

Tullson, P. C., and Terjung, R. L. (1990). Adenine nucleotide degradation in striated muscle. *Int. J. Sports Med.* 11: S47–55.

Vergara, J., Tsien, R. Y., and Delay, M. (1985). Inositol 1,4,5-trisphosphate: A possible chemical link in excitation–contraction coupling in muscle. *Proc. Natl. Acad. Sci. USA* 82: 6252–6356.

Viires, N., Murciano, D., Seta, J.-P., Dureuil, B., Pariente, R., and Aubier, M. (1988). Effects of Ca^{2+} withdrawal on diaphragmatic fiber tension generation. *J. Appl. Physiol.* 64: 26–30.

Vollestad, N. K., and Sejersted, O. M. (1988). Biochemical correlates of fatigue. *Eur. J. Appl. Physiol.* 57: 336–347.

Volpe, P., Salviati, G., Di Virgilio, F., and Pozzan, T. (1985). Inositol 1,4,5-trisphosphate induces calcium release from sarcoplasmic reticulum of skeletal muscle. *Nature* 316: 347–349.

Whalen, R. G., Toutant, M., Gutler-Browne, G. S., and Watkins, S. C. (1985). Hereditary pituitary dwarfism in mice affects skeletal and cardiac myosin isozyme transitions differently. *J. Cell Biol.* 101: 603–609.

Wheeler, T. J., and Lowenstein, J. M. (1979). Adenylate deaminase from rat muscle. *J. Biol. Chem.* 254: 8994–8999.

Wicks, K. L., and Hood, D. A. (1991). Mitochondrial adaptations in denervated muscle: Relationship to performance. *Am. J. Physiol.* 260: C841–C850.

Williams, H. M., and Ianuzzo, C. D. (1988). The effects of triiodothyronine on cultured neonatal rat cardiac myocytes. *J. Mol. Cell. Cardiol.* 20: 689–699.

Williams, R. S., Salmons, S., Newsholme, E. A., Kaufman, R. E., and Mellor, J. (1986). Regulation of nuclear and mitochondrial gene expression by contractile activity in skeletal muscle. *J. Biol. Chem.* 261: 376–380.

Williams, R. S., Garcia-Moll, M., Mellor, J., Salmons, S., and Harlan, W. (1987). Adaptation of skeletal muscle to increased contractile activity. *J. Biol. Chem.* 262: 2764–2767.

Yamamoto, S., and Greef, K. (1981). Effect of intracellular sodium on calcium uptake in isolated guinea pig diaphragm and atria. *Biochim. Biophys. Acta* 646: 348–352.

Zavecz, J. H., Anderson, W. M., and Adams, B. (1991). Effect of amiloride on diaphragmatic contractility: Evidence of a role for Na^+–Ca^{2+} exchange. *J. Appl. Physiol.* 70: 1309–1314.

12

Oxygen-Derived Free Radicals and the Respiratory Muscles

GERALD S. SUPINSKI and A. ANZUETO

Case Western Reserve University
Metrohealth Medical Center
Cleveland, Ohio

I. Introduction

The toxic effects of exogenous free radical compounds on biological tissues have been known for decades, but the extent to which endogenously generated oxygen-derived free radicals play an important role in mediating tissue damage in many common pathophysiological conditions has only recently been appreciated. It is now recognized, for example, that reestablishment of normal levels of blood flow to ischemic organs can often increase the amount of tissue dysfunction present (Southern, 1988). This "reperfusion" injury is produced largely by hydroxyl radicals formed during the period of reperfusion. Studies have shown that this mechanism may account for tissue injury following ischemia–reperfusion in several vital organs, including the heart, kidney, brain, and intestines (Gaudeul and Duvelleroy, 1984; Baker et al., 1985; Domanska-Janik and Wideman, 1974; Granger et al., 1980). In addition, oxygen-derived free radicals are thought to play a role in mediating tissue injury produced in response to neutrophils, fatty acids, arachidonic acid, hyperoxia, and in response to ionizing radiation (Smith et al., 1989b; Badwey et al., 1984; Kontos and Hess, 1983; White et al., 1989; Yau and Mencl, 1981).

Recent studies have suggested that oxygen-derived free radicals may also mediate or modulate several forms of respiratory muscle dysfunction, including the reductions in muscle contractility observed following periods of strenuous contrac-

349

tion and in response to systemic infections (Reid et al., 1992a,b; Shindoh et al., 1990, 1992; Anzueto et al., 1992; Surell et al., 1992). Although this is an emerging field with a relatively small published literature, a review of this subject matter is important because free radical-mediated respiratory muscle dysfunction may prove to be both common in clinical practice and preventable through the administration of appropriate free radical scavengers.

The purpose of this chapter is to review free radical biology, with an emphasis on the role played by oxygen-derived free radicals in mediating clinically relevant forms of respiratory muscle dysfunction. The first few sections of the chapter describe the chemical species of oxygen free radicals involved in producing tissue injury, the cellular pathways by which these substances are produced, the mechanisms by which free radicals damage cellular constituents, methods of detecting free radicals, and the use of scavengers to block free radical effects. Because free radical-mediated cardiac muscle damage has been more extensively studied than that for limb or respiratory musculature, we also briefly review the literature concerning free radical injury to cardiac muscle. We then discuss the role of free radicals in producing several types of limb and respiratory skeletal muscle dysfunction (that dysfunction produced by ischemia or reperfusion, strenuous contraction, and sepsis). Finally, we discuss the potential for future research into the relation between oxygen-derived free radicals and respiratory muscle function.

II. Biology of Free Radicals

A. Species of Oxygen-Derived Free Radicals

Chemically, any compound or atom with an orbit containing a single unpaired electron is a *free radical* (Grisham and McCord, 1986). By convention, a single dot is often appended to the chemical name if a molecule is a free radical containing a single unpaired electron (e.g., Pb·). Free radicals may be electrically neutral (Pb·), positively charged, or negatively charged (OH⁻·), and may be either organic (ArO·) or inorganic (Pb·) in composition. Free radicals are generally highly reactive, since compounds containing unpaired electrons are energetically unstable. In addition, reaction of one free radical with a nonradical neutral compound can produce a second free radical compound. The second free radical can, in turn, react with additional nonfree radical molecules, initiating a chain of reactions that is terminated only when the free radical product of the chain combines with yet another free radical. In this fashion, a single free radical can chemically modify a large number of compounds. As will be shown later in this discussion, such chain reactions are responsible for producing lipid peroxidation and membrane damage in biological systems in response to free radicals.

Although many free radicals have biologically relevant effects, the most physiologically important are a group of "oxygen-derived" free radicals. This group includes superoxide anion radicals (O_2^-·), that are generated by transfer of a single electron to molecular oxygen (O_2) as well as hydroxyl radicals and singlet oxygen (Freeman and Crapo, 1982). Although hydrogen peroxide has no unpaired electron, it is also customary to include hydrogen peroxide along with the "true" oxygen-derived free radicals when discussing the biological relevance of these molecules. This is because the reaction sequences responsible for generating superoxide and hydroxyl radicals are intimately related to the production and degradation of hydrogen peroxide. In addition to hydrogen peroxide, there are several other toxic, nonradical compounds that can be derived from superoxide and hydroxyl anions and can produce damage in biological systems (e.g., the hypohalous anions including $HOCl^-$) (Klebanoff, 1975). We will briefly discuss the biochemistry of each of these oxygen-derived species.

The superoxide anion plays a central role in the chemistry of oxygen free radicals both because this anion is generated in large quantities by several biological pathways and, also, because this anion serves as the normal precursor for most of the other oxygen-derived free radical compounds. The superoxide radical is an unstable species, having a half-life of a few milliseconds at a neutral pH (Klebanoff, 1980). This molecule spontaneously dismutates to produce H_2O_2 and molecular oxygen (O_2) by the following reaction:

$$2O_2^- \cdot + 2H+ \rightarrow H_2O_2 + O_2 \tag{1}$$

The rate constant for this reaction is relatively high (2×10^2 M/s), with the result that superoxide formation is always accompanied by the formation of hydrogen peroxide (H_2O_2). Superoxide itself can act as an oxidant or reductant, but usually with a low reactivity compared with that of its products (i.e., hydrogen peroxide and hydroxyl radicals). Superoxide anions do not abstract hydrogen from lipid membranes directly, and it cannot directly enter the interior of membrane-bound structures, because these molecules are charged and have a high molecular weight. Nevertheless, this species reacts with and can inactivate a number of cell constituents, including tRNase, RNase, and the NADH–LDH complex (Kellogg and Fridovich, 1977; Lavalle et al., 1973; Fantone and Ward, 1982). In addition, superoxide can cross cell membranes by anion transport channels.

Hydrogen peroxide is produced by the degradation of superoxide anions, according to the foregoing reaction [Eq. (1)]. This reaction is markedly accelerated in the presence of the enzyme superoxide dismutase, with a concomitant increase in the production of hydrogen peroxide. Hydrogen peroxide is a strong oxidant that can damage macromolecules by oxidizing sulfhydryl groups (Lavalle et al., 1973; Stocks and Dormandy, 1971). Unlike superoxide, this latter compound is relatively stable, providing that trace metals (e.g., iron, copper) are not present.

Superoxide radicals and hydrogen peroxide serve as precursors for the formation of hydroxyl radicals by the iron-catalyzed Haber–Weiss reaction:

$$O_2^- \cdot + Fe^{3+} \rightarrow O_2 + Fe^{2+}$$
$$H_2O_2 + Fe^{2+} \rightarrow HO\cdot + OH^- + Fe^{3+} \tag{2}$$

In addition to being catalyzed by free iron and other trace metals, this reaction can proceed in the presence of various iron-containing compounds, including $ADP-Fe^{3+}$, hemoglobin, ferritin, and transferrin (Tien and Aust, 1982; Thomas et al., 1985; Motohashi and Mori, 1983). The hydroxyl ions formed by this reaction are extremely reactive and capable of combining with most organic compounds. Because of this high reactivity, the hydroxyl radical is probably responsible for most radical-mediated cell toxicity in biological systems (Fong et al., 1973). Hydroxyl radicals can oxidize sulfhydryl side groups, forming sulfur-to-sulfur cross-linkages and, thereby, inactivating or altering the function of enzymes and other protein cellular constituents (Carp and Janoff, 1979; Armstrong and Buchanan, 1978; Bielski and Shiue, 1979). This radical also reacts with nucleic acids, damaging DNA and RNA (Van Hemmen and Meuling, 1975). Some carbohydrate moieties (e.g., mucopolysaccharides) are also susceptible to degradation by hydroxyl radicals (Cross et al., 1984).

Probably the most important biological mechanism by which hydroxyl radicals produce cellular damage, however, is by the reaction of these ions with the lipid constituents of cellular membranes (Fridovich, 1978; Fong et al., 1973; Kellogg and Fridovich, 1975; Chance et al., 1979). Membrane lipid peroxidation is initiated by the reaction of a hydroxyl ion with, and removal of a hydrogen ion from, one of the CH_2 groups located adjacent to a double bond in a lipid molecule (lipid molecules are designated by L in the following reaction sequences). Such removal leaves behind an unpaired electron, and produces an alkyl radical (L·):

$$HO· + LH \rightarrow H_2O + L· \tag{3}$$

This alkyl radical can undergo a molecular rearrangement, with formation of a second double bond, conjugated to the first. Such conjugated dienes readily react with oxygen to form peroxyl lipid radicals (LOO·), which can further react with other lipid molecules:

$$L· + O_2 \rightarrow LOO·$$
$$LOO· + LH \rightarrow LOOH + L· \tag{4}$$

The alkyl radical produced by this latter reaction [Eq. (4)] can, in turn, generate additional lipid peroxy radicals, with this cycle repeated multiple times. This cycle can be terminated by reaction of two radicals with each other:

$$L· + L· \rightarrow L-L, \text{ or}$$
$$L· + LOOH \rightarrow LOO-L \tag{5}$$

The net result of these reaction sequences is the extensive peroxidation of lipid molecules and the formation of cross-linkages between lipids. Moreover, the lipid peroxides formed by these reactions can further react with iron-centered complexes $(X-Fe^{2+})$, in the same way that hydrogen peroxide reacts with iron-containing compounds:

$$LOOH + X-Fe^{2+} \rightarrow L=O + X-Fe^{3+} + OH^- · \tag{6}$$

This last reaction generates lipid aldehydes (L=O), such as malondialdehyde and, also, produces a hydroxyl radical, which can then initiate a new round of lipid peroxidation. Extensive peroxidation of membrane lipids in this fashion by hydroxyl radicals results in alterations in membrane permeability (Hicks and Gebicki, 1978). With more severe damage, membrane rupture and cellular death may occur.

Another toxic group of compounds that can be derived from oxygen free radicals are hypohalous acids. Hypohalous compounds (e.g., hypochlorous acid, HOCL) are formed by reactions using hydrogen peroxide and halide anions as substrates and is catalyzed by certain tissue peroxidases (Strauss et al., 1970; Selvaraj et al., 1974):

$$H_2O_2 + CL^- \rightarrow HOCL + OH^- \tag{7}$$

One important catalyst of this reaction is myeloperoxidase (MPO), an enzyme contained in the azurophilic granules of neutrophils (Selvaraj et al., 1980). Activation of neutrophils by complement or by antibody-coated bacteria leads to release of MPO and hydrogen peroxide into the extracellular space (Strauss et al., 1970). Chloride ions in the extracellular medium can then be oxidized by an MPO-catalyzed reaction, producing hypochlorous acid (HOCl). Hypochlorous acid is several times more reactive than hydrogen peroxide, and is capable of oxidizing a wide variety of organic compounds: thereby, damaging cells.

A final oxygen-derived free radical species that may play some role in producing injury in biological systems is singlet oxygen (Van Hemmen and Meuling, 1975). Singlet oxygen (O_2:) is a form of molecular oxygen containing two orbits, each with a single unpaired electron. Singlet oxygen can react with conjugated double bond-containing compounds to produce hydroperoxides (Kellogg and Fridovich, 1975).

B. Sources of Oxygen-Derived Free Radicals

In the foregoing section we have described reaction sequences by which hydrogen peroxide, hydroxyl radicals, hypochlorous acid, and a variety of lipid peroxidation by-products, all can be produced within cells as a consequence of a series of reactions that use superoxide anions as an initial substrate. This section will discuss the cellular pathways by which cells generate superoxide anions; thereby initiating the reaction sequences that ultimately produce tissue injury. These pathways include the generation of superoxide anions by (1) the mitochondrial electron transport chain; (2) the xanthine oxidase-catalyzed conversion of hypoxanthine to xanthine; (3) white blood cell NADPH oxidase; (4) the microsomal P-450 system; (5) several membrane-bound NADH- and NADPH-dependent enzymes; and (6) as a by-product of arachidonic acid metabolism.

Oxygen free radicals are a normal intermediary in mitochondrial oxidative phosphorylation (Turrens and Boveris, 1980). The first step by which oxygen is reduced by the electron transport chain involves the reaction of molecular oxygen with a semiquinone radical, with the formation of superoxide anion radicals:

$$\text{Hydroquinone} + \text{cytochrome } c^{3+} \rightarrow \text{Semiquinone radical} + H^+ \tag{8}$$

$$\text{Semiquinone radical} + O_2 \rightarrow \text{Ubiquinone} + O_2^{-} \cdot {}^{+\,H+} \tag{9}$$

Normally, the electron transport chain reduces oxygen completely (i.e., to form H_2O) by subsequently supplying three additional electrons to these superoxide anions. Approximately 95–99% of oxygen molecules involved in oxidative phosphorylation in normal resting tissues are fully reduced in this fashion. These oxygen molecules remain bound to the enzymes of the oxygen transport chain until fully reduced, and present no danger to cellular structures. The remaining 1–5% of oxygen molecules are not further reduced beyond the ubiquinone step and leave the oxygen transport chain as superoxide anions. The rate of this superoxide anion production or "electron leakage" is proportional to the partial pressure of oxygen in the mitochondria, with a lower rate of production (i.e., 1%) at normal atmospheric concentrations of oxygen (21% O_2) and at a higher rate in the presence of 100% oxygen (Fridovich, 1976). The superoxide anions produced in this fashion can react with mitochondrial membranes and, if present in sufficient quantities, can also damage other cellular structures and even cause cell death. For example, superoxide anions generated by this pathway are thought to play an important role in mediating the lung injury observed following the prolonged inhalation of high concentrations of inspired oxygen (White and Repine, 1985). It has been postulated that the superoxide leakage from this chain may also increase under conditions in which total cellular oxygen utilization increases, for example, during exercise.

Another pathway by which superoxide is generated in living tissues is as a by-product of the xanthine oxidase-catalyzed conversion of hypoxanthine to xanthine and, thence, to uric acid:

$$\text{Xanthine oxidase}$$
$$\text{Hypoxanthine} + H_2O + 2O_2 \rightarrow \text{Xanthine} + 2O_2^{-} \cdot \tag{10}$$

This pathway is thought to play an important role in mediating the free radical generation and cellular damage observed following periods of transient tissue ischemia (Parks and Granger, 1983). It is important to note that free radicals are formed primarily during the period of reperfusion that follows the ischemic episode, an observation that can be accounted for by considering the effects of ischemia and reperfusion on cellular concentrations of the substrates for the foregoing reaction [i.e., Eq. (10)]. During periods of ischemia, oxidative regeneration of ATP from ADP is impaired, and ADP is catabolized by a reaction sequence that culminates with the formation of adenosine:

$$\text{ATP} \rightarrow \text{ADP} \rightarrow \text{AMP} \rightarrow \text{Adenosine}$$

The adenosine produced by this pathway diffuses out of the cells of the ischemic organ (e.g., the heart) and enters adjacent endothelial cells. In the endothelium, adenosine is converted to hypoxanthine.

Xanthine oxidase normally exists in nonischemic healthy cells predominantly as an NAD^+-dependent dehydrogenase (xanthine dehydrogenase) (Parks et al., 1988). This form of the enzyme uses NAD^+ instead of O_2 as the electron acceptor during oxidation of purines and does not produce superoxide or hydrogen peroxide. As endothelial ATP levels decline, cellular calcium-ATPase activity is reduced, and movement of calcium into the cell cytoplasm occurs. This calcium is thought to activate a calcium-dependent protease that converts endothelial xanthine dehydrogenase to xanthine oxidase (Fox et al., 1987; McCord, 1985; Chambers et al., 1985). As a result, as ischemia progresses, endothelial levels of xanthine oxidase and hypoxanthine increase. With reperfusion, molecular oxygen is resupplied to this reaction mixture, driving the conversion of hypoxanthine to xanthine [see Eq. (10)] and causing the formation of large quantities of superoxide anions. Free radicals, generated by these reaction pathways, have been implicated as a mediator of injury resulting from ischemia and reperfusion to various organs including the brain, heart, limb muscle, skin, liver, intestine, and kidney.

The generation of superoxide anions by the xanthine oxidase-mediated conversion of hypoxanthine to xanthine appears to have only deleterious effects on living tissues. Under some circumstances, however, free radical production is useful. For example, free radicals play an important role in defending against infections, and constitute one of the major products of neutrophils. Neutrophils generate superoxide anion radicals and release these anions, along with the enzyme myeloperoxidase (MPO), into the surrounding medium when activated. Superoxide dismutates to form hydrogen peroxide, which serves, in turn, for the myeloperoxidase-catalyzed formation of hypochlorous acid. These reaction products (superoxide, hydrogen peroxide, and hypochlorous acid) then act to damage the targets of the activated white cells. Neutrophils also have an enzyme located on the cell surface, NADPH oxidase, which produces superoxide anions by the following reaction:

$$\text{NADPH oxidase}$$
$$2O_2 + NADPH \rightarrow 2O_2^- \cdot + NADP^+ + H^+ \tag{11}$$

Once released from white cells, however, free radicals act indiscriminantly and can damage whatever cells lie adjacent to neutrophils, including normal tissues. As a result, activated neutrophils can sometimes act as agents producing or amplifying tissue injury initiated by other biophysical mechanisms. For example, activated neutrophils are thought to contribute to the tissue injury associated with ischemia and reperfusion. White cells can attach to endothelium initially damaged by other mechanisms (e.g., by free radicals generated by the xanthine–xanthine oxidase system). These white cells can then be stimulated by other metabolites released as a consequence of ischemia. For example, phospholipase A_2 is activated by the increased cytosolic calcium concentrations present in tissue during ischemia. This lipase releases arachidonic acid from the outer cell membrane, leading to the generation of leukotrienes, chemotaxins, and white cell activators as arachidonic acid is metabolized by cyclooxygenase and lipooxygenase pathways. The resultant activated white cells then release additional free radicals and MPO, amplifying the tissue damage produced by the initial episode of ischemia and reperfusion. As a result, reperfusion injury appears to be mediated by both reactive oxygen metabolites and activated polymorphonuclear leukocytes.

Another important source of free radicals is the microsomal P-450 system, which generates superoxide by an NADPH-dependent reaction. This source of free radicals plays a role in mediating the damage produced by several cellular toxins. This pathway also participates in free radical production and tissue damage in response to oxygen administration.

Free radicals are also produced as a by-product of arachidonic acid metabolism, specifically, as a product of the conversion of prostaglandin (PG) G_2 to PGH_2. This latter reaction sequence is an important source of free radicals in the brain following periods of ischemia (Kontos, 1985).

C. Measurement of Free Radical Generation

Because free radicals, and hydroxyl radicals in particular, are short-lived species with a high reactivity, it is difficult to directly measure the concentrations of these species in organs. As a result, a variety of experimental approaches have been developed to indirectly assess free radical generation in tissues or to infer a role for free radicals in producing a given type of tissue damage. One approach that has been used is to compare the ability of a series of free radical scavengers to prevent a given injury. If, for example, such damage can be prevented by the administration of active superoxide dismutase (which reduces superoxide concentrations), but is unaffected by administration of an appropriate control (i.e., denatured superoxide dismutase), then an argument can be made that superoxide anions are involved in producing that particular form of injury.

Since several oxygen-derived free radicals and free radical breakdown products (e.g., superoxide anion, hydrogen peroxide, and hydroxyl radical) can produce damage, and each of these species is scavenged by different substances, it is common to assess the effects of a battery of free radical scavengers on a given form of damage to determine which free radical species may be implicated in inducing cellular damage. As an example, many studies have examined the response to superoxide dismutase, catalase, and either dimethyl sulfoxide or mannitol. Choice of these particular scavengers is based on the fact that superoxide anions are specifically scavenged by superoxide dismutase, hydrogen peroxide levels are reduced by catalase administration, and hydroxyl radicals are scavenged by compounds such as dimethyl sulfoxide and mannitol. If, for example, superoxide anions per se are responsible for a given form of tissue injury, superoxide dismutase administration will prevent such injury, but dimethyl sulfoxide will have no effect. Similarly, if hydrogen peroxide alone is responsible for inducing injury, substances catalyzing the degradation of hydrogen peroxide (e.g., catalase) will obviate such injury, but hydroxyl radical scavengers should have little effect. If, however, hydroxyl radicals are responsible for inducing injury, then administration of either superoxide or hydroxyl radical scavengers should be efficacious in preventing such injury (Beckman and Freeman, 1986).

A somewhat more direct approach to assessing free radical formation has been to employ assays that measure the reaction products of free radicals with other compounds. One such assay is the measurement of the ferrocytochrome *c* formed after incubation of ferricytochrome *c* with a solution suspected of containing or generating superoxide anions (Taylor and Townsley, 1986):

$$\text{Ferricytochrome } c + O_2^- \cdot \rightarrow \text{Ferrocytochrome } c + O_2$$

The amount of ferrocytochrome formed by this reaction is proportional to the concentration of superoxide present.

Other assays based on this same concept include (1) assessment of the reduction of nitroblue tetrazolium by superoxide anions, (2) measurement of hydrogen peroxide production by determining the rate of formation of the cytochrome *c* peroxidase–hydrogen peroxide complex after adding cytochrome *c* peroxidase to medium containing hydrogen peroxide, (3) measurement of hydrogen peroxide by determining the rate of oxidation of ferrocyanide to ferricyanide, (4) measurement of hydroxyl anion formation by determining the formation of products of the reaction of hydroxyl anions with dimethyl sulfoxide, and (5) assessment of hydroxyl radical formation by determining its reaction with salicylate (Fantone and Ward, 1982; Forman and Boveris, 1982; Bernard et al., 1984; Richmond et al., 1981). This last assay is based on the fact that hydroxyl radicals readily react with aromatic rings, combining with hydrobenzoic acid (salicylic acid) to form 2,3-dihydroxybenzoic acid.

There have been several reports of electrodes designed to specifically measure the concentrations of superoxide anions and of hydrogen peroxide in suspensions (Green et al., 1984). In addition, chemiluminescence techniques have been developed to demonstrate the production of free radicals in solutions (Townsley et al., 1985).

Free radicals can also be assayed by use of spin resonance techniques. The unpaired electrons in free radicals absorb and emit radiation at fixed wavelengths when switching between spin states, producing a characteristic electron spin resonance spectrum. Although hydroxyl and superoxide anion radicals have extremely short half-lives, some of the free radicals produced by reaction of these species with other compounds are longer-lived, and more amenable to detection by spin resonance spectra. Therefore, it is possible to supply the precursors to these more long-lasting radicals (termed spin traps) to a reaction medium containing oxygen-derived free radicals and use electron spin resonance techniques to quantitate the long-lived radicals produced. For example, superoxide anions react with (5,5-dimethyl-1-pyrroline-1-oxide (DMPO) to produce a semistable radical that can be detected by electron spin resonance (Rosen and Freeman, 1984). Similarly, lipid free radicals can be trapped using phenyl-*N-tert*-butylnitrone, whereas hydroxyl anions can be trapped using DMPO.

Most of the techniques listed are most useful for detecting free radical generation in in vitro systems or in media containing suspensions of cells. Spin traps have also been used to detect free radicals (i.e., superoxide anions) in the venous effluents of several organs. It is more difficult, however, to detect free radical formation within whole organs by using these techniques. One approach to indirectly assessing free radical generation in whole organs has been to measure the concentrations of tissue products of free radical reaction with cellular constituents. For example, a number of lipid peroxidation products have been found in a variety of tissues damaged by processes involving free radical generation (Luo and Hultin, 1986). These assayable lipid peroxidation products include conjugated dienes, malondialdehyde, and volatile hydrocarbons (pentane and ethane).

The measurement of conjugated dienes (Brattin et al., 1985), as an index of free radical-mediated lipid peroxidation, is based on the fact the lipids normally do not have any "conjugated" diene bonds, but such a diene bond configuration can result following free radical reaction with membrane lipids. The free radical lipid intermediate rearranges to the energetically more favorable conjugated diene conformation, with either a *cis–trans* or a *trans-trans* geometry:

"Normal"   lipid   Conjugated   diene

$$-C=CCC=C- \ + \ O_2^{-\cdot} \ \rightarrow \ -C=CC=C- \ + \ H_2O_2 \tag{12}$$

Conjugated diene bonds have light absorbance at 242- and 233-nm wavelengths permitting the spectrophotometric detection of compounds containing these bonds (Corogin et al., 1989).

The thiobarbituric acid assay has also been used extensively to measure tissue lipid peroxidation breakdown products (Ohkawa, 1979). Malondialdehyde is usually used to calibrate this assay, and these thiobarbituric acid reaction products (TBAR) are often expressed as "malondialdehyde" levels. It is clear, however, that thiobarbituric acid reacts with several substances other than malondialdehyde, including other lipid peroxidation products and other cellular constituents. Other assays (fluorescent techniques or high-performance liquid chromatography; HPLC) have been used to measure malondialdehyde levels, and these newer techniques have the advantage of more specifically measuring malondialdehyde.

Lipid peroxides formed by reaction of free radicals with cellular lipids are unstable and can decompose in the presence of iron-containing proteins, liberating pentane and other small, volatile hydrocarbons. The efficacy of iron-containing heme compounds (cytochromes, hematin) in causing lipid hydroperoxide decomposition to volatile hydrocarbons is comparable with the relative ability of these substances to initiate lipid peroxidation in the presence of hydroxyl anions (O'Brien and Rahimtula, 1975). An example of such a reaction is the formation of pentane from linolenic acid:

$$CH_3(CH_2)_4COOH\text{-}R + Fe^{+2} \rightarrow CH_3(CH_2)_4C\text{-}O\cdot R + Fe^{+3} + OH^-$$
$$CH_3(CH_2)_4C\text{-}O\cdot\text{-}R \rightarrow CH_3(CH_2)_3\dot{C}H_2$$
$$CH_3(CH_2)_3\dot{C}H_2 + H \rightarrow CH_3(CH_2)_3CH_3 \ (\text{pentane}) \tag{13}$$

In addition, ethane is produced from the degradation of linoleic acid, octane from oleic acid, pentene and butane from myristoleic acid and heptane and hexane from vaccenic acid. These volatile hydrocarbons readily cross cell membranes, easily dissolve in plasma, and are eliminated in expired air. Hydrocarbon gases present in expired air samples can then be separated and identified by gas–liquid chromatographic techniques (Wispe et al., 1985). Several studies have shown detectable levels of volatile hydrocarbons in the expired gases of humans and animals subjected to stresses known to elicit free radical production. For example, Dillard et al. found more pentane and ethane in the expired gas of rats fed a low vitamin E diet, a condition known to induce free radical formation in tissues, than in the expired gas of rats fed a diet supplemented with high levels of vitamin E (Dillard et al., 1977).

Finally, free radical generation stresses cellular antioxidant defense systems, causing a decrease in reduced glutathione levels, an increase in the concentration of oxidized glutathione (GSSG), and a reduction in cellular levels of vitamin E (Thomas et al., 1985). Demonstration of changes in levels of antioxidant cellular constituents, therefore, provides indirect evidence for free radical generation. In addition, the overall rate of lipid peroxidation can also be monitored by measuring the rate of loss of unsaturated fatty acids from cells.

D. Free Radical Scavengers

There are several natural substances and pharmacological agents that are capable of inactivating oxygen free radicals and, thereby, protecting tissues from the deleterious effects of these compounds. These include superoxide dismutase, catalase, α-tocopherol, dimethyl sulfoxide, dimethylthiourea, N-acetylcysteine, the glutathione–redox system, and mannitol. In addition, some forms of free radical generation can be prevented by the administration of agents that block specific cellular pathways responsible for generating superoxide anions. An example of this latter class of substances is allopurinol, which blocks xanthine oxidase, thereby preventing superoxide formation as a by-product of the metabolism of hypoxanthine to uric acid in the presence of xanthine oxidase. We will briefly review the effects and mechanisms of action of several of these free radical scavengers in this section.

Superoxide dismutase is a naturally occurring constituent of cells that acts to catalyze the dismutation of the superoxide anion radical according to the following equation:

$$2O_2^- \cdot + 2H^+ \rightarrow H_2O_2 + O_2 \tag{14}$$

This enzyme has two forms, a manganese-containing enzyme that is localized to mitochondria and a copper–zinc-containing enzyme found primarily in the cytoplasm (McCord, 1974). Although most of the latter enzyme is located within cells, small amounts of this enzyme (e.g., approximately 5% of the dismutase in the lung) may be located extracellularly. Both molecules have a high molecular weight and penetrate cell membranes poorly, with the result that extracellular superoxide dismutase (SOD) generally does not enter cells, and that SOD contained within cells does not normally leach into the extracellular space.

Since SOD reduces concentrations of potentially toxic superoxide anion radicals, one might think it possible to reduce superoxide-mediated tissue damage by pharmacologically augmenting tissue levels of this enzyme. The capacity of such administration to provide protection from the effects of free radicals is obviously diminished, however, by the short half-life and poor cellular penetrability of intravenously administered SOD.

There are several factors, however, that may facilitate the effects of intravenously administered enzyme scavengers. For one thing, some free radicals can cross cell membranes (e.g., superoxide can be transported through the anion channel to the extracellular space) and scavengers may, in some cases, act principally to destroy these extracellular radicals. Second, in many pathophysiological states, free radical production may be principally localized to the perivascular space and, therefore, would be amenable to inactivation by blood-borne scavengers. For example, free radicals produced by endothelial cells or released by activated neutrophils may be concentrated in the extracellular, perivascular space.

Another method of facilitating the action of intravenously administered superoxide dismutase is by administering either polyethylene glycol-conjugated superoxide dismutase (PEG–SOD) or by encapsulating superoxide dismutase in liposomes (Tamura et al., 1988; Turrens et al., 1984). Conjugation with PEG markedly increases the circulating half-life of SOD (from minutes to days) and may also facilitate entry of these substances into cells. In addition, polyethylene glycol also appears to act as a weak scavenger, reacting with and detoxifying hydroxyl anions (White et al., 1989). Liposomal encapsulation even further increases cellular penetration, since liposomes can be taken into cells by membrane fusion or endocytosis (Yatvin and Lelkes, 1982). Several studies have found that intravenously administered liposomal and PEG-adsorbed forms of SOD are capable of protecting tissue from forms of oxidant-induced injury.

Catalase is an iron-centered enzyme that catalyzes the degradation of hydrogen peroxide to water and molecular oxygen:

$$2H_2O_2 \rightarrow O_2 + 2H_2O \tag{15}$$

This enzyme specifically degrades hydrogen peroxide, and will not decompose organic hydroperoxides (Chance and Boveris, 1979). Catalase is contained in subcellular peroxisomes and, similar to SOD, is a high molecular weight compound, with a short intravenous half-life and an inability to cross cellular membranes. Also like SOD, a polyethylene glycol-adsorbed form of catalase has been developed that has a much longer intravenous half-life, and may prove to be a more effective means of pharmacologically augmenting cellular defenses against hydrogen peroxide. Note that superoxide dismutase and catalase work in tandem to decompose superoxide anions to hydrogen peroxide and, thence, to nontoxic (water and oxygen) molecules.

Another cellular enzyme capable of degrading hydrogen peroxide is glutathione peroxidase. Glutathione peroxidase is a tetrameric selenoprotein that reduces hydrogen peroxide and other organic peroxides at the expense of the oxidation of GSH to glutathione disulfide (GSSG):

$$H_2O_2 + 2GSH \rightarrow GSSG + 2 H_2O$$
$$ROOH + 2GSH \rightarrow GSSG + ROH + H_2O \tag{16}$$

Another set of enzymes, the glutathione S-transferases, can also participate in the reduction of lipid peroxides, but not of hydrogen peroxide.

For glutathione peroxidase to be effective, adequate cellular levels of glutathione (GSH) must be present. In fact, glutathione is normally the most prevalent thiol compound and most abundant (0.5–10 mM) small peptide present in mammalian cells (Deneke and Fanburg, 1989; Meister, 1989; Pascoe and Reed, 1989). Glutathione is a central substrate for the reduction of disulfide linkages of proteins and other molecules, for the synthesis of deoxyribonucleotide precursors, for the protection of cells against the effects of free radicals and of other reactive oxygen intermediates, and it is also a coenzyme for several enzymes (Meister and Anderson, 1983; Meister, 1989; DiMascio et al., 1988; Pascoe and Reed, 1989).

Glutathione disulfide (GSSG), the product of glutathione peroxidase-catalyzed reactions, is a toxic compound. It can react with protein sulfhydryls by a mixed disulfide reaction, potentially altering protein function (Deneke and Fanburg, 1989). This particular substance has been proposed to participate in the modification of enzymatic activity, making cellular thiol–disulfide status an important regulator of metabolic function (Gilbert, 1982; Ji et al., 1988a).

A third enzyme, glutathione reductase, acts to regenerate reduced glutathione from oxidized glutathione, thereby providing additional substrate for the decomposition of hydrogen peroxide by glutathione peroxidase:

$$GSSG + NADPH + H^+ \rightarrow 2GHS + NADP^+$$

Glutathione reductase has the highest rate of NADPH consumption among the various NADPH-dependent enzymes (Reed, 1986).

Another important defense of membranes and plasma lipoproteins against peroxidation is provided by α-tocopherol. α-Tocopherol is often called vitamin E, but chemical characterization has revealed that four different tocopherols have activity in the rat bioassay (Burton and Ingold, 1986). α-Tocopherol is the most active, and it seems to be the most important lipid-soluble antioxidant in humans (the other antioxidants—such as SOD, catalase, glutathione peroxidase, and ceruloplasmin—operate in the aqueous phase of cells or body fluids). Being a hydrophobic molecule, α-tocopherol localizes into the hydrophobic interior of biological membranes or with the phospholipid content of plasma lipoproteins. Vitamin E is thought to act as a nonspecific intracellular antioxidant by donating protons to free radicals that form in lipid membranes, thereby stopping the destructive chain reactions associated with lipid peroxidation. This molecule possesses a hydroxyl (-OH) group the hydrogen atom of which is easily removed.

As a result, peroxy radicals generated during lipid peroxidation react much faster with α-tocopherol than with adjacent polyunsaturated fatty acid side chains or with membrane proteins. The result is production of a nonreactive tocopherol radical:

Tocopherol-OH + lipid-O· → Lipid-O$_2$H + tocopherol

In addition to these naturally occurring antioxidants, there are various other pharmacological agents that can react with the principal oxygen-derived free radicals (Ziment, 1986). For example, *N*-acetylcysteine is capable of reacting with and detoxifying all three of the primary free radical-derived species. *N*-Acetylcysteine also serves as a glutathione precursor and can replete cellular GSH levels decreased by reaction of glutathione with free radicals. Unlike catalase and superoxide dismutase, however, *N*-acetylcysteine has other actions on cells that are unrelated to its activity as a free radical scavenger. For example, this compound can alter blood flow to some organs, and some of its therapeutic effects may be linked to this action (Harrison et al., 1991).

Dimethyl sulfoxide is a powerful hydroxyl radical scavenger that has a long half-life, a small molecular weight, and good tissue penetrability. Unlike *N*-acetylcysteine, dimethyl sulfoxide (DMSO) does not also scavenge superoxide anions or hydrogen peroxide. Like *N*-acetylcysteine, however, DMSO has effects on cells that are unrelated to its actions as a hydroxyl anion scavenger (Taylor and Townsley, 1986; Neulieb and Neulieb, 1990). Dimethylthiourea and mannitol are also good hydroxyl radical scavengers that, like DMSO, have additional actions unrelated to their effects as scavengers (Fox, 1984). Several analogues of glutathione and *N*-acetylcysteine that appear to be very active scavengers or glutathione precursors have been synthesized. However, these compounds have been used only recently for experimental and clinical work and have only limited availability.

It is also possible to reduce the free radical burden of an organ by blocking the cellular pathways responsible for free radical generation. This last approach to reducing free radical concentrations is pathway-dependent, and agents capable of blocking one source of free radicals will be ineffective against other sources. A good example of this latter type of agent is allopurinol, which blocks xanthine oxidase and, thereby, prevents superoxide generation as the result of hypoxanthine metabolism (DeWall et al., 1971).

The response to allopurinol, however, is fairly variable for ischemia–reperfusion forms of free radical-mediated injury. For example, allopurinol, was ineffective in preventing cardiac injury in dogs caused by ischemia and reperfusion when administered shortly before or at the time of reperfusion (Reimer and Jennings, 1985). The variation in the response to allopurinol is probably the result of several factors. For one thing, oxipurinol, the principal metabolite of allopurinol, appears to produce a far more potent inhibition of superoxide production by xanthine oxidase than allopurinol per se (Spector, 1988). Several hours may be required to convert allopurinol to oxipurinol and, thereby, achieve maximal inhibition of xanthine oxidase. Second, there appears to be marked variation in the xanthine dehydrogenase enzyme levels in different species and different tissues and, also, variability in the rate of conversion of xanthine dehydrogenase to xanthine oxidase. For example, xanthine dehydrogenase is abundant in the hearts of cows (Jarasch et al., 1981) and rats (Hammond and Hess, 1985), but the myocardium in pigs (Das et al., 1987) and rabbits (Downey et al., 1987; Weiss and LoBublio, 1982) lacks this enzyme. In addition, xanthine oxidase-mediated generation of free radicals is only one of the mechanisms by which free radicals are generated during ischemia and reperfusion. Specifically, administration of pterinaldehyde, a specific inhibitor of the conversion of xanthine dehydrogenase to xanthine oxidase, only partially decreased free radical production in enterocytes studied in vitro following deoxygenation–reoxygenation (Riva et al., 1987).

It is also possible to prevent some forms of free radical-mediated tissue damage through the administration of desferoxamine (Fligiel et al., 1984). This agent acts by chelating iron and preventing hydroxyl radical formation by the iron-catalyzed Fenton reaction. Although this approach does nothing to prevent superoxide anion or hydrogen peroxide formation, hydroxyl radicals are the most reactive and toxic oxygen-derived free radical species, and are generally the species most responsible for inducing tissue injury.

III. Free Radical-Mediated Injury in Cardiac Muscle

Although there has been only limited examination of the role of free radicals in producing limb and respiratory muscle dysfunction, extensive study has been made of free radical-mediated damage as a mechanism of myocardial dysfunction following periods of myocardial ischemia. These studies have shown that a form of cardiac damage, akin to that observed following myocardial ischemia, can be produced by free radical-generating solutions, that cellular markers of free radical-mediated lipid peroxidation can be found in the heart following periods of ischemia–reperfusion, and that cardiac damage resulting from ischemia–reperfusion can be reduced by treating hearts with free radical scavengers. This section will review this work and, in addition, will discuss the postulated mechanisms by which free radical-mediated cardiac dysfunction is produced.

Several studies have examined the effect of various free radical-generating solutions on myocardial function. For example, Ytrehus et al. (1987) found that infusion of a mixture of hypoxanthine–xanthine oxidase into the isolated rat heart produces severe myocardial cell damage, with organelle disruption, cellular swelling, and cell death. This group also found that myocardial damage produced in this fashion could be prevented by adding superoxide dismutase and catalase to the infusion containing the free radical-generating solution. Other studies have examined the effects produced by incubation of isolated cardiac cells or subcellular fractions in free radical-generating solutions. For example, incubation of rat myocardial membranes with any one of several free radical-generating solutions (iron–ascorbate, copper and *t*-butylhydroperoxide, soybean lipooxygenase, linoleic acid hydroperoxide; Parinandi et al., 1991) resulted in an increase in cardiac thiobarbituric acid-reactive products and a loss of extractable phospholipids in cardiac membranes. These free radical-generating solutions also produced a loss of membrane peptides and the accumulation of high molecular weight material in membranes. This last finding suggests that cardiac membrane proteins may form high molecular weight adducts with peroxidized membrane phopholipids following exposure to free radicals, causing alterations in membrane integrity and function.

More to the point of demonstrating a role for free radicals in mediating myocardial injury, a host of studies have detected the by-products of free radical reaction with tissue constituents in myocardium following ischemia–reperfusion. Both Rao et al. (1983) and Das et al. (1986) found an accumulation of lipid peroxides in the heart during periods of transient ischemia, including an increase in malondialdehyde levels. In keeping with these findings, Gauduel and Duvelleroy (1984) found that reperfusion of the hypoxic heart was associated with the release of malondialdehyde into the venous effluent. In addition to malondialdehyde, conjugated dienes have been demonstrated in the myocardium following ischemia–reperfusion (Romaschin et al, 1987). Spin resonance techniques have also been used to detect free radical formation following reperfusion of ischemic myocardium. By using electron spin resonance, Zweier et al. (1987a,b,c) have shown that both oxygen- and carbon-containing free radicals are present within the myocardium after ischemia–reperfusion. In addition, several studies employing isolated heart preparations have detected free radicals in the venous effluent of these preparations following cycles of ischemia and reperfusion by using spin traps (e.g., dimethyl-pyroline oxide) (Kramer et al., 1987). Addition of superoxide dismutase to the medium perfusing these hearts prevented the appearance of free radicals in the effluent.

Detection of free radicals or free radical products in the heart following ischemia and reperfusion does not, however, prove a pathophysiological relation between free radical generation and tissue injury. Such evidence has been provided, however, by studies showing that administration of free radical scavengers or xanthine oxidase inhibitors attenuates or prevents the cardiac injury produced by ischemia–reperfusion (Gauduel and Duvelleroy, 1984; Shlafer et al., 1982a,b; Casale et al., 1983; Gallagher et al., 1986; Johnson et al., 1987; Shatner et al., 1976; Akizuki et al., 1985; Menasche et al., 1986; Vander et al., 1987; Zweier et al., 1987d). Studies have found evidence that such administration can provide protection against the effects of ischemia–reperfusion on cardiac contractility, on reperfusion arrhythmias, and on histological and biochemical correlates of myocardial injury. Of some importance, one such study found that administration of polyethylene glycol-adsorbed superoxide dismutase (PEG–SOD) resulted in a considerable reduction in the amount of damaged myocardium followed transient ischemia, and that this salvage was long-lasting (Tamura et al., 1988). This finding of long-lasting salvage suggests that scavenger treatment does not simply delay injury following cardiac reperfusion, but prevents it. The long circulating half-life of PEG–SOD may have been partially responsible for the long-lasting beneficial effects observed in this particular study.

A plausible mechanism to account for the effects of transient ischemia on the heart has recently been formulated (Lefer et al., 1991). According to this theory, ischemia–reperfusion initially evokes free radical generation that damages endothelium (xanthine oxidase-mediated degradation of hypoxanthine may play a role in this initial free radical production). As the result of this damage, production of endothelium-derived relaxation factor (EDRF) is reduced, producing vasoconstriction. White cells may then attach to and be activated by the damaged endothelium, eliciting release of additional free radicals from these cells, producing vascular plugging and additional ischemia, and inducing additional endothelial dysfunction. Cardiac muscle damage results from both the direct (damage to myocardial fibers) and indirect (alterations in microvascular blood flow) consequences of this free radical release and vascular dysfunction.

Several pieces of experimental data support this theory. For example, in one experiment, transient myocardial ischemia was induced in cats by occluding coronary arteries; coronary rings were excised at various time points from these animals, and coronary vascular reactivity in response to acetylcholine (a vasodilator that depends upon EDRF for its effectiveness) was assessed from these rings (Lefer et al., 1991). In these experiments, indices of EDRF release by endothelium decreased after reperfusion, with reductions in acetylcholine responsiveness correlating with the production of superoxide anions. Superoxide dismutase infusion protected animals from the effects of reperfusion, preserving EDRF-dependent vasodilation. When nitrous oxide (a substance that directly relaxes vascular smooth muscle) was administered to rings excised after reperfusion, this substance was capable of inducing coronary vasodilation with or without scavenger administration. This latter piece of evidence indicates that smooth-muscle responsiveness per se was unaffected by ischemia–reperfusion, and reductions in vasodilation were a consequence of free radical-mediated alterations in EDRF metabolism in this experimental model.

Similar findings have been found using other experimental preparations. With a perfused rat heart preparation, one group found minimal defects in the coronary response to acetylcholine following ischemia without reperfusion, but large defects (a 80% reduction in acetylcholine responsiveness) when ischemia was followed by reperfusion (Lefer et al., 1991). Superoxide dismutase administration completely prevented this reduction in acetylcholine responsiveness (i.e., EDRF-dependent vasodilation) following ischemia–reperfusion. Reperfusion with a solution having a low oxygen content did not, however, elicit a fall in EDRF-dependent vasodilation. In addition, a period of perfusion of the coronary bed at constant flow with hypoxemic solutions, followed by reoxygenation, produced effects that were comparable with those induced by ischemia–reperfusion per se. Superoxide dismutase also prevented the dysfunction caused by hypoxemia–reoxygenation in this preparation.

Studies have also shown an important role for white cells as mediators of myocardial dysfunction following ischemia–reperfusion. Mullane et al. (1984) found that occlusion of the left anterior descending artery for 1 h resulted in subsequent leukocyte adhesion to the coronary endothelium and myocardial infiltration of neutrophils. Engler et al. (1986) found that Leukopac filter-induced neutrophil depletion performed before myocardial ischemia–reperfusion had a significant effect on postischemic myocardial function, decreasing edema and arrhythmias. Simpson et al. (1988) found that administration of a monoclonal antibody that binds to leukocyte cell adhesion-promoting glycoprotein (MO1) also reduced infarct size. Romson et al. (1983) found that neutrophil depletion (using neutrophil antiserum) before occlusion of the left anterior descending coronary artery, decreased the size of the resulting myocardial infarct by 45–50%. In addition, administration of a monoclonal antibody to cd18 (an antibody to the β-chain of a protein mediating white cell adhesion to endothelium) reduced vasoconstriction in the heart following ischemia–reperfusion and also reduced endothelial dysfunction. Moreover, infusion of activated white cells into the coronary bed produced a reduction in acetylcholine-dependent relaxation in subsequently excised coronary rings.

Although these results would suggest that white cells produce myocardial injury and potentiate endothelial dysfunction, that the onset of endothelial dysfunction following ischemia–reperfusion precedes myocardial neutrophil accumulation and myocardial necrosis suggests that white cells potentiate, but do not initiate, the vascular dysfunction following myocardial ischemia–reperfusion.

There appear to be several subcellular sites within myocardial cells that are particularly affected by the effects of ischemia–reperfusion. Obviously, cell membranes are particularly susceptible to damage by free radicals (Kukreja et al., 1988; 1989). Moreover, Romaschin et al. (1990) found that lipid peroxidation was more pronounced in the sarcolemma than in mitochondria or in the sarcoplasmic reticulum following ischemia–reperfusion. These authors speculate that this occurs because the sarcolemma has a higher phospholipid/protein ratio and a higher polyunsaturated fatty acid content than mitochondrial or sarcoplasmic reticulum membranes. Even so, these other cellular structures are also susceptible to free radical-mediated damage. For example, free radicals have been reported to attenuate sarcoplasmic reticulum function and alter calcium transport in the isolated heart (Kukreja et al.; 1989; Kagan, 1988).

IV. Free Radical-Mediated Injury in Skeletal Muscle

Free radicals have been postulated to play a role in mediating several types of skeletal muscle dysfunction, including dysfunction induced by transient severe ischemia, strenuous contractions, and systemic infections. In the following sections we will review each of these types of dysfunction, discussing the potential for free radical-mediated respiratory muscle dysfunction caused by these stresses.

A. Free Radical Skeletal Muscle Injury: Ischemia–Reperfusion Injury

The most-studied, best-established type of free radical-mediated skeletal muscle damage is that observed following periods of transient severe ischemia. The impetus for intensive experimental examination of this issue was that this particular stress occurs frequently in various clinical situations (e.g., during transient embolic occlusion, during certain forms of trauma, or during periods of severe hypotension). The remainder of this section will describe the type of muscle injury induced by this stress, the evidence that free radicals mediate this form of damage, and the potential mechanisms by which free radicals are produced and induce damage. We will consider the possibility that this type of injury may, under very specific conditions, contribute to respiratory muscle dysfunction.

There are several alterations in muscle physiology that have been described following periods of transient ischemia. Probably the best-recognized alteration is that some capillaries fail to reperfuse after extended periods of skeletal muscle ischemia and the magnitude of this "no reflow" phenomenon actually worsens for some time after the restoration of blood flow (Sanderson et al., 1975; Bagge et al., 1980; Braide et al., 1984; Strock and Majno, 1969). In addition to producing these increases in vascular resistance, ischemia and reperfusion also elicit an increase in vascular permeability, causing a movement of fluid and protein from the vascular space and into the muscle interstitium (Diana and Lauglin, 1974; Korthius et al., 1985; Sparks et al., 1984). More prolonged ischemia can produce alterations in cellular morphology, reductions in muscle contractility, and cell death.

Korthius et al. (1985, 1988) have shown that the vascular injury produced by ischemia–reperfusion in skeletal muscle is free radical-mediated and can be prevented by administering any one of a number of free radical scavengers (dimethyl sulfoxide, catalase, superoxide dismutase, desferoxamine). The fact that each of these scavengers, and dimethyl sulfoxide, in particular, were effective is in keeping with the concept that the free radical species primarily responsible for inducing ischemia–reperfusion injury in skeletal muscles is the hydroxyl radical. It has been suggested that skeletal muscle injury from this stress is at least partly due to free radicals generated by xanthine oxidase-mediated conversion of hypoxanthine to uric acid. Traditionally, however, skeletal muscle had been thought to be relatively protected from the effects of ischemia, because the skeletal muscle isoform of xanthine dehydrogenase is not as readily converted to xanthine oxidase as in other tissues. Such relative protection would seem to be physiologically appropriate, since skeletal muscles are often made transiently ischemic during normal function as the result of elevations in intramuscular pressure during tension generation. More recent data indicate, however, that limb skeletal muscle levels of xanthine oxidase in some species can rise with ischemia, with the implication that the generation of free radicals by the xanthine oxidase–hypoxanthine reaction system may play some role in mediating postischemic injury to skeletal muscle as well as to other tissues (Smith et al., 1989a).

One of the tissue elements known to be damaged by free radical production in reperfused tissues is the vascular endothelium. In fact, it is possible that free radical generation in muscle following ischemia–reperfusion occurs almost entirely in the vascular endothelium, and that muscle dysfunction is either the result of alterations in muscle perfusion or reflects muscle membrane damage produced by free radicals that have diffused from vascular sites of origin. White cell adhesion to this damaged endothelium can lead to vascular plugging, reducing tissue blood flow, and the initiation of additional cycles of ischemia and reperfusion. Alternatively, free radicals may also be generated within muscle fibers, and may induce dysfunction by producing lipid peroxidation of intracellular organelles. In agreement with this latter possibility, ischemia–reperfusion of skeletal muscle has been shown to alter muscle fiber sarcoplasmic reticulum and mitochondrial structure and function.

In keeping with the proposal that white blood cells play an important role in mediating ischemia–reperfusion-induced injury in skeletal muscle, Korthius et al. (1988) have shown that white cell depletion reduces the muscle damage produced by subsequent ischemia–reperfusion. To further evaluate this concept, Smith et al. (1989b) measured myeloperoxidase activity, an index of white cell activity, in skeletal muscle biopsies taken before ischemia, after 4 h of ischemia, and after 1 h of reperfusion. Tissue levels of reduced glutathione, superoxide dismutase, and catalase were also measured. Reperfusion induced a 26-fold increase in tissue myeloperoxidase activity and a 50% decrease in glutathione levels; superoxide dismutase and catalase levels were not changed by ischemia–reperfusion in this study. These later data suggest that ischemia–reperfusion is associated with release of a white cell-derived enzyme (myeloperoxidase) capable of generating free radicals into skeletal muscle.

There are many clinical conditions in which limb muscle ischemia can be sufficiently severe and prolonged to induce free radical-mediated muscle damage. It is not at all clear, however, that blood flow to the respiratory muscles is ever reduced to a comparable degree. This is because the diaphragm is well supplied by a complex network of arteries and is unlikely to sustain complete ablation of its blood supply for a protracted time (Comtois et al., 1987). There are several factors, however, that may influence the susceptibility of the respiratory muscles to this form of injury and may make it possible for xanthine oxidase-induced free radical generation to occur. For one thing, one report found that xanthine oxidase levels in the diaphragms of several species of animals were slightly higher than those in the heart, and these levels were approximately tenfold higher than those in limb skeletal muscle (Khalidi and Chaglassian, 1965). Second, muscle production of hypoxanthine is a function of not only the degree of muscle ischemia, but also of the level of muscle contractile activity. Specifically, hypoxanthine release from muscle during shock is substantially greater in working than in resting muscle (Chaudry et al., 1974, 1976). This should be of special importance relative to the respiratory muscles, for which rhythmic contraction is an obligatory activity throughout life. In keeping with this concept, Ketai et al. (1990) found that hypoxanthine release from the limb and resting diaphragm was relatively small, despite a large increase in arteriovenous gradients of lactate across these tissues. In breathing dogs, however, there was a surprisingly large increase in hypoxanthine release by the diaphragm during shock, with arteriovenous gradients exceeding those observed across the liver or kidney, and manyfold higher than those for limb muscle. This finding is important because it indicates that the diaphragm may produce large amounts of the substrate (hypoxanthine) necessary for generating free radicals by the xanthine oxidase reaction in the presence of ischemia.

In addition, complete cessation of blood flow may not be required to elicit ischemia–reperfusion injury. Specifically, one recent study found that partial ischemia is capable of eliciting ischemia–reperfusion injury in the intestine (Parks et al., 1982), and it is possible that subtotal ischemia could also induce injury in the respiratory muscles. Such subtotal respiratory muscle ischemia could occur clinically as the result of severe systemic hypotension, and it could be potentiated by regional vascular disease within these muscles. Moreover, cardiac studies have indicated that oxygen delivery, rather than blood flow per se, is the critical issue determining the generation of free radicals in tissues. As a result, the development of what may be more appropriately termed free radical-mediated "deoxygenation–reoxygenation" muscle injury should be influenced by the level of arterial oxygen content and tissue metabolic activity, as well as by the level of blood flow. Because of these factors, it is possible that free radical-mediated respiratory muscle damage may occur in clinical conditions in which oxygen tensions within respiratory muscle are transiently reduced to very low levels as a result of some combination of hypoxemia, muscle activity, atherosclerotic vascular disease, and systemic hypotension.

To characterize the type of diaphragmatic injury that might be induced by severe transient reductions in oxygen delivery, one recent study examined the effects produced by sustained perfusion of the diaphragm at low arterial pressures (Supinski et al., 1992). These studies were performed in anesthetized dogs using an in situ diaphragmatic strip preparation. Comparison was made between three groups of experiments, including a control group in which no diaphragm ischemia was produced, a group in which phrenic arterial pressure was reduced to 41 mm Hg for 3 h followed by a 1-h period of reperfusion, and a group given the free radical scavenger dimethyl sulfoxide before ischemia–reperfusion. When compared with the control group of animals, studies in which diaphragm ischemia–reperfusion was produced had significant alterations in diaphragm vascular and contractile function. Specifically, following ischemia–reperfusion the hyperemic phrenic vascular response to transient arterial occlusion was appreciably reduced, and the phrenic flow achieved during high-intensity, rhythmic contractions was appreciably lower than that seen in normal, nonischemic, control animals. Although ischemia–reperfusion did not appear to induce significant alterations in diaphragmatic strength, diaphragm strip fatigability was significantly increased following ischemia–reperfusion. This study also found that administration of a hydroxyl radical scavenger, dimethyl sulfoxide, prevented all the deleterious effects of ischemia–reperfusion. Animals subjected to diaphragm ischemia–reperfusion after dimethyl sulfoxide administration had normal fatigability and normal vascular responses to transient arterial occlusion.

B. Limb Skeletal Muscle Damage Caused By Strong Contractions

Skeletal muscle tension-generating ability decreases following sustained or repeated contractions of high intensity. Under normal physiological circumstances, most of this reduction in tension-generating capacity is due to rapidly reversible forms of muscle fatigue (e.g., alterations in neuromuscular transmission, alterations in cellular phosphate concentrations). With some regimens of contraction, however, long-lasting muscle dysfunction can result. It has been postulated that this latter reduction in muscle contractility may represent a form of muscle injury, reversing only after time-consuming repair of damaged organelles.

It can be argued that at least two forms of long-lasting, slowly reversible muscle dysfunction may exist. A series of recent experiments have shown that eccentric muscle contractions (i.e., contraction during muscle lengthening, as can occur in some leg muscles during downhill running), can produce a form of muscle injury that requires days for recovery (Armstrong et al., 1983). This form of injury is associated with an influx of inflammatory cells into muscle, histological evidence of muscle fiber and myofibrillar degradation, and increases in plasma levels of creatine kinase and lactate dehydrogenase. It has been suggested that free radical-mediated lipid peroxidation of muscle organelles, including damage to muscle membranes, may account for this type of exercise-induced damage (Jenkins, 1988). One report found that free radicals play an important role in inducing this form of muscle injury (Zerba et al., 1990), and it is possible that these free radicals may be a product of the white cells infiltrating muscles following eccentric contractions.

For the inspiratory muscles, however, there is little evidence that intense eccentric contractions ever occur, and there is no evidence that inspiratory muscle injury can be produced by such a mechanism. A second type of long-lasting limb skeletal muscle dysfunction following strenuous contractions has been described, however, and there is evidence for the development of a similar form of dysfunction following intense diaphragmatic contractions. This latter form of contractile dysfunction is characterized by a selective long-lasting reduction in the tension generated in response to low-frequency stimulation. This alteration has been termed "low-frequency" fatigue, and is thought to represent a long-lasting reduction in excitation–contraction coupling. This phenomenon can be produced by concentric muscle contractions (i.e., contractions during which the muscle shortens as it contracts) and may require several days to reverse following a strenuous bout of exercise (Aldrich, 1988). It has been postulated that this latter form of low-grade, long-lasting muscle dysfunction following strenuous contractions is also free radical-mediated. The remainder of this section will review the possible mechanisms by which such dysfunction may be produced and the available data indicating that free radicals may cause contractile dysfunction in limb muscles following exercise. The next section will review free radical generation in the respiratory muscles during strenuous contraction.

There is no evidence for white cell infiltration of muscle following concentric contractions, and an alternative source of free radicals is required to account for any muscle injury that may accompany this form of contraction. In theory, however, there are several potential sources of oxygen-derived free radicals in contracting muscle. For one thing, sarcoplasmic reticulum membranes of skeletal muscle are known to contain NADPH-dependent enzyme systems that can generate oxygen-derived free radicals as a reaction by-product (Duncan and Rudge, 1988). It is conceivable that increased membrane metabolic activity could trigger generation of oxygen free radicals at membrane sites during muscle contraction.

In addition, as explained in detail in an earlier section, the electron transport chain normally produces small amounts of superoxide anion radicals under resting conditions, and it is possible that muscle contraction may be accompanied by an increased production of superoxide anion radicals from this pathway. Strenuous exercise can produce a severalfold increase in oxygen utilization and, hence, in the activity of the oxidative phosphorylation pathways. This increased oxygen usage, in turn, could be accompanied by a concomitant increase in superoxide generation (i.e., an increase in the magnitude of the electron "leak" from this pathway; Boveris et al., 1972, 1976; Sjodin et al., 1990). Although mitochondrial membranes contain substances, such as vitamin E, that act as antioxidant defenses, it is possible that muscle superoxide production during strenuous exercise may be great enough to overwhelm these defense systems. Unscavenged superoxide anion radicals could react with and damage intramuscular components directly, or could serve as a substrate for the formation of toxic hydroxyl ion radicals.

Various pieces of experimental data are consistent with the possibility that free radicals may be generated in skeletal muscles following strenuous contractions by these latter mechanisms. Specifically, Davies et al. (1982) found an increase in electron paramagnetic resonance (EPR) signals (an index of free radical production) in rat limb skeletal muscle following a bout of strenuous, fatiguing exercise. Subsequent studies have found evidence for the production of other markers of free radical formation in muscle during exercise. Lew et al. (1985) found that rats exercised by running to exhaustion had increases in plasma levels of glutathione, and that the reduced GSH/GSSG ratio was decreased in plasma, liver, and skeletal muscle. This indicates an increase in oxidized glutathione levels in these tissues during strenuous exercise. Several additional studies have described decreases in skeletal muscle GSH, increases in skeletal muscle GSSG, and other evidence of activation of the GSH redox cycle in animals after exhaustive exercise (Ji and Fu, 1992; Lang et al., 1987; Salminen and Vihko, 1983; Pyke et al. (1986). Other work has described alterations in blood GSSG levels in humans following exercise (Gohil et al., 1988), suggesting increased formation of active superoxide during prolonged exercise. In keeping with these findings, Brady et al. (1979) found an increase in muscle thiobarbituric acid-reactive substances (malondialdehyde levels) following exercise. In addition, Gee and Tappel (1981) have shown an increase in expired air concentrations of pentane, a by-product of free radical-mediated lipid peroxidation, following strenuous limb muscle exercise.

If free radicals produced in limb muscle during exercise are responsible for producing cellular damage that reduces muscle tension-generating ability, then it should be possible, in theory, to increase such damage by reducing cellular concentrations of naturally occurring free radical scavengers. In keeping with such a concept, cellular antioxidant defense systems can be impaired in certain nutritional deficiencies, predisposing to free radical-mediated damage (Quintanilha, 1984; Dillard et al., 1982). This has most dramatically been shown for other forms of free radical-mediated tissue injury. For example, Tierney et al. (1977) found an increase in mortality occurred in vitamin E-deficient rats during hyperoxic exposure. In addition, Kann et al. (1964) found that hemolysis and lipid peroxide formation occurred only in the vitamin E-deficient animals when vitamin E-deficient and control mice were exposed to hyperoxia.

Conceptually, similar observations have been made for muscle following exhaustive exercise. For example, muscle degeneration and dystrophic changes are found in muscles from vitamin E-deficient rats (Jager, 1972). In addition, Davies et al. (1982) found that prolonged feeding of animals with a diet deficient in vitamin E resulted in an increased susceptibility of limb muscles to fatigue. Moreover, vitamin E-deficient rats had a greater postexercise fragility of lysosomal membranes, accumulation of free radicals in muscle, increased lipid peroxidation, and a loss of sarcoplasmic reticulum integrity in this study. Gohil et al. (1986) also found that the endurance capacities of vitamin E-deficient rats were significantly reduced when compared with control animals. In addition, in vivo lipid peroxidation, as measured by expired ethane and pentane production, has been shown by a number of different authors to be increased in vitamin E-deficient rats (Dillard et al., 1977; Herschberger and Tappel, 1982; Kivits et al., 1981).

Since selenium is an cofactor for glutathione peroxidase, one might also expect alterations in exercise tolerance in animals made selenium-deficient if free radical-mediated damage was an important determinant of exercise capacity (Ji et al., 1988b). Lang et al. (1987) examined this issue and found that experimentally induced selenium deficiency decreased glutathione peroxidase activity in muscle, increased total muscle glutathione, increased muscle cytochrome oxidase activity, and increased muscle ubiquinone content. These authors also found a large increase in GSSG levels in selenium-deficient rats, indicating pronounced oxidation of glutathione. However, selenium deficiency had no effect on muscle endurance capacity, suggesting that the residual selenium-dependent glutathione peroxidase activity may have been sufficient to prevent impairment of endurance capacity.

In theory, if free radical-mediated damage were responsible for producing muscle dysfunction following exercise, it should be possible to reduce such damage by maneuvers that augment cellular concentrations of scavengers. In keeping with this concept, Barclay and Hansel (1991) found fatigue rates could be reduced in an electrically stimulated canine limb muscle preparation by preceding contractions with the administration of either allopurinol, desferoxamine, or the free radical scavenger dimethyl sulfoxide. These data suggest that free radicals, generated by a xanthine oxidase-dependent reaction, were responsible for contributing to the development of the muscle dysfunction resulting from rhythmic contractions in this particular experimental model. These authors further postulate that high-intensity contractions may induce a form of relative ischemia in limb muscle, with flows that are lower than those required to maintain optimum function. This relative ischemia may then induce free radical generation in a fashion similar to that induced by ischemia–reperfusion in other organs (i.e., by the xanthine oxidase-catalyzed metabolism of hypoxanthine).

Finally, if muscle endurance is, in part, a function of cellular susceptibility to free radical damage, then training-induced alterations in muscle antioxidant levels may play an important role in training-induced alterations in exercise capacity. In fact, studies have demonstrated an decreased susceptibility to oxidant-induced injury in limb muscles following training. For example, trained mice have reduced lipid peroxidation in muscles following strenuous exercise, with less evidence of fiber necrosis and inflammation (Vihko et al., 1978). In addition, Salminen and Vihko (1983) examined lipid peroxidative capacity in the red and white skeletal muscles of control and endurance-trained mice. These authors found endurance training decreased lipid peroxidation rate in vitro in both muscle types. Catalase activity and vitamin E content were not increased by endurance exercise in this study, however, making it difficult to account for the reduced susceptibility to lipid peroxidation on the basis of alterations in these particular defenses.

Also in keeping with the concept of training-induced alterations in muscle susceptibility to peroxidation, Nuttal and Jones (1968) found that exercise produced a decrease in total thiol groups in the skeletal muscle mitochondria from rats, with a smaller reduction during exercise performed after training. Trained rats also have a smaller increase in plasma products of lipid peroxidation than untrained rats following exercise (Alessio and Goldfarb, 1988).

In human runners, there is also evidence of a relation between training intensity and the level of plasma indices of lipid peroxidation. Robertson et al. (1991) found a significant negative correlation between the level of fitness of trained runners, gauged by measurements of Vo_{2max}, and an index of lipid peroxidation. Specifically, as weekly training intensity increased in these runners, maximum oxygen uptake increased, plasma creatine kinase activity rose, and plasma levels of thiobarbituric-reactive substances decreased.

The influence of prolonged exercise on muscle lipid peroxidation may be complex, however. Since exercise per se generates free radicals, and training may affect muscle susceptibility to free radical generation, the net effect of continuous exercise could, in theory, vary depending on the relative balance between these two factors. With some high levels of prolonged exertion, adaptive responses may be inadequate and cellular antioxidant levels may become depleted. In keeping with such a possibility, one study found that prolonged exercise was associated with a decrease in the muscle mitochondrial vitamin E/ubiquinone ratio (Gohil et al., 1987). Other studies have also suggested that muscle stores of antioxidants can become relatively depleted during some long-term muscle-training regimens (Chance et al., 1979).

C. Free Radical-Mediated Injury in the Respiratory Muscles: Respiratory Muscle Fatigue

Although diaphragm fatigue is thought to be an important factor contributing to the development of respiratory insufficiency in patients with lung disease, the cellular mechanisms by which fatigue develops remain poorly understood. Several mechanisms by which diaphragm fatigue may be produced have been postulated (Bellemare and Bigland-Ritchie, 1987; Roussos and Moxham, 1985). It is thought that respiratory loading can elicit activation of reflex neural pathways that act at the level of the central nervous system to decrease efferent motor outflow, acting to prevent muscle overuse. Such a reduction in drive, however, may act concomitantly to reduce muscle force-generating capacity, producing a form of "central" fatigue. In addition, there is evidence that respiratory loading may sometimes cause "transmission" fatigue, reducing the transmissibility of action potentials across the neuromuscular junction and along the sarcolemmal membrane. Respiratory loading may also induce forms of rapidly reversible "peripheral" fatigue, similar to those produced in limb muscle during strenuous contraction; that is, alterations in the intracellular processes involved in contraction (excitation–contraction coupling, actin–myosin cross-bridge cycling, alterations in muscle energy metabolism). As in limb muscles, peripheral fatigue may be mediated by several different processes, including the deleterious effects produced by alterations in intracellular levels of hydrogen and phosphate ions (Fabiato and Fabiato, 1978).

Also, as in limb muscle, some forms of respiratory muscle dysfunction resulting from strenuous contractions are long-lasting and are difficult to account for on the basis of alterations in neural reflexes, neuromuscular transmission, or cellular alterations in hydrogen or phosphate ion levels. Since evidence suggests that long-lasting limb muscle dysfunction resulting from strenuous regimens of contraction may be partly mediated by oxygen-derived free radicals, it would seem logical to believe that the respiratory muscles may also be susceptible to similar forms of dysfunction. Several recent lines of evidence support such a possibility: (1) infusion of a free radical-generating solution into the diaphragm produces a form of contractile dysfunction akin to that observed with fatigue; (2) lipid peroxidation by-products and other indices of free radical generation have been detected in the respiratory muscles in both in vivo and in vitro models of respiratory muscle fatigue;

(3) free radical scavenger administration reduces the rate of development of diaphragm fatigue both in vitro and in vivo; and (4) experimental manipulations that reduce cellular antioxidant defenses (e.g., vitamin E depletion or reductions in GSH levels) increase the susceptibility of the diaphragm to fatigue. The following paragraphs will review each of these lines of evidence.

Several studies have examined the pattern of myocardial injury induced by infusion of a free radical-generating solution into the heart. In an analogous fashion, Nashawati et al. (1993) recently examined the susceptibility of the diaphragm to damage by a free radical-generating solution and characterized the effects of this intervention on diaphragmatic blood flow and contractile activity. This study was performed using an in situ canine diaphragmatic strip preparation in which the phrenic artery supplying this strip was cannulated and perfused with arterialized blood. Comparison was made between four groups of experiments in which different solutions were infused into the diaphragm, including saline, a free radical-generating solution (iron-ADP complexes), a mixture of iron–ADP and superoxide dismutase, and a mixture of iron–ADP and denatured superoxide dismutase. The diaphragm's tension and blood flow were monitored during electrically induced diaphragmatic contractions for 15 min before intraphrenic infusions, during the period of infusion, and for 90 min after cessation of infusion. Diaphragmatic tension did not change over time in saline-treated control animals, but fell by 60% by 90 min after cessation of infusion in animals in which the free radical-generating solution iron–ADP was infused. This effect of iron–ADP was largely prevented by concomitant administration of active SOD, but not by denatured SOD. Of note, iron-ADP reduced the tension generated in response to all frequencies of stimulation, but had an especially pronounced effect on the tension generated in response to low frequencies of stimulation. Diaphragmatic blood flow did not change significantly in any of these groups of studies. These data suggest that free radical-mediated diaphragmatic injury can result in a marked reduction in the diaphragm's contractility and, like the long-lasting form of diaphragmatic fatigue, has especially pronounced effects on the tensions generated in response to low frequencies of electrical stimulation.

Lipid peroxidation by-products and other chemical indices of free radical generation have been detected in several models of diaphragmatic fatigue. The most compelling of these studies is that of Anzueto et al. (1992), who found that diaphragmatic levels of malondialdehyde rose in anesthetized rats subjected to large, fatiguing inspiratory resistive loads (Fig. 1). This study also observed a pronounced increase in oxidized glutathione levels following resistive-loaded breathing, and a concomitant reduction in reduced glutathione concentrations (Table 1). These data are important not only because they demonstrate that diaphragmatic fatigue can be associated with lipid peroxidation and, by implication, free radical generation, but also because these findings indicate that free radical-associated diaphragmatic fatigue can occur in response to a normal physiological stress: loaded breathing.

Several other investigators have observed evidence of free radical generation during fatiguing contractions performed using in vitro or in situ electrically

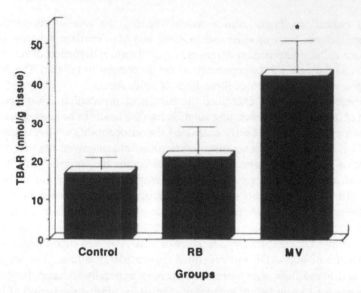

Figure 1   Effect of loaded breathing on thiobarbituric acid-reactive sutstances (TBAR) in the diaphragm. Control animals were not loaded; RB animals had levels determined on the diaphragm immediately after the cessation of loaded breathing; MV animals were loaded, placed on a ventilator for a brief time, and then sacrificed. TBAR, an index of lipid peroxidation, was elevated in the MV group, compared with controls. (From Anzueto et al., 1992.)

Table 1   GSH, GSSG, T-Glu, and GSSG/T-Glu in Diaphragm Tissue[a]

	n	GSH (μmol/g tissue)	GSSG (μmol/g tissue)	T-Glu (μmol/g tissue)	GSSG/T-Glu
Control	7	1081 ± 31	160 ± 21	1426 ± 134	0.22 ± 0.01
RB	6	114 ± 25*	193 ± 16	500 ± 44*	0.77 ± 0.04*
MV	6	184 ± 26*	242 ± 31	721 ± 78*	0.66 ± 0.06*

[a]The table displays diaphragm GSH and GSSG levels for the same experiment described in Figure 1. Control animals were not loaded; RB animals had levels determined on the diaphragm immediately after the cessation of loaded breathing; MV animals were loaded, placed on a ventilator for a brief time, and then sacrificed. Loaded breathing (RB and MV groups) markedly reduced GSH and slightly increased GSSG levels.

Values are means ± SE; n, number of observations; GSH, reduced glutathione; GSSG, glutathione disulfide; T-Glu, total glutathione equivalent.

*$p \leq 0.05$ control vs. RB and MV.

Source: Anzueto et al. (1992).

stimulated diaphragmatic muscle. For example Reid et al. (1992b), who used an intracellular fluorescent probe to detect free radical generation in vitro diaphragmatic strips, found that fluorescent activity increased severalfold in response to electrically induced diaphragmatic contractions (Fig. 2).

Another group of studies have sought to evaluate the role of free radicals in inducing diaphragmatic fatigue by determining the ability of various free radical scavengers, infused into or incubated with diaphragmatic muscle, to attenuate the rate of development of diaphragmatic fatigue. The first of these was a study by Shindoh et al. (1990) that examined the effect of *N*-acetylcysteine on the development of electrically induced fatigue using in situ strips of rabbit diaphragm (Fig. 3). *N*-Acetylcysteine, was chosen for this particular study because this agent is capable of scavenging all three of the major species of oxygen-derived free radicals (i.e., superoxide anion radicals, hydroxyl radicals, and the free radical reaction product hydrogen peroxide). This agent also serves as a glutathione precursor and, thereby, can prevent free radical-mediated depletion of cellular glutathione stores. Alteration in contractile function as a result of rhythmic diaphragmatic stimulation in this study was assessed by examining alterations in the diaphragmatic force–frequency relation over time. *N*-Acetylcysteine reduced the rate of development of diaphragmatic fatigue, but had no effect on the recovery from fatigue. Moreover,

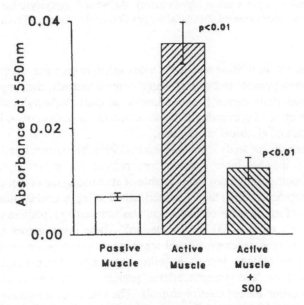

Figure 2 Superoxide production by diaphragm strips in vitro, as detected by measuring cytochrome absorbance. Superoxide production in noncontracting, passive muscle was low, but increased in active muscle. Administration of SOD markedly attenuated superoxide production by active muscle. (From Reid et al., 1992b.)

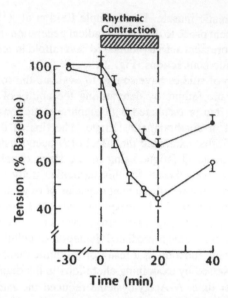

Figure 3 Effect of *N*-acetylcysteine administration on diaphragmatic fatigue. Tracings represent tension over time for electrically stimulated in situ diaphragm strips in rabbits. One group of animals was given saline (open circles), the other *N*-acetyclysteine (solid circles). *N*-Acetylcysteine administration attenuated the development of fatigue. (From Shindoh et al., 1990.)

whereas rhythmic stimulation resulted in a downshift in the force–frequency relation in both *N*-acetylcysteine- and saline-treated control animals, the magnitude of this shift was substantially greater in saline-treated animals. *N*-Acetylcysteine appeared especially effective in preventing reductions in tension development in response to low frequencies of electrical stimulation.

In a more recent study, Supinski et al. (1991a,b) examined the effectiveness with which somewhat more specific free radical scavengers (i.e., superoxide dismutase, dimethyl sulfoxide) were capable of attenuating the rate of diaphragmatic fatigue development. This study was performed using a canine animal model in which fatigue of in situ strips of diaphragm was induced by repetitive electrophrenic stimulation (i.e., trains of 20-Hz stimulation). These investigators also examined the effects of fatigue development and scavenger administration on diaphragmatic malondialdehyde (MDA) levels. Baseline, prefatigue force–frequency curves, phrenic blood flow, and systemic arterial pressures were similar in PEG–SOD-, DMSO-, and saline-treated control animals. The rate of development of diaphragmatic fatigue was much greater, however, in saline-treated control animals than for animals pretreated with either PEG–SOD or DMSO, with tension falling to 22 ± 4, 44 ± 8, and 47 ± 6% of its initial value, respectively, over a 2-h period of electrophrenic stimulation in these three groups of animals. Force–frequency curves shifted downward in all groups, but the magnitude of this shift was much greater in saline controls than for animals to which either of the two free radical scavengers were administered. There were significant increases in diaphragmatic MDA levels following fatigue in saline-treated animals, but no increase in MDA was observed in DMSO- or PEG–SOD-treated animals.

Several conclusions can be drawn from these data. First, under the conditions examined, diaphragmatic MDA formation during fatigue can be prevented by pretreatment with the free radical scavengers PEG–SOD and DMSO. In addition, suppression of MDA formation using free radical scavengers is associated with a significant reduction in the rate of development of diaphragmatic fatigue. The fact that both PEG–SOD and DMSO are effective in preventing MDA formation in the diaphragm and in reducing the rate of development of fatigue is consistent with the notion that hydroxyl radicals play a primary role in diaphragmatic MDA formation and fatigue development. Finally, although free radical scavengers slowed the rate of fatigue development in this study, these agents did not appear to increase the rate of recovery over the first hour following the cessation of contractions. These latter data are also consistent with the notion that the scavengers acted principally to reduce the development of the long-lasting component of fatigue, and had no effect on the rapidly reversible fatigue component, which resolved with equal speed in both scavenger-treated and control animals.

In keeping with this approach, other work has examined the effect of lazaroid administration on diaphragmatic fatigue induced by resistive-loaded breathing in anesthetized animals (A. Anzueto, unpublished observations). Lazaroids (U74006F; Upjohn, Michigan; 21-aminosteroid derivatives) are thought to protect tissues from free radical-mediated damage by inhibiting lipid peroxidation, and these substances have proved effective in protecting several types of tissue from oxidative stress (Hall et al., 1988). When administered to anesthetized rats before resistive loading, lazeroids attenuate diaphragmatic fatigue, increase diaphragmatic tetanic tension generation, and reduce fatigue-induced prolongation of twitch relaxation when compared with nontreated loaded animals.

In yet another study examining these same issues, Reid et al. (1992a) made largely similar observations. They found that in vitro incubation of diaphragm strips with several free radical scavengers (superoxide dismutase, catalase, and dimethyl sulfoxide) resulted in a reduction in the rate at which fatigue developed in response to rhythmic 20-Hz electrical stimulation (Fig. 4). When a similar experiment was performed using a high-stimulation frequency (100 Hz), no protective effect of these scavengers was noted.

This last observation is important, because it indicates that the contribution the free radicals make to the development of diaphragmatic fatigue probably varies, depending on the pattern of muscle activation. It is likely that some patterns of muscle contraction (e.g., that produced in response to high-frequency muscle excitation) result in such rapid development of fatigue that mitochondrial respiration is not maximally engaged and free radical generation is minimal. In theory, such

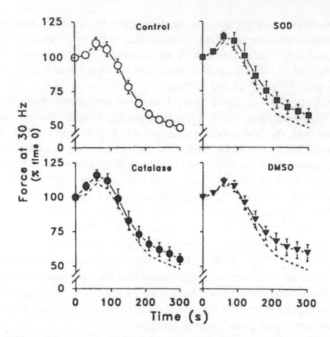

Figure 4 Effect of scavenger administration on diaphragmatic fatigue. Tracings represent tension over time for electrically stimulated in vitro diaphragm strips. Dashed curves represent control force–time relation. Administration of either SOD, catalase, or DMSO attenuated the decline of tension over time. (From Reid et al., 1992a.)

contractions should induce rapid fatigue, recovery might be relatively rapid, and this form of fatigue should have little or no response to free radical scavengers. On the other hand, patterns of contraction producing a slower onset of fatigue may generate greater levels of free radicals, be less reversible with rest, and manifest a greater response to free radical scavengers.

Also in support of a role for free radicals in mediating diaphragmatic fatigue, experimental manipulations that reduce cellular antioxidant defenses (e.g., vitamin E depletion, reductions in GSH levels) increase the susceptibility of the diaphragm to fatigue. For example, Anzueto et al. (1993a) compared the effect of inspiratory resistive breathing on normal rats with vitamin E-deficient rats (comparisons were also made with nonloaded normal and nonloaded vitamin E-deficient groups of rats). Diaphragms from vitamin E-deficient, nonloaded animals developed lower tensions in vitro than diaphragms from normal, nonloaded controls, whereas diaphragms from loaded vitamin E-deficient animals had lower tensions in vitro than either loaded normal animals or vitamin E-deficient nonloaded controls. In addition, GSH/GSSG ratios were very low in loaded, vitamin E-deficient animals, somewhat higher in loaded normal or unloaded vitamin E-deficient animals, and highest in nonloaded normal controls. These data indicate that both vitamin E deficiency and loaded breathing constitute oxidative stress, with the combination of these acting synergistically to impair diaphragmatic function and induce activation of the glutathione redox cycle.

Other studies have examined the effect on the diaphragm of interventions designed to reduce cellular glutathione levels and decrease glutathione peroxidase activity (Morales et al., 1992a,b; Andrade et al., 1992). One such study examined the effect on diaphragmatic function produced by administration of diethylmaleate (DEM), a compound that decreases tissue GSH concentrations. Animals injected with DEM had significantly reduced diaphragmatic levels of glutathione. Moreover, DEM-treated animals had significantly greater reductions in diaphragmatic contractility (manifested as reductions in tension in in vitro studies of excised strips of diaphragm muscle) in response to resistive-loaded breathing than saline-treated control animals. In another study, injection of DL-buthionine-SR-sulfoximine (BSO; an inhibitor of 7-glutamylsynthetase that decreases cellular levels of GSH) potentiated the effect of loaded breathing on the diaphragm's contractility. Specifically, BSO-treated animals had a greater decrement in force-generating ability (i.e., greater reductions in tetanic and twitch tensions) than control animals when subjected to resistive-loaded breathing (Morales et al., 1992b).

Taken together, these various studies provide a strong case that free radicals are generated in the diaphragm during strenuous contractions and that contractile dysfunction mediated by free radicals contributes to the development of diaphragmatic fatigue.

D. Free Radical-Mediated Injury in Muscles During Sepsis

Systemic bacterial infections evoke a complex defensive response designed to both kill invading microorganisms and to protect the body from bacterial products. Many times, however, body tissues are inadvertently damaged as a by-product of this defense. For example, infections are known to elicit a form of skeletal muscle dysfunction in this fashion. The precise mechanism by which infections cause muscle dysfunction remains poorly understood. It is clear that severe, prolonged infection can induce muscle proteolysis and wasting of sufficient severity to cause a major reduction in muscle tension-generating ability. Several humoral substances generated during sepsis (e.g., prostaglandins, TNF, interleukins) have been postulated to act as mediators of this proteolysis, and recent studies suggest that one substance in particular, tumor necrosis factor (TNF), may play an important role (Wilcox and Bressler, 1992; Anzueto et al., 1993b). Higher levels of proteolytic enzymes (i.e., cathepsin and myofibrillar proteinase) have also been detected in limb muscles in some models of sepsis, but not in others.

In the lung and other organs, however, there is increasing evidence that free radicals play a crucial role in mediating a major portion of the tissue damage evoked by infection. In support of this concept, administration of free radical scavengers (i.e., cysteine and glutathione) has reduced the susceptibility of animals to the effects of endotoxic shock, improving survival (Galvin and Lefer, 1978; Cook and DiLuzio, 1973). In addition, one study found that *N*-Acetylcysteine, a glutathione precursor and free radical scavenger, blunted the effects of endotoxin on the lung (Bernard et al., 1984). Specifically, this study found that *N*-acetylcysteine decreased the endotoxin-induced rise in pulmonary artery pressure, prevented changes in cardiac output, and attenuated the change in lung compliance and airway resistance induced by endotoxin. This study also found that *N*-acetylcysteine decreased the chemiluminescence (one index of free radical generation) produced by stimulated granulocytes. Other, more recent, papers have confirmed these findings (i.e., a protective effect against pulmonary damage during sepsis, using superoxide dismutase as a scavenger (Koyami et al., 1992).

There are several potential mechanisms by which infections can elicit free radical generation. First, endotoxin released from bacteria can exert a direct effect on endothelial cells to induce free radical-mediated damage (Brigham et al., 1986). Second, some of the leukocyte products generated in response to endotoxin may lead to free radical generation. For example, tumor necrosis factor, released by macrophages, activates prostaglandin pathways and may induce free radical generation by this means (Marks et al., 1990; Kontos, 1985). Third, neutrophils, activated by complement and other substances (platelet-activating factor, tumor necrosis factor), may release free radicals directly (Till et al., 1982; Ward et al., 1983).

In view of the fact that free radicals seemed to be implicated in promoting lung injury during sepsis, it is plausible that free radical-mediated mechanisms may also play a role in eliciting skeletal muscle dysfunction during infection. In theory, free radicals derived from white cells, produced in response to the direct effects of endotoxin, as a by-product of prostaglandin generation, or in response to other mediators (e.g., TNF), could damage the microvasculator skeletal muscles. This, in turn, could lead to endothelial cell swelling and adherence of white cells to the damaged endothelium. Free radicals can also reduce endothelium-derived relaxation factor (EDRF) levels, causing functional vasoconstriction (Aoki et al., 1989; Rubanyi and Vanhoutte, 1986a,b). It is also possible that free radicals may be produced by and may damage muscle cells directly, causing lipid peroxidation of muscle cellular membranes and other cellular constituents. Finally, it is possible that free radicals may promote muscle proteolysis; the in vitro incubation of proteins with a free radical-generating solution increases their susceptibility to degradation by proteolytic enzymes.

In keeping with these possibilities, there are several recent reports indicating that free radicals play a role in mediating the respiratory muscle dysfunction associated with sepsis. Although it would also seem possible that free radicals could modulate limb muscle dysfunction in response to infection, we are not aware of any studies that have examined this latter issue. The remainder of this section will review those studies that have characterized the respiratory muscle dysfunction that accompanies infections and that have examined the role of free radical generation as a potential mediator of this dysfunction.

It appears that both acute and chronic infections can impair diaphragmatic contractility. For example, Hussain et al. (1986) found that intravenous administration of endotoxin to dogs produced reductions in diaphragmatic pressure generation within several hours. These alterations in contractile function were associated with reductions in diaphragm glycogen stores and increases in the diaphragmatic production of lactate. Boczkowski et al. (1988) found that administration of live streptococci to rats resulted in a reduction in the transdiaphragmatic pressures generated in response to bilateral supramaximal stimulation of the phrenic nerves. Similarly, Shindoh et al. (1992) found that endotoxin administration to rats for 2 days resulted in a reduction in the tension generated in vitro by diaphragmatic strips taken from these animals after sacrifice. Of interest, these investigators found that this model of septic shock reduced the tension generated by the diaphragm in response to a wide range of stimulation frequencies (1–100 Hz), but did not affect twitch kinetics or the twitch/tetanus ratio. Drew et al. (1988) also observed a reduction in the diaphragm's tension-generating ability in rats chronically infected (i.e., infected for weeks) with schistosomiasis.

Shindoh et al. (1992) recently reported the results of a study designed to evaluate the role played by oxygen-derived free radicals in mediating the effects of endotoxin on the diaphragm by determining (1) if endotoxin induces an increase in diaphragm levels of malondialdehyde (MDA), and (2) if it is possible to prevent endotoxin-induced alterations in diaphragmatic MDA levels and contractility by administering PEG–SOD (Fig. 5). Studies were performed on hamsters, with MDA levels and in vitro diaphragmatic contractility assessed using muscle strips excised from the costal diaphragms of freshly sacrificed animals. Four groups of animals were examined in this study, including a group that was injected with endotoxin for 2 days, a group injected with saline, a group injected with both endotoxin and PEG-SOD, and a group given PEG-SOD alone. Diaphragmatic MDA levels for endotoxin-treated animals were significantly higher than levels for control animals (i.e., 71 ± 2 nmol/g and 41 ± 2 nmol/g, respectively), and PEG–SOD administration had the effect of preventing increases of MDA levels in endotoxin-treated animals (MDA concentrations of 46 ± 3 nmol/g in this group). The MDA levels for animals given PEG–SOD alone (43 ± 1 nmol/g) were similar to levels in saline treated controls. Changes in the diaphragm's contractility paralleled alterations in MDA levels, with significantly lower tensions in animals given endotoxin than for animal given either saline, endotoxin plus PEG–SOD, or those given PEG–SOD alone (see Fig. 5). These data suggest that endotoxin administration elicits free radical-mediated lipid peroxidation within the diaphragm, producing contractile dysfunction. Moreover, these results indicate that it is possible to prevent endotoxin-induced diaphragmatic dysfunction by administering a free radical scavenger. In another report, using a similar experimental design, Surell et al. (1992) found that administration of another free radical scavenger, *N*-acetylcysteine, also pre-

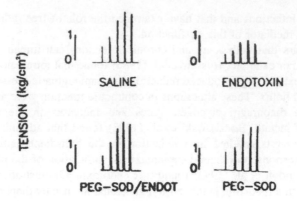

Figure 5 Diaphragmatic force–frequency relation in endotoxin-treated aminals. Tracings represent tension generation in response to sequential stimuilation of in vitro diaphragm strips at 1, 10, 20, 50, and 100 Hz. Data for a strip taken from a saline-treated animal are presented in the upper left corner, for an endotoxin-treated animal in the upper right corner, for an animal given both PEG–SOD and endotoxin in the lower left corner, and for an animal given PEG–SOD alone in the lower right corner. Tension was lower for the strip taken from the endotoxin-treated animal when compared with control; PEG–SOD administration attenuated the effect of endotoxin on the diaphragm. (From Shindoh et al., 1992.)

vented endotoxin-induced diaphragmatic dysfunction secondary to endotoxin (Fig. 6). This latter group also found that this scavenger prevented endotoxin-mediated increases in diaphragmatic malondialdehyde levels.

More recently, Supinski et al. (1993) compared the effects of endotoxin administration on the diaphragm with its effect on the intercostal muscles and examined the effect of several free radical scavengers in protecting these muscles from the effects of endotoxin administration. In this study, diaphragmatic and intercostal musclar function was assessed using muscle strips excised from hamsters after sacrifice. Six groups of animals were studied, including a group injected with endotoxin alone, a saline-treated control group, and three groups given both endotoxin and one of several free radical scavengers [i.e., superoxide dismutase (SOD), PEG–catalase (CAT), and dimethyl sulfoxide (DMSO)]. The sixth group of animals were given both endotoxin and denatured PEG–superoxide dismutase. Endotoxin administration elicited significant and similar reductions in the contractility of both diaphragm and intercostal muscles, as manifested by a reduction in the twitch and tetanic tensions generated by these muscles and by a downward shift in the diaphragms force–frequency curve. The absolute tension generated by intercostal and diaphragm muscles from saline-treated animals also remained higher than the tension of these respective muscles taken from endotoxin-treated animals during in vitro fatigue trials. All three active free radical scavengers tested (PEG–SOD, PEG–CAT, and DMSO) were capable of attenuating the effects of endotoxin on

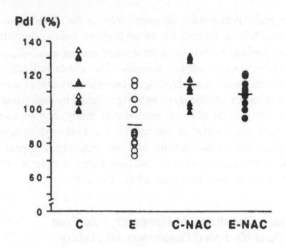

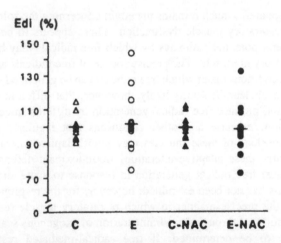

Figure 6 Transdiaphragmatic pressure (Pdi, top panel) and diaphragmatic electromyographic activity (Edi, bottom panel) for control (C), endotoxin-treated (E), control/*N*-acetylcysteine-treated (C-NAC), and endotoxin/*N*-acetylcysteine treated (E-NAC) animals. For the same level of diaphragmatic activation (i.e., Edi was similar in the four groups), there is a reduction in diaphragmatic pressure generation in endotoxin-treated compared with control animals. NAC administration blocked this effect of endotoxin. (Surell et al., 1992.)

the diaphragm and intercostal muscles. Diaphragmatic and intercostal twitch and tetanic tensions for animals given endotoxin and one of these three scavengers were similar to values obtained in saline-treated controls animals and significantly higher than values for endotoxin-treated animals. Fatigue curves for animals given these three active scavengers were also similar to curves in control animals and higher than curves in endotoxin-treated animals. Values for diaphragm and intercostal muscle twitch and tetanic tension for animals given both endotoxin and denatured PEG–SOD were similar to values in endotoxin-treated animals, and significantly lower than for saline-treated control animals. These data indicate that several free radical species (superoxide ions, hydrogen peroxide, hydroxyl ions) play a role in mediating the respiratory muscle dysfunction produced by endotoxin administration. Hydroxyl anions may be the ultimate mediator of injury, and superoxide anions and hydrogen peroxide may serve as precursors for hydroxyl radical formation. In addition, both the intercostal muscles and the diaphragm appear to be similarly affected by endotoxin administration, and both types of muscle are protected from these effects by free radical scavenger administration.

V. Future Directions of Research into Free Radical-Mediated Diaphragmatic Injury

As should be apparent, much remains uncertain concerning the role of free radicals in mediating respiratory muscle dysfunction. There appears to be several mechanisms and several potential pathways by which free radicals may be generated and may produce injury in muscle. The precise source of free radicals and the particular physiological conditions under which free radicals can be generated in the respiratory muscles remain unclear. It seems likely, however, that different stresses (loaded breathing, sepsis) produce free radical generation by different mechanisms.

In addition, exercise and other conditions that regularly or continuously increase the workload of these muscles may elicit adaptive alterations in cellular defenses. In turn, these adaptive alterations in antioxidant defenses may provide protection against free radical generation in response to acute stress. The role of such adaptations has not been examined, however, for the respiratory muscles.

Finally, the precise manner in which respiratory muscle responses to acute stress can be modified through the administration of exogenous scanvengers of free radicals needs to be determined. If free radical-mediated respiratory muscle dysfunction is an important determinant of the development of respiratory failure, administration of such substances may provide a means of either preventing or speeding recovery from respiratory failure. Clearly, however, further animal and cellular research must be done in the area of free radical-mediated diaphragm fatigue before human clinical trials can begin.

References

Akizuki, S., Yoshida, S., Chambers, D. E., Parmley, L. F., Yellon, D. M. and Downey, J. M. (1985). Infarct size limitation by the xanthine oxidase inhibitor, allopurinol, in closed-chest dogs with small infarcts. *Cardiovasc. Res.* 19: 686–692.
Aldrich, T. K. (1988). Respiratory muscle fatigue. *Clin. Chest Med.* 9: 225–236.

Alessio, H. M., and Goldfarb, A. H. (1988). Lipid peroxidation and scavenger enzymes during exercise: Adaptive response to training. *J. Appl. Physiol.* 64: 1333–1336.

Andrade, F., Morales, C., Anzueto, A., Levine, S. M., Lawrence, P. A., and Jenkinson, S. G. (1992). Diaphragmatic function after resistive breathing in Se deficient rats. *FASEB J.* 6: A960.

Anzueto, A., Andrade, F. H., Maxwell, L. C., Levine, S. M., Lawrence, R. A., Gibbons, W. J., and Jenkinson, S. G. (1992). Resistive breathing activates the glutathione redox cycle and impairs performance of the rat diaphragm. *J. Appl. Physiol.* 72: 529–534.

Anzueto, A., Andrade, F. H., Maxwell, L. C., Levine, S., Lawrence, R. A., and Jenkinson, S. G. (1993a). Diaphragmatic function after resistive breathing in vitamin E-deficient rats. *J. Appl. Physiol.* (in press).

Anzueto, A., Andrade, F., Greene, K., Levine, S. M., Silmon, J., Roodman, G. D., Maxwell, L. C., Jenkinson, S. G., and Bryan, C. L. (1993b). Diaphragm muscle impairment in mice chronically exposed to tumor necrosis factor-alpha. *Clin. Res.* 40: A854.

Aoki, N., Siegfried, M., and Lefer, A. M. (1989). Anti-EDRF effect of tumor necrosis factor in isolated, perfused cat carotid arteries. *Am. J. Physiol.* 256: H1509–H1512.

Armstrong, D. A., and Buchanan, J. D. (1978). Reactions of O_2^-, H_2O_2, and other oxidants with sulfhydryl enzymes. *Photochem. Photobiol.* 28: 743–755.

Armstrong, R. B., Olgilvie, R. W., Schwane, J. A. (1983). Eccentric exercise induced injury to rat skeletal muscle. *J. Appl. Physiol.* 54: 80–93.

Badwey, J. A., Curnutte, J. T., Robinson, J. M., Berde, C. B., Karnovsky, M. J., and Karnovsky, L. (1984). Effects of free fatty acids on release of superoxide and on change of shape by human neutrophils. *J. Biol. Chem.* 259: 7870–7877.

Bagge, U., Amundson, B., and Lauritzen, C. (1980). White blood cell deformability and plugging of skeletal muscle capillaries in hemorrhagic shock. *Acta Physiol. Scand.* 108: 159–163.

Baker, G. L., Corry, R. J., and Autor, A. P. (1985). Oxygen free radical induced damage in kidneys subjected to warm ischemia and reperfusion: Protective effect of superoxide dismutase. *Ann. Surg.* 202: 628–641.

Barclay, J. K., and Hansel, M. (1991). Free radicals may contribute to oxidative skeletal muscle fatigue. *Can. J. Physiol. Pharmacol.* 69: 279–284.

Beckman, J. S., and Freeman, B. A. (1986). Antioxidant enzymes as mechanistic probes of oxygen-dependent toxicity. In *Physiology of Oxygen Radicals*. Edited by A. E. Taylor, S. Matalon, and P. A. Ward. Bethesda, MD, American Physiological Society, pp. 39–54.

Bellemare, F., and Bigland-Ritchie, B. (1987). Components of diaphragmatic fatigue assessed by phrenic nerve stimulation. *J. Appl. Physiol.* 62: 1307–1316.

Bernard, G. R., Lucht, W. D., Niedermeyer, M. E., Snapper, J. R., Olgetree, M. L., and Brigham, K. L. (1984). Effect of *N*-acetylcysteine on the pulmonary response to endotoxin in the awake sheep and upon in vitro granulocyte function. *J. Clin. Invest.* 73: 1772–1780.

Bielski, B. H. J., and Shiue, G. G. (1979). Reaction rates of superoxide radicals with the essential amino acids. In *Oxygen Free Radicals and Tissue Damage*. New York, Elsevier, pp. 43–56 (*Ciba Found. Symp.* 65).

Boczkowski, J., Dureuil, B., Brangon, C., Pavlovic, D., Murciano, D., Pariente, R., and Aubier, M. (1988). Diaphragmatic function in sepsis. *Am. Rev. Resp. Dis.* 138: 260–265.

Boveris, A. N., Oshino, N., and Chance, B. (1972). Cellular production of hydrogen peroxide. *Biochem. J.* 128: 617–630.

Boveris, A. N., Cadenas, E., and Shopani, A. O. M. (1976). Role of ubiquinone in the mitochondrial generation of hydrogen peroxide. *Biochem. J.* 156: 435–444.

Brady, P. S., Brady, L. J., and Ullrey, D. E. (1979). Selenium, vitamin E, and the response to swimming stress in the rat. *J. Nutr.* 109: 1103–1109.

Braide, M., Amundson, B., Chein, C., and Bagge, U. (1984). Quantitative studies on the influence of leukocytes on the vascular resistance in a skeletal muscle preparation. *Microvasc. Res.* 27: 331–352.

Brattin, W. J., Glende, E. A., Jr., and Recknagel, R. O. (1985). Pathological mechanisms in carbon tetrachloride hepatotoxicity. *J. Free Radical. Biol. Med.* 1: 27–38.

Brigham, K. L., Meyrick, B., Bernard, G. R., Snapper, J. R., Berry, L. C., Tumen, J., and Hussein, A. (1986). Free radicals and arachidonic acid metabolites in endotoxin-induced pulmonary endothelial injury. In *Physiology of Oxygen Radicals*. Edited by A. E. Taylor, S. Matalon, and P. Ward. Bethesda, MD, American Physiological Society, pp. 199–206.

Burton, G. W., and Ingold, K. Y. (1986). Vitamin E: Application of the principles of physical organic chemistry to the exploration of its structure and function. *Acc. Chem. Res.* 19: 194–201.

Carp, H., and Janoff, A. (1979). In vitro suppression of serum elastase inhibitory capacity by reactive oxygen species generated by phagocytosing polymorphonuclear leukocytes. *J. Clin. Invest.* 63: 793–777.

Casale, A. S., Bulkley, G. B., Bulkley, B. H., Flaherty, J. T., Gott, V. L., and Gardner, T. J. (1983). Oxygen free-radical scavengers protect the arrested, globally ischemic heart upon reperfusion. *Surg. Forum* 34: 313–316.

Chambers, D. E., Parks, D. A., and Patterson, G. (1985). Xanthine oxidase as a source of free radical damage in myocardial ischemia. *J. Mol. Cell. Cardiol.* 17: 145–152.

Chance, B., and Boveris, A. (1979). Hyperoxia and hydroperoxide metabolism. In *Extrapulmonary Manifestations of Respiratory Disease*. Edited by E. D. Robin. New York, Marcel Dekker, pp. 185–205.

Chance, B., Sies, H., and Boveris, A. (1979). Hydroperoxide metabolism in mammalian organs. *Physiol. Rev.* 59: 527–605.

Chaudry, I., Sayeed, M., and Baue, A. (1974). Effect of hemorrhagic shock on tissue adenine nucleotides in conscious rats. *Can. J. Physiol. Pharmacol.* 52: 131–137.

Chaudry, I., Sayeed, M., and Baue, A. (1976). Alternations in high-energy phosphates in hemorrhagic shock as related to tissue and organ function. *Surgery* 79: 666–668.

Comtois, A., Gorczyca, W., and Grassino, A. (1987). Anatomy of the diaphragmatic circulation. *J. Appl. Physiol.* 62: 238–244.

Cook, J. A., and DiLuzio, N. R. (1973). Protective effect of cysteine and methylprednisolone in lead acetate–endotoxin induced shock. *Exp. Mol. Pathol.* 17: 127–138.

Corgin, F. P., Bannai, S., and Dessi, M. A. (1989). Conjugated dienes detected in tissue lipid extracts by second derivative spectrophotometry. *Free Radical Biol. Med.* 7: 183–186, 1989.

Cross, C. E., Halliwell, B., and Allen, A. (1984). Antioxidant protection: A function of tracheobronchial and gastrointestinal mucus. *Lancet* 1: 1328–1330.

Das, D. K., Engelman, R. M., Rousou, J. A., Breyer, R. H., Otani, H., and Ledershow, S. (1986). Pathophysiology of superoxide radical as potential mediator of reperfusion injury in pigs. *Basic Res. Cardiol.* 81: 155–166.

Das, D. K., Engelman, R. M., Clement, R., Otani, H., Prasad, M. R., and Rao, P. S. (1987). Role of xanthine oxidase inhibitor as free radical scavenger: A novel mechanism of action of allopurinol and oxypurinol in myocardial salvage. *Biochem. Biophys. Res. Commun.* 148: 314–319.

Davies, K. J. A., Quintanhilha, A. T., Brooks, G. A., and Packer, L. J. (1982). Free radicals and tissue damage produced by exercise. *Biochem. Biophys. Res. Commun.* 1079: 1198–1205.

Deneke, S. M., and Fanburg, B. L. (1989). Regulation of cellular glutathione. *Am. J. Physiol.* 257: L163–L173.

DeWall, R. A., Vasko, K. A., Stanley, E. L., and Kezdi, P. (1971). Responses of the ischemic myocardium to allopurinol. *Am. Heart J.* 82: 362–370.

Diana, J. N., and Lauglin, M. H. (1974). Effect of ischemia on capillary pressure and equivalent pore radius in capillaries of the isolated dog hind limb. *Circ. Res.* 35: 77–101.

Dillard, C. J., Dumelin, E. E., and Tappel, A. L. (1977). Effect of dietary vitamin E on expiration of pentane and ethane by the rat. *Lipids* 12: 109–114.

Dillard, C. J., Litov, R. E., Savin, M. W., Dumelin, E. E., and Tappel, A. L. (1978). Effects of exercise, vitamin E and ozone on pulmonary function and lipid peroxidation. *J. Appl. Physiol.* 45: 927–932.

Dillard, C. J., Kinert, K. J., and Yappel, A. L. (1982). Effects of vitamin E, ascorbic acid, mannitol on alloxan induced lipid peroxidation in rats. *Arch. Biochem. Biophys.* 216: 204–212.

Di Mascio, P., Murphy, M. E., and Sies, H. (1991). Antioxidant defense systems: The role of carotenoids, tocopherols, and thiols. *Am. J. Clin. Nutr.* 53: 1945–2005.

Domanska-Janik, K., and Wideman, J. (1974). Regulation of thiols in the brain. 2. Effect of hypoxia on the activities of cytoplasmic NADPH-producing enzymes in different parts of the rat brain. *Resuscitation* 3: 37–41.

Downey, J. M., Miura, T., and Eddy, T. (1987). Xanthine oxidase is not a source of free radicals in the ischemic rabbit heart. *J. Mol. Cell. Cardiol.* 19: 1053–1060.

Drew, J. S., Farkas, G. A., Pearson, R. D., and Rochester, D. F. (1988). Effects of a chronic wasting infection on skeletal muscle size and contractile properties. *J. Appl. Physiol.* 64: 460–465.

Duncan, C. J., and Rudge, M. F. (1988). Are lysosomal enzymes involved in rapid damage in vertebrate muscles? A study of the separate pathways leading to cellular damage. *Cell Tissue Res.* 253: 447–455.

Engler, R. L., Dahlgren, M. D., Morris, D. D., Peterson, M. A., and Schmis-Shonbein, G. W. (1986). Role of leukocytes in response to acute myocardial ischemia and reflow in dogs. *Am. J. Physiol.* 251: H314–H322.

Fabiato, A., and Fabiato, T. (1978). Effects of pH on the myofilaments and the sarcoplasmic reticulum of skinned cells from cardiac and skeletal muscle. *J. Physiol.* 276: 233–255.

Fantone, J. C., and Ward, P. A. (1982). Role of oxygen-derived free radicals and metabolites in leukocyte-dependent inflammatory reactions. *Am. J. Pathol.* 197: 397–418.

Fligiel, S. E. G., Ward, P. A., Johnson, K. J., and Till, G. O. (1984). Evidence for a role of hydroxyl radical in immune complex-induced vasculitis. *Am. J. Pathol.* 115: 375–382.

Fong, K. L., McKay, P. B., and Poyer, J. L. (1973). Evidence that peroxidation of lysosomal membranes is initiated by hydroxyl free radicals during flavin enzyme activity. *J. Biol. Chem.* 248: 7792–7797.

Forman, H. J., and Boveris, A. (1982). Superoxide radical and hydrogen peroxide in mitochondria. In *Free Radicals in Biology*, Vol. 5. Edited by W. A. Pryor. New York, Academic Press pp. 65–90.

Fox, H. A., Saffiz, J. E., and Corr P. B. (1987). Pathophysiology of myocardial reperfusion. *Cardiol. Clin.* 5: 31–48.

Fox, R. B. (1984). Prevention of granulocyte-mediated oxidant lung injury in rats by a hydroxyl radical scavenger, dimethylthiourea. *J. Clin. Invest.* 74: 1456–1464.

Freeman, B. A., and Crapo, J. D. (1982). Free radicals and tissue injury. *Lab. Invest.* 47: 412–426.

Fridovich, I. (1976). Oxygen radicals, hydrogen peroxide and oxygen toxicity. In *Free Radicals in Biology*, Vol. 1. Edited by W. A. Pryor. New York, Academic Press, pp. 239–277.

Fridovich, I. (1978). The biology of oxygen radicals. *Science* 201: 875–880.

Gallagher, K. P., Buda, A. J., Pace, D., Gerren, R. A., and Shafer, M. (1986). Failure of superoxide dismutase and catalase to alter size of infarction in conscious dogs after 3 hours of occlusion followed by reperfusion. *Circulation* 73: 1065–76.

Galvin, M. J., and Lefer, A. M. (1978). Salutary effects of cysteine on cardiogenic shock in cats. *Am. J. Physiol.* H657–663.

Gauduel, Y., and Duvelleroy, M. A. (1984). Role of oxygen radicals in cardiac injury due to reoxygenation. *J. Mol. Cell. Cardiol.* 16: 459–70.

Gee, D. L., and Tappel, A. L. (1981). The effect of exhaustive exercise on expired pentane as a measure of in vivo lipid peroxidation in the rat. *Life Sci.* 28: 2425–2429.

Gilbert, H. F. (1982). Biological disulfides: The third messenger? *J. Biol. Chem.* 257: 12086–12091.

Gohil, K., Packer, L., DeLumen, B., Brooks, G. A., and Terblanche, S. E. (1986). Vitamin E deficiency and vitamin C supplements in exercise and mitochondrial oxidation. *J. Appl. Physiol.* 60: 1986–1991.

Gohil, K., Rothfuss, L., Lang, L., and Packer, L. (1987). Effect of exercise training on tissue vitamin E and ubiquinone content. *J. Appl. Physiol.* 63: 1638–1641.

Gohil, K., Viguie, C., Stanley, W. C., Brooks, G. A., and Packer, L. (1988). Blood glutathione oxidation during human exercise. *J. Appl. Physiol.* 64: 115–119.

Granger, D. N., Sennett, M., McElearney, P., and Taylor, A. E. (1980). Effect of local arterial hypotension on cat intestinal capillary permeability. *Gastroenterology* 79: 474–480.

Green, M. J., Hill, H. A. O., Tew, D. J., and Walton, N. J. (1984). An opsonized electrode. The direct electrochemical detection of superoxide generated by human neutrophils. *FEBS Lett.* 170: 69–72.

Grisham, M. B., and McCord, J. (1986). Chemistry and cytotoxicity of reactive oxygen metabolites. In *Physiology of Oxygen Radicals*. Edited by A. E. Taylor, S. Matalon, and P. A. Ward. Bethesda, MD, American Physiological Society, pp. 1–18.

Hall, E. D., Yonkers, P. A. and McCall, J. M. (1988). Attenuation of hemorrhagic shock by the non-glucocorticoid 21-aminosteroid, U7400F. *Eur. J. Pharmacol.* 147: 299–303.

Hammond, B., and Hess, M. L. (1985). The oxygen free radical system: Potential mediator of myocardial injury. *J. Am. Coll. Cardiol.* 6: 225–220.

Harrison, P. M., Wendon, J. A., Gimson, A. E. S., Alexander, G. J. M., and Williams, R. (1991). Improvement by acetylcysteine of hemodynamics and oxygen transport in fulminant hepatic failure. *N. Engl. J. Med.* 324: 1852–1857.

Herschberg, L. A., and Tappel, A. L. (1982). Effects of vitamin E on pentane exhaled by rats treated with methyl ethyl ketone peroxide. *Lipids* 17: 686–691.

Hicks, M., and Gibicki, J. M. (1978). A quantitative relationship between permeability and the degree of peroxidation in UFASOME membranes. *Biochem. Biophys. Res. Commun.* 80: 704–708.

Hussain, S. N., Graham, R., Rudledge, F., and Roussos, C. (1986). Respiratory muscle energetics during endotoxic shock in dogs. *J. Appl. Physiol.* 60: 486–493.

Jager, F. C. (1972). Linoleic acid intake and vitamin E requirement in rats and ducklings. *Ann. N. Y. Acad. Sci.* 203: 199–211.

Jarasch, E. D., Grund, C., Bruder, G., Heid, H. W., Keenan, T. W., and Franke, W. W. (1981). Localization of xanthine oxidase in mammary-gland epithelium and capillary endothelium. *Cell* 25: 67–82.

Jenkins, R. R. (1988). Free radical chemistry; relationship to exercise. *Sports Med.* 5: 156–170.

Ji, L. L., and Fu, R. (1992). Responses of glutathione system and antioxidant enzymes to exhaustive exercise and hydroperoxide. *J. Appl. Physiol.* 72: 549–554.

Ji, L. L., Stratman, F. W., and Lardy, H. A. (1988a). Enzymatic down regulation with exercise in rat skeletal muscle. *Arch. Biochem. Biophys.* 263: 137–149.

Ji, L. L., Stratman, F. W., and Lardy, H. A. (1988b). Antioxidant enzyme systems in rat liver and skeletal muscle. Influences of selenium deficiency, chronic training, and acute exercise. Arch. Biochem. Biophys 263: 150–160.

Johnson, D. L., Horneffer, P. J., Dinatale, J. M., Gott, V. L., and Gardner, T. J. (1987). Free radical scavengers improve functional recovery of stunned myocardium in a model of surgical coronary revascularization. *Surgery* 102: 334–340.

Kagan, V. E. (1988). *Lipid Peroxidation in Biomembranes*. Boca Raton, CRC Press.

Kann, H. E., Mengel, C. E., Smith, W., and Horton, B. (1964). Oxygen toxicity and vitamin E. *Aerospace Med.* 35: 840–849.

Kellogg, E. W., and Fridovich, I. (1975). Superoxide, hydrogen peroxide and singlet oxygen in lipid peroxidation by a xanthine oxidase system. *J. Biol. Chem.* 250: 8812–8817.

Kellogg, E. W., and Fridovich, I. (1977). Liposome oxidation and erythrocyte lysis by enzymatically generated superoxide and hydrogen peroxide. *J. Biol. Chem.* 252: 6721–6728.

Ketai, L. H., Grum, C. M., and Supinski, G. S. (1990). Tissue release of ATP degradation products during shock in dogs. *Chest* 97: 220–226, 1990.

Khalidi, V., and Chaglassian, T. (1965). The species distribution of xanthine oxidase. *Biochem. J.* 97: 318–320.

Kivits, G. A. A., Ganguli-Swarttouw, M. A. C. R., and Chist, E. J. (1981). The composition of alkanes in exhaled air of rats as a result of lipid peroxidation in vivo. *Biochim. Biophys. Acta* 665: 559–570.

Klebanoff, S. J. (1975). Antimicrobial mechanisms in neutrophilic polymorphonuclear leukocytes. *Semin. Hematol.* 12: 117–141.

Kelbanoff, S. J. (1980). Myeloperoxidase mediates cytotoxic systems. In *The Reticuloendothelial System: A Comprehensive Treatise*, Vol. 2. Edited by A. J. Sbarra and R. Strauss. New York, Plenum Press, pp. 279–308.

Kontos, H. A. (1985). Oxygen radicals in cerebral vascular injury. *Circ. Res.* 57: 508–516.

Kontos, H. A. and Hess, M. L. (1983). Oxygen radicals and vascular damage. *Adv. Exp. Med. Biol.* 161: 365–75.

Korthius, R. J., Granger, D. N., Townsley, M. I., and Taylor, A. E. (1985). The role of oxygen-derived free radicals in ischemia-induced increases in canine skeletal muscle vascular permeability. *Circ. Res.* 57: 599–609.

Korthius, R. J., Grishman, M. B., and Granger, D. N. (1988). Leukocyte depletion attenuates vascular injury in postischemic skeletal muscle. *Am. J. Physiol.* 254: H823–H827.

Koyam, S., Kabayashi, T., Kubo, K., Sekiguchi, M., and Ueda, G. (1992). Recombinant-human superoxide dismutase attenuates endotoxin-induced lung injury in awake sheep. *Am. Rev. Respir. dis.* 145: 1404–1409.

Kramer, J. H., Arroyo, C. M., Dickens, B. F., and Weglicki, W. B. (1987). Spin-trapping evidence that graded myocardial ischemia alters post-ischemic superoxide production. *Free Radical Biol. Med.* 3: 153–159.

Kukreja, R. C., Okabe, E., Schrier, G. M., and Hess, M. L. (1988). Oxygen radical-mediated lipid peroxidation and inhibition of Ca^{2+}-ATPase activity of cardiac sarcoplasmic reticulum. *Arch. Biochem. Biophys.* 261: 447–457.

Kukreja, R. C., Weaver, A. B., and Hess, M. L. (1989). Stimulated human neutrophils damage cardiac sarcoplasmic reticulum. *Biochim. Biophys. Acta* 990: 198–205.

Lang, J. K., Gohil, K., Packer, L., and Burk, R. F. (1987). Selenium deficiency, endurance exercise capacity, and antioxidant status in rats. *J. Appl. Physiol.* 63: 1532–2535.

Lavalle, F., Michelson, A. M., and Dimitrijevic, L. (1973). Biological protection by superoxide dismutase. *Biochem. Biophys. Res. Commun.* 55: 350–357.

Lefer, A. M., Tsoa, P. S., Lefer, D. J., and Ma, X. (1991). Role of endothelial dysfunction in the pathogenesis of reperfusion injury after myocardial ischemia. *FASEB J.* 5: 2029–2034.

Lew, H., Pyke, S., and Quintanilha, A. (1985). Changes in the glutathione status of plasma, liver, and muscle following exhaustive exercise in rats. *FEBS Lett.* 185: 262–266.

Luo, S., and Hultin, H. (1986). In vitro lipid peroxidation modifies proteins and functional properties of sarcoplasmic reticulum. *J. Bioenerg. Biomembr.* 18: 315–23.

Marks, J. D., Marks, C. B., Luce, J. M., Montgomery, A. B., Turner, J., Metz, C. A., and Murray, J. F. (1990). Plasma tumor necrosis factor in patients with septic shock. *Am. Rev. Respir. Dis.* 141: 94–97.

McCord, J. M. (1974). Free radicals and inflammation: Protection of synovial fluid by superoxide dismutase. *Science* 185: 529–531.

McCord, J. M. (1985). Oxygen-derived free radicals in postischemic issue injury. *N. Engl. J. Med.* 312: 159–163.

Meister, A. (1989). A brief history of glutathione and a survey of its metabolism and functions. In *Glutathione: Chemical, Biochemical and Medical Aspects*, Part A. Edited by D. Dolphin, O. Avramovic, and R. Poulson. New York, John Wiley & Sons, pp. 1–48.

Meister, A., and Anderson, M. E. (1983). Glutathione. *Annu. Rev. Biochem.* 52: 711–760.

Menasche, P., Grousset, C., Gauduel, Y., and Piwnica, A. (1986). A comparative study of free radical scavengers in cardioplegic solutions: Improved protection with peroxidase. *J. Thorac. Cardiovasc. Surg.* 92: 264–271.

Morales, C., Andrade, F., Anzueto, A., Levine, S. M., Maxwell, L. G., and Jenkinson, S. G. (1992a). Diethylmalate impairs diaphragmatic function during inspiratory resistive breathing. *Am. Rev. Respir. Dis.* 145: A671, 1992.

Morales, C., Anzueto, A., Andrade, F., Brassard, J., Levine, S. M., Maxwell, L. C., Lawrence, P. A., and Jenkinson, S. G. (1992b). Diaphragmatic function after glutathione depletion and resistive breathing in rats. *Chest* 102: A585.

Motohashi, N., and Mori, I. (1983). Superoxide-dependent formation of hydroxyl radical catalyzed by transferrin. *FEBS Lett.* 157: 197–199.

Mullane, K. M., Read, N., Salmon, J. A., and Moncada, S. (1984). Role of leukocytes in acute myocardial infarction in anesthetized dogs: Relationship to myocardial salvage by anti-inflammatory drugs. *J. Pharmacol. Exp. Ther.* 228: 510–522.

Nashawati, E., DiMarco, A. F., and Supinski, G. (1993). Effects produced by infusion of a free radical generating solution into the diaphragm. *Am. Rev. Respir. Dis* (in press).

Neulieb, R. L., and Neulieb, M. K. (1990). The diverse actions of dimethyl sulfoxide: An indicator of membrane transport activity. *Cytobios* 63: 139–165.

Nuttall, F. Q., and Jones, B. (1968). Creatine kinase and glutamic oxalacetic transaminase activity in serum: Kinetics of chance with exercise and effect of physical conditioning. *J. Lab. Clin. Med.* 71: 847–54.

O'Brien, P. J., and Rahimtula, A. (1975). Involvement of cytochrome P-450 in the intracellular formation of lipid peroxides. *J. Agric. Food Chem.* 23: 154–160.

Ohkawa, D. (1979). Assay for lipid peroxides in animal tissues by thiobarbituric acid reaction. *Anal. Biochem.* 95:351–358.

Parinandi, N. L., Zwinzinski, C. W., and Schmid, H. H. O. (1991). Free radical-induced alterations of myocardial membrane proteins. 289: 118–123.

Parks, D. A., and Granger, D. N. (1983). Ischemia-induced vascular changes: Role of xanthine oxidase and hydroxyl radicals. *Am. J. Physiol.* 245: G285–G289.

Parks, D. A., Bulkley, G. B., Granger, D. N., Hamilton, S. R., and McCord, J. M. (1982). Ischemic injury in the cat small intestine: Role of superoxide radicals. *Gastroenterology* 82: 9–15.

Parks, D. A., Williams, T. K., and Beckman, J. S. (1988). Converion of xanthine dehydrogenase to oxidase in ischemic rat intestine: A reevaluation. *Am. J. Physiol.* 254: G768.

Pascoe, G. A., and Reed, D. J. (1989). Cell calcium, vitamin E, and the thiol redox system in cytotoxicity. *Free Radical Biol. Med.* 6: 209–224.

Pyke, S., Lew, H., and Quintanilha, A. (1986). Severe depletion in liver GSH during physical exercise. *Biochem. Biophys. Res. Commun.* 139: 926–931.

Quintanilha, A. T. (1984). Effects of physical exercise and/or vitamin E on tissue oxidative metabolism. *Biochem. Soc. Trans.* 12: 403–404.

Rao, P. S., Cohen, M. V., and Mueller, H. S. (1983). Production of free radicals and lipid peroxides in early experimental myocardial ischemia. *J. Mol. Cell. Cardiol.* 15: 713–716.

Reed, D. J. (1986). Regulation of reductive processes by glutathione. *Biochem. Pharmacol.* 35: 7–13.

Reid, M. B., Haack, K. E., Francik, K. M., Volberg, P. A., Kabzik, L., and West, M. S. (1992a). Reactive oxygen in skeletal muscle I. Intracellular oxidant kinetics and fatigue in vitro. *J. Appl. Physiol.* 73: 1797–1804.

Reid, M. B., Shoji, T., Moody, M. R., and Entman, M. L. (1992b). Reactive oxygen in skeletal muscle II. Extracellular release of free radicals. *J. Appl. Physiol.* 73: 1805–1809.

Reimer, H. A., and Jennings, R. B. (1985). Failure of the xanthine oxidase inhibitor allopurinol to limit infarct size after ischemia and reperfusion in dogs. *Circulation* 71: 1069–1075.

Richmond, R., Halliwell, B., Chauhon, J., and Darbre, A. (1981). Superoxide-dependent formation of hydroxyl radicals: Detection of hydroxyl radicals by hydroxylation and aromatic compounds. *Ann. Biochem.* 118: 328–335.

Riva, E., Manning, A. S., Hearse, D. J. (1987). Superoxide dismutase and the reduction of reperfusion-induced arrhythmias: In vivo dose-response studies in the rat. *Cardiovasc. Drugs Ther.* 1: 133–139.

Robertson, J. D., Maughan, R. J., Duthie, G. G., and Morrice, P. C. (1991). Increased blood antioxidant systems of runners in response to training load. *Clin. Sci.* 80: 611–618.

Romaschin, A. D., Rebeyka, I., Wilson, G. J., and Mickel, D. A. G. (1987). Conjugated dienes in ischemic and reperfused myocardium; in vivo chemical signature of oxygen free radical mediated injury. *J. Mol. Cell. Cardiol.* 19: 289–302.

Romaschin, A. D., Wilson, G. J., Thomas, U., Feitler, D. A., Tumiati, L., and Mickle, D. A.

(1990). Subcellular distribution of peroxidized lipids in myocardial reperfusion injury. *Am. J. Physiol.* 259: H116–H123.

Romson, J. L., Hook, B. G., Kunkel, S. L., Abrams, G. D., Schork, A., and Lucchesi, B. R. (1983). Reduction of the extent of ischemic myocardial injury by neutrophil depletion in the dog. *Circulation* 67: 1016–1023.

Rosen, G. M., and Freeman, B. A. (1984). Detection of superoxide generated by endothelial cells. *Proc. Natl. Acad. Sci. USA* 81: 7269–7273.

Roussos, C. H., and Moxham, J. (1985). Respiratory muscle fatigue. In *The Thorax*. Edited by C. Roussos and P. T. Macklem. New York, Marcel Dekker.

Rubanyi, G. M., and Vanhoutte, P. M. (1986a). Superoxide anions and hyperoxia inactivate endothelium-derived relaxing factor. *Am. J. Physiol.* 250: H822–H827.

Rubanyi, G. M., and Vanhoutte, P. M. (1986b). Oxygen-derived free radicals, endothelium, and responsiveness of vascular smooth muscle. *Am. J. Physiol.* 250: H815–H821.

Salminen, A., and Vihko, V. (1983). Endurance training reduces the susceptibility of mouse skeletal muscle to lipid peroxidation in vitro. *Acta Physiol. Scand.* 117: 109–113.

Sanderson, R. A., Foley, R. K., McIvor, G. W. D., and Kirkaldy-Willis, W. H. (1975). Histological response of skeletal muscle to ischemia. *Clin. Orthop. Relat. Res.* 113: 27–35.

Selvaraj, R. J., Paul. B. B., Strauss, R. R., Jacobs, A. A., and Abarra, A. O. (1974). Oxidative peptide cleavage and decarboxylation by the $MPO–H_2O_2–Cl$–antimicrobial system. *Infect. Immun.* 9: 255–260.

Selvaraj, R. J., Zgliczynski, J. M., Paul. B. B., and Sbarra, A. J. (1980). Chlorination of reduced nicotinamide adenine dinucleotides by myeloperoxodase: A novel bactericidal mechanism. *J. Reticuloendothel. Soc.* 27: 31–38.

Shatner, C. H., MacCarter, D. J., and Lillehei, R. C. (1976). Effects of allopurinol, propranolol and methylprednisolone on infarct size in experimental myocardial infarction. *Am. J. Cardiol.* 37: 572–80.

Shindoh, C., DiMarco, A., Thomas, A., Manubay, P., and Supinski, G. (1990). Effect of N-Acetylcysteine on diaphragm fatigue. *J. Appl. Physiol.* 68: 2107–2113.

Shindoh, C., DiMarco, A., Nethery, D., and Supinski, G. (1992). Effect of PEG–superoxide dismutase on the diaphragmatic response to endotoxin. *Am. Rev. Respir. Dis.* 145: 1350–54.

Shlafer, M., Kane, P. F., and Kirsh, M. M. (1982a). Superoxide dismutase plus catalase enhances the efficacy of hypothermic cardioplegia to protect the globally ischemic, reperfused heart. *J. Thorac. Cardiovasc. Surg.* 83: 830–9

Shlafer, M., Kane, P. F., Wiggins, V. Y., and Kirsh, M. M. (1982b). Possible role for cytotoxic oxygen metabolites in the pathogenesis of cardiac ischemic injury. *Circulation* 66(Suppl 1): 185–92.

Simpson, P. J., Todd, R. F., Fantone, J. C., Mickelson, J. K., Griffin, J. D., and Lucchesi, B. R. (1988). Reduction of experimental canine myocardial reperfusion injury by a monoclonal antibody (anti-Mol, anti-CD11b) that inhibits leukocyte adhesion. *J. Clin. Invest.* 81: 624–629.

Sjodin, B., Westing, Y. H., and Apple, F. S. (1990). Biochemical mechanisms for oxygen free radical formation during exercise. *Sports Med.* 10: 236–54.

Smith, J. K., Cardan, D. L., Sadasivan, K. K., and Korthius, R. J. (1989a). Role of xanthine oxidase in postischemic microvascular injury. *FASEB J.* 3: A1401.

Smith, J. K., Grisham, M. B., Granger, D. N., and Korthius, R. J. (1989b). Free radical defense mechanisms and neutrophil infiltration in postischemic skeletal muscle. *Am. J. Physiol.* 256: H789–H793.

Southern, P. A., and Powis, G. (1988). Free radicals in medicine. II. Involvement in human disease. *Mayo Clin. Proc.* 63: 390–408.

Sparks, H. V., Korthius, R. J., and Scott, J. B. (1984). Pharmacology of hemodynamic factors in fluid balance. In *Edema*. Edited by N. C. Staub and A. E. Taylor. New York, Raven Press, pp. 425–439.

Spector, T. (1988). Oxypurinol as an inhibitor of xanthine oxidase-catalyzed of superoxide radical. *Chem. Pharmacol.* 37: 349–352.

Stocks, J., and Dormandy, T. L. (1971). The autooxidation of human red cell lipids induced by hydrogen peroxide. *Br. J. Haematol.* 20: 95–111.

Strauss, R. R., Paul, B. B., Jacobs, A. A., and Sbarra, A. J. (1970). Role of the phagocyte in host–parasite interactions. XXII H_2O_2-dependent decarboxylation and deamination by myeloperoxidase and its relationship to antimicrobial activity. *J. Reticuloendothel. Soc.* 7: 745–761.

Strock, P. E., and Majno, G. M. (1969). Microvascular changes in acutely ischemic rat muscle. *Surg. Gynecol. Obstet.* 129: 1213–1224.

Supinski, G., Stofan, D., Van Lunteren, E., and DiMarco, A. (1991a). Malondialdehyde levels and diaphragm fatigue. *Am. Rev. Respir. Dis.* 143: A366.

Supinski, G., Nethery, D., and DiMarco, A. (1991b). Effect of free radical scavengers on lipid peroxidation in the fatiguing diaphragm. *Am. Rev. Respir. Dis.* 143: A560.

Supinski, G. S., Renston, J., and DiMarco, A. F. (1992). Free radical mediated diaphragmatic injury following ischemia/reperfusion. *Am. Rev. Respir. Dis.* 145: A672.

Supinski, G. S., Nethery, D., and DiMarco, A. F. (1993). Endotoxin induces free radical mediated diaphragm and intercostal muscle dysfunction. Am. Rev. Respir. Dis. (in press).

Surell, C. V., Boczkowsi, J., Pasquier, C., Du, Y., Franzini, E., and Aubier, M. (1992). Effects of *N*-acetylcysteine on diaphragmatic function and malondialdehyde content in *Escherichia coli* endotoxemic rats. 146: 730–734.

Tamura, Y., Chi, L. G., Driscoll, E. M., Jr., Hoff, P. T., Freeman, B. A., Gallagher, K. P., and Lucchesi, B. R. (1988). Superoxide dismutase conjugated to polyethylene glycol provides sustained protection against myocardial ischemia/reperfusion injury in canine heart. *Circ. Res.* 63: 944–959.

Taylor, A. E., and Townsley, M. I. (1986). Assessment of oxygen radical tissue damage. In *Physiology of Oxygen Radicals.* Edited by A. E. Taylor, S. Matalon, and P. A. Ward. Bethesda, MD, American Physiological Society, pp. 19–38.

Thomas, C. E., Morehouse, L. A., and Aust, S. D. (1985). Ferritin and superoxide-dependent lipid peroxidation. *J. Biol. Chem.* 260: 3275–3280.

Thomas, E. I., Grisham, M. B., Melton, D. F., and Jefferson, M. M. (1985). Evidence for a role of taurine in the in vitro oxidative toxicity of neutrophils toward erythrocytes. *J. Biol. Chem.* 260: 3321–3329.

Tien, M., and Aust, S. D. (1982). Comparative aspects of several model lipid peroxidation systems. In *Lipid Peroxides in Biology and Medicine.* Edited by K. Yagi. New York, Academic Press, pp. 23–29.

Tierney, D. F., Ayers, L., and Kasuyama, R. S. (1977). Altered sensitivity of oxygen toxicity. *Am. Rev. Respir. Dis.* 115: 59–64.

Till, G. O., Johnson, K. J., Kunkel, R., and Ward, P. A. (1982). Intravascular activation of complement and acute lung injury. Dependency on neutrophils and toxic oxygen metabolites. *J. Clin. Invest.* 69: 1126–1135.

Townsley, M. I., Taylor, G. E., Korthius, R. J., and Taylor, A. E. (1985). Promethazine or DPPD pretreatment attenuates oleic acid-induced injury in isolated canine lungs. *J. Appl. Physiol.* 59: 39–46.

Turrens, J. F., and Boveris, A. (1980). Generation of superoxide anion by the NADPH dehydrogenase of bovine heart mitochondria. *Biochem. J.* 191: 421–427.

Turrens, J. F., Crapo, J. D., and Freeman, B. A. (1984). Protection against oxygen toxicity by intravenous injection of liposome-entrapped catalase and superoxide dismutase. *J. Clin. Invest.* 73: 87–95.

Vander, H. R. S., Sobotka, P. A., and Ganote, C. E. (1987). Effects of the free radical scavenger DMTU and mannitol on the oxygen paradox in perfused rat hearts. *J. Mol. Cell. Cardiol.* 19: 615–25.

Van Hemmen, J. J., and Meuling, W. J. (1975). Inactivation of biologically active DNA by gamma-ray-induced superoxide radicals and their dismutation products: Singlet molecular oxygen and hydrogen peroxide. *Biochim. Biophys. Acta* 402: 133–141.

Vihko, V., Salminen, A., and Rantamaki, J. (1978). Oxidative and lysosomal capacity in skeletal muscle of mice after endurance training of different intensities. *Acta Physiol. Scand.* 104: 74–81.

Ward, P. A., Till, G. O., Kunkel, R., and Beauchamp, C. (1983). Evidence for role of hydroxyl radical in complement and neutrophil-dependent tissue injury. *J. Clin. Invest.* 72: 789–801.

Weiss, S. J., and LoBublio, A. F. (1982). Phagocyte-generated oxygen metabolites and cellular injury. *Lab. Invest.* 47: 5–18.

White, C. W., and Repine, J. E. (1985). Pulmonary antioxidant defense mechanisms. *Exp. Lung Res.* 8: 81–96.

White, C. W., Jackson, J. H., Abuchowski, A., Kazo, G. M., Mimmak, R. F., Bergen, E., Freeman, B. A., McCord, J. M., and Repine, J. E. (1989). Polyethylene glycol-attached antioxidant enzymes decrease pulmonary oxygen toxicity in rats. *J. Appl. Physiol.* 61: 584–590.

Wilcox, P. G., and Bressler, B. (1992). Effects of tumor necrosis factor alpha on in vitro hamster diaphragm contractility. *Am. Rev. Respir. Dis.* 145: A457, 1992.

Wispe, J. R., Bell, E. F., and Roberts, J. R. (1985). Assessment of lipid peroxidation in newborn infants and rabbits by measurements of expired ethane and pentane: Influence of parenteral lipid infusion. *Pediatr. Res.* 19: 374–379, 1985.

Yatvin, M. B., and Lelkes, P. I. (1982). Clinical prospects of liposomes. *Med. Phys.* 9: 149–175.

Yau, T. M., and Mencl, J. (1981). A study of the peroxidation of fatty acid micelles promoted by ionizing radiation, hydrogen peroxide and ascorbate. *Int. J. Radiat. Biol.* 40: 47–61.

Ytrehus, K., Myklebust, R., Olsen, R., and Mjos, O. D. (1987). Ultrasturctural changes induced in the isolated rat heart by enzymatically generated oxygen radicals. *J. Mol. Cell. Cardiol.* 19: 379–89.

Zerba, E., Komorowski, T. E., and Faulkner, J. A. (1990). Free radical injury to skeletal muscles of young, adult, and old mice. *Am. J. Physiol.* 258: C429–C435.

Ziment, I. (1986). Acetylcysteine: A drug with an interesting past and a fascinating future. *Respiration* 50: 26–30.

Zweier, J. L., Flaherty, J. T., and Weisfeldt, M. L. (1987a). Observation of free radical generation in the post-ischemic heart. *Proc. Natl. Acad. Sci. USA* 84: 1404–1407.

Zweier, J. L., Flaherty, J. T., and Wesifeldt, M. L. (1987b). Direct measurement of free radical generation following reperfusion of ischemic myocardium. *Proc. Natl. Acad. Sci. USA* 84: 1414–1417.

Zweier, J. L., Rayburn, B. K., Flaherty, J. T., and Weisfeldt, M. L. (1987c). Recombinant superoxide dismutase reduces oxygen free radical concentrations in reperfused myocardium. *J. Clin. Invest.* 80: 1728–34.

Zweier, J. L., Rayburn, B. K., Flaherty, J. T., and Weisfeldt, M. L. (1987d) Recombinant superoxide dismutase reduces oxygen free radical concentrations in reperfused myocardium. *J. Clin. Invest.* 80: 1728–34.

Part II

**RESPIRATORY MUSCLES:
MECHANICS AND ENERGETICS**

RESPIRATORY MUSCLES
MECHANICS AND ENERGETICS

13

An Abbreviated History of the Respiratory Muscles from Antiquity to the Classical Age

JEAN-PHILIPPE DERENNE

Groupe Hospitalier Pitié-Salpêtrière
Paris, France

WILLIAM A. WHITELAW

University of Calgary
Calgary, Alberta, Canada

I. Pre-Galenic Era

It is generally acknowledged that scientific medicine originated in ancient Greece in the fifth century BC. Although a corpus of concepts and treatments existed in more ancient civilizations, the Greek revolution in medicine was characterized by a completely new system of interpretations of the diseases and of their causes. The idea that diseases were created by the Gods was abandoned. Instead, the most prominent medical figure of that time, Hippocrates, a physician living in the small island of Cos, proposed that the causes of illnesses were due to the environment (Jouanna, 1992). Hippocrates was the 17th physician of his family and a descendant of Asclepios, prince of Tricca in Thessalia in Northern Greece. The sons of Asclepios were renowned in Greece because they participated in the Trojan War. One of them, Machaon, was one of the warriors hidden in the famous horse and was killed during the fight that destroyed the city. Another, Podalires, survived the war and established himself in Caria, in Asia Minor, where he founded the city of Syria. Some of his descendants moved to the island of Cos, and we still know the names of all of them from Podalires to Hippocrates (Jouanna, 1992). The family was well known, and the young Hippocrates received a complete medical education. It seems that he learned dissection in the same time as reading and writing (Jouanna, 1992). He traveled to Thessalia, but eventually came back to Cos, where he spent the rest of his life.

There are approximately 60 volumes under the name of Hippocrates. They established the basis for scientific inquiry in medicine. They recommended minute and careful clinical examination of the patients. As for respiration, clear descriptions of fast or slow, deep or shallow, free or labored, regular or periodic breathing are described in several books. Hippocratic physicians practiced direct auscultation of the chest and described rales and friction rubs (Jouanna, 1992). They knew how to drain water or pus from the chest (Hochberg). However, their knowledge of anatomy was crude, and their concepts of respiration rather fanciful. The lungs were not connected with breathing; air breathed in went first to the brain, then to the heart. The diaphragm was frequently mentioned, but its role in respiration was not recognized (Duminil, 1983).

Another prominent figure of the time was the physician and philosopher, Empedocles of Agrigentum in Sicily. He introduced the concepts of the division of matter into four elements, out of which everything else was constituted: earth, air, fire, and water, and of the omnipotence of two principles, love (which unifies) and hate (which divides). This system has played a fundamental role in the history of Western thought (Zafiropulo, 1953). In addition, Empedocles introduced the first scientific concept of respiration, comparing the breathing of air to the movements of water produced with a clepsydra, a closed container with a small hole on the top and many tiny ones on the bottom. Water comes in and out of the clepsydra with different positions of the thumb on the upper hole and of water in the lower ones. By analogy, Empedocles proposed that movements of the blood in the vessels caused movements of air through the pores of the skin (Bollack, 1950; Duminil, 1983; Furley and Wilkie, 1984). Although this analogy does not draw on any concept of modern physics, such as pressure, volume, or flow, it is remarkable that it was the first time that a natural human phenomenon was explained on the basis of a comparison with a physical model. It indicated that the understanding of human physical nature could be based not on esoteric or mystical concepts, but rather, on the observation of the physical laws that govern inanimate objects.

Aristotle was the first to link respiration, thoracic organs, and movement. He paid particular attention to anatomy and introduced the concept of the "final purpose." He lived in the fourth century BC in Athens and in Macedonia, where King Philip hired him as a teacher to his son Alexander (The Great). Aristotle was the son of a physician. As a philosopher, his influence was immense, but he was also a biologist. More than a third of his writings deal with biology. He proposed that the use of respiration was to cool the body to prevent the innate heat from becoming excessive, an analogy to a charcoal fire. The mechanism for it was the heart, which was the site of the innate heat. The heart expanded the lungs, and the lungs expanded the thorax. As for the diaphragm, it was just a wall separating the thoracic content ("the better part") from the abdomen ("which exists only for the benefit of the other part"). His theory was to persist for more than 20 centuries and William Harvey himself was still defending it in the second half of the 17th century. However, one must remember that muscles at that time were only flesh. They were not related to the generation of force and movement. Their functions were to protect the bones from injury, to hold tissues together, and to keep the animal warm (Bastholm, 1950).

The notions of a nervous system with brain and nerves and of muscles as agents of force and movement were introduced in the fourth and third century BC by the Greek physicians of Alexandria in Egypt. Herophilus practiced human dissections and is considered to be the father of modern anatomy. Erasistratus performed animal experiments to prove that the lungs were expanded by the thorax and that the respiratory muscles, particularly the diaphragm, were the agents of this movement (Von Staden, 1989). From the third century BC to the second century AD, we know many names of famous physicians who made significant contributions to the understanding of respiratory muscle physiology. Although their writings have disappeared, they were quoted by Galen, who gave them admiring reviews. In the second century AD, Galen was to synthesize their contributions, together with his own discoveries, thereby producing an astoundingly modern work, which was to become a milestone in the history of science.

II. Galen

Galen (129–200) was born in Pergamon in Asia Minor, a city well known at that time for its famous medical school. He studied medicine in several cities and came back to his birth place, where he was appointed a sports medicine doctor working as the physician to the gladiators from age 27–33. He then moved to Rome, where he became the physician of emperors Marcus Aurelius and Commodus.

Galen was a prodigious writer, who left long accounts of his multiple experiments, clinical observations, arguments, and conclusions, many of which are still available today. He performed an extensive systematic series of experiments that first recapitulated those of Erasistratus, and then went on to detail the anatomy and function of all the respiratory muscles. These were mostly done in pigs, alive or dead, and included dissections of muscles, sections of intercostal and phrenic nerves, of the spinal cord at each segmental level, and sections of individual muscles or sets of muscles. He discovered the two layers of intercostal muscles, as well as the innervation of the diaphragm, the other respiratory muscles, and the larynx. Using the loudness of the cries of the pig as an index of respiratory motor output, he calculated the importance of the various muscle groups for respiration. He classified muscles as inspiratory or expiratory and noted which were used for quiet breathing, moderate hyperpnea, and extreme respiratory efforts. He showed more clearly than any of his successors up to recent times that the diaphragm, unaided, expands the lower, but not the upper, rib cage. He also analyzed the interaction between abdominal muscles and diaphragm for expulsive maneuvers and for breathing. He based his differential diagnosis of dyspnea on observations about the recruitment of respiratory muscles.

The experiments, discussions, and conclusions about the diaphragm are largely laid out in two extensive works and are available in fine English translations, *De Anatomicis Administrationibus* and *De Usu Partium*, but what is assumed to be his most comprehensive description, a set of three books on respiration alone, has unfortunately been completely lost, including the details of his work on the intercostal muscles.

The anatomy of the intercostal muscles is described in a book about anatomy of muscles: *De Musculorum Dissectionibus*. Galen explains there are two layers, internal and external, with fibers running obliquely from one rib to the other and crossing to make an *X*. He then separates the intercostal muscles into posterior sections attached to the bony ribs, and anterior sections attached to the cartilaginous ribs, and says the anterior section of the external layer has its fibers running in the direction opposite those of the fibers in the posterior section, and the same is true for the internal layer. (It seems obvious he must have been describing the muscles we call parasternal intercostal muscles as the anterior, intercartilaginous section of the external intercostal. The deep muscle, running criss-cross with the parasternal in the region of the cartilaginous ribs, is presumably the muscle we now call triangularis sterni. It is not, strictly speaking, an intercostal muscle, but might have been difficult to distinguish from one.) He then states that for the interosseus section, the external layer is inspiratory and the internal layer is expiratory, but for the intercartilaginous section, the external layer is expiratory and the internal layer inspiratory.

Unfortunately, the experiments on which this conclusion is based are not described. We can guess how he did them because we know how his experimental logic worked (Debru, 1990), and he gave an extensive description of his techniques in *De Anatomicis Administrationibus*. His analysis of respiratory and other muscle action primarily depended on ablation experiments. In some experiments, he would disable the muscle in question, either by interfering with the nerve, or by sectioning the belly of the muscle. In complementary experiments, he would disable all of the antagonist and synergist muscles to observe the action of one isolated muscle. In his methods book, he tells students they should practice repeatedly until they are able, with one or two sweeps of a knife, to cut through the fibers of one layer of intercostal muscle without injuring the other layer, and to cut both layers of intercostal muscle without incising the pleura. These skills would have enabled him to disable the whole set of external intercostals at once, or just the interosseus part, or just the intercartilaginous part. He also had a technique for reversibly blocking conduction in the intercostal nerves with ligatures, but talked about doing this only at the point where the nerves leave the spinal cord. He could disable the diaphragm by cutting the phrenic nerve, and the neck accessory muscles by sectioning the muscles themselves. He judged the results by watching movements of the chest wall. (In some vivisection experiments, he exposed much of the rib cage by removing the skin to get a better view.) Readers of this chapter may be interested to try to imagine what experiments he actually did, the results he would have obtained, and how he might have come to the conclusions he did about the function of interosseus and intercartilaginous intercostals.

Galen's conclusions agree roughly with current opinion about the function of the interosseus intercostals, although now we are beginning to appreciate that their function depends on the region of the chest they are in, and on the activity of synergistic muscles. The conclusion Galen drew about the intercartilaginous intercostals is the opposite of current thinking.

Galen's account was based purely on description of what happened when muscles acted alone or in concert in various vivisection experiments, occasionally corroborated by observations on patients. He seldom used arguments based on engineering concepts and apparently did not inquire how the forces exerted by muscles produced the observed actions. His achievement in this field was, nevertheless, a monumental one, so much so that his level of understanding would not really be equaled until the 19th century.

III. Middle Ages and Renaissance

The great syntheses of the respiratory pump was not part of the central core of Galen's work that was copied, translated, discussed, and passed on by the Arabs. Only the briefest precis was available through the Middle Ages, a bare description and tally of the number of respiratory muscles and a statement about which were inspiratory and which expiratory. In most accounts, the intercostals were simply listed as both inspiratory and expiratory. Even the idea that the respiratory muscles were the cause of lung expansion got muddled because Galen was not the undisputed authority. Aristotle also required respect from the scholars, and he had said the heart caused the movement of the lungs. No new work, or even repeats of the old dissections and animal experiments, seems to have been performed through the millenium before the 15th century.

The revival of interest in anatomy and physiology in the Renaissance started as a backward, rather than a forward, movement. The European scholars found, translated, and disseminated the books of the Arabs and Greeks. Human autopsies were performed in many universities in the 13th and 14th centuries and a first modern book of anatomy was published in 1316 by Mundinus, although most of it was simply taken from the Arabs. Indeed the autopsies were generally performed by barbers and surgeons, whereas the anatomist was reading Galen, with the assistants between them and the cadaver, and the audience could hardly see anything. Gradually, however, a spirit of discovery made itself felt and the concept that students should perform autopsies *with their own hands* was strongly promoted by the leading anatomist of the first part of the 16th century, Jacques Dubois (Jacobus Sylvius; 1478–1555) of Paris and his German assistant, Gunther of Andernacht (1487–1574) (Baker, 1909). Sylvius had among his students Andreas Vesalius (1514–1564), a brilliant and wealthy young man from Brussels, Belgium. Vesalius stayed 3 years in Paris, studying with Sylvius and also with Jean Fernel (1497–1558), the creator of modern physiology according to Sherrington (Fernel, 1543; Sherrington, 1946). He then moved to Padua and published what was to become a milestone in the history of human anatomy and physiology, the *De Humani Corporis Fabrica* in the same year (1543) as *De Revolutionibus Orbium Coelestium* of Copernicus (Vesalius, 1543).

On the basis of his own vivisections, Vesalius challenged many of Galen's teachings. Among them was his description of diaphragm action. Vesalius claimed that the diaphragm was more fixed in its central part than at the edges, and that, with contraction, it changed from a more hemispheric shape to a more conical one. In his *The Epitome*, Vesalius also stated that the diaphragm dilated the thorax; but he did not clearly explain how this happened (Vesalius, 1949). His fellow and successor, R. Colombo (Columbus) stated that the diaphragm led both inspiration and expiration and that its contraction moved itself upward and tightened the lower ribs (Colombo, 1543).

Leonardo Da Vinci (1452–1519) had little influence on the development of ideas about respiratory muscles because he never completed his long-term project of writing a comprehensive book of anatomy and physiology, and never published it. His notebooks, preserved in various libraries and published in recent times, nevertheless show that he progressed far ahead of his time by combining his artist's appreciation of anatomical detail with his engineer's ideas of the workings of mechanical devices. The notebooks contain more than 30 drawings or diagrams related to respiratory muscles, together with explanations of how they might work (O'Malley and Saunders, 1952).

For Da Vinci it was clear that when the diaphragm muscle contracted, the dome would tend to descend, making a space in the thorax into which the lung would expand. Because he saw the diaphragm joining the inside of the rib cage at an acute angle, rather than tangentially, he also reasoned that if abdominal contents provided any resistance to descent of the dome, there would be tension in the diaphragm that would tend to draw in the lower margin of the rib cage. To explain the paradox that the lower rib cage margin moves out in inspiration, he deduced there must be a separate expanding force exerted on the ribs, and this he attributed to the serratus anterior, which he believed had its origin on the spinal column, and to the scalenes, which in some animals at least and in his drawings extended far down the rib cage. If he was familiar with Galen's claim that the diaphragm unaided could expand the lower rib cage, he must have rejected this hearsay evidence from antiquity by reason of confident logic based on his anatomical facts and engineering principles. Lacking exact information about the geometry of the diaphragm in vivo, the logic is sound, and the conclusion not far from the correct one.

Da Vinci's ideas focused very much on the relation between the diaphragm and abdominal muscles. His analysis indicated that the diaphragm, in descending, displaced abdominal contents, volume for volume, and he described, on the other hand, how the abdominal muscles by contracting would force the diaphragm up into the chest. These qualitative concepts were fully appreciated by Galen, but the quantitative aspect is completely new. Quantification was to be one of the main features of the upcoming scientific revolution led by Galileo (Grmek, 1990). For Da Vinci, inspiration was active, accomplished by diaphragm and rib cage muscles. Expiration was partly passive, owing to reexpansion of abdominal gas squeezed by diaphragm contraction, and partly active owing to contraction of abdominal muscles. The relaxed position was diaphragm up, based on the finding in cadavers. Concerning expulsive maneuvers, he writes in some sections that the diaphragm participates, but in other sections, he argues it is not essential. The reasoning is based on consideration of displacements. He notes that it is possible to expel feces without breathing at the same time. He expects that if diaphragm displacement caused expulsion, there would necessarily be an accompanying inspiration of a volume of air to match the expelled volume of feces.

Another important function of the diaphragm in Da Vinci's physiology was in digestion. The repeated compression and decompression was supposed to cause emptying of the stomach, the pylorus acting as a one-way valve to prevent reverse flow. It is to be certain that this function is accomplished that we choose to breathe mainly with the diaphragm.

Da Vinci's diagrams include one that illustrates his idea that the scalenes, by analogy with the shrouds that support the mast of a ship, could support the neck upright or could raise the upper ribs. He also pointed out that the intercostal muscles, by contracting together on one side of the body, should be able to draw the ribs together and flex the trunk to that side.

IV. Classical Age

The history of respiration in the 17th century was marked by major advances in the theory of the purpose of respiration. The discovery of the circulation of the blood by Harvey; the description of pulmonary capillaries by Malpighi; the demonstrations by Hooke, Highmore, Boyle, and others that insufflation of air into the lungs was necessary for life, but that no visible air appeared in the pulmonary veins; then, the discovery that blood in the pulmonary vein was a different color from blood in the pulmonary arteries, and that some component of air was consumed by respiration, all summed up to point to the reason that ventilation of the lungs was necessary. After another hundred years Lavoisier's discoveries would give the clear link between combustion and metabolism.

Things were less clear in the realm of respiratory muscles and mechanics. In his Lumlean lectures, Harvey recapitulated the medieval compromise between the theories of Galen and Aristotle. The respiratory muscles caused the lungs to expand, but the heart also did so, the efforts of these two motive organs being marvelously coordinated. He also transmitted the ancient lore relating the diaphragm to hysteria and delerium. However, he had clearly made observations of his own during vivisections and challenged Vesalius's concept of how it contracted, giving, instead, a description of a dome flattening as it descended.

The advances in physics and mathematics led by Galileo and Descartes set physiologists of the 17th century in the direction of explaining the respiratory pump with new engineering concepts. Descartes introduced the revolutionary concept of *"Man, a Machine"* (Descartes, 1972), and Steno analyzed muscle action with very complex geometric models, thus introducing a new way to analyze muscle action, which still persists in our times (Steno, 1667; Balsthom, 1950).

In 1676, Caspar Bartholin published *Diaphragmatis Structura Nova*, which contains illustrations showing the direction of muscle fibers, together with a mathematical model. He considered the costal and crural parts of the diaphragm to be different muscles, and showed them as connected mechanically in series. As well, he thought the action of the diaphragm was coupled in series with that of the transversus abdominis, referring to the whole set as a trigastric muscle (Bartholin, 1676). Borelli's book, *De Motu Animalium* (1681–1682) is laid out in a series of propositions similar to Euclid's geometry, and is based on anatomical data plus mathematical models. In it, Borelli introduced the concept of elastic recoil of the rib cage, although he thought it to be expiratory in direction. He considered the shape of the active diaphragm and *could personally observe on an Indian rabbit in pain the diaphragm descending forcefully into the abdomen, exceeding the flat disc configuration and actually becoming caudally convex (Proposition 89)*. He denied that normal spontaneous inspiration could take place without a contribution from the intercostal muscles, arguing as Da Vinci had, that the diaphragm's insertions must pull the ribs inward (Borelli, 1682). He was certain on the basis of his analysis that the only thing either external or internal intercostal muscles could do is draw the ribs together.

Malpighi studied the problem of diaphragm action and concluded, in 1661, that when its muscle fibers contract, the abdominal viscera are pushed downward, the thorax widens, and the lungs are dilated (Anzalone, 1966). Malpighi also found it necessary to take up the fight against a new idea. A major distraction had appeared with the theory that the diaphragm was only an expiratory muscle. Following several other influential authors (Laurentius, 1600; Bauhin, 1620), Ysbrand Diemerbroek compared the diaphragm to *a casting net which is thrown spread abroad into the water, but being drawn up again, is contracted by the inner ropes of its circumference* and stated that *the diaphragm spread abroad in expiration contracts its circumference by its fibers together with the ribs annexed to it, and so returns its loose convexity* (Diemerbroek, 1694). This concept was supported by several other influential writers of the day, and whether or not the diaphragm was inspiratory remained controversial (Swammerdam, 1667; Sylvius, 1679; Bohn, 1686).

John Mayow, who is better known for his contributions to the theory of chemical respiration, also studied mechanics. He emphasized interaction between abdominal contents and diaphragm, pointing out that breathing was difficult if the andomen was too full, impeding downward motion of the diaphragm. He supposed that orthopnea could be explained by feebleness of a diaphragm that could not combat the weight of the viscera in the supine posture, but could move the viscera downward when aided by gravity in the sitting posture. In these discussions he introduced *pressure* for the first time to characterize the effect the viscera had on the diaphragm. He also argued for the hypothesis that muscles could be involved in the production of symptoms, and thought the suffocation of asthma might "be caused by the convulsed intercostal muscles and diaphragm" (Mayow, 1669).

The 17th century was thus marked by the development of mathematics, physics, and chemistry, and by their introduction in the field of biology. Descartes's definition of Man: *De la Machine de Son Corps* illustrates the rising concept of a separation between the soul and the body, which could be explained according to universal laws and models. The 18th century saw the establishment of physiology as an individual discipline. Albrecht von Haller (1708–1777), the most prominent figure of the 18th century, defined *physiology* as anatomy in movement, a conception which would be definitively rejected only in the middle of the 19th century. Yet, he introduced the new concepts of (pain) *sensitivity* and *irritability* (muscle excitability), which both could hardly be related to the anatomical configuration of the organ (Canguilhem, 1983). In that sense, the 18th century is more a transition between the 17th (introduction of physical and chemical models in biology) and the 19th century when function was no longer related to the gross anatomy of the organs. In fact, the major advances in respiration were linked to the discovery of respiratory gases—carbon dioxide and oxygen—and with the formulation of the chemical laws of respiration by Lavoisier at the end of the century.

Precise anatomical description of the muscles is found in the textbook of anatomy of the very influential J. B. Winslow (1669–1760), *Exposition Anatomique* (Winslow, 1723). Winslow was a former fellow of Caspar Bartholin. He explained the flattening of the contracting diaphragm by two contradictory movements: shortening of the contracting muscle and outward movement of the ribs to which it is attached, whereas the role of the intercostals was to move the ribs and the sternum upward and to widen the intercostal spaces. Herman Boerhaave (1668–1738) was the teacher of Haller and wrote a major textbook of physiology (*Institutione Medicae*, 1708). He clearly stated that the diaphragm pushed the abdomen and inflated the rib cage. Strapping the abdomen resulted in dyspnea, with a reduction in inspiratory volume, compensated by an increased respiratory frequency. Although he did not provide precise reasons for his thinking, he concluded his description of diaphragmatic action by asserting that *the thorax dilates always and in all directions.* Interestingly, he also stated that *the inferior part of the lung . . . followed diaphragmatic notion: it is here that the expansion is the greatest and the circulation of the blood the fastest,* a notion which would be developed only in the second half of the 20th century (Boerhaave, 1758).

Albrecht von Haller was the great physiologist of the 18th century. A fellow and a successor of Boerhaave in Leyden, he published Boerhaave's works with extensive annotations. He was a scholar with an encyclopedic knowledge of the literature, and his works were written with great care, containing accurate and extensive quotations. He originated the controversial notion that the first rib was the least mobile, which led him to conclude that all the intercostals were inspiratory. He considered that this inspiratory action of the intercostals was more obvious in dyspneic men than in women, and thought that it was not sufficient for healthy men, but that the movement was essential to provide the fulcrum for the diaphragm *so that this muscle uses its force not to bring down the ribs but to pull itself down*. He concluded that *in healthy resting man, the diaphragm is nearly the only muscle acting during respiration*. Thus, it is clear that although Haller described the intercostals as inspiratory, he thought that their main activity was that of fixators of the rib cage and facilitators of diaphragmatic action. In addition to his *Elements of Physiology*, he published a monograph on the diaphragm, *De Diaphragmatis Musculis Dissertatio Anatomica* (Haller, 1738), which included a fine representation of the diaphragm with well-individualized sternal, costal, and crural portions (Fig. 1). Interestingly, he recognized two crural parts on each side: appendices exteriores and interiores. Haller summarized previous authors' opinions and gave an impressive list of contributors, most of whom were totally ignored in other publications. He quoted five authors who considered that the diaphragm was expiratory; two who thought that it was inspiratory, and occasionally expiratory; two who thought that although inspiratory it was not the main agent of inspiration; and no fewer than 34, who considered that it was the main inspiratory muscle. He personally believed that the diaphragm did not drive the rib cage, but was responsible for an increase of the vertical diameter of the thorax, a decrease in abdominal volume, and was the only muscle acting during quiet inspiration. If breathing was more profound, the intercostals would be used, and when *violent* inspiration was to be performed, the scalenes, intercostals, and pectorals would be recruited. He too considered that the diaphragm was involved in various other acts, such as expulsion of feces and urine; compression of the gallbladder; facilitation of digestion, of secretion, and of mobility of the humors in the liver and kidneys; but that it was not involved in vomiting and singultus.

Haller is particularly impressive because of his style and of his encyclopedic knowledge. He was the first to use bibliography in the modern way, with references systematically ordered, described, and discussed with great precision. He did not perform extensive experiments in the field of respiratory muscle mechanics and control, but gave a good and comprehensive review of what was known at the time. His controversies with Hamberger were more due to an opposing opinion on the mathematical and physical models of intercostal muscle action. Hamberger published a complete account of the analysis of respiratory muscle action, essentially devoted to vector analysis of intercostal muscle and rib mechanics, directly derived from the Steno–Borelli conceptual vectorial representation, together with two conflicting contributions of Haller, and eight additional chapters of his own, bringing new insight on his own model (Hamberger, 1749).

By the end of the 18th century, the pattern of modern respiratory muscle

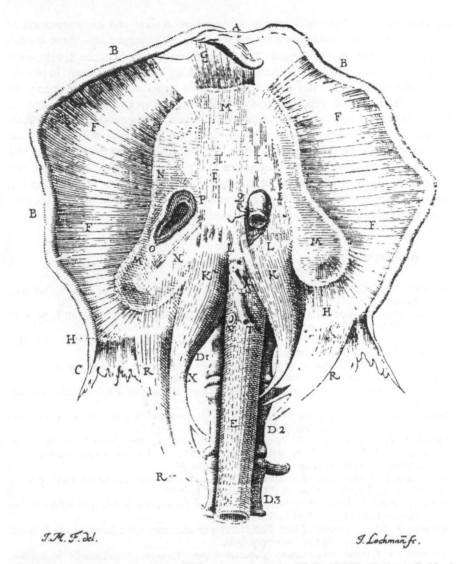

J. H. F. del.   J. Lochman fc.

Figure 1 Representation of the diaphragm according to Haller (1738). Haller individual-ized several parts: costal (F), sternal (G), and divided the crural diaphragm in two (H and R). Haller summarized the current knowledge in the middle of the 18th century.

physiology was thus well established. The main vivisection techniques for whole-animal studies, invented by Galen, had been revived, so that the logic and the experimental means were available for confirming any theoretical conclusion. The process of mathematical or physical modeling, started by Empedocles, had become the major thrust after the introduction of geometric, vectorial analysis by the iatromechanicists. Modern standards of literature review and documentation of discussion had been established by Haller. The 19th century saw these themes developed in considerable degree. The close historical link between development of ideas in physics and their application in physiology suggests that trends in physics and mathematics of the day have been the most important factors in setting the direction and style of thinking and investigation in the area of muscle mechanics. The 19th century saw this theme recur, when the rise of thermodynamics, with its concepts of work and energy were rapidly followed by a major shift to analyzing respiratory mechanics in terms of pressure and volume. Toward the end of the 19th century, this conception of the respiratory pump as a thermodynamic engine, the activity of which could be represented abstractly on a pressure–volume diagram, had the effect of moving the focus of attention away from individual muscles for a considerable time, to return again only in the past 20 years.

References

Anzalone, M. (1966). *Marcello Malpighi e i Suoi Scritti Sugli Organi del Respiro*. Bologna, Tamari.

Aristotle (1956). *Histoire des Animaux* I17, 496b 10sq. *Les Parties des Animaux* III 6, 669a; III 10, 272n; III 10, 273. Paris, Les Belles Lettres.

Baker, F. (1909). The two Sylviuses. An historical study. *Johns Hopkins Hosp. Bull.* 20:1–32.

Bartholin, C. (1676). *Diaphragmatis Structura Nova*. Paris, L. Billain.

Bastholm, E. (1950). *The History of Muscle Physiology*. Copenhagen, E. Munksgaard.

Bauhin, C. (1621). *Theatrum Anatomicum*. Paris, J. T. Debry.

Boerhaave, H. (1758). *Praelectiones Academicae*. Edited and annotated by A. Haller. Leyden, Sumptibus Societatis.

Bohn, J. (1686). Motus diaphragmatis. In *Circulus Anatomicus–Physiologicus seu Oeconomia Corporis Animalis*. Leipzig, p. 86.

Bollack, J. (1969). *Empedocles*. III. *Les Origines, Commentaire 2*. Paris, Les Editions de Minuit.

Borelli G. A. (1681). *De Motu Animalium*. Part II. Roma, A. Bernabo. English translation of chapter VII by R. Borattini Bolchini and G. Ambrogio,

Canguilhem, G. (1983). *Etude d'Histoire et de Philosophie des Sciences*, 5th ed. Paris, Vrin.

Colombo, R. (1543). *De re Anatomica*. Frankfort, M. Lechler.

Debru, A. (1990). *La Pensée* Physiologique. *Doctrines et Langages de la Respiration Chez Galien Dans le Monde Greco–Romain*. Paris.

Descartes, R. (1972). *Treatise of Man*. French text with translation and commentary by T. Steele Hall. Cambridge, Harvard University Press.

Diemerbroeck, I. (1694). *The Anatomy of Human Bodies*. Translated from Latin by W. Salmon. London, Whitwool, pp. 300–304.

Duminil, M. P. (1983). *Le Sang, les Vaisseaux et le Coeur Dans la Collection Hippocratique*. Paris, Les Belle Lettres.

Fernel, J. (1655). *Les Sept Livres de la Physiologie* (1543). Traduit par C. de Saint Germain. Paris, J. Guignard jeune.

Furley, D. J., and Wilkie, J. S. (1984). *Galen on Respiration and the Arteries*. Princeton, Princeton University Press.

Grmek, M. D. (1990). *La Première Révolution Biologique*. Paris, Payot.

Haller, A. von (1738). *De Diaphragmates Musculis Dissertatio Anatomica*. Leyden.

Hamberger, G. E. (1749). *De Respirationis Mechanismo et Usu Genuino Dissertatio*. Iena, C. Croeker.

Hochberg, L. A. *Thoracic Surgery Before the 20th Century*. New York, Vantage Press.

Jouanna, J. (1992). *Hippocrate*. Paris, Fayard.

Laurentius, A. (1600). *Humani Corporis et Singularum Eius Partium Multis Controversÿs et Observationibus Novis Illustra*. Paris, M. Orry.

Mayow, J. (1669). *Tractatus Duo Quorum Prior Agit de Respiratione*. Oxford, Hall and Davis.

O'Malley, C. D., De, C. M., and Saunders J. M. (1952). *Leonardo da Vinci on the Human Body*. New York, H. Schumann.

Sherrington, C. S. (1946). *The Endeavour of Jean Fernel*. Cambridge, Cambridge University Press.

Staden, H. von (1989). *Herophilus: The Art of Medicine in Early Alexandria*. Cambridge, Cambridge University Press.

Steno, N. (1667). *Elementorum Myologiae Specimen*. Florence.

Swammerdam, J. (1738). *Tractatus Physico Anatomico Medicus de Respiratione Usuque Pulmonum*. Leyden, C. Wishoff.

Sylvius II (F. Deleboe) (1679). *Opera Medica*. Amsterdam, D. Elsevier and A. Wolgang.

Vesalius, A. (1543). *De Humani Corporis Fabrica*. Venice, I. Oporini.

Vesalius, A. (1949). *The Epitome*. Translated by L. R. Lind. New York, Macmillan.

Winslow, J. B. (1723). *Exposition Anatomique de la Structure du Corps Humain*. Paris, G. Deprez et J. Desessartz.

Zafiropulo, J. (1953). *Empédocle d'Agrigente*. Paris, Les Belles Lettres.

14

Functional Anatomy of the Chest Wall

DENNIS GORDON OSMOND

McGill University
Montreal, Quebec, Canada

I. Introduction

The human thorax provides an elegant example of the modification of complex anatomical structures to serve one overriding function. Together, the various tissues of the thoracic wall comprise a strong, yet delicately regulated, pump or bellows providing rigidity capable of resisting surrounding pressures, mobility allowing active expansion and aspiration of air, and a resilience that imparts properties of elastic recoil.

The components of the chest wall and their respiratory significance have been recognized since the beginnings of anatomical observation. Many functional correlations, however, remain controversial to the present day. This chapter reviews the basic structure of the chest wall in humans relative to those features that underlie the mechanisms of the thoracic pump.

The general plan of the chest (Fig. 1) is clarified by its evolution and otogeny, detailed in Chapter 5. The separation of a thoracic cavity from the abdomen by a complete muscular diaphragm is a phylogenetically late development, permitting independent chest movements and function. In lower vertebrates, a single body cavity is surrounded by muscle sheets, solely compressive in action. In reptiles and higher forms, the development of rigid bony ribs, located segmentally in the plane of the bony wall muscles, allows the muscles to expand

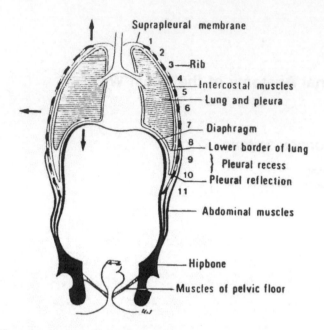

Figure 1   Plan of thoracic wall and body cavities.

the body cavity as well as to compress it. This is facilitated by the evolution of joints between ribs and vertebrae and of a ventral connecting bar, the sternum. In mammals, the development of lungs, originating embryologically from the cervical region, depresses a partition, the diaphragm, representing part of the innermost layer of body wall musculature and creating a separate thoracic cavity. The diaphragm is internal to the ribs at its attachments, continuous with the innermost muscle layer of the abdominal wall (see Fig. 1). The body wall muscles in the plane of the ribs are represented by the intercostal muscles in the thorax. The muscle layer external to the ribs has been modified to form powerful muscles that stabilize the pectoral girdle and arm, and almost completely cloth the external surface of the thoracic cage.

II. Thoracic Shape

Considered as a whole, the adult thorax resembles a truncated cone (Figs. 2–4). Its transverse diameter is greatest at the level of the eighth or ninth rib in the midaxillary line; however, it narrows slightly below that level, and progressively so at higher levels up to the first rib (see Fig. 2). Consequently, below the ninth rib, the inner rib surfaces face somewhat upward, whereas at higher levels they face progressively more downward as well as inward, the first and second ribs facing almost entirely

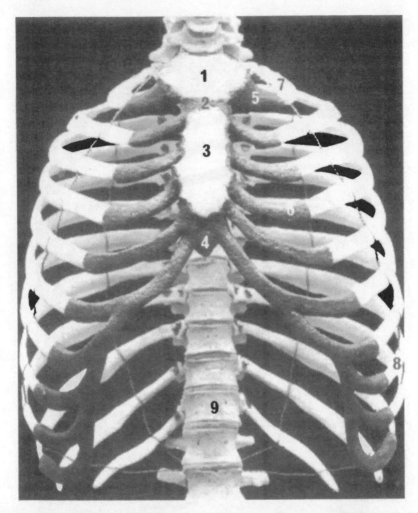

Figure 2 Bones and cartilages of the thoracic wall; anterior view in inspiratory position. 1, Manubrium of sternum; 2, manubriosternal joint (angle of Louis); 3, body of sternum; 4, xiphoid process; 5, first costal cartilage; 6, fourth costal cartilage; 7, first rib; 8, eighth rib; 9, body of 12th thoracic vertebra; 10, spinous process of thoracic vertebra.

downward (see Fig. 1). Anteroposteriorly, the chest is compressed, resulting in an elliptical, rather than circular, profile in horizontal cross section (Fig. 5). This is in marked contrast with quadrupeds, in which a narrow, transversely compressed chest is slung between the forelimbs. With the assumption of the erect posture in humans, the thorax comes to lie within the axis of gravity of the body and is flattened by the invagination of the vertebral column into it. Pronounced paravertebral gutters

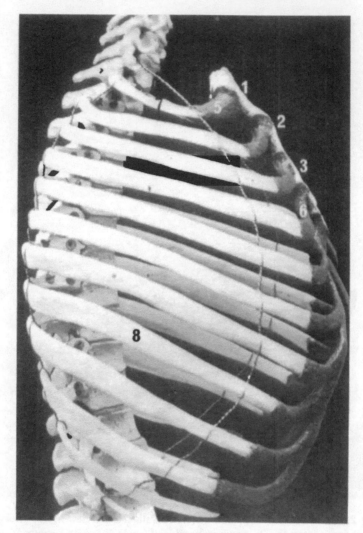

Figure 3 Bones and cartilages of the thoracic wall; lateral view in inspiratory position; numerical identification as in Figure 2.

result, the chest and sternum widen, and the heart rests downward on the diaphragm. These and other structural features must be considered in evaluating experimental work on thoracic mechanisms in laboratory mammals. In vertical dimensions, the length of the thoracic segment of the vertebral column, forming the posterior wall of the thorax, is approximately twice that of the anterior wall formed by the sternum (see Figs. 2 and 3). The inferior border of the chest wall extending forward on each

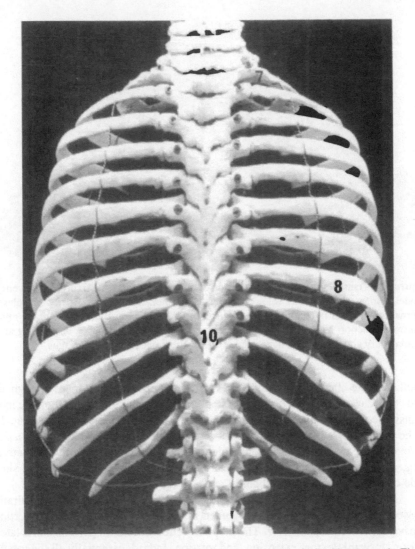

Figure 4 Bones of the thoracic wall; posterior view; numerical identification as in Figure 2.

side from the 12th thoracic vertebra ascends markedly, meeting anteriorly to form the subcostal angle at the lower end of the sternum (see Fig. 2).

The shape of the thoracic cage changes considerably during normal development. Although it is transversely compressed in the fetus, it becomes approximately circular in cross section with the onset of breathing at birth. During the development of standing, locomotion, and the prehensile use of the upper limbs in early

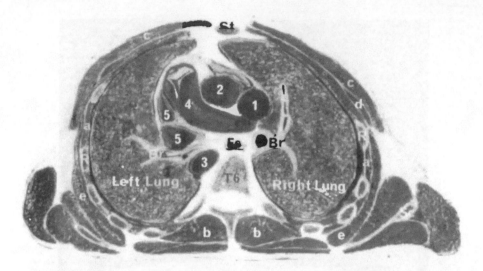

Figure 5 Transverse section through the midthorax at the level of the sixth thoracic vertebra (model). Bones: St, sternum; Sc, scapula; T6, sixth thoracic vertebra; R, rib. Muscles: a, external and internal intercostal; b, erector spinae; c, pectoralis major; d, pectoralis minor; e, serratus anterior. Vessels: 1, superior vena cava; 2, ascending aorta; 3, descending aorta; 4, pulmonary artery; 5, pulmonary vein. Viscera: Br, bronchus; Es, esophagus.

childhood, the chest rapidly undergoes anteroposterior compression, though this tends to occur to a somewhat smaller extent in girls than in boys. The thoracic index (transverse diameter/anteroposterior diameter × 100) increases from less than 100 in the fetus to 130–135 in adults, lower in women than in men. Normal variations in final shape are related to the individual body type, ranging from the relatively long, narrow thorax and acute subcostal angle of the asthenic build to the short, wide chest and more obtuse subcostal angle of the stocky hypersthenic type.

Movements of the thoracic cage are both respiratory and postural. Inspiration is associated with a symmetrical enlargement of the thoracic cage in all axes—vertical, transverse, and anteroposterior. The thoracic vertebral column permits some lateral flexion, forward flexion, extension, and rotation. Indeed, essentially all the rotation of which the vertebral column is capable occurs in the thoracic region. Such spinal movements, transmitted to the ribs, readily produce marked asymmetry of the thoracic cage. Minor degrees of asymmetry may be encountered even at rest, owing to postural habit or "handedness," leading to unequal development of pectoral girdle muscles.

III. Bones, Cartilages, and Joints of the Chest Wall

The thorax is encircled by a series of more or less complete skeletal supports, comprising the thoracic vertebrae, ribs, costal cartilages, and sternum, the form and articulations of which dictate the respiratory movements of the chest wall. Developmentally, these skeletal arches reflect the segmental organization of the trunk. The vertebrae are intersegmental in position, developing from two adjacent somites, whereas the head and neck of the ribs and the intervertebral disks are segmental in origin.

A. Thoracic Inlet

The thoracic inlet or superior boundary of the thorax is surrounded by a strong, unyielding ring formed by the body of the first thoracic vertebra and the flat, wide first rib, which is joined by a thick, short costal cartilage to the superolateral aspect of the manubrium sterni (Fig. 6). From its articulations with the body and transverse process of the first thoracic vertebra, the rib and costal cartilage incline obliquely downward at approximately 45° to the vertical plane. Thus, the level of the inlet drops from the neck of the rib near the upper border of the first thoracic vertebral body posteriorly to the suprasternal notch of the manubrium anteriorly, approximately opposite the lower border of the second thoracic vertebra. The articulation between the first rib and manubrium is a primary cartilaginous joint, the two bones being connected solely by the hyaline costal cartilage, which has irregular, interlocking interfaces with the two bones and a direct continuity of the periosteum and perichondrium (see Fig. 6). No movement occurs across this joint. Moreover, because it is short and thick, and tends to calcify with age, little distortion of the first costal cartilage is normally possible. The manubrium is thus gripped securely by the first ribs and cartilages, the whole arch moving as a single unit. As the first ribs alter their angle of inclination to the vertebra, the movements are transmitted to the manubrium, so that an elevation of the anterior end of the ribs produces a slight forward swinging of the lower end of the manubrium.

The space bounded by the thoracic inlet is kidney-shaped and relatively small (see Fig. 6). It measures only approximately 5 cm anteroposteriorly in the midline, where it is indented by the thoracic vertebra, and approximately 10 cm transversely at its widest point.

Below the thoracic inlet, the successive skeletal segments change in form and dimensions. The vertebral bodies enlarge progressively throughout the thoracic region. In horizontal cross-sectional profile, they change from the shallow, elliptical shape of the cervical vertebrae above to the deep, rounded profile of lumbar vertebrae below, the "typical" midthoracic vertebra being heart-shaped (Fig. 7). From the first vertebra downward, the transverse processes become swept backward to point more posteriorly, carrying the ribs with them. Consequently, the neck and posterior part of the shaft of successive ribs point more acutely backward, forming the wall of an increasingly deep paravertebral gutter (see Figs. 5 and 7). The angle between the axis of the neck of the rib and the sagittal plane opens out from 118°, for the first rib, to 136° in the midthorax (see Fig. 7). The increasing depth of the paravertebral gutter is associated with a more pronounced curvature of the ribs at

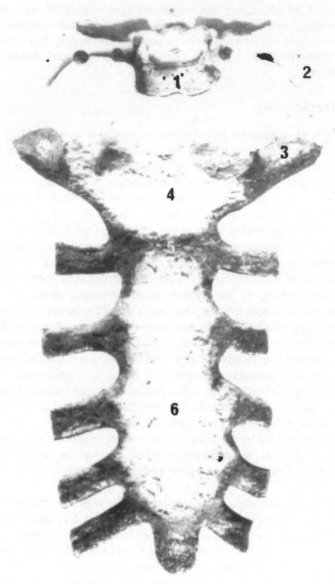

Figure 6 The thoracic inlet and sternum. 1, First thoracic vertebra; 2, first rib; 3, first costal cartilage; 4, manubrium; 5, manubriosternal joint; 6, body of sternum.

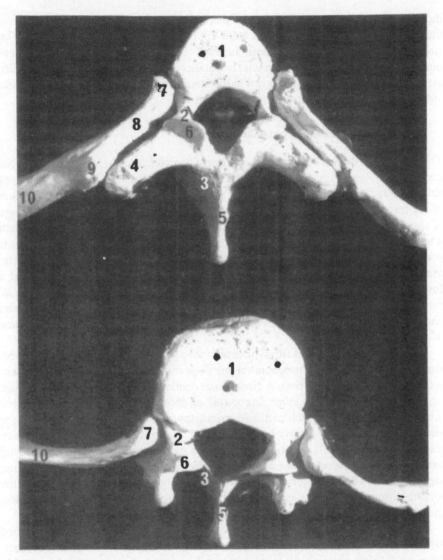

Figure 7 Upper thoracic vertebra (above) and 12th thoracic vertebra (below) with adjacent parts of the respective ribs. Vertebra: 1, body; 2, pedicle; 3, lamina; 4, transverse process; 5, spinous process; 6, superior articular process. Rib: 7, head; 8, neck; 9, tubercle; 10, shaft.

their angles in the floor of the gutter. Otherwise, the ribs increase progressively in their length and radius of curvature from the first to the seventh (see Fig. 2). The ribs pass obliquely around the chest, inclined at approximately 45° to the vertical plane. However, they are not precisely parallel with one another. The obliquity increases slightly from the first down to the ninth or tenth ribs. Thus, the intercostal spaces are somewhat wider in front than behind.

B. Vertebrosternal Costal Arches

The first seven ribs and costal cartilages form a complete arch between the vertebrae and sternum (see Figs. 2 and 3). The shape of the arches, however, changes substantially at different levels. The first two costal cartilages continue the direction of the respective ribs, passing slightly downward to the sternum; the third cartilage is approximately horizontal, the fourth ascends somewhat, and the fifth to seventh angulate upward increasingly sharply after continuing the direction of their respective ribs for an inch or so. Consequently, although each of the latter skeletal arches is inclined generally downward and forward, its lateral convexity lies at a lower level than the plane between its two ends. The implications for chest wall movement are discussed in the following. The shafts of the third to seventh ribs show a progressively marked twist about their length, reflecting the sinuous course of the rib around the chest.

Each costal cartilage is firmly inserted into a pit on the end of the respective rib shaft, forming a series of costochondral junctions situated along a line passing downward and laterally from the first. A direct tissue continuity between bone and cartilage prevents movement at these joints. In contrast, all chondrosternal joints below the first are synovial. The tip of each cartilage articulates with a cartilaginous facet on the sternum, surrounded by synovial membrane and a fibrous capsule. The second such joint is divided internally by a horizontal fibrous partition into two separate synovial cavities, whereas the remainder are single, reflecting their relation to the developing sternum, as noted later. Because of the mobility of the chondrosternal joints and the torsion permitted by the resilient costal cartilages, particularly the longer, lower ones, the vertebrosternal ribs below the first can move relative to the sternum.

The sternum develops embryologically from a cartilaginous model formed after the midline fusion of two vertical mesenchymal bars in the ventral body wall. Five ossification centers appear from above downward at approximately monthly intervals between the fifth and ninth months of intrauterine life. No ossification occurs in the lowest tip, which remains cartilaginous throughout life as the flexible xiphoid process, projecting into the anterior abdominal wall. At birth, five bony segments, sternebrae, are separated from one another by cartilaginous plates. Each plate is connected laterally to the tip of a corresponding costal cartilage by fibrous tissue, which forms an intra-articular disk dividing the chondrosternal joint into two synovial cavities. The lower three cartilaginous plates usually become ossified during childhood, puberty, and at approximately 21 years, respectively, as sternal elongation ceases, forming a single sternal body. Simultaneously, the associated intra-articular disks break down, and the chondrosternal joints become single cavities. However, the cartilage between the upper two sternebrae develops a central fibrous tissue plate, continuous laterally with the intra-articular disk of the second chondrosternal joint, which persists thereafter. A thin layer of hyaline cartilage remains between the sternal bone and the fibrous tissue plate. Thus, the articulation between the adult manubrium and body of the sternum is a secondary cartilaginous joint. In common with other such symphyses, its structure confers permanence and appreciable mobility. The manubriosternal joint rarely ossifies, even in old age (8%). It persists as a pliable hinge joint, permitting variable angulation between the manubrium and body of the sternum. This sternal angle (angle of Louis) forms a readily palpable landmark, situated approximately level with the lower border of the fourth thoracic vertebral body and leading laterally to the second costal cartilage. Occasionally, the first two sternebrae may fuse to form an unusually long manubrium, the sternal angle then being aligned with the third costal cartilage.

C. Vertebrochondral Costal Arches

The eighth to tenth costal elements do not completely encircle the thorax. The costal cartilages turn upward, taper, and articulate near their tip by a small synovial joint with the cartilage immediately above, permitting some lateral movement, as noted later. The cartilage tip usually remains palpable and is often readily movable. The succession of overlapping cartilages, from the seventh to tenth, compose the costal margin.

D. Floating Ribs

The lowest two ribs are short and only slightly curved. They terminate freely in a short, pointed cartilaginous tip. Thus, these last two intercostal spaces, unlike any others, are not closed anteriorly, but communicate directly with the abdominal wall.

E. Thoracic Outlet

The thoracic outlet or inferior thoracic aperture is large and uneven in shape (see Fig. 2). From the midline xiphisternal joint at the level of the lower border of the ninth thoracic vertebral body, the costal margins diverge downward and laterally to their lowest points, the tenth costal cartilages, opposite the third lumbar vertebra. Here, they are approximately only 4 in. from the iliac crest. The inferior thoracic aperture is completed posteriorly by the anterior ends of the last two intercostal spaces, the inferior border of the 12th rib, and the body of the 12th thoracic vertebra.

F. Articulations Between Ribs and Vertebrae

Movements of the thoracic cage are permitted, and their characteristics are largely determined by a series of synovial joints between the ribs and vertebrae. Although the articular areas are small, the joints are reinforced by strong ligaments which confer such stability that dislocation occurs only under exceptional circumstances. Thoracic compression usually results in rib fracture, rather than joint displacement.

Costovertebral Joints

Typically, the head of a rib articulates with the bodies of two adjacent vertebrae, being attached by an intra-articular fibrous disk to the intervertebral disk between them (see Figs. 7 and 8). Two sloping, concave fibrocartilage-covered facets on the head of the ribs, above and below the bony interarticular crest that gives attachment to the intra-articular disk, are separated by small synovial cavities from articular demifacets covered with fibrocartilage on the bodies of the two adjacent vertebrae. These constitute the costovertebral joints. Each joint capsule is strengthened anteriorly by the radiate ligament, extending medially as three bands from the head of the rib to the intervertebral disk and the bodies of vertebrae above and below, respectively (see Fig. 8).

Exceptional articulations occur in the uppermost and lower joints. The first rib articulates solely with a complete facet on the body of the first thoracic vertebra (see Fig. 6). The synovial cavity is single, there being no intra-articular ligament. Similarly, the lowest two ribs articulate solely with their respective vertebrae by single synovial joints (see Fig. 7). The vertebral facets for these joints are situated farther back than the joints above, being on the pedicles, rather than on the body of the vertebra (Fig. 9). The ninth and tenth facets are also mainly on the pedicles. All rib articulations, nevertheless, are with the same embryological component of the vertebra, the neural arch. This gives rise to the part of the adult vertebral body that carries the facets for the costovertebral joints, the pedicles, transverse processes, laminae, and spinous process. The embryological centrum gives rise to the rest of the vertebral body.

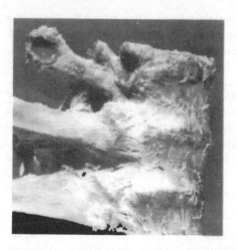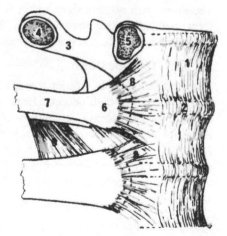

Figure 8 Dissection of costovertebral joints. 1, Body of vertebra covered by anterior longitudinal ligament; 2, intervertebral disk; 3, transverse process; 4, articular facet for tubercle of rib; 5, articular facet for head of rib; 6, head of rib; 7, neck of rib; 8, radiate ligament; 9, superior costotransverse ligament.

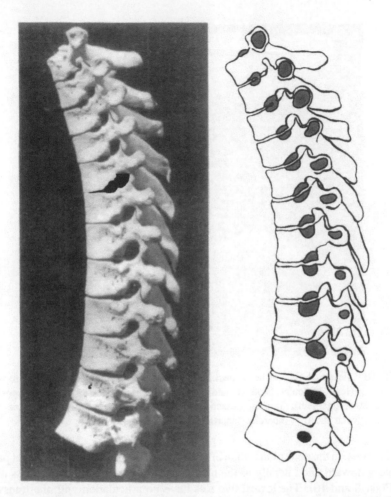

Figure 9   Thoracic vertebral column. The articular facets for ribs on vertebral bodies and transverse processes are shown as black areas in the diagram (right panel).

Costotransverse Joints

The tubercle of the rib displays a medial facet that articulates by a synovial encapsulated joint with a similar facet on the transverse process of the respective thoracic vertebra (Figs. 9 and 10). Three powerful extracapsular ligaments strengthen each joint. Extending back to the transverse process at the same level as the rib, the posterior costotransverse ligament passes from the roughened posterior surface of the neck of the rib to a triangular hollow on the front of the transverse process, and the lateral costotransverse ligament connects a well-defined lateral part of the tubercle of the rib to the tip of the transverse process (see Figs. 7 and 10). From a prominent

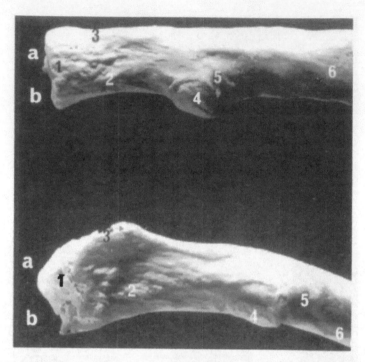

Figure 10   Posterior view of head, neck, and tubercle of upper rib (above) and lower rib (below). 1, Head (articular facets a and b); 2, neck (area of attachment of posterior costotransverse ligament); 3, crest (attachment of superior costotransverse ligament); 4, tubercle; articular facet; 5, tubercle; nonarticular facet; 6, shaft.

superior crest on the neck of the rib, a broad superior costotransverse ligament passes obliquely upward and laterally to the undersurface of the transverse process above (see Figs. 8 and 10). The lowest two ribs have no articulation with the transverse processes, which are represented only by low tubercles (see Figs. 7 and 9). Scattered costotransverse fibrous tissue permits considerable mobility of these ribs.

Important differences are seen between the upper and lower costotransverse joints. The transverse processes project laterally and somewhat backward from the junction of pedicle and lamina of the vertebra, becoming shorter from above downward (see Figs. 7 and 9). On the upper seven processes, the large articular facets face forward and are deeply concave, the facets on the rib tubercles being correspondingly convex and lying in a vertical plane (see Figs. 9 and 11). In contrast, on the transverse processes of the lower vertebrae, the facets are smaller and flattened, and face mainly upward. The rib facets are similarly flat and lie in a horizontal plane on the undersurface of the bone. The seventh transverse process and rib usually represent a transition between the axes and form of the upper and lower costotransverse joints.

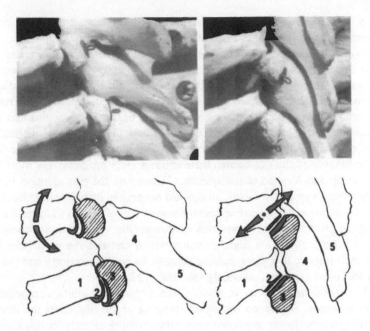

Figure 11 Form and movements of upper costotransverse joints (left) and lower costotransverse joints (right). 1, Rib shaft; 2, tubercle of rib; 3, transverse process; 4, lamina; 5, spinous process.

IV. Movements of the Thoracic Cage

The thoracic wall has so far been considered as if midway through tidal respiration. This "neutral" respiratory position reflects the combined effects of muscle tone, the physical properties of the chest wall and its contents, and gravity. From this position, the skeletal components of the chest move more extensively toward full inspiration than toward full expiration.

Respiratory movements of the thoracic cage are produced by the cumulative effects of small movements of the ribs at each of the costovertebral joints, much magnified anteriorly. The axes of movement are complex and controversial. In general, however, the movements change from above downward, reflecting successive changes in articular surfaces, rib axes, and attachments.

At the *thoracic inlet*, the first ribs hinge about an axis running along their neck, their convex tubercle rotating within the concavity of the costotransverse joint. In inspiration, the ribs become more horizontal. Their anterior end moves forward and upward, but only slightly laterally. The manubrium sterni moves with them, its resulting angulation being compensated by hinging at the manubriosternal joint.

Although movement of the inlet may be slight in tidal respiration, the vital capacity is associated with an extensive vertical displacement of 3–5 cm at the suprasternal notch, 2–4 cm in inspiration, and about 2 cm in expiration.

Below the thoracic inlet, the ribs of the *vertebrosternal costal arches* continue to move mainly by rotation around the long axis of their neck, becoming less oblique in inspiration, thereby expanding the thoracic cavity anteroposteriorly and elevating the thoracic cage anteriorly (see Figs. 11 and 12). In addition, however, from above downward, an increase in the transverse diameter of the thorax occurs and becomes more pronounced. This results from several factors: (1) Because of the increasingly backward sweep of the transverse processes, and thus the axes of the necks of the ribs, the hinging of the ribs carries their anterior ends progressively more laterally as well as up and forward in inspiration. (2) Because the ribs increase in size and curvature from above downward, an upward hinging in inspiration replaces the ribs around the thorax at any given horizontal plane by ribs of greater transverse diameter. (3) Particularly toward the lower ribs of this region, an additional component is added to rib movement—a slight eversion which elevates the most lateral part of the rib shaft relative to a plane passing through its head posteriorly and the anterior end of its costal cartilage, anteriorly (see Fig. 12).

The costal cartilages move freely at the sternocostal joints, compensating for changes in sternal angulation. However, hinging of the ribs alters the direction of the cartilages, the lower angulated ones straightening slightly in inspiration. The resulting torsion and elastic recoil of the cartilages assists in returning the chest wall to the neutral position.

The ribs and cartilages of the *vertebrochondral costal arches* bounding the costal margin anteriorly exhibit the foregoing movements, eversion tending to increase in the lower ribs, plus the addition of another gliding component. Because of the shape and inclination of the costotransverse articular facets, the rib tubercles

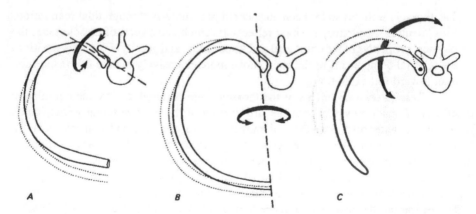

Figure 12   Scheme of axes and directions of movement of (A) upper ribs ("pump-handle" movement), (B) lower ribs ("bucket-handle" movement), and (C) lowest ribs ("caliper" movement). Inspiratory positions are indicated by broken lines. See text for details.

can glide, rather than rotate, against the transverse process (see Fig. 11). Thus, in deep inspiration, the rib tubercles glide backward, up, and medially, swinging the anterior ends of the ribs horizontally outward away from each other (see Fig. 12). This further emphasizes the transverse expansion of the chest, whereas the forward movement of the anterior end of the ribs (which would otherwise be produced by the hinging and lessened obliquity of the ribs) is largely negated by their outward and backward movement resulting from the costotransverse gliding.

The seventh rib and costal cartilage usually represent a transition in axes of movements between the vertebrosternal and vertebrochondral arches.

The last two, or sometimes three, *floating ribs*, lacking costotransverse joints, have a potentially free mobility around a wide range of axes through the head of the rib (see Fig. 7). In practice, the movements of these ribs are restricted by muscular fixation rather than by articular constraints. Their ability to flare open and backward in inspiration is well marked.

Deep inspiration may be associated with extension of the *thoracic vertebral column*, thereby reducing the thoracic curvature and producing movements of the attached ribs. This has the effect of increasing the angulation between successive ribs, widening the intercostal spaces anteriorly, and adding a further component to the vertical enlargement of the thoracic cavity.

V. Muscles and Fascia of the Thoracic Wall

Layers of muscle and fascia between the skeletal elements form a thin, continuous wall around the thoracic cavity.

A. Intercostal Muscles

In the plane of the ribs, two layers of muscle and fascia span each intercostal space. The muscle fibers of the two layers run approximately at right angles to each other, both layers being thicker behind than in front (see Figs. 1 and 13).

The *external intercostal* muscle layer begins posteriorly at the tubercles of the ribs, just lateral to and in the plane of the superior costotransverse ligaments. Near the costochondral junctions, it is replaced by a fibrous transparent aponeurosis, the anterior intercostal membrane, which extends to the anterior end of the intercostal space. The muscle fibers run parallel to each other, downward and forward from the sharp interior border of the rib above, to the rounded superior border of the rib below.

The *internal intercostal* muscle layer begins posteriorly as the posterior intercostal membrane on the inner aspect of the external intercostal muscle. From approximately the angle of the rib, the internal intercostal muscle passes forward continuously to the anterior end of the intercostal space. Parallel muscle fibers run upward and forward from the superior border of the rib and costal cartilage below, to the floor of the subcostal groove of the rib and the edge of the costal cartilage above.

Thus, the intercostal spaces contain two functional layers of muscles laterally, and a single layer both anteriorly and posteriorly (Fig. 13). The internal intercostal muscle, unlike the external one, may be considered to have two parts: intercostal and interchondral. In the lower vertebrosternal spaces, the different directions taken by these two parts of the intercostal space have raised the controversial possibility that the actions of the two regions of the internal intercostal muscle may differ from one another.

The respiratory significance of the external and internal intercostals has long been controversial. Electromyographic studies in humans generally support the historical view that, in accordance with their anatomical orientation, the external intercostals and interchondral part of the internal intercostals can function in inspiration, whereas the interosseus parts of the internal intercostals are expiratory.

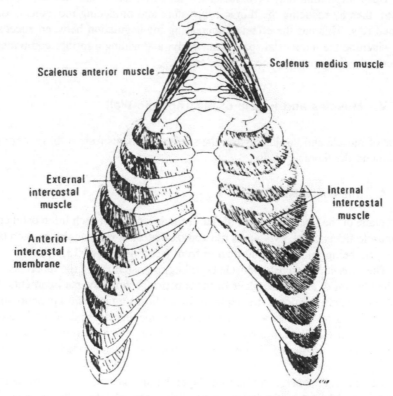

Scalenus anterior muscle

Scalenus medius muscle

External intercostal muscle

Internal intercostal muscle

Anterior intercostal membrane

Figure 13 Intercostal and scalene muscles. On the left side of the chest, the external intercostal muscle and anterior intercostal membrane have been removed to reveal the internal intercostal muscle, whereas the left scalenus anterior has been removed to display the scalenus medius.

However, the pattern of activity depends greatly on the depth of respiration; the precise mechanism by which these muscles move the ribs and their contribution to respiratory volume changes remain uncertain, as detailed in Chapter 19.

As well as their putative action in moving the ribs, the intercostals appear to have other functions in respiration. From their slight, generalized activity throughout respiration, it may be surmised that the tone of the two muscle layers acting at right angles to each other is important in maintaining the soft-tissue tension between adjacent pairs of ribs, as the latter change position and distance from one another. No noncontractile tissue would be capable of performing such a function. Intercostal muscle activity appears to help resist pressure changes across the chest wall, as evidenced by the retraction of intercostal spaces and reduced power of sucking and blowing observed during flaccid paralysis of intercostal muscles. The intercostal muscles are by no means confined to respiratory functions. They are highly active in postural movements of the chest wall, notably in approximating the ribs during lateral flexion of the trunk.

Internal to the plane of the ribs, representing fragments of the deepest muscle layer of the body wall, are the three components of the *transversus thoracis* muscle. The *sternocostalis* muscle radiates from an attachment on the back of the lower third of the sternum, xiphoid process, and adjacent costal cartilages. Muscular slips pass upward and laterally, inserting into each costal cartilage from the second to sixth. The muscle is, therefore, fan-shaped, the upper fibers being almost vertical, the lowest almost horizontal, in line with the transversus abdominis muscle immediately below. Both of the other two components of this muscle layer in the chest run in the direction of the intercostal part of the internal intercostal muscles and vary in their degree of development. The *subcostal* muscles are located posteriorly, best developed in the lower spaces. They pass across the inner surfaces of two or three ribs and intercostal spaces. The *innermost intercostal* muscles are also more developed in the lower spaces than above, but are situated laterally. They are attached to the inner surfaces of adjacent ribs and may be distinguished from the internal intercostals by the intervening neurovascular plane that transmits the intercostal nerves, vessels, and their branches.

Completing the thoracic wall, a thin layer of areolar connective tissue, the endothoracic fascia, covers the rib periosteum and intercostal spaces internally. The parietal pleura lies directly against the fascia, which provides a cleavage plane, permitting the costal pleura to be stripped away readily from the chest wall.

All the foregoing muscles of the intercostal spaces receive both their efferent and afferent innervation from the intercostal nerves, anterior primary rami of the 1st–11th thoracic spinal nerves. The same nerves give sensory branches to the highly sensitive parietal pleura.

B. Suprapleural Membrane

The superior thoracic aperture is closed on each side over the apex of the lung by a strong, unyielding thickening of endothoracic fascia, the suprapleural membrane

(Sibson's fascia; see Fig. 1). The membrane is attached to the sharp inner border of the first rib and to the anterior border of the transverse process of the seventh cervical vertebra (see Fig. 6). It becomes indistinct toward the midline, where the trachea, esophagus, and neurovascular structures pass between the superior mediastinum and the neck. The suprapleural membrane has been considered to represent an aponeurosis of a small muscle, the *scalenus minimus* (pleuralis), which frequently arises from the transverse process of the seventh cervical vertebra, radiating to be attached to the suprapleural membrane and the inner border of the first rib.

C. Diaphragm

The floor of the thoracic cavity is closed by a thin musculotendinous sheet of complex structure and development. The diaphragm, as a whole, is attached peripherally around the complete boundary of the inferior thoracic aperture, from which at first it passes upward almost vertically, ascending high into the thoracic cavity to its two cupolae (see Figs. 1 and 14). These are located in the neutral

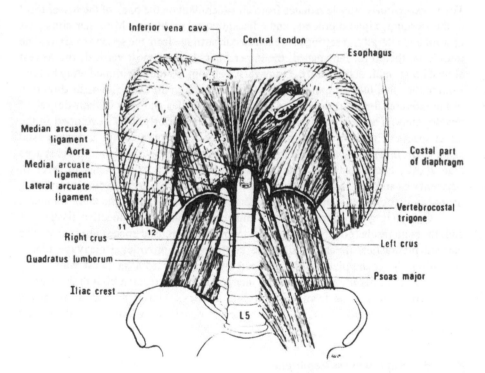

Figure 14 Origin of the diaphragm from the lumbar vertebrae and arcuate ligaments; quadratus lumborum muscle. The diaphragm is shown in schematic coronal section. The positions of the 11th and 12th ribs are indicated in broken outline.

respiratory position at a level in the midclavicular planes of about the fourth intercostal space on the right and the fifth rib on the left, approximately opposite the tenth thoracic vertebra. The level may vary by more than one vertebra above or below this, however, being lower in asthenic than hypersthenic individuals.

From its origins, the diaphragm at first lies in direct contact with the inner aspects of the ribs and the intercostal spaces. Only at higher levels does an angle open up between the diaphragm and chest wall, in which is located the lower limit of the parietal pleura, the costodiaphragmatic pleural recess, and above that, the thin inferior border of the lower lobe of the lung (see Fig. 1). Thus, in the midaxillary line during quiet respiration, the diaphragm lies in contact with the chest wall up to the tenth rib and with the costodiaphragmatic recess from the tenth to eighth ribs, whereas it is related to the lung only above that point.

The central tendon of the diaphragm is thin, strong, and roughly trilobed (Fig. 15). One lobe projects posterolaterally on each side, the left being somewhat narrower than the right. The central part is fused above with the fibrous pericardial sac, both structures at this point being derived from the embryonic septum transversum.

The muscle of the diaphragm, all of which inserts into the central tendon, falls into two main components, sternocostal and vertebral, according to its site of origin. From the back of the xiphoid process and lower end of the sternum, paramedian sternal slips pass almost horizontally backward into the central tendon

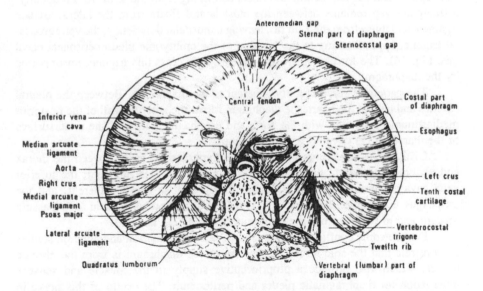

Figure 15 Inferior thoracic outlet from below, showing the attachments and form of the diaphragm.

(see Fig. 15). Separated from the sternal portion by a small gap, the sternocostal triangle, the individual slips arise from the inner aspects of each costal cartilage from the cartilage from the 7th to the tip of the 12th. This muscle, representing part of the innermost phylogenetic layer of the body wall, is in the same plane as the transversus abdominis muscle, of which the slips of origin pass horizontally forward into the abdominal wall from the same costal attachments as the diaphragm. The costal fibers of the diaphragm converge onto the anterior, lateral and, to some extent, posterior borders of the central tendon, increasing progressively in length around the chest and from front to back (see Fig. 15).

The vertebral part of the diaphragm arises from the crura and aponeurotic arcuate ligaments (see Fig. 14). The crura are strong, tapering tendons attached vertically to the anterolateral aspects of the bodies and intervertebral disks of the first three lumbar vertebrae on the right and two on the left. An ill-defined, fibrous thickening arching between the two crura forms the median arcuate ligament. A tendinous medial arcuate ligament passes from the crus on each side across the psoas major muscle to the tip of the transverse process of the first lumbar vertebra. From this point, a lateral arcuate ligament then runs to the 12th rib, crossing the quadratus lumborum muscle (see Fig. 14). The medial and lateral arcuate ligaments are firmly adherent to the posterior body wall, fused to the psoas sheath and the anterior lamella of the lumbar fascia in front of the quadratus lumborum, respectively. Muscle fibers arising from the crura and along the arcuate ligaments pass upward to insert into the posterior border of the central tendon, to some extent overlapping and passing behind the fibers ascending from the 12th rib. Frequently, a triangular gap remains between the most lateral fibers from the lateral arcuate ligament and those from the 12th rib, leaving a muscular deficiency, the vertebrocostal trigone, approximating to the position of the embryonic pleuroperitoneal canal (see Fig. 14). The lower border of the pleura may cross this trigone, unsupported by the diaphragm.

The parietal pleura is tightly adherent to the diaphragm. Between the pleural cavities and behind the heart, the diaphragm forms the anterior wall of the posterior mediastinum, in contact with the aorta and esophagus. Much of the undersurface of the diaphragm is covered with peritoneum.

Of the many structures traversing the diaphragm to pass between the thorax and abdomen, the aorta passes behind the median arcuate ligament, the inferior vena cava perforates the central tendon to which it is firmly adherent, and the esophagus is encircled by muscle, clasped by a continuous muscle loop passing upward and to the left from the right crus (see Figs. 14 and 15).

Despite some conflicting observations, nerve stimulation and ablation studies demonstrate that the sole motor innervation of the diaphragm is from the phrenic nerves, which also provide a proprioceptive supply to the muscle and sensory innervation for diaphragmatic pleura and peritoneum. The origin of this nerve in humans is from the third to the fifth cervical spinal segments, representing the level of cervical somites from which myotomes contribute to the embryonic septum transversum before its subsequent caudal displacement by the expanding lungs and pleural cavities. The main contribution is from the fourth cervical segment. Branches are given off from the front of the respective cervical nerves close to their exit from the spinal canal in the neck. Occasionally, the fibers from the fifth segment reach the phrenic nerves low in the neck or upper thorax as an accessory phrenic nerve, a branch from the nerve to the subclavius muscle. The phrenic nerves perforate the diaphragm. The right nerve passes either with or just lateral to the inferior cava, whereas the left passes through muscle alone as it runs off the side of the pericardial sac. The nerves radiate from these points often as three main branches on the undersurface of the diaphragm, passing anteriorly, laterally, and posteriorly. The peripheral parts of the diaphragm arise embryologically from the pleuroperitoneal folds and from tissue excavated locally from the body wall. As a result, a peripheral band of the costal part of the diaphragm and the crura are innervated by the lower six or seven intercostal nerves. However, this nerve supply appears to be only proprioceptive to the muscle and sensory to pleura and peritoneum.

The diaphragm moves during inspiration, descending relative to the vertebral column to increase the vertical dimensions of the thoracic cavity. The range of vertical movement over the resting tidal volume is about 1.0–1.7 cm, the domes moving more than the central tendon in the midline, increasing to as much as 10 cm (commonly 4–5 cm) over vital capacity volume. The latter corresponds to changes in level of approximately three vertebral bodies (right dome, T8–11; left dome, T9–12). The abdominal viscera displaced by diaphragmatic descent are accommodated by a simultaneous protrusion of the anterolateral abdominal wall and a widening of the upper abdominal cavity.

In considering its mode of action, the two main muscle components of the diaphragm can be distinguished from one another. The vertebral part, arising from the fixed origin of the lumbar vertebrae, can produce movements of only the diaphragm itself, depressing the posterior border of the central tendon. The sternocostal part, arising from a mobile origin that actually rises during inspiration, may exert inspiratory effects on the thoracic cage as well as the diaphragm. Contracting against intra-abdominal pressure and viscera, the sternocostal part of the diaphragm exerts an upward pull on the ribs at the costal margin, thereby helping to move them up, out, and back, as dictated by the plane of their joints. In chronic airway obstruction, in which the diaphragm cupolae are permanently low, the sternocostal muscle fibers are generally more horizontal than usual and may contribute to an inward movement of the costal margin during inspiratory effort.

D. Abdominal Wall

The abdominal cavity is bounded by anterior and posterior longitudinal muscles, which connect the thoracic cage to the pelvis and are contained within strong fascial sheaths, together with three muscle sheets that encircle the remainder of the abdomen (Figs. 16–18). Anteriorly, the *rectus abdominis* covers the external surface of the

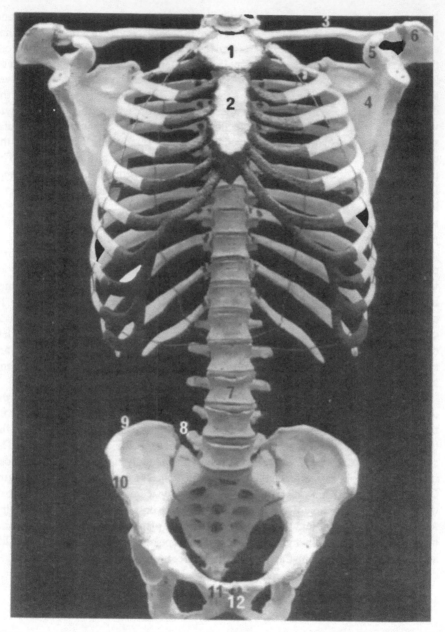

Figure 16 Bones of the trunk and pectoral girdle. 1, Manubrium of sternum; 2, body of sternum; 3, clavicle; 4, body of scapula; 5, coracoid process of scapula; 6, acromion of scapula; 7, body of third lumbar vertebra; 8, transverse process of fifth lumbar vertebra; 9, iliac crest; 10, anterior superior iliac spine; 11, pubic tubercle; 12, pubic symphysis.

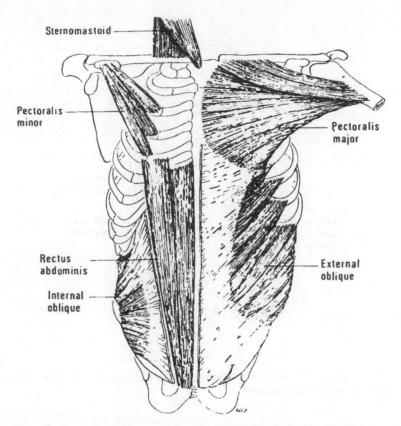

Figure 17 Pectoral and abdominal muscles. On the right side of the body, the pectoralis major and external oblique muscles have been removed.

thoracic cage as it passes vertically downward from its horizontal line of attachment to the fifth, sixth, and seventh costal cartilages (occasionally also the third and fourth) to its tapering tendinous attachment to the pubis (see Figs. 16 and 17). The rectus sheath encloses much of the muscle and is derived from aponeuroses of the three lateral muscles. Posteriorly, the *quadratus lumborum* muscle passes upward and medially as a flat sheet from the iliolumbar ligament and iliac crest below, to the lower border of the medial half of the 12th rib and the transverse processes of the first four lumbar vertebrae (see Fig. 14). It is enclosed in the anterior and middle layers of lumbar fascia, which meet at its lateral edge to give attachment to the lateral abdominal muscles. External to the plane of the ribs, the *external oblique* muscle arises by separate fleshy slips from the lower eight ribs, well above the costal margin, and directly covers the lower ribs and intercostal spaces (see Fig. 17). Its fibers radiate downward to the iliac crest and inguinal ligament, and medially to the midline from the xiphoid process to

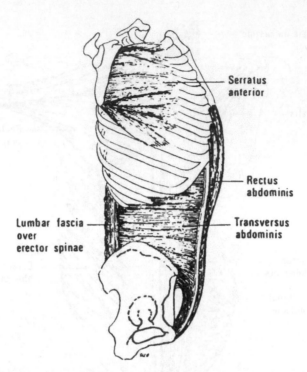

Figure 18 Lateral view of serratus anterior and abdominal muscles after removal of external and internal oblique muscles.

the pubis. In the plane of the ribs, the *internal oblique* muscle passes from the lumbar fascia, iliac crest, and lateral part of the inguinal ligament to an extensive attachment along the costal margin and to an aponeurosis contributing to the rectus sheath down to the pubis (see Fig. 17). Internal to the ribs arises the *transversus abdominis* muscle, interdigitating with the slips of origin of the diaphragm within the costal margin (see Fig. 18). Fibers run horizontally forward from this origin and from the lumbar fascia, iliac crest, and lateral part of the inguinal ligament, to a midline aponeurosis forming the anterior wall of the rectus sheath.

The anterior and lateral abdominal muscles are innervated segmentally from the lower six thoracic nerves, and also from the first lumbar nerve for the internal oblique and transversus. The quadratus lumborum is innervated by the 12th thoracic and first three or four lumbar spinal nerves.

In respiratory function, the muscles of the anterolateral abdominal wall are unequivocal muscles of expiration and antagonists to the diaphragm. Quiet expiration is predominantly the result of passive elastic recoil of the lungs and chest wall. In deep expiration, however, strong contractions of the oblique and transversus abdominis muscles constrict and compress the abdomen. This increases intra-abdominal pressure, helping elevate the relaxing diaphragm, while simultaneously depressing the ribs to which they are attached and compressing the lower thoracic cage. Strong contractions of the abdominal muscles occur in voluntary forced expiration, including coughing, sneezing, and phonation, together with contractions of the muscular pelvic floor (see Fig. 1). The rectus abdominis is also active in lumbar flexion, moving the anterior thoracic cage toward the pubis.

The quadratus lumborum muscle contracts synergistically with the diaphragm, exerting a downward force on the 12th rib and preventing any tendency for the vertebral part of the diaphragm to pull the 12th rib upward. This not only provides a fixed point of origin for the lateral fibers of the vertebral part of the diaphragm, but may even slightly depress the 12th rib in inspiration, helping to open up the costodiaphragmatic recess. The quadratus lumborum muscle, fixing the 12th rib, shows a precisely similar rhythmicity in activity as the diaphragm, including a carryover into early expiration. Thus, the quadratus lumborum and vertebral part of the diaphragm may be regarded as a single functional unit in these respects.

E. Back Muscles

The postvertebral extensor muscles cover the chest wall between the spinous processes of the vertebrae and the posterior angle of the ribs (Fig. 19). The most lateral part of this muscle group, iliocostalis and longissimus, runs vertically across the ribs, whereas the other components run between parts of the vertebrae of various levels. The muscle group is covered posteriorly by the thoracolumbar fascia, the bony attachments of which create a surface elevation at the angle of the ribs. Reflecting the varying width of the extensor muscle group, the posterior angle is farthest from the midline, usually at the eighth rib; it moves progressively more medially at lower and higher levels until it is virtually in line with the tubercle of the first rib, which thus lacks an angle (see Figs. 4 and 19). All muscles deep to the thoracolumbar fascia are innervated by dorsal primary rami of spinal nerves.

The function of the postvertebral muscles is primarily postural, maintaining the erect position against gravity. They show little, if any, rhythmic activity in quiet respiration. Late in forced inspiration they may contract, to extend the vertebral column. The muscle group is more active in forced expiration, however. To some extent, activity of the longissimus and iliocostalis parts may directly assist expiration by depressing the lower ribs. Much of the expiratory activity of the back muscles, however, represents a synergistic effect, counterbalancing the tendency to vertebral flexion that would otherwise be produced by the contraction of the abdominal wall muscles.

F. Muscles Moving or Fixing Ribs from Extracostal Attachments

Important muscles descend from the head and neck to the thoracic inlet. The *scalenus anterior* is a straplike muscle, converging from its upper attachment to the anterior

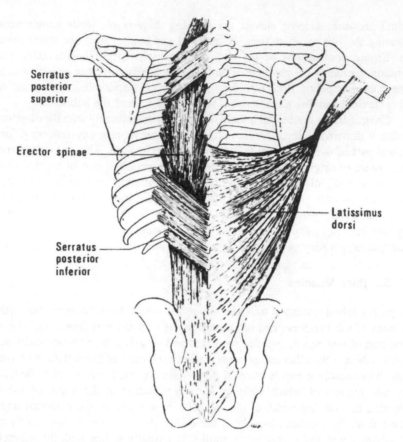

Serratus posterior superior

Erector spinae

Serratus posterior inferior

Latissimus dorsi

Figure 19   Superficial and deep muscles of the back.

tubercles of the transverse processes of the third to sixth cervical vertebrae, to be inserted by a narrow tendon into the scalene tubercle on the upper surface and inner border of the first rib in front of the groove for the subclavian artery (see Fig. 13). The *scalenus medius* is a powerful muscle passing from the posterior tubercles of all the cervical vertebrae to a large roughened area on the upper surface of the first rib between the tubercle and the subclavian artery, as well as to the second rib (*scalenus posterior*); (see Fig. 13). The scalenes are innervated by ventral rami of the cervical nerves (anterior, C4–6; medius, C3–8). The scalene muscles exhibit a spontaneous rhythmic activity during normal inspiration, proportional to the depth of ventilation, thus meeting the criterion of primary respiratory muscles. Their action, deduced from their attachments, is to fix or elevate the thoracic inlet. The mechanical advantage and large mass of these muscles pulling up on the first rib suggest that the power of this action may be considerable. However, the relative contribution of the scalenes and intercostals to chest wall movements is disputed (see Chap. 19).

The scalenes may also contract strongly during forced voluntary expiration, as in coughing. This probably represents an antagonistic action, limiting excessive downward displacement of the thoracic cage by the expiratory muscles, as well as a protective effect, preventing herniation of the lung apex through the thoracic inlet into the root of the neck. Presumably, the contraction includes the deep fibers of scalenus minimus, increasing the tension of the suprapleural membrane.

Superimposed on their respiratory activities, the scalenes have prominent postural functions, controlling cervical flexion.

The *sternocleidomastoid* muscle descends from the mastoid process and adjacent superior nuchal line on the skull to a pointed tendinous attachment to the front of the upper part of the manubrium sterni and a muscular sheet along the upper surface of the medial third of the clavicle (see Fig. 17). The several parts of this muscle receive motor innervation from the spinal accessory nerve (cervical spinal segments, 1–5) and additional proprioceptive fibers from the cervical plexus (C-2).

The sternomastoid shows electromyographic activity, even in normal deep inspiration, contracting most strongly toward the end of the movement. For action from a fixed skull and cervical vertebral column, it is well placed to produce a powerful elevation of the sternum in inspiration, with accompanying elevation of the ribs.

Three sets of muscles pass obliquely from the vertebrae to the ribs posteriorly and can thus move the ribs. The *levatores costarum* are triangular muscles passing downward and laterally from a pointed origin on the tips of the transverse process of the seventh cervical and upper 11 thoracic vertebrae to the upper surface of the next rib below from its tubercle to angle. The *serratus posterior superior* and *inferior* are thin sheets of muscle passing obliquely from spinous process to ribs, located in the plane between the thoracolumbar fascia and the muscles of the pectoral girdle (see Fig. 19). The serratus posterior superior arises in the midline from the lower ligamentum nuchae, the spinous processes and supraspinous ligaments of the seventh cervical and upper two thoracic vertebrae, and inserts just lateral to the angle of the second to fifth ribs. The serratus posterior inferior also attaches to four vertebrae and ribs, but is opposite in direction from the superior muscle; it passes upward and laterally from the spinous processes of vertebrae T11–12 and L1–2 to the lower four ribs. On anatomical grounds, in humans, the levatores costarum and serratus posterior superior may be able to elevate and retract the ribs in inspiration, and the serratus posterior inferior may help either to fix the lower ribs for diaphragmatic contraction in inspiration or to depress the ribs in expiration. Further electromyographic and functional evidence is required to assess their respiratory importance.

A series of powerful muscles moving the pectoral girdle and upper arm on the trunk form the outermost covering of the thoracic cage. Although not of prime concern in respiratory movements, their attachments to the ribs give a theoretical ability to move the thoracic cage when the upper limb is fixed. In passing around the chest wall, they may compress it and mold its form. The *serratus anterior* is attached in a curvilinear fashion by a series of digitations to each of the upper eight ribs from which it converges onto the medial border of the scapula (see Fig. 18). In line with its attachments, similar digitations from the lower four ribs contribute to the *latissimus dorsi*. Other parts of this large, powerful muscle arise from the spines of the lower six thoracic vertebrae, lumbar fascia, and iliac crest, converging to a narrow, flat tendon attached to the shaft of the humerus (see Fig. 19). Also attached to the humerus at this level is the *pectoralis major* tendon, converging from a wide origin on the sternum, upper six costal cartilages, and medial third of the clavicle (see Fig. 17). On a deeper plane, *pectoralis minor* passes from the third, fourth, and fifth ribs (or second, third, and fourth) near the costochondral junction to the coracoid process of the scapula (see Fig. 17).

Thus, the ribs and intercostal spaces are covered externally almost completely by powerful muscles concerned primarily with the functions of the upper limb and abdomen (see Figs. 17–19). In particular, the broad muscle sheets of the serratus anterior and latissimus dorsi, on the one hand, and the external oblique, on the other, envelop much of the anterolateral chest wall. Their contiguous attachments produce a horizontal line on the ribs, the anterior angle, on either side of which the rib surface is molded by the differing direction of contraction and pressure of the respective muscle.

When the pectoral girdle and upper limb are fixed by trapezius, rhomboids, and shoulder muscles, the pectoralis major and minor and the subclavius can elevate the ribs. Contractions occur in respiratory distress, accelerating the rate of inspiration, but only inconstantly in normal deep respiration. Although the attachments of the latissimus dorsi and serratus anterior would suggest the possibility of some similar accessory inspiratory action, observed activities have been variable. However, because they surround and embrace the chest wall, together with the external oblique muscle of the abdomen, they can assist expiratory compression. In particular, the latissimus dorsi is prominently active in coughing.

G. Coordinated Muscular Action and the Thoracic Pump

The major contributions to changes in thoracic volume are made by the diaphragm, in concert with the abdominal muscles, lowering and raising the thoracic floor. Simultaneous movements of the bony thoracic cage are slight in quiet respiration, but increase progressively as maximum ventilation is achieved, with a concurrent increase in activity of the intercostals and the other muscles attached to the thoracic cage.

As detailed in later chapters, the role of individual respiratory muscles in the pattern of muscular activity that regulates thoracic volume and pulmonary ventilation is still often controversial, despite the extensive use of experimental techniques, including electromyography, muscle stimulation, and denervation. Such conflicting views may at times reflect species differences; methodological constraints, such as difficulty in the localization of muscle recordings and stimulation to discrete muscle groups; and physiological factors, including the use of anesthesia and the surgical opening of body cavities. There is also the possibility of alternative interpretations of the experimental data.

It is evident from many examples in the foregoing anatomical discussion that the detection of electromyographic activity in an individual respiratory or accessory muscle during a particular movement does not necessarily mean that the muscle is acting as the primary muscle, directly responsible for producing that movement. The muscle contraction might represent either a synergistic action, preventing the occurrence of some other undesirable movement, or a paradoxical effect, regulating or restraining a movement that is actually being produced by other antagonistic muscles the actions of which are entirely opposite to its own. Conversely, the production of a certain movement by stimulation of an individual muscle does not necessarily demonstrate that the muscle would produce the same effect under physiological conditions when all other synergistic and antagonistic muscle groups are simultaneously active.

An accurate appreciation of the anatomical components of the chest wall interpreted in the light of these functional principles, forms the basis for experimentally evaluating the mechanisms of the thoracic pump.

Acknowledgments

The illustrations were drawn by Ms. Margot Oeltzschner, and the photographic plates were prepared by Mr. A. Graham.

Bibliography

Basmajian, J. V. (1974). *Muscles Alive: Their Functions Revealed by Electromyography*; 3rd ed. Baltimore, Williams & Wilkins.

Basmajian, J. V. (1980). *Grant's Method of Anatomy by Regions Descriptive and Deductive*, 10th ed. Baltimore, Williams & Wilkins.

Breathnach, A. S. (1965). *Frazer's Anatomy of the Human Skeleton*, 6th ed. London, Churchill.

Campbell, E. J. M., Agostoni, E., and Davis, J. N. (1970). *The Respiratory Muscles: Mechanics and Neural Control*, 2nd ed. London, W. B. Saunders.

Cherniack, R. M., Cherniack, L., and Naimark, A. (1972). *Respiration in Health and Disease*, 2nd ed. London, W. B. Saunders.

Duvall, E. N. (1962). *Kinesiology: The Anatomy of Motion*. Englewood Cliffs, NJ, Prentice-Hall.

Gardner, E. D., Gray, D. J., and O'Rahilly, R. (1975). *Anatomy, A Regional Study of Human Structure*, 4th ed. Philadelphia, W. B. Saunders.

Hamilton, W. J., and Simon, G. (1971). *Surface and Radiological Anatomy for Students and General Practitioners*, 5th ed. Baltimore, Williams & Wilkins.

Hollinshead, W. H. (1971). *Anatomy for Surgeons*, Vol. 2: *The Thorax, Abdomen, and Pelvis*, 2nd ed. New York, Hoeber-Harper.

Keith, A., Sir (1948). *Human Embryology and Morphology*, 6th ed. London, Edward Arnold.
Last, R. J. (1978). *Anatomy: Regional and Applied*. London, Churchill.
MacConaill, M. A., and Basmajian, J. V. (1977). *Muscles and Movements: A Basis for Human Kinesiology*, 2nd ed. Huntington, NY, R. E. Krieger.
Warwick, R., and Williams, P. L., eds. (1973). *Gray, H., Anatomy: Descriptive and Applied*, 35th ed. Edinburgh, Longman.

15

The Act of Breathing

PETER T. MACKLEM

Respiratory Health Network of Centres of Excellence
McGill University
Montreal, Quebec, Canada

I. Introduction

In the modern era, our first real understanding of the act of breathing came when Rahn et al. (1) published their classic paper of the pressure–volume curves of the respiratory system, lungs, and chest wall. From the relaxation curve of the respiratory system, it became possible to calculate the pressures required by the respiratory muscles to change lung volume from its equilibrium position—functional residual capacity (FRC)—at which the pressure difference across the system [mouth pressure (Pm) relative to body surface pressure] during relaxation with the glottis open is zero. The pressures at volumes greater than FRC must be produced by inspiratory muscles, whereas those below FRC must be developed by expiratory muscles.

II. Partitioning of Pressure and Displacements

A. Pressures

The second major contribution came from the publication of Agostoni and Rahn (2) when they partitioned the pressure drop across the respiratory system into its component parts: (1) Pm relative to pleural pressure (Ppl) or transpulmonary pressure

(PL); (2) Ppl pressure relative to abdominal pressure (Pab), which they recognized was transdiaphragmatic pressure (Pdi); and (3) Pab relative to body surface pressure, which they pointed out was the pressure that displaced the abdominal wall. This remarkable contribution introduced measurement of the pressure developed by the diaphragm or the transdiaphragmatic pressure (Pdi) developed during contraction or passive stretching of the diaphragm. As a result of this work, the diaphragmatic contribution to the pressures developed during breathing could be quantified for the first time. By convention Pdi is now usually expressed as a positive value Pab − Ppl, rather than Ppl − Pab.

B. Displacements

Konno and Mead (3) made the third major contribution when they partitioned the volumes displaced by the abdomen and rib cage. They provided evidence that, within defined limits, both the rib cage and abdomen behaved as separate compartments, each with a single degree of freedom. A single degree of freedom means that it is possible to measure the change in a single dimension of the rib cage and abdomen and solve for changes in all other dimensions. In other words, provided that the signals are appropriately calibrated, measuring a single rib cage or abdominal dimension could be interpreted in terms of the volumes displaced by rib cage and abdominal motion.

III. Elastic Properties of Rib Cage and Abdomen

Because during relaxation Ppl drives the rib cage while Pab displaces the abdomen, Konno and Mead (4) combined their partitioning of volume with Agostoni and Rahn's partitioning of pressure and described the static pressure–volume curves of the rib cage and abdomen. For the first time, the elastic work of displacing these compartments could be measured. Furthermore, they pointed out that the stiffening of the chest wall at low lung volumes, described by Rahn et al., was due to stiffening of neither the rib cage nor abdomen at low lung volumes (both compartments, in fact, become more compliant as volume diminishes), but was due to passive tension developed across the diaphragm, which resisted further stretching exponentially as volume decreased progressively below FRC.

These contributions set the stage for a virtual explosion of new knowledge about the act of breathing in the subsequent 25 years. This new knowledge has arisen from (1) partitioning the pressures developed by the diaphragm, the non-diaphragmatic inspiratory muscles, and the expiratory muscles during breathing; (2) understanding the forces applied to the rib cage by the inspiratory muscles and the pressures in the pleural and peritoneal cavities; (3) a better understanding of how the diaphragm and other inspiratory muscles act to inflate the respiratory system; (4) determining whether the various muscles and parts of muscles were linked in parallel or in series; (5) measurements of chest wall and rib cage distortions, the pressure costs of these distortions; and finally, (6) the development of a two-compartment rib cage model to study the distortability of the rib cage and how the distortions contribute to the act of breathing.

IV. The Diaphragm and Its Parts

Mead and Loring (5–7) pointed out that a substantial fraction of the internal surface of the rib cage was apposed directly to the pleural surface of the diaphragm. They called this the *area of apposition* and postulated that Ppl in this zone would be somewhere between Pab and 0.5 Pab. As Pab becomes positive during inspiration with diaphragmatic contraction and shortening, whereas Ppl over the surface of the lung falls, the pressure acting on the rib cage in the area of apposition should tend to expand it, whereas Ppl over the lung-apposed part of the rib cage would tend to deflate it. They also postulated that the costal fibers of the diaphragm, which run axially in humans and perpendicular to the costal margin (i.e., cephalodorsally) in dogs, would have a direct action to displace the rib cage cranially over and above the expanding action of the pressure in the area of apposition. This they called the *insertional component* of Pdi.

Subsequently, DeTroyer et al. (8,9) showed, in dogs, that the direct stimulation of the costal fibers produced an inflationary action on the lower rib cage. When the abdomen was opened, preventing an increase in Pab, costal stimulation no longer inflated the lower rib cage. Its inflationary action was restored when a pneumothorax was introduced and pleural pressure changes were prevented by inserting wide-bore tubing through an intercostal space bilaterally. They concluded that (1) Pab did indeed expand the lower rib cage, confirming the postulate of Loring and Mead (7); (2) the insertional component of Pdi was responsible for the rib cage inflation in the absence of changes in Pab and Ppl; (3) Ppl had a deflationary action on the rib cage that counteracted the inflationary action of the insertional component of Pdi.

When they stimulated the crural fibers with the abdomen closed, they found that there was no action on the rib cage, even though Pab increased and the anterior abdominal wall moved outward. When the abdomen was opened, crural contraction had a deflationary action on the rib cage, but, when the pneumothorax was introduced, the rib cage was no longer displaced. They concluded that (1) the crural part of the diaphragm had no direct action on the rib cage because it was not attached to it, whereas the costal part did because it was attached at the costal margin; the actions of the crural part were indirect through the effect of crural contraction on Pab and Ppl. (2) With the abdomen closed, the effect of the rise in Pab was cancelled by the fall in Ppl, whereas when Pab no longer changed, Ppl acting alone, caused the rib cage to deflate; when neither Ppl nor Pab changed, there could be no action of the crural part of the rib cage because the pressures that mediated its action no longer changed.

They found that the upper two cervical segments of the phrenic nerve innervated the costal fibers, whereas the crural part was primarily innervated by the lowermost segment, thereby confirming the results of Sant'Ambrogio et al. (10). Because the two muscular parts of the diaphragm have different embryological origins, different anatomical origins, different cervical segmental innervation, and different actions, they proposed that the diaphragm was composed of two distinct muscles, the crural diaphragm and the costal diaphragm.

Regardless of whether or not it is correct to consider the diaphragm as being composed of two muscles, it is clear that the two parts have separate actions. This being so, it is important to know the mechanical linkage between the two parts to understand how the diaphragm as a whole works (11). If the two parts are linked mechanically in parallel, the forces and pressure they develop are additive, but the displacements or length changes are not. The tension developed in one part will not be transmitted to the other. In a parallel linkage, the total transdiaphragmatic pressure is the sum of the pressures developed by each part, and the tensions developed by each part can be quite different. On the other hand, if the two parts are linked mechanically in series, then the total displacements resulting from shortening of the muscle will be the sum of the length changes in each part, whereas the tension developed in one part will be transmitted to the other. With both parts developing equal tension, even if one part remains inactivated (when the tension that develops is due to passive stretching), the pressure applied to an external structure will not be the sum of the pressures developed by each part. Each part develops the same pressure, which is equal to the pressure applied to the external structure.

Because crural contraction has no direct action on the rib cage, it would seem that tension is not transmitted through the central tendon from the crural to the costal part (12). It would also appear that, with costal contraction, tension is not transmitted to the crural part either. This can be inferred from the observation that during vomiting and eructation, the costal fibers contract, increasing abdominal pressure and generating a large pressure gradient from stomach to esophagus. The crural fibers that surround the esophagus at the esophagogastric junction remain inactivated, allowing stomach contents to flow down the pressure gradient and enter the esophagus. If the crural fibers were passively stretched by costal contraction, this should have a sphincterlike action on the esophagus and delay or prevent transmission of gastric contents from stomach to esophagus. Thus, a parallel mechanical linkage of costal and crural parts of the diaphragm is important physiologically for two reasons.

1. Diaphragmatic strength is increased; therefore, the diaphragm is better able to handle large loads and has longer endurance than it would with a series linkage.
2. Vomiting and eructation are not impaired by transmission of costal tension to the crural fibers.

The mechanical parallel linkage requires that the abdomen can sustain substantial pressure gradients. Duomarco and Rimini proposed that the abdomen behaved mechanically as a bag of liquid with a vertical hydrostatic pressure gradient (13). If so, pressures should equilibrate in the peritoneal cavity at the speed of sound. If this were to occur, the tension developed in one part of the diaphragm should be transmitted to the other, not through the central tendon, but through the agency of Pab. If during isolated crural contraction, for example, Pab were to rise substantially under the costal fibers, the resulting transdiaphragmatic pressure gradient would displace the costal part into the thoracic cavity, stretching the fibers and causing passive tension and an axial cephalad force acting at the costal margin. In contrast to the predictions arising from the Duomarco and Rimini hypothesis, it has been shown that with isolated contraction of the costal and crural part, substantial static abdominal pressure gradients exist (12,14). Indeed, when part of the abdominal viscera is removed and replaced by an equal volume of liquid, changes in Pab become everywhere equal in the abdomen, and the actions of the costal and crural parts become identical (14). Under these circumstance, the two parts probably remain linked in parallel, but with transmission of tension from one part to the other, as would occur with two muscles in parallel, but linked by a connection that went over a pulley.

The clinical counterpart of this situation is ascites. It is unknown whether ascites interferes with vomiting and eructation.

V. The Nondiaphragmatic Inspiratory Rib Cage Muscles

The most important nondiaphragmatic inspiratory muscles of the rib cage appear to be the parasternals and scalene muscles (15,16). The parasternals arise from the lateral margin of the sternum and insert into the upper border of the second to sixth ribs. They contract with every inspiration, and it is difficult, if not impossible, to suppress their contraction voluntarily, although this can be achieved during a Meuller maneuver. Their action is to diminish the angle between the lateral border of the sternum and the upper border of the ribs. Because ribs two through six are rather firmly attached to the sternum as well as the spine, contraction of the parasternals causes the so-called bucket-handle motion of the rib cage.

The scalenes, which originate from the cervical vertebrae and insert into the upper border of the first two ribs, also contract with each inspiration in humans. They act to decrease the angle between the anterior border of the spinal column and the superior border of the first two ribs. Because these ribs are attached to all others by intercostal muscle and fascia, lifting them will lift the whole rib cage in the so-called pump-handle motion.

The parasternals, when acting alone, act to displace the sternum caudally. This action is antagonized by scalene contraction. During inspiration, these muscles are coordinated in a way such that the sternum either remains stationary in the axial direction or undergoes a cephalad displacement.

The levator costae muscles, arising from the spine and inserting into the superior border of the ribs posteriorly, also act as inspiratory muscles. Their importance in humans is poorly understood because of their inaccessibility. In dogs their action during quiet breathing appears to be small (17,18).

The external intercostals run in the same general direction as the scalenes. One might consider these muscles as one large muscle, divided into segments by the ribs, in which each segment is separately innervated and can be separately activated. As the direction of the fibers (for which the posterior border is considered the origin) is ventral and caudal, it is evident that, acting as a single unit, they will have an inflating action on the rib cage (19,20). However, they are inconsistently activated during quiet breathing and, as minute ventilation increases, the pattern of activation is from above downward (i.e., the superior external intercostals are activated first, followed by progressively increasing caudal activation) as ventilation increases (21).

When considered as an individual muscle in each interspace, Hamberger proposed that the balance of forces would be in an inspiratory direction (22). However, he did not consider the relative impedances to motion of the rib cage in the cephalad and caudal directions. These should be determined largely by active or passive tension in the abdominal muscles vis-à-vis the scalene and the sterno-cleidomastoid muscles (23). At high lung volumes, with the ribs elevated, the passive tension in the abdominal muscles should increase, increasing the impedance to cephalad rib cage motion, whereas at low lung volumes, with the rib cage deflated, the passive tension in the salenes and sternocleidomastoids should increase impedance to caudal displacement of the rib cage. As the action of the external intercostals in a single interspace is unquestionably to decrease the distance between the two ribs, whether this will have a net inspiratory or expiratory action on the whole rib cage will depend not only on the balance of forces, as analyzed by Hamberger, but also on the relative impedances to rib cage motion in the cephalad and caudal directions and the number of interspaces activated (12,13).

Indeed, there is direct evidence in dogs that external intercostal muscle contraction in one or more, but not all, interspaces acts in an inspiratory direction at low lung volumes and in an expiratory direction at high lung volumes (23). Similarly, contraction of the abdominal muscles might change the external intercostals into expiratory muscles, whereas the inspiratory action of these muscles might be augmented by the normal inspiratory contraction of the scalene muscles. The sternocleidomastoid, which lifts the sternum when it contracts and is an accessory inspiratory muscle, may also assist the inspiratory action of the external intercostals.

In addition to their respiratory actions the intercostal muscles are thought to play an important postural role in stretching and twisting (24). Indeed, this may be even more important than their respiratory actions, at least during quiet breathing.

VI.   Interactions Between the Diaphragm and the Inspiratory Rib Cage Muscles

An important key to understanding how the diaphragm and inspiratory rib cage muscles are coordinated and how they interact is the realization that these two separate muscle groups are antagonistic to the abdomen and upper rib cage, but act in the same direction on the lower rib cage and the lung. When the diaphragm contracts by itself, Pab increases and, in the absence of simultaneous contraction of the abdominal muscles, the abdominal wall is displaced outward. As Ppl decreases, and in the absence of contraction of the inspiratory rib cage muscles, the upper rib cage is displaced inward (25). When the inspiratory rib cage muscles contract by themselves, they expand the upper rib cage, causing a fall in Ppl that is transmitted across the flaccid diaphragm to the abdomen. Therefore, Pab also falls, and the abdominal wall is displaced inward.

The joint inflating action of these muscles on the lung is reflected in the magnitude of change in PL during inspiration. The antagonistic action on the abdomen is reflected in the resulting change in Pab when both muscle groups contract simultaneously. This results in a greater ΔPL/ΔPab ratio than that which occurs with a pure diaphragmatic contraction (25). With a pure rib cage muscle inspiration, ΔPL/ΔPab is negative. In this way the PL–Pab diagram can be used to quantify the pressures developed by the diaphragm and provide a qualitative description of the relative degree of recruitment of the diaphragm vis-à-vis the other inspiratory muscles. Proportionately equal recruitment of diaphragm and rib cage muscles results in increasing Pdi and PL with constant ΔPL/ΔPab. Proportionately greater recruitment of rib cage muscles increases ΔPL/ΔPab, whereas preferential diaphragm recruitment decreases ΔPL/ΔPab. In addition any action of the expiratory muscles to decrease end-expiratory lung volume, or of the inspiratory muscles to increase end-expiratory lung volume, can be detected by the end-expiratory PL. Use of this diagram has shown that, as ventilation increases owing to chemical stimulation or exercise, the inspiratory rib cage muscles are recruited to a proportionately greater extent than the diaphragm (26,27).

It should be realized that there are limitations to the use of the PL–Pab diagram. It applies only under quasi-static conditions or dynamically when the time constants of lung and chest wall are identical (25). In effect, this frequently limits its usefulness to points of zero flow at end-expiration and end-inspiration.

VII. The Pressures Applied to the Rib Cage

To understand the act of breathing, one must know the pressures that act on and displace the compartments of the respiratory system during breathing. For the lung and the abdomen, the situation is straightforward. The PL, which under most conditions equals –Ppl, changes the volume of the lung, and Pab displaces the abdomen. The situation for the rib cage is more complex because it is exposed to both Ppl and Pab, and both the costal part of the diaphragm and the rib cage muscles are attached to it. The net action, therefore, is an appropriately weighted sum of Pab, Ppl, xPdi, and Prcm, where xPdi is the insertional component of Pdi (7) for which $1 > x > 0$, and Prcm is the pressure developed on the rib cage by the rib cage muscles.

To complicate matters further, these pressures are applied to different parts of the rib cage. The insertional component of Pdi is applied at the costal margin to ribs seven through twelve. At FRC, the ventral ends of these ribs are in the area of apposition. A fraction of Pab is applied to the rib cage in this zone (28,29), which extends laterally approximately at the level of the xiphisternum (5,30). Pleural pressure acts on the rib cage area that is in apposition to the costal surface of the lungs, cephalad to the area of apposition. Prcm is applied to ribs one through six. These ribs are entirely in the lung-apposed part of the rib cage. As the interspace between the sixth and seventh ribs toward the midline anteriorly is at the level of the xiphisternum, it can be seen that Pab and xPdi act on the same ribs, and these are the ribs that are only loosely attached to the sternum by rather long and flexible costal cartilages. On the other hand, Ppl and Pcrm act on ribs one through six that are fairly tightly attached to the sternum. There seems to be little overlap in the geographic site of action of Ppl and Prcm, on the one hand, and Pab and xPdi, on the other.

Because the pressures act on separate geographic sites, with pure diaphragmatic contraction, ΔPab and xPdi act to expand the lower rib cage, whereas ΔPpl acts to deflate the upper rib cage. Indeed, in quadriplegia, the upper rib cage paradoxically moves inward during inspiration, whereas during phrenic stimulation, the lower rib cage expands and the upper rib cage moves paradoxically inward (31). Thus diaphragmatic contraction distorts the rib cage systematically, and the pressure cost of this distortion must be known if one wishes to analyze the pressures and forces acting on the ribs in any rigorous way.

VIII. The Two-Compartment Rib Cage Model

The geographically separate sites at which different pressures and different agencies act on the rib cage led D'Angelo and Agostoni to propose that the rib cage might be considered as consisting of two compartments: the lung-apposed part of the rib cage (the pulmonary rib cage, RCp) and the diaphragm-apposed part (the abdominal rib cage, RCa) (32). Subsequently, Decramer and colleagues (33) measured the dimensions of RCp and RCa in dogs during relaxation, when Pab equals Ppl and xPdi and Prcm are zero. Thus the pressures acting on RCp and RCa are the same. This is defined as the undistorted configuration of the rib cage. When they stimulated the phrenic nerves they produced marked rib cage distortion. The RCp deflated, whereas RCa expanded. The relations between the dimensions of RCp and Ppl and RCa and Pab were very close to those during relaxation. They concluded that in supine anesthetized dogs the rib cage was remarkably flexible and that the resistance to bending was small (32).

Ward et al. extended this model and applied it to humans (33). They showed that, in upright, awake subjects, the human rib cage was much less flexible than in dogs and that the resistance to bending was substantial. They demonstrated this by showing that changes in RCp and RCa dimensions during diaphragmatic twitches, produced by bilateral transcutaneous supramaximal phrenic nerve shocks, were considerably less than during relaxation for the same changes in Ppl and Pab. By comparing these relationships during relaxation and diaphragmatic twitch contractions, they were able to estimate the pressures (Plink) applied to RCp and RCa by the distortion and the inherent resistance to bending of the rib cage. They also developed an index of distortion and constructed graphs of Plink versus distortion. The pressure producing distortion is given as the difference between the pressure acting on RCa and that acting on RCp when the diaphragm is the only muscle contracting. This pressure difference is given by: $Pab + xPdi - Ppl = (x + 1)Pdi$. Thus, Pdi is directly proportional to the pressure that produces distortion, and the plot of distortion versus Pdi is an index of rib cage distortability. Note that the pressure that produces distortion and the pressure that results from distortion are different.

The pressure resulting from distortion in which RCa expands more than RCp, acts to pull RCp with it, thereby decreasing Ppl. Similarly, a deflation of RCp when the diaphragm contracts alone, restricts the expansion of RCa. The Plink, acting to decrease Ppl, also acts to expand the lung. Thus, the rib caged resistance to distortion is inflationary when RCa expands.

During quiet breathing, the rib cage distorts systematically from its relaxation configuration so that, through the mechanical linkage between the two rib cage compartments, RCa acts to expand RCp, which along with simultaneous contraction of the rib cage muscles, counteracts the deflationary action of ΔPpl. The pressures developed by these muscles, and the fall in Ppl resulting from distortion, each provide about 50% of the pressure required to expand the lungs and RCp during quiet breathing. To state these relations in a more rigorous way one may describe the pressures acting on RCp and RCa under equilibrium conditions when the inherent elastic recoil pressure of RCp and RCa (Prc,p and Prc,a resp.) must be exactly equal and opposite to the pressures acting on the two rib cage compartments from external agencies. Thus, during relaxation when all muscle pressures are zero:

Ppl = Prc,p and
Pab = Prc,a

By using these equations, one can then measure Prc,p and Prc,a as a function of the dimensions of RCp and RCa.

During isolated diaphragmatic contractions

Ppl + Plink = Prc,p

This is true because the only action the diaphragm has on RCp is indirectly by distortion and the resulting restoring pressure, Plink. For RCa:

Pab + Plink + xPdi = Prc,a

If one measures the rib cage dimensions Prc,p and Prc,a are known. As Ppl and Pab are also known, one can solve for Plink. During quiet tidal breathing

Ppl + Plink + Prcm = Prc,p

If one measures distortions during quiet breathing, and the relation between distortion and Plink is known, this equation can be solved for Prcm.

If one breathes in such a way that there is no rib cage distortion, then Plink becomes zero and the following holds,

Pab + xPdi = Prc,a

and one can solve for xPdi. Ward et al. showed that this was about 25% of Pdi and that x was independent of the magnitude of Pdi (32).

IX. Summary and Conclusions

The partitioning of the pressure differences across different parts of the respiratory system, the measurement of transdiaphragmatic pressure, and the methodology to describe the volume displacements of the rib cage and abdomen have proved to be major advances in our understanding of the act of breathing. These advances opened up the way to quantifying the action of different groups of respiratory muscles and the actions of different parts or different muscles within a group. They allowed determination of how the various muscle groups are mechanically linked, which is essential to understand how they are coordinated to produce displacements and forces.

The complexity of the pressures and forces acting on the rib cage was a major stumbling block in understanding how that compartment was displaced in anything other than qualitative terms. The realization that the diaphragm, abdominal pressure, pleural pressure, and the pressure resulting from rib cage muscle contraction, all played a role, was a major advance. The further realization that the first two and the last two acted on quite separate areas of the rib cage led to the concept that the rib cage consisted of two compartments. By analyzing the pressures acting on these compartments, their displacements, and their distortions, it has now become possible to quantify the pressures developed by the rib cage muscles, the insertional component of transdiaphragmatic pressure, the distortability of the rib cage, and the restoring pressures resulting from distortion.

Quantification of these parameters has as yet been accomplished only during quiet breathing in the upright posture. The stage is now set to measure them under a variety of physiological conditions, such as posture, exercise, loaded breathing, and pathological conditions. When this is done, we will have a much more complete picture of the act of breathing.

References

1. Rahn, H., Otis, A. B., Chadwick, L. E., and Fenn, W. O. (1946). The pressure volume diaphragm of the thorax and lung. *Am. J. Physiol.* 146: 161–178.
2. Agostoni, E., and Rhan, H. (1960). Abdominal and thoracic pressures at different lung volumes. *J. Appl. Physiol.* 15: 1087–1092.
3. Konno, K., and Mead, J. (1967). Measurement of the separate volume changes of rib cage and abdomen during breathing. *J. Appl. Physiol.* 22: 407–422.

4. Konno, K., and Mead, J. (1968). Static volume–pressure characteristics of the rib cage and abdomen. *J. Appl. Physiol.* 24: 544–548.
5. Mead, J. (1979). Functional significance of the area of apposition of diaphragm to rib cage. *Am. Rev. Respir. Dis.* 119(Part 2): 31–32.
6. Mead, J., and Loring, S. H. (1982). Analysis of volume displacement and length changes of the diaphragm during breathing. *J. Appl. Physiol. Respir. Environ. Exerc. Physiol.* 53: 750–755.
7. Loring, S. H., and Mead, J. (1982). Action of the diaphragm on the rib cage inferred from a force–balance analysis. *J. Appl. Physiol. Respir. Environ. Exerc. Physiol.* 53: 756–760.
8. DeTroyer, A., Sampson, M., Sigrist, S., and Macklem, P. T. (1981). The diaphragm: Two muscles. *Science* 213: 237–238.
9. DeTroyer, A., Sampson, M., Sigrist, S., and Macklem, P. T. (1982). Action of costal and crural parts of the diaphragm on the rib cage in dog. *J. Appl. Physiol. Respir. Environ. Exerc. Physiol.* 53: 30–39.
10. Sant'Ambrogio, G., Frazier, D. T., Wilson, M. F., and Agostoni, E. (1963). Motor innervation and pattern of activity of cat diaphragm. *J. Appl. Physiol.* 18: 43–46.
12. Decramer, M., DeTroyer, A., Kelly, S., Zocchi, L., and Macklem, P. T. (1984). Regional differences in abdominal pressure swings in dogs. *J. Appl. Physiol. Respir. Environ. Exerc. Physiol.* 57: 1682–1687.
13. Duomarco, J. L., and Rimini, R. (1947). *La Presion Intra-abdominal en el Hombre*. Buenos Aires, El Ateneo.
14. Zocchi, L., Garzaniti, N., Newman, S., and Macklem, P. T. (1987). Effect of hyperinflation and equalization of abdominal pressure on diaphragmatic action. *J. Appl. Physiol.* 62: 1655–1664.
15. DeTroyer, A., and Sampson, M. G. (1982). Activation of the parasternal intercostals during breathing efforts in man. *J. Appl. Physiol.* 52: 524–529.
16. DeTroyer, A., and Estenne, M. (1984). Co-ordination between rib cage muscles and diaphragm during quiet breathing in humans. *J. Appl. Physiol.* 57: 889–906.
17. DeTroyer, A., and Farkas, G. A. (1989). Inspiratory function of the levator costae and external intercostal muscles in the dog. *J. Appl. Physiol.* 67: 2614–1621. Levatores costae active but action is small
18. DeTroyer, A. (1991). Inspiratory elevation of the ribs in the dog: Primary role of the parasternals. *J. Appl. Physiol.* 70: 1447–1455.
19. Loring, S. H., and Woodbridge, J. A. (1991). Intercostal muscle action inferred from finite-element analysis. *J. Appl. Physiol.* 70: 2712–1718.
20. Loring, S. H. (1992). Action of human respiratory muscles inferred from finite element analysis of rib cage. *J. Appl. Physiol.* 72: 1461–1465.
21. Whitelaw, W. A., and Teroah, T. (1989). Patterns of intercostal muscle activity in humans. *J. Appl. Physiol.* 67: 2082–2094.
22. Hamberger, G. E. (1927). *De Respiratoinis Mechanismo Iena.*
23. DeTroyer, A., Kelly, S., Macklem, P. T., and Zin, W. A. (1985). Mechanics of intercostal space and actions of external and internal intercostal muscles. *J. Clin. Invest.* 75: 850–857.
24. Whitelaw, W. A., Ford, G. T., Rimer, K. P., and DeTroyer, A. (1992). Intercostal muscles are used during rotation of the thorax in humans. *J. Appl. Physiol.* 72: 1940–1944.
25. Macklem, P. T., Gross, D., Grassino, A., and Roussos, C. (1978). Partitioning of inspiratory pressure swings between diaphragm and intercostal/accessory muscles. *J. Appl. Physiol. Respir. Environ. Exerc. Physiol.* 44:200–208.
26. Sheng, Y., Similowski, T., Gauthier, A., Macklem, P. T., and Bellemare, F. (1992). Effect of fatigue on diaphragmatic function at different lung volumes. *J. Appl. Physiol.* 72: 1064–6067.
27. Bye, P. T., Esau, S. A., Walley, K. R., Macklem. P. T., and Pardy, R. L. (1984). Ventilatory muscles during exercise in air and oxygen in normal men. *J. Appl. Physiol. Respir. Environ. Exerc. Physiol.* 56: 464–471.
28. Macklem, P. T., Zocchi, L., and Agostoni, E. (1988). Pleural pressure between diaphragm and rib cage during inspiratory muscle activity. *J. Appl. Physiol.* 65: 1286–1295.

29. Urmey, W. F., Loring, S. H., DeTroyer, A., and Kelly, K. B. (1986). Direct measurement of pleural pressure in the zone of apposition of diaphragm to rib cage in dogs [abstract]. *Anesthesiology* 65: A585.
30. Paiva, M., Verbanck, S., Estenne, M., Poncelet, B., Segebarth, C., and Macklem, P. T. (1992). Mechanical implications of in vivo human diaphragm shape. *J. Appl. Physiol.* 72: 1–6.
31. Ward, M. E., Ward, J., and Macklem, P. T. (1992). Analysis of human chest wall motion using two-compartment rib cage model. *J. Appl. Physiol.* 72: 1338–1347.
32. Agostoni, E., and D'Angelo, E. (1988). Statics of the chest wall. In *The Thorax*. Edited by C. Roussos and P. T. Macklem. New York, Marcel Dekker, 1988, pp. 259–295.
33. Jiang, T. X., Demedts, M., and Decramer, M. (1988). Mechanical coupling of upper and lower canine rib cages and its functional significance. *J. Appl. Physiol.* 64: 620–626.

16

Statics of the Chest Wall*

EDGARDO D'ANGELO and EMILIO AGOSTONI

University of Milan
Milan, Italy

I. Volume–Pressure Relations During Relaxation

A. Respiratory System

Under static conditions, the pressure exerted by the passive respiratory system depends on elastic, surface, and gravitational forces operating on the lung and the chest wall (i.e., rib cage and diaphragm–abdomen). The pressure exerted by the respiratory system is given by the difference between alveolar pressure and body surface pressure. To determine the static relation between the lung volume and the relaxation pressure of the respiratory system (Rohrer, 1916; Rahn et al., 1946), the subject inspires or expires a volume of air and then relaxes against an obstructed airway, and the pressure across the obstruction is measured. Since there is no flow, the pressure in the mouth or in a nostril equals alveolar pressure. Then the subject breathes in or out maximally from a spirometer so that the volume at which the pressure was measured can be related to one extreme of the vital capacity. This volume must be corrected for the compression or expansion of the gas in the respiratory system caused by the change of pressure during relaxation. When these

---

*This chapter is in part based on "Statics of the respiratory system" by Agostoni and Mead (1964) and "Statics" by Agostoni (1970b).

measurements are made at several volumes, the volume–pressure curve during relaxation is obtained. This method may not be applied to all subjects and some training is necessary.

The volume–pressure curve of the relaxed respiratory system, with the trunk erect, is shown in Figure 1, along with the spirogram showing the pulmonary subdivisions. The volume at zero pressure is the resting volume of the respiratory system; it usually corresponds to the end of a spontaneous expiration during quiet breathing. The horizontal distance from the curve to the ordinate at zero pressure indicates the pressure exerted by the passive structure of the system at a given lung volume. Conversely, this distance indicates the pressure that the respiratory muscles must exert to maintain that lung volume with open airways. This is true only if the shape of the chest wall is the same when the respiratory muscles are relaxed as when they are active at the same lung volume. In fact, the energy of the passive structures of the system is minimum for the configuration occurring during relaxation; whenever, at the same lung volume, this configuration is changed, the energy of the passive structure is increased (Agostoni et al., 1965a). To the extent that contraction of the respiratory muscles deforms the respiratory system relative to its relaxed configuration at a given volume, the pressure exerted by the muscles is larger than that indicated by the volume–pressure diagram. The extra pressure

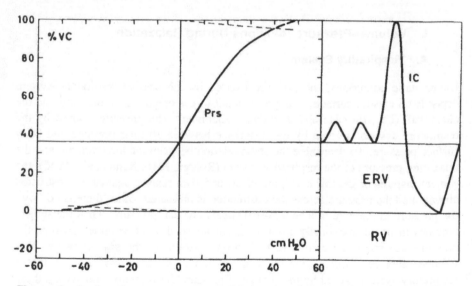

Figure 1 Static volume–pressure curve of the total respiratory system during relaxation in the sitting posture, with a spirogram showing the subdivisions of lung volume. The slanting broken lines indicate the volume change during relaxation against an obstruction caused by gas compression at TLC and expansion at RV. The curve was extended to include the full vital capacity range by means of externally applied pressures. (From Rohrer, 1916, as modified by Agostoni and Mead, 1964.)

exerted by the muscles, however, is difficult to assess (see later discussion). The slope of the static volume–pressure curve gives the compliance of the respiratory system (Crs): it is maximum in the midlung volume range (at which we normally breathe), being about 2% of vital capacity (VC) per centimeter H_2O, or 0.1 L/cm H_2O in an average-sized man.

To overcome the difficulty of voluntary relaxation, the volume–pressure relation of the relaxed respiratory system in the tidal volume range may be estimated with the method proposed by Heaf and Prime (1954). With the subject breathing spontaneously, the pressure at the airway opening is raised above that acting on the body surface (positive pressure breathing): if the subject is relaxed at the end of expiration, the relation is obtained by measuring the change in end-expiratory lung volume and the applied pressure. The relation obtained by this method over the tidal volume range is usually similar to that obtained during voluntary relaxation (Heaf and Prime, 1956; Johnson and Mead, 1963; Cherniack and Brown, 1965; Mognoni et al., 1965). On the other hand, the volume–pressure curve obtained by Rahn et al. (1946) from the end-expiratory values during positive and negative pressure breathing was different from that obtained during voluntary relaxation. This difference seemed related to the fact that, in their experiments during positive (PPB) and negative (NPB) pressure breathing, the head and neck were not exposed to the same pressure as the rest of the body surface (Rahn et al., 1946; Johnson and Mead, 1963). However, as the volume–pressure curve obtained during voluntary relaxation with closed glottis is equal to that with open glottis, the pressure across the cheeks and the neck does not seem to influence the results (Mognoni et al., 1965). In fact, in some subjects, the volume–pressure curve determined from the end-expiratory values during PPB and NPB was different from that obtained during voluntary relaxation, even if in the former case the head and neck were exposed to the same pressure as the rest of the body (Agostoni, 1962; Mognoni et al., 1965). The different results may partly relate to the period of PPB, because the activity of the expiratory muscles seems to appear only after some minutes of PPB (Agostoni, 1970b).

Involuntary respiratory muscle activity may influence the elastic properties of the chest wall. Indeed, submaximal neuromuscular blockade reduces the functional reserve capacity (FRC) in seated humans (DeTroyer and Bastenier-Geens, 1979). In addition, evidence has been presented suggesting the existence of tonic diaphragmatic muscle activity at end expiration in supine humans (Muller et al., 1979). The effects of general anesthesia, muscular paralysis, and their combination on the static mechanical properties of the respiratory system are dealt with in Chapter 55.

B. Chest Wall

The chest wall and the lung are placed in series; therefore, the algebraic sum of the pressure exerted by the two parts gives the pressure of the respiratory system

(Pw + PL = Prs). On the other hand, the change in volume of each part must be equal (except for shifts of blood volume) and must be equal to that of the respiratory system (ΔVw = ΔVL = ΔVrs). Static Prs is the difference between alveolar pressure and body surface pressure; hence, when the latter is atmospheric: PA = Pw + PL. Since Pw is generally taken to indicate the pressure exerted by the relaxed chest wall, when the respiratory muscles are active PA = Pw + PL + Pmus. Under static conditions the pressure exerted by the lung is the difference between alveolar pressure and pleural surface pressure (PL = PA − Ppl). The pressure exerted by the chest wall is the difference between pleural surface pressure and body surface pressure (Pw = Ppl − Pbs). The chest wall pressure may be obtained either indirectly by subtracting the pressure exerted by the lung from that exerted by the respiratory system, or directly from Ppl measurements. In fact, when the subject is relaxed (with closed airways to keep a static condition): PA = PL + Pw, since PL = PA − Ppl, substituting, Pw = Ppl. Moreover, Ppl = PA − PL, and Ppl = Pmus + Pw when the muscles are active. PA may be made equal to zero when holding a given lung volume with open airways, then Ppl = −PL. Pmus may be made equal to zero by relaxing the muscles with the airways closed, then Ppl = Pw. Ppl in humans is usually obtained from esophageal pressure measurements.

The static volume–pressure curves of the relaxed chest wall and of the lung, with trunk erect, are shown in Figure 2. At the resting volume of the respiratory system the chest wall recoils outward, with a pressure equal to that by which the

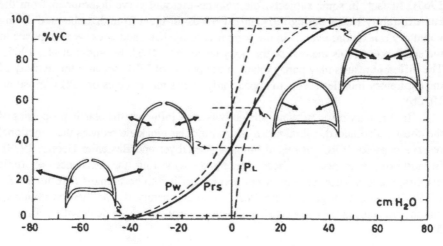

Figure 2 Static volume–pressure curves of the lung (PL), chest wall (Pw), and total respiratory system (Prs), during relaxation in the sitting posture. The static forces of the lung and the chest wall are pictured by the arrows in the side drawings. The dimensions of the arrows are not to scale; the volume corresponding to each drawing is indicated by the horizontal broken lines. (From Rahn et al., 1946, as modified by Agostoni and Mead, 1964.)

lung recoils inward. The resting volume of the lung is below 0% of the VC. That of the chest wall is about 55% of the VC (Agostoni and Mead, 1964). At values higher than this volume, both the chest wall and the lung recoil inward, whereas at those lower than this volume the chest wall recoils outward; hence, the lung and the chest wall behave like two opposing springs. According to Turner and associates (1968), the compliance of the chest wall decreases slightly above 80–90% VC, and the resting volume of the chest wall is higher than indicated in the foregoing. In the tidal volume range, the compliance of the chest wall and that of the lung are about the same. Since the chest wall and the lung are placed in series, the sum of the reciprocals of lung and chest wall compliances equals the reciprocal of the compliance of the respiratory system: $1/C_L + 1/C_w = 1/C_{rs}$.

The static volume–pressure relationships have been represented as single lines, suggesting that static pressures depend on volume alone. In fact, these pressures differ depending on the previous volume history of the respiratory system. For example, static pressures tend to be lower after deep inspirations and higher after deep expirations. As a result, static curves obtained as volume is changed in progressive steps from minimum (RV) to maximum (TLC) levels and back again, are loops, rather than single lines. One consequence is that FRC will be higher when reached during deflation from TLC than during inflation from RV. Loops, such as those shown in Figure 3, are called *hysteresis loops*. "Hysteresis is the failure of a system to follow identical paths of response upon application and

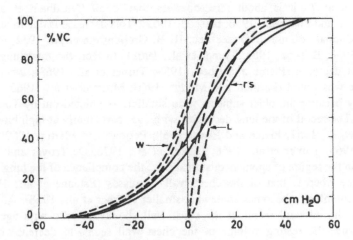

Figure 3 Quasistatic volume–pressure hysteresis of the respiratory system. Volume shifts were produced by gradually changing pressure at the mouth relative to that at the body surface, a complete cycle taking approximately 1 min, during which the subject attempted to relax his respiratory muscles as completely as possible. The volume changes were measured with a body plethysmograph. Pleural pressure was estimated from esophageal pressure measurements. (Modified from Agostoni and Mead, 1964.)

withdrawal of a forcing agent" (Landowne and Stacy, 1957). Static or quasistatic (i.e., long-term) elastic hysteresis is a common phenomenon exhibited by the various tissues of the body (Remington, 1955) and by such nonbiological materials as metals and rubber. In the respiratory system, it depends on viscoelasticity, such as stress adaptation (i.e., a rate-dependent phenomenon), and on plasticity (i.e., a rate-independent phenomenon). Hysteresis occurs both in the lung and in the chest wall (Butler, 1957; Sharp et al., 1967; Van de Woestijne 1967). In the lung, it is mainly due to surface properties and alveolar recruitment–derecruitment (Gil and Weibel, 1972), whereas in the chest wall, it seems mainly related to muscles and ligaments, because both skeletal muscles (Buchtal and Rosenfalck, 1957) and elastic fibers (Remington, 1957) exhibit hysteresis.

For analytical purposes, in the volume–pressure diagrams, pleural surface pressure has been and will be dealt with as a single value (i.e., as if it were uniformly distributed). Under physiological conditions, however, pleural surface pressure varies at different sites because of the effects of gravity on the lung and the chest wall and because of the different shapes of these two structures (Agostoni, 1972). Therefore, it is important to keep in mind that the balance between the lung and the chest wall under physiological conditions results from a wide distribution of pressures (Agostoni, 1972).

The static behavior of the respiratory system, lungs, and chest wall, changes throughout life. The peculiar features at birth and during growth are dealt with in Chapter 25. From young adulthood the vital capacity decreases almost linearly with age; at 70 it is about three-quarters that at 30 (Needham et al., 1954; Pemberton and Flanagan, 1956; Briscoe, 1965). This decrease is due to an increase of the residual volume (RV) (see Sec. III.B; Greifenstein et al., 1952; Pierce and Ebert, 1958; Briscoe, 1965; Turner et al., 1968). In fact, the total lung capacity does not decrease (Pierce and Ebert, 1958; Turner et al., 1968); when a small decrease was found (Permutt and Martin, 1960; Mittman et al., 1965), this was probably because the older subjects were smaller, as pointed out by Turner et al. (1968). The recoil of the lung decreases with age, particularly at high lung volume (Frank et al., 1957; Pierce and Ebert, 1958; Permutt and Martin, 1960; Mittman et al., 1965; Turner et al., 1968; Gibson et al., 1976; De Troyer and Yernault, 1980). In the region of spontaneous breathing, the compliance of the lung increases with age, whereas that of the chest wall decreases (Estenne et al., 1985): the overall compliance becomes somewhat smaller (Turner et al., 1968). At low lung volume, the outward recoil of the chest wall should increase with age. On the other hand, the resting volume of the chest wall seems to decrease in elderly subjects; hence, the volume–pressure curve of the chest wall should become less steep with age, pivoting around a point at about midlung volume, at which its recoil remains the same (Turner et al., 1968). Therefore, the increase of FRC with age found by most investigators (Greifenstein et al., 1952; Frank et al., 1957; Pierce and Ebert, 1958) is mainly due to the decrease of lung recoil and is less marked than that of RV (Turner et al., 1968).

C. Effects of Gravity and Posture

The volume–pressure curves considered so far refer to the erect trunk. That of the lung does not change appreciably with posture, whereas that of the chest wall does, mainly because of the effect of gravity on the abdomen. From the statics point of view, the abdomen can be likened to a container filled with liquid (Duomarco and Rimini, 1947). When a human is in the upright posture and the respiratory muscles are relaxed, the abdomen behaves as a container in which part of its lateral wall is distensible. The pressure in the upper part of such a container is negative (Kelling, 1903). Experimental evidence for this behavior of the abdomen in humans was provided by Duomarco and Rimini (1947).

The level at which the abdominal pressure is equal to ambient pressure, the *zero level*, depends on the equilibrium among the elastic forces of the abdominal wall, diaphragm, rib cage, lung, and the gravitational force of the abdominal contents. From the data of Duomarco and Rimini (1947), it can be estimated that, in the erect posture, the zero level at the end of a normal expiration (i.e., at the resting volume of the respiratory system), is about 3–4 cm beneath the diaphragmatic dome. The pressure just beneath the dome of the diaphragm is approximately what one would expect to find at the surface of the lungs above the diaphragm.

In supine subjects, the zero level corresponds to the ventral wall of the abdomen (Duomarco and Rimini, 1947). The diaphragm is then distended by the pressure exerted by the abdominal contents. It is generally held that during the last part of expiration there is no electrical activity of the diaphragm either in humans (Taylor, 1960) or in anesthetized animals (Fink et al., 1958; Sant'Ambrogio et al., 1963), although tonic diaphragmatic activity has been observed in supine humans (Muller et al., 1979). If one assumes no activity, it seems probable that in the supine position the diaphragm balances with its own elasticity the pressure exerted by the abdominal contents. The zero level in the prone position corresponds to the dorsal wall of the abdomen, and when the subject is lying on one side, it is midway between the two sides (Duomarco and Rimini, 1947). The zero level is expected to shift with lung volume and to a different degree in the upright and supine postures.

Since the volume of gas in the human abdomen is normally negligible, compared with the total lung volume, the volume of the abdomen can be considered constant when its pressure is changed. Therefore, the values of abdominal pressure at different lung volumes may be represented in the volume–pressure diagram of the respiratory system (Agostoni and Rahn, 1960). The pressure on the abdominal side of the diaphragm (Pab) may be estimated from gastric pressure (Agostoni and Rahn, 1960). This widely accepted approach was questioned by Decramer et al. (1984), who found that the changes in pressure measured by balloons or saline-filled catheters anchored under the costal and crural diaphragm and between intestinal loops differed from the changes in gastric pressure during some maneuvers. During relaxation, however, the changes in pressure under the costal and crural diaphragm were similar to those in gastric pressure (Zocchi et al., 1987). Moreover, Mead et al. (1990), on the basis of gastric and rectal pressure measurements, confirmed that the abdomen behaves as an essentially hydrostatic system during relatively slow maneuvers. They showed that the loss in the transmission of pressure is about 5%. In the abdomen there are organs, such as the liver and the spleen, anchored by ligaments, which do not behave as liquid. The occurrence of these organs beneath the diaphragm might have relevance for the mechanical action of the diaphragm (see Chap. 22), but does not prevent the essential hydrostatic behavior of the abdominal contents as a whole. Finally, the finding that the shape of the dorsal part of the diaphragm in supine subjects fits with the Laplace law supports the essential fluid behavior of the abdominal contents (Paiva et al., 1992).

In the upright posture, during relaxation, the transdiaphragmatic pressure (Pdi = Ppl − Pab) is nil above the resting volume of the respiratory system, whereas it increases progressively below the resting volume (Fig. 4, left). The hydrostatic pressure applied on the abdominal surface of the diaphragm changes markedly with lung volume. At residual volume, the zero level is some 20 cm below the diaphragmatic dome. At about 55% VC, which is the resting volume of the chest wall, the zero level is at the top of the abdominal cavity. At higher volume, the zero level is above the top of the abdomen (i.e., the pressure on the abdominal surface of the diaphragm is higher than atmospheric). In the upright posture, gravity acts in the inspiratory direction on the abdomen–diaphragm and in the expiratory direction on the rib cage. The hydrostatic effect of the abdomen is greater at small than at large volumes, because at large volumes the height of the abdomen is less, and its wall is stiffer. When a subject at FRC turns from the sitting to the standing position, the ribs move down and in, whereas the lung volume remains essentially the same. The rib cage cross section at the xiphoid level is reduced to approximately that in the seated posture when the lung volume is lowered to about 16% VC (Agostoni et al., 1966b), whereas the decrease at the angle of Louis is insignificant (E. Agostoni and E. D'Angelo, unpublished observations). Therefore, gravity in the standing posture modifies mainly the caudal part of the rib cage, acting through the stretched abdominal wall and the subatmospheric pressure of the upper part of the abdomen.

In the supine posture (see Fig. 4, right), changes in Pab over the VC are nearly half those occurring in the upright posture; the shift of the zero level with lung volume is accordingly smaller. In the supine posture at full inflation, the dorsoventral diameter of the abdomen is about 18 cm, and the zero level of Pab is close to the ventral abdominal wall; hence, the average hydrostatic pressure applied to the abdominal surface of the diaphragm should be about 9 cm H_2O. This value is similar to that of the pressure acting on the thoracic side of the diaphragm during relaxation against an obstructed airway at full VC; therefore, at this lung volume the pressure across the central part of the diaphragm should be approximately nil. In the supine posture gravity has a marked expiratory action on the abdomen–diaphragm, and a complex action on the rib cage. Indeed, when moving from the sitting to the supine posture, the cross section of the rib cage increases at the xiphisternal level (Vellody et al., 1978;

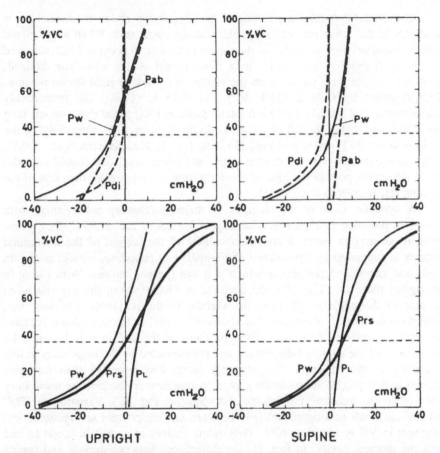

UPRIGHT   SUPINE

Figure 4 Pressure contributed by the various parts of the respiratory system in the sitting and supine posture. The upper diagrams show the volume–pressure relations of the chest wall and the pressures contributed by the diaphragm and abdomen. The circles indicate the resting volume of the respiratory system. The horizontal broken line indicates the resting volume of the respiratory system in the sitting posture. The lower diagrams show the volume–pressure relations of the chest wall, lung, and total respiratory system. (Modified from Agostoni and Mead, 1964.)

D'Angelo, 1981), but decreases at the angle of Louis (D'Angelo, 1981). As a consequence of gravity, the compliance of the chest wall and, hence, that of the total respiratory system, in the midvolume range, increases as one changes from the upright to the supine position (see Fig. 4). When a subatmospheric pressure of 55 cm H_2O is applied to the abdomen caudally to the iliac crest of a supine subject, the volume–pressure curve of his or her respiratory system during relaxation becomes almost equal to that in the sitting posture (Zechman et al., 1967).

In the lateral posture the action of gravity on the abdomen–diaphragm is expiratory in the lower part and inspiratory in the upper one. When anesthetized paralyzed subjects were moved from the supine to the lateral posture, FRC increased by 0.63 L (Rehder et al., 1971). In a more recent study, when anesthetized, paralyzed subjects were moved from the supine to the left or right lateral posture, FRC increased by 0.79 L (15% VC) and 0.93 L (17% VC), respectively (Hedenstierna et al., 1981). In the left lateral posture, FRC of the right (upper) lung was 2.20 L and that of the left lung 0.85 L. In the right lateral posture, FRC of the left lung was 2.09 L and that of the right lung 1.12 L (Hedenstierna et al., 1981). In evaluating the differences between upper and lower lung, one should consider that in the supine posture the FRC of the right lung is 11% greater than that of the left lung (Hedenstierna et al. 1981).

A synoptic view of the changes in major pulmonary subdivisions with posture is provided in Figure 5. The largest variations are in FRC; they occur between postures in which a considerable part of the weight of the abdominal contents is supported by the anterior abdominal wall (standing, sitting, prone on hands and knees) and postures in which it is not (prone, supine). With tilting in the sagittal plane (see Fig. 5B), the decrease in FRC is about linearly related to the sine of the angle of tilt from the vertical to the horizontal position, but, beyond the horizontal, it is reduced or abolished. Thus, in the head-down posture, the expiratory effect of the hydrostatic pressure of the abdomen is lessened by the stiffness of the stretched diaphragm and compensated by the inspiratory action of gravity on the rib cage. The relatively larger FRCs for tall than for short subjects in the upright, but not in the supine posture further illustrate the inspiratory effect of gravity mediated through the abdomen (see Fig. 5C). Variations in TLC and RV are small and significant only between upright posture and recumbency; reduction in VC is less than 10%. They relate mainly to a shift in blood to and from the thoracic cavity. In fact, (1) the differences between upright and supine VC are smaller after applications of tourniquets to the extremities (Hamilton and Morgan, 1932; Asmussen et al., 1939; Dow, 1939; Mills, 1949) or immersion in water (Hamilton and Mayo, 1944); (2) VC changes with ambient temperature according to the expected movements of blood from the thorax to the extremities and vice versa (Glaser, 1949; Rahn et al., 1949); and (3) the VC increases more in the supine than in the upright posture when the same Valsalva maneuver near maximal inspiration is performed immediately before the VC measurements (Bahnson, 1951; Fowler et al., 1951).

The displacement of the volume–pressure curve of the relaxed chest wall that occurs when a sitting subject is submerged up to the xiphoid or to the shoulders (Agostoni et al., 1966a; Hong et al., 1969; Craig and Dvorak, 1975) is shown in Figure 6. The changes occurring during submersion to the xiphoid reflect the lack of downward pull produced by the gravitational field on the abdomen. Hence, the broken curve of Figure 6 should approximate the volume–pressure curve of the relaxed chest wall when gravity-free; it should be displaced about 1 cm H_2O to the

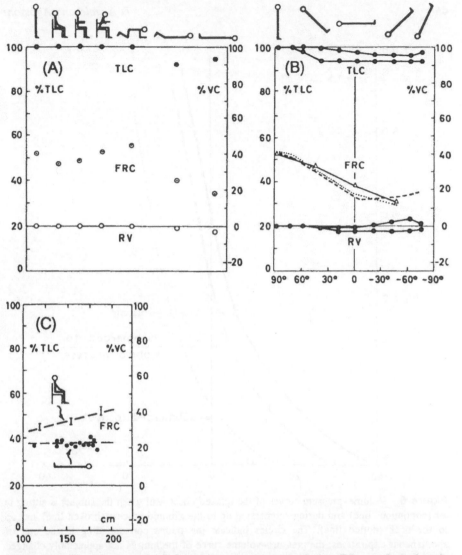

Figure 5 The pulmonary subdivisions in various postures, during tilting, and as a function of body height. In instances during which RV was not determined, it was assumed to be 20% of TLC in the upright posture. The data were obtained from the following sources: (A) Standing (Wade and Gilson, 1951; J. Mead, unpublished observation); seated erect (Craig, 1960; Hurtado and Fray, 1933; Withfield et al., 1950); seated erect, arms supported (Craig, 1960); seated leaning forward, arms supported (Craig, 1960); on hands and knees (Craig, 1960); prone (Moreno and Lyons, 1961); supine (Craig, 1960; Dittmer and Grebe, 1958; Hurtado and Fray, 1933; Moreno and Lyons, 1961; Withfield et al., 1950). (B) Triangles (Wade and Gilson, 1951); all the remaining points were obtained by J. Mead. The dotted (supported at shoulders) and broken lines (supported by ankles) are average values for five subjects. The TLC and RV values are for individual subjects. (C) Seated (Cook and Hamann, 1961); the ranges are the standard error for groups of ten subjects; the broken line is drawn by eye; supine (Morse et al., 1952; Robinson, 1938). (From Agostoni and Mead, 1964.)

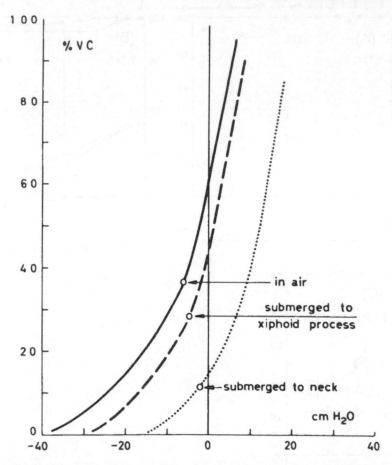

Figure 6 Volume–pressure curves of the relaxed chest wall when the subject is sitting in air (continuous line) and during submersion up to the xiphoid process (broken line) and up to the neck (dotted line). The circles indicate the points corresponding to the end of spontaneous expirations; the pressure–volume curve of the lung is not appreciably changed during submersion and, therefore, the volume–pressure curve of the relaxed respiratory system during submersion undergoes the same shift as that of the chest wall. The volume differences at the upper end of the curves are partly due to the larger compression of the gas and partly to the reduction of the upper limit of the VC occurring during submersion. (From Agostoni et al., 1966a.)

left because of the lack of shoulder weight (Craig, 1960). Accordingly, the expiratory reserve volume when gravity-free should decrease by about 8% of the VC.

Recently Liu and associates (1991) assessed the effects of gravity on the rib cage and the abdomen by measuring the change in the gravitational potential energy caused by the displacements of the rib cage and abdomen with changing lung volume. The subject seated or lay supine on a force platform, and the vertical forces as well as the changes in rib cage and abdominal volume were measured. The vertical force was integrated twice relative to time, and then multiplied by the gravitational acceleration to obtain the changes in gravitational potential energy. By analyzing the data after the model of Wilson (1988), which simply depicts the chest wall as a linear elastic body with 2 degrees of freedom, Liu and co-workers obtained the gravitational pressure acting on the rib cage and the abdomen as the derivative of the gravitational potential energy relative to the corresponding volume change. Within the limits in which the model of Wilson is applicable, it was concluded that (1) in the seated posture the gravitational force is expiratory on the rib cage and inspiratory on the abdomen, the magnitude of both being $\sim$8 cm H_2O; (2) in the supine posture, the gravitational force is expiratory both on the rib cage and abdomen, its magnitude being $\sim$9 cm H_2O; and (3) gravity increases rib cage and abdominal elastance, contributing essentially the same amount independently of posture and type of action. Unfortunately, it is unlikely that these results could be used to predict the effects of acceleration or changes in gravity on the chest wall, as pointed out by Liu et al. (1991); but their indications should be qualitatively valid. As far as the erect posture is concerned, these indications agree with those formulated on the basis of the results obtained with changing body orientation or partial immersion experiments.

The foregoing predictions on the effects of gravity on the statics of the respiratory system in erect subjects have been confirmed by Edyvean et al. (1991) through measurements obtained during 20-s periods of microgravity in an aircraft flying parabolic trajectories. They found that in microgravity FRC decreased by 244 $\pm$ 31 ml (i.e., about 8% VC) owing to a larger decrease in abdominal volume and a smaller increase in rib cage volume. On the other hand, under identical experimental conditions, Paiva and associates (1989) observed larger changes in FRC (413 $\pm$ 70 ml; i.e., about 10% VC) that were entirely due to a decrease in abdominal volume, whereas Baumgarten et al. (1980) and Michels et al. (1979) did not find conclusive evidence for changes in FRC or chest wall dimension. These discrepancies might relate to changes in tonic activity of the respiratory muscles and rib cage shape during the parabolic flight (Estenne et al., 1992), as well as to the method of restraint of the subject (Edyvean et al., 1991). Moreover, in line with Liu et al.'s (1991) prediction, abdominal compliance increased in microgravity (Paiva et al., 1989; Edyvean et al., 1991). Rib cage compliance was not measured directly in these studies; it seems, however, that, at variance with Dechamps et al.'s (1988) prediction, rib cage compliance should have decreased, because tidal volume, dynamic lung compliance, tidal Pw and Pab swings, and end-inspiratory rib cage muscle activity were the same as those under conditions of normal gravity (Paiva et al., 1989; Edyvean et al., 1991; Estenne et al., 1992).

During submersion to the shoulders, the end-expiratory volume is reduced to about 11% of the VC (see Fig. 6). The volume decrease produced by this submersion is almost entirely (5/6) due to the displacement of the abdomen–diaphragm, partly because of the higher hydrostatic pressure acting on the abdomen and partly because of diaphragm–rib cage interaction (see Section I.D). The diaphragm at the end of expiration is displaced craniad nearly as far as at full expiration under normal conditions and is essentially relaxed (Agostoni et al. 1966a; Reid et al., 1986). The pressure difference between water and abdominal contents should be positive according to Agostoni et al. (1966a) and essentially nil according to Reid et al. (1986). The average hydrostatic pressure acting on the chest wall is about 20 cm H_2O (Jarret, 1965; Agostoni, et al., 1966a). A subject completely immersed in the head-up posture chooses, however, to breathe at a pressure lower than the average pressure acting on the chest wall, to avoid the discomfort produced by the stretching of the pharynx and of the cheeks (Thompson and McCally, 1967). In the supine subject, submerged to the ventral wall, the average hydrostatic pressure acting on the chest wall is 6–7 cm H_2O (Hong et al., 1960; Jarret, 1965; Craig and Dvorak, 1975).

As previously pointed out (see Section I.B), pleural surface pressure is not uniform, but it has been considered uniform to undertake the analysis in terms of volume–pressure diagrams. A scheme of the probable distribution of the pressure on the pleural surface at the resting volume of the respiratory system in the upright and lateral postures is given in Figure 7, taking into account the effect of gravity on both the lung and the chest wall. In the upright posture the lung facing the diaphragmatic dome recoils inward, with a pressure that is probably 3–4 cm H_2O (i.e., nearly equal to the pull of the abdominal weight; Duomarco and Rimini, 1947; Agostoni and Rahn,

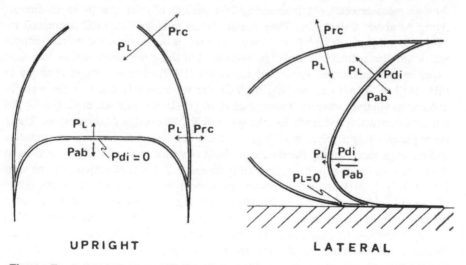

Figure 7 Scheme of the probable distribution of pressures in the respiratory system at the end of a spontaneous expiration in the upright and lateral postures. This scheme takes into account the effect of gravity both on the chest wall and on the lung, and is based on data from humans and animals (From Agostoni, 1970b.)

1960). The superior part of the lung recoils inward, with a pressure that is probably about 10 cm H_2O; the superior part of the rib cage balances the lung recoil with an equal outward recoil. In the lateral position the recoil of the lung in the lowermost part is probably nil, and the lowermost part of the chest wall behaves as a rigid structure under this condition. The upper part of the lung recoils inward, with a pressure that should be about 6 cm H_2O; this recoil is balanced by the opposite one of the superior part of the rib cage. The relaxed diaphragm in the upper part is pulled cranially by the lung recoil and caudally by the abdominal pressure that is subatmospheric. In the lower part, both the lung and the abdominal contents distend the diaphragm cranially, the latter progressively more than the former (Agostoni, 1970b).

D. Rib Cage, Diaphragm, and Abdominal Wall

Lung volume changes occur because of the displacement of the rib cage and of the diaphragm. From this viewpoint, these two structures may be considered to operate in parallel, hence:

$$\Delta Vw = \Delta Vrc,L + \Delta Vdi$$

where $\Delta Vrc,L$ is the volume displaced by the pulmonary part of the rib cage (i.e., that facing the lung). These volumes were obtained by Wade (1954) from measurements of the changes in rib cage circumference and of the displacements of the dome of the diaphragm relative to its insertion on the rib cage over the inspiratory capacity and the expiratory reserve volume. He assumed the volume–displacement relationships of the rib cage and of the diaphragm to be linear and equal in the supine and standing posture, that is

$$\Delta V_L = a\Delta Crc + b\Delta Hdi = \Delta Vrc,L + \Delta Vdi$$

where ΔCrc and ΔHdi are the changes in circumference of the rib cage and in the position of the diaphragm dome, respectively. From the two equations in the two postures, he obtained a and b. Although experimental evidence for a linear relation between axial displacement of the diaphragm and the dependent volume contribution has been recently provided in the standing posture (Verschakelen et al., 1992), Wade's assumption remains questionable. Agostoni et al. (1965b) used a geometric approach to estimate roughly the volume contributed by the change in the dimensions of the pulmonary part of the rib cage as a function of lung volume in the standing, sitting, and supine postures. The volume contributed by the diaphragm displacement was obtained by subtraction from the lung volume change. This approach also involves questionable assumptions, particularly on the motion of the upper part of the rib cage and of the boundary between rib cage and abdomen. Since the results were similar in the two approaches, although the assumptions differed, it seems possible that the errors involved are not marked. Since Wade did not provide data at relaxation and as a function of lung volume, the estimates of Agostoni et al. were used to illustrate the first approach to this matter (Fig. 8, thin lines). These estimates indicate the following features: (1) the volume contributed by the diaphragm

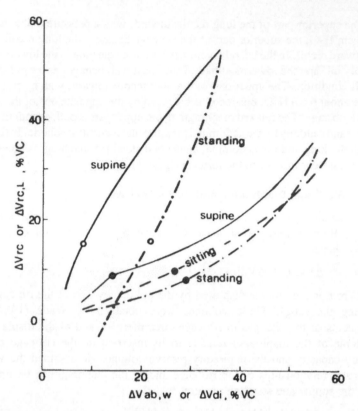

Figure 8 Thin lines: relation between the volume, expressed as percentage VC, contributed by the displacement of the pulmonary part of the rib cage ($\Delta Vrc,L$) and of the diaphragm (ΔVdi) during relaxation in the supine (continuous line), sitting (dashed line), and standing posture (dash-dotted line): closed symbols refer to the resting volume of the relaxed respiratory system. (From data by Agostoni et al., 1965b.) Thick lines: relation between the volume contributed by the displacement of the rib cage (ΔVrc) and of the abdominal wall ($\Delta Vab,w$) during relaxation in the supine (continuous line) and standing posture (dash-dotted line): open symbols refer to the resting volume of the relaxed respiratory system. (From data by Konno and Mead, 1967, 1968.)

displacement is greater than that contributed by the displacement of the pulmonary part of the rib cage; (2) the volume contributed by the pulmonary part of the rib cage at FRC is about the same in the supine and sitting posture, and only slightly smaller in the standing one; therefore, changes in FRC with posture are essentially due to displacement of the diaphragm (see Sec. I.C); (3) the relation between the volume contributed by the pulmonary part of the rib cage and that contributed by the diaphragm is shifted to the right on turning from the supine to the erect posture, indicating a volume displacement from the rib cage to the diaphragm.

Konno and Mead (1967) looked for a method that could allow measurements of the volume displacements of the chest wall by the two pathways, avoiding any assumption. They measured the simultaneous motion of several points on the rib cage and on the abdominal wall at iso-lung volume, keeping fixed the spinal attitude and disregarding a relatively narrow region at the boundary between rib cage and abdomen. They did this at several lung volumes over the VC and showed the following interesting features: (1) there is a unique relation between the displacement of any two points on the rib cage or on the rib cage and on the abdominal wall at any lung volume; (2) if the displacements of the rib cage are plotted against those of the abdominal wall, the iso-lung volume lines are essentially straight, parallel, and equidistant for equal lung volume increments; (3) the volume–displacement relation of each part can then be obtained graphically by moving one part and keeping the other fixed, these relations being nearly linear; (4) from the foregoing relations the volumes contributed by the displacements of the rib cage and of the abdominal wall over the VC may be determined. Konno and Mead partitioning may, therefore, be formulated as follows:

$$\Delta Vw = a'\Delta Drc + b'\Delta Dab = \Delta Vrc + \Delta Vab,w$$

where ΔD indicates the changes in diameter and $\Delta Vab,w$ the volume contributed by the displacement of the abdominal wall proper. Konno and Mead (1967) approach does not measure the displacement of the diaphragm: indeed, part of the volume displaced by the diaphragm is not shared by the abdominal wall, because of the lifting and expansion of the rib cage (Wade, 1954). Hence, the volume displacement of the abdominal wall ($\Delta Vab,w$, Konno and Mead approach) should be smaller than that of the diaphragm (ΔVdi, Wade or Agostoni et al., approach) by the volume displaced by the diaphragm not shared by the abdominal wall. Conversely, the volume displacement of the whole rib cage (ΔVrc, Konno and Mead approach) should be greater than that of the pulmonary part of the rib cage by the same amount. Konno and Mead approach is similar to that of Wade, since it also implies a system with two moving parts operating in parallel—the rib cage and the abdominal wall—both having a linear volume–displacement relation. Moreover, the data of Konno and Mead (1967, 1968) confirm some conclusions reached with the approach of Agostoni et al. (1965b). Namely, that the volume of the rib cage, or of its pulmonary part, at FRC is nearly the same in all postures, in spite of different lung volumes, and that the relation between the volume contributed by the two parts over the VC shifts rightward on turning from the supine to the erect posture (see Fig. 8 thick lines). A comparison between the volume partitioning obtained by the two approaches (thick and thin lines, respectively) as a function of lung volume shows that the fraction of the volume displaced by the diaphragm not shared by the abdominal wall is roughly 0.5 over most of the VC (see Fig. 8).

The first attempt to partition the static volume–pressure curve of the chest wall into those of its component parts (Agostoni and Mead, 1964) used the volume contributions provided by Wade (which were the only data available) and was based on an oversimplification. Namely, the force interactions between diaphragm and rib cage as well as any vertical pressure gradient were neglected. The volume–pressure curves of the pulmonary part of the rib cage and of the abdomen–diaphragm at relaxation shown in Figure 9 are based on this oversimplification, but the volume contributions provided by Wade have been substituted with those provided by Agostoni et al. (1965), which refer to relaxation and are expressed as a continuous function of lung volume. The compliance of the pulmonary part of the rib cage and of the diaphragm decreases progressively below FRC, whereas that of the abdominal wall is nearly constant over the VC. After one turns from the sitting to the supine posture, the volume–pressure curves of the pulmonary part of the rib cage and of the abdominal wall shift to the right; the latter more markedly, suggesting a greater expiratory effect of gravity on this compartment. Moreover, the volume–pressure curve of the pulmonary part of the rib cage does not change its shape with posture, whereas those of the diaphragm and of the abdominal wall do. The smaller compliance of the latter in the erect posture seems essentially due to (1) postural tonus of the abdominal muscles (Strohl et al., 1981), and (2) greater distortion of the abdominal wall in the erect posture owing to the greater top to bottom difference in Pab.

Mead (1981) and Mead and Loring (1982) reconsidered both the partitioning of volume contribution and the oversimplified approach based on the rib cage and diaphragm operating in parallel. The former revision was started with the aim of obtaining better information on the volume displaced by the diaphragm (see Chap. 23), but was soon involved in the latter. Mead (1981) and Mead and Loring (1982) proposed a model of the chest wall in which the lung volume displaced by the diaphragm corresponds on the body surface to the displacement of the abdominal wall plus that of the abdominal part of the rib cage, which is a definition closer to that of Wade (1954) and Agostoni et al. (1965b). Partitioning of the volume of the chest wall is summarized here by the following equations that, in a first approximation, apply to all the approaches mentioned:

$$\Delta Vw = \Delta Vrc,L + \Delta Vdi = \Delta Vrc + \Delta Vab,w$$
$$\Delta Vdi = \Delta Vrc,ab + \Delta Vab,w$$
$$\Delta Vrc = \Delta Vrc,L + \Delta Vrc,ab$$

Mead (1981) and Loring and Mead (1982) took into account that the diaphragm operates in series with the rib cage as a pressure generator (see Chap. 22), in general tending to move the ribs out and up. Moreover, they defined, with more precision, the pressure acting on the rib cage, since this structure is facing both the lungs and the abdominal contents. According to them, the effective pressure of the passive rib cage should be given by:

$$Prc = (1 - f)Pw + fPab - kPdi$$

where f is the fraction of the internal surface of the rib cage not facing the lung (see Chap. 23) and k, which includes the pertinent geometrical features, is the fraction

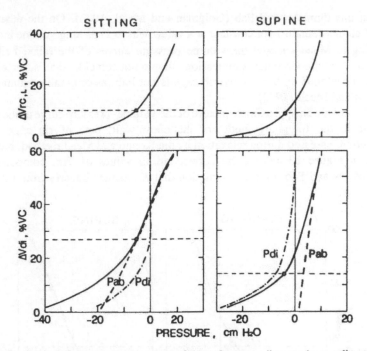

Figure 9 Static volume–pressure curves of the pulmonary rib cage (upper diagrams) and of the abdomen–diaphragm (lower diagrams) during relaxation in the sitting (left diagrams) and supine posture (right diagrams) considering the abdomen–diaphragm in parallel with the rib cage (see text). Data of volume contribution of the pulmonary rib cage (ΔVrc,L) and diaphragm (ΔVdi) are from Agostoni et al. (1965b), those of pressure of the chest wall (Pw), diaphragm (Pdi), and abdomen (Pab) from Agostoni and Mead (1964). The horizontal broken line indicates the volume at FRC.

of transdiaphragmatic pressure acting on the rib cage. When Pdi = 0 and, hence, Pw = Pab, as in the erect posture at or above FRC, Prc = Pw, which was the primitive definition of the pressure developed by the passive rib cage. On the other hand, when Pdi ≠ 0, as in the erect posture below FRC or in the supine posture over most of the VC, Prc should be higher than Pw and closer to Pab, the smaller the lung volume, since f increases with decreasing lung volume. Indeed, considering that Pdi = Pw − Pab and setting $K = f + k$:

$$Prc = (1 - K)Pw + KPab$$

it appears that Prc = Pab when $K = 1$, as it could be near RV, owing to the cranial position of the diaphragm. Some support to this model is provided by the finding that abdominal compression in relaxed upright subjects (greater Pab at any given lung volume) markedly changes the relation between the anteroposterior diameter of the rib cage at the xiphoid level and Pw, but does not substantially change that between this diameter and Pab (Goldman and Mead, 1973). On the other hand, since K cannot remain 1 (or constant at a value near to 1) as lung volume increases, according to Mead's model the volume–pressure curves of the relaxed rib cage, with and without abdominal compression, should not coincide; that is, the effective pressure developed by the passive rib cage is not Pab, as originally maintained by Goldman and Mead (1973).

To provide an approximate picture of the volume–pressure curve of the relaxed rib cage in the foregoing model of the chest wall, data of rib cage volume contribution, assessed during relaxation by the Konno and Mead method, have been plotted in Figure 10 against the corresponding values of Prc, computed from measured Pw and Pab, on the assumption that K changes linearly from 0.9 to 0.2

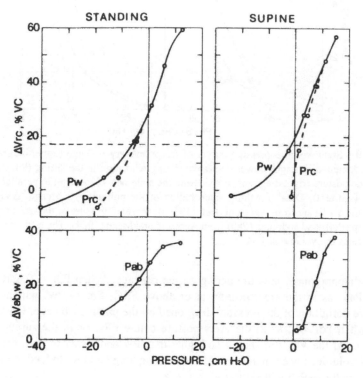

Figure 10 Static volume–pressure curves of the rib cage (upper diagrams) and of the abdominal wall (lower diagrams) during relaxation in the standing (left diagrams) and supine posture (right diagrams) according to the Mead's model of the chest wall (see text). Data of volume contribution of the rib cage (ΔVrc) and abdominal wall (ΔVab,w) as well as of pressure of the chest wall (Pw) and abdomen (Pab) are from Konno and Mead (1968), whereas the effective pressure developed by the passive rib cage (Prc) was computed using the equation Prc = $(1 - K)$Pw + KPab, on the assumption that K varied linearly from 0.9 to 0.2 over the VC in both postures (see text). The horizontal broken line indicates the volume at FRC.

between RV and TLC, both in the standing and supine postures. The progressive decrease of the compliance of the rib cage occurring at low lung volume in the Agostoni and Mead model does not occur in Mead's model. Thus, the stiffness of the chest wall at RV should not be due to both the rib cage and the diaphragm, but essentially to the latter, particularly in the supine posture. Similar to the Agostoni and Mead model, there is a rightward displacement of the curve on turning from the erect to the supine posture, but the rib cage compliance in the supine posture becomes progressively higher than in the standing posture with the decrease in lung volume. This feature should be taken with reservation because the values of K are not known with precision, particularly in the supine posture. On the other hand, it seems likely that the compliance of the relaxed rib cage at midlung volume is larger in the supine than in the standing posture, because an equal compliance would imply a value of K in the supine posture half of that in the standing posture, which does not seem possible.

The volume–pressure curve of the abdominal wall is also shown in Figure 10. It shifts rightward on turning from the standing to the supine posture, and its slope is larger in the supine posture. The larger compliance of the abdominal wall in the supine posture is, in part, only apparent, being the consequence of having used the pressure on the abdominal side of the diaphragm, rather than the average pressure acting on the wall. This is immaterial in the supine posture, but not in the erect one, because, with the descent of the diaphragm, the zero level of abdominal pressure rises, whereas the height of the abdominal cavity decreases. If we assume, for example, that between RV and TLC: (1) the height of the abdominal cavity decreases from 45 to 40 cm, because of the descent of the diaphragm (9 cm) and the concomitant lift of the rib cage (4 cm); (2) the average height of the abdominal wall increases from 30 to 34 cm; (3) the subdiaphragmatic pressure increases from −15 to 12 cm H_2O, and the vertical gradient of abdominal pressure is 1 cm H_2O/cm vertical distance, then the average pressure acting on the abdominal wall should be 15 and 35 cm H_2O at RV and TLC, respectively. That is, the change in pressure in the standing posture would be only 20 instead of 27 cm H_2O; therefore, the compliance of the abdominal wall would be higher. The remaining difference with the compliance in the supine posture should be due to the factors previously mentioned, namely postural muscle tonus and greater distortion of the abdominal wall in the erect posture.

According to the partitioning of the volume of the chest wall made by Mead and Loring (1982), the volume displaced by the diaphragm should be approximately similar to that determined by Agostoni et al. (see foregoing). Hence, the volume–pressure curves of the diaphragm in the erect and supine posture, according to the Mead and Loring model, are similar to those illustrated in Figure 9. The foregoing attempt to illustrate the features of the model for the chest wall proposed by Mead (1981) is justified by the theoretical and practical relevance of the model itself. On the other hand, the difference between Prc and Pw shown in Figure 10 is likely overestimated for the following reasons: (1) this difference increases with the increase in the change of K used to compute these curves, and the value of change used in the foregoing is likely overestimated according to inferences by Loring and Mead (1982) for the head-up posture; (2) as pointed out by Mead (1981), both in the horizontal and erect posture, only part of the abdominal pressure should be transmitted to the rib cage when the diaphragm is under tension, although, in dogs in the supine and lateral postures, ΔPdi in the zone of apposition seems essentially nil in the tidal volume range (Agostoni et al., 1988; Urmey et al., 1988); (3) the tension of the abdominal wall has an effect on the ribs opposite that of the diaphragm. The foregoing overestimation, however, might be compensated by another factor that has been neglected and that displaces Prc to the right. Namely, in the erect posture, owing to the hydrostatic gradient of the abdomen, the average pressure acting on the abdominal part of the rib cage is higher than the subdiaphragmatic pressure, which has been used to compute Prc in Figure 10.

Some other models of the chest wall (Macklem et al., 1983; Hillman and Finucane, 1987; Boynton et al., 1991) have been proposed in addition to that of Mead and Loring; yet it can be shown (Boynton et al., 1991) that, in all of them, the same force balance equations apply for the rib cage and the abdominal compartment, respectively. To the extent that in these models $\Delta Vab,w$ is thought to be a unique function of Pab, it is implicitly assumed that the rib cage and the abdominal wall can move independently (i.e., they are mechanically uncoupled). This, in turn, allows the compliances of the rib cage and the abdomen to be obtained as the ratio between the changes in compartmental volume, ΔVrc and $\Delta Vab,w$, and pressure, ΔPrc and ΔPab, respectively (see Fig. 10). Indeed, some results suggest that coupling between the rib cage and the abdominal wall can be ignored. In seated subjects immersed in water up to the xiphoid process, Agostoni et al. (1966a) observed that the end-expiratory values of rib cage circumference and pleural surface pressure fell along the relation between these parameters obtained during relaxation in air, and Estenne et al. (1985) found that rib cage strapping in seated normal subjects markedly reduced rib cage compliance, but did not affect abdominal compliance. Deschamps et al. (1988) specifically addressed the problem of passive rib cage–abdominal wall coupling by observing the changes in the ΔVrc–Pw and $\Delta Vab,w$–Pw relationships caused by a constant load applied to the rib cage in seated, relaxed subjects. They analyzed the results using the model of Wilson (1988), and concluded that coupling between the rib cage and the abdominal wall is small. To the extent that the press used to apply the load might have caused distortion of the rib cage, beside rib cage displacement, Deschamps et al.'s estimates could involve some errors.

Current models of the human chest wall (Mead and Loring, 1982; Loring and Mead, 1982; Macklem et al., 1983; Hillman and Finucane, 1987; Boynton et al., 1991) assume that both the relaxed rib cage and the abdomen move with 1 degree of freedom over most of the vital capacity. This assumption is based on the aforementioned observations of Konno and Mead (1967). Forces acting on relatively large fractions of the rib cage surface, such as $(1 - f)$ Pw or fPab, are thus considered to affect the rib cage motion (and, hence, the apparent volume–pressure relation of the relaxed rib cage) in the same way as those acting on small areas of the rib cage surface, such as diaphragmatic tension. On the other hand, one would expect distortion of the relaxed rib cage to take place whenever Pw ≠ Pab and, hence, Pdi ≠ 0, as in the supine posture or in the erect posture below FRC. Indeed, contraction of the diaphragm produces marked distortions of the rib cage in tetraplegic subjects breathing quietly within the normal range of lung volumes both in the supine and seated posture (Zechman et al., 1967; Mortola and Sant'Ambrogio, 1978), as it occurs during electrophrenic stimulation both in animals (D'Angelo and Sant'Ambrogio, 1974) and men (Danon et al., 1979). Actually, distortion of the rib cage can occur also in normal subjects during voluntary and involuntary respiratory acts (D'Angelo, 1981; Crawford et al., 1883; McCool et al., 1985), and the pattern of motion of the relaxed rib cage during immersion in seated subjects (Reid et al., 1986) suggests that rib cage flexibility is fairly large. In the dog, the relations between indexes of pulmonary rib cage motion and Pw (D'Angelo and Sant'Ambrogio, 1974; Jiang et al., 1988) as well as between indexes of abdominal wall motion and Pab (Jiang et al., 1988), obtained during isolated diaphragm contractions, fall close to their respective relaxation lines, thereby indicating high rib cage flexibility (D'Angelo et al., 1973) and, hence, negligible mechanical coupling between pulmonary and abdominal rib cage compartments. Distortion, therefore, should be confined to a band along the boundary between the two rib cage compartments not much wider than that between the rib cage and the abdominal wall when these structures are moved away from their relaxation lines by the action of the respiratory muscles during the iso-volume maneuver (Konno and Mead, 1967). If this were also true for the human rib cage, volume–pressure relations for the pulmonary and abdominal rib cage compartment could be readily obtained once satisfactory criteria for partitioning ΔVrc into ΔVrc,L and ΔVrc,ab are established. In paralyzed dogs in the lateral posture, Pab is the factor having the greatest influence on the dispacement of the abdominal rib cage in the volume range near FRC (Agostoni et al., 1988; Jiang et al., 1988). The effect of the insertional traction of the diaphragm becomes relevant at low volume, whereas that of the mechanical linkage with the pulmonary rib cage becomes prevalent at large volume, the other factors being negligible (Agostoni et al., 1988). If coupling between the pulmonary and abdominal rib cage were rather loose, the progressive decrease in chest wall compliance with decreasing lung volume below FRC (see Fig. 4) would reflect a decrease in compliance both of the diaphragm and of the pulmonary rib cage, as suggested by the volume–pressure curves in Figure 9, rather than that of the diaphragm alone, as indicated by the volume–pressure relations in Figure 10, which are based on the assumption of a rigid rib cage. Ward and associates (1992) modified the model of Macklem et al. (1983) by incorporating a two-compartment rib cage, and attempted to evaluate the strength of the coupling between the pulmonary and abdominal rib cage by assessing rib cage distortion and Pw changes at iso-lung volume during electrophrenic stimulation in seated subjects. They concluded that this coupling should ensure transmission of a substantial fraction of the force acting on the abdominal rib cage to the pulmonary rib cage, but pointed out the several theoretical and technical limitations of their approach. Of major concern here is that this approach cannot provide information on the coupling between the relaxed pulmonary and abdominal rib cage for most experimental conditions. Indeed, their approach can be used only in the erect posture and at a lung volume above FRC, because the motion–pressure relations of the pulmonary and abdominal compartments of the relaxed undistorted rib cage (i.e., when Pw = Pab) are instrumental to their analysis.

II. Volume–Pressure Relations During Static Muscular Efforts

A. Alveolar Pressure

The maximum static inspiratory and expiratory pressures exerted for 1–2 s in the lung at different volumes in the upright posture are shown in Figure 11. The outer solid lines of this diagram represent the volume–pressure relations of the system during maximum inspiratory and expiratory efforts. The horizontal distance between these curves and the relaxation curve gives the net pressure exerted by the contraction of the respiratory muscles (broken lines). Similar curves are obtained if, instead of performing the effort against the obstructed airways, the subject, starting from full inspiration or expiration, breathes into or out of containers of different capacity (Cook et al., 1964). The expiratory pressures are larger when the chest is inflated, whereas the inspiratory pressures are larger when it is deflated. This behavior, besides being influenced by the mechanical features of the passive structures

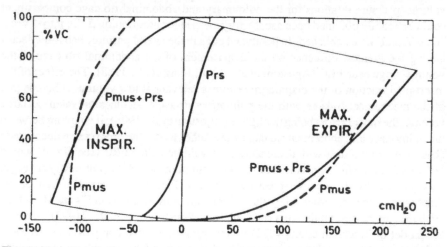

Figure 11 Lung volume against alveolar pressure during maximum static inspiratory and expiratory efforts and during relaxation in the sitting posture. The broken lines indicate the pressure contributed by the muscles. (From Rohrer, 1916, as modified by Agostoni and Mead, 1964.)

involved, by the action of the antagonist muscles (see later), and by a hypothetical inhibition of the efforts, depends on the mechanical advantage and the force–length relation of the agonist muscles. The length of the expiratory muscles increases with lung volume, and the opposite occurs for the inspiratory muscles. There are few data comparing maximal pressures upright and supine. In ten normal men, no difference was found in the maximal expiratory pressures at TLC (225 cm H_2O standing, 226 cm H_2O supine) or maximal inspiratory pressures at RV (118 cm H_2O both standing and supine) (R.E. Hyatt, personal communication). Comparison should also be made at midlung volume because changes in rib cage cross section in various postures suggest that the length of rib cage muscles at FRC should be different at similar lung volumes (standing–sitting) or almost the same at different lung volumes (sitting–supine) (Agostoni, 1970a; see Chap. 22).

The pressure exerted by children is nearly the same as that of adults at most lung volumes. This has been related to the smaller radius of curvature of the rib cage, of the diaphragm, and of the abdominal wall in the children (Agostoni and Mead, 1964; Cook et al., 1964). In fact, according to Laplace law, if the radius of curvature of the wall is small, thin muscles with a small force may exert pressures as great as those exerted by thick muscles of a wall with a greater radius. Human newborn may lower the intrathoracic pressure to -70 cm H_2O to overcome the high resistance to the first breath (Karlberg, 1957). Only on the expiratory side at large lung volumes is the maximum pressure exerted by adults markedly greater than that of children. This could be due to the greater development of accessory expiratory muscles in adults or to reflex inhibition (see later). Women do not develop as high maximum pressures as do men of similar age (Cook et al., 1964). Some of this difference seems due to the difference in strength of the accessory muscles (Ringqvist, 1966). Maximum inspiratory pressures in the Korean diving women are significantly greater than in a control group, whereas the maximum expiratory pressures are about the same. The greater development of inspiratory muscles is probably related to the condition of negative-pressure breathing that these women undergo daily while in water between dives (Song et al., 1963). Ventilatory muscle strength and endurance can be increased by appropriate training programs (Leith and Bradley, 1976). As far as static efforts are concerned, after 5 weeks of strength training (about 30 min each day for 5 days a week), maximum pressure increased by 55%. The decrease of the maximum respiratory pressures with age, their difference between sexes, and their scattering among subjects, parallel those observed for the maximum strength of other groups of muscles in the body (Ringqvist, 1966).

The values given in Figure 11 do not necessarily represent the maximum that the inspiratory and expiratory muscles can exert, because antagonist muscles may be active, particularly during expiratory efforts (see following Sec. II.B). In this case the pressure exerted by the agonists could be higher than that estimated from alveolar pressure changes. Moreover, pressure measurements do not give information about the muscle forces deforming the chest wall. The values of maximum pressure are obtained by voluntary efforts in the laboratory and might not represent the effect of a maximum contraction of the muscles involved (see following section). The maximum values of pressure found in more recent years (Agostoni and Rahn, 1960; Cook, et al., 1964; Milic-Emili et al., 1964; Ringqvist, 1966; Black and Hyatt, 1969) are higher than most of those given in the older literature (see Ringqvist, 1966). Owing to the gas compliance, the pressure swings during inspiratory or expiratory efforts are smaller than they would have been if the system had been filled with liquid. Because of the dependence of gas compliance on absolute pressure, differences in pressure swings may become very large if the same efforts are performed at low ambient pressure. At high altitude, therefore, the volume–pressure diagram is very much curtailed, although the actual mechanics of the chest are not changed (Rahn et al., 1946).

During partial neuromuscular blockade, the maximum pressures exerted by the respiratory muscles are reduced comparatively less than the maximum force of other muscles, such as those involved in hand grip and head lift; moreover, maximum expiratory pressures are reduced more than inspiratory ones (Johansen et al., 1964; Jorgensen, et al., 1966; Saunders et al., 1978; Gal and Goldberg, 1981). In seated subjects, the decreases in VC were greater than predicted on the basis of the percentage changes of maximum pressures and the volume–pressure curve of the relaxed respiratory system: it has been suggested that, with partial paralysis, changes in lung volume partly reflect unequal distribution of muscle weakness and a decreased ability to change rib cage dimensions (Saunders et al., 1978). On the other hand, in supine subjects, the changes in VC during submaximal neuromuscular blockade were consistent with those predicted (Gal and Goldberg, 1981).

B. Abdominal and Thoracic Pressures

Transthoracic pressure measurements give only the resultant of the action of agonist and antagonist groups of muscles when they act simultaneously. A separation of the contribution of inspiratory and expiratory muscles may be done only at the abdominal boundary of the respiratory system through transdiaphragmatic and transabdominal pressure measurements. The pressures on the thoracic and abdominal side of the diaphragm at different lung volumes during static inspiratory, expiratory, and expulsive efforts are shown in Figure 12. During maximum inspiratory efforts, the abdominal pressure in most trained subjects remains roughly as at relaxation. Up to about 60% VC, the transdiaphragmatic pressure remains about the same or decreases slightly as the volume increases; above this volume the transdiaphragmatic pressure decreases progressively. Therefore, the maximum transdiaphragmatic pressure (horizontal distance between solid and broken lines) is similar to the maximum transthoracic pressure (horizontal distance between solid line and ordinate at zero pressure). On the other hand, in untrained subjects the abdominal pressure increases often at large lung volumes (De Troyer and Estenne, 1981), because of abdominal muscle contraction as revealed by electromyography (Mills, 1950;

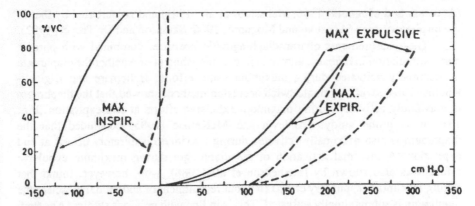

Figure 12 Lung volume against pressure above (continuous line) and below (broken line) the diaphragmatic dome during maximum static inspiratory, expiratory, and expulsive efforts. (Modified from Agostoni and Mead, 1964.)

Campbell, 1952; Campbell and Green, 1953; Delhez et al., 1959). In these subjects, the transdiaphragmatic pressure is roughly the same at all lung volumes; therefore, at large lung volumes, it becomes progressively higher than the transthoracic pressure. This suggests that the diaphragm may exert more pressure when the abdominal muscles contract (see following).

During a moderate expiratory effort above resting volume, the transdiaphragmatic pressure is nil (Agostoni and Rahn, 1960), but during maximum effort there is an abdominal–thoracic pressure difference (see Fig. 12). Since, at these volumes, one would not expect the diaphragm to be passively distended, this pressure should be due to diaphragmatic contraction, as was confirmed by electromyographic findings (Agostoni et al., 1960). With decreasing lung volumes, the pressure contributed by diaphragm contraction increases progressively (Agostoni and Torri, 1962).

During expulsive efforts the muscles of the abdominal wall contract more vigorously than during maximum expiratory efforts, and the diaphragm also increases its activity. Pab reaches its maximum and Ppl becomes smaller than during maximum expiratory efforts, indicating, in this instance, that the stronger action of the muscles of the abdominal wall on the rib cage is more than balanced by diaphragmatic contraction. The pressure differences between maximum expulsive and expiratory efforts decrease with lung volume, becoming nil at RV. At large and midlung volumes, the values of Pdi are generally higher during maximum expulsive than inspiratory efforts, indicating that the diaphragm yields the largest abdominal–thoracic pressure difference when the lower ribs are pulled down and in by the contraction of the muscles of the abdominal wall (Agostoni and Mead, 1964). Indeed, the lateral diameter of the rib cage at the xiphoid level, relative to its iso-lung volume value during relaxation, is reduced by the activity of the expiratory muscles

(Agostoni and Mognoni, 1966; Melissinos et al., 1981) and is increased by that of the inspiratory ones (Agostoni and Mognoni, 1966; Sampson and De Troyer, 1982).

The measurements of transdiaphragmatic pressure, combined with phrenic nerve stimulation in humans, allowed direct establishment of whether the diaphragm is maximally activated during maximum static efforts. Bellemare and Bigland-Ritchie (1984), with the single-twich occlusion method, showed that the diaphragm is maximally activated during maximum expulsive efforts at end expiration (Fig. 13). In a similar study, Gandevia and McKenzie (1985) concluded that the diaphragm is also maximally activated during maximum inspiratory efforts at end expiration. A maximal activation of the diaphragm during maximum expulsive efforts was also shown by Hershenson et al. (1988), who, however, found that during maximum inspiratory efforts (without recruitment of abdominal muscles) the diaphragm is submaximally activated. This is in line with previous studies (Agostoni and Mead, 1964; La Porta and Grassino, 1985) and their own findings that Pdi is greater during maximum expulsive than during inspiratory efforts, except near RV. On the other hand, the difference in Pdi between the two maneuvers could be partly due to the different shape of the diaphragm (see foregoing).

Hershenson et al. (1988) formulated the hypothesis that, during maximum efforts, the differences in muscle strength (or mechanical advantage) require that the activation of the stronger muscle be submaximal to prevent change in

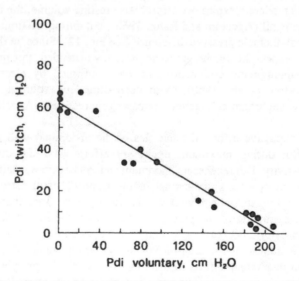

Figure 13 Transdiaphragmatic pressure produced by single, supramaximal twitches to phrenic nerves superimposed to graded expulsive efforts vs. transdiaphragmatic pressure produced by these expulsive efforts at FRC. (Modified from Bellemare and Bigland-Ritchie, 1984.)

thoracoabdominal configuration, which would lengthen the weaker and shorten the stronger muscle. In the maximum inspiratory efforts, the diaphragm would be submaximally activated because it can lower Ppl more than the other inspiratory muscles. Indeed, with negative body surface pressure applied to the rib cage, they found that Ppl becomes 22 cm H_2O more subatmospheric during maximum inspiratory efforts at 40% VC. In line with their hypothesis, they also found that, at volumes above FRC, the electrical activity of the abdominal muscles and the Pab (see also Agostoni and Rahn, 1960) is greater with closed than with open glottis (i.e., keeping alveolar pressure atmospheric) during maximum expulsive efforts. Finally, they confirmed an earlier finding of Milic-Emili et al. (1964): namely, that below 20% VC, the diaphragm can develop a greater pressure than the abdominal muscles, and it is also submaximally activated during maximum expulsive efforts. According to their data, and at variance with those in Figure 12, Pdi during maximum expulsive efforts reaches a maximum (about 200 cm H_2O) at midlung volume.

Hillman et al. (1990), from fluoroscopic examination of the diaphragm during maximal diaphragmatic inspiratory efforts, with or without superimposed maximum expulsive efforts, concluded that diaphragmatic length is greater during the combined maximum efforts and that this was responsible for the associated larger Pdi. Moreover, from the records of changes in configuration of the rib cage and abdomen, they inferred that the diaphragm is being stretched for all the duration (3–5 s) of the combined maximum efforts, and suggested that pliometric contraction of the diaphragm provides an additional explanation for the larger Pdi during this maneuver. It is unclear, however, whether a pliometric contraction of the diaphragm was really occurring throughout the combined efforts, because their records do not show an increasing Pdi during this period, and the reported changes in chest wall configuration do not necessarily imply lengthening of the diaphragm.

To investigate whether dynamic changes in diaphragm length during maximal inspiratory or expulsive maneuver could account for the smaller transdiaphragmatic pressure during the former maneuver, Gandevia et al. (1992) used digital sequential radiography. They found that the diaphragm length decreased by about 20% during maximal inspiratory efforts, whereas it was essentially unchanged during maximal expulsive efforts with glottis open. The smaller transdiaphragmatic pressure achieved during maximal inspiratory efforts, therefore, seems to be due to the smaller length of the diaphragm during this maneuver.

III. Factors Limiting the Volume Extremes

A. Upper Volume Extreme

Mills (1950) proposed that glottis closure is the main factor limiting the expansion of the lung. However, Mead and associates (1963) found that only one in six normal subjects closed the upper airways at the end of maximum inspiration. A balance between the passive opposing force, which rises markedly at both volume extremes, and the driving force of the agonist muscles, which decreases at both extremes (see Figs. 11 and 12), seems the factor setting the upper volume limit in those subjects in whom, at the end of maximum inspiration, the abdominal muscles do not contract (Mead et al., 1963). Some subjects, however, contract the abdominal muscles at full inspiration, as shown by their marked electrical activity (Mills, 1950; Campbell, 1952; Campbell and Green, 1953; Delhez et al., 1959). This contraction antagonizes the action of inspiratory muscles, although it partly improves the action of the diaphragm (see Chap. 22). Hence, when there is a contraction of the abdominal muscles, the limit to the upper volume extreme seems set also by the contraction of the antagonist muscles. It is difficult to assess whether the decrease of the force of the agonist muscles at large volume depends on only mechanical disadvantage or also on a reflex inhibition of the effort (Agostoni, 1970b). Marked increases of TLC have been reported to occur during acute asthmatic attacks (Woolcock and Read, 1966; Anderson et al., 1972; Freedman et al., 1975; Peress et al., 1976), although subsequent studies have shown that most of these increases are due to technical artifacts (Brown et al., 1978; Shore et al., 1982; Stanescu et al., 1982). These increases are accompanied by a loss of lung recoil and, in one subject, an increase of strength of the inspiratory muscles was found (Peress et al., 1976). Finally, small, but significant, increases in TLC were found in normal subjects breathing 6% CO_2; the mechanism was unclear, but since lung recoil was unaltered, changes in the chest wall were most likely responsible (Rodarte and Hyatt, 1973).

B. Lower Volume Extreme

In young, normal humans, RV is determined by a static balance between the pressure exerted by the expiratory muscles and that exerted by the passive structures of the chest wall plus the contraction of antagonist muscles. The patency of most airways at RV is shown by the following findings: (1) at full expiration esophageal pressure is 1–2 cm H_2O below atmospheric (Mead and Milic-Emili, 1964); and (2) a positive expiratory pressure suddenly applied to the respiratory system at or near RV produces a sudden expiration of a volume of air greater than that which could be squeezed from the intrathoracic airways. Thus, maximum expiration is performed quickly and, at full expiration, a condition of no-flow may be kept for several seconds (Leith and Mead, 1967). In the dependent part of the lung at RV, pleural pressure is positive and, therefore, airways are likely closed in this part, even in the upright posture (Milic-Emili et al., 1966; Burger and Macklem, 1968; Rodarte et al., 1977). The closure of the airways in the dependent part could be thought to elicit an inhibition of the expiratory motoneurons and an excitation of the inspiratory ones, thereby preventing a further collapse of the lung, but no experimental evidence supports this hypothesis (Agostoni, 1970b). As shown, both by the electrical activity of the diaphragm (Agostoni and Torri, 1962; Delhez et al., 1964) and by the transdiaphragmatic pressure being higher than at relaxation (Agostoni and Rahn,

1960; Milic-Emili et al., 1964; see Fig. 12), this muscle is contracted at RV. The mechanism leading to the marked contraction of the diaphragm seems related to the simultaneous activity of the abdominal muscles, rather than to a reflex, because this contraction is negligible when the lung volume is reduced to the same extent by an external force, as during submersion or breathing from a tank in which the pressure is kept subatmospheric (Agostoni et al., 1966a).

In elderly humans the static balance described before does not occur because expiration at low lung volume proceeds so slowly that it is ended by an abrupt inspiration before the expiratory flow has ceased and, therefore, before the static balance is achieved (Leith and Mead, 1967). In elderly subjects, the airway flow resistance is high and a positive pressure applied suddenly to the respiratory system at or near RV does not appreciably affect the expiratory flow at the mouth; the expiratory flow is effort-independent because of dynamic compression of the airways, whereas alveolar pressure is effort-dependent and may be markedly positive (Leith and Mead, 1967). In elderly subjects, airway closure occurs over a much greater portion of the lung than in young subjects (Davis et al., 1980). Airway closure, however, only indirectly affects the setting of RV. When airway closure involves a large fraction of the lung, the still open units will have to be at a volume lower by the same amount that the closed units are at higher volume. Hence, the open units reach a flow-limiting condition. The transition from the static RV of young to the flow-time limited RV of elderly subjects occurs, therefore, by decreasing whole lung maximum flow (no closure) and by trapping larger and larger volume of gas in closed units, thereby forcing the remaining open units to operate at correspondingly lower regional volumes and maximum flow (Davis et al., 1980).

References

Agostoni, E. (1962). Diaphragm activity and thoracoabdominal mechanics during positive pressure breathing. *J. Appl. Physiol.* 17: 215–220.

Agostoni, E. (1970a). Kinematics. In *The Respiratory Muscles. Mechanics and Neural Control.* Edited by E. J. M. Campbell, E. Agostoni, and J. Newson-Davis. London, Lloyd-Luke, pp. 23–47.

Agostoni, E. (1970b). Statics. In *The Respiratory Muscles. Mechanics and Neural Control.* Edited by E. J. M. Campbell, E. Agostoni, and J. Newson-Davis. London, Lloyd-Luke, pp. 48–79.

Agostoni, E. (1972). Mechanics of the pleural space. *Physiol. Rev.* 52: 57–128.

Agostoni, E., and Mead, J. (1964). Statics of the respiratory system. In *Handbook of Physiology*, Section 3. Respiration. Vol. 1. Edited by W. O. Fenn and H. Rahn. Washington, DC, American Physiological Society, pp. 387–409.

Agostoni, E., and Mognoni, P. (1966). Deformation of the chest wall during breathing efforts. *J. Appl. Physiol.* 21: 1827–1832.

Agostoni, E., and Rahn, H. (1960). Abdominal and thoracic pressures at different lung volumes. *J. Appl. Physiol.* 15: 1087–1092.

Agostoni, E., and Torri, G. (1962). Diaphragm contraction as a limiting factor to maximum expiration. *J. Appl. Physiol.* 17: 427–428.

Agostoni, E., Sant'Ambrogio, G., and Del Portillo Carrasco, H. (1960). Electromyography of the diaphragm in man and transdiaphragmatic pressure. *J. Appl. Physiol.* 15: 1093–1097.

Agostoni, E., Mognoni, P., Torri, G., and Ferrario-Agostoni, A. (1965a). Static features of the passive rib cage and abdomen–diaphragm. *J. Appl. Physiol.* 20: 1187–1193.

Agostoni, E., Mognoni, P., Torri, G., and Saracino, F. (1965b). Relation between changes of rib cage circumference and lung volume. *J. Appl. Physiol.* 20: 1179–1186.

Agostoni, E., Gurtner, G., Torri, G., and Rahn, H. (1966a). Respiratory mechanics during submersion and negative-pressure breathing. *J. Appl. Physiol.* 21: 251–258.

Agostoni, E., Mognoni, P., Torri, G., and Miserocchi, G. (1966b). Forces deforming the rib cage. *Respir. Physiol.* 2: 105–117.

Agostoni, E., Zocchi, L., and Macklem P.T. (1988). Transdiaphragmatic pressure and rib motion in area of apposition during paralysis. *J. Appl. Physiol.* 65: 1296–1300.

Anderson, S. D., McEvoy, J. D. S., and Bianco, S. (1972). Changes in lung volumes and airway resistance after exercise in asthmatic subjects. *Am. Rev. Respir. Dis.* 106: 30–37.

Asmussen, E., Christensen, E. H., and Sjostrand, T. (1939). Uber die Abhangigkeit der Lungenvolumen von der Blutverteilung. *Skand. Arch. Physiol.* 82: 193–200.

Bahnson, H. T. (1951). *The Effect of a Valsalva Maneuver upon Changes in the Vital Capacity Volume of the Lung.* AF Tech. Report 6528. Wright-Patterson AFB, Dayton, Ohio, pp. 518–521.

Baumgarten, R. J. V., Baldrighi, G., Vogel, H., and Thumler, R. (1980). Physiological response to hyper and hypogravity during rollercoaster flight. *Aviat. Space Environ. Med.* 51: 145–154.

Bellemare, F., and Bigland-Ritchie, B. (1984). Assessment of human diaphragm strength and activation using phrenic nerve stimulation. *Respir. Physiol.* 58: 263–277.

Black, L. F., and Hyatt, R. E. (1969). Maximal respiratory pressures: Normal values and relationship to age and sex. *Am. Rev. Respir. Dis.* 99: 696–702.

Boynton, B. R., Barnas, G. M., Dadmun, J. T., and Fredberg J. J. (1991). Mechanical coupling of the rib cage, abdomen, and diaphragm through their area of apposition. *J. Appl. Physiol.* 70: 1235–1244.

Briscoe, W. A. (1965). Lung volumes. In *Handbook of Physiology*, Section 3. Respiration. Vol. 2. Edited by W. O. Fenn and H. Rahn. Washington, DC, American Physiological Society, pp. 1345–1379.

Brown, R., Ingram, R. H., Jr., and McFadden, E. R., Jr. (1978). Problems in the plethysmographic assessment of changes in total lung capacity in asthma. *Am. Rev. Respir. Dis.* 118: 685–692.

Buchtal, F., and Rosenfalck P. (1957). Elastic properties of striated muscle. In *Tissue Elasticity*. Edited by J. W. Remington. Washington, DC, American Physiological Society, pp. 73–93.

Burger, E. J., Jr., and Macklem P. (1968). Airway closure: Demonstration by breathing 100 percent O_2 at low lung volumes and by N_2 washout. *J. Appl. Physiol.* 25: 139–148.

Butler, J. (1957). The adaptation of the relaxed lungs and chest wall to changes in volume. *Clin. Sci.* 16: 421–433.

Campbell, E. J. M. (1952). An electromyographic study of the role of the abdominal muscles in breathing. *J. Physiol. (Lond.)* 117: 222–233.

Campbell, E. J. M., and Green J. H. (1953). The variations in intra-abdominal pressure and the activity of the abdominal muscles during breathing; a study in man. *J. Physiol. (Lond.)* 122: 282–290.

Cherniack, R. M., and Brown, E. (1965). A simple method for measuring total respiratory compliance: Normal values for man. *J. Appl. Physiol.* 20: 87–91.

Cook, C. D., and Hamann, J. F. (1961). Relation of lung volumes to height in healthy persons between the ages of 5 and 38 years. *J. Pediatr.* 59: 710–714.

Cook, C. D., Mead, J., and Orzalesi, M. M. (1964). Static volume–pressure characteristics of the respiratory system during maximal efforts. *J. Appl. Physiol.* 19: 1016–1022.

Craig, A. B., Jr. (1960). Effects of position on expiratory reserve volume of the lungs. *J. Appl. Physiol.* 15: 59–61.

Craig, A. B., Jr., and Dvorak, M. (1975). Expiratory reserve volume and vital capacity of the lungs during immersion in water. *J. Appl. Physiol.* 38: 5–9.

Crawford A. B. H., Dodd D., and Engel L. A. (1983). Change in rib cage shape during quiet breathing, hyperventilation and single inspirations. *Respir. Physiol.* 54: 197–209.

D'Angelo, E. (1981). Cranio-caudal rib cage distortion with increasing inspiratory airflow in man. *Respir. Physiol.* 44: 215–237.

D'Angelo, E., and Sant'Ambrogio, G. (1974). Direct action of the contracting diaphragm on the rib cage in rabbits and dogs. *J. Appl. Physiol.* 36: 715–719.

D'Angelo, E., Michelini S., and Miserocchi G. (1973). Local motion of the chest wall during passive and active expansion. *Respir. Physiol.* 19: 47–59.

Danon, J., Druz W. S., Goldberg, N. B., and Sharp J. T. (1979). Function of isolated paced diaphragm and cervical accessory muscles in C1 quadriplegics. *Am. Rev. Respir. Dis.*, 119: 909–919.

Davis, C., Campbell, E. J. M., Openshaw, P., Pride, N. B., and Woodroof, G. (1980). Importance of airway closure in limiting maximal expiration in normal man. *J. Appl Physiol.* 48: 695–701.

Decramer, M., De Troyer, A., Kelly, S., Zocchi, L., and Macklem, P. T. (1984). Regional differences in abdominal pressure swings in dogs. *J. Appl. Physiol.* 57: 1682–1687.

Delhez, L., Petit, J.-M., and Milic-Emili J. (1959). Influence des muscles expirateurs dans la limitation de l'inspiration. (Etude electromyographique chez l'homme). *Rev. Fr. Etud. Clin. Biol.* 4: 815–818.

Delhez, L., Troquet, J., Damoiseau, J., Pirnay, F., Deroanne, R., and Petit, J.-M. (1964). Influence des modalites d'execution des maneuvres d'expiration forcee et hyperpression thoraco-abdominale sur l'activite electrique du diaphragme. *Arch. Int. Physiol. Biochem.* 72: 76–94.

Deschamps, C., Rodarte, J. R., and Wilson T. A. (1988). Coupling between rib cage and abdominal compartments of the relaxed chest wall. *J. Appl. Physiol.* 65: 2265–2269.

De Troyer, A., and Bastenier-Geens, J. (1979). Effects of neuromuscular blockade on respiratory mechanics in conscious man. *J. Appl. Physiol.* 47: 1162–1168.

De Troyer, A., and Estenne, M. (1981). Limitation of measurements of transdiaphragmatic pressure in detecting diaphragmatic weakness. *Thorax* 36: 169–174.

De Troyer, A., and Yernault, J. C. (1980). Inspiratory muscle force in normal subjects and patients with interstitial lung disease. *Thorax* 35: 92–100.

Dittmer, D. S., and Grebe, R. M., eds. (1958). *Handbook of Respiration.* Philadelphia, W. B. Saunders, pp. 28–40.

Dow, P. (1939). The venous return as a factor affecting the vital capacity. *Am. J. Physiol.* 127: 793–795.

Duomarco, J. L., and Rimini, R. (1947). *La Presion Intrabdominal en el Hombre.* Buenos Aires, El Ateneo.

Edyvean, J., Estenne, M., Paiva, M., and Engel L. A. (1991). Lung and chest wall mechanics in microgravity. *J. Appl. Physiol.* 71: 1956–1966.

Estenne, M., Yernault, J. C., and De Troyer A. (1985). Rib cage and diaphragm–abdomen compliance in humans: Effects of age and posture. *J. Appl. Physiol.* 59: 1842–1848.

Estenne, M., Gorini, M., Van Muylem, A., Ninane V., and Paiva M. (1992). Rib cage shape and motion in microgravity. *J. Appl. Physiol.* 73: 946–954.

Fink, B. R., Ngai, S., and Holaday D. A. (1958). Effect of air flow resistance on ventilation and respiratory muscle activity. *JAMA* 168: 2245–2249.

Fowler, R. C., Guillet, M., and Rahn, H. (1951). *Lung Volume Changes with Positive and Negative Pulmonary Pressures.* AF Tech. Report 6528. Wright-Patterson AFB, Dayton, Ohio, pp. 522–528.

Frank, N. R., Mead, J., and Ferris, B. G., Jr. (1957). The mechanical behaviour of the lungs in healthy elderly persons. *J. Clin. Invest.* 36: 1680–1687.

Freedman, S., Tattersfield, A. E., and Pride, N. B. (1975). Changes in lung mechanics during asthma induced by exercise. *J. Appl. Physiol.* 38: 974–982.

Gal, T. J., and Goldberg, S. K. (1981). Relationship between respiratory muscle strength and vital capacity during partial curarization in awake subjects. *Anesthesiology* 34: 141–147.

Gandevia S. C., and McKenzie D. K. (1985). Activation of the human diaphragm during maximal static efforts. *J. Physiol. (Lond.)* 367: 45–56.

Gandevia S. C., Gorman, R. B., McKenzie D. K., and Southon F. C. G. (1992). Dynamic changes in human diaphragm length: Maximal inspiratory and expulsive efforts studied with sequential radiography. *J. Physiol. (Lond.)* 457: 167–176.

Gibson, G. J., Pride, N. B., O'Cain, C., and Quagliato, R. (1976). Sex and age differences in pulmonary mechanics in normal nonsmoking subjects. *J. Appl. Physiol.* 41: 20–25.

Gil, J., and Weibel, E. R. (1972). Morphological study of pressure–volume hysteresis in rat lungs fixed by vascular perfusion. *Respir. Physiol.* 15: 190–213.

Glaser, E. M. (1949). The effect of cooling and warming on the vital capacity, forearm and hand volume, and skin temperature of man. *J. Physiol. (Lond.)* 109: 421–429.

Goldman, M. D., and Mead, J. (1973). Mechanical interaction between the diaphragm and rib cage. *J. Appl. Physiol.* 35: 197–204.

Greifenstein, F. E., King, R. M., Latch, S. S., and Comroe, J. H., Jr. (1952). Pulmonary function studies in healthy men and women 50 years and older. *J. Appl. Physiol.* 4: 641–648.

Hamilton, W. F., and Mayo. J. P. (1944). Changes in the vital capacity when the body is immersed in water. *Am. J. Physiol.* 141: 51–53.

Hamilton, W. F., and Morgan, A. B. (1932). Mechanism of the postural reduction in vital capacity in relation to orthopnea and storage of blood in the lungs. *Am. J. Physiol.* 99: 526–533.

Heaf, P. J. D., and Prime, F. J. (1954). The mechanical aspects of artificial pneumothorax. *Lancet* 2: 468–470.

Heaf, P. J. D., and Prime, F. J. (1956). The compliance of the thorax in normal human subjects. *Clin. Sci.* 15: 319–327.

Hedenstierna, G., Bindslev, L., Santesson, J., and Norlander D. P. (1981). Airway closure in each lung of anesthetized human subjects. *J. Appl. Physiol.* 50: 55–64.

Hershenson, M. B., Kikuchi, Y., and Loring S. H. (1988). Relative strengths of the chest wall muscles. *J. Appl. Physiol.* 65: 852–862.

Hillman, D. R., and Finucane, K. E. (1987). A model of the respiratory pump. *J. Appl. Physiol.* 63: 951–961.

Hillman, D. R., Markos J., and Finucane K. E. (1990). Effect of abdominal compression on maximum transdiaphragmatic pressure. *J. Appl. Physiol.* 68: 2296–2304.

Hong, S. K., Ting, E. Y., and Rahn, H. (1960). Lung volumes at different depths of submersion. *J. Appl. Physiol.* 15: 550–553.

Hong, S. K., Cerretelli, P., Cruz, J. C., and Rahn, H. (1969). Mechanics of respiration during submersion in water. *J. Appl. Physiol.* 27: 535–538.

Hurtado, A., and Fray, W. W. (1933). Studies of total pulmonary capacity and its subdivisions. III. Changes with body posture. *J. Clin. Invest.* 12: 825–832.

Jarrett, A. S. (1965). Effect of immersion on intrapulmonary pressure. *J. Appl. Physiol.* 20: 1261–1266.

Jiang, J. X., Demedts M., and Decramer M. (1988). Mechanical coupling of upper and lower canine rib cages and its functional significance. *J. Appl. Physiol.* 64: 620–626.

Johansen, S. H., Jorgensen, M., and Molbech, S. (1964). Effect of tubocurarine on respiratory and nonrespiratory muscle power in man. *J. Appl. Physiol.* 19: 990–994.

Johnson, L. F., Jr., and Mead, J. (1963). Volume-pressure relationships during pressure breathing and voluntary relaxation. *J. Appl. Physiol.* 18: 505–508.

Jorgensen, M., Molbech, S., and Johansen, S. H. (1966). Effect of decamethonium on head lift, hand grip, and respiratory muscle power in man. *J. Appl. Physiol.* 21: 509–512.

Karlberg, P. (1957). Breathing and its control in premature infant. In *Physiology of Prematurity*. Edited by J. T. Lanman. New York, Macy, pp. 77–150.

Kelling, G. (1903). Untersuchungen uber die Spannungzustande der Bauchwand, der Magen und der Darmwand. *Z. Biol.* 44: 161–258.

Konno, K., and Mead, J. (1967). Measurement of the separate volume changes of rib cage and abdomen during breathing. *J. Appl. Physiol.* 22: 407–422.

Konno K., and Mead, J. (1968). Static volume–pressure characteristics of the rib cage and abdomen. *J. Appl. Physiol.* 24: 544–548.

Landowne, M., and Stacy, R. W. (1957). Glossary of terms. In *Tissue Elasticity*. Edited by J. W. Remington. Washington, DC, American Physiological Society, pp. 191–201.

Laporta D., and Grassino, A. (1985). Assessment of transdiaphragmatic pressure in humans. *J. Appl. Physiol.* 58: 1469–1476.

Leith, D. E., and Bradley, M. (1976). Ventilatory muscle strength and endurance training. *J. Appl. Physiol.* 41: 508–516.

Leith, D. E., and Mead, J. (1967). Mechanisms determining residual volume of the lungs in normal subjects. *J. Appl. Physiol.* 23: 221–227.

Loring, S. H., and Mead, J. (1982). Action of the diaphragm on the rib cage inferred from force–balance analysis. *J. Appl. Physiol.* 53: 756–760.

Liu, S., Wilson, T. A., and Schreiner K. (1991). Gravitational forces on the chest wall. *J. Appl. Physiol.* 70: 1506–1510.

Macklem, P. T., Macklem D. M., and De Troyer A. (1983). A model of inspiratory muscle mechanics. *J. Appl. Physiol.* 55: 547–557.

McCool F. D., Loring S. H., and Mead J. (1985). Rib cage distortion during voluntary and involuntary breathing acts. *J. Appl. Physiol.* 58: 1703–1712.

Mead, J. (1981). Mechanics of the chest wall. In *Advances in Physiological Sciences*, Vol. 10. Edited by I. Hutas and L. A. Debreczeni. Oxford, Pergamon Press, pp. 3–11.

Mead, J., and Loring, S. H. (1982). Analysis of volume displacement and length changes of the diaphragm during breathing. *J. Appl. Physiol.* 53: 750–755.

Mead, J., and Milic-Emili, J. (1964). Theory and methodology in respiratory mechanics with glossary of symbols. In *Handbook of Physiology*, Section 3. Respiration. Vol 1. Edited by W. O. Fenn and H. Rahn. Washington, DC, American Physiological Society, pp. 363–376.

Mead, J., Milic-Emili, J., and Turner, J. M. (1963). Factors limiting depth of a maximal inspiration in human subjects. *J. Appl. Physiol.* 18: 295–296.

Mead, J., Yoshino K., Barnas, G. M., and Loring S. H. (1990). Abdominal pressure transmission in humans during slow breathing maneuvers. *J. Appl. Physiol.* 68: 1850–1853.

Melissinos, C. G., Goldman, M., Bruce, E., Elliot E., and Mead J. (1981). Chest wall shape during forced expiratory maneuvers. *J. Appl. Physiol.* 50: 84–93.

Michels, M. D., Friedman, P. J., and West J. B. (1979). Radiographic comparison of human lung shape during normal gravity and weightlessness. *J. Appl. Physiol.* 47: 851–857.

Milic-Emili, J., Orzalesi, M. M., Cook, C. D., and Turner, J. M. (1964). Respiratory thoracoabdominal mechanics in man. *J. Appl. Physiol.* 19: 217–223.

Milic-Emili, J., Henderson, J. A. M., Dolovich, M. B., Trop, D., and Kaneko, K. (1966). Regional distribution of inspired gas in the lung. *J. Appl. Physiol.* 21: 749–759.

Mills, J. N. (1949). The influence upon the vital capacity of procedures calculated to alter the volume of blood in the lungs. *J. Physiol. (Lond.)* 110: 207–216.

Mills, J. N. (1950). The nature of the limitation of maximal inspiratory and expiratory efforts. *J. Physiol. (Lond.)* 111: 376381.

Mittman, C., Edelman, N. H., Norris, A. H., and Shock, N. W. (1965). Relationship between chest wall and pulmonary compliance and age. *J. Appl. Physiol.* 20: 1211–1216.

Mognoni, P., Torri, G., and Agostoni, E. (1965). Confronto della relazione volume–pressione del sistema respiratorio ottenuta con diversi procedimenti. *Atti Accad. Naz. Lincei* 38: 925–928.

Moreno, F., and Lyons, H. A. (1961). Effect of body posture on lung volumes. *J. Appl. Physiol.* 16: 27–29.

Morse, M., Schultz, F. W., and Cassels, D. E. (1952). The lung volume and its subdivisions in normal boys 10–17 years of age. *J. Clin. Invest.* 31: 380–391.

Mortola, J. P., and Sant'Ambrogio, G. (1978). Motion of the rib cage and the abdomen in tetraplegic patients. *Clin. Sci. Mol. Med.* 54: 25–32.

Muller, N., Valgyesi, G., Becker, L., Bryan, M. H., and Bryan, A. C. (1979). Diaphragmatic muscle tone. *J. Appl. Physiol.* 47: 279–284.

Needham, C. E., Rogan, M. G., and McDonald, I. (1954). Normal standard for lung volumes, intrapulmonary gas mixing and maximum breathing capacity. *Thorax* 9: 313–325.

Paiva, M., Estenne, M., and Engel, L. A. (1989). Lung volumes, chest wall configuration, and pattern of breathing in microgravity. *J. Appl. Physiol.* 67: 1542–1550.

Paiva, M., Verbanck, S., Estenne, M., Poncelet, B., Segebarth, C., and Macklem, P. T. (1992). Mechanical implications of in vivo human diaphragm shape. *J. Appl. Physiol.* 72: 1407–1412.

Pemberton, J., and Flanagan, E. G. (1956). Vital capacity and timed vital capacity in normal men over forty. *J. Appl. Physiol.* 9: 291–296.

Peress, L., Sybrecht, G., and Macklem, P. T. (1976). The mechanism of increase in total lung capacity during acute asthma. *Am. J. Med.* 61: 165–169.

Permutt, S., and Martin, H. B. (1960). Static pressure–volume characteristics of lungs in normal males. *J. Appl. Physiol.* 15: 819–825.

Pierce, J. A., and Ebert, R. V. (1958). The elastic properties of the lungs in the aged. *J. Lab. Clin. Med.* 51: 63–71.

Rahn, H., Otis, A. B., Chadwick, L. E., and Fenn, W. O. (1946). The pressure–volume diagram of the thorax and lung. *Am. J. Physiol.* 146: 161–178.

Rahn, H., Fenn, W. O., and Otis, A. B. (1949). Daily variations of vital capacity, residual air and expiratory reserve including a study of the residual air method. *J. Appl. Physiol.* 1: 725–736.

Reid, M. B., Loring, S. H., Banzett, R. B., and Mead, J. (1986). Passive mechanics of upright human chest wall during immersion from hips to neck. *J. Appl. Physiol.* 60: 1561–1570.

Rehder, K., Hatch, D. J., Sessler, A. D., Marsh, H. M., and Fowler, W. S. (1971). Effects of general anesthesia, muscle paralysis, and mechanical ventilation on pulmonary nitrogen clearance. *Anesthesiology* 35: 591–601.

Remington, J. W. (1955). Hysteresis loop behavior of the aorta and other extensible tissues. *Am. J. Physiol.* 180: 83–95.

Remington, J. W., ed. (1957). *Tissue Elasticity.* Washington, DC, American Physiological Society.

Ringqvist, T. (1966). The ventilatory capacity in healthy subjects. *Scand. J. Clin. Lab. Invest.* 18, Suppl.: 88.

Robinson, S. (1938). Experimental studies of physical fitness in relation to age. *Arbeitsphysiologie* 10: 251–323.

Rodarte, J. R., Burgher, L. W., Hyatt, R. E., and Rehder, K. (1977). Lung recoil and gas trapping during oxygen breathing at low lung volumes. *J. Appl. Physiol.* 43: 138–143.

Rodarte, J. R., and Hyatt, R. E. (1973). Effect of acute exposure to CO_2 on lung mechanics in normal man. *Respir. Physiol.* 17: 135–145.

Rohrer, F. (1916). Der Zusammenhang der Atemkrafte und ihre Abhangigkeit vom Dehnungszustand der Atmungsorgane. *Pflugers Arch. Ges. Physiol.* 165: 419–444.

Sampson, M. G., and De Troyer, A. (1982). Role of intercostal muscles in the rib cage distortion produced by inspiratory loads. *J. Appl. Physiol.* 52: 517–523.

Sant'Ambrogio, G., Frazier, D. T., Wilson, M. F., and Agostoni, E. (1963). Motor innervation and pattern of activity of cat diaphragm. *J. Appl. Physiol.* 18: 43–46.

Saunders, N. A., Rigg, J. R. A., Pengelly, L. D., and Campbell, E. J. M. (1978). Effect of curare on maximum static PV relationships of the respiratory system. *J. Appl. Physiol.* 44: 589–595.

Sharp, J. T., Johnson, F. N., Goldberg, N. B., and Van Lith P. (1967). Hysteresis and stress adaptation in the human respiratory system. *J. Appl. Physiol.* 23: 487–497.

Shore, S., Milic-Emili, J., and Martin, G. (1982). Reassessment of body plethysmographic technique for the measurement of thoracic gas volume in asthmatics. *Am. Rev. Respir. Dis.* 126: 515–520.

Song, S. H., Kang, D. H., Kang, B. S., and Hong S. K. (1963). Lung volumes and ventilatory responses to high CO_2 and low CO_2 in the ama. *J. Appl. Physiol.* 18: 466–470.

Stanescu, D. C., Rodenstein, D., Cauberghs, M., and Van de Woestijne, K. P. (1982). Failure of body plethysmography in bronchial asthma. *J. Appl. Physiol.* 52: 939–948.

Strohl, K. P., Mead, J., Banzett, R. B., Loring, S. H., and Kosch, P. C. (1981). Regional differences in abdominal muscle activity during various maneuvers in humans. *J. Appl. Physiol* 51: 1471–1476.

Taylor, A. (1960). The contribution of the intercostal muscles to the effort of respiration in man. *J. Physiol. (Lond.)* 151: 390–402.

Thompson, L. J., and McCally, M. (1967). Role of transpharyngeal pressure gradients in determining intrapulmonary pressure during immersion. *Aerospace Med.* 38: 931–935.

Turner, J. M., Mead, J., and Wohl, M. E. (1968). Elasticity of human lungs in relation to age. *J. Appl. Physiol.* 25: 664–671.

Urmey, W. F., De Troyer, A., Kelly, K. B., and Loring S. H. (1988). Pleural pressure increases during inspiration in the zone of apposition of diaphragm to rib cage. *J. Appl. Physiol.* 65: 2207–2212.

Van de Woestijne, K. P. (1967). Influence of forced inflation on the creep of lungs and thorax in the dog. *Respir. Physiol.* 3: 78–89.

Vellody, V. P., Nassery, M., Druz, W. S., and Sharp, J. T. (1978). Effect of body position change on thoracoabdominal motion. *J. Appl. Physiol.* 45: 581–589.

Verschakelen, J. A., Deschepper, K., and Demedts, M. (1992). Relationship between axial motion and volume displacement of the diaphragm during VC maneuvers. *J. Appl. Physiol.* 72: 1536–1540.

Wade, O. L. (1954). Movements of the thoracic cage and diaphragm in respiration. *J. Physiol. (Lond.)* 124: 193–212.

Wade, O. L., and Gilson, J. C. (1951). The effect of posture on diaphragmatic movement and vital capacity in normal subjects with a note on spirometry as an aid in determining radiological chest volumes. *Thorax* 6: 103–126.

Ward, M. E., Ward, J. W., and Macklem, P. T. (1992). Analysis of human chest wall motion using a two-compartment rib cage model. *J. Appl. Physiol.* 72: 1338–1347.

Wilson, T. A. (1988). Mechanics of compartmental models of the chest wall. *J. Appl. Physiol.* 65: 2261–2264.

Withfield, A. G. W., Waterhouse, J. A. H., and Arnott, W. M. (1950). The total lung volume and its subdivisions. A study in physiological norms. I. Basic data. *Br. J. Soc. Med.* 4: 1–25.

Woolcock, A. J., and Read, J. (1966). Lung volume in exacerbations of asthma. *Am. J. Med.* 41: 259–273.

Zechman, F. W., Musgrave, F. S., Mains, R. C., and Cohn, J. E. (1967). Respiratory mechanics and pulmonary diffusing capacity with lower body negative pressure. *J. Appl. Physiol.* 22: 247–250.

Zocchi, L., Garzaniti, N., Newman, S., and Macklem P. T. (1987). Effect of hyperinflation and equalization of abdominal pressure on diaphragmatic action. *J. Appl. Physiol.* 62: 1655–1664.

17

Dynamics of the Respiratory System

EDGARDO D'ANGELO

University of Milan
Milan, Italy

JOSEPH MILIC-EMILI

Meakins-Christie Laboratories
McGill University
Montreal, Quebec, Canada

I. Introduction

We will first describe the driving pressures that generate the breathing movements. Next we will discuss the dynamic forces that develop in opposition to the driving pressures, the static forces having been described in Chapter 16. Finally, the dynamic performance of the respiratory system will be briefly considered. Because the dynamic performance of the respiratory system depends on both lung and chest wall, both components will be considered. This review is focused on recent advances of respiratory dynamics. Detailed accounts of earlier literature can be found elsewhere (Mead and Agostoni, 1964; Rodarte and Rehder, 1986).

II. The Driving Pressures

The potential range of pressures available to produce the breathing movements are shown in Figure 11 of Chapter 16, which depicts the relations between lung volume and maximal voluntary static inspiratory and expiratory pressures in normal adults. In theory, the maximal mechanical work potentially available for a breathing cycle is given by the area subtended by those curves (Rahn et al., 1946). For male adults it amounts to 20–30 cal; however, this potential work is never realized during the actual breathing movements. Agostoni and Fenn (1960) demonstrated that the maximal work that a subject can achieve during a forced inspiration decreases with increasing flow, in line with the force–velocity relationship of muscle. Other mechanisms also contribute to limit the maximal work per breath, such as the speed of activation of the respiratory muscles and gas compressibility (Jaeger and Otis, 1964).

During a 15-s maximal voluntary ventilation, the respiratory mechanical power output in normal young adults amounts to 485 cal/min (Hesser et al., 1981). In this study, however, volume changes were measured at the mouth; hence, thoracic gas compression was ignored. If measurements are made in a body plethysmograph, the maximal power output increases to 613 cal/min (range, 500–860 cal/min) (J. Milic-Emili, unpublished observations). The latter measurements did not include the elastic work caused by distortion of the chest wall which, during maximal voluntary ventilation, is probably substantial (Goldman et al., 1976). In view of the large power potential of the respiratory muscles, the mechanical power output required during quiet breathing seems rather puny, amounting to less than 0.2% of maximum. During maximal exercise ventilation, the corresponding value is about 20% (Milic-Emili, 1991).

III. The Opposing Pressures

The breathing movements involve several factors, which include (1) elastic forces within the lung and chest wall; (2) resistive forces offered by the airways to gas flow and by the chest wall tissues; (3) viscoelastic forces caused by stress adaptation units within the thoracic tissues (lung and chest wall); (4) plastoelastic forces that cause "quasi-static hysteresis," as reflected by differences in static elastic recoil pressure of the lung and chest wall between inflation and deflation; (5) inertial forces; (6) gravitational forces that may be considered as part of inertial forces, but in practice, are included in the measurements of elastic forces; (7) compressibility of thoracic gas; and (8) distortion of the chest wall from its passive (relaxed) configuration.

Items (1) and (6) are considered in Chapter 16, item (8) is dealt with in Chapter 22, and item (5) will not be considered, because, under most physiological conditions, it is probably negligible (Mead, 1956).

A. Airway and Chest Wall Resistance

Rohrer was the first to estimate the airway flow resistance (1915). Lacking a method for direct measurement of the resistance offered by gas flowing through the airways (Raw), he undertook the formidable task of estimating it by applying the laws governing the flow of gas through tubes to postmortem measurements of the dimension of the airways. Based on these estimates he described the following relationships, which are known as Rohrer's equations:

$$\text{Pres} = K_1\dot{V} + K_2\dot{V}^2 \tag{1}$$

and

$$\text{Raw} = K_1 + K_2\dot{V} \tag{2}$$

where Pres represents the pressure dissipations within the airways owing to gas flow ($\dot{V}$), and K_1 and K_2 are constants. Equation (2) is obtained by dividing both sides of Eq. (1) by $\dot{V}$. Although the specific physical connotations assigned by Rohrer (1915, 1985) to his constants are no longer accepted, Eqs. (1) and (2) are still used because they provide a close empirical description of experimental results (Mead and Agostoni, 1964).

In 1927, Rohrer's pupils, von Neergaard and Wirz (1927) introduced the first method designed for measuring Raw (i.e., the interrupter method). This method was popular until the late 1950s, when it was abandoned in clinical practice because of controversies in the interpretation of the results and, more importantly, because of the introduction of the body plethysmographic method for measuring Raw (Dubois et al., 1956).

Body Plethysmography

With use of the body plethysmography technique, Briscoe and Dubois (1958) have shown that airway conductance (Gaw, the reciprocal of Raw) changes approximately linearly with changes in lung volume, reflecting changes in dimensions of the conducting airways. This method, however, has the disadvantage that almost all body plethysmographs are designed to be used only at rest, in a seated position. These limitations have recently led to a revival of the interrupter technique, which can be readily applied in different body postures, both at rest and during increased ventilation (e.g., exercise). Furthermore, the interrupter technique is particularly suited for use in mechanically ventilated patients, in whom the upper compliant airways are bypassed by intubation (Jaegger, 1982). In nonintubated patients, supporting the cheeks enables correct estimation of the interrupter resistance, provided that airway resistance is not too high (Bates et al., 1987b). The interrupter technique is described in some detail in the following section. A more complete review is provided elsewhere (Bates and Milic-Emili, 1991).

Interrupter Technique

Interrupter Resistance

As originally described by von Neergaard and Wirz (1927), to obtain interrupter resistance (Rint), subjects breathed through a mouthpiece assembly consisting of a pneumotachograph to register flow and a manometer to determine the pressure in the mouthpiece (Pao). When the distal end of the circuit was briefly occluded during the breathing cycle, airflow fell suddenly to zero, whereas Pao changed rapidly to a new value. The rapid change in Pao following occlusion was considered by von Neergaard and Wirz to represent the resistive pressure difference (ΔPres) existing between the mouth and the alveoli before airflow interruption. Accordingly, dividing ΔPres by the immediately preceding $\dot{V}$, Rint was obtained and was assumed to represent airway resistance (Rint = Raw = ΔPres/$\dot{V}$).

Partitioning of Interrupter Resistance

In 1954, on theoretical grounds, Mead and Whittenberger (1954) suggested that Rint should include a chest wall component (Rint,w), as well as a lung component (Rint,L) reflecting mainly Raw. However, in their experiments on spontaneously breathing normal subjects, the rapid airway occlusions were not associated with changes in esophageal pressure (Pes), which should reflect Rint,w. They reasoned that the expected changes in Pes were obscured by the distortion of the chest wall following interruptions. Indeed during the occlusions they observed a paradoxical displacement of the anterior aspect of the rib cage. This argument is not supported by the results obtained by D'Angelo et al. (1991). As shown in Figure 1, in mechanically ventilated, anesthetized, paralyzed subjects in whom there is no distortion of the chest wall during flow interruption, there is still no appreciable immediate change in Pes following airway occlusion. These results could be taken as supporting the notion that, in humans, Rint,w is negligible. On the other hand, this could also reflect that in the foregoing studies the immediate changes in Pes following airway interruption were attenuated by the relatively long occlusion time of the airway shutter (40–120 ms), as well as being obscured by the cardiac artifacts. Recently, Rint,w was assessed in 12 mechanically ventilated, normal, anesthetized, paralyzed subjects, using a rapid shutter (closing time: 10–15 ms) (D'Angelo et al., 1994). Furthermore, 30–40 test breaths were ensemble-averaged in each subject to allow for the cardiac artifacts. With this analysis, Rint,w averaged (SD) 0.4 ± 0.1 cm H_2O s L^{-1} at flows between 0.24 and 1.12 L s^{-1}, amounting to about 27% of total Rint (Rint,rs = Rint,L + Rint,w). Since the latter did not include the resistance of the upper airways, because the measurements of Rint,rs were based on tracheal pressure, it follows that, in intact normal subjects, Rint,w should represent less than 27% of Rint,rs. This is supported by the results of Liistro et al. (1989), who found in normal subjects that the values Rint,rs were close to those of Raw measured with the body plethysmographic technique. In patients with chronic obstructive pulmonary disease (COPD) (Guérin et al., 1993) and with adult respiratory distress syndrome (Eissa et al., 1991a,b) in whom Raw is substantially increased, Rint,w appears to represent a negligible fraction of Rint,rs. By contrast, in patients with ischemic and valvular heart disease, Auler et al. (1987) found values of Rint,w amounting to about 1 cm H_2O s L^{-1}.

In experimental animals (dogs, cats), Rint,w represents a large fraction of Rint,rs (Kochi et al., 1988; Similowski et al., 1989). The reason for this discrepancy with humans is unclear. In humans, as well as in all animal species studied, Rint,w

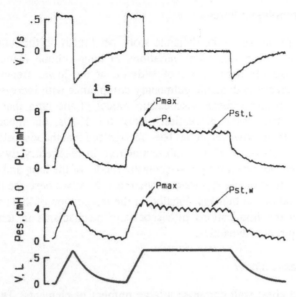

Figure 1 (From top to bottom) Records of flow ($\dot{V}$), changes in transpulmonary pressure (PL), esophageal pressure (Pes), and lung volume (V) in a normal, anesthetized, paralyzed subject in whom during constant-flow inflation ($\dot{V} = 0.55$ L s^{-1}) the airway was suddenly occluded at a V of 0.6 L. After flow interruption, there is an immediate drop in PL from Pmax to P_1, followed by a slow decay to a plateau value that represents static pulmonary end-inspiratory elastic recoil pressure (Pst,L). Dividing Pmax–P_1 by the flow immediately preceding the occlusion yields the interrupter resistance of the lung (Rint,L), which essentially reflects airway resistance (Raw). There is no evident immediate change in Pes after airway occlusion, but only a slow decay to Pst,w. The slow pressure decays (P_1–Pst,L and Pmax–Pst,w) reflect dissipation of viscoelastic energy stored in the pulmonary and chest wall tissues during inspiration. For further information see text.

appears to be independent of volume and flow (i.e., Rint,w = constant). The volume-independence of Rint,w is inconsistent with the predictions of Grimby et al. (1968).

In theory, Rint,L (and, hence, Rint,rs) could include a component of lung tissues. However, when using the alveolar capsule technique in open-chest dogs (Bates et al., 1988b; 1989) and rats (Saldiva et al., 1992) the pulmonary tissues do not contribute appreciably to Rint,L.

In the past, the human values of chest wall "resistance" reported in the literature (~ 1 cm H_2O s L^{-1}; see Mead and Agostoni, 1964) were higher than those of D'Angelo et al. (1994). It should be stressed, however, that previous estimates must have included substantial contributions by viscoelastic pressure dissipations (D'Angelo et al., 1991). Such contributions, however, do not represent "true" flow resistance, although they are included in the "lumped" measurements of total chest wall (Rw) and pulmonary (RL) resistance (see Sec. IV.D).

B. Viscoelastic Forces

In 1955, Mount measured the dynamic work per breath on the lung (Wdyn,L) in open-chest rats, using sinusoidal variations in lung volume (Mount, 1955). To explain the relatively high values of Wdyn,L at the lower frequencies and the progressive decrease in dynamic pulmonary compliance with increasing frequency, he proposed a four-parameter viscoelastic model of the lung that "confers time dependency of the elastic properties." Until the 1970s, his model was largely ignored. Since then, however, it has been recognized that the viscoelastic properties of the respiratory system play a substantial role in respiratory dynamics. In this section, we first provide a simple viscoelastic model of the lung and chest wall that is useful for understanding respiratory dynamics. Next we describe the viscoelastic pressure dissipations in humans. Finally, in the last section of this chapter, we will briefly review the implications of viscoelastic mechanisms in terms of various aspects of respiratory dynamics.

Viscoelastic Model

The lungs and chest wall comprise a large number of elements. This complexity, coupled with the necessity to explain respiratory dynamics under physiological and pathological conditions, has generated the need for relatively simple models that can mimic the mechanical behavior of the respiratory system. From the pioneering work of Mount (1955), Bates and associates (1987a) have proposed the eight-parameter spring-and-dashpot model of the respiratory system shown in Figure 2. The

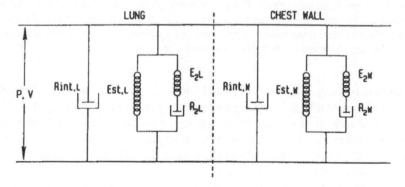

Figure 2   The eight-parameter spring-and-dashpot viscoelastic model for interpretation of respiratory mechanics. Respiratory system consists of interrupter resistance of lung (Rint,L = airway resistance) and chest wall (Rint,w) in parallel with (1) Est,L and Est,w and (2) series spring-and-dashpot bodies (E$_2$ and R$_2$, respectively) of lung and chest wall that represent viscoelastic (*stress adaptation*) units. The distance between the two bars is analogous to lung volume (V), and tension between the bars is analogous to pressure applied to the respiratory system (P).

model consists of two submodels, the lungs and chest wall, which are arranged mechanically in parallel because they both undergo the same volume changes. The lung submodel consists of a dashpot representing Raw ($=$ Rint,L) arranged in parallel with a Kelvin body, which consists of a spring representing static elastance (Est,L), in parallel with a Maxwell body, that is a spring (E_2,L) and a dashpot (R_2,L) arranged serially. The latter, together with the corresponding time constant (τ_2,L $= R_2$,L/E_2,L), accounts for the viscoelastic properties of the lung. Similarly, the chest wall comprises a resistance (Rint,W) and a Kelvin body consisting of static chest wall elastance (Est,W) and corresponding viscoelastic parameters (E_2,W and R_2,W, τ_2,W). It should be stressed (1) that currently the precise structural basis of the viscoelastic parameters in Figure 2 is poorly understood, and (2) that the model is clearly too simplistic to be a true representation of the respiratory system. More complex models have been proposed (Hildebrandt, 1970; Fredberg and Stamenovic, 1989). Nonetheless, the model in Figure 2 is useful, because it mimics and explains several aspects of respiratory dynamics, as will be seen from the following. Also, the viscoelastic units might be functionally important to the extent that they would tend to smooth stress distribution within the thoracic tissues, thereby minimizing local distortion during sudden displacements (Barnas et al., 1989), and reduce regional differences in ventilation distribution caused by time constant inequality.

Viscoelastic Pressure Dissipations

Figure 1 illustrates the *rapid airway occlusion method* (RAO) for determining (1) the interrupter resistance, (2) the viscoelastic pressure dissipations (Pvisc), and (3) the static recoil pressure (Pst) of lung and chest wall. The RAO method is essentially a modification of the interrupter technique, in the sense that airway occlusions are maintained for 4–5 s, not only the 0.2 s, proposed by von Neergaard and Wirz (1927). In this representative example, a normal anesthetized, paralyzed subject was inflated with constant-flow (0.55 L s^{-1}) to a lung volume of 0.6 L. At this lung volume the airway was rapidly occluded, resulting in an immediate drop of transpulmonary pressure (PL) from Pmax to P_1 which represents the pressure dissipations within the airways (see under Sec. III.A on partitioning of Rint). This was followed by a slow decay of PL to an apparent plateau that was achieved in about 3 s. This plateau pressure was taken as representative of Pst,L, whereas P_1–Pst,L should reflect viscoelastic pressure dissipations within the lung. Similarly, the slow drop in Pes from P_1 to Pst,W should represent viscoelastic pressure dissipations within the chest wall. This phenomenon is commonly referred to as *stress relaxation* (Hoppin et al., 1986).

Stress relaxation is consistent with the model in Figure 2. Indeed, when the model is subjected to a "flow interruption" maneuver, by suddenly halting the relative movement of the two horizontal rigid bars, the springs E_2 which during the movements were under tension, will return to their equilibrium lengths. In terms of this model, the difference between P_1 and Pst represents the tension offered by the springs E_2 before airway occlusion; hence, the postinterruption pressure decay from P_1 to Pst in Figure 1 should be interpreted as the relaxation of springs E_2, resulting in resistive energy dissipation into the dashpots R_2. Thus, the amount of relaxation of tension depends on the degree of stretch of springs E_2 at the time of flow interruption.

By using the technique of rapid flow interruption during constant flow inflation, it has been possible to determine the values of E_2, R_2, and τ_2 of the lung and chest wall in both animals (Similowsky et al., 1989; Shardonofsky et al., 1991) and humans (D'Angelo et al., 1989, 1991, 1992). The average values of the viscoelastic parameters obtained on 18 normal, anesthetized, paralyzed humans are provided in Table 1. Over the volume range studied (up to 1 L above FRC), Est,L and Est,w amounted to 8.2 ± 1.7 and 6.3 ± 1.1 cm H_2O L^{-1}, respectively. Thus, on average, $E_{2,L}$ and $E_{2,w}$ amounted, respectively, to 39 and 26% of the corresponding static elastances. The viscoelastic time constants of the lung and chest wall were considerably longer than the *standard* mechanical time constant of the respiratory system ($\tau,rs = Rint,rs/Est,rs$) which amounted to about 0.15 s.

IV. Dynamic Performance

A. Time Dependency of Elastance and Resistance

The viscoelastic elements within the lung and chest wall confer time-dependency of elastance and resistance. Indeed, at high respiratory frequencies (f), the springs E_2 in Figure 2 will oscillate so fast that there will be insufficient time for their tension to be dissipated through the dashpots R_2. By contrast, at low frequencies, the dashpots R_2 are given time to move and dissipate the elastic energy stored in E_2. In the limit, as frequency tends to zero, the springs E_2 should remain at fixed length (i.e., resting length at which tension is zero). This implies that the dynamic lung and chest wall elastances (Edyn) should increase with increasing f. At high frequencies, Edyn should approach the corresponding values of Est + E_2.

During sinusoidal breathing, the contribution of viscoelastic properties (ΔE) to dynamic elastance should change with frequency according to the following function (D'Angelo et al., 1991):

Table 1 Average Values ($\pm$SD) of Viscoelastic Parameters of 18 Anesthetized, Paralyzed, Normal Humans

	R_2 (cm H_2O L^{-1})	E_2 (cm H_2O L^{-1})	τ_2 (s)
Lung	3.44 ± 0.97	3.21 ± 1.14	1.13 ± 0.36
Chest wall	2.12 ± 0.58	1.66 ± 0.37	1.30 ± 0.34

Source: D'Angelo et al. (1991).

$$DE = \frac{\omega^2 \tau_2^2 \, E_2}{(1 + \omega^2 \tau_2^2)} \tag{3}$$

where ω is angular frequency $(2\pi f)$.

Figure 3 shows the relation of ΔE_L and ΔE_W to frequency computed according Eq. (3), using the average values of the constants in Table 1. Also shown on the right ordinates of Figure 3 is dynamic elastance (Edyn = ΔE + Est), expressed as a fraction of corresponding Est. As predicted by the viscoelastic model, Edyn,L and Edyn,W increase with frequency, approaching plateau values (Est + E_2) at frequency of about 0.5 Hz. At these frequencies, on average, Edyn,L is about 38% higher than Est,L, and the corresponding increase for the chest wall is about 26%. This implies that, in normal subjects, there is more marked frequency-dependence of elastance than previously thought (Otis et al., 1956).

During sinusoidal breathing, the effective pulmonary and chest wall tissue resistance (ΔR) owing to viscoelastic mechanisms should decrease with frequency, according to the following function (D'Angelo et al., 1991):

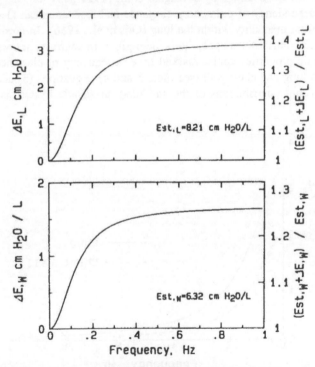

Figure 3 Relation of ΔE of lung (top) and chest wall (bottom) to respiratory frequency computed according Eq. (3) using average values of E_2 and τ_2 in Table 1. Also shown on right ordinates are the changes in dynamic elastance (Est + ΔE), expressed as a fraction of Est. (From D'Angelo et al., 1991.)

$$DR = \frac{R_2}{(1 + \omega^2\tau_2^2)} \tag{4}$$

Figure 4 illustrates the relationship of ΔR_L and ΔR_W with frequency computed according Eq. (4), using the average values of the viscoelastic constants in Table 1. ΔR_L and ΔR_W decrease with increasing frequency, becoming negligible at $f >$ 0.5 Hz.

Time-dependency of pulmonary and chest wall elastance and resistance has been also described, using forced oscillation techniques, by several investigators in awake, relaxed, normal humans (Hantos et al., 1986; Barnas et al., 1987, 1989), as well as in spontaneously breathing patients with obstructive lung disease (Grimby et al., 1968). According to the linear model in Figure 2 and Eq. (4), R_L and R_W at high frequencies should reflect $R_{int,L}$ and $R_{int,W}$, respectively. In this connection, the values of R_W obtained with the forced oscillation technique in relaxed, normal subjects by Barnas et al. (1987) and in spontaneously breathing subjects by Wohl et al. (see Grimby et al., 1968) at frequencies between 2 and 9 Hz were close to the values of $R_{int,W}$ obtained by D'Angelo et al. (1994).

Time-dependency of pulmonary elastance and resistance can also be caused by time-constant inequality within the lung (Otis et al., 1956). In normal subjects, however, such contributions appear to be negligible. In contrast, in normal humans the viscoelastic properties confer marked time-dependency of elastance and resistance to both lung and chest wall (see Figs. 3 and 4). Equations (3) and (4) do not take into account contributions of the so-called quasistatic hysteresis. However,

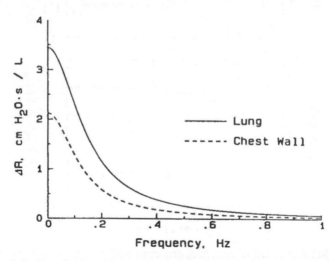

Figure 4 Relation of ΔR of lung and chest wall to respiratory frequency computed according Eq. (4) using average values of constants R_2 and τ_2 in Table 1. (From D'Angelo et al., 1991.)

during tidal breathing, these are normally rather small (Shardonofsky et al., 1990; Jonson et al., 1993).

In patients with pulmonary disease, time constant inequality within the lung probably contributes substantially to the observed increase in the magnitude of time-dependency of both elastance and resistance (Eissa et al., 1991a,b; Guérin et al., 1993).

At frequencies used during quiet breathing ($\sim$ 0.2 Hz), the values of ΔR of both lung and chest wall are high; hence, the dynamic work of breathing is relatively large (D'Angelo et al., 1991; Milic-Emili, 1991). But the energy cost of this phenomenon should be negligible. By contrast, the increase of Edyn,L and Edyn,w with increasing frequency has more profound implications. Indeed, at $f > 0.5$ Hz the elastic work of breathing should increase by about 30%, according to Figure 3. The increases of Edyn,w and particularly of Edyn,L with increasing rate of breathing are of considerable functional significance both during relaxed and forced expiration (see Section IV.C).

B. Work of Breathing

In open-chest rats, Mount (1955) measured the relation between the dynamic pulmonary work per breath (Wdyn,L) and frequency during sinusoidal cycling at fixed tidal volume. His results suggested that, in rats, the viscoelastic component of Wdyn,L was relatively large at low frequencies. The same is true in humans, for both the lung and chest wall. This is shown in Figure 5 (top), which depicts the predicted relations between respiratory frequency and the viscoelastic work of the lung and chest wall. The viscoelastic component (Wvisc) of the dynamic work per breath was computed at fixed VT of 0.47 L, according to the following equation (Milic-Emili, 1991):

$$\text{Wvisc} = \frac{0.5\pi^2 R_2 V_T^2 f}{(1 + 4\pi^2 f^2 \tau_2^2)} \tag{5}$$

Figure 5 (top) shows that, at $f > 0.15$ Hz, the viscoelastic work per breath for both lung and chest wall decreases with increasing frequency. This is predictable in view of the progressive decrease of ΔR with increasing frequency (see Fig. 4). Figure 5 (bottom) shows the frequency dependence of Wdyn,L, which is the sum of Wvisc and the work attributable to airway resistance (Wres,L). The latter was computed according to the classic equation of Otis et al. (1950):

$$\text{Wres,L} = 0.5\pi^2 K_1 V_T^2 f + 1.33\pi^2 K_2 V_T^3 f^2 \tag{6}$$

where K_1 and K_2 are Rohrer's constants. In computing Wres,L, we used the average values of K_1 and K_2 obtained by D'Angelo et al. (1991) on 18 anesthetized, paralyzed, normal subjects, that is 1.85 cm H_2O s L^{-1} and 0.43 cm H_2O s^2 L^{-2}, respectively. In agreement with the observations on rats by Mount (1955) and on awake humans by Cavagna et al. (1962), at low frequencies, Wvisc,L contributes substantially to Wdyn,L, but its relative contribution becomes negligible at $f > 0.5$

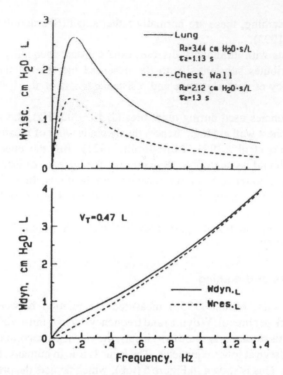

Figure 5 (Top) Relation of viscoelastic component of dynamic work per breathing cycle (Wvisc) of lung and chest wall to respiratory frequency computed according Eq. (5) for tidal volume of 0.47 L, using average values of constants R_2 and τ_2 in Table 1. (Bottom) Relation of total dynamic pulmonary work per breath (Wdyn,L) and airway resistive work (Wres,L) to respiratory frequency. Wres,L was computed according Eq. (6), using the average values of K_1 and K_2 of D'Angelo et al. (1991). Wdyn,L was obtained by adding Wvisc,L to Wres,L. (From D'Angelo et al., 1991.)

Hz. Figure 5 (bottom) also shows that, at low frequencies, the relation between Wdyn,L and f cannot be described simply in terms of Eq. (6), as pointed out by Mount (1955). Neglecting Rint,w (see under Section III.A on the partitioning of Rint), the viscoelastic work of the chest wall (see Fig. 5, top) should reflect its total dynamic work. However, during volume cycling there may be some additional dynamic work attributable to plastoelastic mechanisms, as reflected by differences in static elastic recoil pressures of the lung and chest wall between lung inflation and deflation (i.e., the so-called quasistatic hysteresis). However, with low tidal volumes, such as those used in Figure 5 (0.47 L), this work component should be very small (Shardonofsky et al., 1990; Jonson et al., 1993).

Although the viscoelastic properties of the lung and chest wall appear to contribute appreciably to the total dynamic work only at relatively low frequencies, their contribution to elastic work should increase progressively with increasing frequency, reflecting the increase of dynamic elastance with increasing frequency (see Fig. 3).

C. Expiratory Flow

Although the dynamic work attributable to airway resistance represents energy that is dissipated as heat, part of the elastic energy stored during inspiration in springs E_2 can be recovered during expiration to overcome expiratory airway resistance. Indeed, at $f > 0.5$ Hz, virtually all of the elastic energy stored in springs E_2 during inspiration should be available as expiratory-driving pressure (see Fig. 3). Thus, during increased ventilation (e.g., muscular exercise), some of the requirements for increased expiratory flow rates are intrinsically met by the increase in $E_{dyn,L}$ and $E_{dyn,W}$ because of the higher frequencies. Since the elastic energy stored in the lung and chest wall is greater with rapid than with slow inspirations, lung deflation should be faster following rapid inflation. Augmentation of the expiratory-driving pressure through a viscoelastic mechanism was originally described by Mortola et al. (1985), who found that passive lung deflation was slower if the expiration was preceded by an end-inspiratory hold. This phenomenon, which has been confirmed in several subsequent studies (Eissa et al., 1991b; Guérin et al., 1993), can be readily explained by the fact that, during end-inspiratory hold, the effective elastic recoil pressures of the lung and chest wall decrease progressively owing to stress relaxation. Indeed, as shown in Figure 1, the peak expiratory flow after a 5-s end-inspiratory breathhold was substantially less than during the preceding control expiration in which there was no end-inspiratory hold.

Viscoelastic mechanisms have important effects both on relaxed expiration and on forced expiratory maneuvers.

Relaxed Expiration

The first mechanical model of the respiratory system was introduced by Otis and associates (1950). It consisted of a single compartment of constant elastance (E_{rs}) served by a pathway of constant resistance (R_{rs}) and, hence, is characterized by a single time constant ($\tau_{rs} = R_{rs}/E_{rs}$). From this model, Brody (1954) theorized that the time-course of volume (V) during passive expiration should be described by a single exponential function:

$$V(t) = V_0 \cdot e^{-t/\tau_{rs}} \tag{7}$$

where t is time and V_0 is initial volume above the relaxation volume of the respiratory system.

Equation 7 is the kernel of various methods for measurement of respiratory mechanics, such as that based on the addition of known expiratory resistances (McIlroy et al., 1963) and the "single-breath method" of Zin et al. (1982). However,

Bates et al. (1985) have shown that, in anesthetized, paralyzed dogs, the time course of volume during passive expiration following inflation with a 5-s breathhold, can better be described in terms of a double-exponential function:

$$V(t) = A \cdot e^{-t/\tau'} + B \cdot e^{-t/\tau''} \tag{8}$$

This behavior, which was attributed to viscoelastic mechanisms, has also been observed in normal, anesthetized, paralyzed humans (Chelucci et al., 1991). With a different approach, Jonson et al. (1993) have also concluded that the time course of volume decay during passive expiration in anesthetized, paralyzed, normal humans can be adequately explained by the viscoelastic model in Figure 2. It should be stressed that τ' is a complex parameter that does not correspond to τrs in Eq. (7) (Bates et al., 1986; 1988a). Similarly, τ'' does not correspond to τ_2 (= R_2/E_2). At any rate, these results, together with Eq. (8) indicate that respiratory mechanics cannot be readily assessed during relaxed expiration.

Forced Expiration

Figure 3 implies that, under dynamic conditions, the effective elastic recoil pressure of the lung can exceed the static elastic pressure as a result of the additional elastic pressure (ΔP_L) stored in spring E_2,L (see Fig. 2). Therefore, the maximal flows during forced expiration should be greater when the maneuver is perfomed following a rapid lung inflation (with a concomitant increase in ΔP_L) and without an end-inspiratory pause (to avoid dissipation of this energy into dashpot R_2,L), than after a slow inflation or forced expiration preceded by an end-inspiratory pause. This has been confirmed recently in experiments on normal humans (D'Angelo et al., 1993). As shown by the example in Figure 6, expiratory flows were lower during forced expired vital capacity (FVC) maneuver, following a slow inspiration with a 5-s end-inspiratory pause than after a rapid inspiration without an end-inspiratory pause.

D. Total Elastance and Resistance

Otis et al. (1950) introduced a single-compartment model of the respiratory system that consisted of a constant elastance (E) served by a pathway of constant flow resistance (R). It is based on the assumption that the mechanical properties of the respiratory system are independent of lung volume and flow, and that inertial factors are negligible. Accordingly, the single-compartment mechanical model could be represented by a single first-order differential equation:

$$P(t) = EV(t) + R\dot{V}(t) \tag{9}$$

where at any instant t, $P(t)$ is the forcing pressure that produces volume displacement $V(t)$ from the relaxation volume and instantaneous flow $\dot{V}(t)$. The model has been used in several studies to predict various aspects of respiratory dynamics and to compute the elastance and resistance of the respiratory system (see Otis, 1964). A

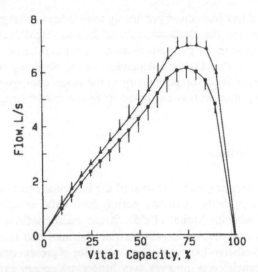

Figure 6 Mean values of expiratory flow obtained in a subjet during forced expired vital capacity maneuvers following slow inspirations with end-inspiratory pause (squares) and rapid inspirations without end-inspiratory pause (triangles). Each point is the mean of 11–15 measurements. Bars are SD. (Modified from D'Angelo et al., 1993.)

similar equation forms the basis of the "elastic subtraction method" for determining pulmonary resistance (R) and elastance (E) (Mead and Whittenberger, 1953). In a variety of ways, this method has been, and still is, commonly used to determine RL and EL (see Peslin et al., 1992). However, during slow breathing, RL and EL should include substantial viscoelastic contributions, which are very sensitive to quite small changes in respiratory frequency (see Fig. 3) and duration of inspiration (D'Angelo et al., 1989, 1991, 1992). Thus, unless the breathing pattern is fixed, the values of elastance and resistance obtained with the foregoing methods are not comparable. In short, owing to viscoelastic behavior (see Fig. 2) in the low-frequency range, the resistance and elastance of the lung and chest wall, and, hence, also Rrs and Edyn,rs, represent "lumped" values that are highly time-dependent. By contrast, at frequencies above 0.5 Hz, the viscoelastic contributions to Rrs become negligible, whereas Edyn,rs approaches a fixed value (= Est,rs + E_2,rs), as shown in Figure 3. In other words, at f > 0.5 Hz the respiratory system effectively behaves as a single-compartment system, consisting of an essentially fixed elastance served by Rint,rs = Raw + Rint,w. Accordingly, for f > 0.5 Hz, Eq. (9) can be rewritten:

$$P(t) = (Ers,st + E_2,rs) \, V(t) + (Raw + Rint,w)\dot{V}(t) \tag{10}$$

Since Raw is flow-dependent [see Eq. (2)], Eq. (10) can be rewritten into:

$$P(t) = (Ers,st + E_2,rs) \, V(t) + (Rint,w + K_1)\dot{V}(t) + K_2\dot{V}(t)^2$$

These equations differ from those previously used (Mead and Agostoni, 1964; Otis, 1964) mainly because the elastance includes E_2,rs. Viscoelastic behavior has not been taken into account in the past because, in normal lungs, the distribution of ventilation was considered to be independent of the breathing frequency, whereas the frequency-dependence of pulmonary compliance and resistance observed in patients with lung disease was attributed to time-constant inequality (Otis et al., 1956; Mead, 1961).

V. Conclusions

In recent years, there has been a revival of the interrupter technique, which can be applied in different body positions during both tidal breathing and increased ventilation. In line with Mount (1955), it has been confirmed that viscoelastic mechanisms confer frequency-dependence of elastance and resistance to the lung and chest wall. Resistive-like viscoelastic behavior is present only at relatively low respiratory frequencies and involves very little extra energy expenditure from the respiratory muscles. In contrast, the increase in pulmonary and chest wall elastance with increasing respiratory frequency implies substantially increased inspiratory elastic work of breathing. As a result of viscoelastic behavior (1) the time course of volume during the passive expiration is characterized by a biexponential, rather than by a monoexponential function, and (2) the maximal expiratory flows are markedly dependent on the previous volume history of the lungs.

References

Agostoni, E., and Fenn, W. O. (1960). Velocity of muscle shortening as a limiting factor in respiratory air flow. *J. Appl. Physiol.* 15: 349–353.

Auler, J. O. C., Jr., Zin, W. A., Caldeira, M. P. R., Cardoso, W. V., and Saldiva, P. H. N. (1987). Pre- and postoperative inspiratory mechanics in ischemic and valvular heart disease. *Chest* 92: 984–990.

Barnas, G. M., Yoshiro, K., Loring, S. T. L., and Mead, J. (1987). Impedance and relative displacements of relaxed chest wall up to 4 Hz. *J. Appl. Physiol.* 62: 71–81.

Barnas, G. M., Yoshino, K., Stamenovic, D., Kikuchi, Y., Loring, S. H., and Mead, J. (1989). Chest wall impedance partitioned into rib-cage and diaphragm-abdominal pathways. *J. Appl. Physiol.* 66: 350–359.

Bates, J. H. T., and Milic-Emili, J. (1991). The flow interruption technique for measuring respiratory resistance. *J. Crit. Care* 6: 227–238.

Bates, J. H. T., Decramer, M., Chartrand, D., Zin, W. A. Boddener, A., and Milic-Emili, J. (1985). Volume–time profile during relaxed expiration in the normal dog. *J. Appl. Physiol.* 59: 732–737.

Bates, J. H. T., Decramer, M., Chartrand, D., Zin, W. A., Boddener, A., and Milic-Emili, J. (1986). Respiratory resistance with histamine challenge by single-breath and forced oscillation methods. *J. Appl. Physiol.* 61: 873–880.

Bates, J. H. T., Brown, K., and Kochi, T. (1987a). Identifying a model of respiratory mechanics using the interrupter technique. In *Proceedings of the Ninth American Conference I.E.E.E. Engineering Medical Biology Society*, pp. 1802–1803.

Bates, J. H. T., Sly, P. D., Kochi, T., and Martin, J. G. (1987b). The effect of a proximal compliance on interrupter measurements of resistance. *Respir. Physiol.* 70: 301–312.

Bates, J. H. T., Baconnier, P., and Milic-Emili, J. (1988a). A theoretical analysis of interrupter technique for measuring respiratory mechanics. *J. Appl. Physiol.* 64: 2204–2214.

Bates, J. H. T., Ludwig, M. S., Sly, P. D., Brown, K., Martin, J. G., and Fredberg, J. J. (1988b). Interrupter resistance elucidated by alveolar pressure measurement in open-chest normal dogs. *J. Appl. Physiol.* 65: 408–414.

Bates, J. H. T., Abe, T., Romero, P. V., and Sato, J. (1989). Measurement of alveolar pressure in closed chest dogs during flow interruption. *J. Appl. Physiol.* 67: 488–492.

Briscoe, W. A., and DuBois, A. B. (1958). The relationship between airway resistance, airway conductance and lung volume in subjects of different age and body size. *J. Clin. Invest.* 37: 1279–1285.

Brody, A. W. (1954). Mechanical compliance and resistance of the lung–thorax calculated from the flow recorded during passive expiration. *Am. J. Physiol.* 178: 189–196.

Cavagna, G., Brandi, G., Saibene, F., and Torelli, G. (1962). Pulmonary hysteresis. *J. Appl. Physiol.* 17: 51–53.

Chelucci, G. L., Brunet, F., Dall'Ava-Santucci, J., Dhainaut, J. F., Paccaly, D., Armaganidis, A., Milic-Emili, J., and Lockhart, A. (1991). A single-compartment model cannot describe passive expiration in intubated, paralysed humans. *Eur. Respir. J.* 4: 458–464.

D'Angelo, E., Calderini, E., Torri, G., Robatto, F., Bono, D., and Milic-Emili, J. (1989). Respiratory mechanics in anesthetized-paralyzed humans: Effects of flow, volume and time. *J. Appl. Physiol.* 67: 2556–2564.

D'Angelo, E., Robatto, F. M., Calderini, E., Tavola, M., Bono, D., Torri, G., and Milic-Emili, J. (1991). Pulmonary and chest wall mechanics in anesthetized paralyzed humans. *J. Appl. Physiol.* 70: 2602–2610.

D'Angelo, E., Calderini, E., Tavola, M., Bono, D., and Milic-Emili, J. (1992). Effect of PEEP on respiratory mechanics in anesthetized paralyzed humans. *J. Appl. Physiol.* 73: 1736–1742.

D'Angelo, E., Prandi, E., and Milic-Emili, J. (1993). Dependence of maximal flow–volume curves on time-course of preceding inspiration. *J. Appl. Physiol.* 75: 1155–1159.

D'Angelo, E., Prandi, E., Tavola, M., Calderini, E., and Milic-Emili, L. (1994). Chest wall interrupter resistance in anesthetized paralyzed subjects. *J. Appl. Physiol.* 77: 883–887.

DuBois, A. B., Botelho, S. Y., and Comroe, J. H., Jr. (1956). A new method for measuring airway resistance in man using a body plethysmograph: values in normal subjects and in patients with respiratory disease. *J. Clin. Invest.* 35: 322–326.

Eissa, N. T., Ranieri, V. M., Corbeil, C., Chassé, M., Braidy, J., and Milic-Emili, J. (1991a). Effects of positive end-expiratory pressure, lung volume, and inspiratory flow on interrupter resistance in patients with adult respiratory distress syndrome. *Am. Rev. Respir. Dis.* 144: 538–543.

Eissa, N. T., Ranieri, V. M., Corbeil, C., Chassé, M., Robatto, F. M., Braidy, J., and Milic-Emili, J. (1991b). Analysis of behavior of the respiratory system in ARDS patients: Effects of flow, volume, and time. *J. Appl. Physiol.* 70: 2719–2729.

Fredberg, J. J., and Stamenovic, D. (1989). On the imperfect elasticity of lung tissue. *J. Appl. Physiol.* 67: 2408–2419.

Grimby, G., Takishima, T., Graham, W., Macklem, P., and Mead, J. (1968). Frequency dependence of flow resistance in patients with obstructive lung disease. *J. Clin. Invest.* 47: 1455–1465.

Guérin, C., Coussa, M.-L., Eissa, N. T., Corbeil, C., Chassé, M., Braidy, J., Matar, N., and Milic-Emili, J. (1993). Lung and chest wall mechanics in mechanically ventilated COPD patients. *J. Appl. Physiol.* 74: 1570–1580.

Hantos, Z., Daroczy, B., Suki, B., Galgoczy, G., and Csendes, T. (1986). Forced oscillatory impedance of the respiratory system at low frequencies. *J. Appl. Physiol.* 60: 123–132.

Hesser, C. M., Linnarsson, D., and Fagraeus, L. (1981). Pulmonary mechanics and work of breathing at maximal ventilation and raised air pressure. *J. Appl. Physiol.* 50: 747–753.

Hildebrandt, J. (1970). Pressure–volume data of cat lung interpreted by a plastoelastic linear viscoelastic model. *J. Appl. Physiol.* 28: 365–372.

Hoppin, F. G., Stothert, J. C., Greaves, I. A., Lai, Y.-L., and Hilderbrandt, J. (1986). Lung recoil: Elastic and rheological properties. In *Handbook of Physiology*, Section 3, The Respiratory System, Mechanics of Breathing, Vol. 3. Bethesda, MD, American Physiological Society, pp. 195–216.

Jaeger, M. J. (1982). Effect of the cheeks and the compliance of alveolar gas on the measurement of respiratory variables. *Respir. Physiol.* 47: 325–340.

Jaeger, M. J., and Otis, A. B. (1964). Effects of compressibility of alveolar gas on dynamics and work of breathing. *J. Appl. Physiol.* 19: 83–91.

Jonson, B., Beydon, L., Brauer, K., Manson, C., Valid, S., and Grytzell, H. (1993). Mechanics of respiratory system in healthy anesthetized humans with emphasis on viscoelastic properties. *J. Appl. Physiol.* 75: 132–140.

Kochi, T., Okubo, S., Zin, W. A., and Milic-Emili, J. (1988) Chest wall and respiratory system mechanics in cats: Effects of flow and volume. *J. Appl. Physiol.* 64: 2636–2646.

Liistro, G. D., Stanescu, D., Rodenstein, D., and Veriter, C. (1989). Reassessment of the interruption technique for measuring flow resistance in humans. *J. Appl. Physiol.* 67: 933–937.

McIlroy, M. B., Tierney, D. F., and Nadel, J. A. (1963). A new method of measurement of compliance and resistance of lungs and thorax. *J. Appl. Physiol.* 18: 424–427.

Mead, J. (1956). Measurement of inertia of the lungs at increased ambient pressure. *J. Appl. Physiol.* 9: 208–212.

Mead, J. (1961). Mechanical properties of lungs. *Physiol. Rev.* 41: 281–330.

Mead, J., and Agostoni, E. (1964). Dynamics of breathing. In *Handbook of Physiology*, Section 3, Respiration, vol. 1. Edited by W. O. Fenn and H. Rahn. Washington, DC, American Physiological Society, pp. 411–427.

Mead, J., and Whittenberger, J. L. (1953). Physical properties of human lungs measured during spontaneous respiration. *J. Appl. Physiol.* 5: 779–796.

Mead, J., and Whittenberger, J. L. (1954). Evaluation of airway interruption technique as a method for measuring pulmonary air-flow resistance. *J. Appl. Physiol.* 6: 408–416.

Milic-Emili, J. (1991). Work of breathing. In *The Lung: Scientific Foundations*. Edited by R. G. Crystal, J. B., West, P. J. Barnes, N. S. Cherniack, and E. R. Weibel. New York, Raven Press, pp. 1065–1075.

Mortola, J. P., Magnante, D., and Saetta, M. (1985). Expiratory pattern of newborn mammals. *J. Appl. Physiol.* 58: 528–533.

Mount, L. E. (1955). The ventilation flow-resistance and compliance of rat lungs. *J. Physiol. (Lond.)* 127: 157–167.

Otis, A. B. (1964). The work of breathing. In *Handbook of Physiology*, Section 3. Respiration, Vol. 1. Edited by W. O. Fenn and H. Rahn. Washington, DC, American Physiological Society, pp. 463–476.

Otis, A. B., Fenn, W. O., and Rahn, H. (1950). The mechanics of breathing in man. *J. Appl. Physiol.* 2: 592–607.

Otis, A. B., McKerrow, C. B., Bartlett, R. A., Mead, J. McIlroy, M. B., Selverstone, N. J., and Radford, E. P. (1956). Mechanical factors in distribution of pulmonary ventilation. *J. Appl. Physiol.* 8: 427–443.

Peslin, R., Felicio da Silva, J., Chabot, F., and Duvivier, C. (1992). Respiratory mechanics studied by multiple linear regression in unsedated ventilated patients. *Eur. Respir. J.* 5: 871–878.

Rahn, H., Otis, A. B., Chadwick, L. E., and Fenn, W. O. (1946). The pressure–volume diagram of the thorax and lung. *Am. J. Physiol.* 146: 161–178.

Rodarte, J. R., and Rehder, K. (1986). Dynamics of respiration. In *Handbook of Physiology*, Section 3. The Respiratory System, Vol. 3, Mechanics of Breathing. Edited by P. T. Macklem and J. Mead. Washington, DC, American Physiological Society, pp. 131–144.

Rohrer, F. (1915). Der Stromungswiderstand in den menschlichen Atemwegen und der Einfluss der unregelmassigen Verzweigung des Bronchialsystems auf den Atmungsverlaud verschiedenen Lungenbezirken. *Arch. Gesamte Physiol. Mens. Tiere* 162: 225–299.

Rohrer, F. (1925). Physiologie der Atembewegung. In *Handbuch der normalen und pathologischen Physiologie*, Vol. 2. Edited by A. T. J. Bethe, G. von Bergmann, G. Embden, and A. Ellinger. Berlin, Springer-Verlag, pp. 70–127.

Saldiva, P. H. N., Zin, W. A., Santos, R. L. B., Eidelman, D. H., and Milic-Emili, J. (1992). Alveolar pressure measurement in open-chest rats. *J. Appl. Physiol.* 72: 302–306.

Shardonofsky, F. R., Sato, J., and Bates, J. H. T. (1990). Quasi-static pressure–volume hysteresis in the canine respiratory system in vivo. *J. Appl. Physiol.* 68: 2230–2236.

Shardonofsky, F. R., Skaburskis, M., Sato, J., Zin, W. A., and Milic-Emili, J. (1991). Effects of volume history and vagotomy on pulmonary and chest wall mechanics in cats. *J. Appl. Physiol.* 71: 498–508.

Similowski, T., Levy, P., Corbeil, C., Albala, M., Pariente, R., Derenne, J. P., Bates, J. H. T., Jonson, B., and Milic-Emili, J. (1989). Viscoelastic behavior of lung and chest wall in dogs determined by flow interruption. *J. Appl. Physiol.* 67: 2219–2229.

von Neergaard, K., and Wirz, K. (1927). Die Messung der Strömungswiederstande in der Atemwege des Menschen, insbesondere bein Asthma und Emphysema. Z. Klin. Med. 195: 51–82.

Zin, W. A., Pengelly, L. D., and Milic-Emili, J. (1982). Single-breath method for measurement of respiratory system mechanics in anesthetized animals. *J. Appl. Physiol.* 52: 1266–1271.

18

Kinematics of the Chest Wall

MICHAEL E. WARD

McGill University
Montreal, Quebec, Canada

PETER T. MACKLEM

Respiratory Health Network of Centres
  of Excellence
McGill University
Montreal, Quebec, Canada

I. Introduction

Kinematics is the branch of mechanics that deals with pure motion without reference to the masses or forces involved. We define the *chest wall* as those parts of the body that surround the lung and that move with breathing. The chest wall consists of two parts, the rib cage and abdomen, the motion of which can be observed and measured. Chest wall kinematics has, therefore, primarily been concerned with measuring rib cage and abdominal motion. The term kinematics, however, also applies to the theory of mechanical mechanisms for converting one kind of motion to another. Since the chest wall may be considered a mechanical contrivance for converting one kind of motion (shortening of the respiratory muscles) to another (ventilation of the lungs), a complete understanding of the topic requires knowledge of how shortening of individual respiratory muscles is converted into rib cage and abdominal motion, and how this, in turn, influences the shape and volume of the lungs.

Failure of the chest wall to efficiently perform its function will limit ventilation and, therefore, survival, despite normal lung and respiratory muscle function. A change in chest wall shape away from the minimum energy configuration during inspiration increases the energy required for its inflation (Agostoni, 1964; Goldman et al., 1973). In addition to influencing the work of inflation directly, changes in

515

the function of the chest wall may alter the manner in which the ventilatory muscles interact with each other (Zocchi et al., 1987). Shifts of the ventilatory load to a part of the system not designed to accommodate it will hasten the development of respiratory failure. Dynamic alterations of the configuration of the chest wall during breathing also change the pattern of intrapulmonary gas flow, potentially interfering with gas exchange (Liu et al., 1990).

Despite the central role of the chest wall in maintaining ventilation, our understanding of the kinematics of the chest wall and the mechanisms responsible for its efficient functioning has evolved slowly. This has largely been due to the difficulty in making direct measurements in human subjects. The difficulty in recording chest wall motion arises from two sources. First, the motion of the chest wall is complex; the rib cage is easily distorted and rarely moves as a compartment with a single degree of freedom (Ward et al., 1992) and, during abdominal muscle contraction, the shape of the abdomen depends on which particular abdominal muscles are active. Second, dynamic recordings introduce problems related to the frequencies over which measurement devices must be able to respond; inadequate frequency response characteristics lead to loss of the signal. Devices adequate for recording static dimensions, therefore, have proved unsuitable for recording dimensions that are continuously changing (see Chap. 36). In addition, since the shape of the rib cage reflects the loads to which it is subjected during locomotion as well as by environmental factors, there exists marked interspecies variation in rib cage shape (Krahl, 1986). The mechanical properties of the human rib cage reflect influences unique to human environmental adaptation; therefore, an acceptable animal model is not available, eliminating an important source of experimental data on which to base theoretical analyses.

II. Movement of the Ribs

There has long been disagreement about the manner in which the ribs move. For many years it was accepted that each rib moved around the axis of its neck (Luciani, 1911; Ganong, 1965; Pean et al. 1991). Others challenged this view and postulated that a second axis of rotation was necessary to explain the motion of the ribs as visualized radiographically. This rotation was hypothesized to be on either an anteroposterior axis (Campbell, 1958; Last, 1959), to account for the "bucket-handle" motion (angle α, Fig. 1), or a vertical axis (Polgar, 1949; Grant et al., 1965), to account for the "pump-handle" motion (angle β, Fig. 1) of the rib cage. The controversy becomes even more complex when the anatomical differences among ribs is considered. The costal cartilage of the first rib is far stiffer than that of the rest of the ribs and is attached to the sternum by means of a primary cartilaginous, rather than synovial joint (Warwick et al., 1980). As a result, the first costal ring moves as a rigid body, with rotation about the manubriosternal joint and with some translation at the first costovertebral joint (Haines, 1946; Saumarez, 1986b). It is

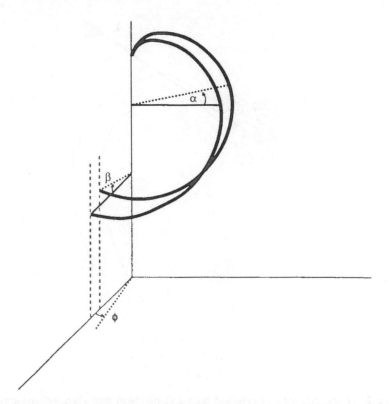

Figure 1 Three-dimensional representation of rib motion. Angle α is subtended by the arc describing the bucket-handle motion and angle β by that describing the pump-handle motion of the rib. Angle ϕ is the angle formed between the sagittal plane and a line between the anterior rib end and the costovertebral joint.

also recognized that the lower six ribs have different articulations than the upper six ribs (Warwick et al., 1980) and are less intimately associated with the sternum, owing to their long costal cartilages. These differences in their mechanical constraints suggest that the upper and lower ribs are likely to differ in the manner in which they move during the respiratory cycle.

The issue appeared resolved when Jordanoglou (1969, 1970) performed vector analysis of the motion of points fixed to the skin overlying the ribs. During tidal breathing, the spatial vectors for different points along a given rib were found to be almost parallel, indicating that the most important movement of the ribs is monoaxial rotation around the costal neck (Fig. 2). The vectors were parallel down to the ninth rib, suggesting that this pattern of movement applied equally to the upper and lower ribs. Greater lateral expansion of the lower ribs than of the upper ribs was observed and attributed to the more posterior angulation of the necks of the lower ribs (Agostoni, 1964; Jordanoglou, 1969). Saumarez (1986c) has recently

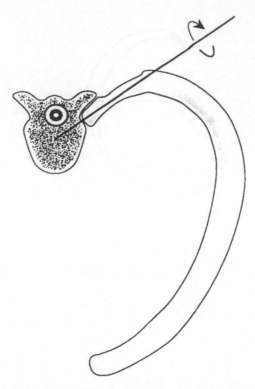

Figure 2 Transverse view of vertebral body and rib. Note that when the costotransverse joint is not oriented perpendicular to the sagittal plane (it is actually oriented anteriorly, superiorly, and medially), monoaxial rotation about the rib neck (axis a) would necessitate lateral translation of the anterior rib end and an increase in the angle ϕ. This motion is severely restricted for the upper ribs because of their attachments to the sternum.

pointed out, however, that rotation on a single axis, with the restriction that the sternocostal junction remains in the sagittal plane, requires the axis to be perpendicular to that plane. This creates an inconsistency, since at least some of the costal necks are not perpendicular to the sagittal plane. A posterior angulation of the rib neck so that the angle between it and the sagittal plane is greater than 90° will lead to the lateral and anterior parts of the rib moving away from the midline when the neck rotates (see angle ϕ, Fig. 1). The movement of a point on such a rib will describe a plane inclined to the sagittal and requires an axis of rotation normal to this second plane. The rib ends, therefore, would have to rotate about an axis that is not parallel to that around which the lateral aspect of the rib rotates.

From a detailed analysis of the geometry of the upper six ribs, vertebrae, costovertebral joints, and sternum, Saumarez (1986c) fit the ribs systematically through a wide range of motion, subject to the constraints imposed by the anatomy of the costovertebral and costotransverse joints and the requirement that the rib tip fit the sternum. The degree of misfit at the costovertebral joints was calculated as the volume between the displaced joint surfaces and the vertebral facets. The path of minimum costovertebral joint misfit was found to correspond to simultaneous rotation about the axis of the costotransverse joint and about an axis oriented perpendicular to the vector normal to the two costovertebral facets that compose the remaining articulations of each costovertebral joint. Deviation from this path requires a further axis oriented 90° to the first two axes. Rotation about this axis would involve a large degree of misfit at the costovertebral and costotransverse joint surfaces, suggesting that only small deviations are likely to be tolerated (Fig. 3). This investigator hypothesized that the path of minimum misfit may correspond to the relaxation characteristic of the rib cage. Respiratory muscle contraction may distort the rib cage from this path at the expense of increasing misfit at these joints.

Wilson et al. (1987) subsequently measured the three-dimensional coordinates of points on ribs 3–7 in two subjects relaxed at functional residual capacity (FRC) and at total lung capacity (TLC) by spatial reconstruction of computed tomographic

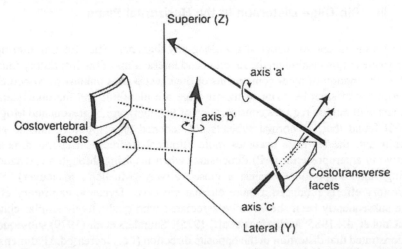

Figure 3 Schematic diagram of rib motion relative to the vertebral body. The articulation between the rib and the vertebra consists of three facets, the costotransverse joint and the two costovertebral surfaces. Rotation around axes a and b corresponds to the motion calculated to result in minimum misfit at the articular surfaces. Rotation about axis a (the axis of the costotransverse joint) would cause the rib end to move upward and laterally. Simultaneous rotation about a second axis, axis b (the axis at right angles to the vectors normal to the costovertebral facets) is required if the rib tip is to remain in contact with the sternum. A further axis of rotation (axis c), perpendicular to axes a and b, was postulated to permit deviation from the trajectory of minimum misfit. Such rotation would result in inferior movement of the tip of the rib and superior movement of its lateral border. (Adapted from Saumarez, 1986a.)

(CT) images. They found that the plane of these ribs at TLC could be described by rotation of the plane at FRC around an axis angled approximately 35° to the midsagittal plane. The radii of the rotational arcs required to fit the data at TLC, however, were larger than those at FRC, also suggesting the necessity for an additional axis of rotation.

Kenyon et al. (1991) have presented a model that incorporates these details. In this model, the ribs are represented as curves and described mathematically as polynomials. They are positioned by the polar coordinates of the costochondral joint relative to the rib (pump-handle motion) and the amount of rotation about the line of the costochondral joint (bucket-handle motion). A further axis of rotation in the vertical plane accounts for outward rib displacement for ribs not attached directly to the sternum or manubrium. Comparison of plots generated by the computer model with the actual radiographs showed errors approaching the limits of radiographic resolution for the orientation of the ribs and the positions of the vertebrae, sternum, and manubrium. The predictive value of the model was, furthermore, not altered following midline sternotomy.

III. Rib Cage Distortion in the Horizontal Plane

The rib cage is able to change shape along any diameter. The effect of altering rib cage shape in this fashion on the function and interactions of the inspiratory muscles and on the motion of other components of the chest wall is unknown. Nonetheless, descriptions of such behavior of the rib cage are plentiful, and the understanding of chest wall motion requires consideration of this literature. Agostoni and Mognoni (1966) found that, in normal subjects not coached on respiratory muscle group recruitment, the rib cage becomes more elliptical (increase in lateral dimension relative to anteroposterior (AP) dimension) when inspiring through a resistance or during static inspirations against a closed airway (Mueller's maneuver). Static expiratory efforts produced a more circular rib cage. Dynamic expiratory efforts have subsequently been shown to be associated with qualitatively similar changes (McCool et al., 1985; Melissinos et al., 1975). Saunders et al. (1979) subsequently demonstrated that distortion in the opposite direction (i.e., increased AP dimensions relative to lateral dimension) occurred if the maneuver were performed primarily with the rib cage intercostal and accessory muscles. Sampson and Detroyer (1982) measured the AP rib cage diameter at the level of the fourth interspace and the lateral rib cage diameter at the level of the sixth interspace. They found that subjects could be subdivided on the basis of whether they recruited their parasternal muscles in response to the imposition of inspiratory resistive or to elastic loads. Those in whom no increase in parasternal electromyograph (EMG) activity was recorded experienced deformation of the rib cage, with an increase in lateral relative to AP diameter. Subjects who recruited their parasternal muscles maintained the normal rib cage shape. In addition, Ringel et al. (1985) demonstrated that the voluntary emphasis of particular muscle groups can result in different patterns of movement in a given subject. A given change in rib cage shape, therefore, may be as much a result of behavioral influences as it is of automatic compensatory adjustments in the pattern of respiratory muscle activation. McCool et al. (1985) measured the AP and lateral diameters of the lower rib cage during quiet breathing, rebreathing, reading, and during various voluntary respiratory maneuvers. They also concluded that changes in pleural pressure over the surface of the lung apposed rib cage shape cannot be the only determinant of rib cage shape. In addition to different direct actions of the inflationary muscles, however, they suggest that differing changes in abdominal pressure may accompany different patterns of respiratory muscle recruitment. This may contribute to the shape of the lower rib cage by changing the pleural pressure in the zone of diaphragmatic apposition.

IV. Movement of the Spine

Vertical displacements of the rib cage partly depend on the movement of the ribs and partly on extension and flexion of the vertebral column. Mead et al. (1985) demonstrated that flexion and extension of the spine could produce changes in chest wall volume equivalent to approximately one-half of the vital capacity. They argued, however, that such movements of the spine probably do not contribute importantly to changes in lung volume, since expansion of the chest wall axially is accompanied by simultaneous inward displacement of the of the rib cage and anterior abdominal wall. During breathing efforts, changes in the attitude of the spine appear to occur mainly at high lung volumes. For example, Wade (1954) found vertical displacement of the xiphisternal junction to occur mainly near TLC, and Agostoni et al. (1965) found the vertical distance between the rib cage and pelvis to increase by about 4 cm over the inspiratory capacity, with the greatest changes occurring at large lung volumes. Elevation of the ribs during inspiration in the absence of spinal extension will result in progressive misfit of the chondrosternal joints, since the ribs are of different lengths and their relation to each other will change as they rise. Saumarez (1986a) has calculated the degree of misfit at the chondrosternal junction and found that by rotating the vertebral bodies in the sagittal plan, a position can be found that allows the tips of the costal cartilages to fit their chondrosternal joints perfectly. Kenyon et al. (1991) found the angle subtended by the spine to change by 12° from RV to TLC. This angle change was restricted after sternotomy and contributed, along with reduced rib motion, to the postoperative change in vital capacity. Spinal mobility, therefore, appears to be important in the normal functioning of the chest wall.

V. Movement of the Diaphragm

Measurements of the movement of the diaphragm relative to the rib cage have been made since the advent of radiography. Wade (1954) found the displacement of the diaphragmatic dome to average 9.5 cm standing and supine over the vital capacity, with displacements of 5.5 and 7.7 cm over the inspiratory capacity and tidal displacements of 1.5 and 1.7 cm standing and supine, respectively.

Motion and shape are tightly linked. Marshall (1962) proposed that the diaphragm converts force into pressure according to the law of Laplace, by which the pressure differences across a curved membrane is related to the tension within the membrane and its radii of curvature. At low lung volumes, the diaphragmatic radius would be small; therefore, a given tension would result in a substantially greater transdiaphragmatic pressure than at higher lung volumes, when the radius of curvature was large. Although Marshall's ideas gave fresh insight into the relation between diaphragmatic force and function, there are several problems about the role of the Laplace law in the relations between diaphragmatic shape, force development, and its conversion to transdiaphragmatic pressure.

The first problem is that the determinants of diaphragmatic shape are poorly understood. Whitelaw (1987) found that the relaxed human diaphragmatic radius of curvature was greater at the apex than at the sides, consistent with more dependent regions being exposed to a hydrostatic gradient in abdominal pressure and a smaller, gravitationally determined, gradient in pleural pressure. This author proposed that, with contraction, the ratio of transdiaphragmatic pressure to force would tend to remain constant, rather than diminish as volume increased, because under these conditions, the radius of the apex in coronal section would diminish, whereas that at the sides would increase. This would be true if free fluid were in contact with the diaphragm on both sides. The abdominal contents, however, are not a fluid and neither is the lung. Although there is a gravitationally determined gradient in abdominal pressure that is close to hydrostatic, regional changes in abdominal pressure are not well transmitted and are not everywhere equal (Decramer et al., 1984b). The inequality (which is static) must be due to elastic elements under tension within the abdomen, preventing the transmission of pressure. Therefore, the abdominal contents do not behave as a fluid. Neither do the lungs. The shear modulus of the lung, which determines how easy it is to deform, may be sufficiently low at low lung volumes that the lung does not impose its shape on the diaphragm. With increasing lung volume, however, the shear modulus increases monotonically, and it appears likely that, at high volumes, the lung does impose its shape on the diaphragm. Paiva et al. (1992) found that the three-dimensional shape of the dorsal half of the human diaphragm in supine subjects relaxed at functional residual capacity, as determined by magnetic resonance imaging (Fig. 4), could be explained by the Laplace law. At higher lung volumes at which the lung is difficult to distort, however, the diaphragm does not conform to the shape predicted by the Laplace law.

A second problem is related to the nature of the contracted diaphragm. Two assumptions are implicit in the application of the Laplace law to relate diaphragmatic shape to function. The first is that the contracted diaphragm does not resist bending. There are no published data on the bending moment of the contracted diaphragm,

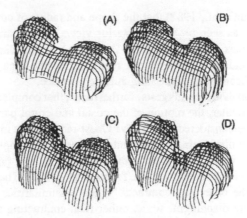

Figure 4 Three-dimensional reconstruction of diaphragm of four subjects using magnetic resonance imaging. (A), (B), (C), and (D) represent images from different subjects. (Adapted from Paiva et al., 1992.)

although preliminary findings (Gauthier et al., personal communication) indicate that in vitro diaphragmatic strips bent at a slight angle, but otherwise unrestricted, show no tendency to straighten when stimulated. The other implicit assumption is that both the relaxed and the contracted diaphragm are isotropic. It seems inherently unlikely that the stress–strain characteristics of the diaphragm, either active or passive, are the same in the direction of the fibers, compared with the orthogonal direction. Furthermore, Pean et al. (1991) have demonstrated, using radiopaque markers and biplane cinefluorography in dogs, that shortening varies along different axes of measurement, and that regional variations in area change during contraction were primarily due to differences in length change perpendicular to the major axis of shortening.

Finally, much of the surface of the diaphragm is in the area of its apposition to the rib cage where the fibers run axially and the application of the Laplace law is unclear. Most of the change in diaphragmatic area during contraction occurs in this region. The surface in contact with the rib cage diminishes markedly between functional residual capacity and total lung capacity, whereas the surface area and shape of the lung-apposed diaphragm changes little. This observation forms the basis for the second school of thought concerning diaphragmatic motion: that the diaphragm behaves as a piston, with most of the fiber shortening occurring in the axial direction, peeling off the inner surface of the rib cage while maintaining its cylindrical shape as it descends. This proposal was supported by the findings of Kim et al. (1976), who calculated the radius of diaphragmatic curvature from the ratio of tension (strain gauge) to transdiaphragmatic pressure during diaphragmatic contraction in dogs. Little change occurred in this parameter up to a lung volume 600 cm^3 above functional residual capacity. It is also compatible with later observations (Braun et al., 1982) that the shape and radius of curvature of the dome of the diaphragm, as seen on anteroposterior views, is unchanged during its tidal descent. Nevertheless, not all the force developed by the diaphragm is directed axially, because muscle fibers are not restricted to the area of apposition, but constitute a significant area of the lung-apposed surface.

Experimental evidence suggests, furthermore, that complex patterns of motion may occur. In particular, the motion of the costal and crural parts of the diaphragm should probably be considered separately. Chest radiographs in supine dogs reveal a dorsal and caudal displacement of the anterior part of the diaphragm during costal contraction and a ventral and caudal displacement of the posterior part of the diaphragm during crural contraction (DeTroyer et al., 1982). The relaxed part moves very little when the other part contracts. These dissimilarities are relevant to the motion of the entire diaphragm, since, rather than contracting as a unit, these two muscles differ in the timing and extent of their contraction. Crural shortening has been noted to be greater than that of the costal part during tidal breathing (Newman et al., 1984), hypercapnia (Road et al., 1986), and airway occlusion (Easton et al., 1987), and Easton et al. (1987) found crural shortening to predominate at the onset of inspiration. Furthermore, the mechanical linkage between these parts appears to change with changes in lung volume (Decramer et al., 1984a). Pean et al. (1991) found diaphragmatic area to decrease during contraction in the crural and midcostal regions. In contrast, near the central tendon and the rib cage insertions, the area decreased to a much smaller extent and even occasionally increased.

Although the foregoing experiments were performed on dogs, asymmetrical contraction patterns are also evident from fluoroscopic studies in humans. Verschakelen et al. (1989) found axial descent of the diaphragm to be greatest at its posterior aspect and least for its anterior section. Froese and Bryan (1974) reported that nondependent regions descended preferentially during passive inflation, when the diaphragm was paralyzed, whereas, during active inspiration, the dependent regions descended more. More detailed information concerning the shape of the diaphragm is available in one subject during static breath holds at functional residual capacity and 1 L above this volume (Whitelaw et al., 1989). These data are considered in detail in Chapter 23. Briefly, the right diaphragm in this subject was longer at rest and shortened more than the left. The posterior aspect of the diaphragm retained its resting two-humped shape while in the contracted state, whereas it became tented anteriorly by its attachment to the sternum.

VI. Movement of the Abdomen

The motion of the anterior abdominal wall has generally been observed to conform to its relaxation relation with intra-abdominal pressure, at least during quiet breathing (Grimby et al., 1976; Ward et al., 1992). The tendency for the abdominal wall to maintain its relaxed configuration and the incompressibility of the abdominal contents justified the classic concept that abdominal motion reflects diaphragmatic motion (Grassino et al., 1978; Grimby et al., 1976; Konno et al., 1967). Mead and Loring (1982) have challenged this idea, pointing out that the volume displaced by the diaphragm may be accounted for by the lower rib cage, as well as the free abdominal wall. More recently, Decramer et al. (1986) studied the relation between abdominal cross-sectional area and costal and crural diaphragmatic length in dogs. They found that shortening of the crural, but not the costal, part was correlated with abdominal movement. If the motion of the diaphragm were largely that of a piston, the length of the crural part would be expected to depend on the degree of diaphragmatic descent (and volume displacement). The inspiratory shortening of the costal diaphragm, however, would bear a linear relation to diaphragmatic volume displacement only if the lower rib cage remained immobile, which it does not.

Abdominal muscle contraction, may displace the trajectory of the abdominal wall away from its relaxation relation with abdominal pressure. During strong contraction of the abdominal muscles, the cross section of the abdomen becomes more rounded (Konno and Mead, 1967). Contraction of these muscles during increased ventilation, either voluntarily or by hypercapnia, shifts the relation between lung volume and abdominal anteroposterior diameter to the left (i.e., higher lung volume at a given abdominal diameter) to the extent that, at end-expiration, this dimension approaches values reached at residual volume in some subjects (Agostoni and Torri, 1967).

VII. Integrated Movement of the Chest Wall

The simplest model of chest wall motion, and the first exploited, is a two-compartment system, whereby volume changes must involve expansion of the rib cage compartment, the abdominal compartment, or both. The rib cage and abdomen are assumed to move with only a single degree of freedom (i.e., to conform to their relaxation characteristics). Although this appears to be gross oversimplification, if the ribs are constrained to conform to their path of minimum misfit, the abdomen remains relaxed, and the spinal attitude is fixed (Smith and Mead, 1986), the use of this model is not unreasonable. Konno and Mead (1967) demonstrated that, in fact, these conditions are met over a limited range of volume changes during spontaneous breathing (Fig. 5). This observation allowed measurement of the elastic properties of the rib cage and abdomen (Konno and Mead, 1968) and has formed the basis of most models proposed to explain the actions of the respiratory muscles and their contributions to changes in lung volume (Loring and Mead, 1982; Goldman and Mead, 1973; Macklem et al., 1978, 1982; Hillman and Finucane, 1987; Petroll et al., 1990) (see Chaps. 19 and 22).

The limitations of this approach, however, have long been recognized. Crawford et al. (1983) found the cross-sectional areas of the upper (axilla) and lower (lower costal margin) rib cages to move during quiet breathing in close, but not

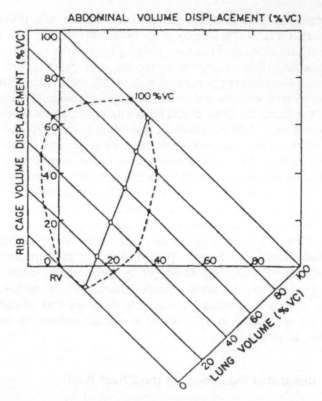

Figure 5 Changes in chest wall configuration described by volumetric displacement of rib cage and abdominal wall in the upright posture. Displacements are expressed as a percentage of the total displacement over the vital capacity (VC) relative to the active state at residual lung volume (RV). Solid lines with open symbols indicate relaxed configuration. Surfaces enclosed by dashed line symbols illustrate a range of possible configurations produced by submaximal contraction of rib cage and abdominal musculature. Constant volume isopleths (solid lines and solid symbols) define displacements at lung volumes indicated. (From Smith and Loring, 1986.)

exact, approximation to their relation at relaxation. McCool et al. (1985) used linearized magnetometers to monitor the relative anteroposterior displacements of the upper (angle of Louis) and lower (fifth rib) rib cages. They found that, although during quiet breathing the relation between these two diameters described a curve close to that during relaxation, the system was easily distorted by changing the muscle groups recruited during inspiration. Isolated contraction of the diaphragm during diaphragm pacing does not drive the rib cage on its passive characteristic (Danon et al., 1979). Recently, electromyographic studies have confirmed that the parasternal intercostal muscles become active during all but the smallest volume changes, and that the absence of rib cage muscle activation alters the inspiratory configuration of the rib cage (DeTroyer and Sampson, 1982; DeTroyer et al., 1984; Sampson et al., 1982). In dogs, Jiang et al. (1984) demonstrated that during isolated diaphragm contraction the relation between the motion of the upper (lung-apposed) rib cage and esophageal pressure and the lower (abdomen-apposed) rib cage and abdominal pressure fell close to their respective relaxation lines. This finding indicates that there is little resistance to bending between rib cage compartments in dogs. The loose mechanical coupling between pulmonary and abdominal rib cage compartments in dogs was confirmed by Krayer et al. (1988), who used dynamic spatial reconstruction of computed tomographic images. Such evidence suggests that unitary behavior of the rib cage is the result of the highly coordinated action of the inspiratory muscles, rather than inherent rigidity. It is apparent, therefore, that further insights into the nature of inspiratory muscle action require more sophisticated models of chest wall motion.

Primiano (1982) developed a model of the chest wall that incorporated a factor to account for changes in the action of the diaphragm on the rib cage caused by varying degrees of rib cage flexibility. Although this permitted description of normal- and paradoxical-breathing patterns, no estimates of the flexibility of the rib cage or any method of determining it was proposed. Agostoni and D'Angelo suggested division of the rib cage into a pulmonary compartment, apposed along its inner surface to the lung (RCp), and an abdominal compartment, apposed along its inner surface to the diaphragm (RCa) (Agostoni et al., 1988). This concept was incorporated into a mathematical model by Ben-Haim and Saidel (1990). Their analysis of chest wall mechanics in adult humans, however, assumes a rigid linkage between rib cage compartments.

A model of chest wall mechanics that incorporates these concepts has recently been presented (Ward et al., 1992). In this model, the human rib cage is divided at the level of the xiphoid process into pulmonary and abdominal compartments (Fig. 6). The characteristics of this model and its implications are discussed in detail in Chapter 16. Briefly, the important inspiratory rib cage muscles were assumed to be the scalenes and parasternal muscles (DeTroyer et al., 1983; DeTroyer, 1991). The former are inserted into ribs 1 and 2; the latter into ribs 2–6, inclusively. These ribs are tightly linked to the sternum by short costal cartilages. The sixth rib attaches to the sternum at its ventral end, and its lower border corresponds to the line dividing the pulmonary from the abdominal compartments. Thus, the direct actions of the major inspiratory rib cage muscles are almost exclusively on RCp. The costal part of the diaphragm originates from the lower end of the sternum and from ribs 7–12, inclusively. These ribs are only loosely linked to the sternum by longer cartilaginous extensions. The area of diaphragmatic apposition to the rib cage (Aap) at functional residual capacity (FRC) extends cranially to about the level of the xiphisternum. Thus, the action of the diaphragm is almost exclusively on RCa. In the seated human, this level corresponds roughly to the top of the zone of diaphragmatic apposition to the rib cage. The intercostal muscles that insert onto RCa are unlikely to have an important effect on inspiratory chest wall motion, at least during quiet

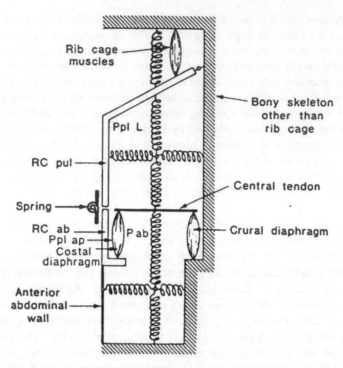

Figure 6 Diagram illustrating the mechanical model of the chest wall incorporating a two-compartment rib cage, the mechanical linkages of the rib cage muscles, the elastic properties of the respiratory system, and the agencies acting to displace and distort the rib cage. For further description see text. (Adapted from Ward et al., 1992.)

breathing or slow inspirations, as they are usually electrically silent during these maneuvers. In humans, the internal intercostal muscles are active only during expiration (Koepke et al., 1958). The external intercostals below the fourth interspace become active late in inspiration with increasing ventilation, but are inactive during quiet breathing (Whitelaw and Feroah, 1989; Koepke et al., 1958; Primiano, 1982; Taylor, 1960), and their inflationary effect decreases caudally (Budzinska et al., 1989). De Troyer and Farkas (1990) found that, even in the cranial interspaces, most of the shortening of the external intercostal muscle could be attributed to the simultaneous contraction of the corresponding parasternal. Motion of the abdomen is assumed to be independent of rib cage motion, as is consistent with available experimental evidence (Boynton et al., 1989).

Figure 6 is a mechanical diagram of the model in lateral projection. The structure shaped like an inverted hockey stick with a detached handle represents the rib cage. The RCp extends to the upper level of the costal fibers and is apposed to the lung. The pressure at its inner surface is the pleural pressure over the surface of the lung PPl,L. With contraction of the rib cage muscles, it is displaced upward and anteriorly, rotating around the hinge at its attachment to the rest of the bony skeleton. It is connected to RCa by a spring that resists deformation. The RCa is represented by the handle of the hockey stick and is directly apposed to the costal fibers. The pressure over its inner surface is the pleural pressure in the zone of diaphragmatic apposition (Ppl,ap). The spring above RCp represents the elastic properties of the rib cage; the springs between RCp, the rest of the skeleton, and the central tendon represent the elastic properties of the lung; the springs between the central tendon, the skeleton, and the anterior abdominal wall represent the elastic properties of the abdomen.

The motion of RCp and RCa are not independent. As a consequence of their linkage, motion of one compartment relative to the other exerts a force on the other compartment that contributes to the pressure change (Plink) and, therefore, to the volume change within that compartment. The magnitude of this force (and of Plink) depends on the degree to which the rib cage is distorted from its neutral position (defined during relaxation when the pressure differences across each part are equal), and the strength of the mechanical linkage between compartments.

When the diaphragm contracts in isolation, Pab increases, displacing the abdominal wall anteriorly. The Pab is transmitted (with or without some gain change) to the inner surface of RCa as Ppl,ap and results in displacement of RCa anteriorly and cranially. At the same time, Ppl,L falls, tending to displace RCp inward and altering the position of RCp relative to RCa, thereby distorting the rib cage. The spring exerts a pressure, Plink, on both compartments that acts to minimize the distortion. The inward motion of RCp and the outward motion of RCa are, therefore, limited to an extent dependent on the strength of their mechanical linkage.

Isolated contraction of the rib cage muscles (parasternals, scalenes, levators costae, and upper external intercostal muscles) results in anterior and cranial displacement of RCp. At the same time, Ppl,L falls. Since the diaphragm is relaxed, this pressure change is transmitted to the abdominal compartment and acts to displace the anterior abdominal wall inward. Transmission of Pab to Ppl,ap exerts an inward force on RCa distorting the rib cage from its relaxation configuration and producing a pressure, Plink, on both compartments, acting to limit their motion relative to one another. The displacement of RCa, therefore, depends on the relative magnitudes of Ppl,ap and Plink.

During normal inspirations both diaphragm and rib cage muscles contract. Since the net effect of the direct actions and the pressures generated by isolated contraction of these muscle groups is antagonistic on RCa and on the anterior abdominal wall, the motion of the chest wall compartments resulting from their simultaneous activation will depend on the degree of muscle recruitment. This is particularly true for RCa, the motion of which is influenced by its mechanical linkage to RCp, by the insertional component of Pdi, and by Pab. When both RCp and the anterior abdominal wall move in the same direction, however, displacement of RCa is no longer ambiguous.

Calculations of rib cage distortability (the relation between distortion and Plink, the inflationary pressure exerted by the rib cage muscles on RCp during spontaneous breathing, and the insertional component of Pdi, using the foregoing model have recently been reported for normal subjects (Ward et al., 1992). The human rib cage is much less distortable than that observed in dogs. As a result, the small distortions that accompany spontaneous breathing result in a substantial inflationary force being applied to RCp. The Plink in these subjects contributed approximately 50% of the inflationary pressure and was approximately equal to the pressure change attributable to the rib cage muscles. Also, in contrast with previous findings in dogs, the insertional component of Pdi was approximately 40% of the total Pdi, and this ratio was not influenced by lung volume over the tidal range.

References

Agostoni, E. (1964). Action of respiratory muscle. In *Handbook of Physiology*. Edited by W. O. Fenn and H. Rahn. Washington, DC, American Physiological Society, pp. 377–386.

Agostoni, E., and Mognoni, P. (1966). Deformation of the chest wall during breathing efforts. *J. Appl. Physiol.* 21: 1827–1832.

Agostoni, E., and Torri, G. (1967). An analysis of the chest wall motions at high values of ventilation. *Respir. Physiol.* 3: 318–332.

Agostoni, E., Mognoni, P., Tossi, G., and Ferrario-Agostoni, A. (1965). Static features of the passive rib cage and abdomen-diaphragm. *J. Appl. Physiol.* 20: 1187–1193.

Agostoni, E., Zocchi, L., and Macklem, P. T. (1988). Transdiaphragmatic pressure and rib motion in area of apposition during paralysis. *J. Appl. Physiol.* 65: 1296–1300.

Ben-Haim, S. A., and Saidel, G. M. (1990). Mathematical model of chest wall mechanics: A phenomenological approach. *Ann. Biomed. Eng.* 18: 37–56.

Boynton, B. R., Glass, G., Frantz, I. D., and Fredberg, J. J. (1989). Rib cage vs. abdominal displacement in dogs during forced oscillation to 32 Hz. *J. Appl. Physiol.* 67: 1472–1478.

Braun, N. M. T., Narinder, S. A., and Rochester, D. F. (1982). Force–length relationship of the normal human diaphragm. *J. Appl. Physiol.* 53: 405–412.

Budzinska, K., Supinski, G., and DiMarco, A. F. (1989). Inspiratory action of separate external and parasternal intercostal muscle contraction. *J. Appl. Physiol.* 67: 1395–1400.

Campbell, E. J. M. (1958). *The Respiratory Muscles and the Mechanics of Breathing*. London, Lloyd–Luke.

Crawford, A. B., Dodd, D., and Engel, L. A. (1983). Changes in rib cage shape during quiet breathing, hyperventilation and single inspirations. *Respir. Physiol.* 54: 197–209.

Danon, J., Druz, W. S., Goldberg, N. B., and Sharp, J. T. (1979). Function of the isolated paced diaphragm and the cervical accessory muscles in C1 quadriplegics. *Am. Rev. Respir. Dis.* 119: 909–918.

Decramer, M., DeTroyer, A., Kelly, S., and Macklem, P. T. (1984a). Mechanical arrangement of costal and crural diaphragms in dogs. *J. Appl. Physiol. Respir. Environ. Exerc. Physiol.* 56: 1484–1490.

Decramer, M., DeTroyer, A., Kelly, S., Zocchi, L., and Macklem, P. T. (1984b). Regional differences in abdominal pressure swings in dogs. *J. Appl, Physiol.* 56: 1682–1687.

Decramer, M., Xi, J. T., Reid, M. B., Kelly, S., Macklem, P. T., and Demedts, M. (1986). Relationship between diaphragm length and abdominal dimensions. *J. Appl. Physiol.* 61: 1815–1820.

DeTroyer, A. (1991). Inspiratory elevation of the ribs in the dog: Primary role of the parasternals. *J. Appl. Physiol.* 70: 1447–1455.

DeTroyer, A., and Decramer, M. (1985). Mechanical coupling between the ribs and sternum in the dog. *Respir. Physiol.* 59: 27–34.

DeTroyer, A., and Estenne, M. (1984). Coordination between rib cage muscles and diaphragm during quiet breathing in humans. *J. Appl. Physiol. Respir. Environ. Exerc. Physiol.* 57: 899–906.

DeTroyer, A., and Farkas, G. (1990). Linkage between parasternals and external intercostals during resting breathing. *J. Appl. Physiol.* 69: 509–516.

DeTroyer, A., and Sampson, M. G. (1982). Activation of the parasternal intercostals during breathing efforts in human subjects. *J. Appl. Physiol. Respir. Environ. Exerc. Physiol.* 52: 524–529.

DeTroyer, A., Sampson, M., Sigrist, S., and Macklem, P. T. (1982). Action of costal and crural parts of the diaphragm on the rib cage in dog. *J. Appl. Physiol. Respir. Environ. Exerc. Physiol.* 53: 30–39.

DeTroyer, A., Kelley, S., and Zin, W. A. (1983). Mechanical action of the intercostal muscles on the ribs. *Science* 220: 87–88.

Easton, P. A., Fitting, J. W., and Grassino, A. E. (1987). Costal and crural diaphragm in early inspiration: Free breathing and occlusion. *J. Appl. Physiol.* 63: 1622–1628.

Froese, A. B., and Bryan, A. C. (1974). Effects of anesthesia and paralysis on diaphragmatic mechanics in man. *Anesthesiology* 41: 242–255.

Ganong, W. F. (1965). *Review of Medical Physiology*, 2nd ed. Oxford, Blackwell Scientific Publications.

Goldman, M. D., and Mead, J. (1973). Mechanical interaction between the diaphragm and rib cage. *J. Appl. Physiol.* 35: 197–204.

Grant, J. C. B., and Basmajian, J. V. (1965). *Grant's Method of Anatomy*, 7th ed. Edinburgh, Livingstone.

Grassino, A., Goldman, M. D., Mead, J., and Sears, T. A. (1978). Mechanics of the human diaphragm during voluntary contraction: Statics. *J. Appl. Physiol. Respir. Environ. Exerc. Physiol.* 44: 829–839.

Grimby, G., Goldman, M. D., and Mead, J. (1976). Respiratory muscle action inferred from rib cage and abdominal V. P. partitioning. *J. Appl. Physiol.* 41: 739–751.

Haines, R. W. (1946). Movements of the first rib. *J. Anat.* 80: 94–100.

Hillman, D. R., and Finucane, K. E. (1987). A model of the respiratory pump. *J. Appl. Physiol.* 63: 951–961.

Jordanoglou, J. (1969). Rib movement in health, kyphoscoliosis and ankylosing spondylitis. *Thorax* 24: 407–414.

Jordanoglou, J. (1970). Vector analysis of rib movement. *Respir. Physiol.* 10: 109–120.

Kenyon, C. M., Pedley, T. J., and Higenbottam, T. W. (1991). Adaptive modeling of the human rib cage in median sternotomy. *J. Appl. Physiol.* 70: 2287–2302.

Kim, M. J., Druz, W. S., Dannon, J., Machnach, W., and Sharp, J. T. (1976). Mechanics of the canine diaphragm. *J. Appl. Physiol.* 41: 369–382.

Koepke, G. H., Smith, E. M., Murphy, A. J., and Dickinson, D. G. (1958). Sequency of action of the diaphragm and intercostal muscles during respiration. *Arch. Phys. Med. Rehabil.* 39: 426–430.

Konno, K., and Mead, J. (1967). Measurement of the separate volume changes of rib cage and abdomen during breathing. *J. Appl. Physiol.* 22: 407–422.

Konno, K., and Mead, J. (1968). Static volume–pressure characteristics of the rib cage and abdomen. *J. Appl. Physiol.* 24: 544–548.

Krahl, V. E. (1986). Anatomy of the mammalian lung. In *Handbook of Physiology*, Section 3. Respiration. Vol. 1. Washington, DC, American Physiological Society, pp. 231–284.

Krayes, S., Decramer, M., Vetterman, J., Rittman, E. L., and Kehder, K. (1988). Volume quantification of chest wall motion in dogs. *J. Appl. Physiol.* 65: 2213–2220.

Last, R. J. (1959). *Anatomy Regional and Applied*, 2nd ed. London, Churchill.

Liu, S., Margulies, S. S., and Wilson, T. A. (1990). Deformation of the dog lung in the chest wall. *J. Appl. Physiol.* 68: 1979–1987.

Loring, S. H., and Mead, J. (1982). Action of the diaphragm on the rib cage inferred from a force–balance analysis. *J. Appl. Physiol. Respir. Environ. Exerc. Physiol.* 53: 756–760.

Luciani, L. (1911). *Human Physiology*. London, Macmillan, p. 408.

Macklem, P. T., Gross, D., Grassino, A., and Roussos, C. (1978). Partitioning of inspiratory pressure swings between diaphragm and intercostal/accessory muscles. *J. Appl. Physiol. Respir. Environ. Exerc. Physiol.* 44: 200–208.

Macklem, P. T., Macklem, D. M., and DeTroyer, A. (1983). A model of inspiratory muscle mechanics. *J. Appl. Physiol. Respir. Environ. Exerc. Physiol.* 55: 547–557.

Marshall, R. (1962). Relationships between stimulus and work of breathing at different lung volumes. *J. Appl. Physiol.* 17: 917–921.

McCool, F. D., Loring, S. H., and Mead, J. (1985). Rib cage distortion during voluntary and involuntary breathing acts. *J. Appl. Physiol.* 58: 1703–1712.

Mead, J., and Loring, S. (1982). Analysis of volume displacement and length changes of the diaphragm during breathing. *J. Appl. Physiol.* 53: 750–755.

Mead, J., Smith, J. C., and Loring, S. H. (1985). Volume displacements of the chest wall and their mechanical significance. In *The Thorax*. Edited by C. Roussos and P. T. Macklem. New York, Marcel Dekker, pp. 370–372.

Melissinos, C. G., Goldman, M. D., Bruche, E., Elliott, E., and Mead, J. (1975). Chest wall shape during force expiratory manoeuvres. *J. Appl. Physiol.* 39: 608–618.

Newman, S., Raod, J., Bellemare, F., Clozel, J. P., Lavigne, C. M., and Grassino, A. E. (1984). Respiratory muscle length measured by sonomicrometry. *J. Appl. Physiol.* 56: 753–764.

Paiva, M., Verbanck, S., Estenne, M., Poncelet, B., Segebarth, C., and Macklem, P. T. (1992). Mechanical implications of in vivo human diaphragm shape. *J. Appl. Physiol.* 72: 1407–1412.

Pean, J. L., Chuong, C. J., Ramanathan, M., and Johnson, R. L. (1991). Regional deformation of the canine diaphragm. *J. Appl. Physiol.* 71: 1581–1588.

Petroll, W. M., Knight, H., and Rochester, D. F. (1990). A model approach to assess diaphragmatic volume displacement. *J. Appl. Physiol.* 69: 2175–2182.

Polgar, F. (1949). Studies on respiratory mechanics. *AJR* 61: 637.

Primiano, F. P., Jr. (1982). Theoretical analysis of chest wall mechanics. *J. Biomech.* 15: 919–931.

Ringel, E. R., Loring, S. H., Mead, J., and Ingram, R. H., Jr. (1985). Chest wall distortion during resistive inspiratory loading. *J. Appl. Physiol.* 584: 1646–1653.

Road, J., Newman, S., and Grassino, A. (1986). Diaphragm length and breathing pattern changes during hypoxia and hypercapnia. *Respiration* 65: 39–53.

Sampson, M. G., and DeTroyer, A. (1982). Role of intercostal muscles in the rib cage distortions produced by inspiratory loads. *J. Appl. Physiol. Respir. Environ. Exerc. Physiol.* 52: 517–523.

Saumarez, R. C. (1986a). An analysis of possible movements of human upper rib cage. *J. Appl. Physiol.* 60: 678–689.

Saumarez, R. C. (1986b). Automated optical measurements of human torso surface movements during breathing. *J. Appl. Physiol.* 60: 702–709.

Saumarez, R. C. (1986c). An analysis of action of intercostal muscles in human upper rib cage. *J. Appl. Physiol.* 60: 690–701.

Saunders, N. A., Kreitzer, S. M., and Ingram, R. H. (1979). Rib cage deformation during static inspiratory efforts. *J. Appl. Physiol.* 46: 1071–1075.

Smith, J. C., and Loring, S. H. (1986). Passive mechanical properties of the chest wall. In *Handbook of Physiology*, Section 3. The Respiratory System, Vol. 3, Part 2. Edited by P. T. Macklem and J. Mead. Bethesda, MD, American Physiological Society, pp. 429–442.

Smith, J. C., and Mead, J. (1986). Three degree of freedom description of movement of the human chest wall. *J. Appl. Physiol.* 60: 928–934.

Taylor, A. (1960). The contribution of the intercostal muscles to the effort of respiration in man. *J. Physiol.* 151: 390–401.

Verschakelen, J. A., Deschepper, K., Jiang, T. X., and Demedts, M. (1989). Diaphragmatic displacement measured by fluoroscopy and derived by Respitrace. *J. Appl. Physiol.* 67: 694–698.

Wade, O. L. (1954). Movements of the thoracic cage and diaphragm in respiration. *J. Physiol.-(Lond.)* 124: 193–212.

Ward, M. E., Ward, J. W., and Macklem, P. T. (1992). Analysis of chest wall motion using a two compartment rib cage model. *J. Appl. Physiol.* (in press)

Warwick, R., and Williams, P. L. (1980). *Gray's Anatomy.* New York, Churchill Livingstone, pp. 275–291.

Whitelaw, W. A. (1987). Shape and size of the human diaphragm in vivo. *J. Appl. Physiol.* 62: 180–186.

Whitelaw, W. A., and Feroah, T. (1989). Patterns of intercostal muscle activity in humans. *J. Appl. Physiol.* 67: 2087–2094.

Wilson, T. A., Krayer, K., Hoffman, E. A., Whitney, C. G., and Rodarte, J. R. (1987). Geometry and respiratory displacement of human ribs. *J. Appl. Physiol.* 62: 1872–1877.

Zocchi, L., Garzaniki, N., Newman, S., and Macklem, P. T. (1987). Effect of hyperventilation and equalization of abdominal pressure on diaphragmatic action. *J. Appl. Physiol.* 62: 1655–1664.

19

Actions of the Respiratory Muscles

ANDRÉ DE TROYER

Erasme University Hospital
Brussels School of Medicine
Brussels, Belgium

STEPHEN H. LORING

Beth Israel Hospital
Harvard Medical School
Boston, Massachusetts

I. Introduction

The mechanical action of any skeletal muscle is essentially determined by the anatomy of the muscle and by the structures it has to displace when it contracts. The respiratory muscles are morphologically and functionally skeletal muscles, and their task is to displace the chest wall rhythmically to pump gas in and out of the lungs. An understanding of the actions of the respiratory muscles, therefore, requires a clear understanding of their anatomy and of the mechanics of the chest wall.

The present chapter will thus begin with a discussion of the basic mechanical structure of the chest wall in humans. It will next analyze the actions of the muscles that displace the chest wall. For the sake of clarity, the functions of the different muscles will be analyzed separately. Thus, we will summarize sequentially what is known about the actions of the diaphragm, the muscles of the rib cage, and the muscles of the abdominal wall. It must be appreciated, however, that all these muscles normally work together in a coordinated manner, and we will draw attention to some of the most critical aspects of their mechanical interdependence.

II. The Chest Wall

The chest wall in mammals can be thought of as consisting of two compartments, the rib cage and the abdomen, separated from each other by a thin musculotendinous structure, the diaphragm. Expansion of the lungs can be accommodated by expansion of the rib cage compartment, the abdominal compartment, or both compartments simultaneously.

The respiratory movements of the abdominal compartment are relatively stereotypical. Indeed, if one neglects the 100–300 ml of abdominal gas volume, the abdominal contents are virtually incompressible. Therefore, any local inward displacement of its boundaries results in an equal outward displacement elsewhere. Furthermore, in humans, many parts of the container are, in the present context, virtually immobile. These are the spine dorsally; the pelvis caudally; and the iliac crests, which nearly meet the rib cage laterally. The parts of the abdominal container that can be displaced, therefore, are largely limited to the ventral abdominal wall and the diaphragm. Consequently, when the diaphragm contracts during inspiration (see following), its descent usually results in an outward displacement of the ventral abdominal wall; conversely, when the abdominal muscles contract, they generally cause an inward displacement of the belly wall, which results in a cranial motion of the diaphragm into the thoracic cavity.

In contrast, the rib cage is a complicated structure, consisting of a series of skeletal arches that are constituted by the thoracic vertebrae, the bony ribs, the costal cartilages, and the sternum. These skeletal supports are connected by joints and ligaments that limit the respiratory movements of the structure, such that the respiratory motion of the ribs can be resolved into two kinds of rotation: (1) a "bucket-handle" rotation about the rib's spinal and sternal articulations, and (2) a "pump-handle" rotation about the transverse axis, passing through the ribs' articulations with the vertebral bodies and the transverse processes (Fig. 1). In the upper portion of the rib cage, the plane of each rib (i.e., the plane defined by three points widely distributed on the arc of the rib) slopes from the back downward toward the front, but projects from the midline nearly horizontally to the side (Wilson et al., 1987). Consequently, when the lateral aspects of the upper ribs move cranially in inspiration, their ventral ends move anteriorly (pump-handle motion), but their lateral displacement is small. In contrast, the planes of the lower ribs project not only downward from back to front but also downward from the midline toward the side (Wilson et al., 1987). Therefore, when these ribs move cranially during inspiration, they have significant lateral as well as anterior displacements.

There is another significant difference between the ribs in the upper portion of the rib cage and those in its lower portion. Although the ventral ends of the ribs are joined to the sternum by cartilaginous attachments and articulations throughout the rib cage, these attachments are shorter and more restrictive for the upper ribs than for the lower ones. Hence, the upper ribs tend to move as a unit with the sternum, whereas the lower ribs have greater freedom to move independently (De Troyer and Decramer, 1985; De Troyer et al., 1986). Thus significant deformations of the rib cage can occur under the influence of muscle contractions and pressures, as will be apparent throughout this chapter.

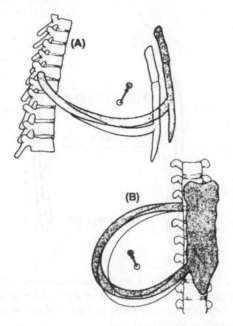

Figure 1 Diagram illustrating the pump-handle (A) and bucket-handle (B) rotations of the ribs in the human rib cage. In both panels, the sternum and one rib are shown before and after rib cage expansion (stippled).

III. The Diaphragm

A. Functional Anatomy

The diaphragm is anatomically unique among skeletal muscles in that its muscle fibers radiate from a central tendinous structure (the central tendon) to insert peripherally into skeletal structures. The crural (or vertebral) portion of the diaphragmatic muscle inserts on the ventrolateral aspect of the first three lumbar vertebrae and on the aponeurotic arcuate ligaments, and the costal portion inserts on the xyphoid process of the sternum and the upper margins of the lower six ribs. From their insertions, the costal fibers run cranially so that they are directly apposed to the inner aspect of the lower rib cage (Fig. 2). Although the old literature has repeatedly suggested the possibility of an intercostal motor innervation of some portions of the diaphragm, it is now clearly established that its only motor supply is through the phrenic nerves.

Functionally, the diaphragm can be considered as an elliptical cylindroid, capped by a dome. The dome of the diaphragm corresponds primarily to the central tendon, and the cylindrical portion corresponds to the muscle directly apposed to the inner aspect of the lower rib cage, the so-called zone of apposition of the

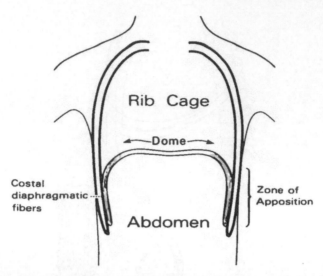

Figure 2 Frontal section of the chest wall at end-expiration, illustrating the functional anatomy of the diaphragm. Note the orientation of the costal diaphragmatic fibers at their insertion on the ribs; these fibers run cranially and are apposed directly to the inner aspect of the lower rib cage (zone of apposition).

diaphragm to the rib cage (Mead, 1979). In standing humans at rest, the height of this zone in the midaxillary line is about 6–7 cm, and the zone of apposition occupies about 25–30% of the total internal surface area of the rib cage. As the diaphragm contracts during inspiration, however, its muscle fibers shorten, and the axial length of the apposed diaphragm diminishes so that the dome of the diaphragm descends relative to its costal insertions. The height of the zone of apposition in normal subjects actually decreases by about 1.5 cm during quiet inspiration. In contrast, the dome of the diaphragm remains relatively constant in size and shape during breathing. Thus, the most important change in diaphragmatic shape, the one responsible for most of the diaphragmatic volume displacement during breathing, is a piston-like axial displacement of the dome related to the shortening of the apposed muscle fibers (Mead and Loring, 1982).

B. Action of the Diaphragm

When tension increases within the diaphragmatic muscle fibers, a caudally oriented force is thus applied on the central tendon, and the dome of the diaphragm descends. This descent has two effects. First, it expands the thoracic cavity along its craniocaudal axis. Hence, pleural pressure falls and, depending on whether the airways are open or closed, lung volume increases or alveolar pressure falls. Second, it produces a caudal displacement of the abdominal visceral mass and an increase in abdominal pressure; this, in turn, results in an outward motion of the ventral abdominal wall.

In addition, because the muscle fibers of the costal diaphragm also insert onto the upper margins of the lower six ribs, they also apply a force on these ribs when they contract; this force, in fact, is equal to the force exerted on the central tendon. As previously emphasized, these diaphragmatic muscle fibers are apposed to the rib cage and are oriented cranially. The force applied on the lower ribs, therefore, is oriented cranially and has the effect of lifting the ribs and rotating them outward. The fall in pleural pressure and the increase in abdominal pressure that results from the diaphragmatic contraction, however, also act to displace the rib cage.

C. Action of the Diaphragm on the Rib Cage

When the diaphragm in anesthetized dogs is selectively activated by electrical stimulation of the phrenic nerves, the upper ribs move caudally and the cross-sectional area of the upper portion of the rib cage decreases (D'Angelo and Sant'Ambrogio, 1974; Jiang et al., 1988). In contrast, the cross-sectional area of the lower portion of the rib cage increases. When a bilateral pneumothorax is introduced, isolated contraction of the diaphragm causes a greater expansion of the lower rib cage, but the dimensions of the upper rib cage now remain unchanged (D'Angelo and Sant'Ambrogio, 1974). It appears, therefore, that the diaphragm has two opposing effects on the rib cage when it contracts. On the one hand, it has an expiratory action on the upper rib cage, and that this action is abolished by a pneumothorax indicates that it is primarily due to the fall in pleural pressure. On the other hand, the diaphragm also has an inspiratory action on the lower rib cage, which, in the dog, prevails over the expiratory effect of pleural pressure.

The cross-sectional shape of the rib cage in humans differs markedly from that in the dog. In the dog, as in many quadrupeds, the dorsoventral diameter of the rib cage is greater than the transverse diameter, whereas in humans, the transverse diameter is greater. Measurements of thoracoabdominal motion in subjects with traumatic transection of the lower cervical cord have shown, however, that these differences in rib cage shape do not fundamentally alter the effects of isolated diaphragmatic contraction (Mortola and Sant'Ambrogio, 1978; Estenne and De Troyer, 1985). Figure 3 illustrates the pattern of chest wall motion in such a subject in the seated posture. The expansion of the abdomen during inspiration is associated with an expansion of the lower rib cage. However, there is also a decrease (paradoxical motion) of the anteroposterior diameter of the upper rib cage. A similar pattern is observed during phrenic nerve pacing in subjects with transection of the upper cervical cord (Danon et al., 1979; Strohl et al., 1984) and during transcutaneous stimulation of the phrenic nerves in normal subjects (A. De Troyer and M. Estenne, unpublished observations). Thus, as in the dog, the diaphragm acting alone in seated humans has both an expiratory action on the upper rib cage and an inspiratory action on the lower rib cage, and this inspiratory action is such that the

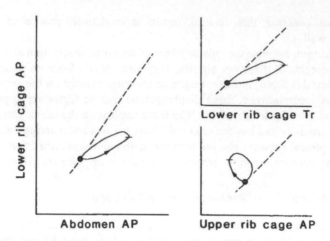

Figure 3 Pattern of chest wall motion in a C-5 tetraplegic subject breathing at rest in the seated position; this subject was breathing only with his diaphragm. Broken lines represent the relaxation curves of the thoracoabdominal system (left panel) and the rib cage (right panels). Closed circles correspond to end-expiration, and solid loops represent tidal volume cycles; arrows indicate the direction of the loops and mark the inspiratory phase, and small horizontal lines mark the end of inspiration. AP, anteroposterior diameter; Tr, transverse diameter. Note that the abdomen expands more than the lower rib cage relative to the relaxed thoracoabdominal configuration (left panel), that the lower rib cage expands predominantly along its transverse diameter (upper right panel), and that the upper rib cage AP diameter decreases during inspiration (lower right panel). (Adapted from Estenne and De Troyer, 1985.)

lower rib cage expands more along its transverse diameter than its anteroposterior diameter (see Fig. 3). The diaphragm thus distorts the lower rib cage in humans to a more elliptical shape.

Theoretical and experimental work has confirmed that the inspiratory action of the diaphragm on the lower rib cage partly results from the force the muscle applies on the ribs by way of its insertions (*insertional force*; De Troyer et al., 1982; Loring and Mead, 1982). This inspiratory action of the diaphragm, however, is also related to its apposition to the rib cage. The zone of apposition makes the lower rib cage, in effect, part of the abdominal container, and measurements in dogs have established that, during breathing, the changes in pressure in the pleural recess between the apposed diaphragm and the rib cage are almost equal to the changes in abdominal pressure (Urmey et al., 1988). Pressure in this pleural recess rises, rather than falls, during inspiration, thereby indicating that the rise in abdominal pressure is truly transmitted through the apposed diaphragm to expand the lower rib cage. This mechanism of diaphragmatic action has been termed the *appositional force*, and its magnitude depends on the size of the zone of apposition and on the rise in abdominal pressure. Clearly, for a given diaphragmatic contraction, the appositional force is greater when the rise in abdominal pressure and the zone of apposition are larger. The greater area of apposed diaphragm at the sides of the rib cage, compared with that at the front, presumably accounts for the fact that the diaphragm in humans has a greater expanding action on the transverse than on the anteroposterior diameter of the lower rib cage (Estenne and De Troyer, 1985).

The inspiratory action of the diaphragm on the lower rib cage is thus related to a combination of two (insertional and appositional) forces. However, the insertional force applies to only the costal portion of the muscle. The crural portion has no direct attachments to the ribs, and so its action on the lower rib cage depends on only the balance between the inspiratory effect of abdominal pressure (appositional force) and the expiratory effect of pleural pressure. As a result, the crural diaphragm, when selectively stimulated, has a smaller inspiratory action on the lower rib cage than the costal diaphragm (De Troyer et al., 1981, 1982).

It must also be appreciated that the resistance provided by the abdominal contents to diaphragmatic descent is a primary determinant of the action of the diaphragm on the rib cage. If this resistance is high (i.e., if abdominal compliance is low), the dome of the diaphragm descends less, the zone of apposition remains significant in size throughout inspiration, and the rise in abdominal pressure is larger. Therefore, for a given diaphragmatic activation, the appositional force tending to expand the lower rib cage is increased. A dramatic illustration of this phenomenon is provided by tetraplegic subjects given external abdominal compression. In these subjects, when a passive, mechanical support to the abdomen is provided by a pneumatic cuff or an elastic binder, the expansion of the lower rib cage during inspiration is accentuated (Danon et al., 1979; Strohl et al., 1984). Conversely, if the resistance provided by the abdominal contents is small (if the abdomen is very compliant), the dome of the diaphragm descends more easily, so that the decrease in size of the zone of apposition is larger and the rise in abdominal pressure is smaller. This probably accounts for the fact that tetraplegic subjects have a smaller expansion of the lower rib cage in the supine posture, in which abdominal compliance is high, than in the seated posture in which abdominal compliance is lower (Mortola and Sant'Ambrogio, 1978; Estenne and De Troyer, 1985; Danon et al., 1979; Strohl et al., 1984). If the resistance provided by the abdominal contents were to disappear, not only would the zone of apposition be suppressed, but also, the contracting diaphragmatic muscle fibers would become oriented transversely inward at their insertions onto the ribs. In this condition, the insertional force would have an expiratory, rather than inspiratory, action on the lower rib cage. Indeed, when a dog is eviscerated, the diaphragm causes a decrease, rather than an increase in lower rib cage dimensions (D'Angelo and Sant'Ambrogio, 1974; De Troyer et al., 1982; Duchenne, 1867).

D. Influence of Lung Volume

The balance between pleural pressure and the insertional and appositional forces of the diaphragm is also markedly affected by changes in lung volume. As lung volume decreases below functional residual capacity (FRC), the zone of apposition increases in size (Mead and Loring, 1982), and the fraction of the rib cage exposed to pleural pressure decreases. As a result, the appositional force increases, while the effect of pleural pressure diminishes, so that the inspiratory action of the diaphragm on the rib cage is enhanced. Conversely, as lung volume increases, the zone of apposition decreases in size, and a larger fraction of the rib cage becomes exposed to pleural pressure. Hence, the diaphragm's inspiratory action on the rib cage diminishes (D'Angelo and Sant'Ambrogio, 1974; De Troyer et al., 1982; Loring and Mead, 1982). When lung volume approaches total lung capacity, the zone of apposition all but disappears (Mead and Loring, 1982), and the diaphragmatic muscle fibers become oriented internally as well as cranially. As in the eviscerated animal, the insertional force of the diaphragm is then expiratory, rather than inspiratory, in direction. These two effects of increasing lung volume account for the inspiratory decrease in the transverse diameter of the lower rib cage in subjects with emphysema and severe hyperinflation (Hoover's sign).

Although the diaphragm contracting alone causes distortion of the rib cage at all lung volumes, normal humans breathing at rest expand the rib cage without distortion (Fig. 4). Thus, during inspiration, the anteroposterior and transverse diameters of the lower rib cage increase proportionately and synchronously, and the anteroposterior diameter of the upper rib cage increases as well. This implies that, even during resting breathing, normal humans contract other muscles that expand the upper rib cage and increase the anteroposterior diameter of the lower rib cage.

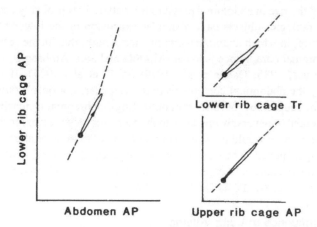

Figure 4   Pattern of chest wall motion in a normal subject breathing at rest in the seated position. Same conventions as in Figure 3. Note that the chest wall, including the entire rib cage, moves on its relaxed configuration.

IV. The Neck Muscles

A. Functional Anatomy

The sternocleidomastoids in humans descend from the mastoid process to the ventral surface of the manubrium sterni and the medial third of the clavicle, and the scalenes comprise three bundles that run from the transverse processes of the lower five cervical vertebrae to the upper surface of the first two ribs. Such anatomical insertions suggest that these muscles can oppose the expiratory action of the diaphragm on the upper rib cage and, indeed, isolated contraction of the sternocleidomastoids or the scalenes in the dog causes a marked cranial displacement of the sternum and the ribs and a significant increase in the rib cage anteroposterior diameter (De Troyer and Kelly, 1984).

B. Action of the Sternocleidomastoids

The action of the sternocleidomastoids in humans has been inferred from measurements of chest wall motion in subjects with transection of the upper cervical cord (Danon et al., 1979; De Troyer et al., 1986). In these subjects, the diaphragm, the scalenes, the intercostals, and the abdominal muscles are paralyzed, but the sternocleidomastoids, the motor innervation of which largely depends on the 11th cranial nerve, are spared and contract forcefully during unassisted inspiration. When breathing spontaneously, these subjects exhibit a marked inspiratory cranial displacement of the sternum and a large inspiratory expansion of the upper rib cage, particularly in its anteroposterior diameter (Fig. 5). The transverse diameter of the upper rib cage (not shown in the figure) also increases during inspiration, whereas the transverse diameter of the lower rib cage decreases.

The pattern of rib cage motion observed in high tetraplegics thus confirms that the sternocleidomastoids in humans can largely counteract the action of the diaphragm on the upper rib cage. In normal subjects breathing at rest, however, the sternocleidomastoids are inactive, being recruited only when ventilation increases substantially, or when the inspiratory muscle pump is abnormally loaded (Campbell, 1955; Raper et al., 1966; Delhez, 1974). Therefore, these muscles cannot account for the expansion of the upper rib cage that takes place normally during quiet inspiration.

C. Action of the Scalenes

Earlier electromyographic studies had suggested that the scalenes are also inactive in normal humans breathing at rest (Campbell, 1955). As a result, these muscles, together with the sternocleidomastoids, have traditionally been considered as "accessory" muscles of inspiration. These earlier electromyographic measurements, however, were obtained with surface electrodes, a technique that is too insensitive to detect signals of low amplitude arising from small or deeply located muscles.

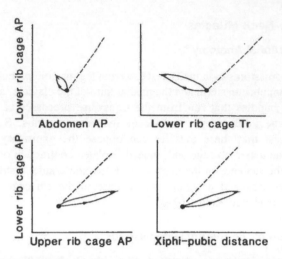

Figure 5 Pattern of chest wall motion during spontaneous breathing in a C1–2 tetraplegic subject. Same conventions as in Figure 3. Note that during inspiration the abdomen moves inward (upper left panel), the lower rib cage transverse diameter decreases (upper right panel), and the upper rib cage AP diameter (lower left panel) and the xiphipubic distance (which reflects the axial motion of the sternum—lower right panel) increase disproportionately more than the lower rib cage AP diameter. (From De Troyer et al., 1986.)

More recent studies, using concentric needle electrodes, have established that, in fact, unlike the sternocleidomastoids, the scalenes in normal humans are invariably active during inspiration (Raper et al., 1966; Delhez, 1974; De Troyer and Estenne, 1984). Seated normal subjects cannot breathe without contracting the scalenes, even when they reduce tidal volume considerably (De Troyer and Estenne, 1984).

There is no clinical setting that causes paralysis of all the inspiratory muscles without also affecting the scalenes. Therefore, the isolated action of these muscles on the human rib cage cannot be precisely defined. Two observations, however, indicate that the scalenes have a significant inspiratory effect during resting breathing. First, the inward inspiratory displacement of the upper rib cage characteristic of tetraplegia is usually not observed when the scalene function is preserved after the lower cervical cord transection (Estenne and De Troyer, 1985). To the extent that the scalenes are innervated from the lower five cervical segments, persistent inspiratory contraction of the scalenes is frequently encountered in subjects with a cervical cord transection at the C-7 level or below. In such subjects, the anteroposterior diameter of the upper rib cage tends to remain constant or to increase slightly during inspiration. Second, when normal subjects attempt to inspire with the diaphragm alone, there is a marked, selective decrease in scalene inspiratory activity associated with either a clear-cut reduction in the inspiratory increase in anteroposterior diameter of the upper rib cage or an inspiratory decrease (paradoxical motion) in this diameter (De Troyer and Estenne, 1984). Thus, there is no reason for using the qualifying adjective "accessory" in describing the scalenes. These muscles in humans are primary muscles of inspiration, and their contraction is an important determinant of the expansion of the upper rib cage during breathing.

In contrast to humans, however, dogs generally do not use the scalenes during resting breathing. These muscles behave like the sternocleidomastoids and remain electrically silent during inspiration, even during breathing against high inspiratory mechanical loads (De Troyer et al., 1994). Nevertheless, all the ribs in the dog, including those situated in the rostral portion of the rib cage, move cranially during inspiration, providing evidence that the intercostal muscles may also play a primary role in displacing the ribs cranially and in expanding the rib cage.

V. The Intercostal Muscles

A. Functional Anatomy

The intercostal muscles are two thin layers of muscle fibers occupying each of the intercostal spaces. They are termed *external* and *internal* because of their surface relations, the external being superficial to the internal. The external intercostals extend from the tubercles of the ribs dorsally to the costochondral junctions ventrally, and their fibers are oriented obliquely caudad and ventrally from the rib above to the rib below. Near the costochondral junctions, the external intercostals are replaced by a fibrous aponeurosis, the anterior intercostal membrane, which extends to the ventral ends of the intercostal spaces. In contrast, the internal intercostals extend from the angles of the ribs dorsally to the sternocostal junctions ventrally, and their fibers run obliquely caudad and dorsally from the rib above to the rib below. Thus, although the intercostal spaces contain two layers of intercostal muscle fibers in their lateral portion, they contain a single muscle layer in their ventral and dorsal portions. Ventrally, between the sternum and the chondrocostal junctions, the only fibers are those of the internal intercostal muscles; these are particularly thick in this region of the rib cage, where they are conventionally called the *parasternal intercostals*. Dorsally, from the angles of the ribs to the vertebrae, the only fibers come from the external intercostal muscles. These latter, however, are duplicated by a spindle-shaped muscle that runs in each interspace from the tip of the transverse process of the vertebra to the angle of the rib below; this muscle is the *levator costae*. All the intercostal muscles are innervated by the intercostal nerves.

B. Actions of the Intercostal Muscles on the Ribs

The action of the intercostal muscles has been a source of controversy throughout medical history (Beau and Maissiat, 1843; Duchenne, 1867; Luciani, 1911). The external and internal intercostal muscles have successively been perceived as being (1) all expiratory; (2) all inspiratory; (3) both inspiratory and expiratory, acting simultaneously; (4) either inspiratory or expiratory, depending on the interspace; or (5) only regulating the tension of the intercostal space. A detailed examination of these various theories is irrelevant to this chapter. The theory of Hamberger (1749), however, deserves a special mention because its conclusions have long provided the basis for conventional thinking in that area.

This theory is based on geometrical considerations and can be summarized as follows (Fig. 6): When an intercostal muscle contracts in one interspace, it pulls the upper rib down and the lower rib up. However, as the fibers of the external intercostal slope obliquely caudad and ventrally from the rib above to the one below, their lower insertion is more distant from the center of rotation (the vertebral articulations) of the ribs than the upper one. Hence, when this muscle contracts, the torque acting on the lower rib is greater than that acting on the upper rib, and its net effect is to raise the ribs. The orientation of the levator costae is similar to that of the external intercostal, so that its action should also be to raise the ribs. In contrast, the fibers of the internal intercostal run obliquely caudad and dorsally from the rib above to the one below. Therefore, their lower insertion is less distant from the center of rotation of the ribs than the upper one. As a result, when this muscle contracts, the torque acting on the lower rib is smaller than that acting on the upper rib, such that its net effect is to lower the ribs to which this muscle is attached. The parasternal intercostals are part of the internal intercostal layer, but their action is referred to the sternum, rather than to the vertebral column; therefore, by similar arguments, their contraction should raise the ribs. Thus, Hamberger concluded that the orientations of the muscle fibers should make the external intercostals, the levator

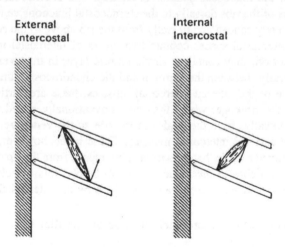

Figure 6 Diagram illustrating Hamberger's theory. In each panel, the hatched area represents the spine and the two bars oriented obliquely represent two adjacent ribs. The intercostal muscles are depicted as single bundles, and the torques acting on the ribs during contraction of these muscles are represented by arrows. See text for further explanation.

costae, and the parasternal intercostals inspiratory in their action on the ribs, whereas the interosseous portion of the internal intercostals should be expiratory in its action on the ribs.

As recently emphasized by Saumarez (1986) and by Wilson and De Troyer (1993), however, the Hamberger theory is incomplete and cannot entirely describe the actions of the intercostal muscles on the ribs for two major reasons. First, the Hamberger model is planar, whereas the real ribs are curved. As a result, the changes in length of the intercostal muscles during a given rotation of the ribs (and, hence, the mechanical advantage and action of these muscles on the ribs) vary as a function of the position of the muscle fibers along the rib. Thus, whereas the Hamberger theory predicts that a cranial rotation of two adjacent ribs produces equal shortening of all external intercostal fibers situated between the two ribs and equal lengthening of all internal intercostal fibers, the curvature of the ribs causes changes in muscle length that are greatest in the dorsal region, decrease progressively as one moves around the rib cage, and are reversed as one approaches the sternum. The second reason is that the Hamberger theory is based on the idea that all the ribs rotate by equal amounts around parallel axes, so that the distance between adjacent ribs remains constant. In fact, the radii of curvature of different ribs are different, increasing from the top downward, and the rotations of the different ribs in the dog have been shown to be different as well (Margulies et al., 1989). As a result, in addition to the changes in muscle length caused by the Hamberger mechanism and by the curvature of the ribs, there is a change in muscle length owing to the changes in distance between the ribs. Indeed, measurements of the respiratory changes in intercostal muscle length in anesthetized dogs have shown that, whereas the parasternal intercostals and levator costae invariably shorten a significant amount during inspiration (Decramer and De Troyer, 1984; De Troyer and Farkas, 1990; van Lunteren and Cherniack, 1986), the external intercostals and internal interosseous intercostals in the lateral aspects of the rib cage show small and variable changes in length; in the rostral interspaces, both muscles, in general, shorten during inspiration, but in the caudal interspaces, both muscles often lengthen during inspiration (Decramer et al., 1986).

The Hamberger theory thus does not explain important features of intercostal muscle mechanics. Nevertheless, many electromyographic recordings from intercostal nerves and muscles in anesthetized cats (Bronk and Ferguson, 1935; Sears, 1964; Bainton et al., 1978; Greer and Martin, 1990; Hilaire et al., 1983) and dogs (De Troyer and Ninane, 1986a; De Troyer and Farkas, 1989) have clearly established that three groups of intercostal muscles are electrically active during the inspiratory phase of the breathing cycle; these are the parasternal intercostals, the external intercostals, and the levator costae (Fig. 7). Of interest, the inspiratory activation of the external intercostals takes place mostly in the dorsal region of the rostral interspaces (Bainton et al., 1978; Greer and Martin, 1990), where these muscles are thickest and have the greatest inspiratory mechanical advantage (Wilson and De Troyer, 1993). Furthermore, when either the parasternal intercostal or the levator

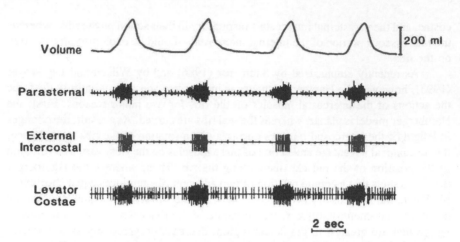

Figure 7 Pattern of electrical activation of the parasternal intercostal, external intercostal, and levator costae muscles of the third interspace in a representative dog breathing quietly in the supine posture. The trace of lung volume is also shown (increase upward). Note that the three muscles are active during inspiration. (From De Troyer and Farkas, 1989.)

costae in a given interspace is selectively activated by electrical stimulation, it causes cranial displacement of the ribs into which it inserts (De Troyer and Kelly, 1982; De Troyer and Farkas, 1989). In addition, when the diaphragm and the parasternal intercostals in dogs are denervated so that the external intercostals and levator costae are the only muscles active during inspiration, the ribs move cranially (De Troyer and Farkas, 1989). An inspiratory cranial displacement of the ribs is similarly seen in animals in which the diaphragm, external intercostals, and levator costae have been paralyzed and the parasternal intercostals are the only muscles active during inspiration (A. De Troyer and T. A. Wilson, unpublished observations). All these observations thus clearly demonstrate that the parasternal intercostals, the external intercostals, and the levator costae have an inspiratory action on the rib cage.

Loring and Woodbridge (1991), using a finite-element analysis of intercostal muscle action, have recently confirmed the inspiratory action of the parasternal intercostal, external intercostal, and levator costae muscles on the rib cage. They have further emphasized, however, that these muscles produce different patterns of rib cage expansion. In their model, the forces generated by the external intercostals caused a large pump-handle motion of the ribs about their spinal ends, with little or no bucket-handle rotation, whereas the forces generated by the parasternal intercostals and levator costae produced both a pump-handle motion and a bucket-handle rotation. Thus the external intercostals produced large cranial motion of the ribs and sternum, with little or no lateral expansion of the rib cage, whereas the parasternal intercostals and levator costae produced a marked lateral rib cage expansion as well. In contrast, when contracting in all interspaces simultaneously, the internal interosseous intercostals produced a caudal, pump-handle motion of the ribs (Loring and Woodbridge, 1991). Indeed, in spontaneously breathing animals, the internal intercostals are active only during the expiratory phase of the breathing cycle (Bainton et al., 1978; De Troyer and Ninane, 1986a), and their activation is confined to the caudal interspaces, where they have a greater expiratory mechanical advantage (Wilson and De Troyer, 1993).

C. Respiratory Function of the Different Intercostal Muscles

In Quadrupeds

As previously pointed out, anesthetized and unanesthetized dogs do not use the scalene and sternomastoid muscles during breathing (De Troyer et al., 1994). In this animal, the inspiratory motion of the ribs and the expansion of the upper two-thirds of the rib cage thus result entirely from the concerted actions of the parasternal intercostals, external intercostals, and levator costae. The following observations suggest, however, that these muscles differ substantially in their relative contributions to inspiration.

1. In anesthetized dogs and cats, the cranial motion of the ribs during inspiration occurs together with a caudal displacement of the sternum (Da Silva et al., 1977; De Troyer and Kelly, 1982; De Troyer and Decramer, 1985). This pattern of motion is due to the contraction of the parasternal intercostals (De Troyer and Kelly, 1982). Indeed, selective activation of these muscles causes the sternum to move caudally, whereas both the external intercostals and the levator costae tend to displace the sternum cranially (De Troyer and Farkas, 1989; Loring and Woodbridge, 1991).

2. Measurements of the respiratory changes in parasternal muscle length in supine or prone dogs at rest have demonstrated that, when the internal intercostal nerve in a single interspace is sectioned at the chondrocostal junction such that the parasternal intercostal in this interspace is selectively denervated, the normal inspiratory shortening of the muscle is virtually abolished (Fig. 8; De Troyer et al., 1988; De Troyer and Farkas, 1993). At the same time, the inspiratory shortening of the external intercostal in the same interspace also decreases markedly, even though the inspiratory activation of this muscle is increased (De Troyer and Farkas, 1990). In contrast, when the external intercostal muscle in a single cranial interspace is selectively denervated, the inspiratory shortening of this muscle is reduced, but the inspiratory activation and shortening of the parasternal intercostal in this interspace remains unchanged. In other words, the inspiratory shortening of the parasternal intercostals results from the muscles' own activation, whereas the inspiratory shortening of the cranial external intercostals is due to the activation of both the parasternal and the external intercostals.

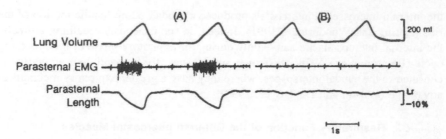

Figure 8 Electromyographic (EMG) activity and respiratory changes in length recorded from the third right parasternal intercostal muscle in a supine dog breathing quietly. (A) Control; (B) after section of the third right internal intercostal nerve at the chondrocostal junction and selective denervation of the muscle. Respiratory changes in muscle length are expressed as percentage change relative to the muscle length during relaxation (Lr); downward deflections indicate muscle shortening. Note that during control, the parasternal is electrically active and shortens with inspiration. In contrast, after selective denervation and suppression of the inspiratory electromyographic activity, the parasternal inspiratory shortening has virtually disappeared. (From De Troyer et al., 1988.)

3. When the canine parasternal intercostals are selectively denervated in all interspaces, the inspiratory cranial motion of the ribs is reduced by 60% (De Troyer, 1991a). This procedure, however, promotes a marked increase in the inspiratory activation of both the external intercostals and the levator costae, which minimizes the reduction in the inspiratory rib motion. In contrast, when the parasternal intercostals are left intact and the external intercostals in all interspaces are sectioned, the activation of the parasternal intercostals is unaltered and the inspiratory cranial displacement of the ribs is reduced only minimally (De Troyer, 1991a).

These observations taken together thus indicate that, in the anesthetized dog, the parasternal intercostals play a larger role than the external intercostals and levator costae during eupnea, being responsible for the caudal displacement of the sternum and most of the cranial motion of the ribs. Yet, Budzinska et al. (1989) and Wilson and De Troyer (1993) have shown that the canine external intercostals and levator costae can produce large falls in airway pressure when they contract forcefully. This apparent discrepancy has led to the suggestion that these muscles constitute primarily a reserve system (De Troyer, 1991a), and indeed electromyographic recordings from the different intercostal muscles in anesthetized cats (Corda et al., 1965; Shannon and Zechman, 1972), rabbits (Sant'Ambrogio and Widdicombe, 1965), and dogs (De Troyer, 1991b) have shown that, when the inspiratory airflow resistance is suddenly increased or the endotracheal tube is occluded at end-expiration for a single breath, the rate of rise of external intercostal and levator costae activity increases markedly. This facilitation of activity results from the activation of the muscle spindles, which are known to be abundantly distributed in these muscles (Duron et al., 1978; Hilaire et al., 1983). In contrast, the parasternal intercostals, like the diaphragm, are poorly supplied with muscle spindles (Duron et al., 1978), so that they do not show any facilitation of activity (De Troyer, 1991b). Rib cage strapping similarly produces a selective increase in the activation of the external intercostals and levator costae (M. Cappello and A. De Troyer, unpublished observations), thus suggesting that, in loading conditions, the contribution of these muscles to the inspiratory displacement of the rib cage increases relative to that of the parasternal intercostals. Measurements of the changes in external intercostal length and rib displacement during step-increases in inspiratory airflow resistance have suggested, however, that the mechanical effectiveness of this reserve, "load-compensating" system is relatively small (De Troyer, 1992).

In Humans

Even though it is technically difficult to make entirely selective recordings from the individual intercostal muscles in humans, it is now clearly established that as with quadrupeds, normal humans breathing at rest have inspiratory activity in the parasternal intercostals and in the external intercostals of the most rostral interspaces (Delhez, 1974; De Troyer and Sampson, 1982; Taylor, 1960; Whitelaw and Feroah, 1989). Activity in the external intercostals, however, appears to be less consistent and to involve fewer motor units than activity in the parasternal intercostals (Delhez, 1974; Taylor, 1960; Whitelaw and Feroah, 1989). This would suggest that in humans, as in quadrupeds, the contribution of the parasternal intercostals to resting breathing is greater than that of the external intercostals.

However, it is uncertain whether the parasternal intercostals in humans play as large a role in displacing the rib cage during breathing as they do in the dog. The respiratory changes in parasternal intercostal length are unknown, and it is difficult to predict how selective denervation of these muscles would affect the pattern of rib cage motion. As previously emphasized, however, humans at rest also show invariable inspiratory activity in the scalenes (Delhez, 1974; De Troyer and Estenne, 1984; Raper et al., 1966), and the sternum moves cranially, rather than caudally, during inspiration. In addition, although voluntary inhibition of the scalenes is associated with an increased parasternal activation, it causes a marked reduction or a disappearance of the normal inspiratory increase in the anteroposterior dimension of the upper rib cage (De Troyer and Estenne, 1984). Therefore, it appears that in humans the parasternal intercostals play a smaller role than the scalenes in producing the inspiratory rib cage expansion.

The reason for this difference between dogs and humans is unclear, but Loring and Woodbridge (1991) and Loring (1992) have pointed out that there is a major difference between the orientation of the ribs in the dog and in humans. In the dog, the ribs project ventrally in a direction nearly perpendicular to the spine. In contrast, the ribs in humans run ventrally and caudally from the spine. Therefore, the muscles that produce a preponderant pump-handle motion (i.e., the scalenes) might be more effective at increasing lung volume in humans than in the dog; conversely, the muscles producing a preponderant bucket-handle rotation (i.e., the parasternal intercostals) would be more effective on the lung in the dog.

D. Nonrespiratory Function of the Intercostal Muscles

De Troyer et al. (1985) have previously speculated that the external and internal interosseous intercostals might play important roles in postural movements. Indeed, the anatomical insertions and fiber orientations of these muscles would make them ideally suited to twist the rib cage. Thus contraction of the external intercostals on one side of the sternum would rotate the ribs in a transverse plane, so that the upper ribs would move forward while the lower ribs would move backward. In contrast, contraction of the internal intercostals on one side of the sternum would move the upper ribs backward and the lower ribs forward. In agreement with this idea, Decramer et al. (1986) have shown that the external and internal interosseous intercostal muscles show large, reciprocal changes in length during rotations of the thorax in anesthetized dogs. When the animal's trunk was twisted passively to the left, the external intercostals on the right side of the chest and the internal interosseous intercostals on the left side were observed to shorten considerably. At the same time, the external intercostals on the left side and the internal intercostals on the right side lengthened. The opposite pattern was seen when the animal's trunk was passively rotated to the right, with a substantial shortening of the right internal and left external intercostals and a marked lengthening of the left internals and right externals. Thus, the length of these muscles changed in the way expected if they were producing the rotations.

Recent electromyographic studies with bipolar fine-wire electrodes in normal humans have confirmed that the external and internal interosseous intercostals are very actively involved in rotations of the thorax (Whitelaw et al., 1992). Thus, the external intercostals on the right side of the chest were activated when the trunk was rotated to the left, whereas they were silent when the trunk was rotated to the right. Conversely, the internal intercostals on the right side of the chest were activated only when the trunk was rotated to the right. Active use of these muscles during such postural movements is consistent with their abundant supply of muscle spindles (Duron et al., 1978).

VI. The Triangularis Sterni

The preceding sections of this chapter have largely focused on the inspiratory muscles, which displace the respiratory system above its relaxation (equilibrium) volume. Several studies, however, have recently indicated that expiration is also frequently an active process. Mammalian quadrupeds, in particular, use expiratory muscles to displace the respiratory system below its relaxation volume, and the triangularis sterni appears to play a prominent role in this process.

A. Functional Anatomy

The triangularis sterni, also called *transversus thoracis* or *sternocostalis*, is a flat muscle that lies deep to the sternum and the parasternal intercostals. As shown in Figure 9, its fibers originate from the dorsal aspect of the caudal half of the sternum and insert into the inner surface of the chondrocostal junctions of ribs 3–7. The muscle receives its motor supply from the intercostal nerves, and its selective stimulation causes a marked caudal displacement of the ribs with a cranial motion of the sternum (De Troyer and Ninane, 1986b). As would be expected from the orientation of the muscle fibers, the isolated action of the triangularis sterni is thus opposite to that of the parasternal intercostals.

B. Respiratory Function

Various electromyographic studies in supine anesthetized dogs have shown that the triangularis sterni is active during expiration, its activity alternating with that of the parasternal intercostals (Fig. 10; De Troyer and Ninane, 1986b; van Lunteren et al., 1988b). During expiration, the canine triangularis sterni, in fact, shortens a substantial amount below its in situ resting length (Ninane et al., 1986, 1989), so that the ribs are pulled caudally, the parasternal intercostals are stretched, and the

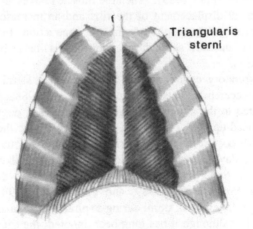

Triangularis
sterni

Figure 9 Dorsal aspect of the ventral wall of the rib cage in the dog, illustrating the insertions of the triangularis sterni muscle on both sides of the sternum. Note that the most cranial portion of the sternum and the first two ribs have been reflected; the triangularis sterni has no insertions there.

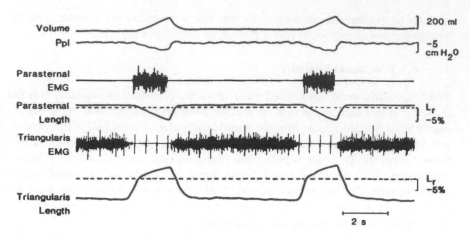

Figure 10 Electromyographic (EMG) activity and respiratory changes in length of the parasternal intercostal and triangularis sterni muscles in a dog breathing at rest in the supine posture. Same conventions as in Figure 8. Note that during expiration, the triangularis sterni is electrically active and shortens below its relaxation length (Lr), (broken line); at the same time, the parasternal intercostal is stretched above its Lr. At end-expiration, relaxation of the triangularis sterni causes the muscle to lengthen toward Lr. The parasternal intercostal then becomes electrically active and shortens below Lr, thereby stretching the triangularis sterni above its Lr.

rib cage is deflated below its resting position (De Troyer and Ninane, 1986b; Ninane et al., 1986; Warner et al., 1989). When the muscle relaxes at end-expiration, there is a passive cranial displacement of the ribs and an increase in rib cage volume preceding the onset of the inspiratory muscle contraction. In supine dogs, phasic activation of the triangularis sterni during expiration is thus an important determinant of rib cage motion.

Phasic expiratory contraction of the triangularis sterni is also observed in anesthetized or decerebrate cats (van Lunteren et al., 1988a; Hwang et al., 1989) and is not limited to the supine posture. In anesthetized dogs a change from the supine to the head-up (De Troyer and Ninane, 1987) or the prone (Farkas and Schroeder, 1990) posture elicits an increased expiratory activation of the muscle, suggesting that it plays an even larger role in displacing the rib cage during breathing in these postures. Recordings in chronically instrumented dogs (De Troyer and Ninane, 1986b; Smith et al., 1989) and cats (Duron, 1981) have shown that contraction of the triangularis sterni during expiration also takes place in conscious animals (Fig. 11). Although it has long been ignored, the triangularis sterni must, therefore, be considered as a primary muscle of breathing in quadrupeds: it shares the work of breathing with the inspiratory muscles and helps the parasternal intercostals produce the rhythmic inspiratory expansion of the rib cage.

Normal humans, in contrast, do not contract the triangularis sterni when

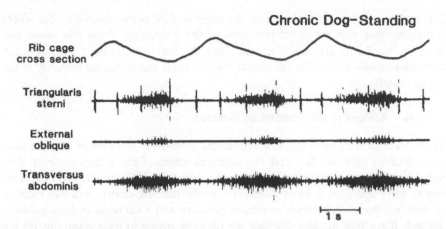

Figure 11 Electrical activity of the triangularis sterni, external oblique, and transversus abdominis muscles in a standing, unanesthetized dog at rest. The respiratory changes in rib cage cross section are also shown (increase upward). Note that the triangularis sterni contracts in phase with expiration (decrease in rib cage cross section). Note also the expiratory contraction of the external oblique and the transversus abdominis; the activity detected in the transversus abdominis is much larger in amplitude and starts much earlier than that recorded from the external oblique. The rectus abdominis (not shown here) was silent.

breathing at rest in the supine posture (De Troyer et al., 1987) and, although triangularis expiratory activity is recorded in many standing subjects (Estenne et al., 1988), its mechanical significance is probably small.

VII. The Abdominal Muscles

A. Functional Anatomy

The four abdominal muscles that have significant respiratory function in humans constitute the ventrolateral wall of the abdomen. The *rectus abdominis* is the most ventral of these muscles. It originates from the ventral aspect of the sternum and the 5th, 6th, and 7th costal cartilages, and it runs caudally along the whole length of the abdominal wall to insert into the pubis. This muscle is enclosed in a sheath formed by the aponeuroses of the other three muscles. The most superficial of these is the *external oblique*. It originates by fleshy digitations from the external surface of the lower eight ribs, well above the costal margin, and directly covers the lower ribs and intercostal muscles. Its fibers radiate caudally to the iliac crest and inguinal ligament and medially to the linea alba. The *internal oblique* lies deep to the external oblique. Its fibers arise from the iliac crest and inguinal ligament, and they diverge to insert on the costal margin and an aponeurosis contributing to the rectus sheath down to the pubis. The *transversus abdominis* is the deepest of the muscles of the lateral abdominal wall. It arises from the inner surface of the lower six ribs, where it interdigitates with the costal insertions of the diaphragm. From this origin and from the lumbar fascia, the iliac crest, and the inguinal ligament, its fibers run circumferentially around the abdominal visceral mass and terminate ventrally in the rectus sheath.

B. Actions of the Abdominal Muscles

These four muscles have important functions as rotators and flexors of the trunk. As respiratory muscles, they have two principal actions. First, as they contract, they pull the abdominal wall inward and produce an increase in abdominal pressure. This causes the diaphragm to move cranially into the thoracic cavity, and this motion, in turn, results in an increase in pleural pressure and a decrease in lung volume. Second, these four muscles displace the rib cage owing to their insertions on the ribs. These insertions would suggest that the action of all abdominal muscles is to pull the lower ribs caudally and to deflate the cage, another expiratory action. Measurements of rib cage motion during separate stimulation of the four abdominal muscles in supine dogs have shown, however, that this action is more complex than conventionally thought (De Troyer et al., 1983).

C. Action of the Abdominal Muscles on the Rib Cage

As anticipated, isolated contraction of the canine rectus abdominis results in a caudal displacement of the sternum and the ribs and causes a decrease in the rib cage anteroposterior and transverse diameters. In contrast, there is no significant rib cage motion during isolated contraction of the internal oblique or the transversus abdominis in the dog. In the external oblique, there is even a cranial displacement of the ribs and sternum, with an increase in the lower rib cage diameters. After evisceration, however, every abdominal muscle (including the external oblique) causes a caudal displacement of the ribs and sternum and a decrease in rib cage diameters (De Troyer et al., 1983).

These observations clearly indicate that the abdominal muscles have two opposing effects on the rib cage. On the one hand, in relation to their attachments, the obliques and rectus tend to pull the ribs caudally and to deflate the rib cage. This insertional, expiratory force is the only acting component after evisceration. On the other hand, the abdominal muscles also have an inspiratory action on the rib cage, and that this action is removed by evisceration indicates that it is primarily related to the rise in abdominal (and pleural) pressure. As previously discussed (see Fig. 2), there is a large zone where the diaphragm is directly apposed to the rib cage, which allows abdominal pressure to be transmitted to the lower rib cage. Thus, the rise in abdominal pressure that takes place when the abdominal muscles contract acts to expand the lower rib cage. Furthermore, the diaphragm, when forced cranially, is stretched, and this passive diaphragmatic tension tends to raise the lower ribs as an active diaphragmatic contraction does ("insertional" force). Both of these mechanisms oppose the expiratory force that the abdominal muscles exert on the lower ribs by way of their insertions (De Troyer et al., 1983).

The action of the abdominal muscles on the rib cage in humans should also be determined by the balance between the insertional, expiratory force of the muscles and the inspiratory force related to the rise in abdominal pressure. The difference between the cross-sectional shape of the rib cage in humans, compared with the dog, however, markedly affects the insertional force of the abdominal muscles. As in the dog, isolated contraction of the rectus abdominis in humans produces a marked caudal displacement of the sternum and a large decrease in the rib cage anteroposterior diameter (Mier et al., 1985). However, the rectus abdominis in humans also causes a small increase in the rib cage transverse diameter. Similarly, the external oblique in humans causes a small caudal displacement of the sternum and a marked decrease, rather than an increase, in the rib cage transverse diameter (Mier et al., 1985). The isolated actions of the internal oblique and transversus abdominis muscles on the human rib cage are unknown.

D. Respiratory Function of the Abdominal Muscles

Regardless of the rib cage displacements that are introduced when they contract, the abdominal muscles are primarily expiratory muscles through their action on the diaphragm and the lung, and they play important roles in activities such as coughing and speaking. The action of these muscles, however, enables them to assist inspiratory muscles as well. The horse breathing at rest provides a dramatic illustration of this phenomenon (Koterba et al., 1988). As shown in Figure 12, this animal displays a biphasic airflow pattern during both expiration and inspiration. As in all animal species, the first part of expiration is essentially passive, owing to the relaxation of the inspiratory muscles. As expiration proceeds, however, there is a strong contraction of the abdominal muscles, which deflates the respiratory system below its relaxation volume and generates a second peak of expiratory airflow. At the onset of the subsequent inspiration, the abdominal muscles relax, allowing the diaphragm to descend passively as the respiratory system returns toward its relaxation volume; this phenomenon accounts for the first peak of inspiratory airflow. After inspiratory flow diminishes, the inspiratory muscles contract producing a second peak of inspiratory flow. This effect is similar to that produced by the canine triangularis sterni, which causes the ribs to move cranially before the onset of parasternal inspiratory contraction.

Although such a biphasic flow pattern is a rather characteristic feature of the horse, the observation that the transversus abdominis in supine anesthetized dogs shortens during expiration below its in situ relaxation length and lengthens during inspiration above its relaxation length (Ninane et al., 1988; Arnold et al., 1988) indicates that this animal uses a similar strategy of breathing. This similarity is even more obvious when the dog is tilted head-up or prone (De Troyer and Ninane, 1987;

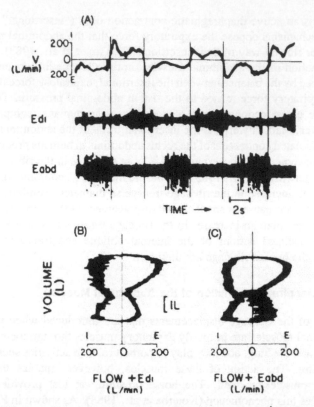

Figure 12 Strategy of breathing in the horse. (A) Traces of flow ($\dot{V}$), electromyogram of the diaphragm (Edi), and electromyogram of the abdominal internal oblique muscle (Eabd) versus time. Note the lag in onset of Edi relative to the onset of inspiratory flow, as well as the lag in onset of Eabd relative to the onset of expiratory flow. (B) The corresponding flow–volume loop, in which the raw Edi signal has been electrically added to the flow tracing; note that most of the Edi signal is in the second phase of inspiration. (C) The same flow–volume loop with the raw Eabd signal electrically added to the flow tracing; note here that the Eabd signal is confined to the second phase of expiration. (From Koterba et al., 1988.)

Farkas et al., 1989; Farkas and Schroeder, 1993). In these postures, the relaxation of the abdominal muscles at end-expiration accounts for 50–60% of the animal's tidal volume.

Adult humans at rest do not employ such a breathing strategy. The abdominal muscles (like the triangularis sterni) are silent in the supine posture and, although most subjects show abdominal muscle activity in the standing posture, this activity is principally tonic, unrelated to the phases of respiration (Delhez, 1974; Floyd and Silver, 1950; Druz and Sharp, 1981; Strohl et al., 1981; De Troyer, 1983). This difference from quadrupeds, however, disappears when the demand placed on the respiratory pump is increased by exercise, by CO_2-enriched gas mixtures, or by increased inspiratory mechanical loads. Under these conditions, most subjects develop rhythmic expiratory contraction of the abdominal muscles (Campbell, 1952; Strohl et al., 1981; Martin and De Troyer, 1982), thereby suggesting that the abdominal muscles in humans may also reduce the work done by inspiratory muscles.

There are marked differences in the recruitment of the different abdominal muscles. During CO_2-induced hyperpnea or during breathing against inspiratory mechanical loads, adult humans recruit the transversus abdominis during expiration well before activity can be recorded from either the rectus abdominis or the external oblique (De Troyer et al., 1990). Similarly, in anesthetized dogs breathing at rest, the transversus abdominis frequently contracts in concert with the triangularis sterni during expiration, whereas the rectus abdominis and external oblique are usually inactive (Gilmartin et al., 1987; Ninane et al., 1988). Unanesthetized dogs exhibit a similar pattern (De Troyer et al., 1989). Among the canine abdominal muscles, however, the rectus has the greatest expiratory action on the rib cage (see foregoing). On the other hand, the rectus runs axially from the rib cage to the pelvis, whereas the transversus constitutes a muscle sheet that is transversely oriented and surrounds the abdominal cavity almost completely. The transversus, therefore, should be the most effective abdominal muscle in increasing abdominal pressure. The differences in the frequency with which the different abdominal muscles are used thus support the idea that the action of these muscles on abdominal pressure is more important to the act of breathing than their action on the rib cage.

VIII. Conclusions

Whether in humans or in quadrupeds, the diaphragm is not the only important contracting muscle as previously thought. The diaphragm acting alone expands the abdomen and the lower rib cage, particularly along its transverse diameter, but it causes an inward displacement of the cranial half of the rib cage. The expansion of this portion of the rib cage is thus accomplished by other inspiratory muscles. Among these, the scalenes (in humans) and the parasternal intercostals (in quadrupeds) play a predominant role. The external intercostals and levator costae probably contribute little to resting breathing; owing to their abundant supply in muscle spindles, these muscles might be a reserve, load-compensating system.

Additional muscles, in particular the triangularis sterni and the transversus abdominis, are also frequently involved in the act of breathing. These muscles are usually considered to be expiratory because they displace the respiratory system below its relaxation volume. By relaxing at end-expiration, however, these muscles cause passive inspiration, reducing the load on the inspiratory muscles. This mechanism operates all the time in quadrupeds, but it may also be observed in humans, in particular when the load imposed on the respiratory muscle pump is increased. Thus, moving the chest wall during breathing is a complex, integrated process that involves many muscles. The control mechanisms that promote coordinated use of these different muscles are critically important to maintaining both the work of breathing and the alveolar ventilation within acceptable limits.

References

Arnold, J. S., Haxhiu, M. A., Cherniack, N. S., and Van Lunteren, E. (1988). Transverse abdominis length changes during eupnea, hypercapnia, and airway occlusion. *J. Appl. Physiol.* 64: 658–665.

Bainton, C. R., Kirkwood, P. A., and Sears, T. A. (1978). On the transmission of the stimulating effects of carbon dioxide to the muscles of respiration. *J. Physiol. (Lond.)* 280: 249–272.

Beau, J. H. S., and Maissiat, J. H. (1843). Recherches sur le mécanisme des mouvements respiratoires. *Arch. Gen. Med.* 1: 265–295.

Bronk, D. W., and Ferguson, L. K. (1935). The nervous control of intercostal respiration. *Am. J. Physiol.* 110: 700–707.

Budzinska, K., Supinski, G., and DiMarco, A. F. (1989). Inspiratory action of separate external and parasternal intercostal muscle contraction. *J. Appl. Physiol.* 67: 1395–1400.

Campbell, E. J. M. (1952). An electromyographic study of the role of the abdominal muscles in breathing. *J. Physiol. (Lond.)* 117: 222–233.

Campbell, E. J. M. (1955). The role of the scalene and sternomastoid muscles in breathing in normal subjects. An electromyographic study. *J. Anat.* 89: 378–386.

Corda, M., Eklund, G., and von Euler, C. (1965). External intercostal and phrenic α motor responses to changes in respiratory load. *Acta Physiol. Scand.* 63: 391–400.

D'Angelo, E., and Sant'Ambrogio, G. (1974). Direct action of contracting diaphragm on the rib cage in rabbits and dogs. *J. Appl. Physiol.* 36: 715–719.

Danon, J., Druz, W. S., Goldberg, N. B., and Sharp, J. T. (1979). Function for the isolated paced diaphragm and the cervical accessory muscles in C_1 quadriplegics. *Am. Rev. Respir. Dis.* 119: 909–919.

Da Silva, K. M. C., Sayers, B. M. A., Sears, T. A., and Stagg, D. T. (1977). The changes in configuration of the rib cage and abdomen during breathing in the anaesthetized cat. *J. Physiol. (Lond.)* 266: 499–521.

Decramer, M., and De Troyer, A. (1984). Respiratory changes in parasternal intercostal length. *J. Appl. Physiol.* 57: 1254–1260.

Decramer, M., Kelly, S., and De Troyer, A. (1986). Respiratory and postural changes in intercostal muscle length in supine dogs. *J. Appl. Physiol.* 60: 1686–1691.

Delhez, L. (1974). *Contribution Électromyographique à l'Étude de la Mécanique et du Contrôle Nerveux des Mouvements Respiratoires de l'Homme.* Liège, Belgium, Vaillant-Carmanne.

De Troyer, A. (1983). Mechanical role of the abdominal muscles in relation to posture. *Respir. Physiol.* 53: 341–353.

De Troyer, A. (1991a). The inspiratory elevation of the ribs in the dog: Primary role of the parasternals. *J. Appl. Physiol.* 70: 1447–1455.

De Troyer, A. (1991b). Differential control of the inspiratory intercostal muscles during airway occlusion in the dog. *J. Physiol. (Lond.)* 439: 73–88.

De Troyer, A. (1992). The electromechanical response of canine inspiratory intercostal muscles to increased resistance: The cranial rib cage. *J. Physiol. (Lond.)* 451: 445–461.

De Troyer, A., and Decramer, M. (1985). Mechanical coupling between the ribs and sternum in the dog. *Respir. Physiol.* 59: 27–34.

De Troyer, A., and Estenne, M. (1984). Coordination between rib cage muscles and diaphragm during quiet breathing in humans. *J. Appl. Physiol.* 57: 899–906.

De Troyer, A., and Farkas, G. A. (1989). Inspiratory function of the levator costae and external intercostal muscles in the dog. *J. Appl. Physiol.* 67: 2614–2621.

De Troyer, A., and Farkas, G. A. (1990). Linkage between parasternals and external intercostals during resting breathing. *J. Appl. Physiol.* 69: 509–516.

De Troyer, A., and Farkas, G. A. (1993). Mechanics of the parasternal intercostals in prone dogs. Statics and dynamics. *J. Appl. Physiol.* 74: 2757–2762.

De Troyer, A., and Kelly, S. (1982). Chest wall mechanics in dogs with acute diaphragm paralysis. *J. Appl. Physiol.* 53: 373–379.

De Troyer, A., and Kelly, S. (1984). Action of neck accessory muscles on rib cage in dogs. *J. Appl. Physiol.* 56: 326–332.

De Troyer, A., and Ninane, V. (1986a). Respiratory function of intercostal muscles in supine dog: An electromyographic study. *J. Appl. Physiol.* 60: 1692–1699.

De Troyer, A., and Ninane, V. (1986b). Triangularis sterni: A primary muscle of breathing in the dog. *J. Appl. Physiol.* 60: 14–21.

De Troyer, A., and Ninane, V. (1987). Effect of posture on expiratory muscle use during breathing in the dog. *Respir. Physiol.* 67: 311–322.

De Troyer, A., and Sampson, M. G. (1982). Activation of the parasternal intercostals during breathing efforts in human subjects. *J. Appl. Physiol.* 52: 524–529.

De Troyer, A., Sampson, M., Sigrist, S., and Macklem, P. T. (1981). The diaphragm: Two muscles. *Science* 213: 237–238.

De Troyer, A., Sampson, M., Sigrist, S., and Macklem, P. T. (1982). Action of costal and crural parts of the diaphragm on the rib cage in dog. *J. Appl. Physiol.* 53: 30–39.

De Troyer, A., Sampson, M., Sigrist, S., and Kelly, S. (1983). How the abdominal muscles act on the rib cage. *J. Appl. Physiol.* 54: 465–469.

De Troyer, A., Kelly, S., Macklem, P. T., and Zin, W. A. (1985). Mechanics of intercostal space and actions of external and internal intercostal muscles. *J. Clin. Invest.* 75: 850–857.

De Troyer, A., Estenne, M., and Vincken, W. (1986). Rib cage motion and muscle use in high tetraplegics. *Am. Rev. Respir. Dis.* 133: 1115–1119.

De Troyer, A., Ninane, V., Gilmartin, J. J., Lemerre, C., and Estenne, M. (1987). Triangularis sterni muscle use in supine humans. *J. Appl. Physiol.* 62: 919–925.

De Troyer, A., Farkas, G. A., and Ninane, V. (1988). Mechanics of the parasternal intercostals during occluded breaths in the dog. *J. Appl. Physiol.* 64: 1546–1553.

De Troyer, A., Gilmartin, J. J., and Ninane, V. (1989). Abdominal muscle use during breathing in unanesthetized dogs. *J. Appl. Physiol.* 66: 20–27.

De Troyer, A., Estenne, M., Ninane, V., Van Gansbeke, D., and Gorini, M. (1990). Transversus abdominis muscle function in humans. *J. Appl. Physiol.* 68: 1010–1016.

De Troyer, A., Cappello, M., and Brichant, J. F. (1994). Do the canine scalene and sternomastoid muscles play a role in breathing? *J. Appl. Physiol.* 76: 242–252.

Druz, W. S., and Sharp, J. T. (1981). Activity of respiratory muscles in upright and recumbent humans. *J. Appl. Physiol.* 51: 1552–1561.

Duchenne, G. B. (1867). *Physiologie des Mouvements.* Paris: Baillière.

Duron, B. (1981). Intercostal and diaphragmatic muscle endings and afferents. In *Regulation of Breathing*, Part 1. Edited by T. F. Hornbein. New York, Marcel Dekker, p. 473–540.

Duron, B., Jung-Caillol, M. C., and Marlot, D. (1978). Myelinated nerve fiber supply and muscle spindles in the respiratory muscles of cat: Quantitative study. *Anat. Embryol.* 152: 171–192.

Estenne, M., and De Troyer, A. (1985). Relationship between respiratory muscle electromyogram and rib cage motion in tetraplegia. *Am. Rev. Respir. Dis.* 132: 53–59.

Estenne, M., Ninane, V., and De Troyer, A. (1988). Triangularis sterni muscle use during eupnea in humans: Effect of posture. *Respir. Physiol.* 74: 151–162.

Farkas, G. A., and Schroeder, M. A. (1990). Mechanical role of expiratory muscles during breathing in prone anesthetized dogs. *J. Appl. Physiol.* 69: 2137–2142.

Farkas, G. A., and Schroeder, M. A. (1993). Functional of significance of expiratory muscles during spontaneous breathing in anesthetized dogs. *J. Appl. Physiol.* 74: 238–244.

Farkas, G. A., Estenne, M., and De Troyer, A. (1989). Expiratory muscle contribution to tidal volume in head-up dogs. *J. Appl. Physiol.* 67: 1438–1442.

Floyd, W. F., and Silver, P. H. S. (1950). Electromyographic study of patterns of activity of the anterior abdominal wall muscles in man. *J. Anat.* 84: 132–145.

Gilmartin, J. J., Ninane, V., and De Troyer, A. (1987). Abdominal muscle use during breathing in the anesthetized dog. *Respir. Physiol.* 70: 159–171.

Greer, J. J., and Martin, T. P. (1990). Distribution of muscle fiber types and EMG activity in cat intercostal muscles. *J. Appl. Physiol.* 69: 1208–1211.

Hamberger, G. E. (1749). *De Respirationis Mechanismo et usu Genuino.* Jena, Germany.

Hilaire, G. G., Nicholls, J. G., and Sears, T. A. (1983). Central and proprioceptive influences on the activity of levator costae motoneurones in the cat. *J. Physiol. (Lond.)* 342: 527–548.

Hwang, J. C., Zhou, D., and St. John, W. M. (1989). Characterization of expiratory intercostal activity to triangularis sterni in cats. *J. Appl. Physiol.* 67: 1518–1524.

Jiang, T. X., Demedts, M., and Decramer, M. (1988). Mechanical coupling of upper and lower canine rib cages and its functional significance. *J. Appl. Physiol.* 64: 620–626.

Koterba, A. M., Kosch, P. C., Beech, J., and Whitlock, T. (1988). Breathing strategy of the adult horse (*Equus caballus*) at rest. *J. Appl. Physiol.* 64: 337–346.

Loring, S. H. (1992). Action of human respiratory muscles inferred from finite element analysis of rib cage. *J. Appl. Physiol.* 72: 1461–1465.

Loring, S. H., and Mead, J. (1982). Action of the diaphragm on the rib cage inferred from a force–balance analysis. *J. Appl. Physiol.* 53: 756–760.

Loring, S. H., and Woodbridge, J. A. (1991). Intercostal muscle action inferred from finite-element analysis. *J. Appl. Physiol.* 70: 2712–2718.

Luciani, L. (1911). Circulation and respiration. In *Human Physiology*, Vol 1. London, Macmillan, pp. 411–415.

Margulies, S. S., Rodarte, J. R., and Hoffman, E. A. (1989). Geometry and kinematics of dog ribs. *J. Appl. Physiol.* 67: 707–712.

Martin, J. G., and De Troyer, A. (1982). The behavior of the abdominal muscles during inspiratory mechanical loading. *Respir. Physiol.* 50: 63–73.

Mead, J. (1979). Functional significance of the area of apposition of diaphragm to rib cage. *Am. Rev. Respir. Dis.* 119: 31–32.

Mead, J., and Loring, S. H. (1982). Analysis of volume displacement and length changes of the diaphragm during breathing. *J. Appl. Physiol.* 53: 750–755.

Mier, A., Brophy, C., Estenne, M., Moxham, J., Green, M., and De Troyer, A. (1985). Action of abdominal muscles on rib cage in humans. *J. Appl. Physiol.* 58: 1438–1443.

Mortola, J. P., and Sant'Ambrogio, G. (1978). Motion of the rib cage and the abdomen in tetraplegic patients. *Clin. Sci. Mol. Med.* 54: 25–32.

Ninane, V., Decramer, M., and De Troyer, A. (1986). Coupling between triangularis sterni and parasternals during breathing in dogs. *J. Appl. Physiol.* 61: 539–544.

Ninane, V., Gilmartin, J. J., and De Troyer, A. (1988). Changes in abdominal muscle length during breathing in supine dogs. *Respir. Physiol.* 73: 31–42.

Ninane, V., Baer, R. E., and De Troyer, A. (1989). Mechanism of triangularis sterni shortening during expiration in dogs. *J. Appl. Physiol.* 66: 2287–2292.

Raper, A. J., Thompson, W. T., Jr., Shapiro, W., and Patterson, J. L., Jr. (1966). Scalene and sternomastoid muscle function. *J. Appl. Physiol.* 21: 497–502.

Sant'Ambrogio, G., and Widdicombe, J. G. (1965). Respiratory reflexes acting on the diaphragm and inspiratory intercostal muscles of the rabbit. *J. Physiol. (Lond.).* 180: 766–779.

Saumarez, R. C. (1986). An analysis of action of intercostal muscles in human upper rib cage. *J. Appl. Physiol.* 60: 690–701.

Sears, T. A. (1964). Efferent discharges in alpha and fusimotor fibres of intercostal nerves of the cat. *J. Physiol. (Lond.)* 174: 295–315.

Shannon, R., and Zechman, F. W. (1972). The reflex and mechanical response of the inspiratory muscles to an increased airflow resistance. *Respir. Physiol.* 16: 51–69.

Smith, C. A., Ainsworth, D. M., Henderson, K. S., and Dempsey, J. A. (1989). Differential responses of expiratory muscles to chemical stimuli in awake dogs. *J. Appl. Physiol.* 66: 384–391.

Strohl, K. P., Mead, J., Banzett, R. B., Lehr, J., Loring, S. H., and O'Cain, C. F. (1984). Effect of posture on upper and lower rib cage motion and tidal volume during diaphragm pacing. *Am. Rev. Respir. Dis.* 130: 320–321.

Strohl, K. P., Mead, J., Banzett, R. B., Loring, S. H., and Kosch, P. C. (1981). Regional differences in abdominal muscle activity during various maneuvers in humans. *J. Appl. Physiol.* 51: 1471–1476.

Taylor, A. (1960). The contribution of the intercostal muscles to the effort of respiration in man. *J. Physiol. (Lond.)* 151: 390–402.

Urmey, W. F., De Troyer, A., Kelly, K. B., and Loring, S. H. (1988). Pleural pressure increases during inspiration in the zone of apposition of diaphragm to rib cage. *J. Appl. Physiol.* 65: 2207–2212.

van Lunteren, E., and Cherniack, N. S. (1986). Electrical and mechanical activity of the respiratory muscles during hypercapnia. *J. Appl. Physiol.* 61: 719–727.

van Lunteren, E., Cherniack, N. S., and Dick, T. E. (1988a). Upper airway pressure receptors alter expiratory muscle EMG and motor unit firing. *J. Appl. Physiol.* 65: 210–217.

van Lunteren, E., Haxhiu, M. A., Cherniack, N. S., and Arnold, J. S. (1988b). Rib cage and abdominal expiratory muscle responses to CO_2 and esophageal distension. *J. Appl. Physiol.* 64: 846–853.

Warner, D. O., Krayer, S., Rehder, K., and Ritman, E. L. (1989). Chest wall motion during spontaneous breathing and mechanical ventilation in dogs. *J. Appl. Physiol.* 66: 1179–1189.

Whitelaw, W. A., and Feroah, T. (1989). Patterns of intercostal muscle activity in humans. *J. Appl. Physiol.* 67: 2087–2094.

Whitelaw, W. A., Ford, G. T., Rimmer, K. P., and De Troyer, A. (1992). Intercostal muscles are used during rotation of the thorax in humans. *J. Appl. Physiol.* 72: 1940–1944.

Wilson, T. A., and De Troyer, A. (1993). Respiratory effect of the intercostal muscles in the dog. *J. Appl. Physiol.* 75: 2636–2645.

Wilson, T. A., Rehder, K., Krayer, S., Hoffman, E. A., Whitney, C. G., and Rodarte, J. R. (1987). Geometry and respiratory displacement of human ribs. *J. Appl. Physiol.* 62: 1872–1877.

20

Volume Displacements of the Chest Wall and Their Mechanical Significance

JERE MEAD

Harvard School of Public Health
Boston, Massachusetts

JEFFREY C. SMITH

University of California
Los Angeles, California

STEPHEN H. LORING

Beth Israel Hospital
Harvard Medical School
Boston, Massachusetts

I. Introduction

Central to the study of the nature and function of the respiratory pump is analysis of the volume displacements produced by movements of the major structures of the chest wall. In this chapter, we consider the manner in which these displacements can be measured and related to lung volume change and respiratory muscle action and can also be used to estimate the mechanical work done by respiratory muscles. We draw heavily on two articles (Mead and Loring, 1982; Loring and Mead, 1982), which present the major ideas that are further developed here.

II. Degrees of Freedom of the Respiratory System and the Partitioning of Body Surface Displacements

In theory, volume displacements of the chest wall can be inferred from analysis of the geometry of the structure, or from measurements of a limited number of linear displacements at discrete points on the external surfaces of the chest wall. The complicated shapes of the chest wall surfaces make a geometric analysis extremely difficult (Agostoni et al., 1965; Agostoni, 1970), but analysis of linear displacements has been satisfactory (Konno and Mead, 1967; Mead et al., 1967). These latter approaches are based on considerations of the degrees of freedom of the chest wall, and here we provide a summary of the principles involved. Detailed discussions of the experimental techniques commonly used to measure the surface displacements are presented elsewhere (Mead et al., 1967; Loring and Bruce, 1986).

The surfaces of the chest wall are those of the body cavity, so that analysis of chest wall volume displacements involves considerations of the manner in which the surfaces of the body cavity move. The body wall has three ways to move and displace volume: (1) by rib cage expansion or contraction, (2) by expansion or contraction of the anterior abdominal wall, and (3) by flexion–extension of the spine. Each of these movements represents a single degree of freedom of the chest wall, to the extent that each can be represented and measured in terms of a single variable. For example, displacements of the rib cage and anterior abdominal wall can be represented by anteroposterior dimensions of these structures (Konno and Mead, 1967); and movements of the spine can be represented by changes in the axial dimension of the chest wall from measurements of the distance between points on the anterior surface near the xiphisternum and pubic symphysis (J. Smith and J. Mead, unpublished observations).

The adequacy of a single-variable representation of these movements has been tested experimentally by examining the relationships between these variables for various patterns of displacement. For example, at constant lung volume and with the attitude of the spine fixed, volume displacements of the rib cage and anterior abdominal wall must be equal and opposite; the relationship between the representative variables must be single-valued so that an x–y plot of these variables forms a single, negatively sloped line. It is readily demonstrated that such single-valued relationships are obtained experimentally with measurements of anteroposterior diameters or with transverse cross sections (Mead, 1974; Loring and Bruce, 1986). Furthermore, these variables are easily calibrated and expressed in terms of volume displacements by several methods. The relationships between these displacements are commonly depicted graphically by plotting the rib cage displacements on the ordinate and abdominal displacements on the abscissa (Konno–Mead diagram) (see Fig. 3). If the relative sensitivity of the variables to volume change is adjusted so that the relationships at constant lung volume have slopes of -1, then an inspiration with a positive slope of 1, for example, would represent a breath in which the rib cage and anterior abdominal wall displacements contribute equally to the volume expansion. Thus, the slope of the relationship indicates the relative volume contributions of the two degrees of freedom.

When the attitude of the spine is fixed, the two-degrees-of-freedom description is sufficient to specify the volume displacements under a variety of conditions of passive or active forcing of the system (Loring and Bruce, 1986). If the attitude of the spine varies, then a three-degrees-of-freedom description is required. The adequacy of this representation is tested by examining the relationships at constant lung volume between the single variable representing the attitude of the spine (e.g., xiphi–pubic distance) and the sum of the variables representing displacements of the rib cage and abdominal wall. When these latter variables are adjusted to equal sensitivity and examined graphically as a function of a signal proportional to xiphi–pubic distance, a family of nearly parallel, single-valued lines at different lung volumes is readily obtained (Fig. 1). Furthermore, the variable for spinal attitude can be directly interpreted in terms of volume displacements. That the isovolume relationships are nearly single-valued demonstrates the adequacy of single-variable representations of the major modes of movement of the chest wall and also demonstrates that the major degrees of freedom have been described. When the relative sensitivities of the variables to volume change are adjusted to be equal, the relative contributions of the three degrees of freedom to the total volume displacement of the system can be measured.

Changes in the attitude of the spine are relatively small during ordinary breathing; hence, this third degree of freedom does not contribute importantly to the volume displacements during breathing. Furthermore, although movements of the spine can cause substantial displacements of the chest wall (see Fig. 1), they probably do not cause significant changes in lung volume. This is attributable to the nature of the displacements produced by spinal flexion and extension. Spinal

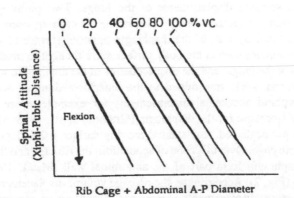

Figure 1 Demonstration of a third degree of freedom of the chest wall in a standing subject. Displacements of the rib cage and anterior abdominal wall are measured by changes in anteroposterior (AP) diameters. Attitude of the spine is represented by the distance between points on the chest wall's anterior surface near the xiphisternum and pubic symphysis (xiphi–pubic distance). The sensitivity to volume change of the signals for the AP diameters was adjusted so that the sum of the signals is zero during an isovolume maneuver produced at fixed spinal attitudes. Then, at fixed increments of the vital capacity, measured spirometrically, the subject slowly flexed and extended his spine between comfortable extremes, and the nearly linear and nearly single-valued isopleths were obtained. The associated volume displacement between these extremes, as indicated by the rib cage–abdominal sum, was approximately one-half of the vital capacity. (From Smith and Mead, 1986.)

extension, which expands the chest wall axially, is accompanied by a simultaneous inward displacement of the rib cage and anterior abdominal wall; spinal flexion shortens the axial dimension of the chest wall and causes outward displacements of the rib cage and abdominal wall. As a result, movements of the spine distort the shape of the chest wall, but have little effect on lung volume. Furthermore, a wide range of rib cage and abdominal wall displacements is possible at a fixed spinal attitude, without any sense that muscular effort is required to maintain the position of the spine fixed. Thus, it is subjectively easy to breathe by displacing the rib cage and anterior abdominal wall without changing spinal attitude, and equally easy to move the spine without changing lung volume. The details of the mechanics by which these respiratory and postural movements are functionally isolated remain to be clarified.

III. Relationship Between Body and Lung Surface Displacements

The relative ease with which body surface displacements could be separated into rib cage and anterior abdominal wall components initially led to an overly simple view of the associated displacements of the lungs. Two pathways for volume displacement were recognized: one by way of the rib cage-apposed surfaces of the lungs, and the other by way of the diaphragm-apposed surface of the lungs. The rib cage displacements seen at the body surface were thought to produce equivalent displacements of the lungs, and the displacements of the diaphragm were considered to be directly and solely transmitted to the anterior abdominal wall. Therefore, inspirations without abdominal displacement, for example, were considered as approximately isometric for the diaphragm (Grassino et al., 1978; Macklem et al., 1978). This view neglected a substantial moving surface—the diaphragm-apposed surface of the rib cage. Over this zone of apposition, the rib cage and the immediately underlying diaphragm form part of the abdominal wall (Mead, 1979; Mead and Loring, 1982) (Fig. 2). Accordingly, the rib cage volume displacement, as estimated from body surface displacements, represents a mixture of abdominal and lung displacements. As Mead and Loring (1982) have pointed out, displacement of the rib cage moves the cephalic surfaces of the abdominal cavity axially as well as radially. As the rib cage expands, it moves headward, moving the diaphragm with it and further expanding the abdomen. The total abdominal component of the rib cage volume displacement is significant. Ordinarily, more than half of the rib cage displacement is abdominal, not pulmonary; even at high lung volumes, when the area of the zone of apposition is small, its contribution to abdominal displacement remains substantial.

How then are lung surface and diaphragmatic displacements to be inferred from body surface measurements? The lungs are directly apposed to the rib cage and to the diaphragm and change volume as these surfaces are displaced. The rib

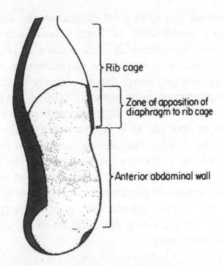

Rib cage

Zone of apposition of
diaphragm to rib cage

Anterior abdominal wall

Figure 2 Schematic diagram of the major components of the body surface that displace volumes during breathing. Zone of apposition of diaphragm to rib cage covers a variable fraction of the rib cage's surface area. At residual volume, it covers approximately one-half of the rib cage surface; with increasing lung voume, diaphragmatic fiber lengths decrease, and the area of the zone of apposition progressively decreases, becoming small near total lung capacity.

cage-apposed surface moves both radially and axially, whereas the diaphragm-apposed surface moves mainly in the axial direction. Axial displacements of the diaphragm-apposed surface of the lungs are caused by two distinct mechanisms: diaphragm length change and diaphragm insertional movement. Length changes result in axial displacements of the diaphragmatic dome relative to its insertions, but the insertions move axially as the rib cage expands, and the entire diaphragm participates in this motion. Thus, the total axial displacement of the diaphragm-apposed lung surface is the sum of shortening and nonshortening components. This distinction is important, because the components have very different implications for lung volume. Axial displacements produced by diaphragmatic shortening alone are associated with equal increases in lung volume. In contrast, an identical axial displacement produced without diaphragmatic shortening (i.e., entirely by rib cage movement) is associated with a smaller change in lung volume. As the rib cage expands and moves cephalad, the diaphragm's insertions on the rib cage move cephalad and outward. The outward displacement tends to flatten the diaphragm, lowering the diaphragm's dome relative to its insertions, so that outward displacement of the rib cage would displace the diaphragm axially, in the inspiratory direction. But the upward component moves the entire diaphragm axially in the expiratory direction.

Clearly the diaphragm's contribution to lung volume change is not resolved in any simple way from analysis of its axial displacements. Another approach is to estimate the rib cage's contribution to lung volume change and obtain the diaphragmatic contribution by subtraction. The volume displaced by the rib cage, estimated from measurements of body surface displacements, is from two-thirds to three-fourths of the total volume change during ordinary breathing (Grimby et al., 1968). At ordinary lung volumes, approximately 60% of this displacement can be assigned to displacement of the rib cage-apposed surface of the lung, and approximately 25% to an opposite axial displacement of the diaphragm-apposed surface (Mead and Loring, 1982). The net displacement of the lung produced by the rib cage, expressed as a fraction of an ordinary tidal volume, is then 0.6(0.67–0.75) minus 0.25(0.67–0.75) (the negative sign reflects the opposite directions of the lung surface displacements), or 0.24–0.29. Thus, nominally, one-fourth of the change in lung volume during an ordinary inspiration can be assigned to the rib cage. The remaining three-fourths of the volume change can be attributed to diaphragm shortening.

IV. Mechanical Actions of the Rib Cage

At first glance, it seems inappropriate to consider the rib cage, which accounts for three-fourths of the volume displaced at the body surface, as producing only one-fourth of the lung volume change. This discrepancy is resolved when it is appreciated that nearly two-thirds of the rib cage's volume displacement either bypasses the lungs (through the zone of apposition), or is transmitted by the lungs, and goes into abdominal displacements. These abdominal displacements are the rib cage's major mechanical contribution to breathing. By means of these displacements, the rib cage makes way for the primary act of the diaphragm, which is to change lung volume: as the rib cage expands, it lowers abdominal pressure and permits a larger fraction of transdiaphragmatic pressure to go into lowering the pleural pressure.

But quite apart from its contribution during phasic respiration, the rib cage has important steady-state functions as well. It serves to moderate other influences of abdominal pressure on respiration and, potentially, to minimize the influence of respiration on abdominal pressure. Abdominal pressure can be increased by the action of abdominal muscles, by external constraints, by ingestion of food or retention of excreta, and by increase in uterine size during pregnancy. The influences of such phenomena on lung volume are smaller than they otherwise would be by virtue of the inspiratory action that the associated increase of abdominal pressure has on the rib cage. This is not obvious until it is noted that abdominal pressure acts on the rib cage at the zone of apposition; this effect is explained in the next section. But, depending on the action of intercostal muscles, the rib cage not only can modulate the action of abdominal pressure on breathing, it can also directly influence abdominal pressure itself. Indeed, this constitutes the abdomen's principal way to accommodate encroachment.

In summary, these ideas indicate that the rib cage is mainly an abdominal pump, and only secondarily a lung pump.

V. Partitioning of Volume Displacements as Related to Muscle Action

Here we simplify analysis of respiratory muscle action by distinguishing three sources of driving pressure: the diaphragm, the muscles of the rib cage (intercostals and accessories), and the muscles of the anterior abdominal wall. First, we consider the volume changes produced by separate actions of the muscles. For these purposes, we develop pathways on the Konno–Mead diagram (Konno and Mead, 1967; Mead, 1974) for various sorts of forcing. In all instances, the forces are considered as being maintained sufficiently to allow quasistatic conditions. The pathways are shown in Figure 3, and their basis is as follows:

The pathways are determined by the relative compliances of the passive parts of the system and the pressures applied to them. The lung is passive in all circumstances, and its volume change depends on its compliance and the change in pleural surface pressure. The volume change of the anterior abdominal wall depends on its compliance and the change in abdominal pressure, whereas that of the passive rib cage depends on its compliance and the change in the pressure applied to it. When the diaphragm is relaxed and under no tension, intrathoracic pressure changes equally above and below the diaphragm, and the passive rib cage is driven by a single pressure change that is equally pleural (ΔPpl) or abdominal (ΔPab). When the diaphragm is actively or passively tensed, the rib cage is exposed to pleural pressure on its lung-apposed surface and to a pressure approximating abdominal pressure on its diaphragm-apposed surface (Mead, 1981). Loring and Mead (1982) have expressed the effect of these pressures on the rib cage with a weighting factor, B. Thus, the sum BPab + (1 − B)Ppl represents a single pressure equivalent, Prc. It should be noted that B is more than simply an expression of pressure partitioning. By rearrangement, Prc becomes Ppl − B(Ppl − Pab), which is seen to equal −BPdi. The term BPdi expresses the total effect of the diaphragm on the rib cage and contains its direct insertional influence as well as its partitioning influence.

In summary, the passively produced volume changes of the lungs, anterior abdominal wall, and rib cage (i.e., ΔVL, ΔVabw, and ΔVrc) can be expressed respectively, as −ΔPplCL, ΔPabCabw, and ΔPrcCrc. (The minus sign in the expression for ΔVL reflects the definition of transpulmonary pressure, which is mouth pressure minus pleural pressure. Mouth pressure being zero, the change in transpulmonary pressure that produces an increase in lung volume is −ΔPpl.) Since lung volume change is the sum of rib cage and anterior abdominal wall displacements (i.e., ΔVL = ΔVrc + ΔVabw), it is always possible to express the volume change of one part of the system in terms of the other two. Accordingly, the volume change of an active component can be expressed in terms of those of the passive components

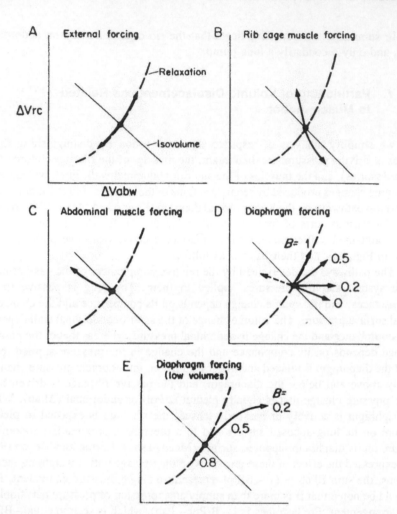

Figure 3 Konno–Mead diagrams showing rib cage and anterior abdominal wall displacements from the relaxed end-expiratory level for various sorts of forcing. The dashed lines represent relaxation characteristics. (A) External forcing, illustrating displacements produced by externally applied pressures, such as produced by respirators. The other examples represent conditions under which only the rib cage muscles (B), abdominal muscles (C), and diaphragm (D,E) are active. Slopes of the displacement pathways (solid lines and arrows) are predicted from the analysis given in the text.

which, in turn, can be expressed in terms of their compliances and the pressures applied to them.

A. External Forcing

Pathways on the Konno–Mead diagram have slopes expressing the relative volume displacements of the rib cage and anterior abdominal wall, $\Delta Vrc/\Delta Vabw$. When the relaxed respiratory system is driven by an externally applied pressure, such as produced by a respirator (see Fig. 3A),

$$\frac{\Delta Vrc}{\Delta Vabw} = \frac{Crc\Delta Prc}{Cabw\Delta Pab} = \frac{Crc(B\Delta Pab + (1 - B)\Delta Ppl)}{Cabw\Delta Pab} \tag{1}$$

In the inspiratory direction, the passive diaphragm is shortened and its tension remains zero. In this case, $\Delta Prc = \Delta Ppl = \Delta Pab$, and $\Delta Vrc/\Delta Vabw$ is given simply by $Crc/Cabw$. That is, the slope of the relaxation characteristic expresses the relative compliance of the rib cage and anterior abdominal wall. For typical values for Crc and Cabw of 0.15 and 0.05 L/cm H_2O, respectively, the slope of the corresponding relaxation characteristic is $+3$.

In the expiratory direction, the diaphragm develops passive tension, and the fraction $\Delta Prc/\Delta Pab$ increases as ΔPpl exceeds ΔPab. Two counteracting influences are any increases in B and decreases in Crc/Cabw, both of which occur with decreasing lung volume; that is, as the surface area of the zone of apposition of diaphragm to rib cage increases, and as abdominal compliance increases. The observation that the slope of the relaxation characteristic in the upright posture actually decreases as lung volume decreases (Konno and Mead, 1967) suggests that these latter factors dominate.

B. Rib Cage Muscle Action

When the muscles of the rib cage are active (see Fig. 3B), ΔVrc can be expressed as $\Delta VL - \Delta Vabw$, which is given by $-CL\Delta Ppl - Cabw\Delta Pab$ or $-(CL\Delta Ppl + Cabw\Delta Pab)$. Accordingly, $\Delta Vrc/\Delta Vabw = -(CL\Delta Ppl + Cabw\Delta Pab)/Cabw\Delta Pab = -[CL(\Delta Ppl/\Delta Pab) + Cabw]/Cabw$. In the inspiratory direction, the expanding rib cage causes the passive diaphragm to shorten, and diaphragmatic tension remains zero. Accordingly, $\Delta Ppl/\Delta Pab = 1$, and for realistic values for the compliances (CL $= 0.2$ and Cabw $= 0.05$ L/cm H_2O), the value of $\Delta Vrc/\Delta Vabw$ is -5. Thus, rib cage expansion results in a paradoxical inward displacement of the anterior abdominal wall. The degree of paradox depends on the compliance of the lungs. In the limit of CL $= 0$ or the equivalent circumstance of complete obstruction of the airway opening, the slope becomes -1.

In the expiratory direction, as the diaphragm is passively tensed, ΔPab exceeds ΔPpl, and $\Delta Vrc/\Delta Vabw$ decreases, approaching -1 as $\Delta Ppl/\Delta Pab$ falls to zero.

C. Abdominal Muscle Action

When the muscles of the anterior abdominal wall are active (see Fig. 3C), ΔVabw can be expressed as ΔVL − ΔVrc, which is seen to be −CLΔPpl − CrcΔPrc or −(CLΔPpl + CrcΔPrc), and ΔVrc/ΔVabw is then CrcΔPrc/−(CLΔPpl + CrcΔPrc). Initially (i.e., before the diaphragm develops tension), ΔPrc = ΔPpl = ΔPab and the expression simplifies to ΔVrc/ΔVabw = −[Crc/(CL + Crc)], which for realistic compliances (CL = 0.2, Crc = 0.15 L/cm H_2O) is = −.43. As in rib cage forcing, the displacements are paradoxical: inward displacements of the abdominal wall result in rib cage expansion. Furthermore, the degree of paradox increases as the lung compliance falls, with the slope approaching −1 as CL approaches 0.

As the diaphragm develops tension, ΔPab exceeds ΔPpl and, as the diaphragm is lengthened, the value of B increases. ΔVrc/ΔVabw increases, approaching −1 as ΔPpl/ΔPab and B approach 0 and 1, respectively.

Thus it is apparent that the effects of rib cage or anterior abdominal wall forcing have the same characteristics. Each results in paradoxical displacements of the other, which are augmented by tension in the diaphragm and by decreasing lung compliance. Increases in impedance of the lung, as from bronchoconstriction or airway obstruction, would have the same effect.

D. Diaphragm Action

To illustrate the actions of the diaphragm (see Fig. 3D), the lungs, rib cage, and anterior abdominal wall are all considered to be driven passively. With the four equations, ΔVL = ΔVabw + ΔVrc, ΔVrc = Crc[BΔPab + (1 − B)ΔPpl], ΔVabw = CabwΔPab, and ΔVL = − CLΔPpl, three unknowns (ΔVL, ΔPab, and ΔPpl) can be eliminated, and an expression for the slope can be obtained that contains only compliance values and B:

$$\frac{\Delta Vrc}{\Delta Vabw} = \frac{B(Crc/Cabw) - (1 - B)(Crc/CL)}{1 + (1 - B)(Crc/CL)} \tag{2}$$

For B = 1, this expression simplifies to Crc/Cabw. The diaphragm acting alone would then drive the respiratory system along its relaxation characteristic.

If the diaphragm had no effect on the rib cage other than through its influence on ΔPpl, B would be zero and ΔVrc/ΔVabw would be given by −Crc/CL/1 + (Crc/CL), which is seen to be identical with that for anterior abdominal wall muscle activity without diaphragmatic tensing. (The direction of action would be opposite, however.) Diaphragmatic contraction in this circumstance would result in paradoxical displacement of the rib cage. The value of B just sufficient to prevent paradox is found by setting ΔVrc/ΔVabw = 0. For the values of compliance given, the value of B in the absence of rib cage displacement would be 0.2 (see Fig. 3E). Loring and Mead (1982) have estimated B to be approximately 0.5 in the resting tidal range. For realistic values of the compliances, $\Delta Vrc/\Delta Vabw$ would then be 0.81. This is substantially greater than 0, but also substantially less than the slope of the relaxation characteristic, and indicates that inspirations approximating the relaxation characteristic require agonist activity of the other respiratory muscles.

From Eq. (2), it can be seen that the slope depends on the lung and anterior abdominal wall compliance, and in a reciprocal manner: for inspirations in which only the diaphragm is active, the relative displacement of the rib cage will decrease as lung compliance decreases. Conversely, the relative displacement of the rib cage increases with reductions in compliance of the anterior abdominal wall.

Note that changes in $\Delta Vrc/\Delta Vabw$ in response to changes in lung compliance, for example, as simulated by elastic loading at the mouth, have different implications depending on the relative contributions of the diaphragm and of rib cage muscles to inspiration. For inspirations produced only by the diaphragm, increases in impedance of the lung will produce a decrease in slope, whereas for an inspiration produced by the rib cage, the slope will increase. A fixed slope in the face of altered impedance would then imply participation of both.

From the preceding discussion, it is apparent that only the diaphragm is capable of driving both the rib cage and abdomen simultaneously in the inspiratory direction (positively sloped characteristic). The other inspiratory acts produce negatively sloped characteristics. A combination of abdominal muscle relaxation and rib cage muscle inspiratory activity could produce a nonparadoxing inspiration. Natural inspirations frequently parallel the relaxation configuration. Such inspirations can be achieved in a variety of ways: for example, by contraction of the diaphragm and muscles of the rib cage, or of the diaphragm and abdominal muscles, or by coordinated contraction of all three.

The foregoing Konno–Mead diagrams illustrate quantitatively the volume displacements of the rib cage and anterior abdominal wall, but this type of graphic analysis does not directly provide information on the associated volume displacements of the diaphragm. Although the lungs and chest wall clearly change volume equally, as we have discussed earlier, only approximately one-third of the volume displacement of the rib cage is directly associated with lung volume change. The remainder results in lung volume change only indirectly by way of the abdomen. This indirect displacement is by way of the diaphragm, which accounts not only for this displacement, but also for any additional displacement of the anterior abdominal wall. The point to be emphasized is that the direct contribution of the diaphragm's displacement to lung volume change is, in most circumstances, large. This is illustrated quantitatively in Figure 4. Figure 4A is a Konno–Mead diagram showing the relative rib cage and anterior abdominal wall displacements for equal tidal volumes produced by various patterns of muscle activity. All but one of the inspirations begin from the relaxed state; the lung volume change corresponds approximately to that during quiet breathing. The bar graphs (see Fig. 4B) partition the volumes. The equal lung and chest wall displacements are partitioned into diaphragm and rib cage components of the lung volume change on the left and rib

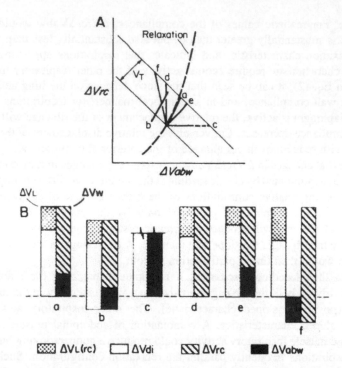

Figure 4 (A) Konno–Mead diagram showing rib cage and abdominal displacements during inspirations of equal lung volume change produced by various patterns of muscle activity. All but one of the inspirations are initiated from the relaxed state. (B) The corresponding volume displacements of the lung and chest wall surfaces are shown. Note the substantial diaphragmatic displacements in all cases.

cage and anterior abdominal wall components of chest wall volume displacement on the right. The latter are derived directly from the Konno–Mead diagram, and the former, from the assumption that one-third of the rib cage displacement measured at the body surface results directly in lung volume change (see foregoing Section III).

Breaths represented by a and b, respectively, fall on, and parallel, the relaxation characteristic. This is commonly true during spontaneous breathing. The breaths represented by c and d are highly artificial, but can be accomplished voluntarily with visual feedback. An inspiration with anterior abdominal wall expansion only (curve c) is possible over only a limited range from the relaxed state, as will become apparent when the abdominal pressure–volume relationship is represented. Curves e and f approximate the relative volume displacements during inspirations in which only the diaphragm (curve e) or rib cage muscles (curve f) are active.

The common feature of the breaths represented in Figure 4 is the substantial direct contribution of the diaphragm's displacement to the lung change. Even when only the muscles of the rib cage are active (breath f), in which the anterior abdominal wall moves inward, the diaphragm shortens, and the diaphragmatic displacement accounts for two thirds of the lung volume change. That the direct contribution of diaphragmatic displacement to lung volume change is large does not necessarily imply, however, that the diaphragm contributes to the mechanical work done. In the example just considered, despite its substantial shortening, the diaphragm would do no work, since the diaphragmatic fibers do not develop tension. The mechanical work done by the respiratory muscles during the breaths illustrated in Figure 4 is analyzed in detail in the following section.

VI. Partitioning of Respiratory Work

In analyzing respiratory work, it is necessary to distinguish the work done by muscles from that done by the structures on which the muscles operate. The muscles are the diaphragm, the rib cage muscles, and the abdominal muscles; the structures are the lungs, the diaphragm itself, the rib cage, and the anterior abdominal wall. In the preceding section, we have defined the volume displacements of these for a tidal volume produced by various patterns of muscle activity in the volume range of normal quiet breathing. Mechanical work, defined by $\int Pdv$, is represented graphically by areas on pressure–volume diagrams, in which these volume displacements are plotted as a function of the appropriate pressures. The pressures developed by muscles are revealed by the pressure differences developed by the structures between the relaxed and active states. This is illustrated in Figure 5A, which shows pleural pressure as a function of lung volume (Campbell diagram). This representation does not distinguish separate muscle actions or separate volume displacements and, as discussed later, is interpretable only in limited circumstances. Nevertheless, it presents one of the classic interpretations of the work of breathing (Margaria et al., 1960), and it develops the conventions to be used in subsequent diagrams. The dashed line corresponds to the relaxation characteristic of the chest wall. The solid line shows the pleural pressure developed by the chest wall during a slowly produced inspiration. The pressure difference between the relaxed and active state is due to muscle action, and the work done by the muscles during the inspiration is represented by the area between the two curves. (In this and the following examples, dynamic pressures are kept small for purposes of clarity, and mainly elastic work is analyzed. Identical arguments apply when full dynamic pressures are included in the analysis.) The work done by the chest wall, as distinguished from the work done by the muscles, consists of two components: one done by the muscles, and the remainder by the elastic recoil of the chest wall. It is defined by the total pressure (i.e., the pressure developed in the relaxed state plus any pressure resulting from muscle action). In Figure 5A, this is the area between the ordinate at zero pressure and the pressure curve.

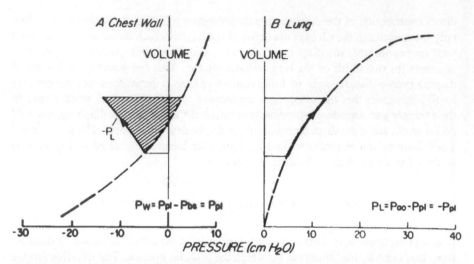

Figure 5 Pressure–volume diagrams for the chest wall (A) and lungs (B), illustrating the work done by the respiratory muscles (obliquely hatched area) and the work done by and on the passive chest wall and lungs (shaded areas) during a slow inspiration, in which the chest wall displacements occur along its relaxation characteristic, such as breath *a* in Figure 4. Pbs, body surface pressure; Pao, airway opening pressure.

  We next need to point out the significance of the sign of the pressure and the direction of the volume change. Areas to the left of the zero pressure ordinate (i.e., at negative pressures) represent work done by the chest wall if the volume is increasing, and work done on the chest wall if the volume is decreasing. Areas to the right of the ordinate represent work done on the chest wall for increasing volumes and by the chest wall for decreasing volumes. Corresponding statements can be made about the work done by muscles: pressures developed by muscles in the negative direction from the relaxation characteristic result in positive work for increasing volumes and negative work for decreasing volumes, and in the positive direction, positive work for decreasing volumes and negative work for increasing volumes.

  Work done by or on the chest wall is done on or by the lungs. Maintaining the sign convention that represents pressure on the mouthward side relative to that on the body surface side of the structure, the corresponding volume–pressure relationships for the lungs (see Fig. B) fall to the right of the ordinate; hence, work is done *on* the lungs during inspiration and *by* the lungs during expiration. In the examples considered in the following (see Figs. 6–9), the inspirations will be identical in terms of lung volume change, and the pressure–volume relationship for the lung holds for these examples. However, the pressure–volume relationship for the chest wall represented in Figure 5 is a valid expression for the combined actions of the respiratory muscles only in the particular circumstance of inspirations that do not depart from the relaxation configuration (e.g., see curve a, in Fig. 4). Spontaneous breathing frequently corresponds fairly closely, or at least parallels, the relaxation configuration; but as illustrated later, this correspondence does not imply fixed patterns of muscle activity. The appropriate volume–pressure relationships for the partitioning of the work of the diaphragm, rib cage, and anterior abdominal wall are developed in Fig. 6.

The pressure developed by the diaphragm, Pdi, by convention, is given by Ppl – Pab. The separate pressures are shown in Figure 6 in the top left panel and Pdi is shown in the right panel. In the volume range of interest, the relaxation

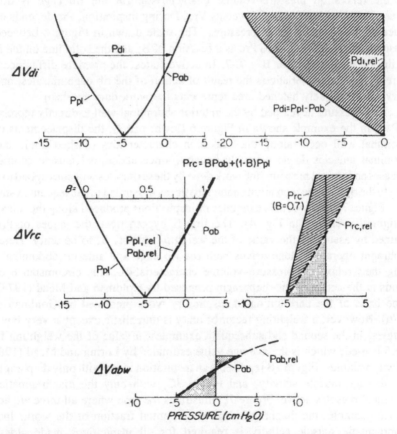

Figure 6 Graphic representation of the work done (obliquely hatched areas) by the separate respiratory muscles, illustrating the approach used for the work analysis in remaining figures: (upper panel) work done by the diaphragm; (middle panel) rib cage muscles; (lower panel) anterior abdominal wall muscles. The total lung volume change is always the sum of the rib cage (ΔVrc) and abdominal (ΔVabw) volume displacements (see Fig. 4). Dashed lines are relaxation pressure–volume characteristics; solid lines represent active characteristics.

pressure of the diaphragm is zero and, hence, corresponds to the zero pressure ordinate on the right. The pressures developed by the diaphragm during inspiration (solid curve) arise from the contractile properties of diaphragmatic muscle elements, and all of the actively developed pressures are negative in sign. The obliquely hatched area between the active curve and the ordinate represents work done by the diaphragm.

The pressure developed by the rib cage, Prc, is approximated by: $Prc = BPab + (1 - B)Ppl$. Abdominal and pleural pressures are shown in Figure 6 (middle panel) on the left, and the corresponding values of Prc are shown on the right. In the relaxed state and in the volume range where $Pdi = 0$, then $Prc = Ppl = Pab$, and the relaxation pressure–volume characteristic for the rib cage is directly represented by either Ppl or Pab versus Vrc. During inspiration, Prc depends on the values of B and the separate pressures. The scale drawn in Figure 6 between the pressures on the left indicates Prc as a function of B, and the solid line on the right, Prc during inspirations for $B = 0.7$. In active states, the pressure difference from the relaxation characteristic is the result of action of the rib cage muscles, and the intervening obliquely hatched area represents the work done by them.

The pressure developed by the anterior abdominal wall is directly represented by Pab. In the example shown in Figure 6 (lower panel), the displacements of the abdominal wall occur along the relaxation characteristics (dashed line), and the abdominal muscles do no work. In general, since abdominal muscle contraction increases abdominal pressure, the work done by these muscles will correspond to areas lying to the right of the relaxation characteristic, as illustrated in subsequent examples.

Figure 7 shows various examples of inspirations produced along the relaxation configuration (line a in Fig. 4). The first is hypothetical: the values of Prc are obtained by assuming the value of the weighting factor, B, to be unity. Here, the diaphragm operating alone drives both the rib cage and anterior abdominal wall along their relaxation pressure–volume characteristics. This circumstance corresponds to the action of the diaphragm proposed by Goldman and Mead (1973) and is the basis of the partitioning of respiratory work presented by Goldman et al. (1976). However, a weighting factor of unity is unrealistic except at very low lung volumes. In the second and subsequent examples, a value of the weighting factor of 0.5 is used, which is the average value estimated by Loring and Mead (1982) at ordinary volumes. Figure 7B represents an inspiration made with only diaphragmatic and rib cage muscle activity, and Figure 7C, with only the diaphragmatic and abdominal muscles active; Figure 7D illustrates the case where all three are active. In each example, the diaphragm does a substantial fraction of the work. Indeed, diaphragmatic muscle activity is required for all inspirations made along the relaxation configuration. This is not true for inspirations that parallel the relaxation configuration. Such inspirations can be achieved by combined action of the rib cage and abdominal muscles, or by combined activity that also involves the diaphragm.

A notable feature of Figure 7 is the variation in the total work required to produce inspirations, all of which would appear to require the same amount of work

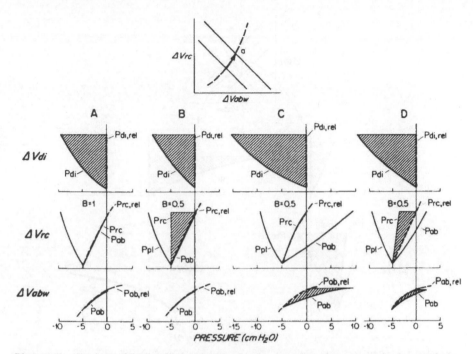

Figure 7 Work partitioning for inspirations made along the relaxation (rel) characteristic. Vertical panel (A) corresponds to the Goldman–Mead hypothesis of diaphragmatic action; namely, that the diaphragm acting alone is capable of driving the chest wall along its relaxation configuration. When the weighting factor, B, is less than unity, coordinated activity of the separate muscles is required: the diaphragm and rib cage muscles in panel (B), the diaphragm and abdominal muscles in panel (C), and all three in panel (D). See text for full explanation.

in the traditional representation of the work of breathing (see Fig. 5). The explanation lies in the fact that none of the muscles (with the exception of the diaphragm in the hypothetical example shown in A) is capable of driving the chest wall without distorting it. To move the chest wall along its relaxation characteristic then requires that work must be done in preventing the distortions. This is most clearly observed when abdominal muscles are active. In panels C and D of Figure 7, it can be seen that the work done by the abdominal muscles is negative in sign; the abdominal displacement is opposite that of the muscles acting alone would produce. The extra work (i.e., the work done in addition to that estimated by the traditional approach) represents work done by the respiratory muscles on one another. Thus, in the example just considered, the abdominal muscles act to prevent the distortion that the diaphragm acting alone would produce.

Inspirations involving only displacements of the rib cage or anterior abdominal wall (Fig. 8) require coordinated contraction of muscles just sufficient to prevent

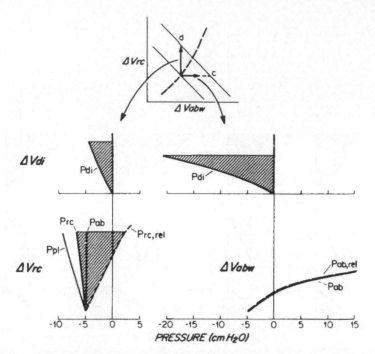

Figure 8 Work partitioning for inspirations in which only the rib cage or anterior abdominal wall move. In each instance, the pressure–volume characteristics for the stationary part are not shown. Volume changes during inspirations produced only by displacement of the anterior abdominal wall are limited for reasons explained in the text.

volume displacements of the stationary part, but such activity does not result in pressure–volume work. Pure rib cage inspirations can be produced by coordinated contractions of the diaphragm and inspiratory muscles of the rib cage. Inspirations involving displacement of only the anterior abdominal wall require coordinated diaphragmatic and expiratory rib cage muscle activity. The magnitude of such inspirations initiated from the relaxed state is limited by the limited distensibility (decreasing compliance) of the anterior abdominal wall and by the mounting antagonist activity required to prevent rib cage expansion.

Inspirations produced by the rib cage muscles alone, or by the diaphragm acting alone, are illustrated in Figure 9. In the former case, transdiaphragmatic pressure remains zero, thus Prc = Ppl = Pab, and the relaxed anterior abdominal wall is displaced in the expiratory direction. This displacement contributes to the work done by the rib cage muscles. Similarly, when the diaphragm acts alone, the associated increase in abdominal pressure directly increases the work done by the diaphragm. Initially, the diaphragm does work on the lung until abdominal pressure becomes positive, and work is then concomitantly done on the anterior abdominal wall.

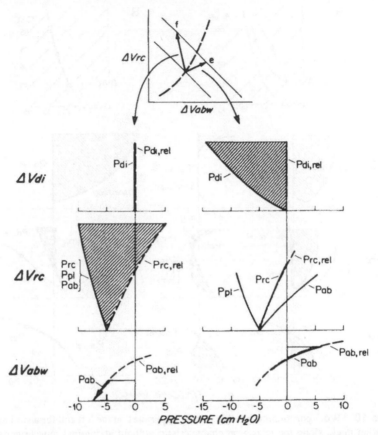

Figure 9 Work partitioning for inspirations in which only the rib cage muscles are active (f) and in which only the diaphragm is active (e). A value of the weighting factor (B = 0.5) is used in computing Prc in (e).

An example of a full respiratory cycle, including realistic dynamic pressures, is shown in Figure 10A. The cycle is diagrammatic, but consistent with observations made during heavy exercise (Grimby et al., 1968). The chest wall configurations lie to the left of the relaxation configurations, and this is mainly due to abdominal muscle activity. The abdominal muscles act as more than simply expiratory muscles; they do negative work during inspiration which is nearly as great as the positive work done during expiration. As a result of their coordinated action with the rib cage muscles, the fluctuations in abdominal pressure are comparatively small. This can be appreciated by comparing this breath with an equal inspiration produced along the relaxation characteristic (see Fig. 10B). The increase in abdominal pressure for such a breath would be substantially greater and, as a result, the work done by

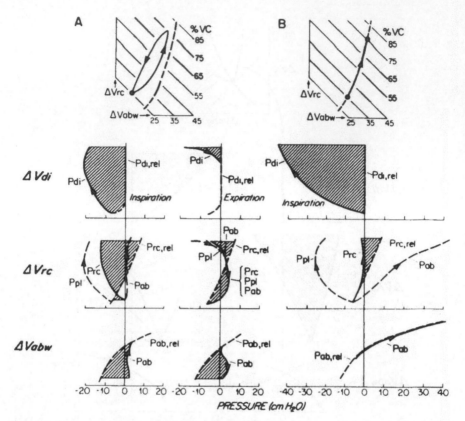

Figure 10 Work partitioning during exercise hyperpnea on the left and for a similarly deep inspiration made along the relaxation characteristic without abdominal muscle activity, on the right. Note the differences in diaphragmatic work required.

the diaphragm would be correspondingly large. Minimization of the work done by the diaphragm may be the key to respiratory muscle coordination during hyperpnea, as has been suggested (Grimby et al., 1968).

From inspection of the foregoing figures, it is apparent that the work done by respiratory muscles during breaths that depart from the relaxation configuration is greater than for breaths that conform to it. It has been previously emphasized that the relaxation configurations represent the minimum energy configurations of the chest wall (Mead, 1974; Goldman et al. 1976); departures from these are associated with distortions of the chest wall that involve additional pressure–volume work (Konno and Mead, 1968).

The main purpose of the preceding discussion has been to illustrate the manner in which mechanical work can be partitioned between the respiratory muscles. One of the major assumptions of the analysis is that shape changes of the rib cage and abdominal wall produced by applied muscle forces are small, and accordingly, that pressure–volume relationships measured in relaxed states of the system continue to define the stored passive elastic energy during active breathing. This approximation is reasonably satisfied during ordinary tidal ventilation, during which the applied forces are relatively small and the rib cage and abdominal wall deform with essentially single degrees of freedom. Significant distortions may occur when the applied muscle forces are large; therefore, the additional energy required to distort the structures should be included in the analysis. Most of the examples presented in this section have developed the analysis for inspiratory work, but the approach is applicable to analysis of expiratory work as well; that is, both any negative work done by the inspiratory muscles during expiration and any positive work done by the expiratory muscles.

VII. Conclusions

Our principal conclusions are several: (1) Diaphragm volume displacements account for the major part (at least two-thirds) of virtually all inspirations. (2) The rib cage acts mainly on the abdomen, and its most important contribution to lung volume change is by way of its abdominal action. (3) The diaphragm does a substantial fraction of inspiratory work, but other inspiratory muscles contribute importantly as agonists, even during quiet breathing.

References

Agostoni, E. (1970). Kinematics. In *The Respiratory Muscles: Mechanics and Neural Control*. Edited by E. M. J. Campbell, E. Agostoni, and J. Newsom Davis. London, W. B. Saunders, pp. 23–47.

Agostoni, E., Mognoni, P., Torri, G., and Saracino, F. (1965). Relation between changes of rib cage circumference and lung volume. *J. Appl. Physiol.* 20:1179–1186.

DeTroyer, A., and Loring, S. H. (1986). Action of the respiratory muscles. In *Handbook of Physiology*, Section 3. The Respiratory System. Volume 3. Mechanics of Breathing. Edited by P. T. Macklem and J. Mead. Bethesda, MD, American Physiological Society, pp. 443–462.

Goldman, M. D., and Mead, J. (1973). Mechanical interaction between the diaphragm and rib cage. *J. Appl. Physiol.* 35:197–204.

Goldman, M. D., Grimby, G., and Mead, J. (1976). Mechanical work of breathing derived from rib cage and abdominal V-P partitioning. *J. Appl. Physiol.* 41:752–763.

Grassino, A., Goldman, M. D., Mead, J., and Sears, T. A. (1978). Mechanics of the human diaphragm during voluntary contraction. Statics. *J. Appl. Physiol.* 44:829–839.

Grimby, G., Bunn, J., and Mead, J. (1968). Relative contribution of rib cage and abdomen to ventilation during exercise. *J. Appl. Physiol.* 24:159–165.

Konno, K., and Mead, J. (1967). Measurement of separate volume changes of rib cage and abdomen during breathing. *J. Appl. Physiol.* 22:407–422.

Loring, S. H., and Mead, J. (1982). Action of the diaphragm on the rib cage inferred from a force–balance analysis. *J. Appl. Physiol.* 53:197–204.

Loring, S. H., and Bruce, E. N. (1986). Methods for study of the chest wall. In *Handbook of*

Physiology, Section 3. The Respiratory System, Volume 3. Mechanics of Breathing. Edited by P. T. Macklem and J. Mead. Bethesda, MD, American Physiological Society, pp. 415–428.

Macklem, P. T., Gross, D., Grassino, A., and Roussos, C. (1978). Partitioning of inspiratory pressure swings between diaphragm and intercostal/accessory muscles. *J. Appl. Physiol.* 44:200–208.

Margaria, R., Milic-Emili, G., Petit, J. M., and Cavagna, G. (1960). Mechanical work of breathing during muscular exercise. *J. Appl. Physiol.* 15:354–358.

Mead, J. (1974). Mechanics of the chest wall. In *Loaded Breathing*. Edited by L. D. Pengelly, A. S. Rebuck, and E. M. J. Campbell. London, Churchill Livingston, pp. 35–49.

Mead, J. (1979). Functional significance of the area of apposition of diaphragm to rib cage. *Am. Rev. Respir. Dis.* 11 (Part 2, Suppl.) 31–32.

Mead, J. (1981). Mechanics of the chest wall. In *Advances in Physiological Sciences*, Vol. 10: *Respiration*. Edited by I. Kutas and L. A. Debreczeni. New York, Pergamon Press, pp. 3–11.

Mead, J., and Loring, S. H. (1982). Analysis of volume displacement and length changes of the diaphragm during breathing. *J. Appl. Physiol.* 53: 750–755.

Mead, J., Peterson, N., Grimby, G., and Mead J. (1967). Pulmonary ventilation measured by body surface movements. *Science* 156: 1383–1384.

Smith, J. C., and Mead, J. (1986). Three degree of freedom description of movement of the human chest wall. *J. Appl. Physiol.* 60: 928–934.

21

Topography of the Diaphragm

WILLIAM A. WHITELAW

University of Calgary
Calgary, Alberta, Canada

I. Introduction

The diaphragm is unlike other muscles in its form and, therefore, in the basis for analysis of its action. Other muscles take the form of fascicles with attachments at either end and produce forces in straight lines that can be represented fairly accurately by vectors with point attachments on bones. Their bulk and direction are easily measured, and they are firm enough to retain the essence of their shape once resected. The diaphragm, on the other hand, is a very thin sheet that acts like a wet handkerchief when separated from its attachments. The force at its peripheral attachment is distributed along a line running around the whole interior of the rib cage. It has no insertion in the usual sense—its fibers end in a central tendon that is not attached to anything rigid and may slip sideways as well as move up and down. The force at its central insertion is balanced largely by pressure distributed across its free surface.

Considerable advances have been made in measuring and analyzing the effects of diaphragmatic contraction, without making reference to the actual shape of the muscle, its attachments, or the forces exerted by them. Instead, the main stream of thought and experiment has depended on abstract theories in which the diaphragm is conceived as a pressure generator consisting of one or two quite formless elements. These interact with each other and the surrounding rib cage, lungs, and abdominal contents through structures or forces that have no more anatomical detail than that of a coefficient in an algebraic equation. So far as the diaphragm is accorded a shape at all, it generally appears in the publications of physiologists as a perfectly hemispheric dome or as a schematic outline intended to illustrate that there exists an area of apposition. This curious tendency to depend on greatly oversimplified idea of the shape of the diaphragm goes back as far as Leonardo da Vinci, who was the first to try to analyze the action of the diaphragm in terms of engineering or mechanics principles. His skills as an artist and familiarity with dissection would have allowed him to draw it in exact anatomical detail, but instead he used sketches in which the muscle appears as a section of a hemisphere—relaxed with a small radius of curvature, contracted with a larger one (O'Malley and Saunders, 1952). It is possible to suppose that Leonardo, whose drawings of the diaphragm occur in note books devoted to understanding mechanisms, chose to consider a structure he could understand, rather than one too complicated for the analysis available to him, even if it was far from an exact representation. The mathematical approaches to analyzing the action of a contractile membrane remain much less accessible to physiologists than those for levers and linear forces. The problem of an asymmetrical, two-humped, nonconical section with fibers out of line with its geometric axes, an irregular tendon, attached to structures with nonuniformly distributed elastic properties and uneven pressures is a challenge still to be answered.

In the next decade, new tools that are now developing should be widely applied, and we should have an entirely new look at diaphragmatic function. It will be based on detailed data about shape, coming from new imaging techniques and measurements of regional length, tension and pressure, and thickness, together with finite element analysis to combine these data. This should tell us with confidence how the diaphragm acts on the rib cage and how it generates pressure. Some surprises may be in store.

This chapter will try to summarize current knowledge about shape and regional diaphragmatic function.

II. Methods for Assessing the Shape of the Diaphragm

The principal reason for the lack of data and, therefore, of interest in the detailed shape of the diaphragm has been that our means of measuring the shape have been very limited.

Anatomy textbooks continue to provide some of the best pictures of the general shape of the diaphragm, but have substantial limitations. Examination of normal shape at autopsy is problematic because the muscle cannot be seen until the lungs are collapsed or the abdomen emptied; maneuvers that change the shape. If the lungs are inflated in the cadavers illustrated, their volume and compliance are unknown and undoubtedly abnormal. Perspective drawings, by their nature, do not lend themselves to quantitative inferences. The pictures show that the diaphragm takes the shape of two domes, with a saddle between, but do not make it easy to appreciate the extent of the area of apposition, the anterior attachments, or the details of curvature of the domes.

Everyday concepts of diaphragmatic shape are based on silhouettes from plain x-ray films, which again have serious limitations. Most of them are taken near total lung capacity, far away from the normal operating length of the muscle at which the shape is of most interest to a physiologist. As well, the state of the diaphragm, whether relaxed or contracted, is not controlled. The diaphragm surface can be appreciated only where it is juxtaposed to air-filled lungs, so that the central portion is hidden by the mediastinum, and the rib cage-apposed portion can be recognized only if markers are placed on the points of diaphragm origin. A silhouette does not necessarily correspond to a plane section through the diaphragm dome, because the silhouette corresponds to the line of highest (i.e., most cranial) points of the diaphragm, whatever plane they happen to be in, and the line of highest points is not likely to be all in one plane. At best, silhouettes show only one section through the diaphragm along the line of highest points, and are incapable of revealing any details of shape elsewhere. Fortunately, the silhouette of the dome in lateral projection corresponds to a line not too different from a sagittal section, at least for the supine subject near functional residual capacity (FRC) (Whitelaw, 1987). Posteroanterior (PA) projections give a more misleading idea of diaphragm shape, partly because the saddle between the domes is obscured by the mediastinum and partly because there are two high points along a midline sagittal section: one between the domes, another at the sternal attachment anteriorly. A striking reminder of the deception produced by this image can be had by measuring the length of the sternum and using the measurement to locate the position of the xiphoid process on a normal total lung capacity (TLC), PA radiograph, in which the sternum is invisible. The lower end of the sternum is several centimeters above the top of the diaphragm silhouette, even though, in fact, the diaphragm is attached directly to it.

Within their limitations, x-ray film silhouettes can yield useful data about the diaphragm's length, radius of curvature, and area of apposition. From radiographs taken especially for the purpose, with subjects relaxed at specified lung volumes, Rochester and co-workers have made measurements of lengths of silhouette lines. By adding radiopaque markers at the points of insertions of the diaphragm into the rib cage margin, they were also able to estimate the width of the zone of apposition and to calculate shortening of the diaphragm's fibers, during change from one volume to another, from measurement of the area of apposition and rib cage expansion, using a geometric model of diaphragmatic volume change (Braun et al., 1982; Petroll et al., 1990a,b; Knight et al., 1990).

Computed tomography (CT) offered the first real promise of detailed information about the diaphragm's shape and continues to improve with advancing technology. Up to now, the respiratory muscle physiologist has been hampered by four technical limitations. First is the time taken to collect the data for one image. Since the diaphragm is normally in continuous motion, clear pictures can be taken only if the scan is made very quickly, 0.1 s or less, or if the subject is able to hold the muscles still for the data collection. In the latter case, the volume, configuration of chest wall, and state of contraction or relaxation of the diaphragm must be monitored, and each slice of a series must be done under the same conditions. The second limitation is that of radiation exposure. To get better definition, many thin slices are required, which puts volunteer subjects at increasing risk of radiation toxicity. The third is that most scanners construct transverse sections, which are the least useful for demonstrating the shape of a dome with a caudocranial axis. This may be partly helped by computer reconstruction, but is still a limitation when a series of sections is taken because, unless the subject can get his lung volume and configuration exactly the same each time, the sections are slightly out of register, and the reconstructed outlines of a sagittal or frontal sections lose definition. Fourth, almost all scanners require the subjects to be horizontal, which prevents the acquisition of data about the shape of the diaphragm in the upright position for which its function has been most studied. New rapid scanners using a spiral track can quickly gather data for a detailed image of a section containing most of the diaphragm and should shortly provide a real breakthrough in this area. The dynamic "spatial reconstrictor," built at Mayo Clinic, can provide excellent images of the diaphragm in experimental animals (Margulies and Rodarte, 1990).

Magnetic resonance imaging (MRI) is also useful. Acquisition of data for one image takes a long time, requiring subjects to be good at breath-holding, but images of sagittal or coronal sections, giving good definition of the diaphragm's shape, can be obtained (Paiva et al., 1992).

III. Measurements of Three-Dimensional Diaphragmatic Shape In Vivo, Relaxed

A. Humans

Several radiologic studies of normal persons and patients have described qualitative features of the diaphragm that can be seen on CT or ultrasound images (Panicek et al., 1988). They report the prevalence and occurrence of the defects called foramina of Bochdalek and Morgagni, the frequent appearance in elderly subjects of both local thickening of the diaphragm (called pseudotumors), and apparent local defects in the musculature (Caskey et al., 1989). Diaphragm slips—the bundles of fibers inserting into each rib—are more prominent in old age, when the dome tends to take on the appearance of a scallop shell, with creases that may indent the liver (Hawkins and Hine, 1991). One study shows detailed images of the anterior attachments of diaphragm to the sternum and ribs (Gale, 1986). It is worth studying because of the complex and unexpected shapes the saddle attachment takes at different volumes, according to whether the saddle is at, above, or below the lower end of the sternum. Clinical radiologic studies are generally hard to interpret from the point of view of tension and length of the diaphragm's segments because the volume or state of contraction of the system while the image is being obtained usually not controlled or specified.

Three sets of measurements of detailed shape of the human diaphragm under defined physiological conditions have been reported. One, using CT, gives the shape relaxed at FRC and during active contraction at the end of a 1-L inspiration, both for the same subject (Whitelaw, 1987; Fig. 1). The second, using MRI, gives the shape at relaxed FRC for four subjects of similar age, height, and build (Paiva et al., 1992; Fig. 2). The data from both studies show the relaxed diaphragm with two domes joined by a saddle that runs from the sternum to the anterior face of the spinal column. The spine makes a considerable posterior indentation in the transverse outline of the thoracic cavity and helps isolate one hemidiaphragm dome from the other. The free surface curves to join the inside of the rib cage tangentially and then runs down the area of apposition to insert at the costal margin. Anteriorly, where the costal margin sweeps up to the end of the sternum, a section of the diaphragm makes an acute angle with the chest wall, with no area of apposition.

In a third study, Gauthier et al. (1994) reconstructed shapes of the diaphragm from MIR in four supine, relaxed subjects at residual volume (RV), functional residual capacity (FRC), FRC plus half inspiratory capacity, and total lung capacity (TLC). As volume increased, rib cage diameter increased, more in the AP than the lateral direction, the area of apposition decreased, and the dome descended. The outline made by the intersection of a coronal plane with the diaphragm seemed to change its shape only a small amount from one volume to another, although the saddle became a little flatter and the radius of curvature of the domes a little greater toward TLC (Fig. 3A). The outlines made by the intersections of sagittal planes with the right and left hemidiaphragm domes showed much greater changes, from nearly round at RV to nearly flat at TLC (see Fig. 3B). There is a sharpness to the anterior part of the curves at FRC+ and TLC that probably results from distortion away from a cylindrical dome shape in the region near the anterior sternal attachment, which is above the dome at TLC. Going from RV to TLC, the posterior part of the dome descends more than the anterior part relative to the sternum. The authors also assessed the area of apposition at various lung volumes, and correlated it with both diaphragm length and with rib cage diameter. As suggested by the theoretical analysis of Petroll and associates (1990a,b), the area of apposition (Aap) decreases with increasing lung volume, mainly because of the shortening of diaphragm fibers, but there is an additional loss of Aap owing to expansion of the rib cage and peeling of the diaphragm away from the ribs.

There are no exact data about the three-dimensional orientation of muscle fibers in the human diaphragm. Observations of excised diaphragms draped over a life-size model of the relaxed supine diaphragm shape (W. A. Whitelaw, unpublished) indicate that the fibers in many places have a slightly spiral orientation, rather than taking the shortest route toward the top of the dome. Posteriorly, for example, there is a gap along the line of insertion of the diaphragmatic fiber into the chest wall, at the location of the foramen of Bochdalek. This creates a triangular

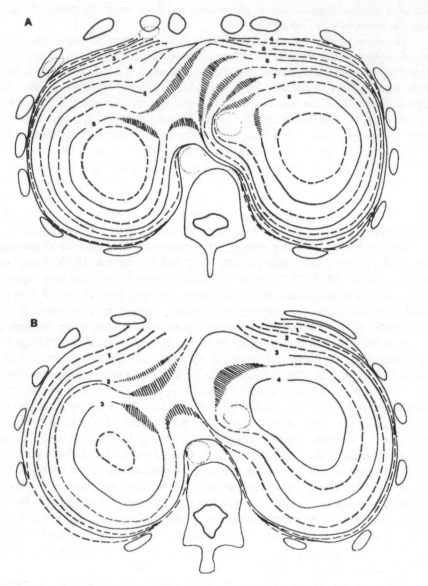

Figure 1 Topographical maps of supine diaphragm, (A) relaxed and (B) contracted, viewed from the thoracic side. Contour lines correspond to transverse planes at 0.5-cm intervals, with 0 at level of lower border of 12th thoracic vertebra. Numbers are centimeters above this plan. Hatched contour lines, regions where exact position of boundary of diaphragm dome was obscured by adjacent structures (e.g., heart and its attachments). Bony silhouettes were taken from a section 5 cm above base (solid lines) and 2 cm above base (dotted lines) in relaxed diaphragm and 2 cm above base on contracted one. Dotted circle near vertebral body is descending aorta; the one in saddle between domes is inferior vena cave. (From Whitelaw, 1987.)

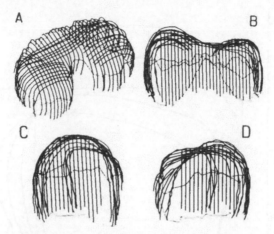

Figure 2 Three-dimensional reconstruction of (A) diaphragm and projections of (B) coronal and (C and D) right and left sagittal slices, respectively. (From Paiva et al., 1992.)

defect in the diaphragm's musculature, with its base on the chest wall and its apex at the central tendon. Fibers on either side of this triangle have a somewhat oblique orientation.

The central tendon itself has the shape of a boomerang, with its two ends pointing posterolaterally (Braun et al., 1982; Fig. 4). Visible patterns of fibrous strands curve across the tendon surface, inviting speculation about lines of force when the muscle is under tension.

B. Dogs

The dog diaphragm more closely resembles a single dome, although by no means circular in its transverse outline. The only detailed three-dimensional data published are shown in Figure 5 from CT images in prone and supine dogs by Margulies and Rodarte (1990). These show a dome, the apex of which is situated anteriorly, closer to the sternum than to the spine in the supine, relaxed condition. The apex moves even closer to the sternum if the dog is placed in the prone position or if lung volume is increased to TLC. The center of the dome is flatter at FRC and more conical at TLC, and it is flatter when the dog is supine than when it is prone. A pneumothorax produces little change at FRC, but at TLC, it allows the diaphragm to become flatter in the center and steeper close to the chest wall.

C. Change in Shape with Active Inspiration

Figure 1 shows the human diaphragm in an active inspiration of moderate degree (1 L), with the rib cage constrained to keep the same AP diameter. The domes

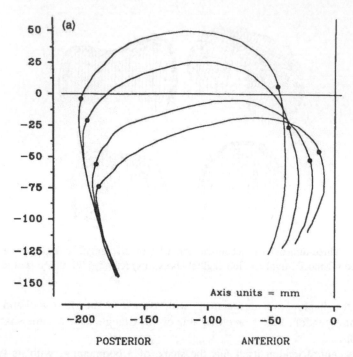

Figure 3 Diaphragm silhouettes at four different lung volumes. Slices chosen were the ones closest to the most cranial part of the diaphragm dome for each respective plane: (a) sagittal plane through left hemidiaphragm dome; (b) midcoronal plane; (c) saggital plane through right hemidiaphragm dome. Dots represent locations of the costophrenic angles for each lung volume. (Personal communication, data from project described in Gauthier et al., 1994.)

descend and flatten. The saddle also flattens as it descends to a level lower than the xiphisternum, where the anterior attachments curve upward to their insertion (Fig. 6). The right dome descends farther than the left. The curvature of the dome cannot be appreciated with any precision from the CT data, and the difference between costal and crural shortening cannot be assessed, because movement of the central tendon cannot be detected by the method.

Information about shape during contraction of the dog diaphragm is contained in the data of Paen et al. (1991), who sewed markers in triangular arrays into the costal diaphragm in three concentric zones, one nearest the rib cage, one next to the central tendon, and a third between the other two. From the positions of these points, measured with biplane cineradiography, they could determine strain vectors in major and minor axes—one along the line of greatest strain, the other perpendicular to the first. In the major axis, which in all cases was radially directed, there was always shortening of about the same degree in each concentric zone. In the minor axis, which

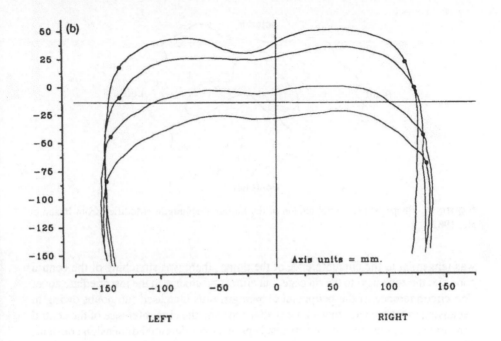

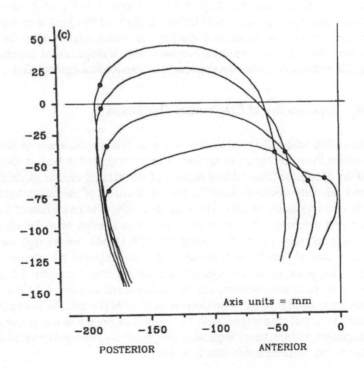

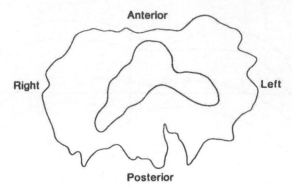

Figure 4 Shape of the central tendon of the human diaphragm. (Modified from Braun et al., 1982.)

was tangential to the circumference of the dome, there was stretching of the central zone and the zone next to the rib cage, but almost no change in the intermediate zone. The circumference of the peripheral diaphragm thus increased (no doubt owing to expansion of the rib cage to which it is attached) and the circumference of the central zone increased, but the zone in between kept its circumferential dimension constant. This implies a change in shape as diagrammed in Figure 7. In this study, the markers were placed quite far anteriorly. A distortion in shape of this kind is conceivable if the dome descends below the anterior attachments, which might pull up the anterior corners in the direction indicated by the arrows. Such a shape can be discerned from studying CT pictures of the human diaphragm's anterior attachments (Gale, 1986).

IV. Topography of Diaphragm Thickness

Two recent dog studies have provided evidence that the thickness of diaphragm muscle varies from one region to another. The method used in both studies was to punch disks of muscle from various regions of the excised muscle of dogs, weigh them, and calculate thickness from the known diameter of the punch hole and an assumed constant muscle density. The main difficulty is to be certain of the length of the excised diaphragm in relation to its unstressed length or its length at FRC. The carefully prepared specimens of Margulies (1991) indicated the right diaphragm was slightly thicker than the left, the anterior costal segment was about 1.4 times as thick as the posterior costal segment, the medial crural segment 1.2 times as thick as the lateral crural segment, and the medial crural segment 1.5 times as thick as the posterior costal segment. Brancatisano et al. (1991) found the same directional differences in costal diaphragm, with the ventral segments twice as thick as the dorsal segments and thickness increasing progressively from posterior to anterior. There are as yet no comparable data from humans.

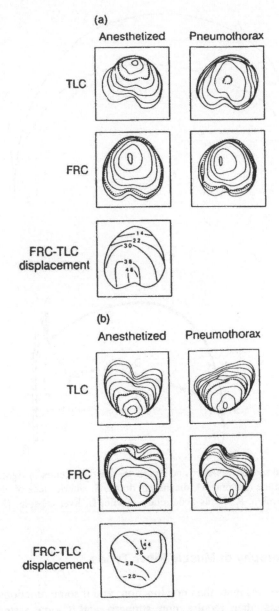

Figure 5 Contour diagrams of diaphragm surface in dog at TLC and FRC in anesthetized and isovolume pneumothorax conditions: (left panel) prone; (right panel) supine. Level lines, outline of diaphragm in a series of 1.6-mm–thick transverse planes with an 8-mm separation. Dashed line, level of a reference location on the spine that remains stationary with changes in lung volume and body position. (From Margulies and Rodarte, 1990.)

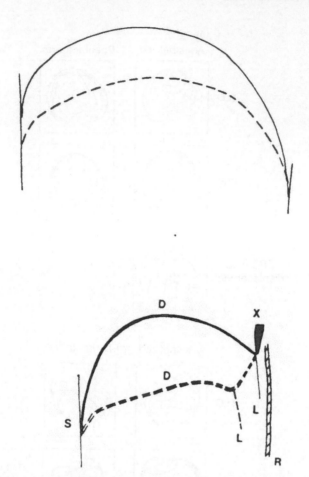

Figure 6   Sagittal sections, relaxed and contracted, through center of right hemidiaphragm dome (top) and midline (bottom). D, diaphragm dome; S, anterior face of vertebral column; X, lower tip of sternum; R, rectus abdominus muscle; L, liver capsule. (From Whitelaw, 1987.)

V.   Topography of Muscle Fiber Types

If the diaphragm serves more than one function, and if some functions require more endurance, whereas others require more strength, and if some parts of the muscle are used preferentially for endurance functions and other parts are used for strength functions, then one might suppose there would be an uneven distribution of fiber types, with slow oxidative fibers more prevalent in some regions and fast, glycolytic fibers in other regions.

Studies have been conducted to look for regional differences in diaphragm

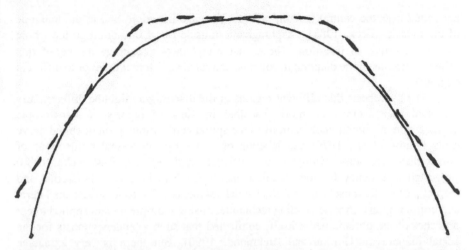

Figure 7 Shape change of anterior dog diaphragm during active contraction, deduced from data of Paiva et al. (1991). Radial diaphragm lengths all shortened in inspiration. Circumference of the parts closest to the central tendon and closest to the rib cage both increased, but circumference of the intermediate zone did not increase. This can be explained by the illustrated shape change from relaxed (solid line) to contracted (dashed line).

composition by muscle fiber types in rats, cats, rabbits, baboons, and infant humans (Davies and Gunn, 1972; Keens et al., 1978; Keens and Ianuzzo, 1979; Kilarski and Sjöström, 1990; Maxwell et al., 1989; Metzger et al., 1985; Sieck et al., 1983, 1987). These studies are difficult to perform and interpret. They have sometimes reported definite differences between regions, but overall, one may conclude that any differences are small and not likely important. Some studies do point to a difference between the abdominal surface and the thoracic surface. The abdominal surface seems to have more oxidative capacity in cats (Sieck et al., 1983) and more type 1 fibers in rats (Metzger et al., 1985) than the thoracic surface. This kind of distribution seems unlikely to have a large mechanical effect. Shortening one side of a muscle more than the other can cause the muscle to bend. If the more oxidative, slower, abdominal face of the diaphragm contracted more in quiet inspiration than the thoracic surface, this might slightly influence the change in shape of the muscle that occurs in the tidal volume range.

VI. Topography of Innervation

The muscle fibers activated by one primary branch of the phrenic nerve or by one phrenic motoneuron are not spread through the whole diaphragm, but are confined to a region covering only 10–15% of the area of the muscle (Hammond et al., 1989; Fournier and Sieck, 1988; Sieck, 1988). In addition, clusters of motor end plates are found near the central tendon, near the rib cage insertion, and in the midzone of the muscle (Sieck, 1988). Diaphragmatic muscle fibers do not all go the whole way from origin to insertion. These anatomical facts encourage the belief that different regions of the diaphragm could be activated at different times or to different degrees.

The hypothesis that different regions of the diaphragm might be differentially activated may seem even more plausible in view of reports of somatotopic organization of phrenic motoneurons in the spinal cord. Stimulation of spinal nerve roots (Duron et al., 1979) and labeling of axons by intravascular injections of horseradish peroxidase (Duron et al., 1979; Rikard-Bell and Bystrzycka, 1980) suggested a tendency for the rostral segments C4–5 to innervate the sternal and medial part of the muscle and for the caudal segments C5–6 to innervate the lateral and crural regions. Precise labeling techniques, using multiple tracers applied to cut branches of the phrenic nerve itself, confirmed that such a tendency exists for the costal diaphragm (Gordon and Richmond, 1990). But there is very extensive intermingling of motoneurons going to different regions of the diaphragm, and motoneurons innervating the crural diaphragm are spread fairly evenly through the three segments. Within both the costal and the crural diaphragm, more ventral fibers tend to be innervated by C-5, more dorsal ones by C-6 (Fournier and Sieck, 1988).

VII. Topography of Activation During Respiration

The diaphragm has different regions (costal and crural grossly and likely subregions as well), the isolated contractions of which produce different mechanical effects (De Troyer et al., 1982). Within any part of the muscle, there are various types of fibers with different mechanical properties. Does the control system make use of regional or microscopic differences in muscle action or muscle properties by selective use of one region or one type of fiber more than another? Some evidence has appeared to indicate it can do so under some circumstances. A difference in activation is hinted at by a difference in fiber types, since slow, oxidative fibers tend to be recruited before fast, glycolytic fibers, according to the "size principle" (Henneman et al., 1965). More direct evidence comes from electromyography and blood flow measurements.

A. Regional Electromyography

It is important to note a major limitation of electromyogram (EMG) and electroneurogram studies of diaphragm activation. They give evidence only about the time course of activity, without any accurate indication of absolute magnitude. Thus, it is not possible to be sure if one region of diaphragm is activated two or three times more than another if both regions have the same time of onset and offset and the same wave shape of activity. This problem is not really resolved by expressing data as percentage of control. Percentage maximum would be better, but it is very difficult to obtain a maximum, uncontaminated, undistorted signal. Studies of diaphragm electrical activity have, by and large, shown synchronous activation with a similar time course for all regions, as if all were controlled in the same way. Similar EMGs are thus seen for the costal and crural diaphragm in both quiet respiration and loaded breathing in dogs (Sant'Ambrogio et al., 1963. Pollard et al., 1985, Van Lunteren et al., 1985) and in human patients with intramuscular electrodes, after abdominal surgery (J.-L. Pansard, unpublished). Interest in the possibility of fine control of different parts of the muscle has driven a number of studies, but these have usually found rather small differences. Henderson-Smart and associates (1982) reported that there was more postinspiratory activity in costal than in crural segments in newborn lambs. Clement and colleagues (1991) found in pigs, after treatment with prostaglandin $F_{2\alpha}$, that crural EMG started earlier than costal, and the burst lasted longer. Riley and Berger (1979) showed quite striking variations in shape of the inspiratory integrated EMG from one part of the diaphragm to another in anesthetized cats. In anesthetized dogs, crural EMG (expressed as percentage control) increased more than costal EMG when animals were turned from supine to head-up or when stimulated with CO_2 (Van Lunteren et al., 1985). In the very particular case of vomiting, there is a dramatic separation of functions of the crural and costal diaphragm. The costal region contracts, while the crural region around the esophagus relaxes (Monges et al., 1978). Inhibition of the part of the crus around the esophageal hiatus can be induced by distending the esophagus, a reflex that is interrupted by cutting the vagus nerve (Oyer et al., 1989). In rapid-eye-movement (REM) sleep, segments of the costal diaphragm of cats are often activated asynchronously, but the significance of this is unclear (Hendricks and Kline, 1991).

Regional differences in activation can be driven by a central pattern generator, or by peripheral reflexes that may adjust α-motor neuron output in responses to local muscle length changes (Cheeseman and Revelette, 1990; Jammes et al., 1986).

B. Regional Blood Flow

Brancatisano et al. (1991) used microspheres to measure regional diaphragmatic blood flow in anesthetized dogs, either paralyzed or breathing spontaneously, with and without inspiratory resistive loads. Flow per unit weight of muscle increased from dorsal to ventral in the costal diaphragm, decreasing again for the most anterior segment (Fig. 8). Present at rest, this flow gradient increased with spontaneous breathing, and increased again with the resistive load. Most of the data came from supine dogs, but in two that were also studied prone the same dorsoventral gradient persisted. No gradient was found within the crural diaphragm, and the mean blood flow per weight for crural and costal segments was the same. In another study, horses increased costal flow more than crural flow when exercising (Manohar, 1990). In conscious sheep, blood flow to the costal region is slightly less than to the crural region (Soust et al., 1987).

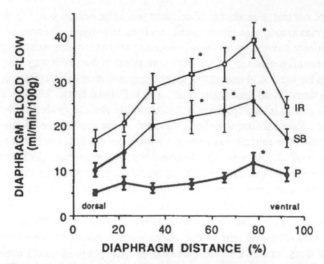

Figure 8   Mean costal diaphragmatic blood flow per unit weight versus diaphragm distance as percentage of maximum during paralysis (P) spontaneous breathing (SB), and inspiratory resistive loading (IR) in all dogs. Each point represents average blood flow per unit weight from two hemidiaphragms. Error bars, SE. Note dorsoventral gradient in blood flow (greater perfusion ventrally) during P (muscle inactive), SB, and IR, and overall increase in blood flow with muscle contraction. (*) significantly different from most dorsal regions ($p <$ 0.0001). (From Brancatisano et al., 1991.)

The implications of differential regional blood flow are as yet unknown. At first glance, the deduction is that more oxygen is consumed per unit mass of the anterior costal diaphragm than of the posterior costal diaphragm. This suggests that the anterior part of the diaphragm is more intensely activated in respiration than the posterior part. Given the difference in thickness between these two parts of the muscle, there is an even more considerable gradient in oxygen consumption per unit surface area of the diaphragm from anterior to posterior. It could be expected, therefore, that the tension generated during active contraction is greater in the anterior segment of the diaphragm than in the posterior segments.

VIII.   Topography of Shortening

A.   Passive Length Changes with Imposed Changes in Lung Volume

Several experiments have been conducted in dogs during which muscle length has been measured in more than one part of the diaphragm, either with sonomicrometers or with radiopaque markers and biplane cineradiography, and volume has been changed and transdiaphragmatic pressure has been measured, all with the muscle relaxed or presumed relaxed. With sonomicrometers Road et al. (1986) found the crural diaphragm was more compliant than the costal diaphragm. That is, its length increased more for a given change in Pdi. During these measurements the abdomen and lower rib cage were encased in a rigid cast, and the diaphragm was stretched by increasing abdominal pressure with a plunger passed through the cast pushing on the anterior abdominal wall. Resting length of the two parts of the diaphragm was measured with the dogs supine and upright at end expiration, and before and after a pneumothorax during posthyperventilation apnea. The optimal length, Lo, was determined later by making active length–pressure curves under 50-Hz supramaximal stimulation. Supine, the costal diaphragm was 105% of Lo and decreased to 102% with a pneumothorax, a change of 3%. The crural diaphragm began at 92% of Lo, and shortened by 8% of Lo after pneumothorax. Turning from supine to head-up, which reduced Pdi and should have eliminated the hydrostatic anteroposterior gradient in Pdi, decreased costal length by 5% and crural by 8%. When diaphragm length was changed by means of continuous positive pressure applied at the airway opening, while the muscle was rendered passive with pancuronium, the crural diaphragm again shortened more than the costal (Road and Leevers, 1989). These measurements all point to a crural segment that is more compliant than the costal segment. It is important to recognize that this conclusion depends on two assumptions. One is that the relation between radial tension and overall Pdi is the same for the crural segment as for the costal segment. The other is that the tension in the circumferential direction is the same for both segments (Griffiths et al., 1992).

Other workers have found comparable results using radiographic techniques. Thus, when passive lengths were referenced either to Lo, determined in excised muscle strips, or to the presumed, relaxed length at TLC, crural diaphragm shortened more than did the costal in inflations from RV to TLC. There were also some differences among ventral middle and dorsal sections of the costal diaphragm (Sprung et al., 1990). All these differences were less marked than those found by Road et al., but inspection of the data of Sprung et al. suggests that the crural diaphragm is most compliant in the region between RV and ERV, which is the region examined by Road et al. (1986, 1989). Above FRC, there is less difference between costal and crural.

Resting FRC supine lengths of the costal and crural diaphragm have been compared in several studies and found to be different (summarized by Margulies et al., 1990). Crural fibers are farther from the optimal length (i.e., about 90% of Lo) compared with costal fibers (about 100% of Lo) (Margulies, 1991). Proceeding from RV, where fibers from all regions are close to Lo (at which they generate their maximum force) to TLC, the shortening of costal fibers seems to be less than for crural fibers, but there is a fairly large amount of scatter between results from different experiments.

These studies have all shown considerable variation from animal to animal, leaving us with very inexact ideas about details of passive behavior of the muscle.

Many differences may be accounted for by experimental details. For example, fibrosis of pleura, peritoneum, or muscle caused by the surgery may change passive properties. But much of the variation and the underlying relations may eventually be explained by the morphology of the muscle. The thickness of the diaphragm may be quite variable either from region to region or, on a small scale, near the measuring devices. Considerable percentage variation in thickness may be very difficult to assess in the thin diaphragm, but can have a major effect on regional length–pressure or length–tension relations. Alterations in shape with volume could have a major effect on the radii of curvature of different regions, and on interdependence of regions. Alterations with volume of the cross-sectional shape of the rib cage to which the fibers are inserted could also affect regional length. And the attachments of mediastinal and abdominal structures can be expected to have more effect on diaphragm shape and local tension at some volumes than at others.

A peculiarity of length–pressure relationships in the diaphragm is that the passive tension at Lo is large, compared with most other muscles in which passive tension usually begins to appear just at Lo. Griffiths and associates (1992) have emphasized that the diaphragm has a prominent connective tissue membrane covering its entire thoracic surface in sheep, horse, cow, rabbit, sea lion, and human. In excised sheep diaphragms, this membrane supports half the passive tension in the muscle at FRC. (They also point out a key detail of experimental procedure. The diaphragm strips must be subjected to stress in two directions at once, longitudinally and transversely, when assessing passive behavior, because if allowed to shrink transversely when being stressed longitudinally, they appear much more compliant than when operating under normal conditions.) This membrane appears to act as a parallel elastic "ligament" that protects the muscle fibers themselves from stress at relaxed FRC. The effect of surgery on properties of this membrane may explain some of the discrepancies between reports on the regional passive length–tension behavior of the diaphragm.

B. Active Length Changes with Respiration

In spite of regional differences in end-expiratory length related to Lo, the amount of shortening of muscle fibers in natural inspiration is the same in all regions (Sprung et al., 1989) and at up to 10 cm H_2O positive end-expiratory pressure (PEEP) (Road and Leevers, 1989). This suggests that any regional differences in mechanical properties of the muscle are compensated by adjustments in the level of activation of the muscle, or that the load on the fibers varies from region to region in such a way that it matches the force–length properties of the muscle locally. Road and Leevers (1989) found that, as lung volume was increased with continuous-positive airway pressure (CPAP) from 0 to 14 cm H_2O in supine, anesthetized, and vagotomized dogs during spontaneous breathing, activation of the diaphragm, assessed by EMG, did not change. End-expiratory length decreased by only 21% (crural) or 13% (costal), but shortening of fibers decreased much more, to 57 and

66% of FRC amount, respectively, so that end-inspiratory length decreased only slightly with volume.

Sprung et al. (1989) noted that during spontaneous breathing there were differences in percentage shortening of distances between adjacent pairs of markers in a row of four or five markers along one radial line in supine dogs. These were consistent in each dog, but differed from dog to dog and region to region of the diaphragm, with no consistent pattern. These could have been artifacts of the method, but they suggest the possibility of some differential activation, even along one line of fibers.

When the human diaphragm contracts in inspiration, according to the one subject studied by CT, the right hemidiaphragm shortens more than the left, and the sagittal meridian lines shorten more than coronal meridian lines (Whitelaw, 1987).

IX. Topography of Tension or Stress

There are almost no reported direct measurements of diaphragm tension. Kim et al. (1976) did measure tension, but did not compare regions.

There are reasons for thinking passive tension is not uniform everywhere. One is the observation of a membrane or ligament covering the surface of the diaphragm, under stretch at FRC, mechanically in parallel with muscle fibers, and responsible for half the passive tension (Griffiths et al., 1992). This ligament seems likely to be more or less isotropic. As the diaphragm contracts actively, tension should be reduced in the membrane, while tension in the diaphragm in the direction of muscle fibers will be supported by the fibers and will increase because of the active contraction. But tension in the circumferential direction depends only on the dimension change and the passive length–tension property of the diaphragm in the circumferential direction. The circumferential dimension may increase, decrease, or remain the same, depending on how rib cage circumference and diaphragm dome shape are altered in inspiration. During contraction, therefore, it can be expected that diaphragmatic tension will be anisotropic.

Stress, which is tension multiplied by cross-sectional area, has been calculated by Margulies et al. (1994) for the passive dog diaphragm with uniform pleural pressure and abdominal pressure following a uniform hydrostatic gradient. The calculation, based on exact shape data and using finite element analysis, shows radial stress to be much greater than circumferential stress.

X. Topography of Transdiaphragmatic Pressure

There are very few measurements that bear on the topography of transdiaphragmatic pressure. It has been assumed, for convenience, that transdiaphragmatic pressure follows a vertical hydrostatic gradient in abdominal pressure of 1 cm H_2O/cm and a vertical pleural pressure gradient of 0.25 cm H_2O/cm. It is known, however, that there are some regional variations in abdominal pressure (Decramer et al., 1984). When Macklem and co-workers (1988) measured transdiaphragmatic pressure in the zone of apposition, they found wide variation in both sign and quantity that did not fit with any simple theory. Their long discussion of the technical problems involved shows the difficulties that will confront further research in this area.

One simple observation implies a considerable anomaly in either trans-diaphragmatic pressure or local tension. The human diaphragm upright at FRC is saddle-shaped. The domes have positive radii of curvature, and must have a positive transdiaphragmatic pressure [according to Laplace's law, see Eq. (2), Section XII]. The saddle has two radii of curvature in opposite directions, and must have a value of $1/R_1 + 1/R_2$ that is small or negative. The transdiaphragmatic pressure in the saddle should be small or negative. Yet the saddle is below the domes in a hydrostatic field, and should have a more positive value of transdiaphragmatic pressure than at the dome. This implies either that structures above or below the diaphragm apply a local force on the saddle, or that there is a considerable tension in the AP fibers with positive curvature that pass through the saddle.

XI. Possible Determinants of the Shape of the Diaphragm's Dome

From a physics point of view, the position of any small segment of the diaphragm under static conditions depends purely on its attachments to surrounding parts of diaphragm, on its attachments to other structures, on the tension in the segment, on the transdiaphragmatic pressure, and on the elastic properties of the segment. The shape of the whole muscle thus ultimately depends on its attachments, on tension within the muscle and its connective tissue sheath, on transdiaphragmatic pressure, and on local forces that might be exerted by, for example, the pericardial attachments, or by friction or shear in places where the lung or liver do not slide easily across the surface.

When tension in the diaphragm and mean transdiaphragmatic pressure are very large in comparison with regional variations in pressure caused by hydrostatic gradients or local deformities, the shape of the muscle overall should be reasonably described by equations relating mean transdiaphragmatic pressure to tension and shape, such as Laplace's law in the form that relates one transmural pressure to one tension and one radius of curvature for the whole muscle (as long as tension is isotropic). Under the conditions of normal breathing near FRC, however, mean transdiaphragmatic pressure may be of the same order as regional variations in pressure. In that event, modeling of the shape–tension–pressure relationship is more complicated and predicts more complicated shapes of the diaphragm dome.

A complete analysis of the mechanics of the diaphragm needs to give the relationships among tension, transdiaphragmatic pressure, muscle fiber length, thickness, and shape for various conditions of load and of activation of muscle fibers. Such an analysis is well beyond reach at present, mainly because we lack the necessary data. Even though information about some factors can be obtained, the simultaneous measurement of all of the key factors has not yet been achieved. In some experiments, shape is assessed, in others pressure, in still others, tension or lengths of one or two segments of muscle. Assumptions are made about the unmeasured variables, and deductions are made. It turns out that many of the assumptions have been invalid, accounting for the variety of conflicting conclusions found in the literature.

Intuitively, it is obvious that the diaphragm, which is squeezed between the lower surface of the lung and heart and the upper surface of the liver, spleen, and stomach, must conform to the shape of these surrounding organs to a degree that depends on the rigidity, or resistance to deformity, of each one. The lung distended to its FRC volume outside the thorax has a concave undersurface, and the liver, by itself, has a convex uppersurface. Both, therefore, have shapes that conform generally to the shape the diaphragm dome would have if the thorax contained only air and the abdomen only water. When the two organs are closely approximated with the diaphragm between, it may be that each is very close to its resting shape. Insofar as their shapes do not match perfectly, each one must exert a distorting force on the other. These forces will show up as an uneven distribution of pressure across the surfaces of the diaphragm or of tension along the ligamentous attachments between the liver, mediastinum, and diaphragm.

We know very little about the resting shape or the deformability of the liver. Experience from the kitchen suggests that the parenchyma is very easily deformable, almost a fluid, but the mechanical characteristics of the organ are likely to be rather different when the capsule is intact, the attachments to vessels and peritoneal ligaments are in place, the blood vessels are under normal pressure, and movement in some directions is constrained by the rib cage and abdominal wall.

The inflated lung keeps its shape when removed from the thorax much better than the liver does when laid on a table, which is partly because the force of gravity has a much less distorting effect on the lung than on the liver. Lai Fook (1979) has shown that the shear modulus of lung increases with lung volume. No attempt has been made to calculate what sort of distribution of surface pressures across the lower surface of the lung would be needed to change its shape in the sense of flattening the diaphragm dome.

From this point of view, it will be of great interest to have measurements of the topography of pressure on both sides of the diaphragm at various volumes, relaxed and during respiratory efforts. The measurement of local surface pressure presents major technical problems, however. Another way to obtain this information will be to examine the topography of very small pleural effusions and ascites collections, since these will permit the organs to return toward to their resting shapes. In a new steady state, the thickness of the effusion will be related to the distance the lung and liver have been drawn away from their resting position to conform to each others' shape. Such data may come from the new generation of scanners.

XII. Relations Between Tension, Shape, and Pressure

Since most of respiratory statics is conceived in the framework of pressure and volume, and these are the measurements most readily available, the diaphragm is characterized as a pressure generator. Transdiaphragmatic pressure is measured. Such variables as strength, degree of activation, tension, and degree of curvature of the diaphragm are estimated from the pressure.

The relation between tension, shape, and transdiaphragmatic pressure (Pdi) is given by the Laplace's formula, which derives from basic principles of physics. Its well known simple form,

$$\Delta P = 2T/R \tag{1}$$

applies to a surface with spherical symmetry. A more general formula is

$$\Delta P = T \left(1/R_1 + 1/R_2 \right) \tag{2}$$

where R_1 and R_2 are the two principal radii required to describe the curvature of a more complicated surface. The formula applies exactly to any point on the surface, but it cannot be used to describe a whole surface, such as the diaphragm, unless the R_1 and R_2 are the same for all points on this surface. It is also important that the formula does not even apply to a single point, unless the tension in the surface is the same in all directions. A convincing calculation of the pressure–tension–shape relation would require integration of local pressure, local shape, and local directional tension over the entire surface. Because such a calculation is beyond that currently possible, given the lack of data about local pressures and local material properties of the diaphragm, calculations up to now have begun with large simplifying assumptions.

One logical approach is to make no attempt to measure shape, or to perform a detailed Laplace's law calculation, but instead, to measure pressure, either measure or estimate tension, and examine the relation

$$P = f \times T \tag{3}$$

where f is a constant or a variable function called a "shape-factor." If it turns out that f is a constant under the experimental conditions in question, the conclusion is drawn that changes in shape do not have an important effect on the diaphragm's function. Conclusions of this kind are sometimes linked with the image of the diaphragm acting like a piston.

One example of this kind of analysis was done by Kim et al. (1976), who made direct measurements of Pdi and tension in costal diaphragm over a large volume range in supine dogs. They found the tension–Pdi relation could all be explained by the length–tension relation of the diaphragm. That is, there was no need to introduce a changing shape factor to account for the loss of Pdi with increase in volume. It was all due to muscle shortening. (In their analysis they assumed the diaphragm contracted isometrically when lung volume was held constant. This has since been shown to be incorrect.)

Hubmayr et al. (1990) measured Pdi and the diaphragm's length during tetanic contractions at different lung volumes, using a radiographic technique with rows of metal markers sewn along the line of muscle fibers. They found that, during 50-Hz supramaximal stimulation, the diaphragm shortened to nearly the same length no matter what the lung volume was. With the same stimulus and nearly the same length, tension should have been nearly the same in all cases. In spite of this, there was a tenfold difference in Pdi between TLC and RV. This strongly suggests that during vigorous diaphragmatic contractions in the dog, there is a very important shape change from one volume to the other, causing a substantial change in the shape factor that relates tension to pressure.

A constant shape factor does not necessarily imply a constant shape, as shown by calculations of the pressure–tension relationship for a cylindrically symmetrical, upright diaphragm, with a hydrostatic gradient in Pdi. As mean Pdi increases, there is a definite progressive change in shape, but the radii of curvature of some parts of the surface increase, whereas others decrease. The net effect is a nearly constant Pdi–tension relation (Whitelaw et al., 1983). The logic of shape-factor analysis depends completely on the assumption that tension is uniform across the whole surface. In fact, there are reasons to believe that tension is not the same at all points in the diaphragm and not even the same in different directions at any one point. And, if the tensions vary across the muscle surface, there is every reason to believe the relationships between tension in one place and tension in another could vary with changes in shape. That is, tension cannot be factored out as implied by Eq. (3), because tension may be modified by a shape factor of its own.

Calculations relating Pdi to tension and shape have been made for shapes more complex than a segment of a sphere and have been compared with experimental observation in two papers. Both calculations used the same assumptions: They assumed that tension is uniform across the surface, that the diaphragm does not resist bending in any way, that there are no sources of local tension owing to ligamentous attachments or shear forces on the pleural or parietal surfaces, and that there is a uniform hydrostatic gradient in Pdi of 0.75 cm H_2O/cm. They then applied Laplace's law [Eq. (2)]. Whitelaw and co-workers (1983) modeled a diaphragm dome in an upright circular cylindrical rib cage (Fig. 9). They calculated shapes of the dome for different combinations of tension and pressure, and compared these with shapes measured from PA radiographic silhouettes of diaphragm domes at FRC. Shapes that matched the observed ones corresponded to Pdi values of between 2 and 5 cm H_2O (at the top of the dome) and tensions of 10–20 g/cm (erroneously labeled dyne/cm in the paper; Fig. 10). The calculated shape was much closer to the observed shape than were best-fit spherical shapes.

Paiva et al. used their three-dimensional images of diaphragms in supine relaxed subjects at FRC to calculate the principal radii of curvature of the hemidiaphragm domes and the sum $1/R = 1/R_1 + 1/R_2$. The law gives:

$$1/R + -0.75/Tdi \, (h - ho) + Pdi.o/Tdi \qquad (4)$$

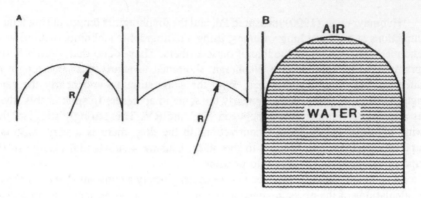

Figure 9 (A) Spherical model of diaphragm shape. (B) Model of diaphragm used in calculations by Whitelaw et al. (1983).

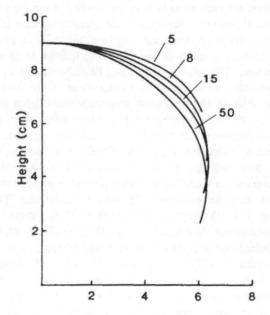

Figure 10 A family of calculated curves describing shape of a passive circular diaphragm dome modeled as in Figure 8, with different tensions, indicated by the numbers (g/cm). (From Whitelaw et al., 1983.)

where *ho* is the height of the diaphragm at the top edge of the free dome; that is, where the diaphragm just touches the anterior chest wall, and *P*di.o is the pressure at that point. Plotting 1/*R* against *h* – *ho* gives the straight line expected if the assumptions are correct, and allows calculation of *T*di and *P*di. The values were 1 and –3.2 cm H_2O for P_{di} and 54 and 32 g/cm for Tdi of the right and left domes, respectively.

These calculations and their agreement with reasonable expectations for pressure and tension and with observed shape give credence to the assumptions made and the validity of the calculation. The results should be treated with caution, however. It is still very possible that the diaphragm is really just conforming to the shape of the surrounding organs: liver, lung, stomach, and spleen. Alternative models of diaphragm shape and tension may give results just as close to the experimental data, which are, as yet, not very precise.

Recent work by Margulies et al. (1994) avoided many of the problems by imaging the relaxed diaphragm in supine dogs that had small pneumothoraces to eliminate regional variations in Ppl and fluid infused into the abdomen to ensure a nearly pure hydrostatic gradient in Pab. They then applied finite element analysis to calculate the stress in small regions of the diaphragm. They found stress to be quite anisotropic—about three times as great along the direction of muscle fibers as perpendicular to them in the plane of the membrane. There was not much variation in stress from region to region.

It makes intuitive sense that the greatest changes in shape and the greatest possible influence of the shape factor should be under conditions of strong contraction of the diaphragm. Maximal contractions are used for experiments for which it is desired to standardize the strength of contraction, but they may produce major distortions of the chest wall and important inaccuracies if the data are presumed to apply to diaphragm function in normal breathing. Shape, no doubt, acts as a very important uncontrolled variable in assessment of diaphragm strength by maximum voluntary effort or by supramaximal stimuli in humans. In dogs, Road and Leevers (1989) found that Pdi-length relations under maximal stimuli were quite different from those of quiet breathing. They considered the possibility that the length–tension curve for the low-grade stimuli of quiet breathing could be quite different from the tetanic curve that is usually assumed to apply, or that an important shape change had altered the tension–pressure relation during tetanic stimulation.

The mechanical principles and assumptions used by Paiva et al. (1992) and Whitelaw et al. (1983) can be applied qualitatively to try to understand the shape changes shown in Figure 5 from Margulies et al. (1990). For the supine dog at FRC, there is expected to be some tension in the diaphragm, and there should be a hydrostatic gradient in Pdi. A supine, cylindrically symmetrical diaphragm should have its most cranial point posteriorly according to the hydrostatic gradient (Fig. 11). The observed anterior location of this point implies that shape is affected by something not considered in the assumptions. This could be the anterior sternal attachments or the surrounding organs. At TLC, tension and Pdi in the relaxed diaphragm must be less than at FRC. The hydrostatic gradient will be relatively

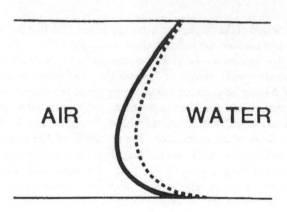

Figure 11   Shape of diaphragm in supine subjects, relaxed (solid line) and contracted (dashed line). (From Whitelaw et al., 1983.)

more important at determining shape, because the variation in Pdi from top to bottom will be a larger percentage of mean Pdi than at FRC. A posterior bulge, therefore, should be even more prominent than at FRC. Similarly, at FRC, at which there is more tension, the diaphragm should be rounder than at TLC, because as tension and Pdi become larger, the hydrostatic gradient becomes less important, and the shape should come closer to the sphere predicted by Laplace's law, for which Pdi is the same everywhere. The data show diaphragmatic shape changes opposite those predicted by these principles. It appears, instead, that the lung is forcing the diaphragm to conform to its shape at TLC, because a pneumothorax changes the diaphragm's shape dramatically. After the pneumothorax, the diaphragm's shape changes qualitatively with volume as predicted by Laplace's law: it is rounder at FRC than TLC and has its most cranial portion slightly more anterior.

The human diaphragm outlines shown in Figure 3 also do not behave as predicted on simple principles. At higher volumes, with lower tensions, it is expected that the hydrostatic gradient would be more important, and the sagittal sections would show an increasingly prominent posterior bulge, but they do not. And during the voluntary contraction of the lower panel of Figure 1, one would expect the dome to be rounder than when it is relaxed, again because the mean Pdi is relatively more important than the hydrostatic gradient; but, in fact, the contracted diaphragm is flatter.

The saddle shape has important implications about how the costal and crural diaphragm might interact. The ratio of curvature in opposite directions allows transdiaphragmatic pressure to be either negative or positive in the saddle. Tension in the AP direction could anchor the position of the central tendon (Fig. 12).

XIII. Perspective

The diaphragm has a complex shape that defies mathematical description. There are reasons to believe that most of the simplifying assumptions one could make in

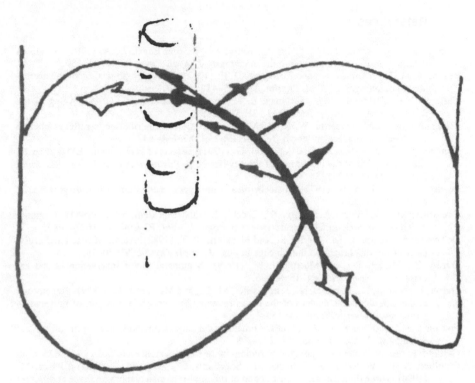

Figure 12 Interaction between tension in medial crural fibers in sagittal plane and tension in transverse direction over domes. Tension across saddle in medial crural fibers (open arrows), similar to tension in a clothesline, can make the saddle effective as an anchor for fibers pulling laterally and upward over domes (solid arrows). (From Whitelaw, 1987.)

analyzing its mechanics, passive or active, are partly invalid. More precise measurements and much more refined calculations will be needed to provide plausible solutions. It is likely that regional variations in tension, thickness, activation, shape, and Pdi are important in diaphragmatic function and will need to be taken into account to make realistic models.

Several very interesting questions about diaphragmatic function may soon be answered by exact measurements and calculations. The whole question of how the "costal" and "crural" portions interact and how they produce their different effects on the rib cage must depend on shape and on distribution of forces applied to the rib cage by the diaphragm's attachments. The significance of the high location of the anterior attachments associated with the upturn of the anterior costal margin found in most mammals should become clear. With a more complete analysis, measurements of shape in physiology and clinical medicine may permit plausible deductions about distribution of pressure or forces on the diaphragm.

References

Brancatisano, A., Amis, T. C., Tully, A., Kelly, W. T., and Engel, L. A. (1991). Regional distribution of blood flow within the diaphragm. *J. Appl. Physiol.* 71: 583–589.

Braun, N. M. T., Arora, N. S., and Rochester, D. F. (1982). Force–length relation of the normal human diaphragm. *J. Appl. Physiol.* 53: 405–412.

Caskey, C. I., Zerhouni, E. A., Fishman, E. K., and Rahmouni, A. D. (1989). Aging of the diaphragm: A CT study. *Radiology* 171: 385–389.

Cheeseman, M., and Revelette, W. R. (1990). Phrenic afferent contribution to reflexes elicited by changes in diaphragm length. *J. Appl. Physiol.* 69: 640–647.

Clement, M. G., Albertini, M., and Aguggini, G. (1991). Effects of PGF$_{2\alpha}$ on the EMG of costal and crural parts of the diaphragm of the newborn pig. *Postaglandins Leuktrienes Essential Fatty Acids* 43: 167–173.

Davies, A., and Gunn, H. (1972). Histochemical fibre types in the mammalian diaphragm. *J. Anat.* 112: 41–60.

Decramer, M., DeTroyer, A., Kelly, S., Zocchi, L., and Macklem, P. T. (1984). Regional differences in abdominal pressure swings in dogs. *J. Appl. Physiol.* 57: 1682–1687.

DeTroyer, A., Sampson, M., Sigrist, S., and Macklem, P. T. (1982). Action of costal and crural parts of the diaphragm on the rib cage in dog. *J. Appl. Physiol.* 53: 30–39.

Duron, B., Marlot, D., and Macron, J. M. (1979). Segmental motor innervation of the cat diaphragm. *Neurosci. Lett.* 15: 93–96.

Duron, B., Marlot, D., Larnicol, N., Jung-Caillol, M. C., and Macron, J. M. (1979). Somatotopy in the phrenic motor nucleus of the cat as revealed by retrograde transport of horseradish peroxidase. *Neurosci. Lett.* 14: 159–163.

Fournier, M., and Sieck, G. C. (1988). Somatotopy in the segmental innervation of the cat diaphragm. *J. Appl. Physiol.* 64: 291–298.

Gale, M. E. (1986). Anterior diaphragm: Variations in the CT appearance. *Radiology* 161: 635–639.

Gauthier, A. P., Verbanck, S., Estenne, M., Segebarth, C., Macklem, P. T., and Paiva, M. (1994). Three dimensional reconstruction of the *in vivo* human diaphragm shape at different lung volumes. *J. Appl. Physiol.* 76: 495–506.

Gordon, D. C., and Richmond, F. J. R. (1990). Topography in the phrenic motoneuron nucleus demonstrated by retrograde multiple labelling techniques. *J. Comp. Neurol.* 292: 424–434.

Griffiths, R. I., Shadwick, R. E., and Berger, P. J. (1992). Functional importance of a highly elastic ligament on the mammalian diaphragm. *Proc. R. Soc. Lond.* 249: 199–204.

Hammond, C. G. M., Gordon, D. C., Fisher, J. T., and Richmond, F. J. R., (1989). Motor unit territories supplied by primary branches of the phrenic nerve. *J. Appl. Physiol.* 66: 61–71.

Hawkins, S. P., and Hine, A. L. (1991). Diaphragm muscular bundles (slips): Ultrasound evaluation of incidence and appearance. *Clin. Radiol.* 44: 154–157.

Henderson-Smart, D. J., Johnson, P., and McClelland, M. E. (1982). Asynchronous respiratory activity of the diaphragm during spontaneous breathing in the lamb. *J. Physiol. Lond.* 327: 377–391.

Hendricks, J. C., and Kline, L. R. (1991). Differential activation within costal diaphragm during rapid eye movement sleep in cats. *J. Appl. Physiol.* 70: 1194–1200.

Henneman, E., Somjen, G., and Carpenter, D. O. (1965). Functional significance of cell size in spinal motoneurons. *J. Neurophysiol.* 28: 560–580.

Hubmayr, R. D., Sprung, J., and Nelson, S. (1990). Determinants of transdiaphragmatic pressure in dogs. *J. Appl. Physiol.* 69: 2050–2056.

Jammes, Y., Mathiot, M. J., Delpierre, S., and Grimaud, C. (1986). Role of vagal and spinal sensory pathways on eupneic diaphragmatic activity. *J. Appl. Physiol.* 60: 479–485.

Keens, T. C., Bryan, A. C., Levison, H., and Ianuzzo, C. D. (1978). Developmental patterns of muscle fibre types in human ventilatory muscles. *J. Appl. Physiol.* 44: 909–913.

Keens, T. C., and Ianuzzo, C. D. (1979). Development of fatigue-resistant muscle fibres in human ventilatory muscles. *Am. Rev. Respir. Dis.* 119: 139–141.

Kilarski, W., and Sjöström, M. (1990). Systematic distribution of muscle fibre types in the rat and rabbit diaphragm: A morphometric and structural analysis. *J. Anat.* 168: 13–30.

Kim, M. J., Druz, W. S., Danon, J., Machnach, W., and Sharp, J. T. (1976). Mechanics of the canine diaphragm. *J. Appl. Physiol.* 41: 369–382.

Knight, H., Petroll, W. M., Adams, J. M., Shaffer, H. A., and Rochester, D. F. (1990). Video fluoroscopic assessment of muscle fiber shortening in the in situ canine diaphragm. *J. Appl. Physiol.* 68: 2200–2207.

Lai-Fook, S. (1979). A continuum mechanics analysis of pulmonary vascular interdependence in isolated dog lobes. *J. Appl. Physiol.* 46: 419–429.

Macklem, P. T., Zocchi, L., and Agostoni, E. (1988). Pleural pressure between diaphragm and rib cage during inspiratory muscle activity. *J. Appl. Physiol.* 65: 1286–1295.

Manohar, M. (1990). Diaphragmatic perfusion hetrogeneity during exercise with inspiratory restive breathing. *J. Appl. Physiol.* 68: 2177–2181.

Margulies, S. S. (1991). Regional variations in diaphragm thickness. *J. Appl. Physiol.*, 70: 2663–2668.

Margulies, S. S., and Rodarte, J. R. (1990). Shape of the chest wall in the prone and supine anesthetized dog. *J. Appl. Physiol.* 68: 1970–1978.

Margulies, S. S., Lei, G. T., Farkas, G. A., and Rodarte, J. R. (1994). Finite element analysis of stress in the canine diaphragm. *J. Appl. Physiol.* 76: 2070–2075.

Maxwell, L. C., Kuehl, T. J., McCarter, R. J. M., and Robotham, J. L. (1989). Regional distribution of fibre types in developing baboon muscles. *Anat. Rec.* 224: 66–78.

Metzger, J., Scheidt, K., and Fritts, K. (1985). Histochemical and physiological characteristics of the rat diaphragm. *J. Appl. Physiol.* 58: 1085–1985.

Monges, H., Salducci, J., and Naudy, B. (1978). Dissociation between the electrical activity of the diaphragmatic dome and crura muscular fibers during esophageal distention, vomiting and eructation. *J. Physiol. (Paris)* 74: 541–554.

O'Malley, C. D., and Saunders, J. B. de C. M. (1952). *Leonardo da Vinci on the Human Body.* Henry Schuman, New York.

Oyer, L. M., Knuth, S. L., Ward, D. K., and Bartlett, D., Jr. (1989). Reflex inhibition of crural diaphragm activity by esophageal distention in cats. *Respir. Physiol.* 77: 195–202.

Paen, J. L., Chuong, C. J., Ramanathan, M., and Johnson, R. J., Jr. (1991). Regional deformation of the canine diaphragm. *J. Appl. Physiol.* 71: 1581–1588.

Paiva, M., Verbanck, S., Estenne, M., Poncelet, B., Segebarth, C., and Macklem, P. T. (1992). Mechanical implications of *in vivo* human diaphragm shape. *J. Appl. Physiol.* 72: 1407–1412.

Panicek, D. M., Benson, C. B., Gottlieb, R. H., and Heitzman, E. R. (1988). The diaphragm: Anatomic patholgic and radiologic considerations, *Radiographics* 8: 385–425.

Petroll, W. M., Knight, H., and Rochester, D. F. (1990a). Effect of lower rib cage expansion and diaphragm shortening on the zone of apposition. *J. Appl. Physiol.* 68: 484–488.

Petroll, W. M., Knight, H., and Rochester, D. F. (1990b). A model approach to assess diaphragmatic volume displacement. *J. Appl. Physiol.* 69: 2175–2182.

Pollard, M. J., Megirian D., and Sherrey, J. H. (1985). Unity of costal and crural diaphragmatic activity in respiration. *Exp. Neurol.* 90: 187–193.

Rikard-Bell, G. C., and Bystrzycka, E. K. (1980). Localization of phrenic motor neucleus in the cat and rabbit studied with horseradish peroxidase. *Brain Res.* 194: 479–483.

Riley, D. A., and Berger, A. J. (1979). A regional histochemical and electrophysiological analysis of the cat respiratory diaphragm. *Exp. Neurol.* 66: 636–649.

Road, J. D., and Leevers, A. M. (1989). Effect of lung inflation on diaphragmatic shortening. *J. Appl. Physiol.* 65: 2383–2389.

Road, J. D., Newman, S., Derenne, J.-P., and Grassino, A. (1986). In vivo force length relationship of canine diaphragm. *J. Appl. Physiol.* 60: 63–70.

Sant'Ambrogio, G., Frazier, D. T., Wilson, M. F., and Agostoni, E. (1963). Motor innervation and pattern of activity of cat diaphragm. *J. Appl. Physiol.* 18: 43–46.

Sieck, G. C. (1988). Diaphragm muscle structural and functional organization, *Clin. Chest Med.* 9: 125–210.

Sieck, G. C., Roy, R. R., Powell, P., Blanco, C. Edgerton, V. R., and Harper, R. M. (1983). Muscle fibre type distribution and architecture of the cat diaphragm. *J. Appl. Physiol.* 55: 1386–1392.

Sieck, G. C., Sachs, R. D., and Blanco, C. E. (1987). Absence of regional differences in the size and oxidative capacity of diaphragm muscle fibres. *J. Appl. Physiol.* 63: 1076–1082.

Soust, M., Walker, A. M., Wilson, F. E., and Berger, P. J. (1987). Origins and regional distribution of blood flow to the respiratory muscles in conscious sheep. *Respir. Physiol.* 67: 283–294.

Sprung, J., Deschamps, C., Hubmayr, R. D., Walters, B. J., and Rodarte, J. R. (1989). In vivo regional diaphragm function in dogs. *J. Appl. Physiol.* 67: 655–662.

Sprung, J., Deschamps, C., Margulies, S. S., Hubmayr, R. D., and Rodarte, J. R. (1990). Effect of body position on regional diaphragm function in dogs. *J. Appl. Physiol.* 69: 2296–2302.

Van Lunteren, E., Haxhiu, M. A., Cherniack, N. S., and Goldman, M. D. (1985). Differential costal and crural diaphragm compensation for posture changes. *J. Appl. Physiol.* 58: 1895–1900.

Whitelaw, W. A. (1987). Shape and size of the human diaphragm in vivo. *J. Appl. Physiol.* 62: 180–186.

Whitelaw, W. A., Hajdo, L. E., and Wallace, J. A. (1983). Relationships among pressure, tension and shape in the diaphragm. *J. Appl. Physiol.* 55: 1899–1905.

22

Chest Wall Mechanics in Newborns

JACOPO P. MORTOLA

McGill University
Montreal, Quebec, Canada

I. Introduction

Records of chest wall movements and spirometric measurements in infants during spontaneous resting breathing reveal several differences from the adult, including two aspects that will be addressed in this review. During inspiration, the infant's thorax does not expand as clearly as in the adult. In fact, during active (rapid-eye-movement; REM) sleep the newborn's rib cage can actually retract during inspiration, and expand during expiration (Fig. 1), following a pattern that is opposite that occurring in the adult. The spirometric record indicates that the end-expiratory level (FRC) is not as stable as in the adult; long expiratory times, or short apneas, which are not rare in the early postnatal period, are often accompanied by an obvious decrease in FRC, whereas rapid breathing increases FRC (Olinsky et al., 1974). [The terms end-expiratory level and functional residual capacity (FRC) are here used interchangeably to indicate the lung volume at end-expiration. Relaxation volume (Vr) indicates the lung volume in relaxed (or passive) conditions.]

These two seemingly unrelated characteristics of the infant's respiration, the paradoxical inward motion of the rib cage in inspiration and the oscillation of the end-expiratory level, find a common basis in the dynamic properties of the chest wall during the early postnatal period. The goal of the present chapter is to review those aspects of neonatal chest wall mechanisms strictly pertinent to the understand-

617

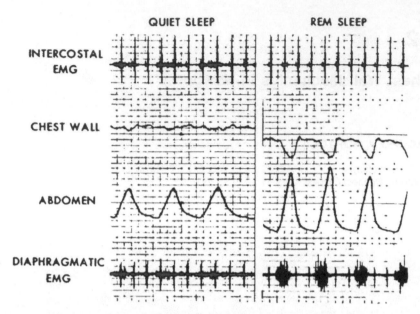

Figure 1 Premature infant during sleep. The anteroposterior diameter of the rib cage (labeled chest wall, measured at the level of the nipple line) and of the abdomen increase with upward deflection of the record. During inspiration, the abdominal dimension increases, whereas the rib cage dimension either changes little (quiet sleep) or decreases (REM sleep). In REM sleep, intercostal activity, measured by surface electrodes, is less than during quiet sleep. (From Muller et al., 1979.)

ing of these two phenomena of infants' breathing; they include the passive structure and function of the chest wall, its dynamic behavior, and some functional properties of the respiratory muscles. Generalities of chest wall mechanics and respiratory muscles are reviewed elsewhere in this volume. Reference to other species will be sought only to complete information not available from human studies; comparative reviews of respiratory mechanics in newborn mammals, including chest wall function, have been recently published (Mortola, 1987, 1991).

II. The Passive Neonatal Chest Wall: Structural and Functional Considerations

From a geometric viewpoint, the major changes in the human thorax with growth are in the cross-sectional shape and the ribs' orientation. With age, the transversal cross section assumes a less rounded, dorsoventrally flattened shape and the dorsoventral orientation of the ribs is progressively more caudal relative to the vertebral attachment (Takahashi and Atsumi, 1955; Howett and Demuth, 1965;

Openshaw et al., 1984). These configurational changes are likely to be contributed by the gravitational pull associated with the standing position; therefore, they are probably less apparent in quadrupeds.

During growth, the end-tidal configuration of the diaphragm follows the changes in thorax shape and the development of the visceral organs; with the progressively more oblique orientation of the ribs, the costal attachments of the diaphragm, relative to the central tendon organ, descend along the body axial direction, enhancing the domelike shape of the muscle and increasing the area of apposition [The apposition area corresponds to the lower region of the rib cage in which the diaphragm is opposed to the rib cage without interposed lung (Devlieger et al., 1991).] This has some functional implications in the translation of muscle force into rib cage expansion and lung inflation. In fact, as the diaphragm contracts, the transmission of abdominal pressure to the lower ribs is larger the greater the appositional area. In the newborn, the small appositional area implies a smaller inspiratory action of the diaphragmatic pressure on the rib cage. In addition, the higher compliance of the abdominal wall does not favor the rise in abdominal pressure. Diaphragmatic efficiency is improved by abdominal loading, such as binding the infant's abdomen (Fleming et al., 1979), or by breathing in the prone position; both decrease abdominal compliance and widen the appositional area (Wolfson et al., 1992), with the effect of improving tidal volume and arterial oxygenation, in comparison with resting breathing in the supine posture (Hutchison et al., 1979; Wagaman et al., 1979). A synergistic activation of the abdominal muscles would also improve the mechanical efficiency of diaphragmatic contraction; however, during unassisted spontaneous breathing, abdominal muscles usually show little activity, or are not active in infants (O'Brien et al., 1980; Kosch and Stark, 1984; South et al., 1987) and, therefore, do not contribute in maintaining a low abdominal compliance and diaphragmatic optimal length. Hence, neonatal breathing in the supine posture requires large diaphragmatic excursions (Laing et al., 1988; Wolfson et al., 1992), possibly contributing to a greater diaphragmatic work (Guslits et al., 1987). During CO_2-induced hyperventilation, the abdominal muscles are recruited (Praud et al., 1991), and probably contribute to the hyperventilation by protecting the length of the diaphragmatic fiber and the mechanical efficiency of its contraction.

The passive compliance of the whole respiratory system (Crs) in infants can be easily measured during artificial ventilation after paralysis or during spontaneous breathing with the multiple occlusion technique (Olinsky et al., 1976; Mortola et al., 1982; Mortola, 1992). [In full-term infants the average Crs value is between 1 and 1.3 ml kg^{-1} cm H_2O^{-1} (reviewed in Mortola, 1992)]. The partitioning of Crs in its lung (CL) and chest wall (Cw) components requires measurements of mean pleural pressure, which are often much more problematic than in the adult and need to be carefully interpreted (LeSouëf et al., 1983; Coates and Stocks, 1991).

Richards and co-workers (Richards and Bachman, 1961; Nightingale and Richards, 1965) found that the Crs value was similar to known values of CL and, therefore, concluded that the human infant's Cw was very high. Their conclusion agrees with later measurements of Cw obtained as the ratio of the change in lung volume and the corresponding change in pleural pressure during artificial inflation of the lung (Reynolds and Etsten, 1966; Gerhardt and Bancalari, 1980). Hence, although in men, Cw and C_L have similar values, in infants Cw is about four to five times higher than C_L (Polgar and Weng, 1979); this difference may become even larger at higher lung volumes, because with lung inflation the recoil of the lung increases more than that of the chest wall. The conclusion of a high Cw/C_L ratio in newborns applies to most of the mammalian species investigated (Mortola, 1987; Davis et al., 1988). The only exception seems to be the pig, a species unusually mature at birth, with a low and constant Cw/C_L ratio throughout postnatal development (Standaert et al., 1991).

From the viewpoint of pulmonary function testing, one practical implication of the very high Cw/C_L ratio in the infant is that measurements of Crs can be interpreted as reflecting C_L, which is convenient because Crs is much more easily measured than C_L (Mortola, 1992). Eventually, during the first three years of life, Cw/C_L ratio decreases (Papastamelos et al., 1995). Some indirect computations would indicate that, in the 5-year-old child, the Cw/C_L ratio is about 1.5–2, and remains approximately steady at about this value throughout adolescence (Sharp et al., 1970).

III. Dynamic Mechanical Behavior

The increase in Cw/C_L ratio, with high Cw, has two important functional implications. First, because the outward pull of the chest on the lung, at any lung volume, is reduced, the static relaxation volume of the respiratory system, Vr, is decreased (Fig. 2). Second, during inspiration, the stability of the chest wall is reduced, contributing to its distortion, thereby compromising the efficiency of diaphragmatic contraction. This latter aspect adds to the aforementioned constraint on diaphragmatic function determined by the small appositional area.

Measurements of Vr have been performed on many newborn species and with different methodologies; in general, per unit of lung weight (LW), Vr is less in newborns than in adults (Fisher and Mortola, 1980). Human infants are probably no exception, since functional residual capacity (FRC), which in infants is dynamically maintained above Vr (see Section IV.B), per unit of LW is smaller than in adult men (Cook et al., 1958). Normalization per body weight (BW) gives mixed results, and could be misleading because of the substantial decrease in LW/BW with growth and because BW includes components extraneous to the mechanical properties of the lung.

Chest wall distortion has been evaluated mostly from measurements of rib cage and abdomen dimensions during breathing. An absence of distortion would occur when chest dimensions during breathing correspond to those observed during artificial lung inflation (i.e., with muscles relaxed); on the other hand, a departure

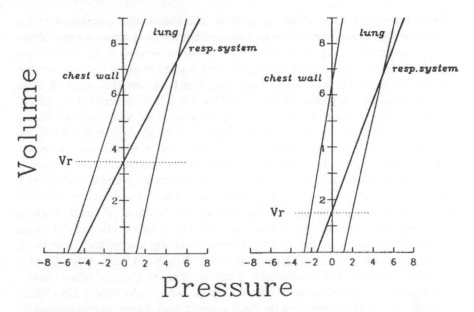

Figure 2 Schematic pressure–volume relations of lung, chest wall, and respiratory system in conditions of low (left panel) or high (right panel) chest wall compliance (Cw). Linear relations have been drawn for simplicity. With higher Cw, the relaxation volume of the respiratory system (Vr) decreases, and so does the mean recoil pressure of the lung at Vr.

from the passive configuration, at any given lung volume, indicates some degree of chest distortion. Occasionally, as during REM sleep, the distortion is obvious, since the rib cage moves inward during inspiration (Knill et al., 1976; Muller et al., 1979; Curzi-Descalova, 1982; Stark et al., 1987) and, therefore, opposite that observed during passive lung inflation. In preterm infants, paradoxical motion of the rib cage occurs even more commonly than in term infants, regardless of sleep state (Davi et al., 1979). With growth, the frequency of rib cage paradoxing decreases (Gaultier et al., 1987) and, in adolescents, the rib cage expands in inspiration also during REM sleep, albeit less than during non-REM sleep or wakefulness (Tabachnik et al., 1981).

The analytical translation of chest wall motion into chest wall volume, and the computation of the magnitude of volume distorted, can be done by calibrating changes in chest wall dimensions with known passive changes in lung volume. In infants, passive conditions can be achieved by occluding the airways during expiration, a maneuver that favors relaxation of the respiratory muscles, or by inflating the infant's respiratory system at different lung volumes with a ventilator (Mortola, 1992). The unavoidable assumption in the analysis is that the motion of the chest region examined is taken as representative of the whole chest, which may be incorrect, especially with marked distortion (Heldt, 1988); in addition, the quantitative assessment of the volumetric distortion of the chest wall, based on body surface move- ments, finds a major complication in the definition of the boundaries between abdo- men and rib cage at the level of the area of apposition. One way to evaluate the total volume distorted by the chest wall during breathing, which circumvents some of these problems, has been proposed in animals and tested in infants (Mortola et al., 1985). Changes in lung volume (V) and abdominal pressure (Pab) were recorded during spontaneous breathing and passive lung inflation; in the absence of distortion, the end-inspiratory Pab–V data points fall on the passive Pab–V relationship. However, at the end of a spontaneous inspiration, V is usually less than expected from the passive curve, indicating that, during breathing, some V was "lost" because of chest wall distortion. In other words, during inspiration some of the pressure generated by the diaphragm, instead of inflating the lungs, distorts the chest wall. A similar analysis can be performed by measuring V and abdominal motion (ab) in place of abdominal pressure (Pab), because, during spontaneous breathing, the infant's abdominal muscles are usually inactive (O'Brien et al., 1980; Kosch and Stark, 1984; South et al., 1987); from the ab–V relationship, it appears that, on average, infants have a volume loss from distortion that is almost as large as their tidal volume (Mortola et al., 1985; Fig. 3). This implies that the diaphragmatic work during rib cage inspiratory

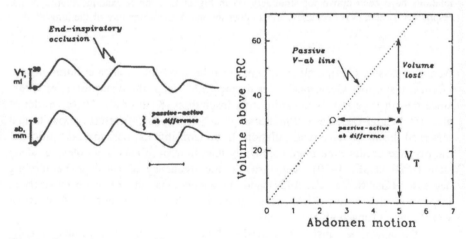

Figure 3 (Left) Records of changes in lung volume (VT) and abdominal anteroposterior dimension (ab) in a spontaneously breathing infants in the supine posture. At end-inspiration the airways are briefly occluded; as lung volume remains constant, ab decreases from the active end-inspiratory point to the passive value. (Right) Abdominal motion–lung volume relation, from the records at left. Extrapolation of the passive line above VT assumes linearity; its accuracy can be verified by occlusions of the periodic, spontaneously occurring, deep inspirations, or by artificially inflating the infant's respiratory system above VT. (Adapted from Mortola et al., 1985.)

paradoxing can be substantially higher than with minimal chest wall distortion, as some estimates from measurements of transdiaphragmatic pressure, abdominal and rib cage motion would indicate (Heldt and McIlroy, 1987; Guslits et al., 1987). To what extent this implies a greater total (i.e., diaphragm plus extradiaphragmatic muscles) cost of breathing has not been thoroughly quantified. In the lamb, which is a precocial species at birth, the oxygen cost of the respiratory muscles during resting breathing was found to be 1.9% of the whole body oxygen consumption (Soust et al., 1989b), a value that is not much higher than that of the adult man.

A distortion not dissimilar to that observed in healthy full-term infants can be observed in adult humans with cervical spinal lesion (tetraplegic patients), who present an obvious inward movement of the upper rib cage in inspiration (Mortola and Sant'Ambrogio, 1978). Therefore, comparison of the motion of the chest between these adult patients and normal subjects clearly stresses the importance of the extradiaphragmatic muscles, namely the intercostals, in limiting chest wall distortion and the consequent volume loss (Mortola et al., 1985). Consequently, the distortion of the chest wall commonly observed in infants is not only the result of the mechanical differences from the adult discussed earlier (small apposition area and high C_W/C_L), but also, and probably mostly, the effect of differences in the inspiratory contribution of the extradiaphragmatic muscles. A corollary of the foregoing is that distortion (and volume loss) is the expected respiratory behavior during contraction of the diaphragm alone; displacement of the chest wall along the relaxation line and absence of volume loss represent "compensated distortion," and not absence of it. In infants with tetraplegia or spinal anesthesia, in whom the diaphragm is presumably the only functioning inspiratory muscle, paradoxing of the rib cage is the consistent finding (Thach et al., 1980; Pascucci et al., 1990). On the opposite end, expansion of the rib cage during inspiration can be seen in conditions of increased respiratory drive to the intercostal muscles, as during CO_2-induced hyperventilation (Hershenson et al., 1989).

The volume lost because of distortion may include part of FRC, especially if, as postulated to occur during REM sleep, chest distortion is accompanied by a major decrease of respiratory muscle tone; this could decrease O_2 stores and possibly increase the vulnerability to asphyxia (Henderson-Smart and Read, 1979; Lopes et al., 1981b). The increased diaphragmatic work required to maintain ventilation during chest distortion has also been considered a potential cause of muscle fatigue (Muller et al., 1979; Heldt and McIlroy, 1987).

IV. Contribution of the Respiratory Muscles to Chest Wall Dynamics

A. Inspiration

The question to be addressed is to what extent the mechanical instability of the neonatal rib cage and its tendency to distortion (see Section III) are contributed by the structural and functional properties of the respiratory muscles. On theoretical grounds, muscle mass and structure, intrinsic mechanical characteristics, resistance to fatigue, and perfusion, all could be factors contributing to differences in respiratory muscle performance and, thereby, to the degree of chest wall stability during development.

Interspecies analysis suggests that the diaphragm mass is a constant proportion of body mass (about 0.35%) in both newborns and adults (Mortola, 1991). Diaphragm mass is proportional to body mass in the growing animal (Davidson, 1968; Lieberman et al., 1972; Powers et al., 1991) as well as among normal adult men of different body weight (Arora and Rochester, 1982). As with other skeletal muscles (Aherne et al., 1971), also in the diaphragm, the increase in muscle mass during postnatal development is almost uniquely owing to muscle fiber hypertrophy (Bowden and Goyer, 1960; Mayock et al., 1987).

The issues of the fatigue of the neonatal respiratory muscles and of its potential contribution to chest distortion and breathing strategies have attracted much attention. In the premature infant and newborn rabbit, the diaphragmatic concentration of type I slow-twitch, high-oxidative (fatigue-resistant) fibers was low (Keens et al., 1978; Le Souëf et al., 1988); this led to the suggestions that muscle fatigue had higher probability of occurring in the newborn than in the adult, and some changes in diaphragm electromyogram (EMG) were eventually interpreted in support of this view (Lopes et al., 1981a). Fiber type concentration, however, is only one aspect of muscle morphology; fiber size and capillarization are other parameters very relevant to muscle performance, and they are known to change drastically during the development of many skeletal muscles, including the diaphragm (Tamaki, 1985; Smith et al., 1989). In contradiction with the original proposition, morphological, biochemical, and functional studies on other species have indicated that the diaphragm is well prepared for high-respiratory work loads, even at young ages (Lieberman et al., 1972; Maxwell et al., 1983; Powers et al., 1991). The diaphragm of the newborn baboon is as fatigue-resistant as that of the adult, and recovers more quickly (Maxwell et al., 1983); in rats and cats the diaphragm resistance to fatigue is actually greater in newborns than in adults (Sieck et al., 1991; Watchko et al., 1992; Trang et al., 1992). A decrease in tonic activity of the inspiratory muscles coincides with the occurrence of periodic breathing (O'Brien, 1985), but this does not mean that the former is the cause of the latter. Changes in the power spectra of the diaphragm EMG, considered signs of muscle fatigue, do not correlate with the infant's episodes of periodic breathing and apneas (Nugent and Finley, 1985). The idea that muscle fatigue is a realistic possibility in the newborn is also contradicted by the observations that ventilation in human infants and other newborn mammals can be maintained much above the resting values for long periods. For example, newborn rats in chronic hypoxic or hypercapnic conditions can sustain a level of ventilation almost double the resting value for several days with no signs of adaptation (Piazza et al., 1988; Rezzonico and Mortola, 1989). In summary, it seems that the possibility that the neonatal respiratory muscles become fatigued has been inappropriately overemphasized. Although it may occur in some pathological conditions (Nichols, 1991), the information presently available does not convincingly indicate that respiratory muscle fatigue represents a potential problem in the newborn any more than it is in the adult.

The magnitude of blood flow to the diaphragm and intercostals was larger (per unit of body, or muscle, weight) in the lamb than in the adult sheep (Soust et al., 1989a). This was interpreted as reflecting the higher metabolic and ventilatory requirements of the newborn, compared with the adult, and the greater needs to stabilize the rib cage in the newborn. As in the adult, with the raise in ventilation respiratory muscle blood flow increases in proportion with the metabolic demands of the muscle (Soust et al., 1989b); only at very fast stimulation rates (100/min), probably higher than the spontaneous-breathing rate of the lamb, the increase in O_2 delivery does not fulfill the O_2 demands of the diaphragm (Nichols et al., 1989).

The intrinsic mechanical properties (force–length and force–velocity relations) of the respiratory muscles have been the object of very few studies in adult species (Sharp and Hyatt, 1986) and, to our knowledge, they have not been examined during the early postnatal period. The shape of the biceps force–length curve in the newborn mouse resembles that of the adult (Goldspink, 1968), but whether this similarity applies to other skeletal muscles and, in particular, to the respiratory muscles, needs to be established.

It is well documented that the inspiratory pressure generated by the newborn's muscles can be very high, up to 70 cm H_2O (reviewed in Mortola, 1977). The inspiratory muscle pressure is the result of the ratio between muscle force, which is directly proportional to the muscle cross section, and the surface over which the force is applied which, in first approximation, is the surface of the thorax. During development, because muscle mass seems to increase in proportion to body mass (see foregoing), muscle cross-sectional area could also increase in proportion to thorax size. Hence, the inspiratory muscles of the newborn can develop respiratory pressures not too different from the adult values, despite the much lower muscle mass. This conclusion would seem to be contradicted by some results in piglets, in which the transdiaphragmatic pressure generated during supramaximal stimulation of the phrenic nerves against occluded airways was progressively larger with the age of the animal (Watchko et al., 1986). It should be noted, however, that even when the airways are occluded and lung volume remains constant, diaphragmatic contraction is not isometric (Newman et al., 1984); hence, the force and trans-diaphragmatic pressure produced by the diaphragm during phrenic stimulation depends on the degree of its shortening, which could be larger in the younger animals because of the greater chest distortion.

B. Expiration

In the broadest functional sense, *respiratory muscles* are all those involved in the control of respiratory flow. This definition is particularly relevant to neonatal respiration, since not only the muscles of the chest, but also those of the larynx play a paramount role in the control of expiratory flow and lung volume.

In the newborn lamb, the thyroarytenoid muscle, a vocal fold adductor, is active in expiration (Harding et al., 1980; Andrews et al., 1985), differently from what is observed in the adult man during undisturbed respiration. The resulting increase in airflow resistance can be extremely high; indeed, momentary complete interruptions of expiratory flow are common in normal infants during the earliest postnatal hours (Fisher et al., 1982; Radvanyi-Bouvet et al., 1982).

As mentioned earlier (see Sec. II), Vr in infants is low because of the high Cw/CL; therefore, the increase in laryngeal resistance during expiration represents a dynamic mechanism oriented in maintaining an elevated mean lung volume; in intubated infants, in whom this mechanism is bypassed, it is ordinary practice to apply a positive end-expiratory pressure (PEEP) of a few centimeters H_2O to avoid lung collapse and respiratory problems (reviewed in Mortola and Fisher, 1988). This degree of PEEP is indeed very similar to the value of end-expiratory pressure spontaneously generated by the infant during the dynamic elevation of functional residual capacity (Mortola et al., 1982). With growth, the end-expiratory volume (FRC) gradually approaches the relaxed value (Vr) (Colin et al., 1989), presumably because of the stiffening of the chest wall and of the decrease in breathing frequency; the former increases Vr (see Fig. 2), whereas the latter reduces the FRC–Vr difference by prolonging the time available for expiration.

The activity of the laryngeal muscles in the regulation of expiratory flow is coupled to the postinspiratory activity of the inspiratory muscles, which in infants lasts for a large fraction of the whole expiratory time (Mortola et al., 1984; Stark et al., 1987; Kosch et al., 1988). This coordination is probably finely tuned (Stark et al., 1987; Kosch et al., 1988), although the details of this control are unknown. Because the primary objective of the integration is likely to be the control of mean lung volume, one may expect the pulmonary vagal afferents to be an important aspect of the regulatory loops, as some observations would suggest (Johnson et al., 1977; Harding, 1980). During REM sleep, the activities of both laryngeal and chest wall muscles decrease in infants and other newborn species (Prechtl et al., 1977; Harding, 1980; Harding et al., 1980; England et al., 1985; Stark et al., 1987), probably contributing to the decrease in lung volume and blood oxygenation observed during this phase of sleep (Henderson-Smart and Read, 1979).

V. Conclusions

The fundamental mechanical characteristic of the newborn's respiratory system is its high Cw/CL ratio; it contributes to the instability of the thorax during inspiration and to the necessity for a dynamic elevation of FRC. Hence, the high Cw can be considered the single most important factor in determining the two peculiarities of neonatal respiration addressed at the onset of this review, the inspiratory thorax paradoxing and the oscillation of the end-expiratory level.

The end-expiratory level is regulated by the coordinated action of thoracic and laryngeal muscles in the control of the expiratory flow. The distortion of the rib cage generated by the contraction of the diaphragm could be compensated by the synergistic contraction of the extradiaphragmatic muscles. Yet, this most often does not occur, for reasons that do not seem to include peculiarities in the structural characteristics of the muscles. The most obvious possibility is that of a different, seemingly less efficient, coordination among inspiratory muscles in the newborn than in adults, but the neural basis for such a conclusion has not been thoroughly investigated. Scattered observations, usually from anesthetized animal preparations, would suggest that the proprioceptive regulation of the intercostal muscles is less developed than in adults (Schwieler, 1968; Trippenbach, 1981). However, the postnatal development of the neural loops responsible for the coordination of the respiratory muscles in wakefulness and sleep has not yet been thoroughly examined; this information would be of obvious importance for a more comprehensive understanding of the contribution of the chest wall to neonatal breathing.

References

Aherne, W., Ayyar, D. R., Clarke, P. A., and Walton, J. N. (1971). Muscle fibre size in normal infants, children and adolescents. An autopsy study. *J. Neurol. Sci.* 14: 171–182.

Andrews, D. C., Fedorko, L., Johnson, P., and Wollner, J. C. (1985). The maturation of the ambient thermal stimulus to breathing during sleep in lambs. In *The Physiological Development of the Fetus and Newborn*. Edited by C. T. Jones and P. W. Nathanielsz. New York, Academic Press, pp. 821–825.

Arora, N. S., and Rochester, D. F. (1982). Effect of body weight and muscularity on human diaphragm muscle mass, thickness, and area. *J. Appl. Physiol.* 52: 64–70.

Bowden, D. H., and Goyer, R. A. (1960). The size of muscle fibers in infants and children. *Arch. Pathol.* 69: 188–189.

Coates, A. L., and Stocks, J. (1991). Esophageal pressure manometry in human infants. *Pediatr. Pulmonol.* 11: 350–360.

Colin, A. A., Wohl, M. E. B., Mead, J., Ratjen, F. A., Glass, G., and Stark, A. R. (1989). Transition from dynamically maintained to relaxed end-expiratory volume in human infants. *J. Appl. Physiol.* 67: 2107–2111.

Cook, C. D., Helliesen, P. J., and Agathon, S. (1958). Relation between mechanics of respiration, lung size and body size from birth to young adulthood. *J. Appl. Physiol.* 13:349–352.

Curzi-Dascalova, L. (1982). Phase relationships between thoracic and abdominal respiratory movement during sleep in 31–38 weeks CA normal infants. Comparison with full-term (39–41 weeks) newborns. *Neuropediatrics* 13(Suppl.): 15–20.

Davi, M., Sankaran, K., MacCallum, M., Cates, D., and Rigatto, H. (1979). Effect of sleep state on chest distortion and on the ventilatory response to CO_2 in neonates. *Pediatr. Res.* 13: 982–986.

Davidson, M. B. (1968). The relationship between diaphragm and body weight in the rat. *Growth* 32: 221–223.

Davis, G. M., Coates, A. L., Papageorgiou, A., and Bureau, M. A. (1988). Direct measurement of static chest wall compliance in animal and human neonates. *J. Appl. Physiol.* 65: 1093–1098.

Devlieger, H., Daniels, H., Marchal, G., Moerman, P., Casaer, P., and Eggermont, E. (1991). The diaphragm of the newborn infant: Anatomical and ultrasonographic studies. *J. Dev. Physiol.* 16: 321–329.

England, S. J., Kent, G., and Stogryn, H. A. F. (1985). Laryngeal muscle and diaphragmatic activities in conscious dog pups. *Respir. Physiol.* 60: 95–108.

Fisher, J. T., and Mortola, J. P. (1980). Statics of the respiratory system in newborn mammals. *Respir. Physiol.* 41: 155–172.

Fisher, J. T., Mortola, J. P., Smith, J. B., Fox, G. S., and Weeks, S. (1982). Respiration in newborns. Development of the control of breathing. *Am. Rev. Respir. Dis.* 125: 650–657.

Fleming, P. J., Muller, N. L., Bryan, M. H., and Bryan, A. C. (1979). The effects of abdominal loading on rib cage distortion in premature infants. *Pediatrics* 64: 425–428.

Gaultier, C., Praud, J. P., Canet, E., Delaperche, M. F., and D'Allest, A. M. (1987). Paradoxical inward rib cage motion during rapid eye movement sleep in infants and young children. *J. Dev. Physiol.* 9: 391–397.

Gerhardt, T., and Bancalari, E. (1980). Chest wall compliance in full-term and premature infants. *Acta Pediatr. Scand.* 69: 359–364.

Goldspink, G. (1968). Sarcomere length during post-natal growth of mammalian muscle fibres. *J. Cell Sci.* 3: 539–548.

Guslits, B. G., Gaston, S. E., Bryan, M. H., England, S. J., Bryan, A. C. (1987). Diaphragmatic work of breathing in premature human infants. *J. Appl. Physiol.* 62: 1410–1415.

Harding, R. (1980). State-related and developmental changes in laryngeal function. *Sleep* 3: 307–322.

Harding, R., Johnson, P., and McClelland, M. E. (1980). Respiratory function of the larynx in the developing sheep and the influence of sleep state. *Respir. Physiol.* 40: 165–179.

Heldt, G. P. (1988). Simultaneous quantification of chest wall distortion by multiple methods in preterm infants. *Am. Rev. Respir. Dis.* 138: 20–25.

Heldt, G. P., and McIlroy, M. M. (1987). Distortion of chest wall and work of diaphragm in preterm infants. *J. Appl. Physiol.* 62: 164–169.

Henderson-Smart, D. J., and Read, D. J. C. (1979). Reduced lung volume during behavioral active sleep in the newborn. *J. Appl. Physiol.* 46: 1081–1085.

Hershenson, M. B., Stark, A. R., and Mead, J. (1989). Action of the inspiratory muscles of the rib cage during breathing in newborns. *Am. Rev. Respir. Dis.* 139: 1207–1212.

Howett, W. F., and DeMuth, G. R. (1965). Configuration of the chest. *Pediatrics* 35: 177–184.

Hutchison, A. A., Ross, K. R., and Russell, G. (1979). The effect of posture on ventilation and lung mechanics in preterm and light-for-date infants. *Pediatrics* 64: 429–432.

Johnson, P., Harding, R., McClelland, M., and White, P. (1977). Laryngeal influences on lung expansion and breathing in lambs [abstract]. *Pediatr. Res.* 11: 1025.

Keens, T. G., Bryan, A. C., Levison, H., and Ianuzzo, C. D. (1978). Developmental pattern of muscle fiber types in human ventilatory muscles. *J. Appl. Physiol.* 44: 909–913.

Knill, R., Andrews, W., Bryan, A. C., and Bryan, H. M. (1976). Respiratory load compensation in infants. *J. Appl. Physiol.* 40: 357–361.

Kosch, P. C., and Stark, A. R. (1984). Dynamic maintenance of end-expiratory lung volume in full-term infants. *J. Appl. Physiol.* 57: 1126–1133.

Kosch, P. C., Hutchison, A. A., Wozniak, J. A., Carlo, W. A., and Stark, A. R. (1988). Posterior cricoarytenoid and diaphragm activities during tidal breathing in neonates. *J. Appl. Physiol.* 64: 1968–1978.

Laing, I. A., Teele, R. L., and Stark, A. R. (1988). Diaphragmatic movement in newborn infants. *J. Pediatr.* 112: 638–643.

Le Souëf, P. N., Lopes, J. M., England, S. J., Bryan, M. H., and Bryan, A. C. (1983). Influence of chest wall distortion on esophageal pressure. *J. Appl. Physiol.* 55: 353–358.

Le Souëf, P. N., England, S. J., Stogryn, H. A. F., and Bryan, A. C. (1988). Comparison of diaphragmatic fatigue in newborn and older rabbits. *J. Appl. Physiol.* 65: 1040–1044.

Lieberman, D. A., Maxwell, L. C., and Faulkner, J. A. (1972). Adaptation of guinea pig diaphragm muscle to aging and endurance training. *Am. J. Physiol.* 222: 556–560.

Lopes, J. M., Muller, N. L., Bryan, M. H., and Bryan, A. C. (1981a). Synergistic behaviour of inspiratory muscles after diaphragmatic fatigue in the newborn. *J. Appl. Physiol.* 51: 547–551.

Lopes, J., Muller, N. L., Bryan, M. H., and Bryan, A. C. (1981b). Importance of inspiratory muscle tone in maintenance of FRC in the newborn. *J. Appl. Physiol.* 51: 830–834.

Maxwell, L. C., McCarter, R. J. M., Kuehl, T. J., and Robotham, J. L. (1983). Development of histochemical and functional properties of baboon respiratory muscles. *J. Appl. Physiol.* 54: 551–561.

Mayock, D. E., Hall, J., Watchko, J. F., Standaert, T. A., and Woodrum, D. E. (1987). Diaphragmatic muscle fiber type development in swine. *Pediatr. Res.* 22: 449–454.

Mortola, J. P. (1987). Dynamics of breathing in newborn mammals. *Physiol. Rev.* 67: 187–243.

Mortola, J. P. (1991). Comparative aspects of respiratory mechanics in newborn mammals. In *Basic Mechanisms of Pediatric Respiratory Disease: Cellular and Integrative.* Edited by V. Chernick and R. B. Mellins. Philadelphia, B.C. Decker, pp. 80–88.

Mortola, J. P. (1992). Measurements of respiratory mechanics. In *Fetal and Neonatal Physiology*, Vol. 1. Edited by R. A. Polin and W. W. Fox. Philadelphia, W.B. Saunders, pp. 813–822.

Mortola, J. P., and Fisher, J. T. (1988). Upper airway reflexes in newborns. In *Respiratory Function of the Upper Airways.* Edited by O. P. Mathew and G. Sant'Ambrogio. New York, Marcel Dekker, pp. 303–357.

Mortola, J. P., and Sant'Ambrogio, G. (1978). Motion of the rib cage and the abdomen in tetraplegic patients. *Clin. Sci. Mol. Med.* 54:25–32.

Mortola, J. P., Fisher, J. T., Smith, B., Fox, G., and Weeks, S. (1982). Dynamics of breathing in infants. *J. Appl. Physiol.* 52: 1209–1215.

Mortola, J. P., Milic-Emili, J., Noworaj, A., Smith, B., Fox, G., and Weeks, S. (1984). Muscle pressure and flow during expiration in infants. *Am. Rev. Respir. Dis.* 129: 49–53.

Mortola, J. P., Saetta, M., Fox, G., Smith, B., and Weeks, S. (1985). Mechanical aspects of chest wall distortion. *J. Appl. Physiol.* 59: 295–304.

Muller, N., Gulston, G., Cade, D., Whitton, J., Froese, A. B., Bryan, M. H., and Bryan, A. C. (1979). Diaphragmatic muscle fatigue in the newborn. *J. Appl. Physiol.* 46: 688–695.

Newman, S., Road, J., Bellemare, F., Clozel, J. P., Lavigne, C. M., and Grassino, A. (1984). Respiratory muscle length measured by sonomicrometry. *J. Appl. Physiol.* 56: 753–764.

Nichols, D. G. (1991). Respiratory muscle performance in infants and children. *J. Pediatr.* 118: 493–502.

Nichols, D. G., Howell, S., Massik, J., Koehler, R. C., Gleason, C. A., Buck, J. R., Fitzgerald, R. S., Traystman, R. J., and Robotham, J. L. (1989). Relationship of diaphragmatic contractility to diaphragmatic blood flow in newborn lambs. *J. Appl. Physiol.* 66: 120–127.

Nightingale, D. A., and Richards, C. C. (1965). Volume–pressure relations of the respiratory system of curarized infants. *Anesthesiology* 26: 710–714.

Nugent, S. T., and Finley, J. P. (1985). Spectral analysis of the EMG and diaphragmatic muscle fatigue during periodic breathing in infants. *J. Appl. Physiol.* 58: 830–833.

O'Brien, M. J. (1985). Respiratory EMG findings in relation to periodic breathing in infants. *Early Hum. Dev.* 11: 43–60.

O'Brien, M. J., van Eykern, L. A., and Prechtl, H. F. R. (1980). Diaphragmatic, intercostal and abdominal muscle tonic EMG activity in normal and hypotonic newborns. In *Ontogenesis of the Brain*, Vol. 3: *The Biochemical, Functional and Structural Development of the Nervous System.* Edited by S. Trojan and F. Stastny. Prague, University Karlova Press, pp. 471–479.

Olinsky, A., Bryan, M. H., and Bryan, A. C. (1974). Influence of lung inflation on respiratory control in neonates. *J. Appl. Physiol.* 36: 426–429.

Olinsky, A., Bryan, A. C., and Bryan, M. H. (1976). A simple method of measuring total respiratory system compliance in newborn infants. *S. Afr. Med. J.* 50: 128–130.

Openshaw, P., Edwards, S., and Helms, P. (1984). Changes in rib cage geometry during childhood. *Thorax* 39: 624–627.

Papastamelos, C., Panitch, H. B., England, S. E., and Allen, J. L. (1995). Developmental changes in chest wall compliance in infancy and early childhood. *J. Appl. Physiol.* 78: 179–184.

Pascucci, R. C., Hershenson, M. B., Sethna, N. F., Loring, S. H., and Stark, A. R. (1990). Chest wall motion of infants during spinal anesthesia. *J. Appl. Physiol.* 68: 2087–2091.

Piazza, T., Lauzon, A.-M., and Mortola, J. P. (1988). Time course of adaptation to hypoxia in newborn rats. *Can. J. Physiol. Pharmacol.* 66: 152–158.

Polgar, G., and Weng, T. R. (1979). The functional development of the respiratory system. From the period of gestation to adulthood. *Am. Rev. Respir. Dis.* 120: 625–695.

Powers, S. K., Lawler, J., Criswell, D., Dodd, S., and Silverman, H. (1991). Age-related changes in enzyme activity in the rat diaphragm. *Respir. Physiol.* 83: 1–10.

Praud, J.-P., Egreteau, L., Benlabed, M., Curzi-Dascalova, L., Nedelcoux, H., and Gaultier, C. (1991). Abdominal muscle activity during CO_2 rebreathing in sleeping neonates. *J. Appl. Physiol.* 70: 1344–1350.

Prechtl, H. F. R., Van Eykern, L. A., and O'Brien, M. J. (1977). Respiratory muscle EMG in newborns: A non-intrusive method. *Early Hum. Dev.* 1/3: 265–283.

Radvanyi-Bouvet, M. F., Monset-Couchard, M., Morel-Kahn, F., Vicente, G., and Dreyfus-Brisac, C. (1982). Expiratory patterns during sleep in normal full-term and premature neonates. *Biol. Neonate* 41: 74–84.

Reynolds, R. N., and Etsten, B. E. (1966). Mechanics of respiration in apneic anesthetized infants. *Anesthesiology* 27: 13–19.

Rezzonico, R., and Mortola, J. P. (1989). Respiratory adaptation to chronic hypercapnia in newborn rats. *J. Appl. Physiol.* 67: 311–315.

Richards, C. C., and Bachman, L. (1961). Lung and chest wall compliance of apneic paralyzed infants. *J. Clin. Invest.* 40: 273–278.

Schwieler, G. H. (1968). Respiratory regulation during postnatal development in cats and rabbits and some of its morphological substrate. *Acta Physiol. Scand.* [*Suppl.*] 304: 3–123.

Sharp, J. T., Druz, W. S., Balagot, R. C., Bandelin, V. R., and Danon, J. (1970). Total respiratory compliance in infants and children. *J. Appl. Physiol.* 29: 775–779.

Sharp, J. T., and Hyatt, R. E. (1986). Mechanical and electrical properties of respiratory muscles. In *Handbook of Physiology*, Section 3, The Respiratory System, Vol. 3, Mechanics of Breathing, part 2. Edited by P. T. Macklem and J. Mead. Bethesda, MD, American Physiological Society, pp. 389–414.

Sieck, G. C., Fournier, M., and Blanco, C. E. (1991). Diaphragm muscle fatigue resistance during postnatal development. *J. Appl. Physiol.* 71: 458–464.

Smith, D., Green, H., Thomson, J., and Sharratt, M. (1989). Capillary and size interrelationships in developing rat diaphragm, EDL, and soleus muscle fiber types. *Am. J. Physiol.* 256: C50–C58.

Soust, M., Walker, A. M., and Berger, P. J. (1989a). Blood flow to the respiratory muscles during hyperpnoea in the newborn lamb. *Respir. Physiol.* 76: 93–106.

Soust, M., Walker, A. M., and Berger, P. J. (1989b). Diaphragm V_{O_2}, diaphragm EMG, pressure–time product and calculated ventilation in newborn lambs during hypercapnic hyperpnoea. *Respir. Physiol.* 76: 107–118.

South, M., Morley, C. J., and Hughes, G. (1987). Expiratory muscle activity in preterm babies. *Arch. Dis. Child.* 62: 825–829.

Standaert, T. A., Wilham, B. E., Mayock, D. E., Watchko, J. F., Gibson, R. L., and Woodrum, D. E. (1991). *Pediatr. Pulmonol.* 11: 294–301.

Stark, A. R., Cohlan, B. A., Waggener, T. B., Frantz, I. D. III, and Kosch, P. C. (1987). Regulation of end-expiratory lung volume during sleep in premature infants. *J. Appl. Physiol.* 62: 1117–1123.

Tabachnik, E., Muller, N. L., Bryan, A. C., and Levison, H. (1981). Changes in ventilation and chest wall mechanics during sleep in normal adolescents. *J. Appl. Physiol.* 51: 557–564.

Takahashi, E., and Atsumi, H. (1955). Age differences in thoracic form as indicated by thoracic index. *Hum. Biol.* 27: 65–74.

Tamaki, N. (1985). Effect of growth on muscle capillarity and fiber type composition in rat diaphragm. *Eur. J. Appl. Physiol.* 54: 24–29.

Thach, B. T., Abroms, I. F., Frantz, I. D. III, Sotrel, A., Bruce, E. N., and Goldman, M. D.

(1980). Intercostal muscle reflexes and sleep breathing patterns in the human infant. *J. Appl. Physiol.* 48: 139–146.

Trang, T. T. H., Viires, N., and Aubier, M. (1992). In vitro functions of the rat diaphragm during postnatal development. *J. Dev. Physiol.* 17: 1–6.

Trippenbach, T. (1981). Laryngeal, vagal and intercostal reflexes during the early postnatal period. *J. Dev. Physiol.* 3: 133–159.

Wagaman, M. J., Shutack, J. G., Moomjian, A. S., Schwartz, J. G., Shaffer, T. H., and Fox, W. W. (1979). Improved oxygenation and lung compliance with prone positioning of neonates. *J. Pediatr.* 94: 787–791.

Watchko, J. F., Mayock, D. E., Standaert, T. A., and Woodrum, D. E. (1986). Postnatal changes in transdiaphragmatic pressure in piglets. *Pediatr. Res.* 20: 658–661.

Watchko, J. F., Brozanski, B. S., O'Day, T. L., Guthrie, R. T., and Sieck, G. C. (1992). Contractile properties of the rat external abdominal oblique and diaphragm muscles during development. *J. Appl. Physiol.* 72: 1432–1436.

Wolfson, M. R., Greenspan, J. S., Deoras, K. S., Allen, J. A., and Shaffer, T. H. (1992). Effect of position on the mechanical interaction between the rib cage and abdomen in preterm infants. *J. Appl. Physiol.* 72: 1032–1038.

23

Respiratory Muscle Blood Flow

ALAIN S. COMTOIS

University of Montreal
Hôpital Notre Dame
Montreal, Quebec, Canada

DUDLEY F. ROCHESTER

University of Virginia Health Sciences Center
Charlottesville, Virginia

I. Introduction

The act of breathing is accomplished by a group of skeletal muscles in the proximity of the chest wall that are collectively known as the respiratory muscles. Functionally, they are classified as the inspiratory and the expiratory muscles. The respiratory muscles are also recruited during other nonrespiratory acts such as speech, cough, posture, and expulsive maneuvers (Detroyer and Loring, 1986).

The inspiratory muscles include the diaphragm, the external intercostal muscles, the parasternal muscles, the scalene muscles, and the sternocleidomastoid muscles (Detroyer and Loring, 1986). On the other hand, the expiratory muscles comprise the abdominal muscles (postural muscles), the internal intercostal muscles, and to some extent in humans, the triangularis sterni muscles (Detroyer and Loring, 1986; Detroyer et al., 1987). Similar to other skeletal muscles, the respiratory muscles are dependent on an adequate energy supply to maintain their rate of contractility against a given load (Bellemare and Grassino, 1982; Bellemare et al., 1983). Their endurance against fatigability, where *fatigability* (fatigue) is defined as the loss in the capacity for developing force that is reversible by rest (NHLBI Workshop Summary, 1990), is a function of continuous regeneration of high-energy phosphate bonds (local supplies of ATP and creatine phosphate) by aerobic and anaerobic pathways (Sjogaard, 1987), as well as exchanges of

633

catabolites with the extracellular milieu (Barclay, 1986). Blood circulation through muscle tissue is thought to be the main vector by which these pathways can fulfill their role of replenishing ATP supplies and catabolite washout (Barclay, 1986; Sjogaard, 1987).

Skeletal muscle blood flow responds to various local factors, such as neural and humoral, and also to mechanical factors that affect the intramuscular vasculature (Barcroft, 1963). As well, blood perfusion through the muscle can be dependent on hemodynamic factors, such as the arterial pressure, the blood volume, and the cardiac output (Barcroft, 1963). Thus, the energy reconstitution of exercising skeletal muscles is dependent on an adequate blood supply to the muscles themselves. If the rate of energy utilization becomes greater than the rate of energy reconstitution, fatigue will develop. The purpose of this chapter is to review the factors known to influence skeletal muscle blood flow and, most particularly, respiratory muscle blood flow, the relation of blood flow and skeletal muscle fatigue, and the relevance of the present work to the current understanding of respiratory muscle function. Most of the chapter will be devoted to studies of diaphragmatic circulation, since most of the research carried in the field of respiratory muscle blood flow has examined circulation through this most important muscle of inspiration.

II. Techniques for Measuring Organ Blood Flow

Numerous methods are available to measure blood flow in organs and within blood vessels. They vary from timed collection of venous blood, to radioactive tracers. All have advantages and disadvantages, and although they all measure blood flow, great care must be taken when interpreting the results obtained by these various methods. Some methods may represent whole-organ blood flow, others may represent nutritive blood flow, and some may represent average flow at a particular instant in time, whereas others may represent instantaneous changes in flow rates (Hudlicka, 1973).

A. Methods for Measuring Instantaneous Blood Flow

Methods that monitor instantaneous changes in flow rate measure whole-tissue blood flow (i.e., shunting and nutritive blood flow through an area of tissue) (Hudlicka, 1973). Early studies of blood flow in skeletal muscles consisted of cannulating veins and measuring timed collection of the venous effluent. Hot wire anemometry consists of cannulating an artery that supplies an organ or a muscle and measures the rate of decay of the volume of blood in a reservoir (connected to the cannula perfusing the artery), which is proportional to the change in electrical resistance caused by the air flowing across (cooling) the hot wires placed over the reservoir

(Anrep et al., 1933; Anrep and Saalfeld, 1935). The change in the electrical resistance represents the blood flow rate through that artery.

Another simpler method to measure diaphragmatic blood flow has recently been used with success by Bellemare et al. (1983). This method consisted of measuring diaphragmatic blood flow by recording the blood-drop count rate from the cannulated left inferior phrenic vein of the diaphragm. Lately, however, electromagnetic and ultrasonic Doppler flowmeters have been used to measure blood flow in arteries supplying the respiratory muscles, most particularly those of the diaphragm (Sharf et al., 1986; Nichols et al., 1988; Hu et al., 1990a). These techniques have the advantage of measuring instantaneous changes in blood flow in the arteries on which they are placed. And in diaphragmatic blood flow studies, the changes observed in phrenic artery blood flow are representative of global changes occurring in the diaphragm, providing, nonetheless, that phrenic nerve stimulation is supramaximal (Nichols et al., 1988).

The electromagnetic flow probes, when placed around a vessel, create a magnetic field around the vessel, and the electrodes incorporated within the probe come in contact with the surface of the vessel (normal to the electric field vector) and record an electromotive force (EMF) that is proportional to the blood flow (Vatner et al., 1970). The ultrasonic pulsed Doppler flowmeters operate in a manner similar to radar systems (Hartley and Cole, 1974; Hartley et al., 1978; Vatner et al., 1970). The single piezoelectric crystal contained in this type of flow probes functions alternately as an emitter and receiver at a certain frequency (69.2 kHz) (Hartley and Cole, 1974). Ultrasounds (20 MHz) are emitted by the crystal and are bounced back by moving erythrocytes within the vessel. In so doing, a Doppler shift is recorded by the crystal that is proportional to the blood flow in the vessel (Hartley et al., 1978). Pulsed Doppler flow probes have the advantage of being smaller and lighter than electromagnetic flow probes, thus producing very little disturbance of the vessel being studied. In addition, they have a stable zero baseline value, which is not true for electromagnetic flow probes, for they depend on good electrode contact on the vessel to maintain a stable zero baseline.

B. Methods for Measuring Capillary Blood Perfusion

Capillary blood flow is measured by using radioactive tracers injected into the organ or tissue of interest. This type of method, however, measures an average flow within a window of time, rather than an instantaneous flow rate (Hudlicka, 1973). There are at least two types of well-known radioactive techniques to measure respiratory muscle blood flow: the inert radioactive-labeled tracer gas method (Rochester and Pradel-Guena, 1973) and the trapping of radioactive labeled microspheres in the microcirculation (Robertson et al., 1977a).

The inert radioactive tracer gas method, like instantaneous methods (electromagnetic and Doppler flowmeters), measures total-organ blood flow (i.e., shunting and nutritive flow through an organ; Hudlicka, 1973). Basically, it consists of measuring the rate of disappearance of a radioactive-labeled inert gas from an organ or tissue. Two approaches can be used with this method. One, in which a bolus of a radioactive tracer is injected directly into the tissue, and the rate of its disappearance is measured with external gamma probes placed directly over the site of injection (Rochester and Pradel-Guena, 1973). Or the other, which is adapted from the Kety–Schmidt (Kety and Schmidt, 1945) nitrous oxide washout technique, also measures the rate of disappearance of a radioactive tracer, but from a cannulated venous vessel in the tissue of interest (Rochester, 1974; Rochester and Bettini, 1976). The Kety–Schmidt approach requires a continuous constant injection of a radioactive tracer into the systemic circulation, performed over a relatively long period (20 min). During this period, simultaneous withdrawals of samples from an arterial source and the cannulated venous vessel are taken; this allows the construction of the *washin* phase, which is proportional to the blood flow rate within the tissue. Blood flow rate can be derived as well without a continuous constant injection of a radioactive tracer, but an additional 20 min of venous sampling must be obtained to construct the *washout* phase of the radioactive tracer, which is proportional to the blood flow rate. The advantage of the inert radioactive tracer gas method is that multiple runs (up to eight) of blood flow measurements can be performed in the same subject. The limitation, however, is that the first approach (washin method) requires exposure of the organ being investigated to allow injection of the radioactive tracer into its tissues, and in the second technique (washout method), is the amount of time taken to measure flow rate (approximately 40 min per run) and the amount of blood drawn.

The trapping of radioactive-labeled microspheres, on the other hand, measures nutritive blood flow (Hudlicka, 1973). The microspheres (15–25 μm) are injected directly into the left ventricle and travel in the systemic arterial circulation. The microspheres become trapped in the microcirculation (capillary bed) of various organs or tissues of interest, and the level of measured radioactivity is proportional to the blood flow rate. This technique requires the timed collection of a sample from a peripheral artery, which allows conversion of radioactivity measurements into blood flow rates. The advantage of this method is that the organ blood flow rate can be expressed as a percentage of the cardiac output, which is interesting when blood flow distribution is a considered factor. The limiting aspects of microspheres, however, are that the number of runs are limited by the amount of different isotopes that can be used, and that they measure blood flow at a particular instant in time.

III. Anatomy of Diaphragmatic Circulation

Various reports on the anatomical description of the diaphragmatic vasculature mention that the diaphragm is perfused by various arterial supplies (Testut, 1921; Greig et al., 1951; Biscoe and Bucknell, 1963; Evans and Christensen, 1979;

McMinn, 1982; Scharf et al., 1986). The most prevalent ones being the inferior phrenic arteries, the intercostal arteries, and the internal mammary arteries; however, these reports also mention that these vessels appear to be terminal vessels, similar to those found in the heart and the central nervous system.

A. Macroscopic Anatomy

The assumption that they are terminal vessels is based on anatomical studies in a wide variety of species. The phrenic arteries of the cat and dog are thought to provide most of the diaphragmatic arterial supply to the crural and the sternal segments, and most of the costal portions of the diaphragm (Biscoe and Bucknell, 1963; Scharf et al., 1986). On the other hand, in dogs and humans, small branches from the intercostal arteries are thought to perfuse the peripheral portions of the diaphragm adjacent to the ribs, whereas the small branches from the internal mammary arteries, named musculophrenic arteries, are thought to perfuse mainly the anterior segment of the diaphragm adjacent to the sternum (Gray, 1980; Scharf et al., 1986).

Even though one study in humans showed that the inferior phrenic arteries anastomosed freely with the other vessels to the diaphragm, the musculophrenic (internal mammary arteries) and lower intercostal arteries, the authors concluded, nonetheless, that the inferior phrenic arteries represented the main source of blood for the diaphragm (Kahn, 1967). The origin in humans of the inferior phrenic arteries is from the aorta or coeliac trunk, with almost equal frequency, whereas in dogs and some other species, they originate either from the superior phrenico-abdominal artery or directly from the abdominal aorta (Greig et al., 1951; Biscoe and Bucknell, 1963; Kahn, 1967; Kanan, 1971; Evans and Christensen, 1979; Scharf et al., 1986). The venous drainage in humans and in other species, including the dog, seems to be performed mostly by the inferior phrenic veins, which empty directly into the inferior vena cava just distal to the site of the hepatic veins on the inferior vena cava (Greig et al., 1951; Rochester, 1974; Rochester and Bettini, 1976; Evans and Christensen, 1979; Bellemare et al., 1983; Martin et al., 1983). Although, in one study in human cadavers, the left inferior phrenic vein terminated in three or four cases into the left side of the left hepatic vein (Bonnette et al., 1983). On the other hand, the intercostal and the internal mammary veins of humans and other species appear to contribute to local venous drainage in their respective area of insertion into the diaphragm (Evans and Christensen, 1979; Gray, 1980; Martin et al., 1983).

Most of these anatomical descriptions, however, were obtained postmortem and are not completely in agreement with some of the physiological findings obtained by investigating the arterial and venous contributions to the diaphragm. In fact, Morgan and Johnson (1980) reported that diaphragmatic work was unaffected by the ligation of the inferior phrenic arteries during both spontaneous breathing at rest and inspiratory resistive loading. This important finding suggested that collateral sources of arterial diaphragmatic supplies were capable of maintaining adequate blood prefusion. Lockhat and co-workers (1985) addressed this issue of collateral sources of the costal and crural diaphragm in the dog. They measured diaphragmatic blood flow with radioactive microspheres during either the occlusion of the internal mammary arteries or the thoracic aorta (i.e., an occlusion of both the inferior phrenic and intercostal arteries). They reported that the occlusion of the internal mammary arteries alone did not affect the diaphragmatic blood flow in either the crural or costal segments, and that only an occlusion of the thoracic aorta (occlusion of inferior phrenic and intercostal arteries) resulted in a decrease of the diaphragmatic blood flow in the crural segment without, however, affecting the costal segment blood flow. Even when they attempted to occlude all of the major arterial supplies (thoracic aorta and internal mammary artery occlusion) crural and costal blood flow was still greater than 25 and 50% of control, respectively. These observations, therefore, suggested that there exist extensive communications between the various arteries supplying the diaphragm.

In fact, these observations were confirmed in a study of the macroscopic anatomy of the diaphragmatic vasculature. In the dog, as indicated in Figure 1, the three major arterial supplies to the diaphragm—the inferior phrenic, the intercostal,

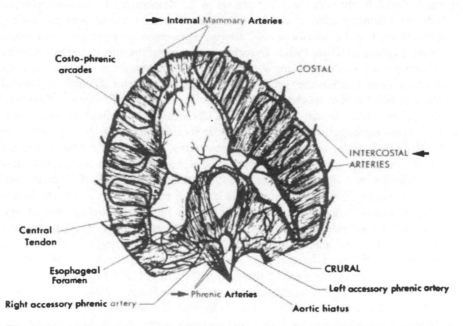

Figure 1   Abdominal view of the diaphragm illustrating the internal arterial circle formed by the head-to-head anastomosis of the phrenic and internal mammary arteries. The branches of the 8th–13th intercostal arteries are shown inserting into the costal and crural periphery and communicating with the internal arterial circle through costophrenic arcades. Dark arrows indicate the three major arterial supplies to the diaphragm. (From Comtois et al., 1987.)

and the internal mammary arteries—formed arterioarterial anastomosis within the muscular leaflet of the diaphragm (Comtois et al., 1987). These authors observed that the ipsilateral inferior phrenic and internal mammary arteries anastomose head to head to form an interior arterial circle along the musculotendinous junction of the central tendon. From the interior arterial circle, vascular ramifications originate and course between muscle fibers toward the diaphragmatic insertion to form head-to-head anastomoses with branches of the 8th–13th intercostal arteries. These head-to-head anastomoses with the intercostal arteries form costophrenic arcades that are found in both costal and crural segments of the diaphragm. This was also observed to be true in the human diaphragm in which the three main arterial sources of the diaphragm formed costophrenic arcades within the muscular leaflet of the diaphragm (Comtois et al., 1988). The venous drainage exhibited a configuration similar to the arterial circulation, with the major difference being in the presence of venous valves in the dog diaphragm, but not in that of the human (Comtois et al., 1987, 1988). An additional point worth noting is that the venous drainage in the dog, under specific conditions of diaphragmatic pacing with open thorax and casted abdomen, appears to be mostly by the intercostal veins (60%), while 25% is through the phrenic veins, and 15% through the internal mammary veins (Hu et al., 1990a).

Extradiaphragmatic arterial anastomoses related to diaphragmatic perfusion are also present in the dog (Fig. 2). They are formed by the anastomosis of the anterior and posterior intercostal arteries that originate from the internal mammary and intercostal arteries, respectively (Comtois et al., 1987). This also appears to hold true for humans, according to various human anatomy textbooks (Gray, 1980; McMinn, 1982). In addition, there are no significant arterial shunts between the left and right hemidiaphragm in either dogs or humans (Hu et al., 1990b; Comtois et al., 1988).

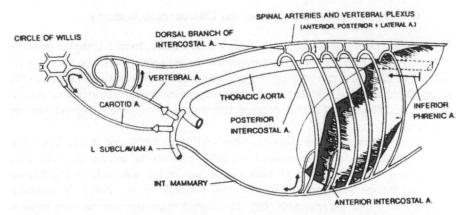

Figure 2 Left view of the extradiaphragmatic anastomosis of major arteries supplying the diaphragm (inferior phrenic arteries, posterior intercostal arteries, and anterior intercostal arteries by internal mammary arteries). (From Comtois et al., 1991.)

B. Microscopic Anatomy

The microcirculation of the diaphragm has also been studied in rats, and as reported by Shraufnagel and colleagues (1983), the branching pattern of the diaphragmatic arterioles and capillaries was identical with the branching pattern of the triceps and intercostal muscles. They concluded, therefore, that there was no evidence to support the premise of a different or more efficient vascular configuration capable of providing a better blood flow during fatigue development when compared with other skeletal muscles. Further examination of the diaphragmatic microcirculation in dogs reveals that the capillary configuration and distribution is similar between costal and crural segments (Reid et al., 1992). This is in agreement with the earlier observations of Boczkowski and colleagues (1990) during which they have shown that the capillary density in the rat diaphragm was similar in the costal periphery when compared with the more central part of the diaphragm adjacent to the central tendon. An interesting point, however, is that, in the dog costal diaphragm, there is a dorsoventral gravity-independent gradient in blood flow, that is not seen in the crural diaphragm (Brancatisano et al., 1991). Since capillary density, configuration, and distribution are similar in both segments, this discrepancy can be explained by the following: The dorsal 80% of the costal diaphragm is 50% thicker than the most ventral portion and, thus, establishes a dorsoventral gradient in thickness that is not observed in the crural diaphragm (Brancatisano et al., 1991). In general, the anatomical evidence of the diaphragmatic microcirculatory bed indicates that it is no different from other highly aerobic muscles. Nonetheless, the diaphragm possesses a unique arrangement by being a partition between the thoracic and abdominal compartments, and this, in itself, can expose the diaphragm to varying pressure swings that can affect blood flow in a manner not seen in other muscles.

C. Physiological Relevance of the Macroscopic Anatomy

The arterial vessels, according to the anatomical studies, form a complex network of costophrenic arcades within their respective hemidiaphragm. These arterio–arterial and veno–venous communications provide a means of perfusing or draining the entire hemidiaphragm from any one of their respective three major arterial or venous vessels: the left and right inferior phrenic, internal mammary, and intercostal arteries and veins.

This anatomical assumption has been verified recently, and it was found that diaphragmatic circulation maintained by only the intercostal arteries was sufficient to maintain the contractility of both costal and crural segments at the fatigue threshold tension time index (TTdi) of 0.20 (Comtois et al., 1991). In addition, perfusion of the diaphragm with only the internal mammary arteries was capable of maintaining the costal, but not the crural, contractility at the same TTdi. Only when all of the arterial supplies to the diaphragm were occluded did costal and crural contractility become compromised. And under those conditions, and similarly to Lockhat and colleagues (1985), attempting to occlude all of the arterial supplies did not abolish the diaphragmatic circulation. In fact, phrenic vein blood flow was 25% of the value observed in the absence of arterial occlusions (control), a value similar to the one observed in the study by Lockhat and colleagues (1985) for the crural circulation under identical conditions of arterial occlusions. One can suggest that most of the shunting responsible for this level of diaphragmatic circulation in the presence of an occlusion of the three main arterial supplies is by the extradiaphragmatic anastomosis which can be provided by the spinal arteries of the vertebral plexus (see Fig. 2; Comtois et al., 1991).

These results, therefore, indicate that the diaphragm has a tremendous capacity to replenish and maintain its blood supply. In addition, the macroscopic anatomical model of costophrenic arcades indicates that the vessels perfusing the diaphragm are not terminal and is consistent with the physiological observations that the diaphragmatic circulation is relatively homogeneous and that the diaphragmatic contractility, at or below the fatigue threshold, is affected only when the arterial supply is severely compromised.

IV. Factors Affecting Skeletal Muscle Blood Flow

Numerous factors affect blood flow through skeletal muscle. These include the arterial pressure, muscle activity, and mechanical aspects, such as the pattern of contraction, the intramuscular pressure, and muscle fiber length. In addition, there are factors related to neural and humoral modulation, and the activation of membrane-bound proteins, such as some specific ionic channels, that become activated under specific conditions such as the development of respiratory muscle fatigue.

A. Perfusion Pressure (Arterial Pressure)

Skeletal muscle blood flow, as with any other organ, is a function of the arterial perfusion pressure (Hobbs and McCloskey, 1987). Factors that affect the arterial perfusion pressure are cardiac output and peripheral vascular resistance, which if expressed mathematically can be represented by the following equation:

$$P = Q \times R \tag{1}$$

where P is the arterial perfusion pressure, Q is the cardiac output, and R is the peripheral vascular resistance. As well, cardiac output and peripheral vascular resistance are affected by several factors that are mediated by neural or humoral vectors. Cardiac output and peripheral vascular resistance, under normal conditions, are influenced by the level of activity or force of contraction of exercising skeletal muscles (Barcroft and Millen, 1939; Barcroft and Dornhorst, 1949; Barcroft, 1963; Bonde-Petersen et al., 1975; Ceretelli et al., 1986). And as in respiratory muscles, they can also be influenced by pathological conditions, such as cardiogenic, septic, or hemorrhagic, shock (Viires et al., 1983; Hussain et al., 1985a; Sharf et al., 1986).

The blood circulation of respiratory muscles, as in skeletal muscles, is influenced by the same following two physical factors: perfusion pressure gradient and vascular resistance (Hussain et al., 1988b). Respiratory muscle blood flow can be expressed by rearranging Eq. (1) as follows:

$$Q_{RES} = \frac{P}{R} \tag{2}$$

where Q_{RES} represents respiratory muscle blood flow, P is the perfusion pressure gradient (arterial pressure minus venous pressure), and R is the vascular resistance of the respiratory muscles. Under normal resting conditions, the perfusion pressure gradient remains relatively constant and vascular resistance can be modified by several factors, which include the following: (1) the level of respiratory muscle activity; (2) the respiratory muscle contraction pattern; (3) mechanical factors, such as respiratory intramuscular pressure and muscle length; and (4) local metabolic, humoral, and neural factors.

B. Respiratory Muscle Activity

The level of respiratory muscle activity is the most important determinant of respiratory muscle blood flow. Numerous studies have demonstrated that respiratory muscle blood flow is a function of minute ventilation. Hyperventilation caused by CO_2 rebreathing or physical exertion (e.g., running on a treadmill) increases diaphragmatic blood flow to approximately 35 ml min^{-1} 100 g^{-1} and 95 ml min^{-1} 100 g^{-1}, respectively (Rochester and Bettini, 1976; Robertson et al., 1977b; Fixler et al., 1976). Nonetheless, the largest increases in diaphragmatic circulation are observed either during high levels of inspiratory, resistive-loaded breathing or during high metabolically demanding phrenic nerve-pacing protocols, during which, under those conditions, respectively, values of approximately 210 and 265 ml min^{-1} 100 g^{-1} have been reported, as shown by the data of Robertson and colleagues in Figure 3 (Robertson et al., 1977a; Buchler et al., 1985a). In a series of various experiments Manohar (1986a,b, 1988) has measured the diaphragmatic circulation in maximally exercising ponies. He reported diaphragmatic blood flow values that ranged from 245 to 265 ml min^{-1} 100 g^{-1}. Under those conditions of maximal exercise, the presence of the potent vasodilator adenosine did not increase diaphragmatic circulation any further, indicating that the diaphragm had reached its maximal vasodilating capacity (Manohar, 1986b). In addition, blood flow values of the principal muscles of propulsion (gluteus medius and biceps femoris) under maximal exercise were similar to those of the diaphragm, ranging from 225 to 255 ml min^{-1} 100 g^{-1} and were unaffected by the presence of adenosine (Manohar, 1986a,b). In fact, the heart was the only organ with higher blood flow values, approximately 600 ml min^{-1} 100 g^{-1}, under near maximal activation (Manohar et al., 1982; Manohar, 1986b).

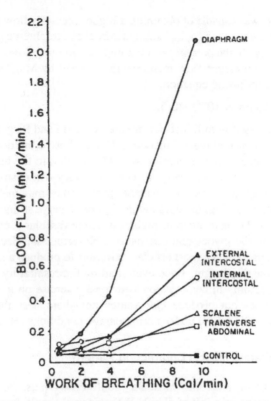

Figure 3 Blood flow to the diaphragm and various other muscles of respiration during spontaneous breathing at rest and graded inspiratory resistances. Note the level of diaphragmatic blood flow in comparison with the other respiratory muscles. Respiratory muscle blood flow was measured by trapping radioactive microspheres. (From Robertson et al., 1977a.)

In a series of elegant experiments, Reid and Johnson (1983) were able to calculate the upper limit of diaphragmatic circulation by producing a maximally vasodilated diaphragmatic vascular bed with infusions of adenosine and nitroprusside while the animals (dogs) breathed 6% O_2 against added inspiratory resistances. Under those conditions the maximal diaphragmatic blood flow (Qdi_{max}) is a parabolic function of the arterial perfusion pressure (Pa) according to the following equation:

$$Qdi_{max} = 1.32 \ Pa^2 + 29.9 \ Pa \times 10^{-4} \tag{3}$$

where Qdi is expressed in milliliters per minute per gram (ml min^{-1} g^{-1}) and Pa is expressed in millimeters mercury (mm Hg). Thus, a normotensive value of 125 mm Hg yields a Qdi_{max} value of 2.44 ml min^{-1} g^{-1} or 244 ml min^{-1} 100 g^{-1}. A value comparable with the range of 210–265 ml min^{-1} 100 g^{-1} was observed by Buchler and colleagues (1985a) during electrical phrenic nerve pacing in dogs. Magder

(1986), however, was capable of obtaining a higher pressure–flow relationship than Reid and Johnson when they applied supramaximal electrophrenic nerve stimulation in anesthetized dogs in the presence of maximal vasodilating doses of nitroprusside. The diaphragmatic pressure–flow relationship obtained by Magder is linear and is expressed by the following equation:

$$Qdi = (3.13 \text{ Pa} \times 10^{-2}) - 0.52 \tag{4}$$

where Qdi is expressed in milliliter per minute per gram and Pa is the mean arterial pressure expressed in millimeters mercury. Under those conditions, the maximal vascular conductance of the diaphragm was 42% of that in the heart. Thus, all of the foregoing studies have one point in common, they demonstrate that maximal activation of the respiratory muscles, whether produced by maximal exercise, severe inspiratory resistive loading, or supramaximal phrenic nerve stimulation, allows the diaphragmatic circulation to attain its highest possible vascular conductance, a value surpassed only by the myocardial circulation. Nevertheless, electrophrenic nerve stimulation appears to be the most efficient stimulus to produce a maximal vascular conductance in the diaphragm, since even loading the respiratory muscles in dogs by left pneumonectomy in combination with peak exercise on a treadmill (6 mph at 25% grade) does not produce Qdi values anywhere near those observed or predicted by Eqs. (3) and (4) under normotensive conditions (Hsia et al., 1992).

C. Respiratory Muscle Contraction Pattern

The sustainability of indefinite muscular contractions must be matched by an appropriate energy supply (blood flow). If the energy supply becomes reduced or interrupted, muscle failure will ultimately occur. Energy supply is interrupted during forceful contractions (Barcroft, 1963). Investigation of limb skeletal muscle has shown that the perfusion of the soleus (Barcroft and Millen, 1939) and of the elbow flexor muscle (Bonde-Petersen et al., 1975) becomes occluded during sustained contractions of 15 and 50% of the muscle's maximal tension, respectively. In their study, Bonde-Petersen and colleagues (1975) also observed that blood flow in the elbow flexors was greatest at 22% of maximal tension, but decreased thereafter as the force developed increased. At levels of 50% of maximal force, blood flow through the elbow flexors was zero. Similar observations were reported by Humphreys and Lind (1963), during which sustained contractions of the hand grip muscles increased blood flow up to tensions of about 40% of the muscle's maximal tension, but decreased thereafter until 70% of the maximal tension was reached. However, the flow at 70% of maximal tension was still greater than that observed at rest.

Even though, in the aforementioned experiments, the absolute blood flow was becoming greater than the blood flow at rest, with an increasing metabolic demand, the endurance time to contractile failure was decreasing, suggesting that the blood flow through the contracting muscle was inadequate and was partly responsible for the development of muscle fatigue (Barcroft, 1963; Humphrey and Lind, 1963; Bonde-Petersen et al., 1975). Therefore, it supported the fact that the relative increase in absolute blood flow was insufficient to meet the energy requirement. In support of this argument, Lind and McNichol (1967) studied the postexercise hyperemia of the hand grip muscles, which, if present, would indicate an inadequate blood supply during the time of contractile activity. They observed that measurements of absolute blood flow values during sustained contraction of the hand grip muscles (up to levels of 30% of maximal tension) was larger than blood flow values seen at rest. However, at tensions of 15% of the maximal tension, a postexercise hyperemia became apparent that increased as higher levels of tension developed. They also reported that the calculated blood flow debt increased exponentially with increasing levels of tension, concluding that blood flow limitation was occurring, at low levels of tension, despite the relative increase in absolute blood flow during the contraction (Lind and McNichol, 1967). This observation suggested that, in skeletal muscle, the absolute increase in blood supply was inadequate to meet the metabolic demand during increased contractile activity.

As mentioned earlier, a rise in respiratory muscle activity increases their absolute blood flow rate (Reid and Johnson, 1983; Robertson et al., 1977a,b,c; Rochester and Pradel-Guena, 1973; Rochester, 1974; Rochester and Bettini, 1976). A common striking feature with these studies is the apparent unlimited capability of the respiratory muscles, and especially the diaphragm, to increase their blood flow. Donovan and colleagues (1979), however, with the use of radioactive-labeled microspheres, demonstrated that the blood flow to the dog diaphragm could, in fact, become limited. These investigators produced sustained isometric contractions at various levels of force by using electrophrenic stimulation of the dog diaphragm. They found increases in absolute blood flow up to transdiaphragmatic pressures (Pdi = gastric pressure – pleural pressure) of 85% of the maximal Pdi, which progressively decreased thereafter, but nevertheless, were still higher than control values. This observation is at variance with those of no apparent limitation to the increase of blood flow in respiratory muscles and, especially, within the diaphragm, but otherwise consistent with those made in other limb skeletal muscles. In fact, a study by Bellemare and colleagues (1983) observed the breath-by-breath variation in blood flow of the dog diaphragm. Diaphragmatic blood flow (Qdi) was measured by counting the blood-drop rate from the catheterized left inferior phrenic vein during bilateral electrophrenic nerve stimulation. These authors reported that Qdi was dependent on the intensity of contraction and the duration of contraction. The intensity of contraction was expressed as the ratio of Pdi over the maximal Pdi (Pdi/Pdi_{max}), and the duration of contraction was expressed as the duty cycle, a ratio of inspiratory time, t_i, over the total time taken for one respiratory cycle, t_{tot} (t_i/t_{tot}). The product of these two ratios was called the tension time index of the diaphragm (TTdi). As shown in Figure 4, Qdi was related by an inverse parabolic function to the TTdi. From their results it was observed that large combinations of Pdi and t_i/t_{tot} could be used, which would limit blood flow and produce postexercise hyperemia.

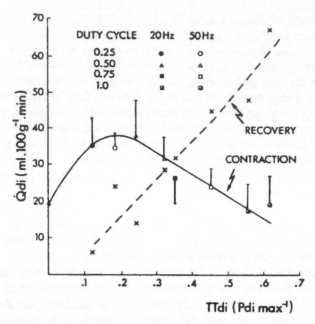

Figure 4 The diaphragmatic blood flow (Qdi) as an inverse parabolic function of the diaphragmatic tension–time index (TTdi) is illustrated by the solid line. The dashed line represents the postexercise hyperemia in relation to the TTdi developed: 20 and 50 Hz represent the electrophrenic nerve stimulation frequency used in combination with the duty cycle to generate various TTdi. Qdi was measured by blood-drop count rate from the catheterized left phrenic vein. (From Bellemare et al., 1983.)

Thus, no single Pdi-critical or t_i/t_{tot}-critical that would produce a limitation in blood flow, but the product of these two parameters yielded a single TTdi-critical that was related to blood flow impediment and caused a postexercise hyperemia. The TTdi-critical for the dog diaphragm was approximately 0.20. Thus, under isometric contractions ($t_i/t_{tot} = 1$) the dog diaphragm performs like other skeletal muscles (i.e., blood flow limitation occurs at 20% of maximal tension).

These observations have been supported as well by another group of investigators. Bark and associates (1987) used a diaphragmatic strip preparation and found that the development of moderate to high levels of diaphragmatic tension (TTdi of 0.30–0.80) during sustained or intermittent rhythmic (15/min) isometric contractions caused a reduction of the blood flow rate. They observed that, during sustained contractions, Qdi became mechanically impeded, possibly by a mechanical compression of the blood vessels between the muscle fibers, but that, during rhythmic contractions, increasing the duty cycle beyond a TTdi greater than 0.30 exerted less restriction on Qdi than during sustained contractions for a similar TTdi (Fig. 5). However, Qdi in their study was completely abolished at 80% of Pdi$_{max}$

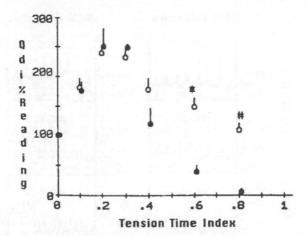

Figure 5 The effect of sustained (closed circles, duty cycle = 1 and tension was varied) and rhythmic (open circles, tension/tension$_{max}$ = 1 and duty cycle varied) isometric contractions on diaphragmatic blood flow (Qdi). Qdi was measured by blood-drop count rate from the catheterized left phrenic vein in a diaphragmatic strip preparation. (From Bark et al., 1987.)

during sustained contractions, a value similar to those reported by other investigators (Donovan et al., 1979; Bellemare et al., 1983). This concept of dynamic blood flow restriction is best illustrated in Figure 6, in which it can be seen that the area of the curve below the blood flow rate trace (i.e., blood volume per breath) is reduced by approximately 25% at a duty cycle of 0.7 and by 62% of Pdi$_{max}$ when compared with the duty cycle of 0.5 at the same Pdi (Hu et al., 1992). This concept of dynamic occlusion is important, since it has been shown in chronic obstructive pulmonary disease (COPD) patients that their respiratory muscle force reserve is greatly reduced, because, under conditions of spontaneous breathing at rest, their breathing pattern is very close to the critical blood flow-limiting TTdi value of 0.20 (Bellemare and Grassino, 1983). This suggests that minor changes in their breathing pattern (increasing the duty cycle, force, or frequency of breathing) could lead them to respiratory muscle fatigue (produced by blood flow limitation) and ensuing hypercapnia.

The effect of Pdi and duty cycle on Qdi has also been reported by other investigators. Buchler and colleagues (1985a) reported that a combination of high breathing frequency (101–160 breaths per minute), produced by electrophrenic nerve stimulation, and high duty cycle (0.75) resulted in a restriction of diaphragmatic blood flow measured with radioactive microspheres. These results suggested that the pattern of contraction was a major determinant of Qdi, for which a high duty cycle allowed very little time for diaphragmatic perfusion during the relaxation phase. In fact, Bark and Scharf (1986) demonstrated that diaphragmatic perfusion

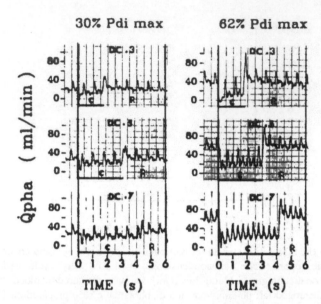

Figure 6 The effect of varying the duty cycle (DC) on the phrenic artery blood flow rate (Qpha) at various levels of transdiaphragmatic pressure (30 and 62% of maximal Pdi) in one animal. Qpha was measured by pulsed Doppler. (From Hu et al., 1992.)

(measured by an electromagnetic blood flow probe around the phrenic artery) occurred mostly during the relaxation phase, an observation supported by another group, during which rhythmic contractions at a constant duty cycle of 0.5 and various Pdis, caused Qdi (measured by an electromagnetic blood flow probe around the phrenic artery) during the contraction phase to reach its zenith at 30% of Pdi_{max} and to decrease thereafter, whereas the relaxation phase blood flow increased curvilinearly up to 90% of Pdi_{max} (Hussain et al., 1989). However, Qdi in their study was related, as observed by Bellemare et al. (1983), by a quadratic function of TTdi ($Qdi = 0.25 + 2.22\,TTdi - 4.02\,TTdi^2$), where Qdi is expressed in milliliters per minute per kilogram of body weight. Similarly, another group of investigators studied the effects of varying the duty cycle at different levels of Pdi. In this study, Qdi (measured by ultrasonic pulsed Doppler) was reported as an inverse parabolic function of the duty cycle and was highest at a t_i/t_{tot} of 0.5, regardless of the Pdi (Hu et al., 1992). Hu and colleagues, nonetheless, observed that even though Qdi peaked at a duty cycle of 0.5, a significant postexercise hyperemia was apparent when the TTdi was greater than 0.20.

In summary, all of the foregoing studies convey similar conclusions: (1) the pattern of contraction (i.e., duration, intensity, and frequency) is a major modulator of Qdi, which is, in fact, linked to the level of respiratory muscle activity; (2) the duty cycle establishes the optimal condition for the best possible flow under the circumstance of either high-intensity contraction or frequency of breathing; (3) the blood flow demand is met mainly during the relaxation period; and (4) blood flow limitation occurs despite the optimal value of Qdi being reached at a duty cycle of 0.5 when the TTdi generated is larger than 0.20, as demonstrated by the presence of a postexercise hyperemia.

D. Mechanical Factors

One of the most significant mechanical factors related to blood flow restriction is the intramuscular pressure acting on the blood vessels between the muscle fibers. Early studies in dogs spontaneously breathing at rest or against occluded airways have demonstrated that left inferior phrenic artery blood flow (measured by hot wire anemometry) was decreased during inspiration, but was restored to the level of the previous expiratory pause during relaxation (i.e., expiration; Anrep et al., 1933; Anrep and Saalfeld, 1935). Blood flow restriction was attributed to blood vessel compression produced by an increase in intramuscular pressure during diaphragmatic contraction. This early observation is in agreement with recent direct measurements of diaphragmatic intramuscular pressure. Several studies have now shown that, during electrophrenic nerve or direct muscle stimulation, the intramuscular pressure in the diaphragm is directly related to its force of contraction (Decramer et al., 1990; Supinski et al., 1990; Hussain and Magder, 1991). Decramer and colleagues (1990), however, have shown that, during spontaneous breathing against inspiratory resistances or upper airway occlusions, the diaphragmatic intramuscular pressure in the costal and crural segment is primarily determined by changes in pleural and abdominal pressure, rather than the tension developed by it, a finding that relates well to the earlier observation by Buchler et al. (1985b), during which they demonstrated that a high negative pleural pressure, developed during sustained diaphragmatic contractions, tends to increase Qdi, whereas a high positive abdominal pressure tends to decrease the flow. They concluded from their observations that a high pleural pressure increased the cross-sectional area, thereby reducing the impedance to diaphragmatic circulation, whereas a high abdominal pressure reduced the arterial perfusion-driving pressure by increasing the intramuscular pressure acting on the blood vessels, thereby producing an effect of Starling resistance (i.e., the driving pressure for blood flow through the diaphragm becomes regulated by the difference in arterial pressure and intramuscular pressure instead of the difference between the arterial and venous pressure). Another finding of mechanical impediment to blood flow in the diaphragm was made by Supinski and colleagues (1986), in which they demonstrated that flow through a diaphragmatic strip was greater at shorter diaphragmatic lengths (90% of Lo) than at longer (110% Lo) during rhythmic isometric contractions. This is an interesting finding that demonstrates that longitudinal stress caused by stretching increases the vascular resistance and contributes in part to other mechanical factors, such as nipping and shearing of blood vessels within muscle tissue (Gray et al., 1967). In fact, Hussain and Magder (1991) have shown that the intramuscular pressure at which the diaphragmatic blood flow during inspiration (contraction phase blood flow measured by electromagnetic blood flowmeter) becomes limited is approximately 50 mm Hg, a pressure much lower than the systemic arterial pressure; thus, the limitation can be partly attributed to a reduction in driving pressure (Starling resistance), as well as to the nipping and shearing of vessels associated with muscle fiber shortening. Nonetheless, the increase in diaphragmatic intramuscular pressure associated with increased force contributes to the rise in diaphragmatic vascular impedance during sustained isometric or intermittent contractions (Supinski et al., 1991).

Thus, overall, the diaphragmatic perfusion is regulated in part similarly to myocardial perfusion; that is, during inspiration (systole) diaphragmatic blood flow is reduced and may even be interrupted with forceful contractions, and it is reestablished during expiration (diastole); however, as expiratory time decreases or force (Pdi) of contraction increases, respiratory muscle blood flow limitation will occur with ensuing contractile failure.

E. Local Metabolic, Neural, and Humoral Factors

Local metabolic factors known to directly influence skeletal muscle blood flow are changes in oxygen and carbon dioxide tension (Hudlicka and el Khelly, 1985). There is no doubt that hypoxia and hypercapnia increases Qdi; nevertheless, most of the previous studies did not dissociate the effects of stimulation on breathing from those affecting the blood vessels directly. One study, in particular, in rabbits subjected to graded hypoxia (PaO_2: 115, 14, 27 mm Hg) with $PaCO_2$ held at 30 mm Hg, or to graded hypercapnia ($PaCO_2$: 30, 42, 65, 78 mm Hg) with PaO_2 kept at 110 mm Hg, demonstrated that respiratory muscle blood flow was proportional to the alterations in arterial blood gas composition during spontaneous breathing, whereas blood flow to limb muscles remained unchanged (Kendrick et al., 1981). When the rabbits were paralyzed, respiratory muscle blood flow fell to about 10% of the spontaneously breathing level and was unaffected by hypoxia or hypercapnia. Thus, it was concluded that hypoxia and hypercapnia per se had no significant effect on respiratory muscle blood flow, other than the one mediated by increased ventilatory activity. More recent studies have now shown that hypoxia has a direct effect on diaphragmatic blood flow (Bark et al., 1986; Hu et al., 1988). One study, in particular, measured diaphragmatic blood flow during constant activation under hypoxia (PaO_2 of 30 mm Hg) and normoxia (Bark et al., 1986). Their results indicated that diaphragmatic blood flow under hypoxia was greater by 20% when compared with normoxic conditions. This suggested that hypoxia had a direct vasodilating effect on the vascular bed that compensated to maintain oxygen delivery at a rate sufficient to maintain oxygen consumption at a level comparable with that observed during normoxia. Furthermore, modest to severe hypoxia (PaO_2 of 30 mm Hg) had no effect on lactic acid production, indicating that the increase in blood flow and oxygen extraction in the respiratory muscles was capable of compensating for the reduced arterial oxygen tension, mostly through a reduction in vascular resistance (Hu et al., 1988).

The mechanism responsible for hypoxic vasodilation, including the liberation of adenosine and other known metabolic mediators, is probably partly produced by the activation of a recently discovered K^+ channel that is inhibited by intracellular ATP (K_{atp}) (Landry and Oliver, 1992). The K_{atp} channels were first reported in cardiac muscle by Noma, and they have since been shown to exist in numerous other tissue types including skeletal and vascular smooth muscle (Noma, 1983; Nichols and Lederer, 1991; Spruce et al., 1985). In vascular smooth muscle of the coronary circulation, they are activated by hypoxia and ischemia and, in skeletal muscle, by the reduction of intracellular ATP or by pH (Daut et al., 1990; Davies et al., 1992). Hypoxia and ischemia reduce the intracellular ATP concentration and increase the probability of activation of the channel. The activation of K_{atp} channels causes the membrane to hyperpolarize, and this is believed to reduce the probability of voltage-dependent Ca^{2+} channels being open, thereby reducing the intracellular free Ca^{2+} and producing a relaxation of vascular smooth muscle. They have now been shown to be activated in vascular smooth muscle of respiratory muscles and contribute in part to active and reactive hyperemia (Vanelli et al., 1994; Vanelli and Hussain, 1994). In fact, Comtois and colleagues (1994) have shown that the time to diaphragmatic failure during phrenic nerve pacing was significantly shorter when K_{atp} channels were inhibited by the sulfonylurea glibenclamide, a specific K_{atp} channel blocker, and this per se was mostly attributed to a reduction in diaphragmatic blood flow produced by a 65% increase in vascular resistance. Thus, there is strong supportive evidence for the contribution of K_{atp} channels to active and reactive hyperemia and as well as to their role in hypoxic vasodilation.

Numerous investigators have now demonstrated the existence of diaphragmatic afferent pathways by type III and IV phrenic nerve fibers. The activation of thin-fiber phrenic afferents by capsaicin has an excitatory effect on arterial pressure, heart rate, and phrenic motoneurons (Revelette et al., 1988; Hussain et al., 1991). Diaphragmatic ischemia produces similar increases in inspiratory motor drive (Teitelbaum et al., 1993). Activation of thin-fiber phrenic nerve afferents also occurs with the injection of K^+ within the diaphragmatic vasculature (Fig. 7) (Supinski et al., 1993). This is an interesting finding, which is more physiological than capsaicin stimulation, and especially since K^+ efflux is known to occur with skeletal muscle exercise (Sjogaard, 1987). There is no doubt that the K^+ efflux occurs through the delayed rectifier channel; nonetheless, the K_{atp} channels have recently been shown to be activated during fatigue development in skeletal muscle (Light et al., 1994). This is also supported by the fact that the presence of a K_{atp} channel inhibitor during diaphragmatic fatigue development reduces the inferior phrenic vein K^+ content by 16% (Comtois et al., 1994). The implication of these observations are interesting and puzzling, because K^+ efflux through K_{atp} channels in the diaphragm could establish a link between the metabolic

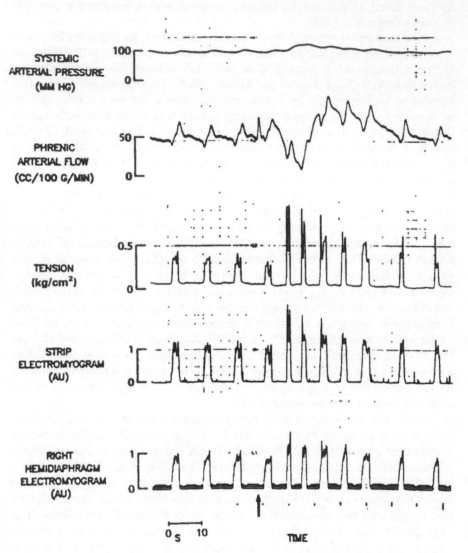

Figure 7 The effect of potassium injection through the left phrenic artery on the mean systemic arterial pressure, left phrenic artery blood flow, left diaphragmatic strip tension, and right and left integrated EMG activity in one animal. Phrenic artery blood flow was measured by Doppler flowmetry in a left diaphragmatic strip preparation. The potassium (0.1 mEq/ml) was injected at the time indicated by the arrow. AU, arbitrary units. (From Supinski et al., 1993a.)

status of the diaphragm (reduction in intracellular ATP and pH, which are the K_{atp} channel activators) and the activation of thin-fiber phrenic nerve afferents by K^+ during fatigue development. The activation of thin-fiber phrenic nerve afferents stimulates the inspiratory drive, a condition unfavorable to sustained breathing during respiratory muscle fatigue development. However, as suggested by Supinski and colleagues (1993a), the excitatory reflex mediated by K^+ activation of thin-fiber phrenic nerve afferents acts to compensate for brief increases in the respiratory work load, and during more sustained loading, inhibitory responses may supervene, overriding this reflex.

The respiratory muscles exhibit a substantial increase in blood flow in response to increased metabolic demands. Recently, the basal release of endothelium-derived relaxing factor (EDRF), identified pharmacologically as nitric oxide (NO), or its release during muscle contraction, has been established as a major contributor to baseline vasomotor tone and to both active and reactive hyperemia in the diaphragm (Hussain et al., 1992; Ward et al., 1993). In exercise-induced vasodilation (active hyperemia), however, the release of NO by the diaphragm is complemented by other mediators of exercise-induced hyperemia, since the inhibition of NO by specific antagonists (L-arginine analogues: L-argininosuccinic acid and N^G-nitro-L-arginine) does not completely reverse the exercise-induced vasodilation. Another contributor to the exercise-induced and reactive hyperemia is through the activation of K_{atp} channels. Jackson has recently shown (1993) that K_{atp} channels contribute to the maintenance of resting arteriolar tone in the hamster cheek pouch and cremaster muscle, a finding further supported by Vanelli and colleagues and other investigators in the diaphragmatic circulation, where they observed the involvement of K_{atp} channels in the response to exercise-induced and reactive hyperemia (Vanelli et al., 1994; Vanelli and Hussain, 1994; Comtois, et al., 1994).

There are other known mediators of exercise-induced hyperemia, such as adenosine, ATP, lactate, H^+, hyperosmolarity, inorganic phosphate, and K^+, that all play substantial roles in skeletal muscle blood flow, and probably in respiratory muscles (Hudlicka and el Khelly, 1985). Thus, not one mediator appears to have prominence over another, but they are all linked together in the modulation of blood flow either during exercise-induced hyperemia or reactive hyperemia.

Last, a salient feature of diaphragmatic circulation, which is similar to other skeletal muscles (Stainsby and Renkin, 1961; Stainsby, 1962), is the ability for autoregulation of this circulation. Hussain and colleagues have shown that the diaphragmatic circulation was autoregulated within the range of 70–120 mm Hg of arterial perfusion pressure (Fig. 8) (Hussain et al., 1988b). Below this range diaphragmatic circulation became linearly related to the arterial perfusion pressure. This characteristic of autoregulation was observed at three levels of inspiratory work. This is an important finding, indicating that the diaphragm can compensate effectively for sudden changes in arterial perfusion pressure or cardiac output (hemorrhagic or cardiogenic shock).

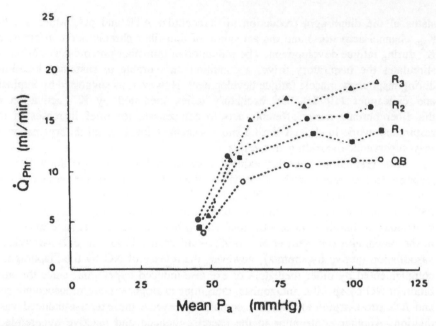

Figure 8 Phrenic artery blood flow (Qphr) as a function of mean arterial blood pressure (Pa) during quiet breathing (QB) and various levels of inspiratory resistances (R_1, R_2, and R_3). Qphr was measured by an electromagnetic flow probe. Arterial pressure was varied by bleeding or reinfusion of heparinized blood. (From Hussain et al., 1988b.)

V. Respiratory Muscle Blood Flow and Contractile Failure

It has been demonstrated by Barcroft and Dornhorst (1949) that blood flow in the human calf muscle increases during strong rhythmic contractions, and that flow during the contraction phase is less than flow between contractions, suggesting, that blood flow could become insufficient during forceful sustained contractions and eventually lead to contractile failure or fatigue. In support of this concept, numerous investigators have shown that the rate of fatigability of the respiratory muscles increases in the face of decreased blood perfusion. Hussain and colleagues have shown that septic shock tremendously reduces the endurance time of the diaphragm to an added respiratory load, and this correlates with a decreased diaphragmatic circulation (Hussain et al., 1985; Hussain and Roussos, 1985). Cardiogenic and hemorrhagic shock produce similar results (Viires et al., 1983; Sharf et al., 1986). Thus, a large amount of evidence supports the concept of increased fatigability with ensuing hypercapnia when the contracting respiratory muscles are challenged by a reduced blood perfusion pressure (Aubier et al., 1981). In fact, under conditions of severe hypotension (50 mm Hg), animals spontaneously breathing at rest develop respiratory muscle failure with ensuing hypercapnia, despite a three- to sixfold increase in diaphragmatic circulation that can require up to 25% of the cardiac output (Viires et al., 1983; Reid and Johnson, 1983; Hussain et al., 1986). This strongly suggests that the increase in respiratory muscle blood flow was inadequate, presumably because of poor perfusion of the microcirculatory bed (i.e., nutritive blood flow). Boczkowski and colleagues (1992) studied the perfusion of the microcirculatory bed of the diaphragm under conditions of septic shock. They observed a reduction in the diameter of second-order arterioles, probably related to arterial hypotension, and an impaired diaphragmatic capillary perfusion. This is an important finding that strongly suggests that the increase in blood flow had reached its maximum level at that given blood pressure and that capillary perfusion was probably impaired by the adherence of granulocytes to endothelial cells (Boczkowski et al., 1992).

It is thought that an adequate blood flow is necessary to maintain constant levels of high-energy phosphate compounds (ATP). Several studies (Dawson et al., 1978; Sjogaard, 1987), however, have demonstrated that ATP stores are not depleted during forceful contractions, suggesting that the contractile proteins do not fail because of a lack of energy stores, but probably because of the build up of metabolic byproducts in the intracellular or extracellular environment (Sjogaard, 1987). This is possibly because inadequate blood perfusion (lack of O_2) may lead the contracting muscle to revert to anaerobic pathways, thereby leading to increased intracellular hydrogen ion concentrations (Mainwood and Cechetto, 1980; Sjogaard, 1987). Activation of glycolitic pathways causes an increase in intracellular hydrogen and phosphate ions that leads to the disruption of membrane events at the sarcoplasmic reticular level. On the other hand, muscle blood flow is involved in the washout of catabolites during muscle activity. It has been demonstrated by Barclay and co-workers (Barclay and Stainsby, 1975) that, in limb muscles, the rate of washout is an important determinant of muscle endurance. The amount of blood volume delivered to a skeletal muscle per unit of time and muscle mass has been shown to be related to its endurance to exercise, both because blood delivers O_2 and nutrients, and because of its ability to washout catabolites generated during contractile activity (Barclay, 1986). This maintains an adequate extracellular environment susceptible to the maintenance of continuous muscle activity. A recent study on the diaphragm, conducted by Supinski and colleagues (1988) supported this argument. They demonstrated that diaphragmatic fatigue could be reversed by increasing diaphragmatic blood flow. In their study, diaphragmatic blood flow was increased by elevating the perfusion pressure of the phrenic artery in a diaphragmatic strip preparation. They concluded that greater flow rates produced an increase in the washout of the catabolites that assisted in the maintenance of an optimal extracellular environment for continued contractile activity. However, it was difficult from their study to determine if the reversal of fatigue was attributed to an increase in oxygen delivery, or to a faster rate of catabolite washout. This question has been addressed recently by Ward and colleagues (1992) when they demonstrated that doubling the diaphragmatic blood flow rate by pump perfusion while maintaining the oxygen delivery constant at the level observed during control (autoperfusion) was capable of delaying, as shown in Figure 9, the onset of fatigue development in the diaphragm. The interesting observation in their study was that fatigue development was delayed by several minutes, but once force decay was initiated, it decayed at a similar rate regardless of the blood flow rate, indicating that other mechanisms of fatigue were now contributing to the development of fatigue; most probably, cellular mechanisms of fatigue, such as the intracellular accumulation of inorganic phosphate and hydrogen ions, two known potent contributors to the loss of muscle contractility (Godt and Nosek, 1989).

Even though increasing the diaphragm blood flow rate by extrinsic means appears to postpone fatigue development, there is now recent evidence indicating that the administration of potent vasodilators in the failing diaphragm has no effect on blood flow and function. This has been demonstrated in a study by Supinski and colleagues (1993) during which administration of the potent NO-liberating vasodilator, sodium nitroprusside, failed to increase diaphragmatic blood flow during fatigue development in the diaphragm, suggesting that under those conditions its vasodilator reserve was completely exhausted. In this example, the treatment of shock is probably better managed by the administration of vasoconstrictors, such as norepinephrine and the sulfonylurea coumpound glibenclamide, which increase the arterial pressure, thus the perfusion pressure, and shunts the residual blood volume toward tissues that are in metabolic need (Hussain et al., 1988a; Landry and Oliver, 1992).

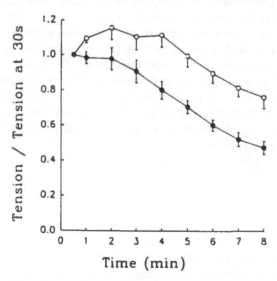

Figure 9   The relationship of diaphragmatic tension as a function of time during control (autoperfusion, closed circles) and pump perfusion (open circles). (From Ward et al., 1992.)

Acknowledgments

Supported by the Medical Research Council of Canada and a Quebec Lung Association grant.

References

Anrep, G. V., Cerqua, S., and Samaan, A. (1933). The effect of muscular contraction upon the blood flow in the skeletal muscle, in the diaphragm and in the small intestine. *Proc. R. Soc. Lond. [Biol.]* 114: 245–357.

Anrep, G. V., and Saalfeld, E. V. (1935). The blood flow through the skeletal muscle in relation to its contraction. *J. Physiol. Lond.* 85: 375–399.

Aubier, M., Trippenbach, T., and Roussos, C. (1981). Respiratory muscle fatigue during cardiogenic shock. *J. Appl. Physiol.* 51: 499–508.

Barclay, J. K. (1986). A delivery-independent blood flow effect on skeletal muscle fatigue. *J. Appl. Physiol.* 61: 1084–1090.

Barclay, J. K., and Stainsby, W. N. (1975). The role of blood flow in limiting maximal metabolic rate in muscle. *Med. Sci. Sports Exerc.* 7: 116–119.

Barcroft, H. (1963). Circulation in skeletal muscle. In *Handbook of Physiology*, Section 2. Circulation. Washington, DC, American Physiological Society, pp. 1353–1385.

Barcroft, H., and Dornhorst, A. C. (1949). The blood flow through the human calf during rhythmic exercise. *J. Physiol.* 109: 402–411.

Barcroft, H., and Millen, J. L. E. (1939). The blood flow through muscle during sustained contraction. *J. Physiol.* 97: 17–31.

Bark, H., and Scharf, S. M. (1986). Diaphragmatic blood flow in the dog. *J. Appl. Physiol.* 60: 554–561.

Bark, H., Supinski, G. S., Bundy, R. J., and Kelsen, S. G. (1986). Effect of acute hypoxia on diaphragmatic muscle contractile function, blood flow, and metabolism. *Am. Rev. Respir. Dis.* 133: A249.

Bark, H., Supinski, G. S., Lamanna, J. C., and Kelsen, S. G. (1987). Relationship of changes in diaphragmatic muscle blood flow to muscle contractile activity. *J. Appl. Physiol.* 62: 291–299.

Bellemare, F., and Grassino, A. (1982). Effect of pressure and timing of contraction on human diaphragm fatigue. *J. Appl. Physiol.* 53: 1190–1195.

Bellemare, F., and Grassino, A. (1983). Force reserve of the diaphragm in patients with chronic obstructive pulmonary disease. *J. Appl. Physiol.* 55: 8–15.

Bellemare, F., Wight, D., Lavigne, C. M., and Grassino, A. (1983). Effect of tension and timing of contraction on the blood flow of the diaphragm. *J. Appl. Physiol.* 54: 1597–1606.

Biscoe, T. J., and Bucknell, A. (1963). The arterial supply of the cat diaphragm with a note on the venous drainage. *Q. J. Exp. Physiol.* 48: 27–33.

Boczkowski, J., Vicaut, E., and Aubier, M. (1990). A preparation for in vivo study of the diaphragmatic microcirculation in the rat. *Microvasc. Res.* 40: 157–167.

Boczkowski, J., Vicaut, E., and Aubier, M. (1992). In vivo effects of *Escherichia coli* endotoxomia on diaphragmatic microcirculation in rats. *J. Appl. Physiol.* 72: 2219–2224.

Bonde-Petersen, F., Mork, A. L., and Nielsen, E. (1975). Local muscle blood flow and sustained contractions of human arm and back muscles. *Eur. J. Appl. Physiol.* 34: 43–50.

Bonnette, P., Hannoun, L., Menegaux, F., Calmat, A., and Cabrol, C. (1983). Etude anatomique de la veine diaphragmatique inferieure gauche. *Bull. Assoc. Anat. (Nancy)* 67: 69–77.

Buchler, B., Magder, S., and Roussos, C. (1985a). Effect of contraction frequency and duty cycle on diaphragmatic blood flow. *J. Appl. Physiol.* 58: 265–273.

Buchler, B., Magder, S., Katsardis, H., Jammes, Y., and Roussos, C. (1985b). Effects of pleural pressure and abdominal pressure on diaphragmatic blood flow. *J. Appl. Physiol.* 58: 691–697.

Brancatisano, A., Amis, T. C., Tully, A., Kelly, W. T., and Engel, L. A. (1991). Regional distribution of blood flow within the diaphragm. *J. Appl. Physiol.* 71: 583–589.

Ceretelli, P., Pendergast, D., Marconi, C., and Piiper, J. (1986). Blood flow in exercising muscles. *Int. J. Sports Med.* 7: 29–33.

Comtois, A., Gorczyca, W., and Grassino, A. (1987). Anatomy of diaphragmatic circulation. *J. Appl. Physiol.* 62: 238–244.

Comtois, A., Hu, F., and Grassino, A. (1988). Anatomy of human diaphragmatic circulation [abstract]. *Am. Rev. Respir. Dis.* 137: 384.

Comtois, A., Hu, F., and Grassino, A. (1991). Restriction of regional blood flow and diaphragmatic contractility. *J. Appl. Physiol.* 70: 2439–2447.

Comtois, A., Sinderby, C., Comtois, N., Grassino, A., and Renaud, J.-M. (1994). An ATP-sensitive potassium channel blocker decreases diaphragmatic circulation in anesthetized dogs. *J. Appl. Physiol.* 77 (in press).

Daut, J., Maier-Rudolph, W., von Beckerath, N., Mehrke, G., Gunther, K., and Goedel-Meinen, L. (1990). Hypoxic dilation of coronary arteries is mediated by ATP-sensitive potassium channels. *Science* 247: 1341–1344.

Davies, N. W., Standen, N. B., and Stanfield, P. R. (1992). The effect of intracellular pH on ATP-dependent potassium channels of frog skeletal muscle. *J. Physiol. Lond.* 445: 549–568.

Dawson, M. J., Guardian, D. G., and Wilkie, D. R. (1978). Muscular fatigue investigated by phosphorous nuclear magnetic resonance. *Nature* 274: 861–866.

Decramer, M., Jiang, T. X., and Reid, M. B. (1990). Respiratory changes in diaphragmatic intramuscular pressure. *J. Appl. Physiol.* 68: 35–43.

De Troyer, A., and Loring S. H. (1986). Action of the respiratory muscles. In *Handbook of Physiology*, Section 3. The Respiratory System. Mechanics of Breathing, Vol. 3. Part 2. Edited by P. T. Macklem, J. Mead, and S. R. Geiger. Bethesda, MD, American Physiological Society, pp. 443–461.

De Troyer, A., Ninane, V., and Gilmartin, J. J. (1987). Triangularis sterni muscle use in supine humans. *J. Appl. Physiol.* 62: 919–927.

Donovan, E., Trippenbach, T., Grassino, A., Macklem, P. T., and Roussos, C. (1979). Effect of isometric diaphragmatic contraction in cardiac output and muscle blood flow [abstract]. Fed. Proc. 38: 1382.

Evans, H. E., and Christensen, G. C. (1979). *Miller's Anatomy of the Dog*, 2nd ed. Philadelphia, W. B. Saunders, pp. 22–323.

Fixler, D. E., Atkins, J. M., Michell, J. H.,and Horwitz, L. D. (1976). Blood flow to respiratory, cardiac, and limb muscles in dogs during graded exercise. *Am. J. Physiol.* 231: 1515–1519.

Godt, R. E., and Nosek, T. M. (1989). Changes of intracellular milieu with fatigue or hypoxia depress contraction of skinned rabbit skeletal and cardiac muscle. *J. Physiol.* 412: 155–180.

Gray, H. (1980). *Anatomy, Descriptive and Surgical*. Philadelphia, Running Press.

Gray, S. D., Carlsson, E., and Staub, N. C. (1967). Site of increased vascular resistance during isometric muscular contraction. *Am. J. Physiol.* 213: 683–689.

Greig, H. W., Anson, B. J., and Coleman, S. S. (1951). Inferior phrenic artery; types of origin in 850 body-halves and diaphragmatic relationship. *Q. Bull. Northwest. Univ. Med. Sch.* 25: 345–350.

Hartley, C. J., and Cole, J. S. (1974). An ultrasonic pulsed Doppler system for measuring blood flow in small vessels. *J. Appl. Physiol.* 37: 626–629.

Hartley, C. J., Hanley, H. G., Lewis, R. M., and Cole, J. S. (1978). Synchronized pulsed Doppler flow and ultrasonic dimension measurement in conscious dogs. *Ultrasound Med. Biol.* 4: 99–110.

Hobbs, S. F., and McCloskey, D. I. (1987). Effects of blood pressure on force production in cat and human muscle. *J. Appl. Physiol.* 63: 834–839.

Hsia, C. C. W., Ramanathan, M., Pean, J. L., and Johnson, R. L., Jr. (1992). Respiratory muscle blood flow in exercising dogs after pneumonectomy. *J. Appl. Physiol.* 73: 240–247.

Hu, F., Comtois, A., and Grassino, A. (1988). Effect of hypoxia on diaphragmatic blood flow [abstract]. *Am. Rev. Respir. Dis.* 137: A321.

Hu, F., Comtois, A., and Grassino, A. (1990a). Contraction dependent modulation in regional diaphragmatic blood flow. *J. Appl. Physiol.* 68: 2019–2028.

Hu, F., Comtois, A., Shadram, E., and Grassino, A. (1990b). Effect of separate hemidiaphragm contraction on left phrenic artery flow and O_2 consumption. *J. Appl. Physiol.* 69: 86–90.

Hu, F., Comtois, A., and Grassino, A. (1992). Optimal diaphragmatic blood perfusion. *J. Appl. Physiol.* 72: 149–157.

Hudlicka, O. (1973). *Muscle Blood Flow. Its Relation to Muscle Metabolism and Function.* Amsterdam, Swets & Zeitlenger.

Hudlicka, O., and el Khelly, F. (1985). Metabolic factors involved in regulation of muscle blood flow. *J. Cardiovasc. Pharmacol.* 7(Suppl. 3): S59–S72.

Humphreys, P. W., and Lind, A. R. (1963). The blood flow through active and inactive muscles of the forearm during sustained hand-grip contractions. *J. Physiol.* 166: 123–135.

Hussain, S. N. A., and Magder, S. (1991). Diaphragmatic intramuscular pressure in relation to tension, shortening and blood flow. *J. Appl. Physiol.* 71: 159–167.

Hussain, S. N. A., and Roussos, C. (1985). Distribution of respiratory muscle and organ blood flow during endotoxic shock in dogs. *J. Appl. Physiol.* 59: 1802–1808.

Hussain, S. N. A., Simkus, G., and Roussos, C. (1985). Respiratory muscle fatigue: A cause of ventilatory failure in septic shock. *J. Appl. Physiol.* 58: 2033–2040.

Hussain, S. N. A., Graham, R., Rutledge, F., and Roussos, C. (1986). Respiratory muscle energetics during endotoxic shock in dogs. *J. Appl. Physiol.* 60: 486–493.

Hussain, S. N. A., Rutledge, F., Roussos, C., and Magder, S. (1988a). Effects of norepinephrine and fluid administration on the selective blood flow distribution in endotoxic shock. *J. Crit. Care* 3: 32–42.

Hussain, S. N. A., Roussos, C., and Magder, S. (1988b). Autoregulation of diaphragmatic blood flow in dogs. *J. Appl. Physiol.* 64: 329–336.

Hussain, S. N. A., Roussos, C., and Magder, S. (1989). Effect of tension, duty cycle, and arterial pressure on diaphragmatic blood flow. *J. Appl. Physiol.* 66: 968–976.

Hussain, S. N. A., Chatillon, A., Comtois, A., Roussos, C., and Magder, S. (1991). Chemical activation of thin-fiber phrenic afferents. 2. Cardiovascular responses. *J. Appl. Physiol.* 70: 77–86.

Hussain, S. N. A., Stewart, D. J., Ludemann, J. P., and Magder, S. (1992). Role of endothelium-derived relaxing factor in active hyperemia of the canine diaphragm. *J. Appl. Physiol.* 72: 2393–2401.

Jackson, W. F. (1993). Arteriolar tone is determined by activity of ATP-sensitive potassium channels. *Am. J. Physiol.* 265: H797–803.

Kahn, P. C. (1967). Selective angiography of the inferior phrenic arteries. *Radiology* 88: 1–8.

Kanan, C. V. (1971). The arterial blood supply to the diaphragm of the camel. *Acta Morphol. Neerl. Scand.* 8: 333–341.

Kendrick, J. E., De Haan, S. J., and Parke, J. D. (1981). Regulation of blood flow to respiratory muscles during hypoxia and hypercapnia. *Proc. Soc. Exp. Biol. Med.* 166: 157–161.

Kety, S. S., and Schmidt, C. F. (1945). The determination of cerebral blood flow in man by the use of nitrous oxide in low concentrations. *Am. J. Physiol.* 143: 53–66.

Landry, D. W., and Oliver, J. A. (1992). The ATP-sensitive K^+ channel mediates hypotension in endotoxemia and hypoxic lactic acidosis in dog. *J. Clin. Invest.* 89: 2071–2074.

Light, P., Comtois, A., and Renaud, J.-M. (1994). The effect of glibenclamide on frog skeletal muscle: Evidence for K_{atp} channel activation during fatigue. *J. Physiol. (Lond.)* 475: 495–507.

Lind, A. R., and McNichol, G. W. (1967). Local and central circulatory responses to sustained contractions and the effect of free or restricted arterial inflow on post-exercise hyperaemia. *J. Physiol.* 192: 575–593.

Lockhat, D., Magder, S., and Roussos, C. (1985). Collateral sources of costal and crural diaphragmatic blood flow. *J. Appl. Physiol.* 59: 1164–1170.

Magder, S. (1986). Pressure–flow relations of diaphragm and vital organs with nitroprusside-induced vasodilation. *J. Appl. Physiol.* 61: 409–416.

Magder, S., Lockhat, D., Luo, B. J., and Roussos, C. (1985). Respiratory muscle and organ blood flow with inspiratory elastic loading and shock. *J. Appl. Physiol.* 58: 1148–1156.

Mainwood, G. W., and Cechetto, D. (1980). The effect of bicarbonate concentration on fatigue and recovery in isolated rat diaphragm muscle. *Can. J. Physiol. Pharmacol.* 58: 624–632.

Manohar, M. (1986a). Blood flow to the respiratory and limb muscles and to abdominal organs during maximal exertion in ponies. *J. Physiol. (Lond.)* 377: 25–35.

Manohar, M. (1986b). Vasodilator reserve in respiratory muscles during maximal exertion in ponies. *J. Appl. Physiol.* 60: 1571–1577.

Manohar, M. (1988). Costal vs. crural diaphragmatic blood flow during submaximal and near-maximal exercise in ponies. *J. Appl. Physiol.* 65: 1514–1519.

Manohar, M., Parks, C. M., Busch, M. A., Tranquilli, W. J., Bisgard, G. E., McPherron, T. A., and Theodorakis, M. C. (1982). Regional myocardial blood flow and coronary vascular reserve in unanesthetized young calves exposed to a simulated altitude of 3500 m for 8–10 weeks. *Circ. Res.* 50: 714–726.

Martin, E. C., Bazzy, A. R., Gandhi, M. R., and Haddad, G. G. (1983). An investigation into the venous drainage of the diaphragm of the sheep. *Invest. Radiol.* 18: 272–274.

McMinn, R. M. H. (1982). *Color Atlas of Human Anatomy.* Chicago, Year Book Medical Publisher.

Morgan, C. D. and Johnson, R. L., Jr. (1980). Alteration of diaphragmatic perfusion and work of breathing by ligation of the inferior phrenic artery [abstract]. *Clin. Res.* 28: 530A.

NHLBI Workshop Summary (1990). Respiratory muscle fatigue. Report of the Respiratory Muscle Fatigue Workshop group. *Am. Rev. Respir. Dis.* 142: 474–480.

Nichols, C. G., and Lederer, W. J. (1991). Adenosine triphosphate-sensitive potassium channels in the cardiovascular system. *Am. J. Physiol.* 261: H1675–H1686.

Nichols, D. G., Scharf, S. M., Traystman, R. J., and Robotham, J. L. (1988). Correlation of left phrenic arterial flow with regional diaphragmatic blood flow. *J. Appl. Physiol.* 64: 2230–2235.

Nichols, D. G., Howell, S., Massik, J., Koehler, R. C., Gleason, C. A., Buck, J. R., Fitzgerald, R. S., Traystman, R. J., and Robotham, J. L. (1989). Relationship of diaphragmatic contractility to diaphragmatic blood flow in newborn lambs. *J. Appl. Physiol.* 66: 120–127.

Noma, A. (1983). ATP-regulated K^+ channels in cardiac muscle. *Nature* 305: 147–148.

Reid, M. B., and Johnson, R. L., Jr. (1983). Efficiency, maximal blood flow, and aerobic work capacity of canine diaphragm. *J. Appl. Physiol.* 54: 763–772.

Reid, M. B., Parsons, D. B., Giddings, C. J., Gonyea, W. J., and Johnson, R. L., Jr. (1992). Capillaries measured in canine diaphragm by two methods. *Anat. Rec.* 234: 49–54.

Revelette, W. R., Jewell, L. A., and Frazier, D. T. (1988). Effect of diaphragm small-fiber afferent stimulation on ventilation in dogs. *J. Appl. Physiol.* 65: 2097–2106.

Robertson, C. H., Jr., Forster, G. H., and Johnson, R. L., Jr. (1977a). The relationship of respiratory failure to the oxygen consumption of, lactate production by, and distribution of blood flow among respiratory muscles during increasing inspiratory resistance. *J. Clin. Invest.* 59: 31–42.

Robertson, C. H., Jr., Pagel, M. A., and Johnson, R. L., Jr. (1977b). The distribution of blood flow, oxygen consumption, and work output among respiratory muscles during unobstructed hyperventilation. *J. Clin. Invest.* 59: 43–50.

Robertson, C. H., Jr., Eschenbacher, W. L., and Johnson, R. L., Jr. (1977c). Respiratory muscle blood flow distribution during expiratory resistance. *J. Clin. Invest.* 60: 473–480.

Rochester, D. F. (1974). Measurement of diaphragmatic blood flow and oxygen consumption in the dog by Kety–Schmidt technique. *J. Clin. Invest.* 53: 1216–1225.

Rochester, D. F., and Bettini, G. (1976). Diaphragmatic blood flow and energy expenditure in the dog. Effect of inspiratory air flow resistance and hypercapnia. *J. Clin. Invest.* 57: 661–672.

Rochester, D. F., and Pradel-Guena, M. (1973). Measurement of diaphragmatic blood flow in dogs from xenon 133 clearance. *J. Appl. Physiol.* 34: 68–74.

Scharf, S. M., Bark, H., Einhorn, S., and Tarasiuk, A. (1986). Blood flow to the canine diaphragm during hemorrhagic shock. *Am. Rev. Respir. Dis.* 133: 205–211.

Schraufnagel, D. E., Roussos, C., Macklem, P. T., and Wang, N. S. (1983). The geometry of the microvascular bed of the diaphragm: Comparison to intercostals and triceps. *Microvasc. Res.* 26: 291–306.

Sjogaard, G. (1987). Muscle fatigue. *Med. Sport Sci.* 26: 98–109.

Spruce, A. E., Standen, N. B., and Stanfield, P. R. (1985). Voltage dependent ATP sensitive potassium channels of skeletal muscle membrane. *Nature* 316: 736–738.

Stainsby, W. N. (1962). Autoregulation of blood flow in skeletal muscle during increased metabolic activity. *Am. J. Physiol.* 202: 273–276.

Stainsby, W. N., and Renkin, E. M. (1961). Autoregulation of blood flow in resting skeletal muscle. *Am. J. Physiol.* 201: 117–122.

Supinski, G. S., Bark, H., Guanciale, A., and Kelsen, S. G. (1986). Effect of alterations in muscle fibre length on diaphragm blood flow. *J. Appl. Physiol.* 60: 1789–1796.

Supinski, G. S., DiMarco, A., Ketai, L., and Altose, M. (1988). Reversibility of diaphragm fatigue by mechanical hyperperfusion. *Am. Rev. Respir. Dis.* 138: 604–609.

Supinski, G. S., DiMarco, A., and Altose, M. (1990). Effects of diaphragmatic contraction on intramuscular pressure and vascular impedance. *J. Appl. Physiol.* 68: 1486–1493.

Supinski, G. S., Dick, T., Stofan, D., and DiMarco, A. F. (1993a). Effects of intraphrenic injection of potassium on diaphragm activation. *J. Appl. Physiol.* 74: 1186–1194.

Supinski, G. S., Stofan, D., Nashawati, E., and DiMarco, A. F. (1993b). Failure of vasodilator administration to increase blood flow to the fatiguing diaphragm. *J. Appl. Physiol.* 74: 1178–1185.

Teitelbaum, J., Vanelli, G., and Hussain, S. N. A. (1993). Thin-fiber phrenic afferents mediate the ventilatory response to diaphragmatic ischemia. *Respir. Physiol.* 91: 195–206.

Testut, L. (1921). *Traité d'Anatomie Humaine*, 7th ed. Librairie Octave Doin, pp. 202–204.

Vanelli, G., and Hussain, S. N. A. (1994). Effects of potassium channel blockers on basal vascular tone and reactive hyperemia of canine diaphragm. *Am. J. Physiol.* 266: H43–H51.

Vanelli, G., Chang, H. Y., Gatensby, A. G., and Hussain, S. N. A. (1994). Contribution of potassium channels to active hyperemia of the canine diaphragm. *J. Appl. Physiol.* 76: 1098–1105.

Vatner, S. F., Franklin, D., and VanCitters, R. L. (1970). Simultaneous comparison and calibration of the Doppler and electromagnetic flowmeters. *J. Appl. Physiol.* 29: 907–910.

Viires, N., Sillye, G., Aubier, M., Rassidakis, A., and Roussos, C. (1983). Regional blood flow distribution in dog during induced hypotension and low cardiac output. *J. Clin. Invest.* 72: 935–947.

Ward, E. M., Magder, S. A., and Hussain, S. N. A. (1983). Role of endothelium-derived relaxing factor in reactive hyperemia in canine diaphragm. *J. Appl. Physiol.* 74: 1606–1612.

Ward, E. M., Magder, S. A., and Hussain, S. N. A. (1992). Oxygen delivery-independent effect of blood flow on diaphragm fatigue. *Am. Rev. Respir. Dis.* 145: 1058–1063.

24

Respiratory Muscle Metabolism

MICHAEL E. WARD and SABAH N. A. HUSSAIN

McGill University
Montreal, Quebec, Canada

I. Oxygen Consumption

Under resting conditions in healthy individuals, the respiratory muscles use little ($\sim 1.5\%$) of the total oxygen consumption (VO_2tot) or cardiac output (Robertson et al., 1977a). This situation is altered, however, when the relation between respiratory muscle metabolic demand and systemic oxygen transport is perturbed. This occurs during exercise, when disease increases the impedance of the respiratory system, and when oxygen delivery is reduced (Anholm et al., 1987; Boutellier et al., 1986; Collett et al., 1985; Oligaiti et al., 1986; Viires et al., 1983; Robertson et al., 1977a; Cala et al., 1991). In normal subjects, respiratory muscle oxygen consumption (VO_2resp) increases linearly with exercise (Cherniack, 1959; Robertson et al., 1977b) because of the increased power output by the respiratory muscles. In patients with pulmonary disease, in contrast, VO_2resp at rest may account for 25% of VO_2tot (Cherniack, 1959; Field et al., 1982). Changes in resting muscle length and recruitment of postural and synergistic accessory muscles, which do not directly contribute to ventilation, furthermore, result in a progressive decrease in respiratory muscle efficiency (VO_2resp/work of breathing) as minute ventilation increases (Cherniack, 1959; Fritts et al., 1959; Rochester et al., 1976). In a theoretical analysis, Riley (1954) has suggested that the degree to which such patients may increase their minute ventilation is limited by oxygen availability. That is, as ventilation increases, an ever-increasing proportion of the additional O_2 uptake is diverted to the respiratory muscles at the expense of O_2 available for nonrespiratory work. A point will be reached beyond which the increase in VO_2resp becomes greater than the increase in Vo_2tot, and further increases in ventilation become detrimental.

This hypothesis has been tested in normal individuals (Aaron et al., 1992). Aaron et al. (1992) found that normal subjects were able to voluntarily mimic maximum exercise work of breathing and respiratory pattern for three to ten times longer than the duration of the maximum exercise. Therefore, although the O_2 cost of exercise hyperpnea is a significant fraction of Vo_2tot, it is not sufficient to cause a critical level of "useful" hyperpnea to be reached in healthy subjects.

In patients with respiratory disease, it remains to be determined whether or not such a condition may occur. During the application of inspiratory resistive loads in humans, McCool et al. (1989) found that the time to failure of a breathing task is closely related to the increase in Vo_2resp and suggested that a critical rate of energy utilization determines the endurance of the inspiratory pump. From the available animal data, however, it appears unlikely that oxygen availability plays a role in limiting respiratory muscle function in the absence of abnormalities in blood flow or blood oxygen content. Manohar (1991) found that, in ponies, the phrenic arteriovenous O_2 content difference remained unchanged during exhaustive exercise. Similarly, direct measurements of diaphragmatic O_2 consumption during resistive loading in animals, have also failed to support this hypothesis. Bazzy et al. (1989) found no decrease in phrenic venous Po_2 during the application of fatiguing inspiratory resistive loads in nonanesthetized sheep. Similarly, Pope et al. (1989b) found that during diaphragmatic fatigue, induced by supramaximal phrenic nerve stimulation in dogs, phrenic venous Po_2 remained above 30 mm Hg, and biochemical evidence of anaerobic metabolism was absent.

In patients with coexistent cardiovascular disease or abnormalities of oxygen-carrying capacity, the situation may be much different. Evidence has recently been presented indicating that impairment of respiratory muscle oxygenation does indeed occur and, at least in patients in whom oxygen delivery is limited by cardiovascular disease, may limit exercise. Mancini et al. (1991), monitored the oxygenation of the serratus anterior muscle using near-infrared spectroscopy and found significant deoxygenation during treadmill exercise in patients with heart failure. Therefore, since the ability of these muscles to function anaerobically is limited (Manohar et al., 1990), their ability to sustain spontaneous ventilation is ultimately limited by their aerobic capacity—the relation between their oxygen transport and metabolic demand. It must be noted, however, that not all of the deleterious effects of inadequate blood flow on respiratory muscle function can be attributed to the reduction in oxygen and plasma-borne substrate delivery (Ward et al., 1992).

In dogs, we have recently compared the relation between systemic O_2 delivery and O_2 consumption with that for the diaphragm during stepwise hemorrhage (Ward et al., 1993). Left diaphragmatic O_2 consumption during rest and during 3 min of continuous (3-Hz) stimulation of the left phrenic nerve, and the O_2 consumption of the remaining non–left-hemidiaphragmatic tissues were measured at each stage of the hemorrhage protocol (Fig. 1). The Vo_2 of the diaphragm

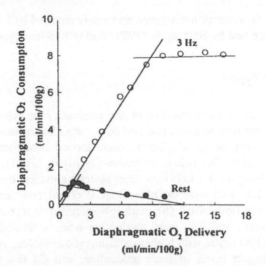

Figure 1 Relations between diaphragmatic O_2 delivery and O_2 consumption with the diaphragm at rest and during 3-Hz stimulation.

during stimulation at this frequency was comparable with that previously recorded during the application of mild resistive loads in intact dogs (Robertson et al., 1977b; Rochester et al., 1976; Reid et al., 1983). Critical diaphragmatic O_2 delivery for the resting diaphragm averaged 0.8 ± 0.16 ml/min/100 g with a critical O_2 extraction ratio of $65.5 \pm 6\%$. In the contracting diaphragm, the critical diaphragmatic O_2 delivery and critical O_2 extraction ratio averaged 5.1 ± 0.9 ml/min/100 g and $81 \pm 5\%$, respectively. The whole-body O_2 delivery at which the O_2 consumption of the resting diaphragm became supply limited was similar to that for the nondiaphragmatic tissues (0.51 ± 0.092 and 0.66 ± 0.08 ml/min/100 g, respectively). Similarly the critical O_2 extraction ratio for the resting diaphragm (0.65 ± 0.08) was not significantly different from the critical O_2 extraction ratio for the nondiaphragmatic tissues (0.62 ± 0.08). In contrast to previous suggestions (Collett et al., 1985), therefore, diaphragmatic oxygenation does not appear to be preferentially preserved during generalized reductions in O_2 delivery. In the contracting diaphragm, supply limitation of O_2 consumption occurred at a higher systemic O_2 delivery (1.1 ± 0.12 ml/min/100 g) than in the rest of the body, despite the increase in O_2 extraction ratio. Therefore, in diseases associated with increased work of breathing and decreased O_2 delivery, the diaphragm may become metabolically impaired before limitation of oxygen consumption is observed systematically.

The maximum O_2 extraction for the contracting diaphragm in the study just described was 0.94 ± 0.022. This value was similar to that recorded for the whole body during the final stages of hemorrhage (0.91 ± 0.02). Similar maximum levels of diaphragmatic O_2 extraction have been previously reported by Scharf et al. (1986) during hemorrhage and by Bark et al. (1988) during hypoxic hypoxia.

II. Fiber Types

The aerobic and anaerobic capacities of the respiratory muscles depend on the characteristics of the muscle fibers that compose them. The mammalian diaphragm comprises three types of muscle fibers, characterized histochemically as slow-twitch oxidative (SO), fast-twitch oxidative–glycolytic (FOG), and fast-twitch glycolytic (FG) (Riley et al., 1979). In other skeletal muscles, these histochemical distinctions correlate well with the physiological characterization of motor units into three types: (1) slow-twitch (S), with low recruitment thresholds, high level of fatigue resistance, and low force production when activated; (2) fast-twitch fatigue-resistant (FR) units, with higher recruitment thresholds, relative resistance to fatigue, and higher levels of force production; and (3) fast-twitch fatiguable (FF), which produce the highest levels of force, have the highest thresholds for recruitment, and are highly susceptible to fatigue (Burke et al., 1971). The fiber composition of the respiratory muscles varies from species to species (Green et al., 1984; Davies and Gunn, 1972). Davies and Gunn (1984) determined the histochemical fiber types present in the diaphragms of adult mice, rats, rabbits, cats, dogs, pigs, horses, and oxen. In smaller animals, with high respiratory rates, the diaphragm has a high proportion of fast-twitch fibers and a preponderantly aerobic metabolism. The diaphragm of larger animals has a majority of slow-twitch fibers and a capacity for combined aerobic and anaerobic metabolism. With microphotometric techniques, Green and associates (1984) studied the differences in concentrations of the aerobic enzyme succinate dehydrogenase (SDH) in type I, IIA, and IIB fibers, based on staining for myofibrillar ATPase (mATPase) activity in the diaphragms of mouse, rat, guinea pig, rabbit, cat, and dog. Large differences in SDH activities were observed between species, with the highest activities in the mouse and rat, intermediate levels in rabbit and guinea pig, and lowest levels in cat and dog. Of significance, since much data concerning diaphragmatic metabolism comes from canine studies, no classic type IIB fibers could be identified in the dog. In adult humans, type I fibers constitute approximately 50–55% of the total in the diaphragm, 65% in the intercostal muscles (Mizuno and Secher, 1989; Keens et al., 1978a), and 40% in the vastus lateralis (Keens et al., 1978a). In humans (Keens et al. 1978a), but not in rats (Nishiyama, 1965), dogs (Reid et al., 1987), or baboons (Maxwell et al., 1983), the intercostal muscles are also inhomogeneous. Mizuno and Secher (1989) studied the histochemical fiber type of the respiratory muscles postmortem in healthy male victims of sudden accidental death. They found that the occurrence of type IIA fibers is greater in expiratory intercostal (~35%) than in the inspiratory parasternal and external intercostal muscles (~17%), but comparable with the diaphragm (~28%).

They propose that the preponderance of these more oxidative fibers reflects adaptation to frequent activation of these muscles during nonrespiratory tasks, such as cough, speech, and postural support, in humans.

Regional heterogeneity in fiber type proportions also exists within the diaphragm itself. It rats, based on enzyme histochemistry, Metzger et al. (1985) found significantly more type I fibers in the costal than in the crural region, and a slightly higher percentage of type Is on the thoracic, relative to the abdominal surface. Consistent variability in the biochemical properties of the rat diaphragm have also been reported. Powers et al. (1990) assayed the activities of the SDH and lactate dehydrogenase (LDH) as representatives of citric acid cycle and glycolytic pathways, respectively, in the rat diaphragm. The SDH activity was 18% less in the crural than in the costal region, whereas LDH activity did not vary significantly among regions. They conclude that the crural region is significantly lower in oxidative capacity than the costal diaphragm. These regional differences may be species-dependent, however. Sieck et al. (1983) also found a higher percentage of SO fibers on the abdominal surface and more FOG and FF fibers on the thoracic surface in the cat diaphragm. These investigators were unable, however, to demonstrate regional differences in fiber type distribution among costal and crural parts of the cat diaphragm, although architectural differences were noted.

The developmental changes in respiratory muscle fiber type composition have been studied in human and nonhuman primates. Keens et al. (1978b) classified diaphragmatic fiber types into type I (slow oxidative) and type II (fast glycolytic) based on histochemical staining for mATPase and nicotinamide adenine dinucleotide tetrazolium reductase (NADH-TR) postmortem in humans from 24 weeks gestation to 59 years of age. Diaphragms from preterm infants were found to have only ~10% type I fibers, increasing at term to ~25%, and to ~55% after 2 years of age. No further increases were found beyond this age. The intercostal muscles underwent parallel developmental changes, increasing in the proportion of type I fibers from ~19%, to ~46%, to ~65%, at each stage, respectively. These authors suggested that, because of the relative paucity of oxidative fibers, the ventilatory muscles of newborn infants are more susceptible to fatigue than those of older subjects, a factor that may contribute to respiratory problems in the neonate. In baboons, however, Maxwell et al. (1983) identified a third intermediate fiber subtype (IIC) in fetal animals. This fiber bears histochemical similarities to type I fibers, including dark staining for NADPH-TR, but is intermediate (exhibiting dark staining following both acid and alkaline preincubation) in its M-ATPase–staining characteristics. Standard M-ATPase staining would classify these fibers as type II, although they are rich in aerobic enzymes. It is unclear whether these fibers represent a transitional stage, or a separate fiber type that atrophies in the immediate postgestational period. Their disappearance soon after birth results in an apparent increase in the proportion of type I fibers. This change, however, does not indicate a lack of aerobic capacity in the neonatal muscle. To the contrary, functional evaluation of contractility and fatigability in the same study indicates that the neonatal baboon diaphragm maintains force generation during repetitive stimulation better than the adult diaphragm and is among the most fatigue-resistant of mammalian skeletal muscles.

III. Substrate Utilization

A. Blood-Borne Substrates

Glucose

Species variability in rate of glucose uptake by the diaphragm is marked. In the resting, isolated rat diaphragm Gorski and Sikorska (1977) recorded a glucose uptake of 25–30 mg g^{-1} h (2.5 μmol g^{-1} min). At acid pH (6.8) the rate of uptake was reduced by 25%. In contrast, the diaphragm of the intact, anesthetized dog exhibits no glucose uptake during quiet breathing. With inspiratory resistive loading, glucose utilization increased in proportion to the increase in Vo_2di such that at a Vo_2di of 100 μl g^{-1} min, glucose uptake was 70–200 nmol g^{-1} min (Rochester and Brisco, 1979; Rochester, 1985). Although species differences in fiber type proportions (see foregoing) explain some of this discrepancy, the availability of substrates other than glucose in the intact dog, in contrast with the isolated rat glucose-perfused rat diaphragm model, has been offered as an alternative explanation (Rochester, 1985). This is likely to be an important factor, since the diaphragm demonstrates substantial ability to alter its pattern of substrate utilization, depending on availability. In fasted rats, diaphragmatic uptake of glucose is less than half that in fed rats, energy requirements being met instead by oxidation of lipid-derived substrates (Issad et al., 1987). This appears to be related to the fact that the diaphragm is continuously active, rather than being a feature specific to this muscle, since similar changes are seen in other muscles (postural muscles and heart) that are active at rest (Issad et al., 1987).

Lactate

The extent of evolution and uptake of lactate from the respiratory muscles has been controversial. In early studies, using the isolated perfused rat diaphragm, Hollanders (1968) and Rowlands (1969) recorded lactate release at a rate of 300 nmol g^{-1} min, which is similar to the in vivo diaphragm under hypoxic conditions. Stimulating the diaphragm at 2 Hz did not change the rate of lactate release, but stimulation at 50 Hz tripled it. The relevance of these findings to the metabolism of the normal diaphragm is uncertain, given the nonphysiological nature of this preparation. In intact spontaneously breathing dogs, moderate increases in work of breathing are not consistently associated with increased lactate release by the diaphragm (Robertson et al., 1977a; Rochester and Biscoe, 1979). As the work load increases, the diaphragm first utilizes lactate as a substrate and, eventually, becomes a net producer of lactate. Rochester and Biscoe (1979) noted a progressive increase in lactate uptake as VO_2di increased from 50 to 170 $\mu l\ g^{-1}$ min, and Robertson et al. (1977a) recorded lactate production of 145 $nmol/g^{-1}$ min during the application of severe inspiratory loads (VO_2di = 240 $\mu l\ g^{-1}$ min). In the study of Rochester and Biscoe (1979), furthermore, no lactate production was observed when phrenic venous PO_2 values exceeded 20 mm Hg.

Bazzy et al. (1991, 1987a,b) demonstrated that inspiratory flow-resistive loads to the point of respiratory failure did not result in increased lactate production. In rabbits, Ferguson et al. (1990a) found that progressive inspiratory threshold loading, to the point of respiratory failure, resulted in no increase in diaphragmatic lactate concentration unless the normal mechanisms that preserve diaphragmatic function are circumvented by phrenic pacing or thoracoabdominal binding. Lactate production during phrenic nerve pacing may, however, be subject to factors not yet fully understood. Pope et al. (1989a) found that an initial period of supramaximal phrenic nerve stimulation resulted in diaphragmatic fatigue and lactate production; however, a second subsequent pacing period, associated with a similar rate of fatigue and VO_2di, did not.

Fregosi and Dempsey (1986) found exhaustive exercise in rats to be associated with an increase in diaphragmatic lactate concentration (similar to the increase in arterial blood and plantaris muscle lactate concentrations) except at VO_2max, at which point the increase in respiratory muscle lactate concentration was less than that in blood or nonrespiratory skeletal muscle. Glycogen depletion was not observed, suggesting that the increase in lactate concentration resulted from an increase in lactate uptake, rather than from lactate production. In ponies, Manohar et al. (1988, 1990) demonstrated that extreme exertion was not associated with lactate evolution by the diaphragm.

During the development of respiratory failure in shock states, in contrast, arterial lactate is increased and mechanical ventilation alleviates some of this increase (Aubier et al., 1982). Excessive production of lactate by these muscles, however, is not the only mechanism that could have contributed to lactic acidemia under these conditions, nor is it the only process that could be potentially improved by eliminating respiratory muscle activation. Reduced hepatic blood flow may have impaired lactate clearance and, since cardiac output was fixed, elimination of respiratory muscle blood flow requirements would alleviate supply-critical conditions in this and other vital organs. Similarly, sites of lactate production, such as nonrespiratory skeletal muscles would become less dependent on glycolytic ATP synthesis as blood flow and oxygen delivery improved. More convincing, however, is the recent report of increased arteriovenous lactate gradient across the phrenic circulation during hemorrhagic shock in dogs (Ketani et al., 1990). Therefore, there may be a difference between the metabolic response to an imbalance between respiratory muscle substrate delivery and metabolic demand, depending on whether supply or demand are primarily affected.

Direct measurement of diaphragmatic lactate production has not been carried out in human subjects. Inspiratory (Eldridge, 1966; Jardim et al., 1981) and expiratory (Freedman et al., 1983) resistive-loading do increase peripheral blood lactate levels in normal volunteers, but only when breathing hypoxic gas mixtures and only to a modest degree. Factors other than increased respiratory muscle lactate production may have contributed to the observed peripheral lactic acidemia.

Free Fatty Acids

Free fatty acids (FFA) are a major source of fuel for skeletal muscles and are the preferred substrate of the resting rat diaphragm (Neptune et al., 1959). Muscle contraction enhances FFA uptake (Fritz et al., 1958) and further reduces glucose utilization (Issad et al., 1987). In humans, the shift toward lipid metabolism appears to be dependent on the availability of oxygen. In normal humans, Mannix et al. (1993) found inspiratory resistive-loading to be associated with a fall in the respiratory exchange ratio, reflecting increased respiratory muscle dependence on lipid-derived substrates, when subjects inspired normoxic gas mixtures, but not during hypoxic gas administration. Labeled palmitate is rapidly taken up by the diaphragm, such that at 10 min, 25% appears as diglyceride and 60% as triglyceride; after 2 h, the distribution of label is 13% as diglyceride and 75% as triglyceride (Herodek, 1968). Reductions in substrate delivery during shock alter the distribution of FFA uptake among the organs. In anesthetized, spontaneously breathing dogs subjected to hemorrhagic shock, Daniel et al. (1983) found that incorporation of radiolabeled palmitate into tissue lipids increased in the diaphragm, whereas in nonactive muscles (sartorius and rectus abdominis), uptake either remained unchanged or fell. Tissue phospholipid levels remained unchanged in the diaphragm, indicating that the uptake of FFA reflects replenishment of tissue stores, rather than phospholipid accumulation. The rectus abdominis, in contrast, demonstrated depletion of muscle phospholipid concentration.

B. Stored Substrates

Glycogen

Glycogen is the primary storage form of carbohydrate in all muscle cells. In isolated rat diaphragm, the incorporation of glucose into glycogen is inversely proportionate to the initial level of glycogen present (Bar and Blanchaer, 1965). Addition of glucose or lactate to the perfusate increases the rate of glycogenesis in fasted animals, the yield from glucose being four times that from lactate (Bar and Blanchaer, 1965). As in other skeletal muscles, insulin increases the rate of glycogenesis (Adolfsson, 1973), an effect that is modified by the initial glycogen level (Wermers et al., 1970); low levels enhancing glycogen synthase activity. The effects of insulin and glucose are also altered by contractile activity; stimulated contraction reduces the rate of increase in glycogen content in response to these stimuli (Wermers et al., 1970). Reciprocal regulation of glycogenolysis occurs in skeletal muscles, increases in glycogen phosphorylase activity being stimulated by catecholamines and by a fall in the ratio of ATP to AMP.

Because of the high capacity for aerobic metabolism, it is unclear to what extent the diaphragm depends on endogenous glycogen as a fuel source during the increases in its activity that are associated with exercise and lung disease. Depletion of glycogen in the diaphragm is correlated with the development of fatigue during direct nerve stimulation, as it is in peripheral skeletal muscles (Ferguson et al., 1990a). In rats, glycogen concentration in the diaphragm falls after prolonged exhaustive swimming (Gorski et al., 1978) and treadmill running (Moore and Gollnick, 1982), and slowly returns to normal over the subsequent 12 h. This suggests that endogeneous glycogen is needed by the respiratory muscles during physiological tasks and that depletion of these stores may contribute to their failure. Evidence conflicting with this view, however, has been presented by Fregosi and Dempsey (1986). These investigators reported a lack of significant glycogen utilization in rat respiratory muscles during normoxic exercise. Only under conditions of extreme metabolic demand, coupled with reduced O_2 transport, did glycogen utilization increase in the diaphragm and intercostal muscles. In contrast with this report, Ianuzzo et al. (1987), who carried out studies in which rats were exposed to a similar normoxic exercise regimen and sacrificed by similar techniques, found a significant reduction (43% of control values) in glycogen content in the diaphragm and intercostal muscles. The reduction occurred in both type I and II fibers. The reason for the discrepancy in the results of these two studies remains unclear.

The role that depletion of intramuscular carbohydrate stores plays in the pathophysiology of respiratory failure is also disputed. Depletion of glycogen has been observed in the fatigued dog diaphragm during hemorrhagic and cardiogenic shock (Aubier et al., 1982; Magder et al., 1985) and at the point of respiratory failure during septic shock (Hussain et al., 1986). When oxygen and blood-borne substrate availability is unrestricted, however, no relation between the development of respiratory failure and glycogen depletion has been demonstrated. Ferguson et al. (1990a) studied the effects of incremental inspiratory threshold loads on the biochemistry and function of the diaphragm in ketamine anesthetized rabbits. They found no evidence of either glycogen depletion or of contractile failure, despite the inability of the animals to continue to initiate inspiratory airflow. In this model, therefore, it appears that central factors or failure of transmission at the neuromuscular junction played a greater role in the pathophysiology of diaphragm failure than did imbalance between substrate availability and the metabolic requirements of the muscle.

Triglycerides

Triglycerides also form an important, although less immediately accessible, form of intramuscular energy storage. Gorski and Sikorska (1977) found that, during swimming, diaphragmatic triglyceride stores did not change in the first hour, a period over which the most rapid depletion of glycogen content was observed. At between 1 and 3 h of exercise, triglyceride levels fell to 65% of control values and then plateaued. Diaphragmatic triglyceride levels had returned to control values after 3 h of recovery in their study. Endogenous triglyceride breakdown appears primarily regulated by catecholamines acting through changes in cyclic AMP levels and involving intracellular calcium concentration (Abumrad et al., 1980). Insulin antagonizes the mobilizing effect of catecholamines.

High-Energy Phosphates

The intramuscular supply of ATP is so small that a contracting muscle would exhaust the available supply in minutes if its concentration were not vigorously defended. In the dog diaphragm, ATP and phosphocreatine concentrations averaged 3.8 μmol/g and 10.2 μmol/g, respectively, during quiet breathing, and 3.3 μmol/g and 12.2 μmol/g, respectively, during resistive loading. When the compensatory mechanisms that protect diaphragm function are bypassed by pacing the phrenic nerve, however, modest depletion of ATP and more severe depletion of phosphocreatine to 73 and 64% of control, respectively, occurred (Rochester, 1985). Similarly, during exercise, Fregosi and Dempsey (1986) found that ATP concentration in rat diaphragm and intercostal muscles was maintained at rest levels during exhaustive exercise under both normoxic and hypoxic conditions. Phosphocreatine levels, however, were markedly depleted. In contrast, when diaphragmatic oxygen and substrate supply are limited, evidence has been presented supporting net ATP catabolism by the diaphragm. Ketani et al. (1990) measured purine nucleotide degradation product (PNDP) concentrations in canine phrenic and peripheral skeletal muscle venous effluent as a marker of net ATP degradation during hypovolemic shock. They found a significant increase in both lactate and PNDP concentrations across the phrenic circulation. Across the hindlimb, however, lactate concentration was elevated, but PNDP concentrations were not. They interpreted these findings to indicate that anaerobic pathways may suffice to maintain ATP levels in resting muscle, whereas in the contracting diaphragm, anaerobic resynthesis of ATP may not keep up with energy requirements.

IV. Training Effects

Although endurance training increases aerobic enzyme and mitochondrial concentrations of skeletal muscle, little change can be demonstrated in the oxidative capacity of the myocardium (Holloszy and Booth 1973). This is attributed to the fact that the myocardium has such a high aerobic capacity that there is no need for further adaptation. The questions arise, therefore, whether or not the diaphragm which, like the heart, is also highly aerobic and continuously contracting, may be trained to an even higher level of endurance and whether or not such training may contribute to an overall improvement in exercise tolerance.

Studies of the effects of both whole-animal endurance training and of specific training of the respiratory muscles have been carried out. In rats, Moore and Gollnick (1982) found an increase in SDH, phosphorylase, hexokinase, and lactate dehydrogenase activities in the diaphragm and plantaris, but not the intercostal muscles, after 8–26 weeks of treadmill exercise training. Similarly, Ianuzzo et al. (1982) found increases in both aerobic and anaerobic enzyme concentrations in the rat diaphragm following 12–16 weeks of treadmill training of a magnitude comparable with that observed in the limb muscles. A further study by Powers et al. (1992) has recently demonstrated age-related and regional variability in the diaphragmatic responses to training. These authors found 10 weeks of treadmill exercise to be associated with increases in aerobic and anaerobic enzyme concentrations in the costal, but not in the crural, diaphragm of young rats. In aging animals, no training-induced increase in aerobic capacity of the costal diaphragm could be identified, although aerobic enzyme levels were higher in older untrained than in young untrained animals. In contrast to some previous studies, these investigators found increased aerobic enzyme concentrations in the intercostal muscles of both young and old trained animals. Also in apparent contradiction to the findings of the study of Powers et al. (1992), Gosselin et al. (1992b) were able to demonstrate an increase in SDH activity in all fiber types in both young and old animals following 10 weeks of treadmill training. The differences in the findings among these studies remains to be adequately explained.

Further insight into the adaptations that the respiratory muscles undergo during the stress of endurance training may be found in studies in which alterations in myosin heavy chain (MHC) subtypes have been quantified (Sugiura et al., 1990; Gosselin et al., 1992a). The MHC composition correlates with velocity of shortening and peak isometric force as well as the relative area occupied by specific fiber types. Thus, slow isoforms are preponderant in oxidative muscles, with large type I fiber populations, whereas the fast isoforms (IIa, IIb, IIc, and IId) are found in glycolytic muscles. Gosselin et al. (1992a) recently reported that treadmill training had no effect on the relative density of fast and slow MHC isoforms in the rat diaphragm, despite increases in SDH activity within the same muscle. The explanation for this apparently contradictory result may be that all fast isoforms are not equally associated with glycolytic energy production. In support of this thesis, Sugiura et al. (1990) have reported an alteration in fast MHC phenotype expression in the diaphragm (and limb muscle) with prolonged swim training, characterized by an increase in IIb and IId isoform concentrations. The increase in aerobic capacity may, therefore, reflect a shift in relative concentration of the fast isoforms, rather than an increase in preponderance of slow MCH isoform.

The diaphragm also exhibits metabolic and functional adaptation to training with resistive loads. Akabas et al. (1989) exposed unanesthetized sheep to inspiratory resistances for 2–4 h/day for 3 weeks. Training produced increases in citrate synthase, 3-hydroxyacyl-CoA dehydrogenase, and cytochrome oxidase in both the costal and crural diaphragm. These changes were associated with functional improvements reflected by a reduction in $Paco_2$ during application of the loads, higher transdiaphragmatic pressures (Pdi), and an ability to sustain this level of Pdi for up to 2 h longer than before the training protocol. Interestingly, increased aerobic capacity of the crural diaphragm, consistently absent in endurance exercise-trained rats, occurred when the respiratory muscles were specifically targeted for training. Presumably, the increased ventilation during exercise did not result in sufficient recruitment of the crural part to induce a training effect. The increased ventilatory load associated with exercise may, therefore, involve a different recruitment pattern for the costal and crural diaphragm than that associated with added inspiratory resistances, a possibility that requires further investigation.

V. Effects of Disease

A. Chronic Obstructive Lung Disease

Metabolic alterations in both respiratory and nonrespiratory muscles have been reported in patients with chronic obstructive pulmnary disease (COPD). In patients who had developed acute respiratory failure, moderate, but significant, reductions in muscle ATP and phosphocreatine and increases in muscle lactate have been found in both intercostal and quadriceps muscles (Gertz et al., 1977). In another series, biopsies of intercostal and latissimus dorsi muscles were performed in patients with COPD undergoing thoracotomy for suspected lung cancer (Campbell et al., 1980). Modest decreases in glycogen, ATP, and phosphocreatine concentrations, and increases in lactate concentrations, were found. The severity of airflow limitation, furthermore, correlated significantly with the severity of the abnormalities in muscle lactate and phosphocreatine levels. The ATP and phosphocreatine levels were also influenced by weight loss and the presence of malignant disease. In contrast, muscle fiber type proportions do not appear predictive of the severity of chronic airflow limitation. In COPD patients undergoing investigative thoracotomy, Sanchez et al. (1982) and Hards et al. (1990) found no relation between any test of pulmonary function and muscle fiber morphometry, although the severity of disease in the patients in these studies was fairly mild.

B. Corticosteroids

Long-term treatment with corticosteroids modifies the clinical picture of many patients with chronic lung disease. Ferguson et al. (1990b) studied the histopathology, biochemistry, and function of the diaphragm in rabbits treated with 10 mg/kg per day of cortisone acetate for 2 weeks. Marked pathological changes, including vacuolization, loss of fiber cross-sectional area, fragmentation, and myonecrosis, in association with decreased endurance, were found in the dia-phragm. Similar, but far milder, changes were also observed in the extensor digitorum longus (EDL). Glycogen levels were significantly elevated in the diaphragm, but were normal in the EDL. Lactate levels were increased to a similar extent in both muscles. Diaphragmatic lactate levels rose further with inspiratory loading in the steroid-treated animals, but not in the controls. Interestingly, the pathological changes involved the diaphragm to a greater extent than the peripheral muscle and affected all fiber types. This contrasts with reports in nonrespiratory muscles that suggest that steroid myopathy is most severe in inactive muscles, particularly those composed primarily of type II fibers (Jaspers and Tischler, 1986; Roy et al., 1985). Although no explanation for this finding has yet been established, it may be that the myopathy associated with steroid use is modified in the respiratory muscles because of the requirement for their continuous rhythmic activity.

VI. Summary

The oxygen consumption of the respiratory muscles is maintained over a wide range of oxygen deliveries owing to adjustment of oxygen extraction. As a result, as long as oxygen delivery is not limited, it remains well oxygenated and, hence, is not limited functionally by the availability of oxidative substrates. This seems to hold true, even during the application of severe inspiratory loads, and the development of respiratory failure under these conditions appears unrelated to metabolic factors occurring in the diaphragm.

When oxygen delivery is limited, during shock or by cardiovascular disease, deoxygenation of the respiratory muscles is demonstrable. The point at which this occurs depends on the metabolic requirements of these muscles, which is a direct function of the load they must overcome to sustain ventilation. At rest, the oxygen consumption of the diaphragm becomes limited at the same oxygen delivery as the whole body, thus any increase in its oxygen requirements will result in it becoming delivery-limited earlier than will be appreciated by measurement of whole-body oxygen extraction.

In the absence of adequate oxygen availability, the ability to enhance energy production through oxidation of free fatty acids results in increased dependence on glucose availability and, ultimately, on the anaerobic metabolism of stored glycogen. The resulting intracellular acidosis further impairs function of the mus-cle and limits the efficacy of energy production by inhibition of glycolytic en-zymes.

The diaphragm, therefore, is resistant to fatigue by merit of mechanical compensatory mechanisms that protect diaphragmatic function and because its oxygenation is protected by the tremendous capacity for enhancement of diaphrag-matic blood flow and oxygen extraction. It is particularly vulnerable, however, when the ability to call on these mechanisms is limited. This is particularly true when the ability to maintain blood flow in proportion to metabolic demand is limited and accounts for the frequency of respiratory failure as the mechanism of death during shock. Although further studies are required to validate the concept, these factors may also play a role in the respiratory limitation of exercise in patients with cardiovascular disease.

References

Aaron, E. A., Seow, K. C., Johnson, B. D., and Dempsey, J. A. (1992). Oxygen cost of exercise hyperpnea: Implications for performance. *J. Appl. Physiol.* 72: 1818–1825.

Abumrad, N. A., Tepperman, H. M., and Tepperman, J. (1980). Control of endogenous triglyceride breakdown in the mouse diaphragm. *J. Lipid Res.* 21: 149–155.

Adolfsson, S. (1973). Glycogen synthesis in rat diaphragm in vivo: A biphasic effect of insulin on glycogen synthetase enzyme. *Acta Physiol. Scand.* 87: 265–273.

Akabas, S. R., Bazzy, A. R., Dimauro, S., and Haddad, G. G. (1989). Metabolic and functional adaptation of the diaphragm to training with resistive loads. *J. Appl. Physiol.* 66: 529–535.

Anholm, J. D., Johnson, R. L., and Ramanathan, M. (1987). Changes in cardiac output during sustained maximal ventilation in humans. *J. Appl. Physiol.* 63: 181–187.

Aubier, M., Viires, N., Syllie, G., Mozes, R., and Roussos, C. (1982). Respiratory muscle contribution to lactic acidosis in low cardiac output. *Am. Rev. Respir. Dis.* 126: 648–652.

Bar, U., and Blanchaer, M. D. (1965). Glycogen and CO_2 production from glucose and lactate by red and white skeletal muscle. *Am. J. Physiol.* 209: 905–909.

Bark, H., Supinski, G., Bundy, R., and Kelson, S. (1988). Effect of hypoxia on diaphragm blood flow, oxygen uptake and contractility. *Am. Rev. Respir. Dis.* 138: 1535–1541.

Bazzy, A. R., Pang, L. M., Akabas, S. R., and Haddad, G. G. (1989). O_2 metabolism of the sheep diaphragm during flow resistive loaded breathing. *J. Appl. Physiol.* 66: 2305–2311.

Boutellier, U., and Farhi, L. E. (1986). Influence of breathing frequency and tidal volume on cardiac output. *Respir. Physiol.* 66: 123–133.

Burke, R. E., Levine, D. N., Zajac, F. E., Tsairis, P., and Engel, W. K. (1971). Mammalian motor units: Physiological–histochemical correlation in three types of cat gastrocnemius *Science* 174: 709–712.

Cala, S. J., Wilcox, P., Edyvean, J., Rynn, M., and Engel, L. A. (1991). Oxygen cost of inspiratory loading: Resistive vs. elastic. *J. Appl. Physiol.* 70: 1983–1990.

Campbell, J. A., Hughes, R. L., Sahgal, V., Frederiksen, J., and Shields, T. W. (1980). Alterations in intercostal muscle morphology and biochemistry in patients with obstructive lung disease. *Am. Rev. Respir. Dis.* 122: 679–686.

Cherniack, R. M. (1959). The oxygen consumption and efficiency of the respiratory muscles in health and emphysema. *J. Clin. Invest.* 38: 494–499.

Collett, P. W., Perry, C., and Engel, L. A. (1985). Pressure–time product, flow and oxygen cost of resistive breathing in humans. *J. Appl. Physiol.* 58: 1263–1272.

Daniel, A. M., Kapadia, B., and MacLean, L. D. (1983). Fatty acid supply and organ phospholipid turnover in two canine shock models. *J. Surg. Res.* 35: 218–226.

Davies, A. S., and Gunn, M. M. (1972). Histochemical fibre types in the mammalian diaphragm. *J. Anat.* 112: 41–60.

Easton, P. A., Fitting, J. W., and Grassino, A. E. (1987). Costal and crural diaphragm in early inspiration: Free breathing and occlusion. *J. Appl. Physiol.* 63: 1622–1628.

Eldridge, F. (1966). Anaerobic metabolism of the respiratory muscles. *J. Appl. Physiol.* 21: 853–857.

Ferguson, G. T., Irvin, C. G., and Cherniack, R. M. (1990a). Relationship of diaphragm glycogen, lactate and function to respiratory failure. *Am. Rev. Respir. Dis.* 141: 926–932.

Ferguson, G. T., Irvin, C. G., and Cherniack, R. M. (1990b). Effect of corticosteroids on diaphragm function and biochemistry in the rabbit. *Am. Rev. Respir. Dis.* 141: 156–163.

Field, S., Kelly, S. M., and Macklem, P. T. (1982). The oxygen cost of breathing in patients with cardiorespiratory disease. *Am. Rev. Respir. Dis.* 126: 9–13.

Freedman, S., Cooke, N. T., and Moxham, J. (1983). Production of lactic acid by respiratory muscles. *Thorax* 38: 50–54.

Fregosi, R. F., and Dempsey, J. A. (1986). Effects of exercise in normoxia and acute hypoxia on respiratory muscle metabolites. *J. Appl. Physiol.* 60: 1274–1283.

Fritts, H. W., Filler, J., Fishman, A. P., and Cournand, A. (1959). The efficiency of ventilation during voluntary hyperpnea: Studies in normal subjects and in dyspneic patients with either chronic pulmonary emphysema or obesity. *J. Clin. Invest.* 38: 1339–1348.

Fritz, L. B., Davis, D. G., Holtrop, R. H., and Dunder, H. (1958). Fatty acid oxidation by skeletal muscle during rest and activity. *Am. J. Physiol.* 194: 377–386.

Gertz, I., Hedenstierna, G., Hellers, G., and Wahren, J. (1977). Muscle metabolism in patients with chronic obstructive lung disease and acute respiratory failure. *Clin. Sci. Mol. Med.* 52: 395–403.

Gorski, J., and Sikorska, J. (1977). Effect of pH and lactate on glucose uptake by red and white skeletal muscle in vitro. *Acta Physiol. Pol.* 28: 441–444.

Gorski, J., Namiot, Z., and Giedroje, J. (1978). Effect of exercise on metabolism of glycogen and triglycerides in the respiratory muscles. *Pflugers Arch.* 377: 251–254.

Gosselin, L. E., Betlach, M., Vailas, A. C., Greaser, M. L., and Thomas, D. P. (1992a). Myosin heavy chain composition in the rat diaphragm: Effect of age and exercise training. *J. Appl. Physiol.* 73: 1282–1286.

Gosselin, L. E., Betlach, M., Vailas, A. C., and Thomas, D. P. (1992b). Training induced alterations in young and senescent rat diaphragm muscle. *J. Appl. Physiol.* 72: 1506–1511.

Green, N. J., Reichmann, H., and Pette, D. (1984). Inter- and intraspecies comparisons of fibre type distribution and of succinate dehydrogenase activity in type I, IIA and IIB fibres of mammalian diaphragms. *Biochemistry* 81: 67–73.

Hards, J. M., Reid, W. D., Pardy, R. L., and Pare, P. D. (1990). Respiratory muscle fiber morphometry: Correlation with pulmonary function and nutrition. *Chest* 97: 1037–1044.

Herodek, S. (1968). Temporal changes in the distribution of labelled palmitic acid in the different lipids of rat adipose tissue, liver and diaphragm. *Acta Biochem. Biophys. Acad. Sci. Hung.* 3: 227–237.

Hollanders, F. D. (1968). The production of lactic acid by the perfused rat diaphragm. *Comp. Biochem. Physiol.* 26: 906–916.

Holloszy, J. O., and Booth, F. W. (1973). Biochemical adaptation to endurance exercise in muscle. *Annu. Rev. Physiol.* 38: 217–232.

Hussain, S. N. A., Graham, R., Rutledge, F., and Roussos, C. (1986). Respiratory muscle energetics during endotoxic shock in dogs. *J. Appl. Physiol.* 60: 486–493.

Ianuzzo, C. D., Noble, E. G., Hamilton, N., and Dabrowski, B. (1982). Effects of streptozotocin diabetes, insulin treatment, and training on diaphragm. *J. Appl. Physiol.* 52: 1471–1475.

Ianuzzo, C. D., Spalding, M. J., and Williams, H. (1987). Exercise-induced glycogen utilization by the respiratory muscles. *J. Appl. Physiol.* 62: 1405–1409.

Issad, T., Penicaud, L., Ferre, P., Kande, J., Baudon, M. A., and Girard, J. (1987). Effects of fasting on tissue glucose utilization in conscious resting rats: Major glucose-sparing effect in working muscles. *Biochemistry* 246: 241–244.

Jardim, J., Farkas, G., Prefaut, C., Thomas, D., Macklem, P. T., and Roussos, C. (1981). The failing inspiratory muscles under normoxic and hypoxic conditions. *Am. Rev. Respir. Dis.* 124: 274–279.

Jaspers, S. R., and Tischler, M. E. (1986). Role of glucocorticoids in the response of rat leg muscles to reduced activity. *Muscle Nerve* 9: 554–561.

Keens, T. G., Bryan, A. C., Levison, H., and Ianuzzo, C. D. (1978a). Developmental pattern of muscle fiber types in human ventilatory muscles. *J. Appl. Physiol.* 44: 905–908.

Keens, T. G., Bryan, A. C., Levison, H., and Ianuzzo, C. D. (1978b). Developmental pattern of muscle fiber types in human ventilatory muscles. *J. Appl. Physiol.* 44: 909–913.

Ketani, L. H., Grum, C. M., and Supinski, G. S. (1990). Tissue release of adenosine triphosphate degradation products during shock in dogs. *Chest* 97: 220–226.

Magder, S. A., Lockhat, D., Luo, B. J., and Roussos, C. (1985). Respiratory muscle and organ blood flow with inspiratory elastic loading and shock. *J. Appl. Physiol.* 58: 1148–1156.

Mancini, D. M., Ferraro, N., Nazzaro, D., Chance, B., and Wilson, J. R. (1991). Respiratory muscle deoxygenation during exercise in patients with heart failure demonstrated with near-infrared spectroscopy. *J. Am. Coll. Cardiol.* 18: 492–498.

Mannix, E. T., Sullivan, T. Y., Palange, P., et al. (1993). Metabolic basis for inspiratory muscle fatigue in normal humans. *J. Appl. Physiol.* 75: 2188–2194.

Manohar, M., and Hassan, A. S. (1990). Diaphragm does not produce ammonia or lactate during high-intensity short-term exercise. *Am. J. Physiol.* 259: H1185–H1189.

Manohar, M., and Hassan, A. S. (1991). Diaphragmatic energetics during prolonged exhaustive exercise. *Am. Rev. Respir. Dis.* 144: 415–418.

Manohar, M., Goetz, T. E., Holste, L. C., and Nganwa, D. (1988). Diaphragmatic O$_2$ and lactate extraction during submaximal and maximal exertion in ponies. *J. Appl. Physiol.* 64: 1203–1209.

Maxwell, L. C., McCarter, R. J. M., Kuehl, T. J., and Robotham, J. L. (1983). Development of histochemical and functional properties of baboon respiratory muscles. *J. Appl. Physiol.* 54: 551–561.

McCool, F. D., Tzelepis, G. E., Leith, D. E., and Hoppin, F. G. (1989). Oxygen cost of breathing during fatiguing inspiratory resistive loads. *J. Appl. Physiol.* 66: 2045–2055.

Metzger, J. M., Scheidt, K. B., and Fitts, R. H. (1985). Histochemical and physiological characteristics of the rat diaphragm. *J. Appl. Physiol.* 58: 1085–1091.

Mizuno, M., and Secher, N. H. (1989). Histochemical characteristics of human expiratory and inspiratory intercostal muscles. *J. Appl. Physiol.* 67: 592–598.

Moore, R. L., and Gollnick, P. D. (1982). Response of ventilatory muscles of the rat to endurance training. *Pflugers Arch.* 392: 268–271.

Neptune, E. M., Sudduth, H. C., Fash, F. J., and Foreman, D. R. (1959). Quantitative participation of fatty acid and glucose substrates in oxidative metabolism of excised rat diaphragm. *Am. J. Physiol.* 196: 269–262.

Nishiyama, A. (1965). Histochemical studies on the red, white and intermediate muscle fibers of some skeletal muscles. I. Succinic dehydrogenase activity and physiological function of intercostal muscle fibers. *Acta Med. Okayama* 19: 177–189.

Oligaiti, R., Atchou, G., and Cerretelli, P. (1986). Hemodynamic effects of resistive breathing. *J. Appl. Physiol.* 60: 846–853.

Pean, J. L., Chuong, C. J., Ramanathan, M., and Johnson, R. L. (1991). Regional deformation of the canine diaphragm. *J. Appl. Physiol.* 71: 1581–1588.

Pope, A., Scharf, S., and Brown, R. (1989a). Diaphragm metabolism during supramaximal phrenic nerve stimulation. *J. Appl. Physiol.* 66: 567–572.

Pope, A., Scharf, S. M., and Brown, R. (1989b). Diaphragm metabolism during supramaximal phrenic nerve stimulation. *J. Appl. Physiol.* 66: 567–572.

Powers, S. K., Lawler, J., Criswell, D., et al. (1990). Regional metabolic differences in the rat diaphragm. *J. Appl. Physiol.* 69: 648–650.

Powers, S. K., Lawler, J., Criswell, D., Lieu, F. K., and Martin, D. (1992). Aging and respiratory muscle metabolic plasticity: Effects of endurance training. *J. Appl. Physiol.* 72: 1068–1073.

Reid, M. B., and Johnson, R. L., Jr. (1983). Efficiency, maximal blood flow, and aerobic work capacity of canine diaphragm. *J. Appl. Physiol.* 54: 763–772.

Reid, M. B., Ericson, G. C., Feldman, H. A., and Johnson, R. L. (1987). Fiber types and fiber diameters in canine respiratory muscles. *J. Appl. Physiol.* 62: 1705–1712.

Riley, D. A., and Berger, A. J. (1979). A regional histochemical and electromyographic analysis of the cat respiratory diaphragm. *Exp. Neurol.* 66: 636–649.

Riley, R. L. (1954). The work of breathing and its relation to respiratory acidosis. *Ann. Intern. Med.* 41: 172–176.

Robertson, C. H., Foster, G. H., and Johnson, R. L. (1977a). The relationship of respiratory failure to the oxygen consumption of, lactate production by, and the distribution of blood flow among respiratory muscles during increasing inspiratory resistance. *J. Clin. Invest.* 59: 31–42.

Robertson, C. H., Pagel, M. A., and Johnson, R. L. (1977b). The distribution of blood flow, oxygen consumption and work output among the respiratory muscles during unobstructed hyperventilation. *J. Clin. Invest.* 59: 43–50.

Rochester, D. F. (1985). Respiratory muscle blood flow and metabolism. In: *The Thorax*. Edited by C. Lenfant and C. Roussos. New York, Marcel Dekker, pp. 393–436.

Rochester, D. F., and Bettini, G. (1976). Diaphragmatic blood flow and energy expenditure in the dog, effects of inspiratory airflow resistance and hypercapnia. *J. Clin. Invest.* 57: 661–672.

Rochester, D. F., and Briscoe, A. M. (1979). Metabolism of the working diaphragm. *Am. Rev. Respir. Dis.* 119: 101–106.

Rowlands, S. D. (1969). The lactic acid production and glycogen content of perfused rat diaphragm. *Comp. Biochem. Physiol.* 30: 183–208.

Roy, R. R., Gardiner, P. F., Simpson, D. R., and Edgerton, V. R. (1985). Glucocorticoid-induced atrophy in different fibre types of selected rat jaw and hindlimb muscles. *Arch. Oral Biol.* 28: 639–643.

Sanchez, J., Derenne, J. P., Dobesse, B., Riquet, M., and Monod, H. (1982). Typology of the respiratory muscles in normal men and in patients with moderate chronic respiratory diseases. *Bull. Eur. Physiopathol. Respir.* 18: 901–914.

Scharf, S. M., Bark, H., Einhorn, S., and Tarasiuk, A. (1986). Blood flow to the canine diaphragm during hemorrhagic shock. *Am. Rev. Respir. Dis.* 133: 205–211.

Sieck, G. C., Roy, R., Powell, P., Blanco, C., Edgerton, V. R., and Harper, R. M. (1983). Muscle fiber type distribution and architecture of the cat diaphragm. *J. Appl. Physiol.* 55: 1386–1392.

Sugiura, T., Morimoto, A., Sakata, Y., Watanabe, T., and Murakami, N. (1990). Myosin heavy chain isoform changes in rat diaphragm are induced by endurance training. *Jpn. J. Physiol.* 40: 759–763.

Viires, N., Sillye, G., Aubier, M., Rassidakis, A., and Roussos, C. (1983). Regional blood flow distribution in dog during induced hypotension and low cardiac output. *J. Clin. Invest.* 72: 935–947.

Ward, M. E., Magder, S. A., and Hussain, S. N. A. (1992). Oxygen delivery-independent effect of blood flow on diaphragm fatigue. *Am. Rev. Respir. Dis.* 145: 1058–1063.

Ward, M. E., Chang, H. Y., and Hussain, S. N. A. (1993). Systemic and diaphragmatic O_2 delivery–O_2 consumption relationships. *J. Appl. Physiol.* (in press).

Wermers, B. W., Cavert, H. M., Harris, J. O., and Quello, C. F. (1970). Glycogen metabolism in perfused contracting white rat hemidiaphragm muscle. *Am. J. Physiol.* 219: 1434–1439.

25

Respiratory Muscle Energetics

CHARIS ROUSSOS

National and Kapodistrian University
   of Athens Medical School
Athens, Greece
McGill University
Montreal, Quebec, Canada

SPYROS ZAKYNTHINOS

Evangelismos Hospital
Athens, Greece

I. Introduction

The hydrolysis of ATP is the primary source of chemical energy for skeletal muscle metabolism, and the rate of hydrolysis varies depending on the intensity of the muscle contraction. Thermodynamic questions thus arise concerning the relationship of energy utilization to mechanical work and to heat production. Insofar as the respiratory muscles behave as other skeletal muscles, some general principles can be inferred; however, the particular requirements of the respiratory muscles warn against the glib assumption that they are the same as all other skeletal muscles. The general problems of muscle energetics are dealt with in several excellent reviews and original works (1–9).

II. Thermodynamics

Skeletal muscle exchanges both energy (work and heat) and matter (e.g., in the form of O_2 and CO_2). Thus it is an open thermodynamic system as opposed to a closed system, such as a piston in a cylinder with heat-conducting walls, in which energy is exchanged (but not matter). During contraction the mechanical events are accompanied and followed by the production of heat. According to the first law of thermodynamics,

$$n\Delta H = Q + W + \Delta(PV) \tag{1}$$

where n is the number of moles of reactant participating in the contraction, ΔH is the change in the molar enthalpy of the chemical reaction, Q is the heat produced, W is the external work performed (e.g., load displacement), and $\Delta(PV)$ is the pressure-volume component of the energy exchanged with the surroundings of the muscle. In a muscle, reactions take place at an almost constant pressure (atmospheric pressure), and thus the term $\Delta(PV)$ reduces to $P\Delta V$. Furthermore, the volume changes are trivial (5), and therefore PV in Eq. (1) can be omitted. Thus muscle can be considered a closed thermodynamic system at a constant pressure and volume (5), and Eq. (1) reduces to

$$n\Delta H = Q + W \tag{2}$$

For a closed system, the conservation equation for the difference of internal energy between two equilibrium states becomes

$$\Delta U = Q + W \tag{3}$$

where ΔU is the change of internal energy of the system between the two stages. From Eqs. (2) and (3) it follows that

$$n\Delta H = \Delta U \tag{4}$$

and consequently in this situation the terms *energy* and *enthalpy* can be used interchangeably in relation to the quantities symbolized by ΔH or ΔU.

A. Heat, Work, and Efficiency

During contraction the change in total enthalpy appears as heat and work in different proportions, depending on the force against which the muscle pulls. One portion of the total energy change performs work (free energy), and another portion is inextricably bound to the material transformation underlying that change and is not available to do work (bound energy or entropy). Theoretically, under optimal conditions, all free energy (G) can be transformed into work, which is conventionally also called maximum work (W_{max}). Therefore, during a reaction the total change in energy for 1 mol of reactant may be expressed as

$$\Delta H = \Delta G + T\Delta S \tag{5}$$

where ΔG is the change in free energy and $T\Delta S$ is the change in bound energy arising from the entropy change (ΔS) that occurs at temperature T (kelvin). Quantitatively, $\Delta S = Q/T$, where Q is the heat in calories that is absorbed in carrying a system reversibly from an initial to a final state through a small temperature change. However, only a fraction of the available free energy is converted into work, whereas the rest is transformed into heat. This fraction is determined by the conditions under which the reaction takes place, and the ratio of work to free energy defines the thermodynamic efficiency (*e*)

$$e = \frac{W}{n\Delta G} \qquad (6)$$

Thus the heat produced during muscular contraction equals the change in entropy plus the heat from the dissipation of free energy

$$\text{heat produced} = (\Delta G - e\Delta G) + T\Delta S$$
$$= \Delta G(1 - e) + T\Delta S \qquad (7)$$

When the muscle is maximally efficient (*e* = 1), the heat produced equals $T\Delta S$, whereas when the muscle does not produce work at all (*e* = 0), the heat produced equals $\Delta G + T\Delta S$.

In practice, the thermodynamic efficiency of a muscle in vivo is extremely difficult to estimate because the value of free energy of ATP is uncertain (10). This difficulty is further complicated by problems in determining energy balance during muscle contraction; a substantial amount of evidence indicates that more heat and work are produced during contraction than can be explained by the observed metabolic reactions (1). Hence for practical purposes the mechanical efficiency (*E*) of muscle contraction has been defined as

$$E = \frac{W}{Q + W} = \frac{W}{n\Delta H} \qquad (8)$$

In this chapter the term *efficiency* refers to *mechanical efficiency* as just defined.

B. Energy Balance

During muscular contraction the heat and work produced are greater than the amount of energy that can be explained by the observed metabolic reactions: observed ($Q + W$) = explained ($Q + W$) + unexplained ($Q + W$). The problem is important because identifying all the chemical reactions involved at the molecular level is central to understanding muscle contraction. Since the work of Hill (6), the subject has been under investigation without resolution. Fortunately, the problem can be approached from a phenomenological point of view by examining the total amount of energy changes observed during muscular contraction and partitioning it among the various processes, such as activation, shortening, tension development, and work performance.

Based on Hill's studies (6) with skeletal muscle, a balance sheet for the energy expenditure during muscle contraction has been established by Mommaerts (8) as

$$U_T = A + W + ax + f(P,t) \qquad (9)$$

where U_T is the total energy expenditure, *A* is the heat of activation, *ax* is the heat associated with shortening (*a* is a constant with units of force and *x* is the distance by which the muscle shortens), and $f(P,t)$ indicates that a component of heat production is related to the intensity and duration of the tension maintained. Equation (9) is expressed in Figure 1. This figure indicates that an unloaded isotonic and an isometric muscle twitch liberate approximately the same total energy in the form of heat. Figure 1 also gives the total energy as a function of the velocity of fiber shortening and gives the heat of shortening, the heat of activation, and the heat of tension and duration. The production of free heat is explained by the interaction of two opposing effects: (1) the decrease in time taken up by the shortening phase due to the duration of the active state and the tension-time index (TTI) and (2) the

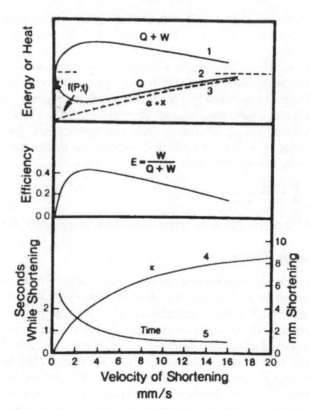

Figure 1 Variation of energy production (top) and efficiency (middle) during muscle twitches at different shortening velocities. Curve 1, total energy as function of velocity of fiber shortening; curve 2, heat production, which is composed of heat of shortening (curve 3), heat of activation, and heat of tension and duration [$f(P,t)$], which is the difference between curves 2 and 3. Energy production is greatest at velocity where greatest amount of work is done (Fenn effect). Interpretation of heat production (bottom) depicts time spent shortening (curve 5) and distance (x) shortened (curve 4). Q, heat; W, work; αx, heat of shortening; E, efficiency. (From Ref. 8.)

amount of shortening, which determines the heat of shortening. The efficiency changes are shown as a function of the velocity of shortening. As the velocity increases, the heat of shortening increases, reaching the largest values at high velocities of shortening when efficiency approaches zero. Conversely, as the velocity of shortening decreases, the displacement decreases, with the work reaching zero during isometric contraction, at which point efficiency is also zero. Between these two extremes there is an optimum efficiency that is ≈30% of the maximum velocity and also ≈30% of the maximum isometric tension. Thus there is no single value of mechanical efficiency for a muscle contraction; it depends mainly on the speed of shortening and on the various experimental conditions (see Sec. V). Figure 1 also shows that the energy output ($Q + W$) is greater when work is performed and is dependent on the amount of work done [Fenn effect (11,12)]. In simple terms, the Fenn effect states that more energy is liberated when a muscle performs work.

C. Energetics and Limitation of Airflow

During isotonic contraction the heat of activation [Eq. (9)] is liberated before the muscle develops tension; for analysis this heat can be ignored because it is not related to contraction but instead is liberated before the muscle develops tension. For simplicity, although it introduces a measurable error in the following analysis, the term $f(P,t)$ can be omitted to clarify the dominant relationships in Hill's equation that relate force, velocity, and the rate of extra energy liberated during muscle shortening.

Hill's fundamental equation is derived from the analysis of extra energy (U_E) liberated during muscle contraction in the form of work and heat (13). When a muscle moves a load (P) over a distance (x), the extra energy liberated as work is Px and as heat is ax (shortening heat):

$$U_E = Px + ax = (P + a)x \tag{10}$$

The rate at which this extra energy is liberated ($\dot{U}_E$) is obtained by differentiating Eq. (10) with respect to time:

$$\dot{U}_E = (P + a)\,dx/dt = (P + a)V \tag{11}$$

where dx/dt equals velocity (V).

Experimentally, $\dot{U}_E$ has an inverse linear relationship to load. With the use of a constant proportionality (b), $\dot{U}_E$ is equated to load ($P_0 - P$), where P_0 equals the maximal force developed during isometric contraction. Hence

$$(P + a)V = b(P_0 - P) \tag{12}$$

This equation can be rearranged algebraically:

$$(P + a)(V + b) = (P_0 + a)b \tag{13}$$

Equation (13) with all the constants on the right resembles the general equation for a hyperbola. When experimental results are plotted as a force-velocity curve, a hyperbolic relationship is found that is almost identical to the relationships obtained by Fenn and Marsh (2) from direct measurements.

Hill's equation indicates that the tension diminishes to zero as the velocity increases to its maximum unloaded value and that the force increases to its isometric value (P_0) as the velocity diminishes to zero. This prediction is best interpreted in terms of the observation that muscles must liberate extra energy when they shorten and do work (11,12). Such a transformation of chemical energy into mechanical energy has a limiting rate, which is proportional to $P_0 - P$, according to Hill's equation. With a limited rate of energy available for work, less tension can be maintained at high velocities of contraction than at low velocities. Agostoni and Fenn (14) have suggested that the velocity of airflow in maximal inspiratory efforts is limited by these metabolic force-velocity requirements. This conclusion is supported by the observation that the alveolar pressure developed during maximum inspiratory efforts is an inverse function of the velocity of airflow. For example, if a maximum inspiration is completed in 1 s, the alveolar pressure is never lower than -40 cm H_2O, whereas during a 1-s maximum inspiratory effort with closed glottis the alveolar pressure falls to -120 cm H_2O (Fig. 2). If this magnitude of alveolar pressure had developed during the inspiration with open glottis, it would have generated a much more rapid airflow. The factors limiting the rate of inspiration therefore seem to be not only the airway, lung, and chest wall resistance, but also the force-velocity or the metabolic properties of the inspiratory muscles. This conclusion, however, depends on the assumption that the respiratory muscles can be equally and maximally excited regardless of airway resistance. Insofar as respiratory muscles behave like other skeletal muscles, this assumption is not unrealistic.

III. Energy Supply

We use the term *energy supply* to indicate the supply of chemical energy to the respiratory muscles from sources available either in the muscles or in the blood.

A. Blood Flow

The classic approach to the measurement of blood flow ($\dot{Q}$) through any organ or tissue is by application of the Fick principle:

$$\dot{Q} = \dot{V}x/(ax - vx) \tag{14}$$

To apply this principal, the uptake or liberation of a substance (x) by the tissues ($\dot{V}x$) is measured and the concentration of x in all the arterial blood (a) entering and all the venous blood (v) leaving the tissue is measured. This approach cannot be applied to the respiratory muscles as a whole because of the number of separate arteries and veins. However, the Fick principle can approximate blood flow to the diaphragm. The history of attempts to estimate the blood flow—and the O_2

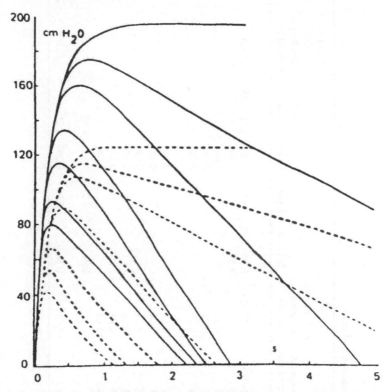

Figure 2 Positive (continuous lines) and negative (broken lines), alveolar pressures versus time from beginning of maximum expiration and inspiration made as quickly as possible against different resistances. Lowest line corresponds to the tests with no added resistance except that of the flowmeter and its connection; intermediate lines correspond to progressively higher resistances, and the top line, to an infinite resistance. Expiratory curve, not completely shown in diagram, intercepts abscissa at 9.5 s, and the two inspiratory ones, respectively, at 5.8 and 10.5 s. (From Ref. 14.)

consumption ($\dot{V}O_2$)—of the respiratory muscles has therefore been dominated by the indirect approach. Techniques for measuring diaphragmatic blood flow have been described in excellent original works (15–36) and are reviewed in Chapter 23. In the present chapter are discussed some aspects of blood flow to the respiratory muscles that we would like to particularly emphasize.

Table 1 summarizes the data on the amount of blood flow received by the various respiratory muscles under different conditions in the dog, pony, sheep, rabbit, and monkey. The respiratory muscles increase their blood flow as the load of breathing increases. This increase is especially prominent in the diaphragm. Perfusion per unit mass of both the diaphragm and other respiratory muscles increases substantially during hyperventilation induced by hypercapnia, hypoxia,

Table 1 Respiratory Muscle Blood Flow Under Various Conditions

	Artificial ventilation	Quiet breathing	Unobstructed hyperventilation	Resistance to inspiratory airflow	Exercise	Hypoxia	Shock	Heat stress	Maximum tetanic electrophrenic stimulation	Intermittent phrenic stimulation
Inspiratory muscles										
Diaphragm	0.04–0.18	0.08–0.25	0.18–0.33	0.52–2.0	0.96–2.45	0.21	0.50	1.71–2.09	0.43	1.39–4.5
External intercostals	0.03	0.07–0.12	0.25	0.68	1.2		0.80			
Scalenes	0.04	0.06–0.08	0.05	0.29			0.04			
Serratus anterior	0.04	0.04–0.08	0.02	0.12			0.04			
Serratus posterior	0.05	0.04	0.03	0.02			0.04			
Expiratory muscles										
Transverse abdominal	0.05	0.05–0.09	0.17	0.23			0.10			
Internal intercostals	0.04	0.04–0.11	0.15	0.54			0.15			
Internal oblique	0.04	0.04–0.07	0.07	0.14			0.08			
External oblique	0.03	0.03–0.04	0.04	0.12			0.04			
Rectus abdominis	0.03	0.03–0.07	0.03	0.02			0.03			
Ileocostalis	0.04	0.04–0.06	0.04	0.03			0.04			
Inspiratory and expiratory intercostal muscles	0.04	0.15			0.43	0.07		0.29		
Control group	0.04–0.06	0.03–0.17	0.04	0.04	0.55	0.05	0.007	0.01	0.01	0.07

Values in ml/g/min.

exercise, or heat stress (19,21,26,27,30) or during an increase in the work of breathing caused by an inspiratory or expiratory resistance to airflow (22,23,28,29).

Effect of Muscle Contractile Activity on Respiratory Muscle Blood Flow

Perhaps the most important determinant of respiratory muscle blood flow is the level of muscle contractile activity. In the dog, blood flow per gram appears to be similar for all respiratory and nonrespiratory muscles during mechanical ventilation (Table 1). In the transition from mechanical ventilation to spontaneous resting ventilation, only the blood flow to the diaphragm and external intercostal muscles increases. At low and moderate levels of ventilation or inspiratory resistive breathing, the relationship of blood flow to work of breathing remains linear for all respiratory muscles. However, as the work of breathing becomes greater than 4 cal/min during high inspiratory resistive breathing, the blood flow to the diaphragm (and to a lesser degree to the intercostals) increases exponentially, reaching a value of ≈2 ml/g/min (Fig. 3). This corresponds to a 25-fold increase over the resting level when the work of breathing increases 15 times. A similar relationship is obtained if the tension-time index (TTI) is used instead of the work of breathing (22,29). This index appears to be a good indicator of muscle energy expenditure (see Sec. II.D). High diaphragmatic blood flow has also been observed during exercise [0.96 ml/g/min (26) or 0.86–2.45 ml/g/min (37)], the increase of blood flow being much higher in the costal than in the crural regions of the diaphragm (Fig. 4), heat stress [2.09 ml/g/min (27)], and intermittent electrophrenic stimulation [1.39 ml/g/min (19) or 2–4 ml/g/min (24,25)].

During breathing against a high expiratory threshold load (20 cm H_2O), the blood flow to the respiratory muscles of dogs increases predominantly to the conventionally defined expiratory muscles (Fig. 3) and particularly to the transverse abdominal muscle (0.70 ml/g/min), followed by the internal obliques (0.40 ml/g/min), internal intercostals (0.30 ml/g/min), and external obliques (0.20 ml/g/min) (28). However, the striking feature is that although the blood flow to the expiratory muscles has been tested only up to 2.5 cal/min of work of breathing, the transverse abdominal muscle receives almost three times more blood flow per gram than the diaphragm during inspiratory resistive breathing for comparable work done on the lung (28,29). These results may indicate that the expiratory muscles are at a mechanical disadvantage compared with inspiratory muscles and require greater tension and energy supply in generating a given pleural pressure. The diaphragm has been clearly shown to receive the largest amount of blood flow per gram, 2.0 ml/g/min during inspiratory resistive breathing, corresponding to 10 cal/min of work of breathing and during severe heat stress (27,29). Despite this, it is not known whether the transverse abdominal muscle or other expiratory muscles are also able to increase their blood flow to the same degree as the diaphragm at comparable metabolic demands.

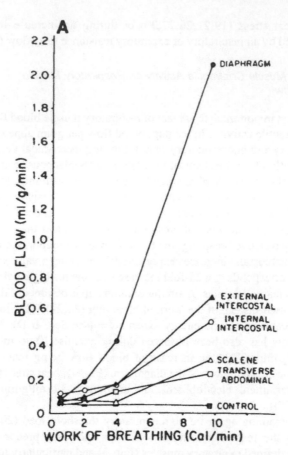

Figure 3 Blood flow to respiratory muscles during inspiratory (A) and expiratory (B) loaded breathing. Note marked increase of diaphragmatic blood flow with increased rate of work of breathing. Transverse abdominal receives largest amount of blood flow at comparable rates of work done on the lung (e.g., 2 cal/min). (From Ref. 29.)

Total blood flow to the respiratory muscles during expiratory threshold loading is much higher at comparable levels of work of breathing (i.e., 2.5 cal/min) than either inspiratory loads or hyperventilation (Fig. 5), reaching 13% of the cardiac output (28). The large fraction of the cardiac output destined for the respiratory muscles represents the combination of an increased blood flow to the muscles and a decreased cardiac output. Inspiratory resistive breathing, however, induces a fourfold increase in the work of breathing (10 cal/min) compared with resting levels, resulting in the total blood flow to the respiratory muscles almost doubling (400 ml/min vs. 230 ml/min during expiratory threshold loading). Nevertheless the blood flow represents ~10% of the cardiac output because the latter remains unchanged (29).

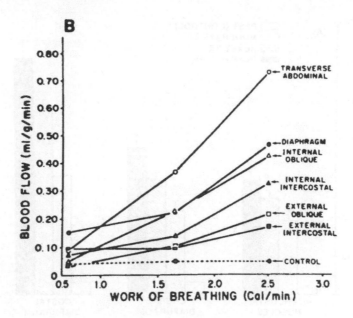

During high rates of work of breathing in dogs, the increase in blood flow to the respiratory muscles is distributed preferentially to the inspiratory or expiratory muscles or both depending on the means of increasing the task of breathing. During hyperventilation induced by CO_2 rebreathing, 45% of the increase in blood flow to the respiratory muscles goes to expiratory muscles and 55% goes to inspiratory muscles; the diaphragm receives 40% of this total increase (30). During inspiratory resistive breathing, 25% of the increase in blood flow goes toward the expiratory muscles, whereas 75% goes toward the inspiratory muscles; the diaphragm receives 50% of this total increase (29). Finally, during expiratory threshold loaded breathing, 80% of the augmented flow goes to the expiratory muscles and 20% to the inspiratory muscles. Furthermore, at low expiratory work loads the internal intercostals receive most of the augmented blood flow, whereas at high expiratory work loads the abdominals are the main recipients (28).

Studies of limb skeletal muscles have shown that limb muscle tension development produces two quite opposite effects on muscle blood flow. First, the increased muscle metabolic activity resulting from contraction leads to the local release of vasoactive substances that relax vascular smooth muscle, producing a reduction in vascular resistance and an increase in muscle blood flow. In addition, muscle tension development results in the compression of intramuscular vessels, increasing vascular resistance and tending to decrease muscle blood flow. Several studies have suggested that moderate to high levels of diaphragm tension development can act to compress the intradiaphragmatic vasculature, limiting the maximum

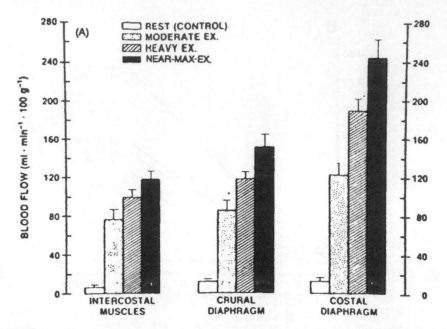

Figure 4   (A) Blood flow to intercostal muscles and crural and costal regions of the diaphragm in healthy ponies at rest and during graded (moderate, heavy, near-maximal) exercise. Note that, although at rest costal and crural phrenic blood flows were similar, during exercise costal blood flow was much higher than crural. (B) Changes in regional and total diaphragmatic fraction of cardiac output in the same experiments. Note that costal diaphragm of ponies received 1.9% of cardiac output during near-maximal exercise, whereas crural diaphragm's shave was 0.3%. Entire diaphragm received 2.21% of the cardiac output, representing an increment of 23.5% above control. (From Ref. 37.)

blood flow that can be achieved during strenuous respiratory muscle contractions (38,39). The magnitude of this compressive effect appears to be a function of the amount and duration of the tension generated during diaphragmatic contraction. At moderate levels of tension development, the magnitude of the decrease in flow resulting from compression during contractions is roughly a linear function of the diaphragmatic TTI, defined as the product of the relative duration of contraction (T_I/T_{TOT}, where T_I is the duration of inspiratory contraction and T_{TOT} is the duration of each breathing cycle), and the relative magnitude of contraction (P/P_{max} where P is the tension generated during contraction and P_{max} is the maximum tension-generating ability of the muscle). Therefore, at moderate levels of tension development (P/P_{max} 20–80%) the net compressive effect of contraction is a function of both the magnitude and duration of tension development. At extremely high levels of tension development (P/P_{max} exceeding 80%), however, diaphragm blood flow appears to stop entirely during contraction, the amount of blood flow depending solely on the

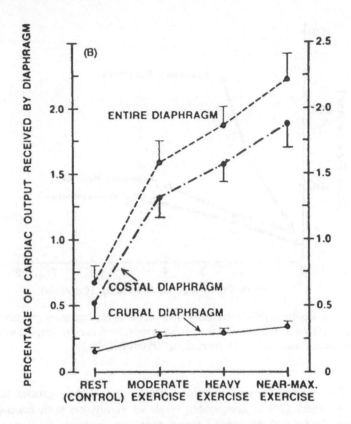

duration of muscle relaxation. As a result, diaphragm blood flow is inversely related to TI/TTOT when tension exceeds 80% of maximum (39).

Autoregulation of Diaphragm Blood Flow

Diaphragmatic blood flow at rest, during exercise, during low O_2 breathing, and during unobstructed hyperventilation has been shown to be related to cardiac output (18,21,23,26), presumably caused by the associated changes in arterial pressure. However, no significant relationship has been established between cardiac output and respiratory muscle perfusion during resistive breathing (22,28,29). This difference may indicate that the respiratory muscles receive the required blood flow according to their energetic demands despite a large variation in cardiac output. The findings of Rous and Gilding (15), who reported that the diaphragm remains well perfused in hemorrhagic shock, support this proposition. Additional evidence favoring this interpretation was found by Viires et al. (31), who demonstrated that when cardiac output was reduced to 30% of control, the blood flow to the respiratory muscles, particularly the diaphragm, increased as the

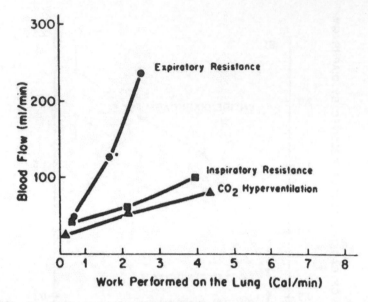

Figure 5 For similar rates of work performed on the lung, expiratory resistance requires a significantly greater total blood flow to respiratory muscles than either inspiratory resistance or hyperventilation induced by CO_2 rebreathing. (From Ref. 30.)

ventilation increased. These blood flow values were slightly greater than those reported by others (30) at comparable levels of ventilation with normal cardiac output (Fig. 6); i.e., as the cardiac output decreases in shock, respiratory muscle blood flow increases, possibly exceeding 20% of the cardiac output (31). Consistent with autoregulation of diaphragmatic blood flow (i.e., the vascular response, which maintains blood flow independent of alterations in perfusion pressure) are also the findings of Hussain et al. (40) and Reid and Johnson (41). In fact, decreasing arterial pressure in steps by controlled hemorrhage, Hussain et al. (40) proved that diaphragmatic blood flow was independent of arterial pressure (i.e., plateau of pressure-flow ventilation) within the normal ranges of arterial pressure during spontaneous unobstructed quiet breathing as well as during inspiratory loading. At lower arterial pressure flow was directly related to pressure (Fig. 7). In tissues that autoregulate, a rise in arterial pressure normally causes increased vascular tone and decreased vascular conductance; blood flow is thereby maintained relatively constant despite changes in perfusion pressure. Reid and Johnson (41) found a negative correlation between diaphragmatic vascular conductance and mean aortic pressure in normoxic animals, consistent with vascular autoregulation in the diaphragm. When vascular tone was abolished with vasodilators, vascular conductance in the diaphragm became a function of perfusion pressure and autoregulation was abolished (Fig. 8). On the contrary, Scharf et al. (42)

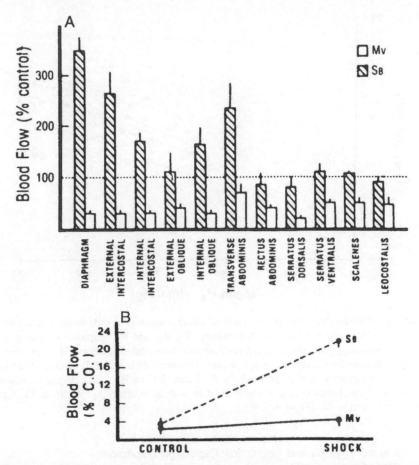

Figure 6 Blood flow to respiratory muscles during low cardiac output (30% of control) in spontaneously breathing (Sb) or mechanically ventilated (Mv) dogs. (A) Respiratory blood flow expressed in percent change from values obtained during quiet breathing (control) with normal circulation (horizontal dotted line). (B) Respiratory blood flow expressed in percent of cardiac output. Note large amount of respiratory blood flow during Sb, amounting to 20% cardiac output compared with 3% of cardiac output during Mv. (From Ref. 33.)

suggested that diaphragmatic blood flow is not autoregulated during hemorrhagic shock. However, the ranges of arterial pressues studied were not large and may not have included pressures sufficiently above the critical pressures for autoregulation. Thus, taken together, the above studies indicate that because of autoregulation, the diaphragm, even when subject to hypotension and low cardiac output, retains the ability to increase its blood flow in response to increased metabolic demands.

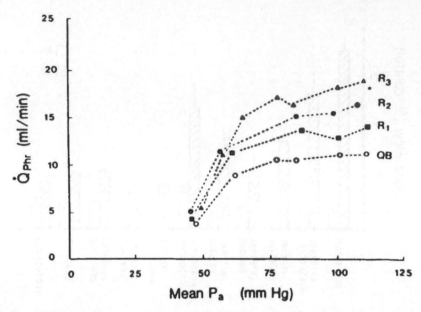

Figure 7   Relationship between mean arterial blood pressure (Pa) and phrenic arterial blood flow (Qphr) from one dog. QB, quiet breathing; R_1, R_2, and R_3, inspiratory loading with resistance increasing peak transdiaphragmatic pressure two-, three- and fourfold, respectively. Note that pressure-flow relations always plateau. However, during quiet breathing, diaphragmatic flow is independent of Pa between Pa of 75 and 120 mm Hg, while during inspiratory loading the Qphr plateau ends at a higher Pa than with quiet breathing. At lower Pa, Qphr is directly related to Pa. (From Ref. 40.)

Effect of Hypoxia and Mechanical Factors on Diaphragm Blood Flow

Several studies have shown that respiratory muscle blood flow increases during systemic hypoxemia (23,43). Adachi and co-workers, for example, found that diaphragm blood flow increased by 198% during exposure to 10% oxygen and by 450% during exposure to 5% oxygen, while intercostal muscle blood flow increased by 30% and 129%, respectively, during exposure to these two levels of inspired oxygen (23). These increases appear to be caused largely by the effect of hypoxemia activating chemoreceptors and thereby increasing respiratory muscle contractile activity by augmenting respiratory drive from the central nervous system. However, it has been shown that even when diaphragm activity is held constant, blood flow increases during hypoxia (44). In addition, hypoxia is recognized as an important component of hyperemia in the working diaphragm (41,44). This latter action of hypoxia is thought to reflect hypoxia's direct effect of eliciting vasodilation of muscle vasculature. In fact, a sharp rise in vascular conductance occurred as

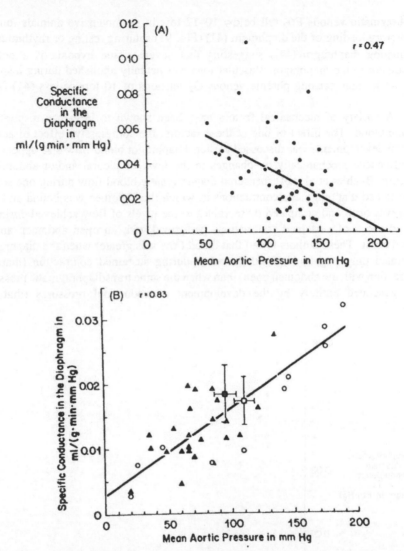

Figure 8 Relationship of vascular conductance in diaphragm to mean aortic pressure (A) in absence of pharmacological vasodilation in normoxic animals and (B) in dogs during pharmacological vasodilation (▲) or when diaphragmatic venous O_2 tension had been lowered to 10 torr or less by arterial hypotension (○). Negative correlation in A consists of diaphragmatic vascular autoregulation, while positive correlation in B indicates abolishment of this autoregulation. (From Ref. 41.)

diaphragmatic venous PO_2 fell below 10–12 torr in normotensive animals during inspiratory loading of the diaphragm (41) (Fig. 9) or during resting or rhythmically contracting diaphragm (44), suggesting that severe tissue hypoxia is a potent vasodilator in the diaphragm. Vascular tone was actually abolished during inspiratory work loads causing phrenic venous O_2 tensions of 10 torr or less (41) (Fig. 8B).

A variety of mechanical factors have been shown to influence respiratory muscle blood. The effect of one of these factors, the compressive effect of active tension development, was discussed earlier. Diaphragm blood flow also appears to be influenced mechanically by changes in the level of pleural and/or abdominal pressure. Buchler et al. (24) measured diaphragmatic blood flow during one series of sustained diaphragmatic contractions in which the abdomen was bound and the chest was open and compared these values to the levels of flow achieved during a second series of sustained contractions performed with an open abdomen and a closed chest. These authors found that blood flow was greater when the diaphragm generated only negative pleural pressures during sustained contraction (that is, contraction with the abdomen open) than when the same transdiaphragmatic pressure was generated entirely by the development of abdominal pressures (that is,

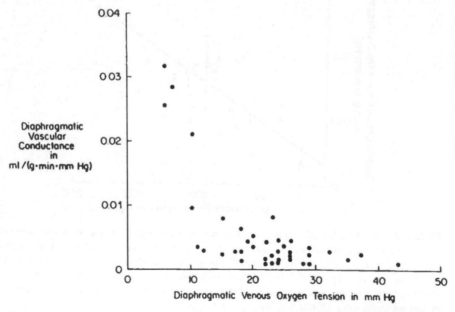

Figure 9 Relationship of diaphragmatic vascular conductance to diaphragmatic venous O_2 tension in normotensive dogs during inspiratory loading of the diaphragm. Note that conductance begins to increase sharply at O_2 tensions below 15 torr, suggesting that severe tissue hypoxia is a strong vasodilator in the diaphragm. (From Ref. 41.)

contraction with the chest open). These results suggest that high abdominal pressures may be transmitted to the diaphragm musculature, compressing intramuscular vessels and increasing vascular resistance, while negative pleural pressures may act to hold intradiaphragmatic vessels open, decreasing vascular resistance. However, during intermittent diaphragmatic contractions, high positive abdominal pressures do not affect total blood flow, since any inhibition of blood flow during the contractile period can be compensated for during the relaxation period between contractions. Another factor that appears to influence the level of diaphragm blood flow mechanically is diaphragm fiber length. Supinski and co-workers have shown that stepwise increases in diaphragm fiber length (from approximately 85 to 110% of Lo, where Lo is the length at which diaphragm tension is greatest during tetanic stimulation) produce progressive reductions in muscle blood flow (45). This was found to be true for the resting diaphragm as well as during rhythmic contractions developing high (tension 80% of maximum) and low (tension 20% of maximum) levels of active tension. These authors have suggested that this effect of length is, at least in part, mechanical in origin. As muscle length increases, intramuscular vessels may be stretched, developing a stress along their longitudinal axis and, as a result, narrowing. Reductions in vascular diameter may, in turn, explain the reduction in diaphragm blood flow resulting from increases in muscle length. This study also found that resting blood flow was a linear function of the passive tension developed in the diaphragm at different muscle fiber lengths, with flow falling as passive tension increased. Because the level of passive tension is an index of the longitudinal stress created in response to stretch, this latter finding is consistent with the possibility that the effect of length on muscle blood flow may be due to increased passive tension development. This finding also suggests that the effects of active and passive tension may in some respects be similar, in that both may result in the application of stresses to the microvasculature that result in a reduction in vessel diameter.

Limits of Blood Flow to the Diaphragm

Quantification of blood flow distribution to the respiratory muscles has revealed that under a variety of conditions and metabolic requirements these muscles, particularly the diaphragm, can increase their perfusion without apparent limits. Furthermore, the highest observed flow per unit weight to the diaphragm, 600 ml/100 g/min (41), is greater than the flow observed in most other skeletal muscles (46–48), even in the heart [$\approx$500 ml/100 g/min (49)].

Reid and Johnson (41) attempted to calculate the maximum blood flow to the diaphragm in dogs by producing a flaccid diaphragmatic vasculature with no possibility of autoregulation by local pressure changes. These authors used large doses of adenosine and nitroprusside while the animals were breathing 6% O_2 against added resistances. The vascular conductance (Gdi), which was linearly related to the rate of diaphragmatic work of breathing before the vasodilation, became a linear function of mean aortic blood pressure ($\bar{P}a$) (Fig. 8B) and was independent of the diaphragmatic work load:

$$Gdi = (1.32\bar{P}a + 29.6) \times 10^{-4} \tag{15}$$

where $\bar{P}a$ is expressed in mm Hg and Gdi is expressed in millimeters per gram per minute per mm Hg. Thus maximal blood flow to the diaphragm ($\dot{Q}di,max$) can be estimated by a modification of Eq. (15):

$$\dot{Q}di,max = (1.32\bar{P}a^2 + 29.6\bar{P}a) \times 10^{-4} \tag{16}$$

where $\dot{Q}di$ is expressed as milliliters per gram per minute. Thus, under conditions in which O_2 availability might limit diaphragmatic work, blood flow to the muscle becomes exquisitely sensitive to changes in arterial blood pressure. Based on Eq. (16), maximal blood flow to the diaphragm in dogs might range from 243 ml/100 g/min at a mean perfusion pressure of 125 mm Hg down to 45 ml/100 g/min at a perfusion pressure of 50 mm Hg. Maximum blood flow to the diaphragm, amounting to 600 ml/100 g/min, was measured by Reid and Johnson (41) in dogs having mean aortic blood pressure equal to 189 mm Hg. [Equation (16) predicts $\approx$530 ml/100 g/min.] Viires et al. (31) have shown that during shock, with a blood pressure of $\approx$50–60 mm Hg, the blood flow to the diaphragm is 50 ml/100 g/min. Comparison of this value with that predicted by Eq. (16) indicates that perhaps in the presence of low cardiac output the diaphragmatic blood flow reaches its maximum level and is governed only by the perfusion pressure. With an arterial pressure of 120 mm Hg, as shown by Robertson et al. (29), the calculated $\dot{Q}di,max$ is $\approx$2.10 ml/min, which is not different from that observed during breathing against high inspiratory resistances (2.07 ml/min). Thus, although the diaphragmatic blood flow did not reach a plateau in the various experimental settings reported, the blood flow in these two conditions (low cardiac output or breathing against a high inspiratory resistance) might approximate the maximum attainable blood flow. In fact, Buchler et al. (25) have shown that during electrophrenic stimulation in dogs at various combinations of intensity, duration, and frequency of contraction while maintaining blood pressure constant at $\approx$120–150 mm Hg, blood flow to the diaphragm reached its maximum of 200–400 ml/100 g/min; this value is comparable to that found by Robertson et al. (29) during high inspiratory resistive breathing. This finding of Buchler et al. supports the notion that in experiments with high inspiratory resistance the diaphragm received its maximum attainable blood flow (106).

Factors that affect the maximum diaphragmatic blood flow, other than the perfusion pressure, may be perivascular pressures during contraction restricting blood flow and/or other mechanical factors previously discussed. These factors may account for at least part of the scatter of data in experiments relating diaphragmatic vascular conductance and aortic blood pressure during maximal vasodilation (Fig. 8B).

Recently, endothelium-derived relaxing factor (EDRF) has been recognized as a major determinant of the changes in vessel diameter in response to changes in blood flow and to a variety of chemical mediators (e.g., ATP, ADP, serotonin, histamine). In addition, it has been shown that in the diaphragm EDRF plays an important role in the regulation of baseline vasomotor tone and its release modulation contributes to the reactive vasodilatory response to transient vascular occlusion (reactive hyperemia) (50). Because vascular occlusion is accompanied by the most dramatic fluctuations in flow likely to be encountered under physiological conditions and because many of the proposed mediators of metabolic control also influence EDRF release (51), it is probable that modulation of EDRF release is one of the underlying mechanisms of maximal vasodilation of the diaphragm when its work is increased during arterial hypotension and/or hypoxemia.

B. Substrate Metabolism

The respiratory muscles are not qualitatively different from other skeletal muscles in terms of substrate metabolism, i.e., glucose, acetoacetate, triglycerides, D-3-hydroxybutyrate, fatty acids, L-lactate, and amino acids (52–54). However, the important feature of the respiratory muscles (particularly the diaphragm), which like the heart have to work continuously to sustain life, is that they function mainly aerobically; because they receive their energy supply in "real time" through their abundant blood flow, the fuel storage in these muscles is of little importance. Thus, taking the stoichiometry for glucose combustion and using only intramuscular glycogen stores, the maximal time (t_{max}) during which the greatest energy yield possible is

$$t_{max} = \frac{6 \text{ glycogen}}{\dot{V}O_2 \text{ max}} = \frac{6 \text{ mmol/kg}}{\text{mmol/kg/min}} \tag{17}$$

The factor "6" stands for the O_2 equivalent. Assuming 60 mmol glycogen (≈ 10 g)/kg and a maximum O_2 consumption ($\dot{V}O_2$ max) of ≈ 20 mmol/kg/min [corresponding to ≈ 45 ml/100 g/min—a value close to the estimated $\dot{V}O_2$ max of the diaphragm (see Sec. III.C)], the muscle will be exhausted in 18 min. This time becomes markedly shorter if lactate is produced and should be contrasted with 100 min calculated for typical skeletal muscles (52). The point meriting emphasis is that glycogen storage, or other forms of fuel storage (e.g., endogenous lipids), are advantageous only during those short periods when the tissue cannot maintain a high capacity for extraction of substrates from the blood. It then depends on energy stores for short periods of high power output, conditions that are much more typical of limb muscles than of respiratory muscles.

How do the respiratory muscles utilize the different substrates at various work rates? Busse (23a) and Rochester and Briscoe (55) found that as the ventilation increases and the diaphragmatic $\dot{V}O_2$ increases up to 10 ml/100 g tissue/min, $\approx 50\%$ of the diaphragm's energy requirements is derived from the oxidation of carbohydrates. For example, a $\dot{V}O_2$ of 10 ml/100 g tissue/min equals 446 μmol O_2/100 g tissue/min. At that level, glucose and lactate utilization levels are 7 and 60 μmol/100 g/min, respectively. The O_2 equivalent, based on 6 mol O_2/mol glucose and 3 mol O_2/mol lactate, is 222 μmol/100 g/min, which accounts for half the total Vo_2. The remainder of the O_2 requirement is probably met by oxidation of free fatty acids—as in other muscles. In fact, Busse (23a) showed that diaphragmatic uptake of free fatty acids range from 2 to 20 μmol/100 g/min until diaphragmatic $\dot{V}o_2$ exceeds 10 ml/100 g/min, at which point utilization of free fatty acids increases approximately threefold. If the oxidation of each mole of oleic acid requires 25.5 mol O_2, the levels of fatty acid utilization reported by Busse (23a) could well meet the remaining half of the diaphragm's requirements.

Most studies indicate that the diaphragm and perhaps the other respiratory muscles are resistant to anaerobic metabolism (29,44,55–60). The very low or zero level of the diaphragmatic lactate production is similar to that of the heart. This strongly suggests that glycolytic pyruvate production is adjusted to its rate of aerobic oxidation. Apparently the diaphragm, unlike other skeletal muscles, does not produce lactate when venous partial pressure of O_2 (Po_2) values fall to 20–30 mm Hg (60–62). Robertson et al. (29) found that when diaphragmatic venous Po_2 is between 15 and 20 mm Hg, diaphragmatic lactate production is insignificant. Similarly, Rochester and Briscoe (55) have shown that diaphragmatic lactate production becomes prominent only when diaphragmatic venous Po_2 falls below 10–20 mm Hg. However, when the respiratory muscles are subjected to a very high power output, they do employ anaerobic metabolism to maintain adequate ventilation before becoming exhausted. Hollanders (63) has demonstrated that the excised perfused diaphragm can produce lactate for a prolonged period. Normal humans breathing 15% O_2, who hyperventilate through inspiratory resistances, increase their blood lactate by 0.4 mM (56). Similarly, normal subjects breathing against very high inspiratory resistances and inhaling either room air or 13% O_2 increase their blood lactate by $\approx$1 mM (57). Although there may be other factors, high blood lactate levels have also been found in patients with severe asthma (64). The exact origin of lactate and the rate of lactate removal by the liver have not been established. However, it is reasonable to suggest that strenuous work by the respiratory muscles may be partly responsible for elevated blood lactate levels.

Assuming that all the glycogen stored in the respiratory muscles is used anaerobically, one can calculate the maximum level of lactic acid produced from glycogen alone. In the presence of 60 mmol glycogen/kg, with the respiratory muscles comprising 15% of the total-body muscle mass or $\approx$4 kg in a 70-kg human, the total amount of lactate that can be produced is 480 mmol. This amount would result in a blood level concentration of $\approx$10 mM lactate if it were evenly distributed in all the body fluids and if it were not utilized. This value could be even higher if other sources of lactate are taken into consideration, e.g., glucose supplied by the circulation and amino acids. However, such high lactate production by the respiratory muscles and high blood lactate concentration can only serve as general guidelines in view of the number of assumptions made. Nonetheless, there are clinical situations that mimic and may approximate these limits. In a patient with cardiorespiratory disease there may be a combination of high ventilation, stiff lungs, arterial hypoxemia, and low cardiac output. The production of lactate by the respiratory muscles may then be significant, whereas the uptake by the liver due to low perfusion is reduced. Aubier et al. (65) subjected two groups of dogs to the same degree of low cardiac output by pericardial tamponade and found that the blood lactate concentration in the spontaneously breathing animals reached 9 mM, a value twice as high as that of the paralyzed and mechanically ventilated dogs (Fig. 10).

C. Oxygen Cost of Breathing

The diaphragm, like the heart and quite probably the other respiratory muscles, obtains its energy almost entirely by oxidative metabolism over a large range of work output. In these organs, enthalpy changes can be closely approximated to $\dot{V}O_2$. Even though the amount of heat liberated per gram of fat oxidized (≈ 9 kcal) is more than twice that per gram of carbohydrate or protein (≈ 4 kcal), the enthalpies expressed as kilocalories per liter of $\dot{V}O_2$ are quite similar for various substrates, i.e., 4.69 kcal for fat, 5.05 kcal for carbohydrate, and 4.60 kcal for protein. This similarity stems from the fact that more O_2 is needed to metabolize a gram of fat than a gram of carbohydrate or protein. Therefore, regardless of the substrate being

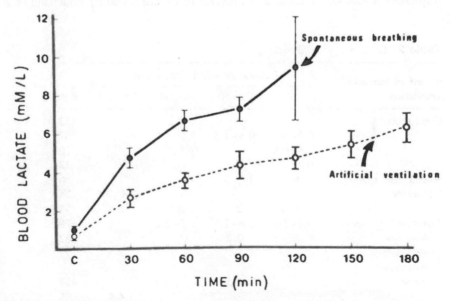

Figure 10 Blood lactate levels in two groups of dogs submitted to low cardiac output. Spontaneously breathing dogs had greater blood lactate concentration than the paralyzed and mechanically ventilated dogs. (From Ref. 65.)

oxidized, the enthalpies of the metabolic reactions responsible for ATP production can be estimated quite well from measurements of $\dot{V}O_2$.

Measurement of Oxygen Cost of Breathing

Direct Approach

The classic method for measuring the $\dot{V}O_2$ of an organ or a region is application of the Fick principle [Eq. 14)]: O_2 consumption ($\dot{V}O_2$) = blood flow ($\dot{Q}$) × arteriovenous O_2 content differences ($CaO_2 - C\bar{v}O_2$). This principle can be applied only if the total blood flow to the organ or tissue can be measured; this is not the case for the respiratory muscles in humans because an estimate of muscle mass is needed to permit expression in terms of absolute blood flow. Using this technique in animals, however, one may extrapolate the findings to humans, assuming that the situations are similar.

During artificial ventilation, when the diaphragm is inactive, the $\dot{V}O_2$ of the diaphragm in dogs is 0.2–0.8 ml $O_2/100$ g/min (21,23,30), which is similar to the values for other resting skeletal muscles (Table 2), whereas during quiet breathing it is 0.5–2.0 ml $O_2/100$ g/min. The diaphragmatic $\dot{V}O_2$ increases as the ventilation and work of breathing increase. Thus during unobstructed hyperventilation the diaphragmatic $\dot{V}O_2$ increases further [1.7–3.0 ml $O_2/100$ g/min (21,30)], whereas the highest levels of diaphragmatic $\dot{V}O_2$ occur during breathing against high respiratory resistances. Indeed, at the highest resistance tested by Robertson et al.

Table 2 Oxygen Cost of Breathing

Means of increasing ventilation	Pulmonary ventilation, L/min				Ref.
	20	20–50	50–100	100–270	
Dead space	1	2	3.2		153
	0.2–0.5	0.5–1.5	0.5–1.5		67
	0.4–0.8		0.5		70
	0.2				72
Added dead space	1	2 –3			66
Voluntary				2.4–7.9	74
	1	2	3	8	75
Voluntary and added dead space	0.4–1.1	0.6–2.3	1.5–3.5		128
		2.2			82
Steady-state voluntary				8.3	77
Exercise		1.5			154
				4.4	76
CO_2	0.3–0.8				154

Values in ml/L ventilation.

(29) the diaphragm consumed 24 ml $O_2/100$ g/min. Similar information is not available for the other respiratory muscles. However, assuming that the increase in the total-body $\dot{V}O_2$ during hyperventilation or resistive breathing is due to the increase in aerobic metabolism of the respiratory muscles, the $\dot{V}O_2$ increase from a control value of $\approx 150–200$ ml O_2/min during respiratory resistive breathing may indicate that the respiratory muscles extracted an extra 50 ml O_2/min. Furthermore, ≈ 25 ml O_2 was taken up by the diaphragm.

Indirect Approach

A different, indirect approach for measuring the $\dot{V}O_2$ pioneered by Liljestrand (66) has been used mainly in humans by several investigators. The total-body $\dot{V}O_2$ and ventilation are measured at rest; ventilation is then increased voluntarily by the addition of dead space or, preferably, by breathing CO_2. By extrapolating the changes in $\dot{V}O_2$ and ventilation, the O_2 cost of breathing can be calculated (Fig. 11). This approach is difficult to apply because the proportion of total $\dot{V}O_2$

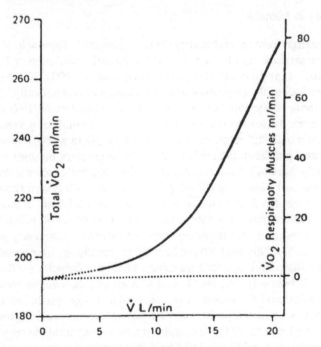

Figure 11 Relation between oxygen consumption and ventilation. The solid curve indicates the total oxygen consumption as measured. The extrapolation of this line to zero ventilation determines the level of the horizontal broken line, which indicates the magnitude of the oxygen consumption used for functions other than breathing. The vertical distance between this horizontal line and the curve represents the oxygen cost of breathing, as indicated by the scale of ordinates on the right. (Data from Refs. 66 and 95.)

of the respiratory muscles is small (only 1–2%). Physiologically it is difficult to achieve conditions at rest during which the basal (nonrespiratory) $\dot{V}O_2$ is sufficiently stable (± 1–2%), and at high levels of ventilation, nonrespiratory muscles may become active. Furthermore, $\dot{V}O_2$ may increase in other tissues, notably the heart. Analytically this method is also difficult to assess, again because of the small $\dot{V}O_2$ of the respiratory muscles. Thus with the classic open-circuit method the inspired-expired O_2 difference (5%) at rest with a minute ventilation of 7 L/min falls to $\approx 0.5\%$ at 70 L/min, so an analytical error of $\pm 0.05\%$ causes a 10% error in the estimate of total $\dot{V}O_2$—10 times the likely $\dot{V}O_2$ of the respiratory muscles. Campbell et al. (67) sought to overcome this analytical difficulty by using a modification of the Benedict-Roth closed-circuit method for measuring $\dot{V}O_2$ (68,69). This approach, however, has its own problem, notably that fluctuations in FRC make the slope of the spirometric trace (i.e., $\dot{V}O_2$) difficult to determine precisely. In addition the circuit—spirometer, CO_2 absorber, and air space—increases the respiratory cost at high ventilation.

Studies in Humans

Four facts emerge from several studies using Liljestrand's approach. (1) At rest the $\dot{V}O_2$ of the respiratory muscles is ≈ 0.25–0.5 ml/min/L ventilation or 1–2% of basal $\dot{V}O_2$ (a "gain" expressed as $\dot{V}O_2$ produced/O_2 cost of 100). (2) As ventilation increases, the $\dot{V}O_2$ of the respiratory muscles increases hyperbolically. (3) The slope of the hyperbola is variable between subjects. Campbell et al. (67) describe one subject in whom the respiratory $\dot{V}O_2$ was only 0.5 ml/min/L at a ventilation of 80 L/min, which would still represent a gain of ≈ 100. (4) In a few studies of patients with respiratory problems, the resting $\dot{V}O_2$ of the respiratory muscles was increased (approximately doubled), but more important, the hyperbolic increase with increased ventilation was early and steep (67,70). In one subject with severe emphysema (67) the increase exceeded 5 ml/min/L at a ventilation of 15 L/min, a total O_2 cost of breathing of 125 ml/min. This patient had a $\dot{V}O_2$ max of <460 ml/min, partly due to his severely reduced ventilatory capacity and defective pulmonary gas exchange that caused >25% of his total $\dot{V}O_2$ to be used for breathing. Extrapolation of these data indicates that at the subject's maximum breathing capacity (≈ 200 L/min) the gain would fall below 1; i.e., the O_2 cost of a greater increase in breathing would exceed the additional O_2 intake. The conceptual design establishing a level of ventilation beyond which a further increase becomes uneconomic (gain falls below 1) was pioneered by Otis (71); he calculated that a comparable level of ventilation for CO_2 elimination would be ≈ 140 L/min in normal subjects.

The large variation in estimates of O_2 cost of breathing among different investigators and, more important, between subjects in the same series (Fig. 12; Table 2) can be explained either by physiological variation or by experimental differences. The differences observed between subjects may certainly reflect individual variations that become very important in estimating the efficiency of the

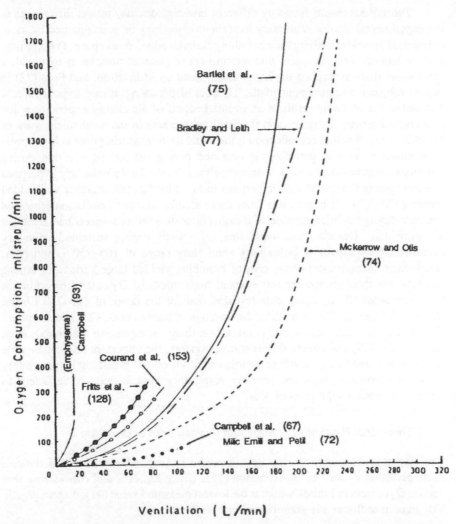

Figure 12 Oxygen cost of breathing at various levels of ventilation. Ventilation is increased either by breathing through a dead space or voluntarily (administering CO_2 to avoid hypocapnia). Note variability among studies and steep slope of patients with emphysema. (From Ref. 79.)

respiratory muscles. The reason for such differences is not known; the variations between subjects may be due to differences in muscle fiber composition. However, such variations may also be explained by the different responses of individuals to high ventilatory tasks. People with a high O_2 cost of breathing may use more muscles, such as postural muscles, that do not necessarily directly inflate the thorax.

The various results found by different investigators may reflect differences in the experimental setting. Voluntary hyperventilation may be accompanied by more extraneous muscular activity than breathing through added dead space. Posture may also be important to the extent that recruitment of postural muscles is involved, a mechanism that can explain the high values found by Milic-Emili and Petit (72) in supine subjects. Measurement of the O_2 cost of breathing during hypocapnia, if allowed to occur, could result in an overestimation of the energy expenditure due to increased airway resistance and the resultant increase in the mechanical work of breathing (73). Another complication is the usual short measuring time at high levels of ventilation; $\dot{V}O_2$ in particular is obtained during periods of <1 min during voluntary hyperventilation (74), within the first 1–3 min during voluntary hyperpnea and rebreathing (75), or during hyperpnea induced by exercise together with added inspired CO_2 (76). It is not clear from these studies whether ventilation remained constant during the brief duration of measurement or whether subjects had achieved a steady state. Despite these arguments, in a study during sustained voluntary normocarbic hyperpnea at pulmonary ventilatory range of 103–250 L/min (77), steady-state measurement of O_2 cost of breathing yielded large variability among subjects, but their grouped results showed high values of O_2 cost of breathing at high ventilation. Their group data revealed that for the range of 103–250 L/min, $\dot{V}O_2$ was 8.31 ml/L. This resembles the findings of Bartlett et al. (75) and Shephard (76) during exercise. Although O_2 cost of breathing varies among individuals even after training (77) and among different investigators, the important and inescapable conclusion is that at high levels of ventilation of O_2 cost of breathing is measurably high. One wonders, however, whether respiratory muscle mass is sufficient to account for such a high level of $\dot{V}O_2$.

Theoretical Predictions of Maximum Oxygen Cost of Breathing

The diaphragm is known to meet its augmented metabolic O_2 needs by increments in its perfusion as well as O_2 extraction (55). Using Eq. (16) and considering that venous O_2 content is 1 ml/dl, which is the lowest measured value (41), diaphragmatic $\dot{V}O_2$ max in milliliter per gram per minute becomes

$$\dot{V}O_2 \text{ max} = (1.32 \, \bar{P}a^2 + 29 \, \bar{P}a) \cdot (Ca_{O_2} - Cv_{O_2}) \times 10^{-4} \tag{18}$$

where Ca_{O_2} is arterial O_2 content and Cv_{O_2} is venous O_2 content expressed as milliliters of O_2 per deciliter of blood. With $\bar{P}a = 120$ mm Hg and assuming that the hemoglobin concentration is 15 g/100 ml blood (≈ 20 ml O_2/dl blood), the maximum $\dot{V}O_2$ by the diaphragm is ≈ 40 ml/100 g/min. This value is substantially greater than the maximum observed (25 ml/100 g/min). We have previously theorized that blood flow reaches the maximum achievable level either during low cardiac output or when breathing against a high inspiratory resistance. Until this level (≈ 2 ml/100 g/min, with an arterial pressure of 120 mm Hg), blood flow to the diaphragm has an approximately linear relationship to O_2 consumption (41) (Fig. 13). Theoretically, $\dot{V}O_2$ max could

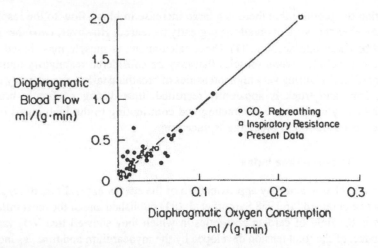

Figure 13 Relationship between diaphragmatic blood flow and O_2 consumption during quiet breathing and during increased work of breathing. Data from the study include normoxic and normotensive control measurements at rest and during increased inspiratory resistive loading (●). For comparison averaged data are included from previous publications (29,30), using graded inspiratory resistance (□) or CO_2 rebreathing (○) to increase O_2 consumption, a regression line is shown for these average data. (From Ref. 41.)

be achieved at a higher load only by increasing CaO_2–CvO_2. We found supportive evidence in animals subjected to severe shock. As suggested (31), the diaphragmatic blood flow in these experiments reached its maximal value at Pa = 50 mm Hg [(Fig. 6); see Sec. III.A]; in addition, the CaO_2–CvO_2 was 18–19 ml/100 ml blood. Thus it is apparent from several studies (21,22,23a,28–31,55) that at low levels of work, the O_2 demands are achieved primarily by increasing CaO_2–CvO_2 with little increase in blood flow; at moderate levels of respiratory work and $\dot{V}O_2$, the O_2 requirements of the diaphragm are met primarily by increased blood flow. However, when the blood flow reaches its maximum, any further increase in $\dot{V}O_2$ appears to be achieved by a further increase in CaO_2–CvO_2.

An estimation of the total mass of the respiratory muscles in dogs shows that these muscles constitute 5–6% of the total-body weight, and this represents ≈ 14–15% of the total-body muscle weight (29), assuming that 40% of the body consists of muscles. Assuming that all inspiratory and expiratory muscles can increase their $\dot{V}O_2$ as much as the diaphragm does [Eq. (18)], the theoretical $\dot{V}O_2$ max of the respiratory muscles for a 20-kg dog is ≈400–500 ml/min and for a 70-kg human is ≈1500–1800 ml/min. To achieve these levels of $\dot{V}O_2$ in humans the blood flow to the respiratory muscles must amount to 8.5 L/min. Yet these values of $\dot{V}O_2$ are of the same magnitude as those observed in normal humans approaching maximum breathing capacity (74,75,77) or breathing through high inspiratory resistances (78,79). This coincidence can be explained, although not proved, by accepting the premise that there is a large increase in blood flow to the respiratory muscles when the work of breathing is greatly increased. However, two other factors should be taken into account. (1) These calculations of muscle mass based on the dog do not include several muscles that may be considered respiratory muscles in humans (80). (2) During very high intensities of breathing tasks, almost every muscle in the arms and trunk is apparently recruited; thus during maximum breathing capacity many muscles are contracting and contributing to the high levels of $\dot{V}O_2$, but their contribution to breathing is uncertain.

D. Tension-Time Index

How can a reliable and easy approximation of the energy expenditure of respiratory muscles be obtained? In 1958 Sarnoff et al. (81) published one of the most influential papers in the field of cardiac energetics in which they showed that $\dot{V}O_2$ varied as the product of the total tension developed by the myocardium and time, as indicated by the area under the curve of the systolic pressure, the so-called tension-time index (TTI). [The term *tension-time index* ($\int T dt$) or mean tension ($\bar{T}$) is traditionally used not only when tension per se, but also pressure (e.g., pleural pressure), is measured. It is calculated as the tension or pressure integrated over a period of 1 min.] They also reported that TTI bore little relation to the external work of the heart and was a better index of myocardial O_2 usage than the peak systolic pressure. Intuitively this latter conclusion is easily understood by considering that in a tetanized skeletal muscle with repetitive stimulation, tension soon plateaus, whereas energy expenditure continues, albeit at a reduced rate. Under such conditions TTI would be the better index and not the peak tension alone.

The importance of the tension developed in respiratory muscle energetics was initially stated by McGregor and Becklake (82). They found a different relationship between work and O_2 cost of breathing ($\dot{V}O_{2rs}$) when they compared unloaded hyperventilation with breathing through a resistance. However, the relationship between force developed by the respiratory muscles and their $\dot{V}O_2$ was the same for the two conditions. These findings suggest that force is a better index of energy consumption of the respiratory muscles than work. Subsequently, the relationship between diaphragmatic $\dot{V}O_2$ and TTI was examined by Rochester and Bettini (22) in dogs during hyperventilation and breathing through a resistance. They found a good correlation between these parameters, indicating that TTI could be a useful index of $\dot{V}O_2$ and therefore of the changes in enthalpy of the respiratory muscles. More recently, Field et al. (83) concluded that, although the TTI of the diaphragm is a good index of $\dot{V}O_2$, over a wide range of respiratory patterns during resistive breathing, work rate ($\dot{W}$) is not. However, in the above studies TTI has not been sufficiently examined under various conditions to assess the validity of this possibility. In fact, in the heart during sympathetic stimulation (84), hypothermia (85), and norepinephrine or calcium infusions (86), there is a clear discrepancy between TTI and $\dot{V}O_2$. Subsequently, Collett et al. (87) found in subjects breathing through an inspiratory resistance at constant volume that TTI is a good index of O_2 cost of breathing only when mean inspiratory flow ($\dot{V}$) is constant and that the slope of this relationship between $\dot{V}O_2$ and TTI increases with increasing $\dot{V}$. In addition, they concluded that in contrast to TTI, work rate can predict the energy consumption over a large range of inspiratory flow rates, pressures, and work rates. Furthermore, the same authors (88) proved that during inspiratory resistive breathing against fatiguing loads in which TTI was kept constant, work rate determines endurance. Since the mechanism underlying fatigue has been considered in terms of energetics as an imbalance between energy supply and demand, the above results also indicate that work rate is a better index of O_2 cost of breathing than TTI.

Applying Eq. (9), regarding energy expenditure during muscle contraction, to the respiratory muscles, $\dot{V}O_{2rs}$ during breathing at a constant tidal volume is given by (89)

$$\dot{V}O_{2rs} = K_1 A + K_2 \dot{W} + K_3 TTI \tag{19}$$

where K_1 corresponds to the frequency to contraction and K_2 and K_3 are assumed to be constant, $\dot{W}$ represents work rate, and TTI the development and maintenance of tension. The component of shortening (ax) is omitted here because it is negligible in mammalian muscle at body temperature (90). It is apparent that during isometric contraction, because work equals zero, TTI is an index of O_2 consumption. As previously mentioned, it has been proposed that TTI of the respiratory muscles may reflect their O_2 consumption also under conditions of dynamic contraction (22,82, 83). This implies that the O_2 cost of shortening and performing work may be small in relation to that required for the development and maintenance of tension. However, the results of Engel and co-workers (87–89) indicate that the O_2 cost of performing work at high flow rates is high in comparison to that required for tension development and maintenance.

Since the rate of mechanical work ($\dot{W}$) is the product of TTI and the average airflow ($\dot{V}$), because

$$\dot{W} = \bar{P} V_T f$$

$$= \frac{\bar{P} T_I f}{T_I} V_T \qquad \text{(substituting TTI for } \bar{P} T_I f\text{)}$$

$$= \frac{TTI}{T_I} V_T$$

$$= TTI \, \dot{V} \tag{20}$$

where $\bar{P}$ is mean inspiratory pressure, T_I is inspiratory time, and f is frequency, it follows that

$$\dot{V}O_{2rs} = \frac{\dot{W}}{E} = TTI \, \frac{\dot{V}}{E} \tag{21}$$

where E is mechanical efficiency. The results of Collett et al. (87) are compatible and may be considered as experimental expressions of this equation. Since E was constant (≈ 2), $\dot{V}O_{2rs}$ was found to be linearly related to TTI when $\dot{V}$ remained constant, but the slope of this relationship increased with increasing $\dot{V}$. Furthermore, as pointed out by Roussos and Macklem (90a), for TTI to be proportional to $\dot{V}O_{2rs}$, the ratio of the average airflow (which can be considered an expression of the average velocity of shortening) to the efficiency must remain relatively constant. This implies that E should increase indefinitely with $\dot{V}$, which clearly is not possible because there is a limiting (maximal) value of E. In fact, as Figure 1 shows, the efficiency of skeletal muscle increases rapidly with velocity of shortening until it reaches a maximum at a speed corresponding to about 20% of maximal velocity (8). Beyond this critical velocity, efficiency slowly declines. Therefore, operating on the ascending limb of the efficiency-velocity relationship or within a small range of velocities during daily activities could make the TTI index a good approximation of the energy demands.

IV. Work of Breathing

A. Definitions

External work (W) is performed when a force (F) moves its point of application a length (l). The work then equals Fl, or $Fl \cos a$, if the direction of the force and that of the displacement differs by an angle a. Work is also done by a torque in rotating a shaft, in which case work is the product of the torque times the angular displacement. In a fluid system, work is performed when a pressure (P) changes the volume (V) of the system. Because pressure is force per unit area, force may be replaced by pressure $\times$ area (A), and therefore $W = P\,A\,l$; because $Al = V$, then $W = P\,V$.

When a muscle contracts, it either shortens (miometric contraction), lengthens (pliometric contraction), or does not change its length (isometric contraction). During a miometric contraction the muscle does work on something, and the work so performed is called positive. If a force does work on a contracting muscle, the displacement is opposite to the direction of the force exerted by the muscle, and the latter must lengthen. This is called negative work. Finally, during an isometric contraction, no displacement takes place and therefore no mechanical work is performed.

B. Graphical Analysis of Work

In physical terms, work, in a fluid system, is described by the relation:

$$W = \int P\,dV \tag{22}$$

The work done by the respiratory muscles during a breathing cycle is represented as the area under a pressure-volume curve. The respiratory muscles work against five main types of forces:

1. Elastic forces, which are developed in the tissues of the lung and chest when a change in volume occurs
2. Flow-resistive forces offered by the airways to the flow of gas by the nonelastic deformation of tissue
3. Inertial forces, which depend on the mass of the tissues and gases
4. Gravitational forces, which can be considered as part of the inertial forces but in practice are included in the measurement of elastic forces
5. Distorting forces of the chest wall, observed at relatively high ventilations or when the subject breathes through resistances

In the analysis of the work of breathing, inertial forces are not usually considered because they are probably negligible (91,92), and no experimental estimates of inertial work have been made. Furthermore most of the inertial work done during the accelerative phase of a breathing cycle would be recovered during the decelerative phase.

Elastic and Flow-Resistive Work

In this analysis it is assumed that at all times the respiratory system maintains, at a given lung volume, a configuration identical to that in the relaxed state at the same volume. This makes it easy to understand the work of breathing in terms of the relationship between pleural pressure and lung volume. When the lung volume is held constant with open airways at different levels of inflation, the mirror image of the static pressure-volume curve for the lung is obtained (93) [Fig. 14, left, curve -Pst,L (static pressure of the lung)]. When the airways are closed and the muscles are relaxed, the static pressure-volume curve of the relaxed chest wall is obtained [Fig. 14, left, curve Pst,W (static pressure of the chest wall)]. The horizontal distance between -Pst,L and Pst,W indicates the pressure that the respiratory muscles must

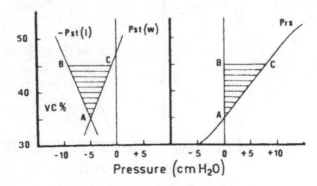

Figure 14 Pressure-volume diagram in terms of pleural pressure (left) and mouth pressure (right). Horizontal hatching, elastic work done by inspiratory muscles during inspiration. (From Ref. 79.)

contribute to maintain the respiratory system at a given volume with open airways, assuming there is no distortion of the chest wall. This pressure corresponds to the pressure given by the static pressure-volume curve of the respiratory system (Prs) during relaxation (Fig. 14, right). The elastic work thus done by the muscles during an inspiration from FRC (point A) equals the area ABCA. The elastic work of breathing may be further analyzed as shown in Figure 15, in which the pressure-volume relationships of the lungs and the thorax are plotted separately in both panels. The elastic work required to increase the volume of the lungs alone is the area ABDEA, whereas the total elastic work required for inspiration is the area ABCA as in Figure 14. Thus, in this example, the elastic work required to inflate the whole system (lungs and thorax) is less than that required to inflate the lungs alone by an amount ACDEA. The extra work is done by the extra energy stored in the thorax, which is released during inspiration and represented by the area AFGBA (Fig. 15, right) and is equal to the area ACDEA. During expiration this energy is transferred without loss from the lungs back to the thorax. At lung volumes greater than those indicated by point H in Figure 15 the counterspringing effect disappears because the elastic forces of both the lungs and the thorax act in the same direction.

During inspiration some pressure must be added to the elastic forces in order to overcome the flow resistance. Curve-Pdyn,L (dynamic pressure of the lung) in Figure 16 (left) is the pathway of pleural pressure relative to atmospheric pressure under dynamic conditions. The horizontal distance between -Pdyn,L and -Pst,L (Fig. 16, left) or Pst,L (Fig. 16, middle) reveals the pressure necessary to overcome the flow resistance of the lungs (airways and tissue). The vertical hatching represents the work required of the inspiratory muscles to overcome the flow resistance of the lung. The broken lines in Figure 16 (left and middle) trace the pathway of the pressure necessary to overcome the flow resistance of the chest wall, and thus the

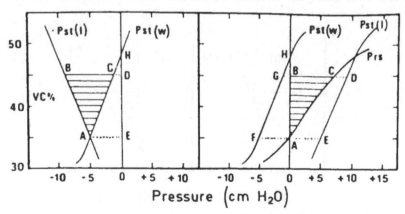

Figure 15 Pressure-volume diagram in terms of pleural pressure (left) and pleural and mouth pressure (right). Horizontal hatching, elastic work done by inspiratory muscles during inspiration. (From Ref. 79.)

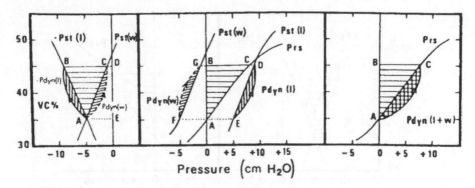

Figure 16 Pressure-volume diagram in terms of pleural pressure (left), pleural and mouth pressure (middle), and mouth pressure (right). Horizontal hatching, inspiratory elastic work; vertical hatching, inspiratory work required to overcome flow resistance of the lung (airways and tissue); oblique hatching, inspiratory work required to overcome flow resistance of the chest wall; cross-hatching, inspiratory work required to overcome the flow resistance of the lung and chest wall. (From Ref. 79.)

horizontal distance between the broken line and Pst,w represents this pressure during an inspiration [$Pdyn,w$ (dynamic pressure of the chest wall)]. The area enclosed between Pst,w and the broken line (oblique hatching) represents the work done by the inspiratory muscles to overcome the flow resistance of the chest wall. However, measurement of the area between Pst,w and the broken line, and thus the flow-resistive work of the chest wall, cannot be obtained directly in a spontaneously breathing subject. Attempts have been made to determine this work in a paralyzed subject during artificial respiration, after subtracting the work of the flow resistance of the lung and airways from the total flow-resistive work [Fig. 16, right, cross-hatching (94)].

During an expiration, if all the respiratory muscles were completely relaxed and the pulmonary and chest wall resistances were equal, expiration would proceed down a line midway between the two static curves in Figure 17 (left) or on the line B-A of Figure 17 (right). In that case all the elastic energy stored in the lung would be used to overcome the flow resistances of the lung and chest wall. In fact, only some of this energy is used for this purpose, as indicated by areas a and b for the lung and chest wall, respectively [or their sum (Fig. 17, right, area c)], whereas the rest of the work is used to overcome the persistent activity of the inspiratory muscles. This is depicted by the horizontal hatching and represents the negative work performed by the inspiratory muscles, which lengthen during expiration.

Now consider the various components of the mechanical work and the exchange of energy between different parts of the respiratory system during the breathing cycle [Figs. 18 and 19 (80)]. An important factor is that the pressure is contributed by the inspiratory muscles when $-Pst,L$ is to the left of Pst,w and by the

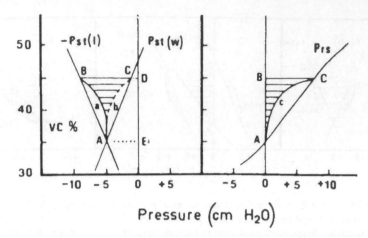

Figure 17 Pressure-volume diagram in terms of pleural pressure (left) and mouth pressure (right). Horizontal hatching, negative work performed by inspiratory muscles during expiration; areas a and b, energy stored in the lung during inspiration and dissipated during expiration to overcome flow resistances of lung and chest wall, respectively (their sum equals area c). (From Ref. 79.)

expiratory muscles when it is to the right. Figures 18 and 19 illustrate breathing cycles at increased ventilation. Both indicate contraction of expiratory muscles, but Figure 18 starts at FRC, whereas Figure 19 commences below FRC. Further development of this analysis is presented in Figure 20, in which the pressure-volume relationships of the respiratory system are depicted during breathing cycles at various lung volumes (95).

Work Due to Chest Wall Distortion

One type of chest wall distortion is that observed in a variety of conditions such as exercise or CO_2 breathing, during which there are volume shifts between the abdomen and the rib cage (96–104). This implies that at all times the configuration of the respiratory system does not correspond to the one obtained during relaxation at the same lung volume (VL). In the absence of a blood volume shift between the periphery and chest wall, all lung volume changes must equal changes in chest wall volume (Vw). Because the lung is in series with the chest wall, $V_L = V_w$. Also the rib cage and abdomen behave as volume-displacing elements in parallel, thus $V_{rc} + V_{ab} = V_w$ and thus $V_L = V_{rc} + V_{ab}$, where Vrc is rib cage volume and Vab is abdominal volume. The important implication of this reasoning is that the volume displacement of the rib cage and abdomen can be independent of one another; indeed, volume displacement of either one can be in a direction opposite to that of overall lung volume change. Hence all inspiratory muscles do not necessarily shorten during inspiration, nor must all expiratory muscles shorten during

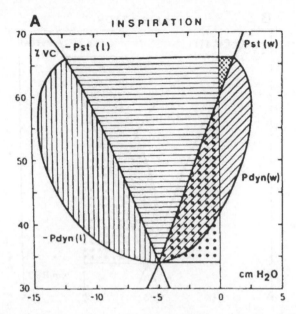

Figure 18 Graphical analysis of work done during a breathing cycle at increased ventilation. Cycle starts at resting volume of respiratory system. (A) Vertical hatching, work done by inspiratory muscles to overcome flow resistance of the lung; horizontal hatching, work done by inspiratory muscles to overcome elastic resistance of the lung; cross-hatching, work done by inspiratory muscles to overcome elastic resistance of the chest wall; oblique hatching, work done by inspiratory muscles to overcome flow resistance of the chest wall; coarse stippling, elastic energy transferred from the chest wall to the lung. (B) Horizontal and cross-hatching, work done by elastic energy of the lung and chest wall, respectively, against persistent activity of inspiratory muscles; fine stippling, work done by elastic energy of the lung to overcome part of flow resistance of the lung; broken hatching, work done by expiratory muscles to overcome rest of flow resistance of the lung (according to representation used; but this energy could be utilized to overcome part of the flow resistance of the chest wall); oblique hatching and solid area, work done by elastic energy of the lung and chest wall, respectively, to overcome flow resistance of the chest wall; coarse stippling, elastic energy transferred from the lung to the chest wall. (From Ref. 80.)

expiration. The second type of chest wall distortion is the deformation of the rib cage itself, which may occur during resistive breathing (including disease). The change in the shape of the rib cage during the breathing cycle is characterized by a phase lag of anteroposterior diameter change relative to the transverse diameter (96,98). However, in the absence of added external respiratory loads, this kind of distortion does not occur in normal subjects to an important degree, even at the values of ventilation achieved during heavy exercise (105).

Goldman et al. (100,101) have estimated the mechanical work of altering the distribution of volume changes between rib cage and abdomen based on measure-

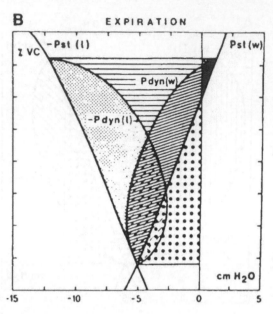

Figure 18   (*Continued*)

ments of rib cage and abdominal volume displacements, changes in lung volume, and estimates of transthoracic pressure (Fig. 21). Figure 21 (top) shows the conventional -Pst,L and Pst,w relaxation pressure volume curves, with lung volume (left ordinate) plotted against the transthoracic pressure (Campbell diagram). In the Goldman analysis the overall lung volume change is distributed between the rib cage and abdomen. Thus the areas representing volume and transthoracic pressure changes are shown schematically for the rib cage (Fig. 21, top, right ordinate) and abdomen (Fig. 21, bottom) individually. The total volume change is identical in both analyses, with an arbitrary distribution of 80% (Fig. 21, top, OZ') and 20% (Fig. 21, bottom, O'X) between the rib cage and abdomen, respectively. It is also assumed that the distribution of volume change shown is the same as that obtained during relaxation at the same volumes. Segment RB represents the path followed by transthoracic pressure as the lung undergoes a volume increase, during which the ΔVrs equals 80% of the total ΔVL. The transthoracic pressure at point C' is identical to that at point C, because both points represent the overall relaxation of the chest wall or of the rib cage, respectively, at the same lung volume. In Figure 21 (bottom), segment RG represents the path of transthoracic pressure during the volume change under consideration, and the transthoracic pressures at points G and E are identical to those at points I and C, respectively. The work done by the inspiratory muscles neglecting the resistive work is given by the sum of the areas of triangles RBC' and RGE. This sum must be identical to the area of triangle RIC,

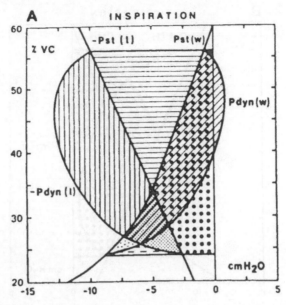

Figure 19 Graphical analysis of work done during a breathing cycle at increased ventilation. Cycle starts below resting volume of respiratory system. (A) Broken hatching, work done by elastic energy of the chest wall to overcome persistent activity of expiratory muscles; fine stippling, work done by elastic energy of the chest wall to overcome part of flow resistance of the lung (gas and tissues); area with small crosses, work done by elastic energy of the chest wall to overcome part of flow resistance of the chest wall; oblique hatching, work done by inspiratory muscles to overcome rest of flow resistance of the chest wall; vertical hatching, work done by inspiratory muscles to overcome part of flow resistance of the lung; horizontal hatching, work done by inspiratory muscles to overcome elastic resistance of the lung; coarse stippling, elastic energy transferred from the chest wall to the lung. (B) Horizontal hatching, work done by elastic energy of the lung against persistent activity of inspiratory muscles; fine stippling, work done by elastic energy of the lung to overcome part of flow resistance of the lung; oblique hatching, work done by elastic energy of the lung to overcome part of flow resistance of the chest wall; vertical broken hatching, work done by expiratory muscles to overcome part of flow resistance of the chest wall; oblique broken hatching, work done by expiratory muscles to overcome part of flow resistance of the lung; horizontal broken hatching, work done by expiratory muscles to overcome elastic resistance of the chest wall; coarse stippling, elastic energy transferred from the lung to the chest wall. (From Ref. 80.)

because all the triangles have the same base (i.e., P from points I–C, B–C′, or G–E), and the sum of heights of triangles RBC′ and RGE ($\Delta V\text{rc} + \Delta V\text{ab}$) equals the height of triangle RIC ($\Delta V\text{L}$). Similarly, the sum of the areas of trapezoids RC′Z′OR and REXO′R must be identical to the area of trapezoid RCZ′OR. Thus there is no difference in the amount of work calculated with the Goldman approach

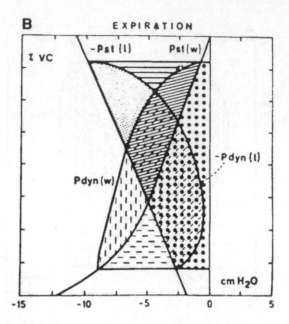

Figure 19   (*Continued*)

compared with the Campbell approach, when both estimates are based on the assumption that the distribution of volume change during breathing is the same as that during relaxation.

With this background in mind, let us now consider an inspiration during which rib cage volume displacement accounts for 100% of the change in lung volume instead of 80% of the total. The Campbell diagram gives the same estimate of inspiratory work as before (Fig. 21, top, triangle RIC), but the rib cage pressure-volume diagram gives a larger estimate, namely, the area of triangle RIC″. Point C″ is obtained by a schematic linear extension of the relaxation pressure-volume curve of the rib cage. It should be emphasized that the compliance of the rib cage (shown in Fig. 21, top) is less than that of the overall chest wall because the compliance of each element in a system of volume-elastic elements, arranged in parallel, must be summed together to give the overall compliance of the systems. This analysis therefore implies that any distribution of volume change between the two chest wall pathways other than that obtained during relaxation results in a distortion of the chest wall from its relaxation characteristics, and extra work is done to overcome the elastic cost of this distortion (104). Thus the elastic work done by the muscles of the chest wall is greater when only one of the two parallel pathways is utilized for a given change in lung volume.

In summary, during breathing at rest the two estimates (Campbell and Goldman approaches) are comparable and are consistent with little or no distortion

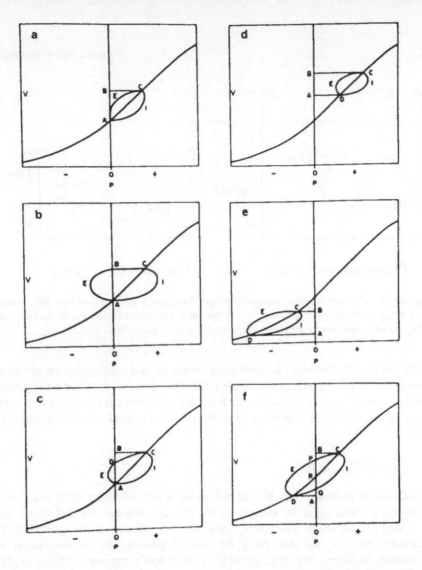

Figure 20 Pressure-volume relationship of respiratory system during breathing cycles at various lung volumes. Various types of work and total mechanical work can be analyzed as:

Cycle	Elastic work	Flow-resistive work	Negative work	Total mechanical work for one breathing cycle
a	ABCA	AICA	BCEAB	AICBA + BCEAB
b	ABCA	AICA + BEAB		AICBEA
c	ABCA	AICA + DEAD	BCDB	AICBDEA + BCDB
d	ABCDA	DICD	BCEDAB	ADICBA + BCEDAB
e	BADCB	CEDC	ADICBA	BCEDAB + ADICBA
f	RBCR + RADR	QICRQ + PEDRP	BCPB + ADQA	DAQICBPED + BCPB + ADQA

(From Ref. 95.)

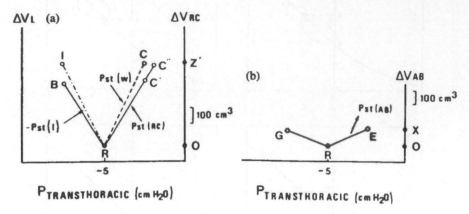

Figure 21 Pressure-volume diagram (Campbell diagram). (a) Lung volume (left ordinate) and rib cage volume (right ordinate) vs. transthoracic pressure. (b) Abdominal volume (right ordinate) vs. transthoracic pressure. For details see text. (From Ref. 101.)

of the chest wall. However, as ventilation increases, and the distribution of volume change can be preferential to one or the other compartment, the Goldman approach implies greater mechanical work. In fact, for ventilation levels achieved during exercise, the Campbell diagram may underestimate the work of breathing by up to 25%.

Partitioning the Work

The Goldman approach (100,101) partitions work into that done along two parallel pathways terminating at the surfaces of the rib cage and anterior abdominal wall. It is tempting to assign work done along the first pathway to the intercostal and accessory muscles and that along the second pathway to the diaphragm and abdominal muscles. But this, as well as Macklem's approach (106), neglects mechanical interaction between the diaphragm and rib cage; it also neglects the role of the rib cage in abdominal displacements. Although the importance of these features is recognized, there is not sufficient agreement about their quantitative aspects to permit definitions of the separate contributions of the respiratory muscles to respiratory work (79,107–112).

C. Theoretical Estimation of Work

Geometrical Estimation

Graphical analysis of the work of breathing indicates that by applying elementary geometry one can obtain the mechanical work of breathing; this approach gives a fairly good estimate of the work of breathing (113). For a system with approximately linear-elastic and flow-resistive properties, the work performed for a given volume and pressure amplitude would lie between the extremes of PV and $1/2$PV, where P and V represent the amplitude of pressure and volume changes, respectively. More precisely, the figure of the minimal area (representing elastic work only; see Fig. 14) approximates a triangle yielding $W = PV/2$. The flow-resistive work of a normal inspiration, by the pressure-volume relationship, is represented by a geometrical figure resembling an ellipse. Thus the work of inspiring a single breath can be approximated by the expression $W = \pi/4 \ PV$. Finally, the figure of the maximal area that could be traced during an inspiration with a square-wave flow pattern produced through a flow resistance would be a rectangle, and in this case $W = PV$.

Mathematical Estimation

The work done by the respiratory muscles can be calculated by using the general form of the equation of motion for breathing (71,94):

$$P_T = \frac{1}{C} V + K_1 \dot{V} + K_2 \dot{V}^2 \tag{23}$$

where P_T is the total pressure difference developed across the system by the respiratory muscles, C is the compliance of the respiratory system (lungs and thorax), V is the displacement from the relaxation volume, $\dot{V}$ is the flow, and K_1 and K_2 are empirical constants. The assumptions involved are that the relaxation curve is linear with a slope C, the pressure required to overcome flow resistance is adequately described by the last two terms, and inertia is negligible.

If the breathing pattern is assumed to follow a sine wave, then

$$\dot{V} = a \sin bt$$

or $\tag{24}$

$$dV = a \sin bt \ dt$$

where a is the amplitude of flow (peak inspiratory + peak expiratory) and $b/2\pi =$ f (frequency of breathing). Experimental justification for this assumption stems from the work of Cooper (114), who found that the external work done by subjects breathing against a resistance was similar to that done by a sine wave pump at corresponding levels of ventilation.

The differential expression for work (W) is $dW = P \ dV$, and by substituting Eqs. (23) and (24) it becomes

$$dW = \frac{1}{C} V \ dV + K_1 a^2 \sin^2 bt \ dt + K_2 a^3 \sin^3 bt \ dt \tag{25}$$

The total work required during a single inspiration (WI) of tidal volume VT and duration π/b is

$$W_I = \frac{1}{2C} V_T^2 + \frac{K_1}{4} \pi^2 f V_T^2 + \frac{2K_2}{3} \pi^2 f^2 V_T^3 \tag{26}$$

The mechanical work of inspiration per unit time ($\dot{W}I$), i.e., the mechanical power, is obtained by multiplying Eq. (26) by the frequency of breathing:

$$WI = \frac{1}{2C} fVT^2 + \frac{K_1}{4} \pi^2 f^2 VT^2 + \frac{2K_2}{3} \pi^2 f^3 VT^3 \tag{27}$$

or

$$WI = \frac{1}{2Cf} \dot{V}E^2 + \frac{K_1}{4} \pi^2 \dot{V}E^2 + \frac{2K_2}{3} \pi^2 \dot{V}E^3 \tag{28}$$

where $\dot{V}E$ is the minute ventilation.

If expiration is passive (i.e., no agonist expiratory muscles are used), as during quiet breathing, work in Eqs. 26–28 represents the total positive work of breathing ($\dot{W}T$), either per breath [Eq. (26)] or per minute [Eqs. (27 and 28)], which is the power required for breathing. However, if expiratory muscles contract and all the elastic energy stored in the lung is utilized during expiration to overcome the flow resistance (e.g., at very high ventilation or breathing through a resistance), the positive work per unit time will equal twice the value of the last two terms of Eq. (28):

$$\dot{W}T = 2\left(\frac{K_1}{4} \pi^2 \dot{V}E^2 + \frac{2K_2}{3} \pi^2 \dot{V}E^3\right) \tag{29}$$

It should be emphasized that these equations provide only a method for rough estimation of the total mechanical work of breathing from measurements of C, K_1, and K_2, which may be considered constant only within narrow limits. However, in practice the validity of Eq. (29) is very well supported by the results of Margaria et al. (115), who found that this equation yielded curves closely fitting their experimental measurements relating mechanical work of breathing to ventilation during exercise.

In light of present knowledge, however, the analysis of Otis et al. (94) needs to be modified in two respects: (1) the equation of motion [Eq. (23)] needs to be updated, and (2) the assumption that the flow profiles during inspiration and expiration are both sinusoidal and symmetrical requires clarification (116).

Recent studies (117–119) indicate that the dynamic pressure losses provided by the tissues of the lung and chest wall do not obey ohmic behavior but, instead, exhibit characteristic viscoelastic behavior; hence, nonelastic tissue impedance cannot be included into the constant K_1 of Eq. (23), as was common practice in the past (94,120). Based on a model of viscoelastic behavior of thoracic tissues proposed by Bates et al. (117), the relationship between $\dot{W}_1$ and $\dot{V}$ during sinusoidal cycling is given by (116):

$$WI = \frac{1}{2Cf} \dot{V}E^2 + \frac{K_1}{4} \pi^2 \dot{V}E^2 + \frac{2K_2}{3} \pi^2 \dot{V}E^3 + \frac{R}{4(1 + 4\pi^2 T^2 f^2)} \pi^2 \dot{V}E^2 \tag{30}$$

where R and T are the intrinsic resistance and time constant that characterize the viscoelastic behavior of the stress adaptation units within the thoracic tissues

(117,119), and K_1 and K_2 in this case represent *solely* the resistive properties of the airways. According to Eq. (28), for a given ventilation, $\dot{W}I$ should decrease with increasing frequency solely as a result of decreased elastic work. However, Eq. (30) indicates that increased frequency of breathing reduces the viscoelastic power requirements as well. Figure 22 depicts the relationship between nonelastic $\dot{W}I$ and ventilation for various frequencies of breathing. These computations were made according to Eq. (5) (neglecting the elastic power term), using the average values of the constants K_1, K_2, R, and τ reported by D'Angelo et al. (119). It can be seen that, at any given ventilation, the nonelastic power requirements should increase with decreasing frequency as a result of a greater contribution of the viscoelastic component. At any given respiratory frequency, however, the relative contribution of viscoelastic power to the total nonelastic power output decreases with increasing ventilation because of a disproportionate increase in $\dot{W}I$ resulting from the cubic term in Eq. (30). Since respiratory frequency increases with increasing ventilation, from the analysis in Figure 22 it follows that at ventilations higher than 20–30 L/min

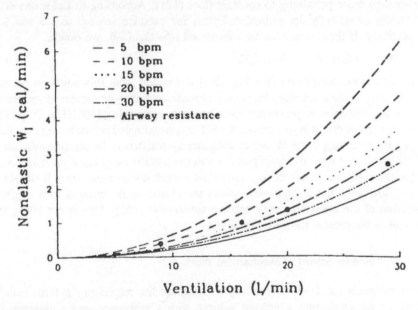

Figure 22 Relationship between nonelastic inspiratory power and ventilation computed according to Eq. (30) using average values of constants of D'Angelo et al. (119): $K_1 = 1.9$ cm H_2O L^{-1} s; $K_2 = 0.52$ cm H_2O L^{-2} s^2; R = 5.86 cm H_2O L^{-1} s; s = 1 s; $\tau = 1$ s. The lower curve (solid line) indicates power output resulting from airway resistance: $\dot{W}I = K_1/4$ $\pi^2 V_E^2 + 2K_2/3 \pi^2 V_E^3$. The broken curves represent total nonelastic inspiratory power output (resistive plus viscoelastic) at various respiratory frequencies (*f*). This analysis pertains to sinusoidal breathing cycles. (Circles) Typical frequencies at different exercise ventilations in normal subjects. (From Ref. 116.)

the viscoelastic component should become negligible provided the frequency is greater than 20 breaths/min. In contrast, at lower ventilations, which are normally associated with $f < 20$ breaths/min, the viscoelastic power is relatively more important (116).

The values of the numerical constants in Eqs. (23) and (30) depend on both the inspiratory flow profile and the duty cycle, that is, the ratio of inspiratory time to total cycle duration (T_I/T_T). In all analyses based on sinusoidal breathing, a T_I/T_T ratio of 0.5 is assumed. Except at rest, the inspiratory flow profile in spontaneously breathing humans is usually nonsinusoidal (121). In fact, during muscular exercise both inspiratory and expiratory flow profiles tend to become rectangular (constant flow), while T_I/T_T is close to 0.5 (121). For constant flow and T_I/T_T of 0.5, the value of the numerical constants in Eq. (29) decreases from 5 (i.e., $2\pi^2/4$) and 13 (i.e., $4\pi^2/3$) to 4 and 8, respectively (121). In fact, the latter are minimal values: Any deviation of flow from constancy increases the value of these constants, thereby increasing the power requirements for a given ventilation. Because in exercise the flow profile is not truly rectangular, the actual values of the constants are necessarily higher than those pertaining to constant flow (121). According to Lafortuna et al. (121), the empirically determined constants for exercise amount to 4.8 and 9.6, respectively. If these constants are substituted into Eq. (29), we obtain

$$\dot{W}_T = 4.8\ K_1\dot{V}_E^2 + 9.6\ K_2\dot{V}_E^3 \tag{31}$$

The viscoelastic component [see Eq. (30)] is omitted from this equation because during exercise the respiratory frequency increases rapidly with increased ventilation and hence viscoelastic pressure losses become negligible (119) (Fig. 22). This analysis implies that at high ventilations $\dot{W}_T$ is approximated by the power expended during the breathing cycle in overcoming airway resistance. In practice this can be readily measured from dynamic plots of volume against esophageal pressure. Such loops necessarily also include any viscoelastic work done on the lung. It should be noted, however, that at high ventilations the elastic work required as a result of distortion of the chest wall may become substantial (101). This is not taken into account in the present theoretical analysis.

D. Measurement of Mechanical Work

The total mechanical work necessary to ventilate the respiratory system may be estimated by ventilating a relaxed subject with a respirator and measuring the differential pressure between the mouth and the body surface (94). This method may be criticized because it is difficult for subjects to relax completely. It will measure the total work only if the subjects are paralyzed. Whether this work is the same as that done by the respiratory muscles is open to question because the pattern of spontaneous breathing may be different from that produced by the respirator, particularly at high ventilation. Nonetheless, the work measured in relaxed subjects might not be very different from that obtained in paralyzed subjects, because Sharp et al. (122) did not find any electrical activity in the intercostal and abdominal muscles during artificial ventilation of relaxed subjects.

There is no method for directly measuring the total mechanical work performed during spontaneous breathing. The catheter balloon technique (123) is the most common method of measuring simultaneous changes in lung volume, preferably measuring changes in rib cage and abdominal volumes separately (100,101), pleural pressure, and gastric pressure [the latter if the Goldman et al. (100,101) approach is adopted]. Thus work is calculated from the area enclosed by the pressure-volume loop. The total work will equal the sum of the elastic work, negative work, and flow resistive work as shown in Figures 14–24. However, with this technique it is not possible to measure flow resistive work done to the thorax, which according to some authors (124,125) can account for 28–36% of the total mechanical work. Similarly, it is not possible to estimate the elastic work done on the chest wall and the negative work performed unless the compliance of the thorax is taken into account, which is a difficult task.

The compressibility of a gas is another factor that may give rise to an incorrect estimation of the work of breathing if the changes in volume are measured at the mouth (126). The volume change actually produced by the respiratory muscles is that occurring in the lungs. However, due to the compressibility of the gas the lung volume change is greater than the volume change measured at the mouth. These differences are very small at sea level in normal subjects. However, during maximum voluntary ventilation the two volumes may differ by as much as 35% (127). Such differences also become significantly large in patients with high flow resistances and elevated FRC, who breathe at high frequencies and during breathing at high altitude (126). Clearly, elastic work will be underestimated if the calculation is based on the tidal volume measured at the mouth (126). Furthermore, work is required to compress alveolar gas at the beginning of expiration and expand it during the first part of the inspiration. Because of phase differences between chest wall movement and flow at the mouth, only a part of the energy stored in the alveolar gas by compression or expansion is available for producing gas flow. The amount of elastic work not utilized to displace the gas is dissipated as heat, balancing an equal amount of work done by the antagonist muscles (126).

E. Work Rate (Power)

During quiet breathing through the nose the work of breathing per minute (rate of work or power) is ≈ 1 cal/min ($= 0.4$ kg m/min $= 4$ J/min $= 0.06$ W) (71,72,124, 128) or ≈ 0.12 cal/L of ventilation. Of this, 0.8 cal/min is the positive work done during inspiration and 0.2 cal/min is the negative work done by the inspiratory muscles during expiration. As implied in Eq. (30), $\dot{W}_I$ for a given ventilation varies markedly with the breathing pattern and it is greater during nose breathing than during mouth breathing because of higher airway resistance (120). In addition, $\dot{W}_I$ tends to increase disproportionately with increasing ventilation as a result of increased nonelastic work rate. Because of this, normal subjects switch from nose to mouth breathing at relatively low levels of exercise ventilation, thereby circumventing a large source of resistance to airflow (116). In all reported studies, as ventilation increases, the positive work of breathing progressively increases, but the range of experimental estimates is large. The work of breathing reported varies greatly for a given ventilation: e.g., for a ventilation of 60–70 L/min the work of breathing reported ranges from 12 to 50 cal or 5 to 20 kg m/min (72,128). The variability may be attributed either to true physiological differences between subjects or to differences in methods of measurement, experimental conditions (e.g., posture, flow resistance of equipment), or methods of interpreting the work of breathing (e.g., some investigators have considered the compliance of the thorax in interpreting their measurements, whereas others did not). A better relationship between the rate of work of breathing and minute ventilation has been found during exercise at various intensities (Fig. 23). The values of power obtained by most investigators refer only to the work measurable by determining the esophageal pressure change and volume at the mouth; therefore, they do not account for all the work of breathing. One can correct this value with a 25% increase by calculating the changes of rib cage and abdominal volumes, as did Goldman et al. (100,101). Thus, at very high levels of ventilation, i.e., 140 L/min, the power is ≈120 cal/min.

The relationship between mechanical power and ventilation during exercise reported by Margaria et al. (115) and Milic-Emili et al. (129) closely fits Eq. (31) (116). In addition, this relationship is the same during rebreathing as during muscular exercise (130). If during exercise a lower respiratory frequency is imposed than that chosen spontaneously, the mechanical power increases (131). This probably reflects, in part, increased viscoelastic power output (Fig. 22) but is probably also caused by the fact that at low frequencies the subjects were forced to mobilize lung volumes below the resting FRC, where the airflow resistance becomes very high (132).

F. Maximal Available Work and Power

The theoretical maximal work available for one breath could be obtained by the area that is defined by the curves relating the maximal pressures that can be developed statically at different lung volumes. For young male adults it amounts to 20–30 cal. However, when flow is allowed to occur, this theoretical work per breath is not obtained. Agostoni and Fenn (14) have shown that the maximal inspiratory work for a breathing cycle is an inverse linear relationship of the mean inspiratory flow rate. This is in keeping with the force-velocity relationship of muscle; the greater the speed of shortening of a muscle, the less force it will develop. The effect of flow on the work obtained has also been studied by Craig (133), who found that when a subject breathes with maximal effort through a resistance so that mean flow is ≈0.3 L/s, 80% of the theoretical maximum work is obtained during inspiration, whereas 70% is obtained during expiration. Other mechanisms, however, also contribute to limit the maximal work per breath; these include (1) the speed of activation of the respiratory muscles

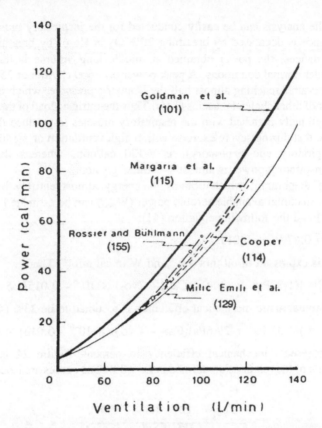

Figure 23 Relationship between rate of mechanical work of breathing and minute ventilation during muscular exercise of various intensities. Solid line indicates 25% greater rate of work of breathing found by Goldman et al. (101), who calculated changes of rib cage and abdominal volume instead of measuring changes of lung volumes at the mouth. (From Ref. 79.)

at the beginning of forced inspirations and expirations, and (2) gas compressibility (116). In terms of maximal inspiratory power output, however, the respiratory system seems to be well designed. In fact, the maximal $\dot{W}$I occurs at an inspiratory flow of 3.6 L/s (14). For TI/TT of 0.5, this should correspond to a ventilation of 216 L/min, which is close to maximal voluntary ventilation (116).

For other skeletal muscles the maximum power is obtained at ≈30% of the maximum isometric tension and velocity of shortening. Thus it is possible to calculate the power of the respiratory muscles at different loads from the pressure-flow relationship [because TTI (or mean inspiratory pressure)·$\dot{V}$ = $\dot{W}$; Eq. (20)]. For the expiratory muscles, the pattern is complicated by the compression of the airways because the internal load of the respiratory system changes markedly.

However, the analysis can be easily conducted for the inspiratory muscles. When flow resistance is decreased by breathing 20% O_2 in He or by breathing through graded resistances, the power obtained at middle lung volume is less than that obtained under normal conditions. A peak power of $\approx$600 cal/min or 250 kg m/min occurs at pressures reaching almost half the isometric pressure, which is not unlike the behavior of other skeletal muscles (134). Thus the intrinsic load of the respiratory system is optimally matched with the respiratory muscles to produce the maximal power. Note that during severe exercise with a high ventilation of $\approx$140 L/min, the power (inspiratory and expiratory), is $\approx$120 cal/min, whereas the available maximum inspiratory power is almost 4–5 times greater.

In the diaphragm, which obtains its energy almost entirely by oxidative metabolism, maximal available aerobic power ($\dot{W}_{max}$) can be estimated by combining Eq. (18) and the following equation (41):

$$\dot{V}O_2 = 0.87 \, \dot{W} + 0.015 \tag{32}$$

where $\dot{V}O_2$ is expressed in ml min^{-1} g^{-1} and $\dot{W}$ in cal min^{-1}. Then

$$\dot{W}_{max} = [(1.32\bar{P}a^2 + 29.6\bar{P}a)(Cao_2 - Cvo_2) \times 10^{-6} - 0.015]1.5$$

or where diaphragmatic mechanical efficiency is assumed to be 23% (41):

$$\dot{W}_{max} = [(1.32 \, \bar{P}a^2 + 29.6\bar{P}a)(Cao_2 - Cvo_2) \times 10^{-6} - 0.015] \times 0.05E \tag{33}$$

where E represents mechanical efficiency in percent. Figure 24 is a graphic representation of the relationship defined in Eq. (33). The curves are isocontent lines

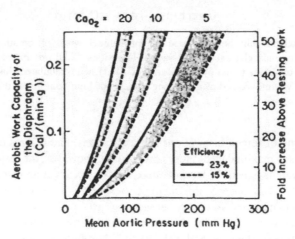

Figure 24 Predicted relationship of inspiratory work capacity to mean aortic pressure, assuming a diaphragmatic venous O_2 content of 1 ml/dl. This relationship is shown at 3 representative arterial O_2 contents (Cao_2) (curves labeled 20, 10, and 5 ml/dl). Shaded region represents an assumed range of mechanical efficiency for diaphragm between 15 and 23%. (From Ref. 41.)

that describe the aerobic work capacities predicted for any given mean aortic pressure at three different arterial O_2 contents, where a venous O_2 content of 1 ml/dl was used to calculate arteriovenous O_2 difference. The shaded region encloses a range of mechanical efficiencies between 15 and 23%. Exercising humans have been shown to elevate their work of breathing as much as 100-fold (72). According to the findings of Reid and Johnson (41), which are graphically represented in Figure 24, elevations in diaphragmatic aerobic work of these magnitudes should be accommodated by the available capacity for O_2 delivery to the diaphragm under normoxic normotensive conditions. However, O_2 availability can become critical with arterial oxyhemoglobin desaturation or during hypotension. For example, for the dog at 23% mechanical efficiency (41), only about a 30-fold increase in diaphragmatic work is possible when, at a mean arterial pressure of 100 mm Hg, O_2 content is 10 ml/dl; only about a 20-fold increase is available when, with an O_2 content of 20 ml/dl, arterial pressure falls to 50 mm Hg. In disease states where elevated ventilatory work is superimposed on a substantial hypoxemia, hypotension, or anemia, O_2 delivery to the diaphragm may become inadequate. When ventilation requires a higher work output than can be supported aerobically, failure will eventually ensue and ventilation will be reduced to a level that can be supported by the O_2 supply plus anaerobic metabolism (41).

V. Efficiency of Breathing

Superficially the concept and determination of the efficiency of the respiratory muscles would seem to be relatively simple. All that is needed is a measurement of the mechanical work of breathing and the energy equivalent of the metabolism ($\dot{V}O_2$) of the respiratory muscles; the ratio then yields the efficiency. The matter is much more complicated, as reflected by the variability in reported efficiency measurements, ranging from 1% to 25% (41,72,82,87,94,128,135–139).

By taking the usual estimate of the efficiency of aerobic exercise involving large muscle groups, as determined by cycle ergometry, a guide to what might be expected of the respiratory muscles is provided; 25% is a good, although slightly high, estimate. In some rhythmic acts, such as hopping, running, and walking, in which the recoil energy is stored in the series-elastic elements of skeletal muscles, the efficiency may be higher (140). It seems unlikely, however, that sufficient velocities, displacements, or oscillation frequencies are reached in the act of breathing to make this mechanism important for the respiratory muscles. Nonetheless, why have most observers reported values for respiratory muscle efficiency on the order of 5–10%? Have they underestimated the mechanical work or overestimated the metabolic cost?

A. Mechanical Work

With the possible exception of the studies of Otis et al. (94), there can be no doubt that mechanical work is underestimated. Work done on the elastic and nonelastic forces of the chest wall is not measured by the usual esophageal balloon technique. In particular, displacement of the heavy abdominal contents may be quite large, and forces due to distortion are not measured.

B. Metabolic Cost

It is difficult to get a steady base line; the basal $\dot{V}O_2$ falls in a completely relaxed subject, and minor changes in posture of the limbs produce changes comparable with the changes in $\dot{V}O_2$ of the respiratory muscles. Any study in which such changes in basal $\dot{V}O_2$ are not controlled will yield falsely low or, more often, high estimates of respiratory muscle $\dot{V}O_2$. Several synergistic muscles may be employed that consume O_2 but do not work during (1) high ventilations, (2) imposed frequency and depth of breathing, (3) breathing against resistance, or (4) disease.

The only conventional study in which efficiency on the order of 20–25% was found was that of Milic-Emili and Petit (72), but their subjects were supine and the esophageal pressure measurements must be suspect (123). Furthermore, they give insufficient information to assess the stability of the basal $\dot{V}O_2$.

A different approach was used by Campbell et al. (136) and by Cain and Otis (135); they measured the increase in $\dot{V}O_2$ needed to sustain ventilation against an external load that did not alter the pattern of breathing and obtained values of $\approx 10\%$. The circumstances of those experiments strengthened these criticisms.

It is not unreasonable to adopt the common-sense view that the true efficiency of the respiratory muscles probably lies in the range of 20–25%; however, from the overall standpoint of physiological economics, the efficiency of breathing is probably $\approx 10\%$ but in disease may fall to 1–2%.

An elegant example of the influence of some of the factors affecting respiratory muscle efficiency can be seen in the results obtained by McGregor and Becklake (82) in an experiment in which the same subjects breathed through resistances or hyperventilated. The authors found that for the same amount of work done, the O_2 cost of breathing was strikingly greater in the resistive-breathing experiment (Fig. 25). These findings gain support because during resistive breathing, apart from the fact that the work of deformation, compression, and decompression increases, muscles are contracting isometrically to maintain the posture or to stabilize the chest wall; thus they consume O_2 but do not directly ventilate the lung. In fact, efficiency of the total respiratory system falls as work of breathing is increased by adding inspiratory resistance (29,139). On the other hand, when O_2 consumption and mechanical work were measured separately for the diaphragm (41), a constant diaphragmatic efficiency of about 23% as inspiratory resistance was increased up to the point of respiratory failure was found (Fig. 26). A possible explanation of this disparity is that, as inspiratory resistive loading progressively increases, diaphragmatic descent accounts for progressively more and rib cage expansion progressively less of the total volume inspired. Nevertheless, O_2 consumption of intercostal and accessory inspiratory muscles of the rib cage continues to increase

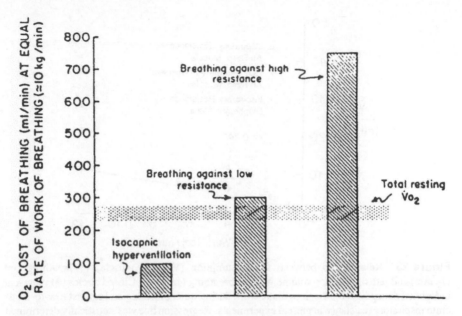

Figure 25 Oxygen cost of breathing at equal (about 10 kg/m/min) work of breathing per minute (power) during isocapnic increases in minute ventilation, breathing against small resistance, and breathing against high resistance. Note the marked difference in O_2 consumption. These results indicate that the mechanical efficiency (work per O_2 cost of breathing) decreases during breathing through resistance. (From Ref. 78.)

(29). At high inspiratory resistive loads the diaphragm accounts for all the inspired volume even though intercostal muscles as well as other nonrespiratory muscles continue to contract and consume O_2 without performing measurable pressure-volume work (41). Hence, even though mechanical efficiency of the diaphragm remains essentially constant, efficiency of the system as a whole declines. In addition, during resistive breathing more fast-twitch muscle fibers may be recruited that are inefficient. Thus, Cala et al. (137) found that $\dot{V}_{O_2}$ during resistive breathing is greater than during breathing against elastic loads for the same amount of work rate and pressure-time product. The most probable explanation is that this difference may be due to preferential recruitment of faster, less efficient muscle fiber in both the inspiratory muscles and those acting as chest wall fixators and stabilizers during breathing against resistive loads (137).

The high efficiencies reported by Milic-Emili and Petit (72) in humans may be attributable in part to the fact that their subjects lay supine, a position in which fewer postural muscles are needed to contract isometrically when stabilizing the thorax. Furthermore, their subjects breathed spontaneously without imposed control of rate or depth. Another consideration may be that in the supine position the diaphragm (the main inspiratory muscle) has greater curvature and longer length;

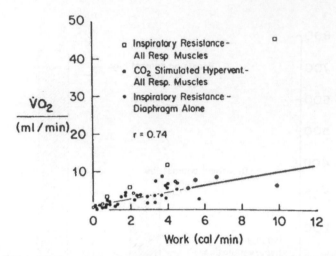

Figure 26 Relationship between O_2 consumption ($\dot{V}O_2$) of muscles of breathing (ml O_2/min) and rate of pressure-volume work of breathing (cal/min). Closed circles (●) represent individual data points for diaphragmatic work during quiet breathing and against low-to-moderate inspiratory resistance in present experiments. Regression line was statistically determined for 36 data points and yielded the following equation: $y = 0.867x + 1.537$, $r = 0.74$. Pressure-volume work and $\dot{V}O_2$ for the present data are those for diaphragm alone. Reciprocal of slope of regression line is proportional to mechanical efficiency of diaphragm. These data are compared in this graph with data from previous studies (19,30) in which $\dot{V}O_2$ of all respiratory muscles is plotted against total work performed on the lung (open symbols). Mechanical efficiency of diaphragm is constant during inspiratory resistive loading, whereas mechanical efficiency of total respiratory system falls. (From Ref. 41.)

thus, for a given pressure to be developed, less excitation is needed and hence less energy is expended. Finally, it is possible that the work of breathing was overestimated by using the esophageal balloon to estimate pressure changes because the balloon lies under the heart in the supine position.

Increased lung volume is another factor that decreases efficiency by increasing $\dot{V}O_2$ (138,139). However, when the work of breathing at high lung volume was normalized for the decrease in maximum inspiratory muscle pressure, efficiency at high lung volume did not differ from that at FRC, suggesting that the fall in efficiency may have been related to the fall in inspiratory muscle strength (138).

As previously reported, the importance of the respiratory muscle fiber composition should not be neglected when interpreting interindividual differences between studies with different experimental procedures (hyperventilation vs. resistive loading or resistive vs. elastic loading). Figure 1 shows that at very low and very high velocities of shortening, muscle efficiency approaches zero. Thus results obtained at different velocities of shortening give different values of efficiency. One now appreciates that the maximum efficiency with which a muscle performs a specific type of work is determined partly by the intrinsic rate of ATP hydrolysis by the contractile proteins. The amount of energy required by a slow red muscle to shorten slowly when moving a heavy load is less than that required by a fast white muscle. The latter has contractile proteins that hydrolyze ATP at a faster rate and therefore performs more economically if shortening rapidly or against a light load. Consequently, the efficiency is optimized if fast-contracting muscles shorten rapidly against light loads. In contrast, slowly contracting muscle fibers are more efficient when they develop tension. The respiratory muscles are rather fast muscles; therefore, their efficiency appears lower when they operate at low speeds (e.g., during resistive breathing).

In summary, the differences that arise in measuring efficiency may be attributed to an overestimation or an underestimation of the work of breathing and/or the O_2 cost of breathing. However, it must be realized that a single value of efficiency does not exist; it varies as a result of numerous factors from a value of zero (i.e., inspiratory effort with closed airways) to a maximum value, which appears to be 20–25% when breathing through external dead space in the supine position.

VI. Physiological Considerations

A. Optimal Breathing Frequency

In the previous section, breathing frequency was implicated as a factor that could affect the energy expenditure. An analytical approach suggests that an optimal breathing frequency should exist for a given level of ventilation. "Optimal" is used to imply the least energy expenditure for a given level of ventilation. Equation (28) shows that elastic power is inversely related to frequency, whereas nonelastic power is independent of frequency. It then follows that for a given ventilation the work of breathing should be lower the higher the frequency. This does not necessarily imply the most economical ventilation; that will rather depend on the efficiency of breathing (and consideration of alveolar ventilation). However, for moderate levels of ventilation (5–35 L/min) and for a range of 5–20 breaths/min, the O_2 cost of breathing diminishes as the frequency increases (66). The decrease in the work of breathing as frequency increases has a limit, however, because Eqs. (29) and (31) predict that with a high ventilation requiring active participation of the expiratory muscles the total work that is only nonelastic is independent of frequency. Milic-Emili et al. (131) have confirmed that at a level of ventilation of 41–130 L/min, the mechanical work of breathing is not affected by frequency over a range of 20–60 breaths/min. Furthermore, by increasing the frequency, for reasons already explained (recruitment of postural muscle), the efficiency may appreciably decrease, thus resulting in an increase in the $\dot{V}O_2$. The increase in frequency therefore becomes less economical.

Apart from the limits in energetics, physiologically there are two other reasons that may set limits for the minimum and maximum frequency of breathing at a given minute ventilation. The lower limit is set by the maximal anatomical tidal volume, whereas the upper one is set by the rate at which the neuromuscular apparatus can generate alternating movements (71). This has been partially confirmed by the experiments of Milic-Emili et al. (131) for a total ventilation of 41–130 L/min, when the tidal volume does not exceed the inspiratory capacity and the frequency of breathing ranges from 20/min to 60/min. When the frequency falls below the value at which the tidal volume exceeds the inspiratory capacity, the work of breathing increases rapidly. Therefore, for any given minute ventilation there appears to be a certain frequency below which Eq. (29) does not hold. Thus the greater the ventilation, the narrower the range of frequencies over which the work required is constant and minimal.

In this analysis the optimal frequency was examined in terms of total minute ventilation. We concluded that at a given minute ventilation the work of breathing decreases and eventually plateaus as frequency increases. Now consider the optimal frequency in terms of alveolar ventilation. Because total minute ventilation ($\dot{V}E$) equals alveolar ventilation ($\dot{V}A$) plus dead-space ventilation ($\dot{V}DS$), it follows that at constant $\dot{V}A$, as frequency increases, total $\dot{V}E$ must increase.

Rohrer (140a) was the first to point out that a given alveolar ventilation should be maintained at some particular optimal frequency. The situation can be approached again through Eq. (28), in which ventilation can be substituted by $\dot{V}A + \dot{V}DS$ or $\dot{V}A + fVDS$, where VDS is volume of the dead space and by assuming that ventilation is passive (71):

$$W = \frac{1}{2C}\left(\frac{\dot{V}A^2}{f} + 2\dot{V}A VDS + fVDS^2\right) + \frac{K_1}{4}\pi^2(\dot{V}A + fVDS)^2 + \frac{2K_2}{3}\pi^2(\dot{V}A + fVDS)^3 \qquad (34)$$

The first term of this equation indicates that the frequency will have two opposing effects on the elastic work: an increasing frequency tends to increase elastic work because the work required for dead-space ventilation is increased, whereas it tends to decrease the elastic work because a smaller tidal volume is required. Thus, because of these opposite effects, an optimum frequency (f_{opt}) exists for minimum elastic work (Fig. 27) and is given by

$$f_{opt} = \dot{V}A/VDS \qquad (35)$$

obtained by differentiating the first term of Eq. (34) with respect to frequency and setting the result equal to zero. It appears from this solution that the optimal frequency of breathing for minimum elastic work occurs when alveolar ventilation equals dead-space ventilation or when the tidal volume equals twice the dead-space volume.

For a given alveolar ventilation the effect of frequency on the nonelastic work will be more pronounced with increasing frequency simply because the total ventilation increases. It follows from Eq. (34) that if only flow-resistive work were involved, the lowest frequency would be most economical (Fig. 27). When flow-resistive and elastic work are both considered, the conditions of minimum

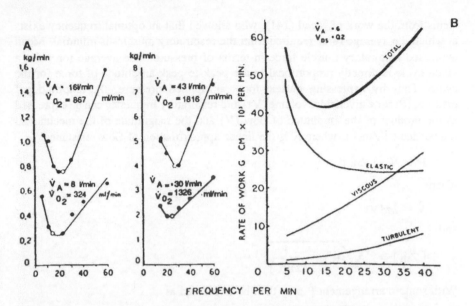

FREQUENCY PER MIN

Figure 27 Mechanical work of breathing as a function of frequency of breathing. (A) Frequency at which minimal work occurs at several constant rates of alveolar ventilation ($\dot{V}_A$). Note that frequency for minimal work increases progressively with increased $\dot{V}_A$. Open circles, frequencies spontaneously chosen by subjects during exercise and corresponding closely at each level of $\dot{V}_A$ with frequency resulting in minimal work. (B) Contribution of elastic and turbulent work to total work of breathing at constant $\dot{V}_A$ and dead space (V_{DS}). Note that as frequency increases, elastic work decreases and reaches a plateau, whereas viscous and turbulent work increase. (A from Ref. 145; B from Ref. 94.)

work become more complex. From Eq. (34), Mead (141) derived this general solution for the conditions of minimal work—optimal frequency (fw_{opt})—making the assumption that as a first approximation, flow resistance can be expressed with a single constant:

$$fw_{opt} = \frac{\sqrt{1 + 4\pi^2 RC\dot{V}_A/V_{DS}} - 1}{2\pi^2 RC} \tag{36}$$

Thus the minimum work frequency is seen in this approximation to be a function of two parameters: the time constant of the mechanical system (RC) and the alveolar ventilation-dead space ratio ($\dot{V}_A/V_{DS}$).

The implication of Eqs. (35) and (36) for a given alveolar ventilation is that the optimal frequency will be lowered by increasing the dead space, the nonelastic resistance, or the compliance. It also appears that for a given dead space, compliance, and resistance the optimal frequency will increase with increasing alveolar ventilation.

A different approach relating optimal frequency to minimal energy expenditure stems from the work of Mead (141), who showed that an optimal frequency exists at which the average force required from the respiratory muscles is minimal. Mead expressed respiratory muscle force in terms of pressure. The average force for a given cycle is directly proportional to the peak-to-peak amplitude of force for the cycle. Thus by expressing muscle force as applied pressure, the amplitude of pressure ($\hat{P}$) for a given tidal volume (V_T) and respiratory frequency can be expressed as the product of the amplitude of flow ($\dot{V}$) and the magnitude of the mechanical impedance ($|Zm|$), where R is the linear approximation of flow resistance:

$$\hat{P} = \dot{V} \cdot |Zm|$$

where

$$\dot{V} = 2\pi f V_T$$

and

$$|Zm| = \sqrt{R^2 + \frac{1}{(2\pi fC)^2}}$$

With some rearrangement $\hat{P}$ may then be expressed as

$$\hat{P} = \frac{V_T\sqrt{(2\pi fRC)^2 + 1}}{C} \tag{37}$$

Reexpressing this equation in terms of alveolar ventilation and volume of dead space and differentiating the resulting expression with respect to frequency yields an equation that, when set equal to zero, yields the following solution for the frequency (fp_{opt}) at which the amplitude of pressure, and hence average muscle force, would be minimum:

$$fp_{opt} = \left(\frac{\dot{V}_A}{V_{DS}}\right)^{1/3} (2\pi RC)^{-2/3} \tag{38}$$

Clearly fp_{opt} is expressed as a function of the same parameters (RC and $\dot{V}_A/V_{DS}$) as was the minimum work frequency. However, the combination of high alveolar ventilation–dead space ratios and low time constant affords a considerable separation between the two frequencies.

Although some studies show that during spontaneous breathing, subjects or animals choose a breathing frequency that corresponds to the minimum work (142–145), in both humans and guinea pigs the optimal frequency during sponta-neous breathing corresponds more closely to that associated with the minimum average force rather than that associated with the minimal work (141,146). Minimal force optimal frequencies are consistently higher than minimal work optimal frequencies.

The relationship existing between breathing frequency and minimal work, from the point of view of physiological mechanics, is difficult to explain. Such regulation requires a complicated integration of information, and under the same condition, work is not the best index of the energy requirement. In contrast, the relationship between force and energy expenditure has been well known for years in other skeletal muscles (147,148), in the heart (149), and in the inspiratory muscles (82). It is therefore sensible, intuitively and teleologically, that the frequency chosen under a variety of conditions coincides with the minimal average force is likely to express the minimal energy expenditure (141). Mead suggested that imposed mechanical changes have an effect when these changes are internal (lung) and the adjustments of frequency are mediated via the vagal afferents. Although this suggestion is elegantly presented, the significance of chest wall or respiratory muscle afferents has not been directly tested. Furthermore, there is good evidence that afferents from the respiratory muscles readily affect the off-switch mechanism of the respiratory controllers (150,151). Thus it seems most likely that both afferents have an important role in choosing the optimal frequency, but the precise mechanisms and the quantitative significance of each afferent(s) under a variety of conditions, particularly under severe respiratory muscle stress or insult (i.e., shock or pulmonary edema), remain unknown.

B. Respiratory Muscle Energetics and Exercise

In Figure 23 the curves obtained by several investigators demonstrate that the relationship between the rate of work of breathing (W) and minute ventilation is curvilinear with an upward concavity. These curves are of ever-increasing slope (dW/dV). This implies that the energy cost of breathing (Urs) per any additional units of air ventilated (dUrs/dV) becomes greater with any increase in ventilation, provided efficiency does not change or diminish.

During exercise, total-body $\dot{V}o_2$ bears a relationship to pulmonary ventilation; during light exercise the relationship is linear, whereas during heavy muscular exercise, pulmonary ventilation increases more than the total-body $\dot{V}o_2$. Thus the relationship between total energy uptake (UT), as is measured by the $\dot{V}o_2$ and $\dot{V}E$, is a curve of ever-decreasing slope (i.e., dUT/dV).

Otis (71) and Margaria et al. (115) have pointed out that when

$$dUrs/dV = dUT/dV \tag{39}$$

any further increase in ventilation will not render more energy available for work other than the work of breathing. This implies that the ventilatory value corresponding to dUrs/dV = dUT/dV will represent the maximum ventilatory value available for useful external work. Any further increase in ventilation will not make more O_2 available without lowering the arterial Po_2 unless the respiratory muscles work anaerobically for any additional ventilation. Margaria et al. (115) depicted these concepts using two subjects (Fig. 28). The values of dUT/dV were obtained by determining the total energy expenditure of the body. The curves corresponding to dUrs/dV were calculated for each subject by dividing the mechanical work of breathing by the mechanical efficiency of breathing, using values of efficiency of

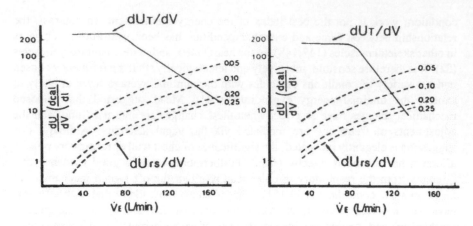

Figure 28 Energy expenditure per volume (dU/dV) as a function of minute ventilation (V̇E) in two subjects. Solid lines (dUT/dV), slope of curve between total energy uptake (UT) and ventilation (V̇E); broken lines (dUrs/dV), slopes of curve between energy consumption of respiratory system (Urs) and ventilation at different values of mechanical efficiency (0.05, 0.10, 0.20, and 0.25). (From Ref. 115.)

0.05, 0.10, 0.20, and 0.25. It appears that in these two subjects the critical ventilation varies from about 105–125 and 130–165 L/min, levels of ventilation that are certainly achieved during exercise. As the ventilation increases with increasing exercise, the efficiency probably progressively drops, partly due perhaps to the recruitment of muscles that do not directly move the thorax (see Sec. V). Thus it may be suggested that at low levels of ventilation the subject operates at the bottom broken line of Figure 28 and progressively moves upward as the workload and ventilation increase. Assuming an efficiency of 10%, the critical ventilation in Figure 28 approaches 100 L/min, which is often observed at high intensities of exercise.

C. Respiratory Muscle Energetics in Health and Disease

Previously the energetics of the respiratory muscles have been approached from a physiologist's point of view; namely, an analytical examination traced the interplay between the energy available for work, the work performed, and the efficiency of the respiratory system. In disease states these physiological considerations can often be met, and this last section identifies the significance of respiratory muscle energetics in the overall economy of the body. Disease states of particular importance are those that compromise the energy supply (i.e., low cardiac output), increase the work of breathing (i.e., hyperventilation, high airway resistance and/or low compliance, and stiffness of the chest wall), and decrease the efficiency (i.e., breathing against high respiratory impedance and metabolic disorders). In practical medicine, shock (152), lung disease with airflow limitation (70), kyphoscoliosis

(124), and obesity (122) are examples of a potential imbalance between energy demands to the respiratory muscles and energy supplies.

Figure 29 combines some theoretical predictions and experimental findings. The lower right quadrant traces the relation of power output as a function of ventilation, using Eq. (28) with constants K_1 and K_2 obtained by Milic-Emili et al. (129). It indicates that for a given ventilation, the work of breathing becomes greater as the airway resistance increases, or for a given work of breathing, the ventilation diminishes as the airway resistance increases. The upper right quadrant shows that for a given rate of work of breathing, i.e., power (e.g., 10 kg/m/min, a value frequently observed in disease), the oxygen consumption will increase as the efficiency decreases from values of 20% as in the supine position (72,75) to 2% (87) or 1% in normal subjects breathing through a resistance or in patients with chronic obstructive pulmonary disease (COPD) (82). The values depicted by N and P represent the relationship obtained during hyperventilation in normal subjects in the upright position, and that obtained from normal subjects breathing through a resistance or from patients with airflow limitation (82), respectively. For this level of work of breathing, patients may require 400 ml of oxygen, which, although a high value, will not be an imminent threat for the body as a whole. However, even a moderate rate of work output will require a considerable amount of the available energy if the cardiac output decreases or if the hemoglobin content and/or its oxygen saturation decreases, of if the tissues are unable to extract oxygen (septic shock). The oxygen cost of breathing is directly related to blood flow by the Fick principle: $\dot{V}_{O_{2rs}} = \dot{Q}(Ca_{O_2} - Cv_{O_2})$, where $\dot{Q}$ represents respiratory muscle perfusion and $(Ca_{O_2} - Cv_{O_2})$ represents the arteriovenous oxygen content difference across the muscle. The left quadrant of Figure 29 plots respiratory muscle blood flow against $\dot{V}_{O_{2rs}}$ at different values of $(Ca_{O_2} - Cv_{O_2})$; clearly, for any given $\dot{V}_{O_{2rs}}$, the smaller the $(Ca_{O_2} - Cv_{O_2})$, as in septic shock, the greater the blood flow. For example, if a patient with severe airway obstruction has a $\dot{V}_{O_{2rs}}$ of 500 ml O_2/min, which corresponds to a minute ventilation ($\dot{V}_E$) of about 15 L/min, respiratory muscle blood flow will be of the order of 4 L/min for high values of $(Ca_{O_2} - Cv_{O_2})$ but will be much larger with lower values of $(Ca_{O_2} - Cv_{O_2})$ as can occur with anemia or hypoxemia. Although such values seem enormous, it has been shown (25,29) that the diaphragm can receive up to 200–400 ml/100 g/min of blood. Assuming similar properties for the other respiratory muscles (which comprise approximately 4–5 kg of a 70-kg man), the above estimate remains within the expectations of the Fick principle. Alternatively, during heavy work of breathing, many nonrespiratory muscles (arm, trunk) are recruited to aid in the ventilatory task, thus consuming oxygen and contributing to the high levels of $\dot{V}_{O_{2rs}}$ whether they move the thorax or not. In addition, if the cardiac output is decreased, as occurs in cardiogenic shock, the respiratory muscles may use a dangerously high proportion of this depressing available energy (31). Therefore, one can follow an imaginary pathway from health to disease: if a given ventilation is needed to maintain a normal P_{CO_2}, large amounts of work of breathing will be required; consequently, a greater amount

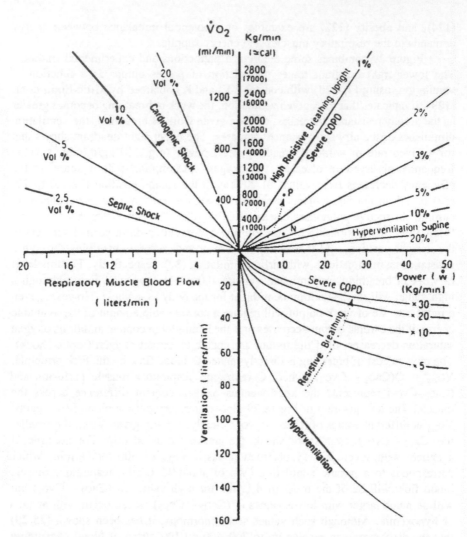

Figure 29 Relationship between respiratory muscle energetics and overall body economy in health and disease. (Left upper quadrant) Graphical solution of Fick principle at various arteriovenous oxygen content differences. (Right upper quadrant) Relationship of respiratory muscle energy expenditure with their power output at different levels of efficiency (1%, 2%, 3%, 5%, 10%, 20%). N, value obtained during hyperventilation in normal subjects in upright position; P, value obtained from normal breathing through resistance or subjects with airflow limitation. (Data from Ref. 129.)

of energy must be supplied. These increasing demands will be further potentiated by reducing the efficiency. Any compromise of available energy will potentiate the significance of these needs of the respiratory muscles.

References

1. Curtin, N. A., and R. C. Woledge. (1978). Energy changes and muscular contraction. *Physiol. Rev.* 58: 690–761.
2. Fenn, W. O., and B. S. Marsh. (1935). Muscular force at different speeds of shortening. *J. Physiol. Lond.* 85: 277–297.
3. Gibbs, C. L. (1974). Cardiac energetics. In: *Mammalian Myocardium*. Edited by G. A. Langer and A. J. Brady. New York: Wiley, pp. 105–133.
4. Gibbs, C. L. (1978). Cardia energetics. *Physiol. Rev.* 58: 174–254.
5. Gibbs, C. L., and J. B. Chapman. (1979). Cardiac energetics. In: *Handbook of Physiology. The Cardiovascular System*. Edited by R. M. Berne and N. Sperelakis. Bethesda, MD: Am. Physiol. Soc., sect. 2, vol. I, chap. 22, pp. 775–804.
6. Hill, A. V. (1964). The variation of total heat production in a twitch with velocity of shortening. *Proc. R. Soc. Lond. Ser. B.* 159: 596–605.
7. Homsher, E., and C. J. Kean. (1978). Skeletal muscle energetics and metabolism. *Annu. Rev. Physiol.* 40: 93–131.
8. Mommaerts, W. F. H. M. (1969). Energetics of muscular contraction. *Physiol. Rev.* 49: 427–508.
9. Wilkie, D. R. (1974). The efficiency of muscular contraction. *J. Mechanochem. Cell. Motil.* 2: 257–267.
10. Wilkie, D. R. (1968). Heat work and phosphorylcreatine break-down in muscle. *J. Physiol. Lond.* 195: 157–183.
11. Fenn, W. O. (1923). A quantitative comparison between the energy liberated and the work performed by the isolated sartorius muscle of the frog. *J. Physiol. Lond.* 58: 175–203.
12. Fenn, W. O. (1924). The relation between the work performed and the energy liberated in muscle contraction. *J. Physiol. Lond.* 58: 373–395.
13. Hill, A. V. (1938). The heat of shortening and the dynamic constants of muscle. *Proc. R. Soc. Lond. Ser. B* 126: 136–195.
14. Agostoni, E., and W. O. Fenn. (1960). Velocity of muscle shortening as a limiting factor in respiratory air flow. *J. Appl. Physiol.* 15: 349–353.
15. Rous, P., and H. P. Gilding. (1929). Studies of tissue maintenance. I. The changes with diminished blood bulk. *J. Exp. Med.* 50: 189–211.
16. Anrep, G. V., S. Cerqua, and A. Samaan. (1933). The effect of muscular contraction upon the blood flow in the skeletal muscle in the diaphragm and in the small intestine. *Proc. R. Soc. Lond. Ser. B* 114: 245–257.
17. Aguggini, G., P. Mognoni, F. Saibene, and M. G. Clement. (1972). Flusso ematico nell'arteria diafragmatica di cane durante iperventilazione (Abstract). *Atti. Congr. Naz. Soc. It. Fisiol.*, 24th, Rome.
18. Rochester, D. F., and M. Pradel-Guena. (1973). Measurement of diaphragmatic blood flow in dogs from xenon 133 clearance. *J. Appl. Physiol.* 34: 68–74.
19. Mognoni, P., F. Saibene, G. Sant'Ambrogio, and E. Camparesi. (1974). Perfusion of inspiratory muscles at different levels of ventilation in rabbits. *Respir. Physiol.* 20: 171–179.
20. Kety, S. S., and C. F. Schmidt. (1945). The determination of cerebral blood flow in man by the use of nitrous oxide in low concentrations. *Am. J. Physiol.* 143: 53–66.
21. Rochester, D. F. (1974). Measurement of diaphragmatic blood flow and oxygen consumption in the dog by the Kety-Schmidt technique. *J. Clin. Invest.* 53: 1126–1221.
22. Rochester, D. F., and G. Bettini. (1976). Diaphragmatic blood flow and energy expenditure in the dog. *J. Clin. Invest.* 57: 661–672.

23. Adachi, H., W. Straus, H. Ochi, and H. N. Wagner, Jr. (1976). The effect of hypoxia on the regional distribution of cardiac output in the dog. *Circ. Res.* 29: 314–319.

23a. Busse, J. (1977). Blood flow and metabolism of the diaphragm of intact dogs. Cologne, West Germany: University of Cologne. Thesis.

24. Buchler, B., S. Magder, H. Katsardis, Y. Jammes, and C. Roussos. (1985). Effects of pleural pressure and abdominal pressure on diaphragmatic blood flow. *J. Appl. Physiol.* 58: 691–697.

25. Buchler, B., S. Magder, and C. Roussos. (1985). Effects of contraction frequency and duty cycle on diaphragmatic blood flow. *J. Appl. Physiol.* 58: 265–273.

26. Fixler, D. E., J. M. Atkins, J. H. Mitchell, and L. D. Horwitz. (1976). Blood flow to respiratory, cardiac, and limb muscles in dogs during graded exercise. *Am. J. Physiol.* 231: 1515–1519.

27. Hales, J. R. S. (1973). Effects of heat stress on blood flow in respiratory and non-respiratory muscle in the sheep. *Pfluegers Arch.* 345: 123–130.

28. Robertson, C. H., Jr., W. L. Eshenbacher, and R. L. Johnson, Jr. (1977). Respiratory muscle blood flow distribution during expiratory resistance. *J. Clin. Invest.* 60: 473–480.

29. Robertson, C. H., Jr., G. H. Foster, and R. L. Johnson, Jr. (1977). The relationship of respiratory failure to the oxygen consumption of, lactic production by, and distribution of blood flow among respiratory muscles during increasing inspiratory resistance. *J. Clin. Invest.* 59: 31–42.

30. Robertson, C. H., Jr., M. A. Pagel, and R. L. Johnson, Jr. (1977). The distribution of blood flow, oxygen consumption, and work output among the respiratory muscles during unobstructed hyperventilation. *J. Clin. Invest.* 59: 43–50.

31. Viires, N., G. Sillye, A. Aubier, G. Rassidakis, and C. Roussos. (1983). Regional blood flow distribution in dog during induced hypotension and low cardiac output. Spontaneous breathing versus artificial ventilation. *J. Clin. Invest.* 72: 935–947.

32. Scharf, S. M., and H. Bark. (1984). Function of canine diaphragm with hypovolemic shock and β-adrenergic blockade. *J. Appl. Physiol.* 56:648–655.

33. Hussain, S. N. A., C. Roussos, and S. Magder. (1988). Autoregulation of diaphragmatic blood flow in dogs. *J. Appl. Physiol.* 64:329–336.

34. Hussain, S. N. A., C. Roussos, and S. Magder. (1989). Effects of tension, duty cycle, and arterial pressure on diaphragmatic blood flow in dogs. *J. Appl. Physiol.* 66:968–976.

35. Hussain, S. N. A., C. Roussos, and S. Magder. (1989). In situ isolated perfused and innervated left hemidiaphragm preparation. *J. Appl. Physiol.* 67:2941–2946.

36. Ward, M. E., S. Magder, and S. N. A. Hussain. (1992). Oxygen delivery-independent effect of blood flow on diaphragm fatigue. *Am. Rev. Respir. Dis.* 145:1058–1063.

37. Manohar, M. (1988). Costal vs. crural diaphragmatic blood flow during submaximal and near-maximal exercise in ponies. *J. Appl. Physiol.* 65:1514–1519.

38. Bark, H., G. S. Supinski, and J. C. La Manna. (1987). Relationship of changes in diaphragmatic muscle blood flow to muscle contractile activity. *J. Appl. Physiol.* 62:291–299.

39. Bellemare, F., D. Wight, and C. M. Lavigne. (1983). Effect of tension and timing of contraction on the blood flow of the diaphragm. *J. Appl. Physiol.* 54:1597–1606.

40. Hussain, S. N. A., C. Roussos, and S. Magder. (1988). Autoregulation of diaphragmatic blood flow in dogs. *J. Appl. Physiol.* 64:329–336.

41. Reid, M. B., and R. L. Johnson, Jr. (1983). Efficiency, maximal blood flow, and aerobic work capacity of canine diaphragm. *J. Appl. Physiol. Respir. Environ. Exercise Physiol.* 54: 763–772.

42. Scharf, S. M., H. Bark, S. Einhorn, and K. A. Tarasiuk. (1986). Blood flow to the canine diaphragm during hemorrhagic shock. *Am. Rev. Respir. Dis.* 133:205–211.

43. Doherty, J. U., and C. Liang. (1984). Arterial hypoxemia in awake dogs. Role of the sympathetic nervous system in mediating the systemic hemodynamic and regional blood flow responses. *J. Lab. Clin. Med.* 104:665–677.

44. Bark, H. S., G. S. Supinski, R. J. Bundy, and S. Kelsen. (1988). Effect of hypoxia on diaphragm blood flow, oxygen uptake, and contractility. *Am. Rev. Respir. Dis.* 138:1535–1541.

45. Supinski, G. S., H. Bark, and A. Guanciale. (1986). Effect of alterations in muscle fiber length on diaphragm blood flow. *J. Appl. Physiol.* 60:1789–1796.
46. Honig, C. R., and C. L. Odoroff. (1981). Calculated dispersion of capillary transit times: significance for oxygen exchange. *Am. J. Physiol.* 240 (Heart Circ Physiol 9): H199–H208.
47. Horstman, D. H., M. Gleser, and J. Delehunt. (1976). Effects of altering O_2 delivery on V_{O_2} of isolated, working muscle. *Am. J. Physiol.* 230: 327–334.
48. Laughlin, M. H., and R. B. Armstrong. (1982). Muscular blood flow distribution patterns as a function of running speed in rats. *Am. J. Physiol.* 243 (Heart Circ Physiol 12): H296–H306.
49. Manohar, M., J. Thurmon, W. J. Tranquilli, M. Devous, M. Theodovakis, R. Shawley, D. Feller, and J. Benson. (1981). Regional myocardial blood flow and coronary vascular reserve in unanesthetized young calves with severe concentric right ventricular hypertrophy. *Circ. Res.* 48: 785–796.
50. Ward ME, S. Magder, and S. N. A. Hussain. (1993). Role of endothelium-derived relaxing factor in reactive hyperemia in canine diaphragm. *J. Appl. Physiol.* 74:1606–1612.
51. Bjornberg, J., U. Albert, and S. Mellander. (1990). Resistance responses in proximal arterial vessels, arterioles and veins during reactive hyperaemia in skeletal muscle and their underlying regulatory mechanisms. *Acta Physiol. Scand.* 139:535–550.
52. McGilvery, R. W. (1975). The use of fuels for muscular work. In: *Metabolic Adaptation to Prolonged Physical Exercise.* Edited by H. Howald and J. R. Poortmans. Berlin: Birkhauser, pp. 12–30.
53. McGilvery, R. W. (1979). Fuel for breathing. *Am. Rev. Respir. Dis.* 119: 85–88.
54. Odessey, R. (1979). Amino acid and protein metabolism in the diaphragm. *Am. Rev. Respir. Dis.* 119: 107–112.
55. Rochester, D. F., and A. M. Briscoe. (1979). Metabolism of the working diaphragm. *Am. Rev. Respir. Dis.* 119: 85–88.
56. Eldridge, F. (1966). Anaerobic metabolism of the respiratory muscles. *J. Appl. Physiol.* 21: 853–857.
57. Jardim, J., G. Farkas, C. Prefaut, D. Thomas, P. T. Macklem, and C. Roussos. (1981). The failing inspiratory muscles under normoxic and hypoxic conditions. *Am. Rev. Respir. Dis.* 124: 274–279.
58. Bazzy, A. R., L. M. Pang, S. R. Akabas, and G. G. Haddad. (1989). O_2 metabolism of the sheep diaphragm during flow resistive loading breathing. *J. Appl. Physiol.* 66:2305–2311.
59. Manohar, M., T. E. Goetz, and D. Nganwa. (1988). Costal diaphragmatic O_2 and lactase extraction in laryngeal hemiplegic ponies during exercise. *J. Appl. Physiol.* 65:1723–1728.
60. Manohar, M., and A. S. Hassan. (1991). Diaphragmatic energetics during prolonged exhaustive exercise. *Am. Rev. Respir. Dis.* 144:415–418.
61. Piiper, J., P. E. Di Prampero, and P. Cerretelli. (1968). Oxygen debt and high-energy phosphates in gastrocnemius muscle of the dog. *Am. J. Physiol.* 215: 523–531.
62. Stainsby, W. N., and H. G. Welch. (1966). Lactate metabolism of contracting dog skeletal muscle in situ. *Am. J. Physiol.* 211: 177–183.
63. Hollanders, F. D. (1968). The production of lactic acid by the diaphragm. *Comp. Biochem. Physiol.* 26: 907–916.
64. Roncoroni, A. J., H. J. A. Adrougué, C. W. De Obrutsky, M. L. Marchisio, and M. R. Herrero. (1976). Metabolic acidosis in status asthmaticus. *Respiration* 33: 85–94.
65. Aubier, M., N. Viires, G. Sillye, and C. Roussos. (1982). Respiratory muscle contribution to lactic acidosis in low cardiac output. *Am. Rev. Respir. Dis.* 126: 648–652.
66. Liljestrand, G. (1918). Untersuchungen über die Atmungsarbeit. *Skand. Arch. Physiol.* 35: 199–293.
67. Campbell, E. J. M., E. K. Westlake, and R. M. Cherniack. (1957). Simple methods of estimating oxygen consumption and efficiency of the muscles of breathing. *J. Appl. Physiol.* 11: 303–308.
68. Benedict, F. (1918). A probable respiration apparatus for clinical use. *Boston Med. Surg. J.* 178: 667–678.

69. Roth, P. (1922). Graphic method for the estimation of the metabolic rate. *Boston Med. Surg. J.* 196: 457.
70. Cherniack, R. M. (1959). The oxygen consumption and efficiency of respiratory muscle in health and emphysema. *J. Clin. Invest.* 38: 494–499.
71. Otis, A. B. (1954). The work of breathing. *Physiol. Rev.* 34: 449–458.
72. Milic-Emili, G., and J. M. Petit. (1960). Mechanical efficiency of breathing. *J. Appl. Physiol.* 15: 359–362.
73. Newhouse, M. T., M. R. Becklake, P. T. Macklem, and M. McGregor. (1964). Effect of alterations in end tidal CO_2 tension on flow resistance. *J. Appl. Physiol.* 19: 745–749.
74. McKerrow, C. B., and A. B. Otis. (1956). Oxygen cost of hyperventilation. *J. Appl. Physiol.* 9: 375–379.
75. Bartlett, R. G., Jr., H. F. Brubach, and H. Specht. (1958). Oxygen cost of breathing. *J. Appl. Physiol.* 12: 413–434.
76. Shephard, R. J. (1966). The oxygen cost of breathing during vigorous exercise. *Q. J. Exp. Physiol.* 57: 336–350.
77. Bradley, M. E., and D. E. Leith. (1978). Ventilatory muscle training and the oxygen cost of sustained hyperpnea. *J. Appl. Physiol. Respir. Environ. Exercise Physiol.* 45: 885–892.
78. Roussos, C., and P. T. Macklem. (1982). The respiratory muscles. *N. Engl. J. Med.* 307: 786–797.
79. Roussos, C. (1985). Energetics. In: Lung Biology in Health and Disease. *The Thorax.* Edited by C. Roussos and P. T. Macklem. New York: Dekker, pp. 437–492.
80. Campbell, E. J. M., E. Agostoni, and J. Newsom Davis (editors). (1970). *The Respiratory Muscles: Mechanics and Neural Control.* Philadelphia: Saunders.
81. Sarnoff, S. J., E. Braunwald, and G. H. Welch, Jr., R. B. Case, W. N. Stainsby, and R. Macurz. (1958). Hemodynamic determinants of oxygen consumption of the heart with special reference to the tension-time index. *Am. J. Physiol.* 192: 148–156.
82. McGregor, M., and M. Becklake. (1961). The relationship of oxygen cost of breathing to respiratory mechanical work and respiratory force. *J. Clin. Invest.* 40: 971–980.
83. Field, S., S. Sanci, and A. Grassino. (1984). Respiratory muscle oxygen consumption estimated by the diaphragm pressure-time index. *J. Appl. Physiol.* 57:44–51.
84. Rayford, C. R., E. M. Khouri, and D. E. Gregg. (1965). Effect of excitement on coronary and systemic energetics in unanaesthetized dogs. *Am. J. Physiol.* 209: 680–688.
85. Monroe, R. G., R. H. Strang, C. G. LaFarge, and J. Levy. (1964). Ventricular performance, pressure-volume relationships, and O_2 consumption during hypothermia. *Am. J. Physiol.* 206: 67–73.
86. Sonnenblick, E. H., J. Ross, Jr., J. W. Covell, G. A. Kaiser, and E. Braunwald. (1965). Velocity of contraction as a determinant of myocardial oxygen consumption. *Am. J. Physiol.* 209: 919–927.
87. Collett, P. W., C. Perry, and L. A. Engel. (1985). Pressure-time product, flow, and oxygen cost of resistive breathing in humans. *J. Appl. Physiol.* 58:1263–1272.
88. Dodd, D. S., S. Kelly, P. W. Collett, and L. A. Engel. (1988). Pressure-time product, work rate, and endurance during resistive breathing in humans. *J. Appl. Physiol.* 64:1397–1404.
89. Dodd, D. S., P. W. Collett, and L. A. Engel. (1988). Influence of inspiratory flow rate and frequency on O_2 cost of resistive breathing in humans. *J. Appl. Physiol.* 65:760–766.
90. Gibbs, C. K., and W. R. Gibson. (1972). Energy production of rat soleus muscle. *Am. J. Physiol.* 223:864–879.
90a. Roussos, C. S., and P. T. Macklem. (1977). Diaphragmatic fatigue in man. *J. Appl. Physiol. Respir. Environ. Exercise Physiol.* 43: 189–197.
91. DuBois, A. B., A. W. Brody, D. H. Lewis, and B. F. Burgess, Jr. (1956). Oscillation mechanics of lungs and chest in man. *J. Appl. Physiol.* 8: 587–594.
92. Mead, J. (1956). Measurement of inertia of the lungs at increased ambient pressure. *J. Appl. Physiol.* 9: 208–212.
93. Campbell, E. J. M. (1958). *The Respiratory Muscles and the Mechanics of Breathing.* Chicago: Year Book.

94. Otis, A. B., W. O. Fenn, and H. Rahn. (1950). The mechanics of breathing in man. *J. Appl. Physiol.* 2: 592–607.
95. Otis, A. B. (1964). The work of breathing. In: *Handbook of Physiology. Respiration.* Edited by W. O. Fenn and H. Rahn. Washington, DC: Am. Physiol. Soc., sect. 3, vol. I, chapt. 17, pp. 463–476.
96. Agostoni, E., and P. Mognoni. (1966). Deformation of the chest wall during breathing efforts. *J. Appl. Physiol.* 21: 1827–1832.
97. Agostoni, E., P. Mognoni, G. Torri, and F. Saracino. (1965). Relation between changes of rib cage circumference and lung volume. *J. Appl. Physiol.* 20: 1179–1186.
98. Agostoni, E., and G. Torri. (1967). An analysis of the chest wall motions at high values of ventilation. *Respir. Physiol.* 3: 318–322.
99. Bergofsky, E. H. (1964). Relative contributions of the rib cage and the diaphragm to ventilation in man. *J. Appl. Physiol.* 19: 698–706.
100. Goldman, M. D. (1972). *Thoracoabdominal Mechanics and the Work of Breathing.* Boston: Harvard School of Public Health, MD thesis.
101. Goldman, M. D., G. Grimby, and J. Mead. (1976). Mechanical work of breathing derived from rib cage and abdominal V-P partitioning. *J. Appl. Physiol.* 41: 752–763.
102. Grimby, G., J. Bunn, and J. Mead. (1968). Relative contribution of rib cage and abdomen to ventilation during exercise. *J. Appl. Physiol.* 24: 159–166.
103. Grimby, G., M. Goldman, and J. Mead. (1976). Respiratory muscle action inferred from rib cage and abdominal V-P partitioning. *J. Appl. Physiol.* 41: 739–751.
104. Konno, K., and J. Mead. (1968). Static volume-pressure characteristics of the rib cage and abdomen. *J. Appl. Physiol.* 24: 544–548.
105. Agostoni, E., P. Mognoni, G. Torri, and G. Miserocchi. (1966). Forces deforming the rib cage. *Respir. Physiol.* 2: 105–117.
106. Macklem, P. T. (1979). A mathematical and graphical analysis of inspiratory muscles action. *Respir. Physiol.* 38: 133–171.
107. Loring, S. H., and J. Mead. (1982). Action of the diaphragm on the rib cage inferred from a force-balance analysis. *J. Appl. Physiol. Respir. Environ. Exercise Physiol.* 53: 756–760.
108. Macklem, P. T., D. Gross, A. Grassino, C. Roussos. (1978). Partitioning of inspiratory pressure swings between diaphragm and intercostal/accessory muscles. *J. Appl. Physiol. Respir. Environ. Exercise Physiol.* 44: 200–208.
109. Macklem, P. T., D. M. Macklem, and A. De Troyer. (1983). A model of inspiratory muscles mechanics. *J. Appl. Physiol Respir. Environ. Exercise Physiol.* 55: 547–557.
110. Macklem, P. T., C. Roussos, J. P. Derenne, and L. Delhez. (1979). The interaction between the diaphragm intercostal/accessory muscles of inspiration and the rib cage. *Respir. Physiol.* 38: 141–152.
111. Mead, J., and S. H. Loring. (1982). Analysis of volume displacement and length changes of the diaphragm during breathing. *J. Appl. Physiol. Respir. Environ. Exercise Physiol.* 53: 750–755.
112. Mead, J., J. C. Smith, and S. H. Loring. (1985). Volume displacements of the chest wall and their mechanical significance. In: *Lung Biology in Health and Disease. The Thorax.* Edited by C. Roussos and P. T. Macklem. New York: Dekker, pp. 369–392.
113. Cook, C. D., J. M. Sutherland, S. Segal, R. B. Cherry, J. Mead, M. B. McIlroy, and C. A. Smith. (1957). Studies of respiratory physiology. III. Measurements of mechanics of respiration. *J. Clin. Invest.* 36: 440–448.
114. Cooper, E. A. (1960). A comparison of the respiratory work done against an external resistance by man and by a sine wave pump. *Q. J. Exp. Physiol.* 45: 179–191.
115. Margaria, R., G. Milic-Emili, J. M. Petit, and G. Cavagna. (1960). Mechanical work of breathing during muscular exercise. *J. Appl. Physiol.* 15: 354–358.
116. Milic-Emili, J. (1991). Work of breathing. In: Crystal RG, West JB et al. eds. *The Lung.* New York: Raven Press, pp. 1065–1075.
117. Bates, J. H. T., K. A. Brown, and T. Kochi. (1990). Respiratory mechanics in the normal dog determined by expiratory flow interruption. *J. Appl. Physiol.* 67:2276–2285.

118. Barnas, G. M., K. Yoshiko, S. T. L. Lorring, and J. Mead. (1987). Impedance and relative displacements of relaxed chest wall up to 4 Hz. *J. Appl. Physiol.* 62:71–81.
119. D'Angelo, E., E. Calderini, G. Torri, F. Robatto, D. Bono, and J. Milic-Emili. (1990). Respiratory mechanics in anesthetized-paralyzed humans: effects of flow, volume and time. *J. Appl. Physiol.* 67:2556–2564.
120. Mead, J., and E. Agostoni. (1964). Dynamics of breathing. In: Femm WO, Rahn H, eds. Handbook of Physiology, Section 3: Respiration, vol. 1. Washington, DC: American Physiological Society, pp. 411–427.
121. Lafortuna, C. L., A. E. Minetti, and P. Mognoni. (1984). Modelling the airflow pattern in humans. *J. Appl. Physiol.* 57:1111–1119.
122. Sharp, J., J. P. Henry, S. K. Sweany, W. R. Meadows, and R. J. Pietras. (1964). The total work of breathing in normal and obese men. *J. Clin. Invest.* 43: 728–739.
123. Milic-Emili, J., J. Mead, and J. M. Turner. (1964). Topography of esophageal pressure as a function of posture in man. *J. Appl. Physiol.* 19: 212–216.
124. Bergofsky, E. H., G. M. Turino, and A. P. Fishman. (1959). Cardiorespiratory failure in kyphoscoliosis. *Med.* Baltimore 38: 263–317.
125. Opie, L. H., J. M. K. Splading, and F. D. Scott. (1959). Mechanical properties of the chest during intermittent positive-pressure respiration. *Lancet* 1: 545–550.
126. Jaeger, M. J., and A. B. Otis. (1964). Effects of compressibility of alveolar gas on dynamics and work of breathing. *J. Appl. Physiol.* 19: 83–91.
127. Milic-Emil, J., M. M. Orzalesi, C. D. Cook, and J. M. Turner. (1964). Respiratory thoracoabdominal mechanics in man. *J. Appl. Physiol.* 19:217–223.
128. Fritts, H. N., Jr., J. Filler, A. P. Fishman, and A. Cournand. (1959). The efficiency of ventilation during voluntary hyperpnea. *J. Clin. Invest.* 38: 1339–1348.
129. Milic-Emili, G., J. M. Petit, and R. Deroanne. (1962). Mechanical work of breathing during exercise in trained and untrained subjects. *J. Appl. Physiol.* 17: 43–46.
130. Milic-Emili, J., J. M. Petit, and R. Deroanne. (1961). Il lavono meccanico della respirazione durante rirespirazione. *Arch. Sci. Biol.* 45:141–153.
131. Milic-Emili, G., J. M. Petit, and R. Deroanne. (1960). The effects of respiratory rate on the mechanical work of breathing during muscular exercise. *Int. Z. Angew. Physiol. Einschl. Arbeitsphysiol.* 18: 330–340.
132. Vincent, M. J., R. Knudson, D. E. Leith, P. T. Macklem, and J. Mead. (1970). Factor influencing pulmonary resistance. *J. Appl. Physiol.* 29:236–243.
133. Craig, A. B., Jr. (1960). Maximal work of one breathing cycle. *J. Appl. Physiol.* 15: 1098–1100.
134. Wilkie, D. R. (1950). The relation between force and velocity in human muscle. *J. Physiol. Lond.* 110: 249–280.
135. Cain, C. C., and A. B. Otis. (1949). Some physiological effects resulting from added resistance to respiration. *J. Aviat. Med.* 20: 149–160.
136. Campbell, E. J. M., E. K. Westlake, and R. M. Cherniack. (1958). The oxygen consumption and efficiency of the respiratory muscles of young male subjects. *Clin. Sci.* 18: 55–64.
137. Cala, S. J., P. Wilcox, J. Edyrean, M. Rynn, and L. A. Engel. (1990). Oxygen cost of inspiratory loading: resistive vs. elastic. *J. Appl. Physiol.* 70:1983–1990.
138. Collett, P. W., and L. A. Engel. (1986). Influence of lung volume on oxygen cost of resistive breathing. *J. Appl. Physiol.* 61:16–24.
139. McCool, E. D., G. E. Tzelepis, D. E. Leith, and F. G. Hoppin. (1989). Oxygen cost of breathing during fatiguing inspiratory resistive loads. *J. Appl. Physiol.* 66:2045–2055.
140. Cavagna, G. A., and M. Kaneko. (1977). Mechanical work and efficiency in level walking and running. *J. Physiol. Lond.* 26: 467–481.
140a. Rohrer, F. Physiologie der Atembewegung. (1925). In: *Handbuch der normalen und pathologischen Physiologie.* Edited by A. T. J. Bethe, G. von Bergmann, G. Embden, and A. Ellinger. Berlin: Springer-Verlag, vol. 2, pp. 70–127.
141. Mead, J. (1960). Control of respiratory frequency. *J. Appl. Physiol.* 15: 325–336.

142. Agostoni, E., F. F. Thimm, and W. O. Fenn. (1959). Comparative features of breathing. *J. Appl. Physiol.* 14: 679–683.
143. Crosfill, M. L., and J. G. Widdicombe. (1961). Physical characteristics of the chest and lungs and the work of breathing in different mammalian species. *J. Physiol. Lond.* 158: 1–14.
144. McIlroy, M. R., R. Marshall, and R. V. Christie. (1954). Work of breathing in normal subjects. *Clin. Sci.* 13: 127–136.
145. Milic-Emili, G., and J. M. Petit. (1959). Il lavoro mecanico della respirazione a varia frequenza respiratoria. *Arch. Sci. Biol. Bologna* 43: 326–330.
146. Clark, J. M., R. D. Sinclair, and J. B. Lenox. (1980). Chemical and nonchemical components of ventilation during hypercapnic exercise in man. *J. Appl. Physiol. Respir. Environ. Exercise Physiol.* 48: 1065–1076.
147. Evans, C. L., and A. V. Hill. (1914). The relations of length to tension development and heat production on contraction in muscle. *J. Physiol. Lond.* 49: 1–16.
148. Hill, A. V. (1925). Length of muscle and the heat and tension developed in an isometric contraction. *J. Physiol. Lond.* 60: 237–263.
149. McDonald, R. H., Jr. (1966). Developed tension: a major determinant of myocardial oxygen consumption. *Am. J. Physiol.* 210: 351–356.
150. Jammes, Y., P. T. P. Bye, R. L. Pardy, and C. Roussos. (1983). Vagal feedback with expiratory threshold load under extracorporeal circulation. *J. Appl. Physiol. Respir. Environ. Exercise Physiol.* 55: 316–322.
151. Remmers, J. E., and I. Marttila. (1975). Action of intercostal muscle afferents on the respiratory rhythm of anesthetized cats. *Respir. Physiol.* 24: 31–41.
152. Aubier, M., T. Trippenbach, and C. Roussos. (1981). Respiratory muscle fatigue during cardiogenic shock. *J. Appl. Physiol. Respir. Environ. Exercise Physiol.* 51: 499–508.
153. Cournand, A., D. W. Richards, R. A. Bader, M. E. Bader, and A. P. Fishman. (1954). The oxygen cost of breathing. *Trans. Assoc. Am. Physi.* 67: 162–173.
154. Nielsen, M. (1936). Die Respirationsarbeit bei Körperruhe und bei Muskul Arbeit. *Skand. Arch. Physiol.* 74: 299–316.
155. Rossier, P. H., and A. Bühlmann. (1959). Dyspnoe und Atemarbeit. *Schweiz. Med. Wochenschr.* 89: 543–548.

Part III

RESPIRATORY MUSCLE CONTROL

26

Control of Respiratory Motor Activity

**THOMAS E. DICK and
ERIK VAN LUNTEREN**

Case Western Reserve University
Cleveland, Ohio

STEVEN G. KELSEN

Temple University School of Medicine
Philadelphia, Pennsylvania

I. Introduction

Respiratory muscles are characterized by their activity pattern, which is correlated with ventilation, and by their mechanical action, which is to influence airflow. These muscles can be classified further as either valvular or pumping muscles, based on their function. Valvular muscles are muscles the activity of which influences airflow resistance. These are the laryngeal, pharyngeal, palatal, and nasal muscles, and consist of both abductors—muscles for which activity decreases airway resistance—and adductors—muscles for which activity increases airway resistance. Generally, abductors are active during inspiration, facilitating airflow and resisting airway collapse (see hypoglossal nerve activity; Fig. 1), whereas adductors are active during early expiration braking airflow (see thyroarytenoid nerve activity; Fig. 1). However, it should be kept in mind that inactivity of abductors is a major contributor to the increase in airway resistance during expiration. Pumping muscles are muscles the activity of which alters thoracic volume and airway pressure. The muscles of the thorax (i.e., chest wall) represent most of the pumping muscles. Thoracic muscles act both as inspiratory muscles that increase thoracic volume and decrease airway pressure (see phrenic nerve activity, Fig. 1); and as expiratory muscles that decrease thoracic volume and increase airway pressure (see triangularis sterni nerve activity, Fig. 1). Abdominal muscles are another set of pumping muscles that can be activated during expiration to decrease thoracic volume. In this chapter, the control and function of the thoracic pumping muscles will be contrasted with those of the airway valvular muscles.

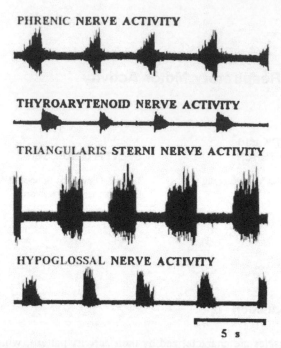

PHRENIC NERVE ACTIVITY

THYROARYTENOID NERVE ACTIVITY

TRIANGULARIS STERNI NERVE ACTIVITY

HYPOGLOSSAL NERVE ACTIVITY

5 s

Figure 1 Representative motor activities of the respiratory cycle. Top trace, phrenic nerve activity associated with inspiration. It has a graded, augmenting ramp profile. Second trace, thyroarytenoid nerve activity associated with stage I expiration or the central postinspiration. The thyroarytenoid muscle is a laryngeal adductor, increasing airway resistance and braking airflow. It has a decrementing profile that appears to last longer than the postinspiratory activity of the phrenic nerve. Third trace, triangularis sterni activity associated with stage II expiration or central expiration. It has an augmenting ramp profile. Bottom trace, middle branch of the hypoglossal nerve associated with inspiration also, but a distinctly different profile, almost decrementing. These recordings were made in a decerebrate, vagotomized cat during eucapnia and normothermia.

Respiratory muscles also participate in other behaviors, most notably posture. In the mid-1970s, the postural function of these muscles was correlated to the number of muscle spindles that the respiratory muscle possessed (Duron, 1973; Duron et al., 1978; Duron and Marlot, 1980). Intercostal muscles participate in both respiration and posture, possess a high concentration of muscle spindles, and have tonic activity that is modulated phasically (Taylor et al., 1960; Parmegianni and Sabattini, 1972; Duron, 1973; Duron et al., 1978; Duron and Marlot, 1980; Dick et al., 1982, 1984). These muscles were contrasted with the diaphragm, parasternal, and triangularis sterni muscles, which have low concentrations of spindles and highly phasic activity (Duron, 1973; Duron et al., 1978; Duron and Marlot, 1980).

The activity of postural muscles that have high concentrations of muscle spindles is heavily influenced by the state of consciousness. During rapid eye movement (REM) sleep, nuchal and hindlimb muscles are quiescent. Similarly, intercostal muscles have decreased activity during REM sleep, whereas diaphragmatic activity continues (Parmeggiani and Sabattini, 1972; Dick et al., 1984). However, this decrease in muscle activity is principally due to active inhibition of motoneurons by brain stem neurons, rather than disfacilitation of motoneurons by decreased excitatory afferent activity from muscle spindles (Glenn et al., 1978; Nakamura et al., 1978). Furthermore, in contrast with the correlation between activity and muscle spindle number, upper airway muscles, such as the genioglossus, are also quiescent during REM sleep (Remmers et al., 1980). This is also due to active inhibition of hypoglossal motoneurons during REM sleep and may lead to obstructive sleep apnea (Sauerland and Harper, 1976; Remmers et al., 1980).

The state of consciousness also influences the brain stem neurons controlling respiration. During REM sleep, breathing is highly variable. Variability in the breathing pattern has been correlated with pontogeniculo-occipital (PGO) waves, large fluctuations in the extracellular field potential caused by synchronous neuronal discharges that occur as isolated events in deep non-rapid eye movement (NREM) sleep and as clusters during REM sleep (Orem, 1980a,b). Medullary respiratory-modulated activity is excited during a PGO wave, but diaphragmatic activity appears to be inhibited, in fact, "fractionated" (Orem, 1980a,b). Thus, influences on respiratory motor activity interact not only at the level of the motoneuron— Sherrington's final common pathway—but also at the level of the brain stem (i.e., the respiratory pattern generator's input to respiratory motoneurons).

This review will examine three distinct influences controlling respiratory motoneurons. These are (1) input from the respiratory pattern generator (see Figs. 1 and 2) and other pattern generators (Fig. 3), (2) intrinsic membrane properties of motoneurons that may shape their response to these inputs, and (3) inputs associated with a state of consciousness (Fig. 4). A detailed description of the respiratory pattern generator is beyond the scope of this review. Indeed, a forthcoming monograph in the *Lung Biology in Health and Disease* series will be devoted to this subject. Moreover, reviews on the control of both spinal and cranial respiratory motoneurons have been published recently (Iscoe, 1988; Monteau and Hilaire, 1991).

II. Respiratory Pattern Generator

Over the last decade, research investigating the neural substrate of the respiratory pattern generator has utilized two distinctly different animal models (for reviews see Berger, 1990; Euler, 1986; Ezure, 1990; Richter et al., 1986, 1992; Feldman, 1986; Feldman et al., 1990; 1991). One is an *in vivo* and the other is an *in vitro* animal model. For the most part, the *in vivo* animal model has been the pentobarbital-anesthetized, paralyzed, vagotomized adult cat, although recently

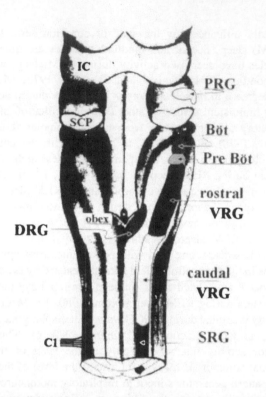

Figure 2 Schematic of the brainstem from a dorsal perspective. Respiratory groups outlined
on the right side. Abbreviations: IC, inferior colliculus; SCP, superior cerebellar peduncle;
C1, dorsal root of the first cervical nerve; DRG, dorsal respiratory group, associated with
the nucleus of the solitary tract in the dorsomedial medulla; PRG, pontine respiratory group,
associated with the medial parabrachial nucleus and Kölliker–Fuse nucleus in the dorsolateral
pons; Böt, Bötzinger complex, expiratory neurons associated with the retrofacial nucleus;
Pre-Böt, pre-Bötzinger, an area between the obex and Bötzinger complex that contains
neurons that may initiate inspiration; VRG, ventral respiratory group, the rostral part contains
bulbospinal inspiratory neurons, and the caudal part contains bulbospinal expiratory neurons;
SRG, spinal respiratory group at the C-1 level which contains preponderantly propriospinal
inspiratory neurons.

adult rats are being utilized more frequently (Ezure et al., 1988; Ellenberger and
Feldman, 1990; Ellenberger et al., 1990; Saether et al., 1987; Schwarzacher et al.,
1991). The *in vitro* animal model is derived from neonatal rat brainstem and spinal
cord tissue, and ranges in size from a 400-μm-thick slice of the medulla to the
complete brainstem spinal cord (Suzue, 1984; Smith and Feldman, 1987; Smith et
al., 1988, 1991; Berger, 1990). These two different experimental models led to two
different hypothetical models regarding the control of respiration. In particular, the
in vivo animal model led to a "network" model and the *in vitro* model led to a

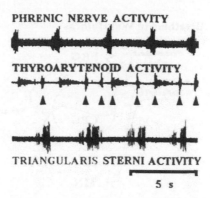

PHRENIC NERVE ACTIVITY

THYROARYTENOID ACTIVITY

TRIANGULARIS STERNI ACTIVITY

5 s

Figure 3 Representative motor activities of the respiratory cycle with repetitive swallowing. Top three traces, phrenic, thyroarytenoid, and triangularis sterni nerve activities, respectively. Swallows are the bursts of thyroarytenoid nerve activity (denoted by the arrow heads). Swallows occurred preponderantly at or near phase transitions, and when they occurred during expiration, triangularis sterni activity was inhibited. Repetitive swallowing was induced by stimulation of the superior laryngeal nerve in a decerebrate cat.

"pacemaker" model. In both these models, neural membrane properties and synaptic connections between neurons generate the rhythm. The difference lies in the degree to which synaptic connections or membrane properties determine the rhythm. In the "network" model, synaptic inhibition mediated through a chloride channel plays a critical role in determining phase duration, whereas in the "pacemaker" model the endogenous bursting properties of a single class of neurons determines rhythm. The former was hypothesized after demonstrating the hyperpolarization of cells during their quiescent phase could be reversed following intracellular chloride injection. The latter was demonstrated by recording repetitive and rhythmic activity in hypoglossal motoneurons after blocking chloride-dependent inhibition with glycine and GABAergic antagonists, bathing the tissue with chloride-free solution, and removing many of the other medullary nuclei hypothesized to be elements of the CPG (Feldman et al., 1990; Smith et al., 1991).

Although it is beyond the scope of this chapter to analyze and to resolve the differences in these models, a major difference between the models is the stage of their development. The in vitro model has employed neonatal tissue (Suzue, 1984). With maturation, the pacemaker may develop as an element within a network (Feldman et al., 1990; Richter et al., 1992). More mature in vitro preparations are dependent on chloride-mediated, inhibitory synaptic connections for a rhythm to be produced (Hayashi and Lipski, 1992). For the purpose of this chapter, we will focus on data from the in vivo model and assume that the respiratory drive potential is formed by a central pattern generator and is transmitted from the medulla to the spinal inter- and motoneurons (Sears, 1964).

Central pattern generators (CPG) are networks of neurons located in the central

(A) Breathing in Wakefulness

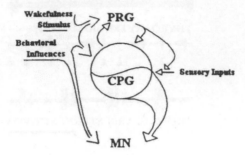

(B) Breathing in NREM Sleep

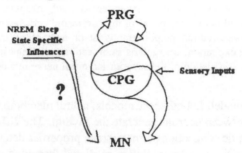

(C) Breathing in REM Sleep

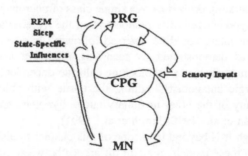

Figure 4 Schematics of the state-dependent influences on breathing. (A) During wakefulness, two distinct effects are present. The "wakefulness stimulus" and behavioral influences act on the respiratory pattern generator (denoted as CPG) and on respiratory motoneurons (denoted as MN). (B) During NREM sleep, the wakefulness stimulus is absent and state-specific NREM influences are highly questionable. (C) During REM sleep, again state influences act at two distinct sites: the CPG and the MN. On the right side of A, B, and C are shown interactions between the pontine respiratory group (PRG) and sensory input. A working hypothesis is that the PRG gates sensory input during different behaviors in wakefulness and during REM sleep. With NREM sleep, this gating phenomenon is diminished, and the CPG is reafferentated.

nervous system (Grillner, 1985; Grillner et al., 1991). Once activated, they elicit rhythmic, repetitive movements (Delcomyn, 1980). These movements are believed to be formed centrally because stereotypic, "fictive" patterns of motor nerve activity are generated in paralyzed, reduced animal preparations in which rhythmic afferent input, including sensory feedback, is absent. The generated patterns of motoneuronal activity depend not only on the connections of neurons in the network, but also on the membrane properties of these neurons (Richter et al., 1992).

As indicated in the foregoing the respiratory pattern generator remains active in both anesthetized in vivo and reduced in vitro preparations. However, many basic issues defining the respiratory CPG itself remain unresolved, for instance, the number of joints that the respiratory CPG controls. In locomotion, a CPG controls the movement at one joint (Delcomyn, 1980) and coupling between segmental CPGs provides the coordinated movement (Grillner et al., 1991). In breathing, it is not clear if one or more than one CPG controls cranial, cervical, thoracic, and lumbar musculature (Richardson and Mitchell, 1982). Another issue is whether the respiratory neuronal network is a separate functional entity, or if neuronal components of the respiratory CPG participate in one or more CPGs (i.e., for swallowing or chewing; Dick et al., 1993; Meyrand et al., 1991). Third, the manner in which the underlying neural mechanisms of the respiratory CPG affects timing of the cycle and amplitude of motor activity (Feldman, 1986); in particular, whether the neurons mediating changes in timing or rhythm differ from those mediating changes in amplitude of motor activity. Finally, it is unknown if the respiratory CPG consists of two or three distinct phases (see Fig. 1). A controversial three-phase model has been proposed (Richter et al., 1986, 1992), but similar data have been interpreted and presented in the classic two-phase model (Ezure, 1990). Peripheral motor activity has been interpreted to represent phases of the CPG; that is, phrenic nerve activity may be representative of the inspiratory phase, thyroarytenoid nerve activity represents the postinspiratory phase, and triangularis sterni nerve activity represents the expiratory phase (see Fig. 1; Hwang et al., 1989; Zhou et al., 1989; St. John and Zhou, 1989, 1990; Oku et al., 1993). However, centrally, these phases are determined by neurons having activities for which correlations with the cycle vary (Orem and Dick, 1983; Orem and Trotter, 1992).

Even though the respiratory CPG remains undefined, its location has been restricted to specific areas of the brain stem where three populations of rhythmically active cells have been recorded in various animal preparations (see Fig. 2) (for reviews see Euler, 1986; Feldman, 1986; Richter et al., 1986, 1992; Ezure, 1990). These populations are located in the dorsomedial and ventrolateral medulla and the dorsolateral pons, and have been referred to as the *dorsal* (DRG), *ventral* (VRG), and *pontine* (PRG) *respiratory groups*, respectively. Within these respiratory groups, various types of respiratory neurons were recorded. Since their original description in 1977 (Berger et al., 1977a, b, c), additional neighboring groups have been identified. Whether or not these neighboring groups should be included in the DRG and VRG is another issue that remains unresolved.

In general, neurons are characterized electrophysiologically by the location of their cell body, activity pattern, projection pattern, and synaptic input. Respiratory neurons are classified similarly. However, cells are labeled on the basis of their activity patterns, because neurons with different firing patterns appear clustered in the same respiratory group, and because projections are identified as whether or not they are activated antidromically from the spinal cord. The onset and offset of activity is defined in relation to phrenic nerve activity, and the envelope of their integrated discharge pattern has been described as augmenting, decrementing, or continuous, depending on whether discharge frequency increases, decreases, or remains the same during a phase of the respiratory cycle (Ezure, 1990). In addition, cells may have burst or sustained activity that starts in one phase and terminates in another. Despite this simple scheme for classifying neurons, similar neural activity has been classified differently by different authors (Richter et al., 1992). For example, neuronal activity that starts discharging immediately after phrenic nerve activity terminates, reaches its peak-firing frequency quickly, and decreases its firing frequency through the early stage of expiration, such as thyroarytenoid nerve activity (see Fig. 1), has been classified as postinspiratory, decrementing expiratory, early expiratory, biphasic expiratory, and even preinspiratory (Richter et al., 1992). The latter two names occur because these cells may discharge immediately before inspiration begins (Richter et al., 1987).

A. Dorsal Respiratory Group

The DRG was defined originally to include various types of inspiratory neurons located in the ventrolateral subnucleus of the solitary tract (nTS) (Berger, 1977; Berger et al., 1977a,b,c). Vagal afferent fibers from slowly adapting pulmonary stretch receptors (SAR) terminate in this subnucleus of the solitary tract and synapse directly on inspiratory-modulated neurons (Averill et al., 1984; Backman et al., 1984; Berger and Averill, 1983; Berger and Dick, 1987). In addition, pump-related or P cells were identified in the ventrolateral subnucleus (Berger, 1977; Berger and Dick, 1987). The P cells do not receive central respiratory drive potential (i.e., do not depolarize with inspiration), but their activity is synaptically driven by vagal afferent fibers innervating SARs so their activity is pump modulated (Berger and Dick, 1987). These cells may be second-order interneurons in the Hering–Breuer reflex (Bonham and McCrimmon, 1990; Bonham et al., 1993).

Since the original description of the DRG, the terminal fields of pulmonary stretch receptor afferent fibers and of additional physiologically identified respiratory afferents have been mapped and found to extend beyond the classically defined DRG. Pulmonary SAR fibers terminate in other subnuclei of the solitary tract (Kalia and Richter, 1985a, b). Furthermore, myelinated fibers from rapidly adapting receptors (RAR) terminate primarily in the dorsal and dorsolateral subnuclei and secondarily in the intermediate subnucleus (Kalia and Richter, 1988a,b). No terminals have been found in the ventrolateral subnucleus (Kalia and Richter,

1988a,b). Similarly, bronchopulmonary C fibers terminate in the medial subnuclei rostral to the obex and in the commissural subnucleus caudal to the obex (Kubin et al., 1991; Bonham and Joad, 1991). In addition to these mechanical and irritant receptors, the chemical receptor afferents projecting from the carotid body in the carotid sinus nerve terminate in the dorsal, dorsolateral, and commissural subnuclei of the solitary tract (Berger, 1979b, 1980; Davies and Kalia, 1981).

Second-order neurons receiving input from these afferent fibers are also located beyond the classically identified DRG. The P cells have been recorded in the medial subnucleus of the solitary tract (Bonham and McCrimmon, 1990). Neurons in the commissural subnucleus have been identified as potentially the second-order neurons of pulmonary RARs (Lipski et al., 1991; Bonham and Joad, 1992). In addition few, if any, inspiratory-modulated neurons have been identified in the ventrolateral nucleus of the solitary tract in the rat (Saether et al., 1987; Ezure et al., 1988). Therefore, because the DRG was defined functionally, it seems reasonable to broaden the definition to include the terminal fields of respiratory afferent fibers, to include their second-order neurons and to include the subnuclei of the nTS associated with these neurons, especially the dorsal, dorsolateral, medial, and commissural subnuclei (see Fig. 2).

The inspiratory neurons in the DRG generally have an augmenting pattern of discharge, but can be distinguished by their onset times and their response to lung inflation (Berger, 1977). Nearly all inspiratory neurons project to the contralateral spinal cord (Berger, 1977) and synapse directly on phrenic motoneurons (Lipski et al., 1983). The activity of DRG inspiratory-modulated neurons can be enhanced by lung inflation, and these neurons may mediate Head's paradoxical reflex, a vagally mediated reflex in which lung inflation increases phrenic nerve activity (DiMarco et al., 1981). In addition, stimulation of the superior laryngeal nerve (SLN), an afferent nerve that terminates in the ventrolateral subnucleus (Bellingham and Lipski, 1992), evokes a short-latency excitation, followed by inhibition in the activity of the contralateral phrenic nerve that may also be mediated by these neurons (Donnelly et al., 1989). Lesions in the DRG diminish inspiratory motor activity in the diaphragm, but have little effect on respiratory frequency (Berger and Cooney, 1982; Speck and Feldman, 1982). Indeed, because extensive lesions affected only motor amplitude, rather than timing, attention has shifted away from the DRG playing a primary role in the generation of the respiratory pattern (compare Berger et al., 1977a,b,c with Richter et al., 1992).

Cells in the medial subnucleus may be necessary for the Hering–Breuer reflex in rats (Bonham and McCrimmon, 1990; Bonham et al., 1993). In this vagal reflex, first described in 1868, lung inflation terminates the inspiratory phase and prolongs the expiratory phase. Synaptic activation of P cells is essential for this reflex (Bonham and McCrimmon, 1990; Bonham et al., 1993).

In summary, the DRG was defined originally as the ventrolateral subnucleus of the solitary tract, but should be defined more broadly to include neurons, such as P cells, that integrate vagal afferent input with the respiratory pattern generator.

Moreover, a primary role of the DRG may be related to mediating reflexes, rather than providing the primary drive to phrenic and intercostal motoneurons.

B. Ventral Respiratory Group

Similar to the DRG, the original definition of the ventral respiratory group (VRG) has become too limiting (see Fig. 2). The original definition included a column of cells located in the ventrolateral medulla that consisted of nucleus ambiguus (nA), nucleus para-ambigualis (nPA), and nucleus retroambigualis (nRA) (Berger et al., 1977a,b,c; Feldman, 1986; Euler, 1986; Cohen, 1979). Vagal motoneurons of the nA innervate muscle of branchiomeric origin (e.g., the larynx) and are excluded from the respiratory pattern generator. The nRA contains both inspiratory and expiratory cell types, which are preferentially distributed, such that inspiratory neurons are preponderant in the rostral nRA and expiratory neurons are preponderant at the caudal end (Merrill, 1974). Many of these neurons composing the rostral and caudal VRG have bulbospinal projections (see Fig. 2).

Since the original description of the VRG, other groups of neurons have been identified at the rostral end of the VRG in the retrofacial nucleus. These are primarily expiratory neurons that have extensive medullary collaterals as well as projections down the spinal cord and have been referred to as the Bötzinger complex. In the neonatal in vitro preparation, successive sectioning of the tissue has led to the identification of a group of cells just caudal to the Bötzinger complex, which is referred to as the pre-Bötzinger complex (Smith et al., 1991). Recordings from these cells in the in vitro preparation indicate the presence of a conditional burster, a pacemakerlike cell that discharges rhythmically and repetitively with depolarizing input. Theoretically, each of these groups of cells have specific functions. For Bötzinger cells, the function has been hypothesized to be extensive inhibition of motor and premotor inspiratory neurons during expiration; and for pre-Bötzinger complex, the neurogenesis of inspiration (Feldman et al., 1990). However, many pharyngeal motoneurons have been characterized in the anatomical location identified as the Bötzinger complex (Grelot et al., 1989a,b; Zheng et al., 1991). The critical role of the pre-Bötzinger neurons in rhythmogenesis may be limited to an early stage of development (see foregoing and Richter et al., 1992). In addition, a second laboratory, using a similar in vitro preparation, has identified another population of inspiratory-initiating neurons slightly more rostral in the retrotrapezoid nucleus (Onimaru and Homma, 1987; Onimaru et al., 1992). These neurons discharge during pre- and postinspiration (Onimaru and Homma, 1987). Furthermore, an analogous population of cells may have been identified in the retrotrapezoid nucleus of the adult cat (Connelly et al., 1990). In summary, these data indicate that, although the exact roles of these neurons remain controversial, neurons in these nuclei are rhythmically active during phase transitions, critical periods in the cycle; therefore, similar to the definition of the DRG, the definition of the VRG should be extended to include these rostral groups that may play a vital role in the neurogenesis of respiration.

In mammals, motoneurons are excluded from rhythmogenesis and, consequently, the VRG (Feldman, 1986). However, the soma of many respiratory motoneurons are near and within the boundaries of the VRG. The upper airway is innervated by motoneurons of the trigeminal, facial, retrofacial, and hypoglossal nuclei, as well as those of the nA (Iscoe, 1988). The motor pools for the upper airway are organized somatotopically and rostrocaudally across nuclei [i.e., facial motoneurons that innervate alae nasi (Bystrzycka and Nail, 1983) versus nA motoneurons that innervate the larynx], and within nuclei [i.e., vagal motoneurons innervating the pharynx are located more rostral in the nA than those innervating the larynx (Davis and Nail, 1984; Yoshida et al., 1984)]. These motoneurons are not critical in generating respiratory rhythm because breathing persists in the absence of their activity, for instance, owing to anesthetics that attenuate activity of upper airway muscles (Sherrey and Megirian, 1977).

Several subtypes of inspiratory neurons in the rostral nRA separate from vagal motoneurons have been recorded in reduced preparations (Merrill, 1974; Smith et al., 1990). Even more variable types have been recorded in the intact, unanesthetized preparation (Orem, 1989; Orem and Dick, 1983, 1990; Orem et al., 1985; Orem and Trotter, 1992, 1993). In the anesthetized preparation, inspiratory neuronal activity displays one of the following patterns: (1) an early-onset, augmenting activity during inspiration; (2) an early-onset, decrementing activity; or (3) a late-onset activity. Inspiratory neurons with early-onset, augmenting activity may be propriobulbar or bulbospinal (premotor). Inspiratory neurons with an early-onset, decrementing firing pattern are propriobulbar and project extensively to the contralateral VRG. Neurons that discharge late in inspiration and cease firing shortly after the inspiratory phase has terminated (late inspiratory neurons) are found in both the DRG and VRG and are most likely propriobulbar cells (Euler, 1986; Feldman, 1986; Richter et al., 1986, 1992; Ezure, 1990).

Expiratory neurons of the caudal nRA have a firing onset that is delayed until after the sharp decline in phrenic nerve activity, and have an augmenting, firing pattern. In the cat, the axons of these neurons project caudally to the contralateral spinal cord, without collaterals in the brain stem. The cells may function as premotor neurons for spinal expiratory motoneurons (Euler, 1986; Feldman, 1986; Richter et al., 1986, 1992; Ezure, 1990).

Distributed within the VRG and Bötzinger complex are a separate class of neurons referred to as postinspiratory neurons (Richter et al., 1986, 1992). These neurons have also been referred to as expiratory decrementing neurons in a two-phase model of the respiratory cycle (Ezure, 1990). The onset of postinspiratory activity occurs with the start of the rapid decline of phrenic nerve activity, reaches peak firing frequency quickly, and decrements through the initial phase of expiratory airflow (Richter et al., 1986). Certainly, subclasses of this class of neurons exist. For example, a subset must activate the motoneurons that innervate upper airway muscles (i.e., the thyroarytenoid muscles; see Fig. 1). Another subset of postinspiratory neurons has been shown to project to the spinal cord. A subset of postinspiratory neurons may interact with early-inspiratory, decrementing neurons to form the primary oscillator generating the respiratory rhythm (Richter et al., 1992).

In summary, the VRG has been proposed to contain the elements that generate the respiratory pattern. Research in the neonatal preparation indicates that at this early stage of development neurons with conditional bursting or pacemakerlike properties underlie respiratory rhythm. As the organism matures, these cells may become imbedded in a network of cells that form the pattern generator evident in adults. In general, membrane properties play an important role in determining the respiratory pattern.

C. Pontine Respiratory Group

Little is known about this group of cells, even though extensive electrical recordings were made in the pons as early as in the medulla (Cohen and Wang, 1959). Respiratory-modulated activity was recorded preponderantly in the dorsolateral pons, specifically the parabrachial nuclei and the Kölliker-Fuse nucleus (Cohen and Wang, 1959; Bertrand and Hugelin, 1971). In the pons, respiratory-modulated activity appears less phasic and less modulated than in the medulla (Cohen and Wang, 1959; Bertrand and Hugelin, 1971).

The role proposed for the PRG in the regulation of respiration is that PRG interacts with vagal afferents to determine phase duration (Feldman and Gautier, 1976). Lesioning the pons in a vagotomized animal results in apneusis, a breathing pattern characterized by prolonged inspiration (Feldman and Gautier, 1976). In addition, the pons may play an important role in determining stability of the respiratory cycle (Oku and Dick, 1992). With placement of discrete lesions in the pons, the breathing pattern becomes more variable and the time necessary for the cycle to return to its steady-state cycle length becomes longer (Oku and Dick, 1992).

Neurophysiological and neuroanatomical evidence suggests interaction between pontine and medullary respiratory groups and even pontine and spinal respiratory groups. Electrical stimulation of the pons inhibits phrenic nerve activity at a latency similar to medullary respiratory neural activity, indicating a pontospinal, in addition to a pontobulbar, projection (Cohen, 1971). Pontospinal projections have been identified by retrograde labeling following injection of horseradish peroxidase in the phrenic motor nucleus (Rikard-Bell et al., 1984). Both the effect from electrical stimulation and the pontospinal projections may result from nonrespiratory neurons; however, in one study, pontospinal projections of respiratory-modulated neurons have been identified tentatively by antidromic activation (Bianchi and St. John, 1982).

D. Spinal Respiratory Groups

Spinal respiratory groups (SRG; see Fig. 2) consist of propriospinal interneurons. The role of these neurons in shaping the respiratory pattern has been underemphasized. With the characterization of the central respiratory drive potential (CRDP; Sears, 1964) and the subsequent identification of monosynaptic connections between medullary respiratory neurons and spinal motoneurons (Lipski et al., 1983), the prevalent thought was that the respiratory pattern was generated in the medulla and transmitted to the motoneurons, and that the motoneurons were slaves to the rhythm. However, evidence in the early 1980s indicated that the monosynaptic connections between medullary neurons and motoneurons were too weak to depolarize respiratory motoneurons above threshold (Davies et al., 1985a,b). Furthermore, a generalized broad-peak synchronization in the cross correlograms between thoracic motoneuronal activities appeared to be aperiodic and, therefore, unique from central respiratory drive, which has a high-frequency periodicity (Kirkwood et al., 1982a,b). This broad-peak synchronization became more evident with the reduction of the central respiratory drive potential (Kirkwood et al., 1984). Subsequently, interneuronal pools in the thoracic spinal cord have been identified, both neuroanatomically and electrophysiologically, that could form the neural substrate for this broad-peak synchronization (Kirkwood et al., 1988, 1993; Schmid et al., 1993). The role that these interneurons play in shaping the respiratory pattern is unknown, but preliminary evidence indicates that many interneurons have inhibitory synaptic connections to motoneurons (Kirkwood et al., 1993).

Two distinct groups of interneurons have been identified in the cervical spinal cord as well (Bellingham and Lipski, 1990; Aoki, 1982; Lipski and Duffin, 1986). First, in the most rostral segments from C-1 to C-3, inspiratory units have been recorded (Lipski and Duffin, 1986). These cells project caudally to both the phrenic motor nucleus and the thoracic spinal cord. However, because few synaptic connections were found, it was concluded that these cells do not act directly on motoneurons, but act through at least a disynaptic pathway (i.e., interneurons; Lipski and Duffin, 1986). The second group of cervical interneurons was identified in the phrenic motor nucleus (Bellingham and Lipski, 1990). These interneurons displayed inspiratory- or expiratory-modulated activity. It was assumed that these neurons synapsed onto phrenic motoneurons (Bellingham and Lipski, 1990).

E. Other Central Pattern Generators

The brain stem also contains other CPGs in addition to the respiratory pattern generator. Chewing and swallowing are examples of other repetitive, rhythmic movements that are generated by CPGs (see Fig. 3). The CPGs for chewing and swallowing must interact with breathing to prevent aspiration of food. The interaction between mastication and respiration, and between swallowing and breathing, has been recorded in humans (Fontana et al., 1992) and in intact unanesthetized animals (McFarland and Lund, 1993). During spontaneous mastication, respiratory rate increased and the masseter muscle was activated preferentially at the phase transitions associated with the onset of inspiration and expiration (Fontana et al., 1992). Consequently, mastication and respiration were coupled in a 2:1 or 3:1 ratio (Fontana et al., 1992). In contrast to chewing, respiratory rate decreased during swallowing. Although swallowing can occur at any point in the respiratory cycle, given a strong enough stimulus, it has a tendency to be initiated in late inspiration (Kawasaki, 1964) and occurs primarily in expiration (Clark, 1920; Kawasaki, 1964; Doty, 1968; Wilson et al., 1981; Nishino et al., 1985; Smith et al., 1989).

The interaction among chewing, swallowing, and breathing has also been studied in reduced animal preparations (see Fig. 3; Dick et al., 1993; Doty, 1951, 1968; Miller and Loizzi, 1974; Miller, 1982; Grelot et al., 1989b). In the reduced preparation, the behaviors are "fictive." Fictive chewing is elicited by cortical stimulation (Rioch, 1934; Amri et al., 1991), and fictive swallowing is elicited by continual stimulation of the SLN, which contains afferent fibers from receptors in the glottal region of the throat (Doty, 1951, 1968; Kawasaki et al., 1964; Miller and Loizzi, 1974; Miller, 1982; Grelot et al., 1989b; König, 1990). Fictive swallows are stereotypic events during which upper airway muscles are activated briefly and consistently in a characteristic pattern, comparable with that observed in eating animals (Doty, 1951, 1968; Kawasaki et al., 1964; Miller and Loizzi, 1974; Miller, 1982).

Fictive swallowing and breathing were elicited concurrently in decerebrate animal preparations (see Fig. 3; Dick et al., 1993). Stimulating the SLN at the threshold stimulus for eliciting swallows evokes the behavior at specific points in the respiratory cycle. Swallows coincided with the phase transitions of the respiratory cycle, indicating entrainment between swallowing and breathing (Dick et al., 1993). The pattern of concurrent swallows at the phase transitions varied from animal to animal, but included swallows occurring at the phase transition between stage I and stage II expiration.

The manner in which central pattern generators are structured or restructured for different behaviors is unknown. Specifically, do elements of the respiratory pattern generator participate in the other pattern generators? In an invertebrate model, restructuring of pattern generators with common elements results in totally different behaviors elicited separately (Meyrand et al., 1991). Similarly, in mammalians during vomiting, respiration stops and reshaping of the pattern generator may occur (Bianchi and Grelot, 1989). However, with swallowing and breathing, there is a confluence; that is, both behaviors occur simultaneously and can appear entrained (see Fig. 3). This suggests that elements of both CPGs are common.

One potential element of the respiratory pattern generator that may play a critical role in integrating these behaviors is the postinspiratory cell. The occurrence of swallows at the phase transitions in the respiratory cycle—the inhibition of stage II expiratory activity, and the prolongation of expiration—together indicate an important role for postinspiratory neurons. First, postinspiratory cells are not inhibited at any phase transition. They are depolarized at the transitions between inspiration and stage I expiration, as well as between stage II expiration and inspiration (Richter et al., 1986). At the phase transition between stage I and -II expiration, postinspiratory cells are not inhibited, but are less excitable because of calcium-dependent membrane properties (Richter et al., 1992). In addition, reflex activation of these postinspiratory neurons terminates inspiration, but also prolongs expiration (Remmers et al., 1986).

The hypothesis that coordination between swallowing and breathing is mediated through postinspiratory motoneurons must be oversimplified, because at least subpopulations of both inspiratory and expiratory neurons are excited during swallowing (Hukuhara and Okada, 1956; Sumi, 1963), and a subpopulation of postinspiratory neurons are inhibited during swallowing (Lawson et al., 1991). In extracellular recordings in decerebrate cats, excitatory and inhibitory responses were observed in both inspiratory and expiratory cells. Approximately 50% of the inspiratory ($n = 18$ of 35 cells recorded) and almost all of the expiratory ($n = 14$ of 17) neurons were excited during swallowing. The excitatory response in inspiratory cells was different from that of expiratory neurons (Sumi, 1963). In both groups, the short burst of activity coincided with the swallow and was evoked independently of the respiratory phase. In inspiratory neurons, activity could precede the swallow and, in expiratory neurons, activity could be prolonged, continuing after the swallow (Sumi, 1963). Clearly, the complete respiratory pattern generator is not inhibited during swallowing, which indicates that the neural network for breathing has been reshaped for swallowing. In preliminary evidence from intracellular recordings, when water was infused into the larynx of an anesthetized swine, respiration ceased and the postinspiratory neuron had a sustained depolarization except for two brief hyperpolarizations that may have coincided with swallows (Lawson et al., 1991). Finally, from recent studies on the interaction among these CPGs, the degree of convergence of these CPGs on upper airway motoneurons themselves is unclear (Amri et al., 1991). In particular, only a fraction of motor units can be activated by more than one CPG, whereas other motor units in the same pool may be activated by only one of these CPGs (Amri et al., 1991). Therefore, although it is clear that breathing and swallowing interact, the interaction of the underlying neurons, even at the motoneuronal level, remains speculative.

III. Intrinsic Properties of Motoneurons

Motoneuronal activity is determined not only by the input a motoneuron receives, but also by its intrinsic cellular properties. Examples of intrinsic cellular properties include synaptic conductance and current, electrotonic attenuation of synaptic current, specific membrane capacitance and resistivity, voltage- and time-dependent conductances, and cell geometry. The expression of these intrinsic properties, especially conductances, is dependent on the pattern of excitation and inhibition a cell receives. These intrinsic properties have been investigated in respiratory motoneurons, although most of the research has been performed in lumbar motoneurons.

Motoneurons are grouped anatomically and functionally into motoneuronal pools (Stuart et al., 1988; Burke, 1987). Anatomically, motoneuronal pools consist of motoneurons that innervate the same muscle. Motoneuronal pools can be partitioned further, for example, by grouping motoneurons that receive similar afferent input, particularly Ia afferent input from muscle spindles (Stuart et al., 1988). Generally, motoneuronal pools contain various types of motor units, a *motor unit* being defined as a single motoneuron and the muscle fibers it innervates. Motor units have been classified according to the contractile properties of their muscle fibers as slow-twitch, fatigue-resistant; fast-twitch, fatigue-resistant; and fast-twitch, fatigable (Burke, 1987). According to Henneman's size principle (Henneman and Mendell, 1981), during graded and progressive recruitment of motor units in a pool, the first motoneurons activated are the smallest, with subsequent recruitment of larger motoneurons. Within a motoneuronal pool, intrinsic properties of motoneurons have been correlated to physiological properties of a motor unit, such as recruitment, size, and contraction characteristics (Zengel et al., 1985; Zajac et al., 1985).

An analysis of how intrinsic properties influence the recruitment pattern of phrenic motoneurons has been performed (Dick et al., 1987; Jodkowski et al., 1987, 1988) and a review has been published recently (van Lunteren and Dick, 1992b). Anatomically, the phrenic motor pool consists of the motoneurons that innervate the diaphragm. However, the diaphragm consists of at least three separate muscles, based on their anatomical insertions: the costal, crural, and sternal diaphragms (Gordon et al., 1989). Furthermore, the muscle fibers of each motor unit have a restricted distribution, such that motor units can be isolated to regions of the diaphragm (Hammond et al., 1989). Nevertheless, in the spinal cord, there is extensive overlap in the distribution of the soma and even more extensive overlap in the dendrites of the motoneurons innervating these separate regions (Gordon and Richmond, 1990).

The distribution of inputs from brain stem central pattern generators may be relatively uniform, or they may be selective for the diaphragmatic motor units. Clearly, some inputs are distributed differentially to the phrenic motor pool. During deglutition, the crural portion of the diaphragm relaxes, allowing food to pass from the esophagus to the stomach (Altshuler et al., 1987). The possibility for differential distribution of CRDP input has been shown for motoneurons recruited early and late in the respiratory cycle (Monteau et al., 1985; Monteau and Hilaire, 1991). However, intrinsic properties also potentially play a critical role in this differential distribution of onset times (Jodkowski et al., 1987, 1988).

Only a portion of diaphragmatic motor units are recruited during resting ventilation (Sieck and Fournier, 1989; Dick and Kelsen, 1989). Apparently, every phrenic motoneuron receives a form of central respiratory drive, although many do not reach threshold (Jodkowski et al., 1987, 1988). For inspiratory motoneurons, CRDP appears as depolarization during inspiration and, in a portion of phrenic motoneurons, as hyperpolarization during expiration (Berger, 1979a). The proportion of motor units depolarizing above threshold appears small during resting ventilation and may consist of only slow-twitch motor units (Sieck and Fournier, 1989). During periods of increased drive, additional motor units are recruited, and only during extreme situations, such as Valsalva maneuvers or aspiration reflexes, do all the motor units appear to be activated (Sieck and Fournier, 1989; Dick and Kelsen, 1989).

The envelope of "leaky-integrated" phrenic multiunit activity appears as a graded ramp. However, this envelope does not necessarily reflect the graded recruitment of motor units, nor a progressive increase in their firing frequency. First, phrenic motor units have a bimodal distribution of onset times (Berger, 1979a; Dick et al., 1987; Donnelly et al., 1985; Hilaire et al., 1972; Iscoe et al., 1976). A portion of phrenic motoneurons are recruited before the first 10% of the inspiratory period and are referred to as "early." Another portion are recruited after the first 20% of the inspiratory period and are referred to as "late." Therefore, according to the hypothesis (Sieck and Fournier, 1989), during resting ventilation, both early- and late-recruited motor units would be slow-twitch motor units, which are present in all three diaphragmatic muscles. Second, the instantaneous firing frequency of phrenic motoneurons does not follow the graded ramp. After an initial increase in firing frequency, a stable firing frequency is reached (Dick et al., 1987).

To hypothesize a role for instrinsic properties in determining recruitment of diaphragmatic motoneurons, it is important to show that the pattern of recruitment could be predicted by the size principle; namely, that smaller motor units were recruited before larger ones (Iscoe et al., 1976; Dick et al., 1987). The recruitment of diaphragmatic motor units is indeed predicted by the size principle (Dick et al., 1987). Thus, the distribution of central respiratory drive and intrinsic properties in the phrenic motor pool is such that recruitment is correlated with cell size.

The differential distribution of central respiratory drive inputs must play a role in determining the bimodal recruitment pattern of phrenic motoneurons (Monteau and Hilaire, 1991). Bulbospinal neurons that discharged late in inspiration projected preferentially to phrenic motoneurons that discharged late in inspiration (Monteau et al., 1985). Additionally, if CRDP includes not only depolarization, but also hyperpolarization, then differential input is clearly noted by the fact that only a portion of phrenic motoneurons are inhibited during expiration (Berger, 1979a). The differential distribution of hyperpolarization plays a critical role in determining which intrinsic properties of the motoneuron are expressed.

Electrophysiological studies have described intrinsic properties as a possible mechanism for determining this biphasic recruitment order of phrenic motoneurons (Jodkowski et al., 1987, 1988). Phrenic motoneurons were recorded intracellularly in anesthetized and paralyzed animals that were hyperventilated to apnea, thereby blocking rhythmic synaptic drive and allowing measurements of passive membrane properties (Jodkowski et al., 1987, 1988). Two types of phrenic motoneurons were identified: (1) those with a high-input resistance and low rheobase, and (2) those with a low-input resistance and high rheobase. In 11 cases, recordings remained stable while carbon dioxide was added to the inspired gas. When apneic threshold was surpassed, activating the respiratory pattern generator and phrenic nerve activity, all the motoneurons were depolarized during the inspiratory phase, four above threshold. These four cells had uniform passive membrane properties, high-input resistance and low rheobase, but had onset times distributed in both early and late periods of inspiration. Thus, even with this small population and the transient nature of this state, it was evident that passive membrane properties that can distinguish slow- from fast-twitch motor units (Zengel et al., 1985) did not distinguish early from late diaphragmatic motor units. These data support the hypothesis that only slow-twitch motor units are recruited during inspiration (Sieck and Fournier, 1989).

In the follow-up study, hyperpolarizing and depolarizing current ramps were injected intracellularly (Jodkowski et al., 1988). If depolarizing ramps were delivered to mimic ramp depolarization during inspiration, phrenic motoneurons began to discharge uniformly when the ramp reached threshold. If a hyperpolarizing ramp preceded the depolarizing ramp, to mimic the sequence of hyperpolarization and depolarization associated with expiratory and inspiratory phases, respectively, then two different behaviors were evident: in one, latency to discharge decreased and cells began to discharge earlier; in the other, onset of activity was delayed, and cells began to discharge later. Again carbon dioxide was increased in the inspired gas and one cell with rebound excitation had an early onset, and another cell, the onset of which was delayed by a preceding hyperpolarization ramp, had a late onset. Thus, different intrinsic properties were associated with the different onset times. Phrenic motoneurons, therefore, are not simply slaves to the respiratory rhythm. They possess different intrinsic properties that allow them to express different firing behaviors to the same input.

In contrast with the phrenic motor nucleus, the hypoglossal motor nucleus seems to have a relatively even distribution of intrinsic membrane properties (Haddad et al., 1990; Viana et al., 1993a, b). This uniform distribution is surprising, because this motor nucleus has mixed targets, and not all motor neurons even receive central respiratory drive. The respiratory activity and, therefore, the respiratory motor units, are clustered in subnuclei located ventrally and medially in the hypoglossal motor nucleus (Lowe, 1981). Cells in this region are depolarized rhythmically with respiration, but in various phases (Withington-Wray et al., 1988; van Lunteren and Dick, 1989, 1992a,b). For example, in a population of 34 hypoglossal motoneurons with respiratory modulated activity, 18 cells were depolarized during inspiration and appeared to be hyperpolarized during expiration, 14 depolarized during inspiration and early expiration, and 4 depolarized during postinspiration and expiration (Withington-Wray et al., 1988). These various activity patterns arose from different synaptic inputs.

A first step to determine if intrinsic properties influence the recruitment pattern of hypoglossal motoneurons is to determine if the recruitment order is predicted by the size principle. The difference in activity profiles (see Fig. 1, square wave versus ramp) does not facilitate the identification of cell size as a distinguishing property. In phrenic nerve activity, a graded ramp reflects a progressive depolarization, which is ideal for an excitatory drive to recruit progressively larger cells. Because of the relation between synaptic current and input resistance, larger cells with lower-input resistance need more synaptic current to attain the same threshold depolarization as smaller cells. With a square wave or step change, cells are either recruited or fail to reach threshold.

In summary, data have been generated on both intrinsic and extrinsic electrophysiological properties of phrenic and hypoglossal motoneurons. Differential distribution of intrinsic properties influences the activity pattern of phrenic motoneurons, whereas differential distribution of synaptic drive determines the activity pattern of hypoglossal motoneurons.

IV. Effect of State of Consciousness on Respiratory Motor Activity

Respiration is state-specific, being different in wakefulness, NREM, and REM sleep (Orem, 1980a,b; Orem and Dick, 1990). These differences arise from an integration of two distinct neural control systems (see Fig. 4). First, breathing is controlled behaviorally (Orem, 1989; Orem and Dick, 1990). During wakefulness breathing interacts with other functions, ranging from vocalization to posture. During NREM sleep, breathing is the most regular and is under metabolic control. However, during REM sleep, breathing is highly irregular, similar to wakefulness, and has been described as under state influences (i.e., a direct state influence on the respiratory pattern generator). Second, the control of skeletal muscle and, consequently, respiratory muscles is state-specific. In REM sleep, motoneurons are actively inhibited. This occurs in the motor pools of most skeletal muscles, independent of muscle spindle content, and results in decreased and even absent muscle tone. The integration of these two effects is best exemplified by comparing medullary respiratory neuronal activity with phrenic motoneuronal activity. During a pontogeniculo-occipital (PGO) wave, a REM-specific event, medullary neurons are excited, whereas phrenic neurons are inhibited (Orem, 1980a,b).

Breathing may stop during sleep. Sleep apneas have been classified into two general groups: obstructive and central. *Obstructive sleep apneas* are identified by cessation of airflow owing to closure of the airway while negative intrathoracic pressures continue. *Central sleep apneas* are identified by cessation of both airflow and development of negative intrathoracic pressure. Mixed apneas include elements from both central and obstructive apneas; namely, breathing stops because of the absence of the development of driving forces, then, when contraction of the diaphragm recurs, the upper airway is obstructed and no airflow occurs. Sleep apneas can occur frequently in both NREM and REM sleep and lead to hypoxemia. The response to sleep apnea is arousal and, consequently, sleep deprivation. There may be multiple underlying neural causes of these events, and we will examine some of the contributing factors.

Probably the best understood factor is the REM sleep influence on skeletal muscle tone. Rapid eye movement sleep atonia arises from the basic brain stem mechanisms controlling this state. This sleep is controlled by neurons in the dorsolateral pons, specifically in the pedunculopontine tegmental (PPT) nucleus (Hobson, 1992). Neurons in this region are active specifically during REM sleep (Hobson, 1992). These cells project to, and excite neurons located in, the medullary and pontine reticular formation. Reticular neurons that contain inhibitory neurotransmitters, such as glycine, project to the spinal cord and even synapse on motoneurons (Holstege and Bongers, 1991). Stimulation of these cells results in inhibition of motoneurons. Spinal interneurons may also play a role in this inhibition (Takakusaki et al., 1989). The inhibitory postsynaptic potentials during REM sleep are strong enough to hyperpolarize the soma; consequently, muscles are atonic and quiescent.

Atonia is particularly evident in the upper airway muscles, especially those of the oropharyngeal region, such as the genioglossus. This may lead to occlusion of the upper airway and obstructive sleep apnea. Low doses of strychnine, an antagonist to glycine, have been administered to reverse the inhibition of hypoglossal motoneurons that occurs during REM sleep (Remmers et al., 1980). Obstructive sleep apneas are attenuated during REM sleep following strychnine (Remmers et al., 1980). An additional detrimental effect of REM sleep atonia has been reported in infants who have highly compliant chest walls. During obstructive sleep apneas, the decreased muscle tone in the chest wall allows the thorax to be sucked in during inspiration. This results in a paradoxical rib cage motion during breathing.

Acetylcholine is the neurotransmitter that has been identified to mediate the activation of reticular neurons by the PPT nucleus, and it appears to act through a muscarinic receptor. This has lead to the development of a carbachol model of REM sleep atonia (Morales et al., 1987a,b). Results from this model have been compared with those obtained in the sleeping cat, and in both, the upper airway is preferentially affected (Orem et al., 1980; Kubin et al., 1992). However, the underlying neural mechanisms of the hyperpolarization of hypoglossal motoneurons may not be the same in both natural and carbachol-induced REM sleep atonia. During natural REM sleep, breathing frequency and variability is comparable with wakefulness, whereas during carbachol-induced muscle atonia, breathing remains regular and slow, much like NREM sleep. This difference is surprising, because one source of the respiratory variability is evident in the carbachol model. Fractionation of diaphragmatic activity—a REM sleep event associated with the PGO wave—occurs in the carbachol model, which does display PGO waves. The frequency of fractionations in diaphragmatic activity has not been reported. Furthermore, in raw records from the carbachol model, only occasional and infrequent epochs of breathing variability appear (Taguchi et al., 1992; Tojima et al., 1992). However, these appear associated with PGO waves. Nevertheless, these data support the contention that, during REM sleep, there must be two mechanisms contributing to sleep apnea. One is the REM sleep atonia, which can lead to obstructive apneas. The other is the instability in the breathing pattern. The high variability in the ventilatory pattern that occurs normally during REM sleep indicates a decrease in the stability of respiratory pattern generator. This may be a critical factor, leading to central sleep apneas.

In NREM sleep, breathing is slow, with a regular periodicity, thus appearing very stable. A principal factor leading to apnea during NREM sleep is thought to be the loss of the "wakefulness stimulus" for breathing (Fink, 1961; Fink et al., 1963; Orem and Dick, 1990). Wakefulness stimulates breathing (see Fig. 4). Hypocapnic humans breathe rhythmically while awake, but become apneic while asleep (Fink et al., 1963). Similarly, in animals, apneic threshold decreases with state, changing from wakefulness to NREM sleep (Phillipson et al., 1977). The neural substrate for the wakefulness stimulus is undetermined, but the effect can be observed most prominently in medullary cells that are poorly correlated with respiration (Orem et al., 1985). When respiratory-modulated neuronal activity is recorded in the unanesthetized, unparalyzed, vagally intact, spontaneously breathing cat, then two general classes of activity are evident: highly modulated, highly correlated activity and poorly modulated, poorly correlated activity (Orem and Dick, 1983; Orem et al., 1985). These data were interpreted such that the highly modulated activity was either part of, or was coupled to, the respiratory pattern generator, whereas the poorly modulated activity integrated nonrespiratory and respiratory inputs. In other words, the poorly correlated cells serve as the interface between the outside world and the respiratory pattern generator. As such, these cells cannot be considered a homogeneous group, although as a group these cells become quiescent during sleep, rather than increasing a phasic respiratory component of their activity. According to the hypothesis, one of the actions of the poorly modulated cells is to quasi-rhythmically activate the respiratory pattern generator. With the absence of this activation the pattern generator becomes totally dependent on chemical drive for its activation. Therefore, with the loss of the wakefulness stimulus, the respiratory system becomes "reafferentated," rather than deafferentated.

The loss of the "wakefulness stimulus" contributes to the pathogenesis of sleep apnea in another way besides disfacilitating the respiratory pattern generator. The wakefulness stimulus is preferentially distributed to upper airway muscles (Orem et al., 1980). Upper airway muscles, even the laryngeal adductors, become quiescent during sleep (Insalaco et al., 1993). With arousal, upper airway muscles, rather than chest wall muscles, appear preferentially activated (Orem et al., 1980).

Only preliminary reports of state-specific effects have appeared concerning control of motor activity during NREM sleep. An augmentation of expiratory muscle activity was apparent in chest wall EMG recordings (Dick et al., 1982). Similar increases in muscle activity were reported for cervical postural muscles (Lydic et al., 1983).

In summary, relative to the state control of breathing, two factors must be considered: (1) state influences on muscle tone and (2) state influence on the respiratory pattern generator. During both REM and NREM sleep, the breathing pattern is destabilized. A present working hypothesis is that this destabilization results from state-related decreases in pontine respiratory activity, since small lesions there destabilize breathing (see Fig. 4).

V. Conclusions

Respiratory muscles are controlled by various respiratory groups distributed in the brain stem and spinal cord. The respiratory pattern generator is probably located rostral to the classically defined ventral respiratory group. Monosynaptic input from the medullary respiratory groups provide the preponderant source of central respiratory drive, but additional sources have been identified, in particular pro-priospinal interneurons.

In addition to the respiratory pattern generator, respiratory muscles are controlled by other pattern generators. During repetitive, rhythmic fictive swallowing, the confluence of patterns was such that the swallowing event occurred preferentially at the phase transitions in the respiratory cycle. This was interpreted to indicate common elements in the two central pattern generators.

Respiratory motoneurons are not simply slaves to the rhythm. They possess intrinsic membrane properties that shape their activity pattern; for instance, onset time and firing frequency. These membrane properties appear to be expressed differentially in phrenic motoneurons, but appear to be distributed uniformly in hypoglossal motoneurons.

The state of consciousness appears to influence respiratory muscle in two ways: directly, through its action on muscle tone, and indirectly, through its action on the respiratory pattern generator. This is especially apparent in the carbachol model of REM sleep, which elicits only the muscle atonia of REM sleep. In this model, respiratory muscle activity decreases, but respiration slows as well. Respiration is not erratic and variable like it is during spontaneous REM sleep.

Acknowledgments

The authors would like to thank Dr. Sharon K. Coles for her critical reading of the manuscript and Ms. Cheryl Gilliam-Walker for her professional preparation of the manuscript. In addition, the preparation of this chapter was supported primarily by HL-42400.

References

Altschuler, S. M., Davies, R. O., and Pack, A. I. (1987). Role of medullary inspiratory neurons in the control of the diaphragm during oesophageal stimulation in cats. *J. Physiol. (Lond.)* 391: 289–298.

Amri, M., Lamkaden, M., and Car, A. (1991). Effects of lingual nerve and chewing cortex stimulation upon activity of the swallowing neurons located in the region of the hypoglossal motor nucleus. *Brain Res.* 548: 149–155.

Aoki, M. (1982). Respiratory-related neuron activities in the cervical cord of the cat. In *Central Neural Production of Periodic Respiratory Movements.* Edited by J. L. Feldman and A. J. Berger. Chicago: Northwestern University Department of Physiology Press, pp. 155–156.

Averill, D. B., Cameron, W. E., and Berger, A. J. (1984). Monosynaptic excitation of dorsal medullary respiratory neurons by slowly adapting pulmonary stretch receptors. *J. Neurophysiol.* 52: 771–785.

Backman, S. B., Anders, C., Ballantyne, D., Röhrig, N., Camerer, H., Mifflin, S., Jordan, D., Dickhaus, H., Spyer, K. M., and Richter, D. W. (1984). Evidence for a monosynaptic connection between slowly adapting pulmonary stretch receptor afferents and inspiratory beta neurones. *Pflugers Arch.* 402: 129–136.

Bellingham, M. C., and Lipski, J. (1990). Respiratory interneurons in the C5 segment of the spinal cord of the cat. *Brain Res.* 533: 141–146.

Bellingham, M. C., and Lipski, J. (1992). Morphology and electrophysiology of superior laryngeal nerve afferents and postsynaptic neurons in the medulla oblongata of the cat. *Neuroscience* 48: 205–216.

Berger, A. J. (1977). Dorsal respiratory group neurons in the medulla of cat: Spinal projections, responses to lung inflation and superior laryngeal nerve stimulation. *Brain Res.* 135: 231–254.

Berger, A. J. (1979a). Phrenic motorneurons in the cat: Subpopulations and nature of respiratory drive potentials. *J. Neurophysiol.* 42: 76–90.

Berger, A. J. (1979b). Distribution of carotid sinus nerve afferent fibers to solitary tract nuclei of the cat using transganglionic transport of horseradish peroxidase. *Neurosci. Lett.* 14: 153–158.

Berger, A. J. (1980). Distribution of the cat's carotid sinus nerve afferent and efferent cell bodies using the horseradish peroxidase technique. *Brain Res.* 190: 309–320.

Berger, A. J. (1990). Recent advances in repiratory neurobiology using in vitro methods. *Am. J. Physiol.* 259: L24–L29.

Berger, A. J., and Averill, D. B. (1983). Projection of single pulmonary stretch receptors to solitary tract region. *J. Neurophysiol.* 49: 819–830.

Berger, A. J., and Cooney, K. A. (1982). Ventilatory effects of kainic acid injection of the ventrolateral solitary nucleus. *J. Appl. Physiol.* 52: 131–140.

Berger, A. J., and Dick, T. E. (1987). Connectivity of slowly adapting pulmonary stretch receptors with dorsal medullary respiratory neurons. *J. Neurophysiol.* 58: 1239–1274.

Berger, A. J., Mitchell, R. A., and Severinghaus, J. W. (1977a). Regulation of respiration (first of three parts). *N. Engl. J. Med.* 297: 92–97.

Berger, A. J., Mitchell, R. A., and Severinghaus, J. W. (1977b). Regulation of respiration (second of three parts). *N. Engl. J. Med.* 297: 138–143.

Berger, A. J., Mitchell, R. A., and Severinghaus, J. W. (1977c). Regulation of respiration (third of three parts). *N. Engl. J. Med.* 297: 194–201.

Bertrand, F., and Hugelin, A. (1971). Respiratory synchronizing function of nucleus parabrachialis medialis: Pneumotaxic mechanisms. *J. Neurophysiol.* 34: 189–207.

Bianchi, A., and Grelot, L. (1989). Converse motor output of inspiratory bulbospinal premotoneurons during vomiting. *Neurosci. Lett.* 104: 298–302.

Bianchi, A., and St. John, W. M. (1982). Medullary axonal projections of respiratory neurons of pontile pneumotaxic center. *Respir. Physiol.* 48: 357–373.

Bonham, A. C., and Joad, J. J. (1991). Neurones in commisural nucleus tractus solitarii required for full expression of the pulmonary C fibre reflex in rat. *J. Physiol. (Lond.)* 441: 95–112.

Bonham, A. C., and McCrimmon, D. R. (1990). Neurones in a discrete region of the nucleus tractus solitarius are required for the Breuer–Hering reflex in rat. *J. Physiol. (Lond.)* 427: 261–280.

Bonham, A. C., Coles, S. K., and McCrimmon, D. R. (1993). Pulmonary stretch receptor afferents activate excitatory amino acid receptors in the nucleus tractus solitarii in rats. *J. Physiol. (Lond.)* 464: 725–745.

Burke, R. E. (1987). Synaptic efficacy and the control of neuronal input–output relations. *Trends Neurosci.* 10: 42–45.

Bystrzycka, E. K., and Nail, B. S. (1983). The source of respiratory drive to nasolabialis motoneurons in the rabbit: An HRP study. *Brain Res.* 266: 183–191.

Clark, G. A. (1920). Deglutition apnea. *J. Physiol. (Lond.)* 54: 59P.

Cohen, M. I. (1971). Switching of the respiratory phases and evoked phrenic responses produced by rostral pontine electrical stimulation. *J. Physiol. (Lond.)* 217: 133–158.

Cohen, M. I. (1979). Neurogenesis of respiratory rhythm in the mammal. *Physiol. Rev.* 59: 1105–1173.

Cohen, M. I., and Wang, S. C. (1959). Respiratory neuronal activity in the pons of cat. *J. Neurophysiol.* 22: 33–50.

Connelly, C. A., Ellenberger, H. H., and Feldman, J. L. (1990). Respiratory activity in retrotrapezoid nucleus in cat. *Am. J. Physiol.* 258: L33–L44.

Davies, J. G. McF., Kirkwood, P. A., and Sears, T. A. (1985a). The detection of monosynaptic connextions from inspiratory bulbospinal neurons to inspiratory motoneurons in the cat. *J. Physiol. (Lond.)* 368: 33–62.

Davies, J. G. McF., Kirkwood, P. A., and Sears, T. A. (1985b). The distribution of monosynaptic connextions from inspiratory bulbospinal neurons to inspiratory motoneurons in the cat. *J. Physiol. (Lond.)* 368: 63–87.

Davies, R. O., and Kalia, M. (1981). Carotid sinus nerve projections to the brain stem in the cat. *Brain Res. Bull.* 6: 531–541.

Davis, P. J., and Nail, B. S. (1984). On the location and size of laryngeal motoneurons in the cat and rabbit. *J. Comp. Neurol.* 230: 13–32.

Delcomyn, F. (1980). Neural basis of rhythmic behavior in animals. *Science* 210: 492–498.

Dick, T. E., and Kelsen, S. G. (1989). Relationship between diaphragmatic activation and twitch tension to superimposed electrical stimulation in the cat. *Respir. Physiol.* 76: 337–346.

Dick, T. E., Parmeggiani, P. L., and Orem, J. M. (1982). Intercostal muscle activity during sleep in the cat: An augmentation of expiratory activity. *Respir. Physiol.* 50: 255–265.

Dick, T. E., Parmeggiani, P. L., and Orem, J. M. (1984). Intercostal muscle activity of the cat in the curled, semiprone sleeping posture. *Respir. Physiol.* 56: 385–394.

Dick, T. E., Kong, F. J., and Berger, A. J. (1987). Correlation of recruitment order with axonal conduction velocity for supraspinally driven diaphragmatic motor units. *J. Neurophysiol.* 57: 245–259.

Dick, T. E., Oku, Y., Romaniuk, J. R., and Cherniack, N. S. (1993). Interaction between central pattern generators for breathing and swallowing in the cat. *J. Physiol. (Lond.)* 465: 715–730.

DiMarco, A. F., von Euler, C., Romaniuk, J. R., and Yamamoto, Y. (1981). Positive feedback facilitation of external intercostal and phrenic inspiratory activity by pulmonary stretch receptors. *Acta Physiol. Scand.* 113: 375–386.

Donnelly, D. F., and Haddad, G. G. (1986a). Effect of graded anesthesia on laryngeal-induced central apnea. *Respir. Physiol.* 66: 235–245.

Donnelly, D. F., Cohen, M. I., Sica, A. L., and Zhang, H. (1985). Responses of early and late onset phrenic motoneurons to lung inflation. *Respir. Physiol.* 61: 69–83.

Donnelly, D. F., Sica, A. L., Cohen, M. I., and Zhang, H. (1989). Dorsal medullary inspiratory neurons: effects of superior laryngeal afferent stimulation. *Brain Res.* 491:243–252.

Doty, R. W. (1951). Influence of stimulus pattern on reflex deglutition. *Am. J. Physiol.* 166: 142–158.

Doty, R. W. (1968). Neural organization of deglutition. In *Handbook of Physiology*, Section 6. The Alimentary Canal, Vol. IV. Motility. Edited by C. F. Code. Bethesda, MD, American Physiological Society, pp. 1861–1902.

Duron, B. (1973). Postural and ventilatory functions of intercostal muscles. *Acta Neurobiol. Exp.* 33: 355–380.

Duron, B., and Marlot, D. (1980). Intercostal and diaphragmatic electrical activity during wakefulness and sleep in normal unrestrained adult cats. *Sleep* 3: 269–280.

Duron, B., Jung-Caillol, M. C., and Marlot, D. (1978). Myelinated nerve fiber supply and muscle spindles in the respiratory muscles of cat: Quantitative study. *Anat. Embryol.* 152: 171–192.

Ellenberger, H. H., and Feldman, J. L. (1990). Subnuclear organization of the lateral tegmental field of the rat. I: Nucleus ambiguus and ventral respiratory group. *J. Comp. Neurol.* 294: 202–211.

Ellenberger, H. H., Feldman, J. L., and Zhan, W. Z. (1990). Subnuclear organization of the lateral tegmental field of the rat. II: Catcholamine neurons and ventral respiratory group. *J. Comp. Neurol.* 294: 212–222.

Euler, C. von (1986). Brain stem mechanisms for generation and control of breathing pattern. In: *Handbook of Physiology*, Section 3. Respiration. Vol. II Control of Breathing. Edited by N. S. Cherniack and J. G. Widdicombe. Bethesda, MD, American Psychological Society, pp. 1–67.

Ezure, K. (1990). Synaptic connections between medullary respiratory neurons and considerations on the genesis of respiratory rhythm. *Prog. Neurobiol.* 35: 429–450.

Ezure, K., Manabe, M., and Yamada, H. (1988). Distribution of medullary respiratory neurons in the rat. *Brain Res.* 455: 262–270.

Feldman, J. L. (1986). Neurophysiology of breathing in mammals. In: *Handbook of Physiology*, Section 1. The Nervous System, Vol. IV. Intrinsic Regulatory Systems In The Brain. Edited by F. E. Bloom. pp. 463–524. Bethesda, MD, American Physiological Society.

Feldman, J. L., and Gautier, H. (1976). The interaction of pulmonary afferents and pneumotaxic center in control of respiratory pattern in cats. *J. Neurophysiol.* 39: 31–44.

Feldman, J. L., Smith, J. C., Ellenberger, H. H., Connelly, C. A., Liu, G., Greer, J. J., Lindsay, A. D., and Otto, M. R. (1990). Neurogenesis of respiratory rhythm and pattern: Emerging concepts. *Am. J. Physiol.* 259: R879–R886.

Feldman, J. L., Smith, J. C., and Liu, G. (1991). Respiratory pattern generation in mammals: In vitro en bloc analyses. *Curr. Opin. Neurobiol.* 1: 590–594.

Fink, B. R. (1961). Influence of cerebral activity in wakefulness on regulation of breathing. *J. Appl. Physiol.* 16: 15–20.

Fink, B. R., Hanks, E. C., Ngai, S. H., and Papper, E. M. (1963). Central regulation of respiration during anesthesia and wakefulness. *Ann. N.Y. Acad. Sci.* 109: 892–900.

Fontana, G. A., Pantaleo, T., Bongianni, F., Cresci, F., Viroli, L., and Sarago, G. (1992). Changes in respiratory activity induced be mastication in humans. *J. Appl. Physiol.* 72: 779–786.

Glenn, L. L., Foutz, A. S., and Dement, W. C. (1978). Membrane potential of spinal motoneurons during natural sleep in cats. *Sleep* 1: 199–204.

Gordon, D. C., and Richmond, F. J. R. (1990). Topography in the phrenic motoneuron nucleus demonstrated by retrograde multiple-labelling techniques. *J. Comp. Neurol.* 292: 424–434.

Gordon, D. C., Hammond, C. G. M., Fisher, J. T., and Richmond, F. J. R. (1989). Muscle-fiber architecture, innervation, and histochemistry in the diaphragm of the cat. *J. Morphol.* 201: 131–143.

Grelot, L., Barillot, J. C., and Bianchi, A. L. (1989a). Central distribution of the efferent and afferent components of the pharyngeal branches of the vagus and glossopharyngeal nerves: An HRP study in the cat. *Exp. Brain Res.* 78: 327–335.

Grelot, L., Barillot, J. C., and Bianchi, A. L. (1989b). Pharyngeal motoneurons: respiratory-related activity and responses to laryngeal afferents in the decerebrate cat. *Exp. Brain Res.* 78: 336–344.

Grillner, S. (1985). Neurobiological bases of rhythmic motor acts in vertebrates. *Science* 228: 143–149.

Grillner, S., Wallen, P., and Viana di Prisco, G. (1991). The lamprey locomotor system—basic locomotor synergy. In *Neurobiological Basis of Human Locomotion*. Edited by M. Shimamura, S. Grillner, and V. E. Edgerton. Tokyo: Japan Scientific Societies Press, pp. 77–92.

Haddad, G. G., Donnelly, D. F., and Getting, P. A. (1990). Biophysical properties of hypoglossal motoneurons in vitro: Intracellular studies in adult and neonatal rats. *J. Appl. Physiol.* 69: 1509–1517.

Hammond, C. G. M., Gordon, D. C., Fisher, J. T., and Richmond, F. J. R. (1989). Motor unit territories supplied by branches of the phrenic nerve. *J. Appl. Physiol.* 66: 61–71.

Hayashi, F., and Lipski, J. (1992). The role of inhibitory amino acids in control of respiratory motor output in an arterially perfused rat. *Respir. Physiol.* 89: 47–63.

Henneman, E., and Mendell, L. M. (1981). Functional organization of motoneuron pool and its inputs. In: *Handbook of Physiology*, Section 1. The Nervous System, Motor Control. Vol. II. Edited by J. M. Brookhart and V. B. Mountcastle. Bethesda, MD, American Physiological Society, pp. 423–507.

Hilaire, G., Monteau, R., and Dussardier, M. (1972). Modalités du recrutement des motoneurons phréniques. *J. Physiol. (Paris)* 64: 457–478.

Hobson, J. A. (1992). Sleep and dreaming: Induction and mediation of REM sleep by cholinergic mechanisms. *Curr. Opin. Neurobiol.* 2: 759–763.

Holstege, J. C., and Bongers, C. M. H. (1991). A glycinergic projection from the ventromedial lower brainstem to spinal motoneurons: An ultrastructural double labeling study in rat. *Brain Res.* 566: 308–315.

Hukuhara, T., and Okada, H. (1956). Effects of deglutition upon spike discharges of neurons in the respiratory center. *Jpn. J. Physiol.* 6: 162–166.

Hwang, J.-C., Zhou, D., and St. John, W. M. (1989). Characterization of expiratory intercostal activity to triangularis sterni activity in cats. *J. Appl. Physiol.* 67: 1518–1524.

Insalaco, G., Kuna, S. T., Catania, G., Marrone, O., Constanza, B. M., Bellia, V., and Bonsignore, G. (1993). Thyroarytenoid muscle activity in sleep apneas. *J. Appl. Physiol.* 74: 704–709.

Iscoe, S. (1988). Central control of the upper airway. In *Respiratory Function of the Upper Airway*. Edited by O. P. Mathew and G. Sant' Ambrogio, New York, Marcel Dekker, pp. 125–192.

Iscoe, S., Dankoff, J., Migicovsky, R., and Polosa, C. (1976). Recruitment and discharge frequency of phrenic motoneurones during inspiration. *Respir. Physiol.* 26: 113–128.

Jodkowski, J. S., Viana, F., Dick, T. E., and Berger, A. J. (1987). Electrical properties of phrenic motoneurons in the cat: Correlation with inspiratory drive. *J. Neurophysiol.* 58: 105–124.

Jodkowski, J. S., Viana, F., Dick, T. E., and Berger, A. J. (1988). Repetitive firing properties of phrenic motoneurons in the cat. *J. Neurophysiol.* 60: 687–702.

Kalia, M., and Richter, D. (1985a). Morphology of physiologically identified slowly adapting lung stretch receptor afferents stained with intra-axonal horseradish peroxidase in the nucleus of the tractus solitarius of the cat: I. A light microscopic analysis. *J. Comp. Neurol.* 241: 503–520.

Kalia, M. and Richter, D. (1985b). Morphology of physiologically identified slowly adapting lung stretch receptor afferents stained with intra-axonal horseradish peroxidase in the nucleus of the tractus solitarius of the cat: II. An ultrastructural analysis. *J. Comp. Neurol.* 241: 521–535.

Kalia, M., and Richter, D. (1988a). Rapidly adapting pulmonary receptor afferents: I. Arborization in the nucleus of the tractus solitarius. *J. Comp. Neurol.* 274: 560–573.

Kalia, M., and Richter, D. (1988b). Rapidly adapting pulmonary receptor afferents: II. Fine structure and synaptic organization of central terminal processes in the nucleus of the tractus solitarius. *J. Comp. Neurol.* 274: 574–594.

Kawasaki, M., Ogura, J. H., and Taklenouchi, S. (1964). Neurophysiologic observation of normal deglutition: I. Its relationship to the respiratory cycle. *Laryngoscope* 74: 1747–1765.

Kirkwood, P. A., Sears, T. A., Tuck, D. L., and Westgaard, R. H. (1982a). Variations in the time course of the synchronization of intercostal motoneurons in the cat. *J. Physiol. (Lond.)* 327: 105–135.

Kirkwood, P. A., Sears, T. A., Stagg, D., and Westgaard, R. H. (1982b). The spatial distribution of synchronization of intercostal motoneurons in the cat. *J. Physiol. (Lond.)* 327: 137–155.

Kirkwood, P. A., Sears, T. A., and Westgaard, R. H. (1984). Restoration of function in external intercostal motoneurons of the cat following partial central deafferentation. *J. Physiol. (Lond.)* 350: 225–251.

Kirkwood, P. A., Munson, J. B., Sears, T. A., and Westgaard, R. H. (1988). Respiratory interneurons in the thoracic spinal cord of the cat. *J. Physiol. (Lond.)* 395: 161–192.

Kirkwood, P. A., Schmid, K., and Sears, T. A. (1993). Functional identities of thoracic respiratory interneurons in the cat. *J. Physiol. (Lond.)* 461: 667–687.

König, S. T., Czachurski, J., and Dembowsky, K. (1990). Inhibition of cardiac sympathetic nerve activity during swallowing evoked by laryngeal afferent stimulation in the cat. *Neurosci. Lett.* 188: 265–268.

Kubin, L., Kimura, H., and Davies, R. O. (1991). The medullary projections of afferent bronchopulmonary C fibres in the cat as shown by antidromic mapping. *J. Physiol. (Lond.)* 435: 207–228.

Kubin, L., Kimura, H., Tojima, H., Pack, A. I., and Davies, R. O. (1992). Behavior of VRG neurons during the atonia of REM sleep induced by pontine carbochol in decerebrate cats. *Brain Res.* 592: 91–100.

Lawson, E. E., Richter, D. W., Czyzyk-Krzeska, M. F., Bischoff, A., and Rudesill, R. C. (1991). Respiratory neuronal activity during apnea and other breathing patterns induced by laryngeal stimulation. *J. Appl. Physiol.* 70: 2742–2749.

Lipski, J., and Duffin, J. (1986). An electrophysiological investigation of propriospinal inspiratory neurons in the upper cervical cord of the cat. *Exp. Brain Res.* 61: 625–637.

Lipski, J., Kubin, L., and Jodkowski, J. (1983). Synaptic action of R_β neurons on phrenic motoneurons studied with spike-triggered averaging. *Brain Res.* 288: 105–118.

Lipski, J., Ezure, K., and Wong She, R. B. (1991). Identification of neuronls receiving input from pulmonary rapidly adapting receptors in the cat. *J. Physiol. (Lond.)* 443: 55–77.

Lowe, A. A. (1981). A neural regulation of tongue movements. *Prog. Neurobiol.* 15: 295–344.

Lydic, R., McCarley, R. W., and Hobson, A. A. (1983). The time course of dorsal raphe discharge, PGO waves, and muscle tone averaged across multiple sleep states. *Brain Res.* 274: 365–370.

McFarland, D. H., and Lund, J. P. (1993). An investigation of the coupling between respiration, mastication, and swallowing in the awake rabbit. *J. Neurophysiol.* 69: 95–108.

Merrill, E. G. (1974). Finding a respiratory function for the medullary respiratory neurons. In *Essays on the Nervous System*. Edited by R. Bellairs and E. G. Gray. Oxford, Clarendon Press, pp. 451–486.

Meyrand, P., Simmers, J., and Moulins, M. (1991). Construction of a pattern-generating circuit with neurons of different networks. *Nature* 351: 60–63.

Miller, A. J. (1982). Deglutition. *Physiol. Rev.* 62: 129–184.

Miller, A. J., and Loizzi, R. F. (1974). Anatomical and functional differentiation of superior laryngeal nerve fibers affecting swallowing and respiration. *Exp. Neurol.* 42: 369–387.

Monteau, R., and Hilaire, G. (1991). Spinal respiratory motoneurons. *Prog. Neurobiol.* 37: 83–144.

Monteau, R., Khatib, M., and Hilaire, G. (1985). Central determination of recruitment order: Intracellular study of phrenic motoneurons. *Neurosci. Lett.* 56: 341–346.

Morales, F. R., Boxer, P., and Chase, M. H. (1987a). Behavioral state-specific inhibitory post-synaptic potentials impinge on cat lumbar motoneurons during active sleep. *Exp. Neurol.* 98: 418–435.

Morales, F. R., Engelhardt, J. K., Soja, P. J., Pereda, A. E., and Chase, M. H. (1987b). Motoneuron properties during motor inhibition produced by microinjection of carbachol into the pontine reticular formation of the decerebrate cat. *J. Neurophysiol.* 57: 1118–1129.

Nakamura, Y., Golberg, L. J., Chandler, S. H., and Chase, M. H. (1978). Intracellular analysis of trigeminal motoneuron activity during sleep in the cat. *Science* 199: 204–207.

Nishino, T., Yonezawa, T., and Honda, Y. (1985). Effects of swallowing on the pattern of continuous respiration in human adults. *Am. Rev. Respir. Dis.* 132: 1219–1222.

Oku, Y., and Dick, T. E. (1992). Phase resetting of the respiratory cycle before and after unilateral pontine lesion in cat. *J. Appl. Physiol.* 72: 721–730.

Oku, Y., Dick, T. E., and Cherniack, N. S. (1993). Phase-dependent dynamic responses of respiratory motor activities following perturbation of the cycle in the cat. *J. Physiol. (Lond.)* 461: 321–337.

Onimaru, H., and Homma, I. (1987). Respiratory rhythm generator neurons in medulla of brainstem–spinal cord preparation from newborn rat. *Brain Res.* 403: 380–384.

Onimaru, H., Homma, I., and Iwatsuki, K. (1992). Excitation of inspiratory neuron by preinspiratory neuron in rat medulla in vitro. *Brain Res. Bull.* 29: 879–882.

Orem, J. (1980a). Medullary respiratory neuron activity: Relationship to tonic and phasic REM sleep. *J. Appl. Physiol.* 48: 54–65.

Orem, J. (1980b). Neuronal mechanisms of respiration in REM sleep. *Sleep* 3: 251–267.

Orem, J. (1989). Behavioral inspiratory inhibition: Inactivated and activated respiratory cells. *J. Neurophysiol.* 62: 1069–1078.

Orem, J., and Dick, T. (1983). Consistency and signal strength of respiratory neuronal activity. *J. Neurophysiol.* 50: 1098–1107.

Orem, J., and Dick, T. (1990). Brainstem respiratory neurons and their control during various behaviors. In: *Brainstem Mechanisms of Behavior.* Edited by W. R. Klemm and R. P. Vertes. New York, John Wiley & Sons, pp. 383–406.

Orem, J., and Trotter, R. H. (1992). Post-inspiratory neuronal activities during behavioral control, sleep, and wakefulness. *J. Appl. Physiol.* 72: 2369–2377.

Orem, J., and Trotter, R. H. (1993). Medullary respiratory neuronal activity during augmented breaths in intact unanesthetized cats. *J. Appl. Physiol.* 74: 761–769.

Orem, J., Dick, T., and Norris, P. (1980). Laryngeal and diaphragmatic responses to airway occlusion in sleep and wakefulness. *Electroencephalogr. Clin. Neurophysiol.* 50: 151–164.

Orem, J., Osorio, I., Brooks, E., and Dick, T. (1985). Activity of respiratory neurons during NREM sleep. *J. Neurophysiol.* 54: 1144–1156.

Parmegianni, P. L., and Sabattini, L. (1972). Electromyographic aspects of postural, respiratory and thermoregulatory mechanisms in sleeping cats. *Electroencephalogr. Clin. Neurophysiol.* 33: 1–13.

Phillipson, E. A., Kozar, L., Rebuck, A. S., and Murphy, E. (1977). Ventilatory and waking responses to CO_2 in sleeping dogs. *Am. Rev. Respir. Dis.* 115: 251–259.

Remmers, J. E., Anch, A. M., deGroot, W. J., Baker, J. P., Jr., and Sauerland, E. K. (1980). Oropharyngeal muscle tone in obstructive sleep apnea before and after strychnine. *Sleep* 3: 447–453.

Remmers, J. E., Richter, D. W., Ballantyne, D., Bainton, C. R., and Klein, J. P. (1986). Reflex prolongation of stage-I of expiration. *Pflugers Arch.* 407: 190–198.

Richardson, C. A., and Mitchell, R. A. (1982). Power spectral analysis of inspiratory nerve activity in the decerebrate cat. *Brain Res.* 233: 317–336.

Richter, D. W., Ballantyne, D., and Remmers, J. E. (1986). How is the respiratory rhythm generated? A model. *News Physiol. Sci.* 1: 109–112.

Richter, D. W., Ballantyne, D., and Remmers, J. E. (1987). The differential organization of medullary post-inspiratory activities. *Pflugers Arch.* 410: 420–427.

Richter, D. W., Ballanyi, K., and Schwarzacher, S. (1992). Mechanisms of respiratory rhythm generation and its modulation by neural control. *Curr. Opin. Neurobiol.* 2: 788–793.

Rikard-Bell, G. C., Bystrzycka, E. K., and Nail, B. S. (1984). Brainstem projections to the phrenic nucleus: An HRP study in the cat. *Brain Res. Bull.* 12: 469–477.

Rioch, J. M. (1934). The neural mechanism of mastication. *Am. J. Physiol.* 108: 168–176.

Saether, K., Hilaire, G., and Monteau, R. (1987). Dorsal and ventral respiratory groups of neurons in the medullar of the rat. *Brain Res.* 419: 87–96.

Sauerland, E. K., and Harper, R. M. (1976). The human tongue during sleep: Electromyographic activity of the genioglossus muscle. *Exp. Neurol.* 51: 160–170.

Schmid, K., Kirkwood, P. A., Munson, J. B., Shen, E., and Sears, T. A. (1993). Contralateral projections of thoracic respiratory interneurones in the cat. *J. Physiol. (Lond.)* 461: 647–665.

Schwarzacher, S. W., Wilhelm, Z., Anders, K., and Richter, D. W. (1991). The medullary respiratory network in the rat. *J. Physiol. (Lond.)* 435: 631–644.

Sears, T. A. (1964). The slow potentials of thoracic respiratory motoneurons and their relation to breathing. *J. Physiol. (Lond.)* 175: 404–424.

Sherrey, J. H., and Megirian, D. (1977). State dependence of upper airway respiratory motoneurons: Functions of the cricothyroid and nasolabial muscles of the unanesthetized rat. *Electroencephalogr. Clin. Neurophysiol.* 43: 218–228.

Sieck, G. C., and Fournier, M. (1989). Diaphragm motor unit recruitment during ventilatory and nonventilatory behaviors. *J. Appl. Physiol.* 66: 2539–2545.

Smith, J., Wolkove, N., Colacone, A., and Kreisman, H. (1989). Coordination of eating, drinking and breathing in adults. *Chest* 96: 578–582.

Smith, J. C., and Feldman, J. L. (1987). In vitro brainstem–spinal cord preparations for study of motor systems for mammalian respiration and locomotion. *J. Neurosci. Methods* 21: 321–333.

Smith, J. C., Feldman, J. L., and Schmidt, B. (1988). Neural mechanisms generating locomotion studied in mammalian brain stem-spinal cord in vitro. *FASEB J.* 2: 2283–2288.

Smith, J. C., Greer, J. J., Liu, G., and Feldman, J. L. (1990). Neural mechanisms generating respiratory pattern in mammalian brain stem–spinal cord in vitro: I. Spatiotemporal patterns of motor and medullary neuron activity. *J. Neurophysiol.* 64: 1149–1169.

Smith, J. C., Ellenberger, H. H., Ballanyi, K., Richter, D. W., and Feldman, J. L. (1991). Pre-Bötzinger complex: A brainstem region that may generate respiratory rhythm in mammals. *Science* 254: 726–729.

Speck, D. F., and Feldman, J. L. (1982). The effects of microstimulations and microlesions in the ventral and dorsal respiratory groups in medulla of cat. *J. Neurosci.* 2: 744–757.

St. John, W. M., and Zhou, D. (1989). Differing control of neural activities during various portions of expiration in the cat. *J. Physiol. (Lond.)* 418: 189–204.

St. John, W. M., and Zhou, D. (1990). Discharge of vagal pulmonary receptors differentially alters neural activities during various stages of expiration in the cat. *J. Physiol. (Lond.)* 424: 1–12.

Stuart, D. G., Hamm, T. M., and Noven, S. V. (1988). Partitioning of monosynaptic Ia EPSP connections with motoneurons according to neuromuscular topography: Generality and functional implications. *Prog. Neurobiol.* 30: 437–447.

Sumi, T. (1963). The activity of brain-stem respiratory neurons and spinal respiratory motoneurons during swallowing. *J. Neurophysiol.* 26: 466–477.

Suzue, T. (1984). Respiratory rhythm generation in the in vitro brain stem–spinal cord preparation of the neonatal rat. *J. Physiol. (Lond.)* 354: 173–183.

Taguchi, O., Kubin, L., and Pack, A. I. (1992). Evocation of postural atonia and respiratory depression by pontine carbachol in the decerebrate rat. *Brain Res.* 595: 107–115.

Takakusaki, K., Ohta, Y., and Mori, S. (1989). Single medullary reticulospinal neurons exert postsynaptic inhibitory effects via inhibitory interneurons upon alpha-motoneurons innervating cat hindlimb muscles. *Exp. Brain Res.* 74: 11–23.

Taylor, A. (1960). The contribution of the intercostal muscles to the effort of respiration in man. *J. Physiol. (Lond.)* 151: 390–402.

Tojima, H., Kubin, L., Kimura, H., and Davies, R. O. (1992). Spontaneous ventilation and respiratory motor output during carbachol-induced atonia of REM sleep in the decerebrate cat. *Sleep* 15: 404–414.

van Lunteren, E., and Dick, T. E. (1989). Motor unit regulation of mammalian pharyngeal dilator muscle activity. *J. Clin. Invest.* 84: 577–585.

van Lunteren, E., and Dick, T. E. (1992a). Breath-to-breath variability in hypoglossal motor unit firing. *Respir. Physiol.* 89: 37–46.

van Lunteren, E., and Dick, T. E. (1992b). Intrinsic properties of pharyngeal and diaphragmatic respiratory motoneurons and muscles. *J. Appl. Physiol.* 73: 787–800.

Viana, F., Bayliss, D. A., and Berger, A. J. (1993a). Calcium conductances and their role in the firing behavior of neonatal rat hypoglossal motoneurons. *J. Neurophysiol.* 69: 2137–2149.

Viana, F., Bayliss, D. A., and Berger, A. J. (1993b). Multiple potassium conductances and their role in action potential repolarization and repetitive firing behavior of neonatal rat hypoglossal motoneurons. *J. Neurophysiol.* 69: 2150–2163.

Yoshida, Y., Mitsumasu, T., Miyazaki, T., Kirano, M., and Kanaseki, T. (1984). Distribution of motoneurons in the brain stem of monkeys innervating the larynx. *Brain Res. Bull.* 13: 413–419.

Wilson, S. L., Thach, B. T., Broulliette, R. T., and Abu-Osba, Y. K. (1981). Coordination of breathing and swallowing in human infants. *J. Appl. Physiol.* 50: 851–858.

Withington-Wray, D. J., Mifflin, S. W., and Spyer, K. M. (1988). Intracellular analysis of respiratory-modulated hypoglossal motoneurons in the cat. *Neuroscience* 25: 1041–1051.

Zajac, F. E., and Faden, J. S. (1985). Relationship among recruitment order, axonal conduction velocity, and muscle-unit properties of type-identified motor units in cat plantaris muscle. *J. Neurophysiol.* 53: 1303–1322.

Zengel, J. E., Reid, S. A., Sypert, G. W., and Munson, J. B. (1985). Membrane electrical
   properties and prediction of motor-unit type of medial gastrocnemius motoneurons in the
   cat. *J. Neurophysiol.* 53: 1323–1344.
Zheng, Y., Barillot, J. C., and Bianchi, A. L. (1991). Are the post-inspiratory neurons in the
   decerebrate rat cranial motoneurons or interneurons. *Brain Res.* 551: 256–266.
Zhou, D., Huang, Q., St. John, W. M., and Bartlett, D., Jr. (1989). Respiratory activities of
   intralaryngeal branches of the recurrent laryngeal nerve. *J. Appl. Physiol.* 67: 1171–1178.

27

Organization and Recruitment of Diaphragm Motor Units

GARY C. SIECK

Mayo Medical School and Mayo Foundation
Rochester, Minnesota

I. Introduction

In skeletal muscles, including the diaphragm, the final element of neural control is the motor unit, each composed of a motoneuron and the muscle fibers it innervates (i.e., the muscle unit; Liddell and Sherrington, 1925; Sherrington, 1992; Fig. 1). These motor units can vary considerably in their physiological, histochemical, and biochemical properties (Burke, 1981; Burke et al., 1973; Enad et al., 1989; Fournier and Sieck, 1988b; Hamm et al., 1988; Martin et al., 1988; Nemeth et al., 1981, 1986; Sieck and Fournier, 1989; Sieck et al., 1989a). It is this heterogeneity of motor unit properties that affords the nervous system a basis for control of muscle force generation during different motor behaviors. At the same time, it is the cumulative contractile and fatigue properties of the motor unit pool that determines the constraints under which the diaphragm muscle responds to the various mechanical demands placed on it during different ventilatory and nonventilatory behaviors.

Until very recently, the physiological properties of diaphragm motor units had never been directly characterized. Instead, the physiological properties of these units were inferred from histochemical analyses of muscle fiber types. However, such inferences can be misleading, as physiological and histochemical properties of motor units display a wide continuous distribution, and there is not always a precise relation between motor unit histochemical and physiological properties across different muscles.

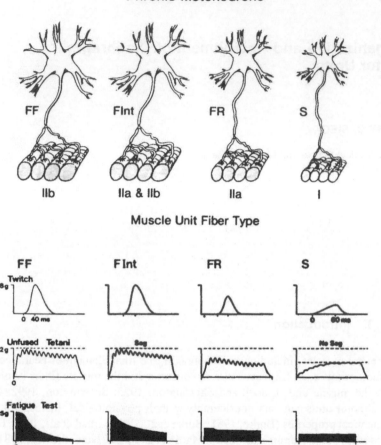

Figure 1 Diaphragmatic motor units comprise a phrenic motoneuron and the muscle fibers it innervates (i.e., the muscle unit). Muscle unit fibers have uniform histochemical-staining profiles for myofibrillar ATPase after alkaline and acid preincubations, such that they can be classified as type I, IIa, or IIb. Mechanical properties of muscle units also distinguish different motor unit types. Fast-twitch units are distinguished from slow-twitch units by the presence of "sag" in unfused tetany. Subclassification of fast-twitch units is based on fatigue resistance to repetitive stimulation.

Therefore, it is important that the physiological and histochemical characteristics of the motor unit population be determined separately for each muscle. However, the characterization of motor unit physiological properties is technically difficult and, perhaps, impractical under every experimental condition. Certainly, it is much easier to examine the histochemical properties of muscle fibers, and there is considerable evidence that the muscle fibers belonging to a single motor unit share a similar histochemical profile. It is this relation between the physiological properties of motor units and the histochemical properties of muscle fibers that has provided the basis and incentive for classifying muscle fiber types. It is thought that if the proportions of muscle fiber types are identified, the distribution of motor unit types can be deduced.

II. Classification of Motor Unit Types

It has proved useful to classify motor units into different types based on a clustering of their isometric contractile properties (Burke, 1981; Burke et al., 1971, 1973). Such a classification of motor unit types has provided an essential framework for describing the orderly recruitment of motor units during various behaviors.

According to the standardized criteria introduced by Burke and his colleagues (Burke et al., 1971, 1973), fast-twitch units in the cat medial gastrocnemius muscle are distinguished from slow-twitch units by the presence (fast) or absence (slow) of "sag" during unfused tetanic activation (see Fig. 1). Isometric twitch contraction time (time to peak twitch force) of these motor units is continuously distributed, but generally corresponds to the classification of slow- and fast-twitch units based on the sag phenomenon. Motor units are further subclassified by their resistance to fatigue during repetitive stimulation at 40 Hz in trains of 330-ms duration, repeated each second for a 2-min period (see Fig. 1). A "fatigue index" (fi) is then calculated as the ratio of the force generated after 2 min of repetitive stimulation to the initial force (i.e., the residual force). With this fatigue test, slow-twitch units (S) are consistently found to be fatigue-resistant (i.e., fi > 0.75). In contrast, fatigability of fast-twitch units is distributed such that three types can be readily classified: fast-twitch, fatigue-resistant (FR; fi > 0.75); fast-twitch, fatigue-intermediate (FInt; 0.25 < fi < 0.75); and fast-twitch, fatigable (FF: fi < 0.25). In the cat medial gastrocnemius muscle, very few FInt motor units are found; thus, a bimodal distribution of fatigability is observed (i.e., FF units are clearly distinguished from S and FR units), suggesting a clustering of motor unit mechanical properties that corresponds to the histochemical classification of muscle fiber types (Burke et al., 1971, 1973).

A. Motor Unit Types in the Diaphragm

Recently, we described the mechanical properties of motor units in the adult cat (Fournier and Sieck, 1988b; Sieck, 1988, 1991a,b) and hamster (Sieck 1991a,b) diaphragms using the standardized physiological criteria described by Burke and colleagues (Burke, 1981; Burke et al., 1971, 1973). As in hindlimb muscles, fast-twitch units in the diaphragm can be distinguished from type S units on the basis of sag during unfused tetany (see Fig. 1), which generally corresponds to the isometric twitch contraction time of the unit. Slow-twitch units in the diaphragm are uniformly fatigue-resistant (fi > 0.75), whereas fast-twitch units show a wide distribution of fatigability (Fig. 2). In general, however, FF units in the diaphragm are not as fatigable as those in hindlimb muscles. Moreover, in both the cat and hamster diaphragms, there is an abundance of FInt units, when compared with the relative absence of these units in most hindlimb muscles (see Fig. 2).

B. Determinants of Motor Unit-Specific Force

The contractile strength (specific force of force per cross-sectional area) of different motor unit types generally corresponds to their classification. For example, type S motor units generate the lowest twitch and maximum tetanic forces of any type, whereas type FF motor units generate the greatest forces, with FInt and FR units being intermediate. It should be stressed that the classification of motor unit types should always be thought of in relative terms, since the absolute forces generated by specific motor unit types can vary markedly across muscles and species (Table 1). For example, the forces generated by type S units in one muscle may be as great as the forces generated by FF units in another muscle. This variation among muscles does not invalidate the usefulness of classifying motor unit types. Instead, it emphasizes the importance of characterizing the contractile properties of motor units for each specific muscle. This is illustrated in the diaphragm. One can still take advantage of the basic framework for modeling diaphragm neuromotor control offered by the classification of motor unit types, in spite of the fact that the contractile and fatigue properties of diaphragm motor units differ from those observed in limb skeletal muscles (see Table 1).

In any muscle, the forces generated by motor units depend on three factors:

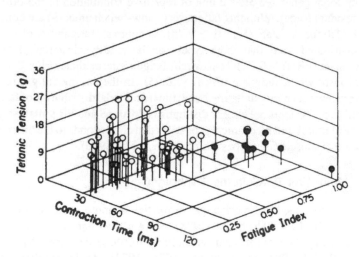

Figure 2 Scatter plot displaying the relation between twitch contraction time (time to peak twitch force), maximum tetanic force, and fatigue resistance (fatigue index is the ratio of force after 2 min of 40-Hz stimulation in 330-ms–duration trains repeated each second to the initial force) for motor units in the cat diaphragm. Filled circles are slow-twitch units and open circles are fast-twitch units.

Table 1 Summary of the Relative Differences in Maximum Tetanic Tension, Innervation Ratio, Cross-Sectional Area, and Specific Tension Among Different Types of Motor Units[a]

Muscle	Unit type	Max tetanic tension	Innervation ratio	Cross-sectional area	Specific tension	Ref.
	S	1.0	1.0	1.0	1.0	
TA	FR	2.5	2.1	1.0	1.2	Bodine et al. (1987)
	FF+FInt	5.5	2.9	1.3	1.4	
	S	1.0	1.0	1.0	1.0	
MG	FR	3.8	0.9	1.2	3.7	Burke (1981)
	FF+FInt	9.4	1.1	2.3	4.0	
	S	1.0	1.0	1.0	1.0	
FDL	FR	4.8	0.7	1.4	4.8	Burke (1981)
	FF+FInt	27.3	1.8	2.6	5.8	
	S	1.0	1.0	1.0	1.0	
SOL	FR	1.9	1.3	1.1	1.2	Chamberlain and Lewis (1989)
	S	1.0	1.0	1.0	1.0	
DIA	FR	2.3	0.9	1.3	1.8	Sieck (1991a);
	FF+FInt	3.6	1.1	1.7	1.9	Sieck and Fournier (1991)

[a]All values are referenced to those of type S units.
Abbreviations: TA, tibialis anterior muscle of cat; MG, medial gastrocnemius muscle of cat; FDL, flexor digitorum longus muscle of cat; SOL, soleus muscle of rat; DIA, diaphragm muscle of cat.

(1) innervation ratio of the unit (i.e., the number of muscle fibers innervated by a motoneuron); (2) total cross-sectional area of muscle unit fibers; and (3) specific force of the muscle unit fibers (i.e., the force generated per unit cross-sectional area) (Burke, 1981). With the introduction of the glycogen-depletion technique to identify muscle unit fibers (Edström and Kugelberg, 1968), it became possible to directly measure these variables (Fig. 3). Yet, only a few studies have reported such direct measurements and usually only for motor units in hindlimb muscles (see Table 1). These limited data do not provide a consistent insight to an underlying mechanism for the differences in force generated by the different motor unit types. For example, in the medial gastrocnemius and flexor digitorum longus muscles of the cat, the greater forces generated by fast-twitch units are primarily related to a greater specific force of type II fibers, and, to a lesser extent, the larger cross-sectional areas of muscle unit fibers (Burke, 1981). In contrast, in the tibialis anterior muscle of the cat (Bodine et al., 1987) and the soleus muscle of the rat (Chamberlain and Lewis, 1989), the greater forces generated by fast-twitch units are primarily related to a greater innervation ratio of these units and, to a lesser extent, the larger cross-sectional areas of muscle unit fibers.

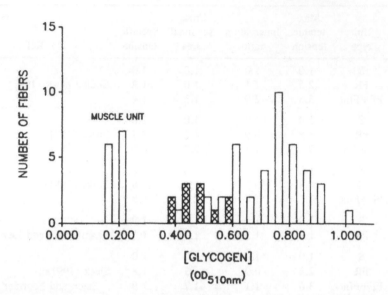

Figure 3   Muscle unit fibers can be identified histochemically using the glycogen-depletion technique. After prolonged repetitive stimulation of a fast-twitch unit in the cat diaphragm, the glycogen content (quantified by microdensitometry; measured optical density, OD, at 510 nm) of the muscle unit fibers were depleted relative to other type II fibers not belonging to this particular unit.

In the cat and hamster diaphragms, FF and FInt units also generate the greatest twitch and tetanic forces, followed in order by FR and S units (see Tables 1 and 2). These differences in motor unit forces in the cat diaphragm are related to a combination of a larger cross-sectional area of type II muscle fibers (comprising fast-twitch muscle units; Sieck et al., 1989a) and a greater specific force of these units (see Table 2). The innervation ratios of the different motor unit types in the cat diaphragm are comparable (see Table 2).

C.   Motor Unit Territories in the Diaphragm

The cat, rat, and hamster diaphragms are innervated somatotopically by two to four segments of the cervical spinal cord (Fournier and Sieck, 1987, 1988a; Laskowski and Sanes, 1987). In the cat diaphragm, the ventral portions of the costal and crural regions are primarily innervated by the C-5 ventral root (with a contribution in some cases from C-4), and the dorsal portions of both regions are primarily innervated by the C-6 ventral root (with an occasional contribution from C-7) (Fournier and

Table 2 Summary of the Contractile and Morphometric Properties of Motor Units in the Cat Diaphragm[a]

Motor unit type	S	FR	FInt	FF
Contractile properties				
Proportion (%)	30	4	25	41
Sag	–	+	+	+
CT (ms)	68 ± 18	42 ± 5	42 ± 7	34 ± 3
P_t (g)	1.5 ± 0.4	2.6 ± 2.0	3.5 ± 2.3	3.3 ± 1.9
P_o (g)	3.9 ± 1.2	8.8 ± 6.0	13.4 ± 7.2	14.4 ± 8.0
Relative force (%)	11	3	31	55
Morphometric properties				
CSA (μm^2)	1324 ± 170	1787 ± 221	2086 ± 510	2347 ± 793
% Total CSA	20	4	27	49
Innervation ratio	245	224	270	256
Specific tension (kg/cm^2)	1.2	2.2	2.2	2.4

[a]Values are means ± 1 standard deviation.
Abbreviations: CT, twitch contraction time; P_t, peak twitch tension; P_o, maximum tetanic tension CSA, fiber cross-sectional area.
Source: Sieck (1991a); Sieck and Fournier (1991).

Sieck, 1988a, 1987); (Fig. 4). Within each of the larger areas innervated by a single ventral root, the fibers constituting single motor units occupy a more restricted territory. Even within a ventral root, a somatotopic pattern is observed, such that motor axons situated more rostrally in the C-5 ventral root innervate muscle unit fibers in the sternocostal or ventral crural regions, whereas axons more caudally situated innervate muscle unit fibers in the midcostal or ventral crural regions. Thus, the territories occupied by diaphragm muscle unit fibers are also somatotopically organized (Fournier and Sieck, 1987).

Laskowski and Sanes (1987) demonstrated a similar somatotopic innervation of the costal region of the rat diaphragm, with C-4 innervating the more ventral portions and C-6 innervating the more dorsal portions. In the rat, C-5 innervates the midcostal region. Recently, we confirmed this somatotopic organization in the innervation of the rat diaphragm, with the additional observation that the C-3 ventral root provides a small contribution to the innervation of the ventral costal region (Sieck et al., unpublished observations). We have also observed a similar somatotopy in the hamster diaphragm, with the phrenic nerve comprising axons originating from C3–C5 (Sieck et al., unpublished observations).

III. Histochemical Classification of Muscle Fiber Types

Although a number of histochemical schemes for classifying muscle fiber types have been proposed over the years, two schemes are most commonly used: one

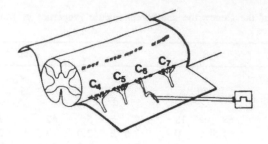

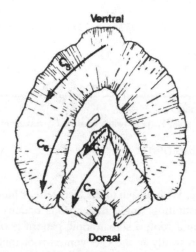

Figure 4   The cat diaphragm is somatotopically innervated by cervical spinal cord segments (C4–C7). The innervation derived from C-5 projects to the ventral portions of the costal and crural regions, and the innervation derived from C-6 projects to the dorsal portions of both regions. This somatotopy was characterized by electrophysiological mapping of electromyographic (EMG) responses evoked by ventral root stimulation and by histochemical examination of the patterns of glycogen depletion elicited by repetitive stimulation of ventral roots. (From Fournier and Sieck, 1988a.)

based on the pH lability of myofibrillar adenosine triphosphatase (mATPase) staining (Brooke and Kaiser, 1970; Brooke et al., 1971), and the second based on the metabolic profile (oxidative and glycolytic enzyme-staining intensities) of muscle fibers (Peter et al., 1972). In both schemes, two fiber types are initially distinguished, based on differences in staining for mATPase after alkaline preincubation (Fig. 5). Muscle fibers that stain lightly for mATPase are classified as type I (Brooke and Kaiser, 1970; Brooke et al., 1971) and, since they comprise the type S motor units, they are also sometimes referred to as slow-twitch fibers (Burke et al., 1971, 1973; Peter et al., 1972). In contrast, fibers that stain darkly for mATPase are

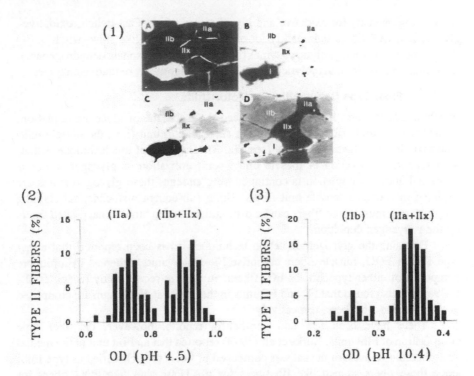

Figure 5 Histochemical classification of muscle fiber types is based on staining profiles for (A) myofibrillar ATPase after alkaline preincubation at pH 9.0 (B) acid preincubations at pH 4.3, (C) pH 4.5 and (D) after paraformaldehyde fixation and alkaline preincubation at pH 10.4. Note that type IIa fibers stained lighter than IIb and IIx in section C, whereas type IIb fibers stained lighter than IIa and IIx in section D. These differences in staining intensity were verified by microdensitometry (measuring OD and normalizing across animals by calculating Z-scores).

classified as type II fibers (Brooke and Kaiser, 1970; Brooke et al., 1971) and, since these fibers comprise the fast-twitch motor units, they are sometimes referred to as fast-twitch fibers (Burke et al., 1971, 1973; Peter et al., 1972).

The two histochemical classification schemes differ in the criteria they use to further subclassify type II or fast-twitch muscle fibers. This difference in classification criteria is important in that the fiber types classified by both schemes are not equivalent. In one scheme (Brooke and Kaiser, 1970; Brooke et al., 1971), type II muscle fibers are further subdivided based on differences in mATPase-staining intensity after preincubation at a pH of 4.5–4.6, at which type IIa fibers remain lightly stained for mATPase, and type IIb fibers stain darkly (see Fig. 5). At this pH, type I fibers also stain darkly for mATPase. In the second scheme, devised by Peter et al. (1972), fast-twitch fibers are further subdivided, based on differences in histochemical-staining intensity for oxidative and glycolytic enzymes. Fast-twitch, oxidative–glycolytic (FOG) fibers stain darkly for oxidative enzymes (like slow-twitch or SO fibers) and darkly for glycolytic enzymes (e.g., α-glycerophosphate dehydrogenase). In contrast, fast-twitch, glycolytic (FG) fibers stain lightly for oxidative enzymes.

A. Fiber-Type Composition of Motor Units

In 1968, Edström and Kugelberg introduced the technique of glycogen depletion, by which the muscle fibers belonging to a single motor unit (i.e., the muscle unit) could be identified histochemically (see Fig. 3). The basis of this technique is that, with repetitive activation of muscle unit fibers, utilization of glycogen stores is promoted and, if stimulation is continued long enough, these glycogen stores are depleted in activated muscle unit fibers. Upon subsequent histochemical staining for glycogen, muscle unit fibers can be distinguished from other nonactivated fibers by their glycogen depletion.

By using the glycogen-depletion technique, it has been reported that either type IIa, or FOG, muscle fibers comprise FR motor units, whereas FF units are composed of either type IIb, or FG, fibers. In a more recent study (Sieck et al., 1989a), we also found that FR and FF units in the adult cat diaphragm are composed of type IIa and IIb fibers, respectively.

There have been few and conflicting reports, however, on fiber type composition of FInt units. Burke et al. (1973) reported that an FInt unit in the medial gastrocnemius muscle of the cat was composed of fibers they classified as type IIab, since these fibers stained like IIb fibers for mATPase, but like FOG fibers for oxidative enzymes. In the tibialis anterior muscle of the cat, Bodine et al. (1987) reported that an FInt unit comprised FG fibers. In the cat diaphragm, we (Sieck et al., 1989a) found that FInt units had a mixed fiber type composition, containing both type IIa and IIb fibers, with oxidative enzyme activities that were intermediate between FF and FR units. The ambiguity in the fiber type composition of FInt motor units most likely reflect the lack of correspondence between the two major histochemical classification schemes. Several studies have shown that the classification of fiber types using these two schemes is not interchangeable (Green et al., 1984; Nemeth and Pette, 1981; Reichmann and Pette, 1982; Sieck et al., 1992). Although type IIa fibers generally have higher oxidative enzyme activities (e.g., succinate dehydrogenase, SDH activity) and most type IIb fibers have lower SDH activity, some type IIb fibers also have higher SDH activities and would thus be classified as FOG. Therefore, we found that differences in oxidative enzyme (SDH) activity provide inadequate positive predictive power to distinguish between type IIa and IIb fibers (Fig. 6 and Table 3). As can be seen from Table 3, type IIb fibers in the rat diaphragm characteristically display lower SDH activity (– Z-scores) and greater cross-sectional areas (+ Z-scores) than type IIa fibers. However, type IIa fibers cannot be reliably discriminated from IIb fibers based on higher SDH activity (+ Z-scores) or smaller cross-sectional areas (– Z-scores).

The lack of correspondence between the two most commonly used classifi-

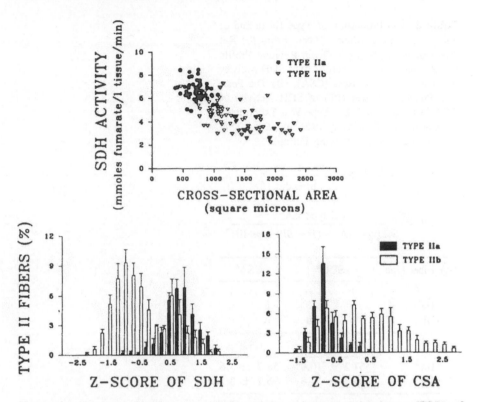

Figure 6 Succinate dehydrogenase (SDH) activity and cross-sectional area (CSA) of muscle fibers in the rat diaphragm were quantified using an image-processing system (cf, Blanco et al., Edgerton, 1988). The distributions of SDH activity and CSA of type IIa and IIb fibers displayed considerable overlap. Generally, larger fibers with lower SDH activity were consistently classified as type IIb. However, smaller fibers with higher SDH activity were not uniquely type IIa.

cation schemes may also reflect the subjective nature of assessing histochemical staining intensities, particularly in assessing the staining intensity of muscle fibers for oxidative enzymes. Recognition of the subjectivity of fiber type classification is very important because of the functional inferences that are drawn. For example, the proportion of higher oxidative fibers (i.e., type I and IIa, or SO and FOG) is thought to directly correlate with the fatigue resistance of a muscle. When these fiber-type proportions change under certain conditions, it is concluded that muscle fatigue resistance has also changed. Yet, whether there is a substantive basis for fiber-type classification has not been demonstrated. Indeed, evidence from our laboratory (Sieck et al., 1986; Sieck et al., 1987, 1992) indicates that, at least in some muscles, there is no reliable quantitative basis for subclassifying fiber types based on differences in oxidative enzyme activity (see Fig. 6 and Table 3).

Table 3 (A) Proportion of Type IIa (a and c) and IIb (b and d) Muscle Fibers From the Rat Diaphragm Displaying a Given Relative Profile (+: Z-score < 0; −: Z-score < 0) of SDH Activity and Cross-Sectional Area (CSA). (B) The Positive Predictive Power (PP) of SDH Activity of CSA in Identifying Fiber Type Was Determined by Calculating Sensitivity (SE) and Specificity (SP) Based on the Following Formula.

$$SE = \frac{a}{a + c} \; ; \; SP = \frac{d}{b + d};$$

$$PP = \frac{SE \text{ type IIA}}{SE \text{ type IIA} + (1 - SP) \text{ type IIB}}$$

(A) Fiber type	SDH[a]		CSA[a]	
	+	−	−	+
IIa	a	c	a	c
IIb	b	d	b	d

(B)	SDH[a]	CSA[a]
IIa	67.2 ± 10.9[b]	58.7 ± 5.6
IIb	95.3 ± 7.8	95.2 ± 8.1

[a]A priori prediction was that SDH activity would be higher and CSA lower in type IIa fibers compared with IIb.
[b]Mean ± SD ($n = 6$) probability (%)
Source: Woolson (1987).

B. Myosin Heavy Chain Phenotype

The myosin heavy chain (MHC) is coded by a highly conserved family of genes consisting of at least six isoforms in mammalian skeletal muscle: (1) embryonic (*MHC-Emb*); (2) neonatal (*MHC-Neo*); (3) slow (*MHC-Slow*); (4) fast type IIa (*MHC-2A*); (5) fast type IIb (*MHC-2B*); and (6) fast type IIx (*MHC-2X*) (Mahdavi et al., 1986; Nguyen et al., 1982; Periasamy et al., 1989). Immunohistochemical procedures have been used to identify the expression of at least some of these different MHC isoforms within muscle fibers. In most adult muscles, MHC phenotype corresponds with the histochemical classification of fiber types based on the pH lability of mATPase (Bar and Pette, 1988; Gorza, 1990; Pierobon-Bormioli et al., 1988; Schiaffino et al., 1988a; Watchko et al., 1992) and, as stated before, these different fiber types comprise motor units with characteristic physiological properties (Burke, 1981; Burke et al., 1971, 1973; Sieck et al., 1989a). The only possible exceptions to this general correspondence are (1) an absence of any unique relationship between histochemically classified type IIc fibers in developing or injured muscle and the expression of MHC-Emb or MHC-Neo; and (2) an ambiguity between the standard histochemical classification of type IIb fibers and a phenotypic distinction between the expression of MHC-2B or MHC-2X isoforms (Bar and Pette, 1988; Gorza, 1990; Pierobon-Bormioli et al., 1988; Schiaffino et al., 1988a; Watchko et al., 1992). Recently, Gorza (1990) demonstrated that fibers composed of the MHC-2X isoform could also be distinguished histochemically from fibers expressing the MHC-2B isoform based on a modified mATPase-staining procedure at pH 10.4. In rat diaphragm muscle, we have recently confirmed, by quantitative analysis, the applicability of this modified histochemical technique (G. C. Sieck, unpublished observations; (see Fig. 5).

Several studies have examined the postnatal differentiation of the different adult MHC isoforms (Butler-Browne et al., 1990, 1982; Hoh et al., 1988; Kelly, 1983; Kelly et al., 1991; Kelly and Rubinstein, 1980; Mahdavi et al., 1986; Narusawa et al., 1987; Pette and Vrbova, 1985; Staron and Pette, 1987; Stockdale and Miller, 1987; Swynghedauw, 1986; Whalen et al., 1981). The etiology of fiber differentiation appears to depend on several factors including (1) the genetic "program" of the specific muscle (i.e., the proportion of fiber types found in the adult); (2) the pattern of innervation, level of activation, or neurotrophic influences; and (3) the hormonal environment (e.g., insulin, thyroid hormone, growth factors, corticosteroids).

C. Influence of Innervation on Myosin Heavy Chain Phenotype and Muscle Contractility

Substantial evidence indicates that innervation or activation history exerts an important influence over the contractile protein composition and metabolic enzyme activities of muscle fibers (Blanco et al., 1991; Buller et al., 1960; Burke, 1981; Burke et al., 1971a, 1973; Edström and Kugelberg, 1968; Enad et al., 1989; Fournier and Sieck, 1986; Hamm et al. 1988; Nemeth et al., 1981, 1986; Pette and Vrbova, 1985; Sieck, 1991a; Sieck and Fournier, 1991; Sieck et al., 1989a,b; Zhan and Sieck, 1992). For example, following prolonged inactivation—induced by tetrodotoxin (TTX), blockade of axonal action potential propagation, or denervation—adult muscle fibers in the rat diaphragm (Carraro et al., 1985; Sieck et al., unpublished observations) and tibialis anterior muscles (Schiaffino et al., 1988b) begin to reexpress MHC-Emb and MHC-Neo isoforms (coexpressed with MHC-Slow). Consistent with these changes in MHC expression, the maximum specific force and maximum unloaded shortening velocity of diaphragm muscle fibers decrease after prolonged inactivation (TTX or denervation-induced) (Zhan and Sieck, 1992; Johnson et al., 1993b). Other recent studies have demonstrated changes in MHC phenotype after prolonged stimulation of muscle (e.g., Pette and Vrbova, 1985).

Further support of the role of innervation in influencing the physiological, histochemical, and metabolic properties of muscle fibers was derived from motor unit studies, in which homogeneous fiber type composition and metabolic enzyme activities of muscle unit fibers have been attributed to the influence of common innervation or activation history (Burke, 1981; Burke et al., 1971, 1973; Edström and Kugelberg, 1968; Enad et al., 1989; Fournier and Sieck, 1986; Hamm et al., 1988; Nemeth et al., 1981, 1986; Sieck et al., 1989a).

During postnatal development, the final proportionate expression of adult slow and fast MHC isoforms is markedly affected by the level of neuromuscular activity (Gauthier et al., 1978; Kelly, 1983; Pette and Vrbova, 1985; Stockdale and Miller, 1987). If neural activation is abolished (e.g., using TTX or denervation), the proportion of fibers expressing MHC-Slow is decreased (Butler-Browne et al., 1982; Dhoot and Perry, 1983; Gauthier et al., 1978), and there is a delay in the differentiation of some fibers, with continued expression of the MHC-Neo isoform (Butler-Browne et al., 1982; Dhoot and Perry, 1983). However, the differentiation of adult fast MHC isoforms (i.e., MHC-2A, MHC-2B, and MHC-2X) is not significantly affected by inactivity or denervation. In recent studies (Zhan et al., 1993; Johnson et al., 1993b), we found that, following transection of the right phrenic nerve at 7 days of age, the expression of MHC-Neo in the denervated diaphragm persists, and the expression of MHC-Slow is reduced. These changes in MHC phenotype transitions are associated with a slowing of maximum unloaded shortening velocity and a decrease in maximum specific force. However, the normal correlations between MHC phenotype transitions and changing contractile properties during postnatal development are completely abolished after denervation (i.e., the effect on MHC phenotype has no predictive influence on diaphragm contractile properties).

D. Influence of Thyroid Hormone on Myosin Phenotype

Increasing evidence indicates that thyroid status (hypo- or hyperthyroidism) influences the expression of MHC isoforms. Although the specific influence of thyroid hormone is age- and muscle-dependent, the general patterns of thyroid effects are apparent (d'Albis et al., 1990). In adult muscles, hypothyroidism consistently increases the expression of the MHC-Slow isoform, whereas the effect on MHC-2A expression varies across muscles (Caiozzo et al., 1991; Diffee et al., 1991; Fitzsimmons et al., 1990; Ianuzzo et al., 1977; Petrof et al., 1992, Sieck et al., 1993; Wilson et al., 1993). It has been suggested that the adult rat diaphragm may be less susceptible to the influence of hypothyroidism than hindlimb muscles (Ianuzzo et al., 1984), but several laboratories, including our own recent studies (Sieck et al., 1993; Wilson et al., 1993), have noted effects of altered thyroid status on the diaphragm's histochemical and contractile properties in the adult (Johnson et al., 1983; Mier et al., 1989; Miyashita et al., 1992).

In developing limb muscles, hypothyroidism alters the intrinsic program for

MHC phenotype transitions, such that the expression of MHC-Neo persists until well after weaning (3–4 weeks of age), the expression of MHC-Slow is promoted, and the expression of MHC-2B is inhibited (Butler-Browne et al., 1984; Gambke et al., 1983). Conversely, hyperthyroidism tends to advance the transition from MHC-Neo to adult fast MHC isoforms and inhibits the expression of MHC-Slow (Butler-Browne et al., 1990; Gambke et al., 1983; Russell et al., 1988). d'Albis and colleagues (1990) reported that, with hypothyroidism in developing rats, the expression of MHC-Neo in muscles persists, but these authors found that hyperthyroidism had no effect on MHC-Neo transitions. In a more recent study (Sieck et al., 1993; Wilson et al., 1993), we also found that, with hypothyroidism, the expression of MHC-Neo in the developing rat diaphragm persists, the relative expression of MHC-Slow increases, and the expression of adult fast MHC isoforms is inhibited. These changes in MHC phenotype are associated with a slowing of maximum shortening velocity and a decrease in the maximum specific force of the diaphragm. However, as with denervations, the effect of hypothyroidism on postnatal MHC phenotype transitions has no predictable influence on diaphragm's contractile properties (i.e., the normally strong correlations between MHC phenotype transitions and muscles' contractile properties are abolished). Hyperthyroidism exerts less of an effect on postnatal MHC phenotype transitions in the rat diaphragm, but we did note a more rapid decrease in the expression of MHC-Neo with age, a decrease in the expression of MHC-Slow, and an increase in the expression of adult fast MHC isoforms, especially MHC-2A. The effects of hyperthyroidism on postnatal changes in contractile properties have not yet been evaluated.

E. Actomyosin Adenosine Triphosphatase Activity and Muscle Fiber Type

The MHC, a major structural component of the myosin cross-bridge, is the site of actin-dependent myosin ATPase (actomyosin ATPase) activity (Wagner, 1981). In adult muscles, the energy costs for contraction of type I fibers (composed of MHC-Slow) are approximately half that of type II fibers (composed of adult fast MHC isoforms) (Crow and Kushmerick, 1982). This difference in energy utilization between fiber types may be related to differences in actomyosin ATPase activity. We recently developed a microdensitometric procedure (quantitative histochemistry) for determining the kinetics of the Ca^{2+}-dependent myosin ATPase (actomyosin ATPase) reaction in individual muscle fibers at physiological pH (i.e., maximum velocity of the reaction and the Michaelis–Menten rate constant) (Blanco and Sieck, 1992). We found that, in the cat and rat diaphragms, actomyosin ATPase activity (maximum velocity of the reaction) is lowest in type I and highest in type IIB fibers, with actomyosin ATPase activity of type IIa and IIx fibers being intermediate. Preliminary studies have shown that actomyosin ATPase activity in type IIc fibers of the neonatal diaphragm is lower than that of adult type II fibers and comparable with type I fibers. These quantitative histochemical results are qualitatively similar to values obtained from biochemical analysis of myofibrillar ATPase activity of muscle homogenates (Baldwin et al., 1978; Belcastro, 1987).

Barany (1967) first reported a correlation between biochemically determined myofibrillar ATPase activity and the maximum shortening velocity of muscles. Subsequently, several studies have shown a correlation between MHC phenotype and the maximum shortening velocity of single, skinned-muscle fibers (Bottinelli et al., 1991; Reiser et al., 1985, 1988a,b; Schiaffino et al., 1988a; Sieck et al., unpublished observations). Fibers expressing MHC-Slow have slower maximum shortening velocities than fibers expressing adult fast MHC isoforms. Among type II fibers, however, no significant differences in maximum shortening velocities have been observed for fibers expressing MHC-2A, 2B, or 2X isoforms. The relation between MHC phenotype and maximum shortening velocity is usually attributed to differences in actomyosin ATPase activity and, thus, a slower cross-bridge cycling rate of type I fibers.

Biochemical studies have shown that the rate of myofibrillar ATPase activity in developing muscle is lower than that in adult muscle (Baldwin et al., 1978; Belcastro, 1987). Accordingly, we (Sieck et al., 1993; Johnson et al., 1993a) and others (Reiser 1988a,b) have found that developing muscle fibers expressing MHC-Neo have slower maximum shortening velocities than adult fast fibers.

Given the differences in actomyosin ATPase activity among adult and neonatal fiber types, it is entirely possible that neonatal fibers might vary from adult fibers in the energy costs for contraction. With lower energy costs, it might also be expected that the neonatal muscle would be more fatigue-resistant, as we and others have observed (Sieck, et al., 1991b; Sieck and Fournier, 1991; Watchko et al., 1992; Watchko and Sieck, in press; Maxwell et al., 1983). With the differentiation of adult fibers (especially type II), energy costs for contraction would increase and fatigue resistance would decrease. It might also be expected that, as the energy costs for contraction increase, the metabolic support for energy production (e.g., oxidative capacity) within muscle fibers would also increase. The rapid growth and increased protein synthesis (structural and contractile proteins) within developing muscle fibers would also require additional metabolic support. Thus, it is not surprising that the SDH activities of the diaphragm's fibers increase during early stages of postnatal development (Sieck and Blanco, 1991; Sieck and Fournier, 1991; Sieck 1991a; Smith et al., 1988).

IV. Neural Control of Muscle Force

In the classic model of neuromotor control proposed by Sherrington (Liddell and Sherrington, 1925; Sherrington, 1929), the forces generated by a muscle during any motor behavior result from the recruitment of variable numbers of motor units, each of which contributes a quantal amount of force to the total. In this model, the central nervous system produces the desired level of force by controlling the temporal and numerical combination of these functional quanta (i.e., motor units). Thus, force can be controlled by changing the number of activated motor units (recruitment coding); or by modifying the discharge frequency of recruited motor units (frequency coding).

The Sherrington model of neuromotor control assumes that, when the motoneuron discharges an action potential, it is propagated to all muscle unit fibers, which are then activated through neuromuscular transmission in an all-or-none fashion. Furthermore, this model implies that each muscle fiber belongs to only one motor unit. These implications, inherent in Sherrington's concept of a quantal organization of neuromotor control, have been subjected to considerable examination and are substantively correct, at least in the normal adult muscle. However, there are important exceptions to these basic assumptions. For example, action potential propagation failure occurs at motor axonal branches (Krnjevic and Miledi, 1958, 1959; Sandercock et al., 1985; Sieck and Fournier, 1990; Fournier et al., 1991). With such neuromuscular transmission failure, not all muscle unit fibers would be activated. Changes in muscle unit EMG waveform or amplitude during repetitive activation may be indicative of axonal branch point failure (Sandercock et al., 1985; Sieck and Fournier, 1990). Neuromuscular transmission failure can also occur during repetitive activation (Aldrich et al., 1986; Fournier et al., 1991; Johnson and Sieck, 1993; Kelsen and Nochomovitz, 1982; Kuei et al., 1990; Sieck and Fournier, 1990; Pagala et al., 1984).

Motor units vary in their susceptibility to neuromuscular transmission failure, such that type FF and FInt units are more susceptible than type S and FR units (Clamann and Robinson, 1985; Sandercock et al., 1985; Sieck and Fournier, 1990). In a recent study (Johnson and Sieck, 1993), we estimated the susceptibility of different diaphragm muscle fiber types (and, by inference, different motor unit types) to neuromuscular transmission failure by comparing glycogen-depletion patterns after repetitive direct muscle stimulation versus phrenic nerve stimulation. It was assumed that, if neuromuscular transmission failure occurred, there would be less glycogen depletion, compared with direct muscle stimulation. Our results indicated that type IIb fibers (FF and FInt motor units) are most susceptible to neuromuscular transmission failure. These results generally agree with our observation that motor unit EMG changes during repetitive stimulation are most pronounced in FF and FInt units, compared with FR and S units (Sieck and Fournier, 1990). The importance of neuromuscular transmission failure in neuromotor control remains to be determined. Clearly, the extent of neuromuscular transmission failure is dependent on stimulus rate (Clamann and Robinson, 1985; Fournier et al., 1991; Johnson and Sieck, 1993; Kuei et al., 1990; Sandercock et al., 1985; Sieck and Fournier, 1990). Perhaps the motoneuron discharge adaptation that occurs during sustained depolarizing current injection (Kernell and Monster, 1982a,b) is a protective mechanism to prevent neuromuscular transmission failure. The stimulus rate required to sustain a given level of motor unit force slows during repetitive stimulation (Botterman, 1986), most likely owing to the prolonged relaxation time of muscle unit fibers.

Another exception to Sherrington's general concept of the motor unit occurs during early postnatal development, when polyneuronal innervation of muscle fibers is prevalent. This suggests that the quantal recruitment of motor units might differ significantly during early postnatal development. Polyneuronal innervation of muscle fibers also occurs after the reinnervation of denervated muscles (Bagust et al., 1974; Dubowitz, 1967; Dum et al., 1985). With polyneuronal innervation, the relative size of motor units is greater and recruitment coding of force generation is less effective.

Regardless of these exceptions to Sherrington's concept of the motor unit, the principles of a quantal organization of motor units and an orderly recruitment of units during motor behaviors form the cornerstones for all current models of neuromotor control of skeletal muscles.

A. Size Principle of Motor Unit Recruitment

In 1957, Henneman hypothesized that susceptibility of neurons to discharge is a function of size, which dictates the intrinsic electrophysiological properties of motoneurons. This "size principle" has been restated over the years, but generally it predicts that the orderly recruitment of motor units is related to the intrinsic electrophysiological properties of motoneurons (Henneman, 1957; Henneman et al., 1965; Henneman and Mendell, 1981). Smaller motoneurons have higher membrane input resistance and, thus, a lower rheobase (i.e., the input current required for evoking repetitive action potential discharge) than larger motoneurons with lower membrane input resistance. Given similar synaptic input currents, smaller motoneurons would thus be recruited before larger motoneurons (Burke, 1981; Fleshman et al., 1981; Henneman and Mendell, 1981; Sypert and Munson, 1981; Zajac and Faden, 1985; Zengel et al., 1985). Support for the size principle has come from comparisons of motor unit recruitment order in relation to axonal conduction velocities (Dick et al., 1987a,b; Henneman et al., 1965; Henneman and Mendell, 1981). Smaller motoneurons have smaller axons (Berger, 1979; Clamann and Henneman, 1976; Webber and Pleschka, 1976) and, thus, slower axonal conduction velocities. Motor units with slower axonal conduction velocities are invariably recruited before larger motoneurons with faster axonal conduction velocities. Smaller motoneurons also innervate type S muscle unit fibers (i.e., type I fibers), which produce lower maximum tetanic force. Accordingly, a relation between motor unit type, motor unit maximum tetanic force, and recruitment order have also been observed (Burke, 1981; Fleshman et al., 1981; Sypert and Munson, 1981; Zajac and Faden, 1985; Zengel et al., 1985). In contrast, larger motoneurons innervate fast-twitch muscle unit fibers, which generate greater tetanic forces. Among the fast-twitch motor units, FR units have the lowest recruitment threshold, followed in rank order by FInt and FF units (Burke, 1981). Thus, the order of motor unit recruitment is directly related to the size (axonal conduction velocity and maximum tetanic force) and fatigue resistance of units.

B. Diaphragmatic Motor Unit Recruitment

Several studies (Dick et al., 1987a,b; Jodkowski et al., 1987) have presented evidence indicating that the order of motor unit recruitment in the diaphragm muscle also depends on the intrinsic electrophysiological properties of phrenic motoneurons. Dick and associates (1987a,b) found that, during spontaneous breathing, phrenic motoneurons in the cat are recruited in an order related to increasing axonal conduction velocity. In light of the demonstrated relation between axonal conduction velocity and phrenic motoneuronal membrane input resistance (Berger, 1979; Webber and Pleschka, 1976), these authors concluded that the size principle predicts the order of diaphragm motor unit recruitment. In the study by Jodkowski et al. (1987), it was reported that two subpopulations of phrenic motoneurons exist in the cat, segregated by differences in membranal input resistance and rheobase. These authors reported that most (i.e., 60%) of those phrenic motoneurons with higher-input resistance and lower rheobase can be recruited during spontaneous hypercapnic breathing. In contrast, none of the phrenic motoneurons with lower-input resistance and higher rheobase are recruited during inspiration, even with end-tidal CO_2 at 7%. These authors suggested that the phrenic motoneurons normally recruited with respiration innervate type S muscle unit fibers (i.e., type I fibers), whereas those not recruited with breathing innervate type F muscle unit fibers (i.e., type II fibers). The proportion of all phrenic motoneurons that they found to be recruited with inspiration (i.e., 23%) approximates the proportion of type S motor units that we found in the cat diaphragm (Fournier and Sieck, 1988b; Sieck, 1988; see Table 2).

An alternative model for diaphragm motor unit recruitment has been presented by Hilaire and co-workers (Hilaire et al., 1983, 1987; Monteau et al., 1985). By using techniques of cross-correlation and spike-triggered averaging, these authors demonstrated that medullary inspiratory neurons that discharge early during inspiration have an increased probability of monosynaptically driving phrenic motoneurons that also display early recruitment during inspiration. Conversely, medullary inspiratory neurons that discharge late in inspiration monosynaptically drive phrenic motoneurons recruited later during inspiration. These results suggested that the recruitment order of diaphragm motor units might be dictated not only by the size and intrinsic properties of phrenic motoneurons, but also by the specific pattern of synaptic input from medullary inspiratory neurons.

In several studies, diaphragm motor units (and phrenic motoneurons) have been classified as "early" or "late," depending on the onset time of their activation during inspiration (Berger, 1979; Donnelly et al., 1985; Hilaire et al., 1983; Iscoe et al., 1976; Monteau et al., 1985). This classification of phrenic motoneurons and diaphragm motor units is useful in that it matches the common classification of medullary and pontine "inspiratory" neurons as early or late. However, there is no objective basis for classifying phrenic motoneurons or diaphragm motor units as early or late, as there is no clear bimodal distribution of onset times for motor unit recruitment. Therefore, it appears that the definition of early and late phrenic motoneurons has been largely arbitrary. There continues to be a debate about whether the order of diaphragm motor unit recruitment depends on the intrinsic size-related electrophysiological properties of phrenic motoneurons (i.e., the size principle) or the extrinsic pattern of synaptic input to phrenic motoneurons (e.g., specific bulbospinal connections). The classification of early versus late phrenic motoneurons (diaphragm motor units) implicitly assumes the latter hypothesis to be correct. However, usually, the distribution of diaphragm motor unit recruitment times relative to inspiratory onset is continuous and not bimodal.

The relation between the order of phrenic motoneuron recruitment and diaphragm motor unit type also remains unknown. If phrenic motoneurons are recruited solely on the basis of premotor connectivity (e.g., early versus late), it is possible that the normal relation between motor unit recruitment and motor unit type (i.e., an orderly progression from type S, FR, FInt, and finally FF units) that is present in other skeletal muscles might not exist in the diaphragm. However, an early recruitment of fatigable units seems unlikely, particularly considering the unique activation requirements of the diaphragm.

In determining how and when diaphragm motor units are recruited during different motor behaviors, the nervous system must be very selective, since some motor units display a greater susceptibility to fatigue with repetitive activation (Fournier and Sieck, 1988b; Sieck and Fournier, 1989; Sieck, 1991a,b). For example, recruitment of type FF motor units would be disadvantageous in accomplishing the sustained force generation required during normal repetitive ventilatory behaviors (eupnea), as the force contribution of FF units would fatigue considerably under such conditions. In contrast, type S and FR motor units are more fatigue-resistant; thus, their recruitment during eupnea would be preferable.

Other motor behaviors of the diaphragm require short-duration bursts of substantial force generation (e.g., sneezing, coughing, or vomiting). In such behaviors, the recruitment of larger motor units that generate greater forces would be required. Among the motor unit population of most mixed skeletal muscles, including the diaphragm, there appears to be an inverse relation between contractile strength and fatigability. Type FF motor units are the largest, generate the greatest force, but are the most susceptible to fatigue (Burke, 1981; Fournier and Sieck, 1988b; Sieck and Fournier, 1989). In contrast, type S motor units are the smallest, generate the least amount of force, and are the most fatigue-resistant. Thus, the combined strength and fatigue characteristics of the diaphragm motor unit population will dictate the constraints on the ventilatory and nonventilatory performances of the whole muscle.

In recent studies (Sieck and Fournier, 1989; Sieck, 1991a,b), we estimated the proportion of the motor unit pool in the cat and hamster diaphragms that would be recruited during different ventilatory and nonventilatory (e.g., sneezing, coughing) behaviors. Diaphragm forces generated during these different behaviors were indexed by measuring transdiaphragmatic pressures (Pdi) and compared with the maximum Pdi (Pdi max) evoked by bilateral phrenic nerve stimulation (tetanic stimulation). We estimated that the Pdi generated during eupnea in the cat amounts to only a small fraction (12%) of Pdi max (Fig. 7). This is comparable with the relative Pdi generated during eupnea in humans (G. C. Sieck, unpublished observations). In contrast, in the hamster diaphragm, eupneic Pdi accounts for approximately 27% of Pdi max (see Fig. 7). Even at the lower motor unit discharge rates normally observed during spontaneous breathing (e.g., 10–30 Hz in unanesthetized cats; Sieck et al., 1984), the diaphragm, in either species, would generate only approximately 60% of its Pdi max if all units were simultaneously recruited (see Fig. 7). Therefore, it is quite clear that not all diaphragm motor units are recruited during normal quiet inspiratory efforts. If, as in other mixed skeletal muscles, type S motor units are recruited first, we estimated that approximately 10–15% of Pdi max could be generated by the maximal activation of these units alone (see Fig. 7). However, at activation rates of 10–30 Hz (Sieck et al., 1984), type S units in both the cat and hamster diaphragm produce only approximately 60–80% of their maximum force (Fournier and Sieck, 1988b). Thus, although most of the required ventilatory force during quiet breathing can be generated by the recruitment of type S units, it would appear that the recruitment of at least some fast-twitch units would be required. The additional recruitment of type FR units would be sufficient to produce the required pressures during normal quiet breathing in both species (see Fig. 7). Thus, from our estimates, it appears likely that very few type FF and FInt units are recruited during normal breathing.

In the cat, when the drive for ventilation is increased by having animals inspire a hypercapnic (5% CO_2)–hypoxic (10% CO_2) gas mixture, Pdi increases to 28% of Pdi max. We estimated that this force level could be generated by the additional recruitment of some FInt units (see Fig. 7). Even during total airway occlusion, the forces generated by the cat (49% of Pdi max) and hamster (43% of Pdi max) diaphragms can be accomplished without the recruitment of FF units, assuming that the recruited units are maximally activated (see Fig. 7). Even if no rate coding of force generation occurs, the diaphragm forces produced during sustained tracheal occlusion would not require the full recruitment of all motor units. This was verified by superimposing bilateral phrenic nerve stimulation during the occluded inspiratory effort. With phrenic stimulation, an additional increment in Pdi is consistently observed during all ventilatory behaviors. Only during expulsive nonventilatory behaviors are maximum forces generated in the cat diaphragm. Interestingly, in the hamster, we were unable to elicit these nonventilatory behaviors. From these results, we conclude that the normal ventilatory requirements of the diaphragm in both species can be met by the recruitment of only fatigue-resistant motor units (type S and FR). Furthermore, these results suggest that many motor units in the adult diaphragm remain relatively inactive during normal ventilation.

Figure 8 compares the model of motor unit recruitment in the cat diaphragm with a similar model for motor unit recruitment in the cat medial gastrocnemius muscle during different locomotor behaviors (Walmsley et al., 1978). As in the diaphragm, the recruitment model in the medial gastrocnemius muscle also predicts

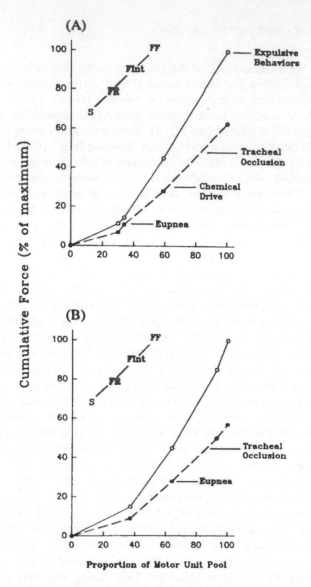

Figure 7 Recruitment models for motor units in (A) the cat and (B) hamster diaphragms are proposed based on the assumption of an orderly recruitment of different motor unit types (based on fatigue resistance). The forces required for different ventilatory and nonventilatory behaviors of the diaphragm were estimated from the transdiaphragmatic pressure (Pdi) measurements referenced to the maximal Pdi generated by bilateral phrenic nerve stimulation. The cumulative forces generated by motor unit recruitment were estimated from the mean forces generated by each unit type and their proportion within the diaphragm. Open circles and solid lines assume unit activation at maximum tetanic force, whereas filled circles and dashed line assume activation at the center frequency of the force–frequency relation of each unit. Note that in each case, eupnic pressures could be generated by the recruitment of only fatigue-resistant units (S and FR). More forceful ventilatory and nonventilatory behaviors would require the recruitment of more fatigable units (FInt and FF).

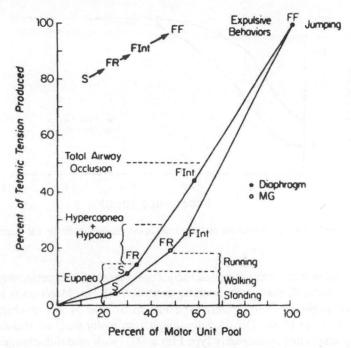

Figure 8 Comparison of motor unit recruitment models in the diaphragm (data from Fournier and Sieck, 1988b) and medial gastrocnemius muscles (data from Walmsley et al., 1978) of the cat during different motor behaviors. These models assume (1) a specific order of motor unit recruitment (i.e., S, FR, FInt, and FF); and (2) complete activation of one motor unit type before the next type is recruited.

that a large fraction of the motor unit pool is employed only infrequently during behaviors of short duration, requiring high levels of force (e.g., jumping). In contrast, all locomotor behaviors of the medial gastrocnemius muscle can be accomplished by the recruitment of fatigue-resistant motor units (i.e., S and FR). Thus, the distribution of motor unit types within any muscle may be a reflection of its functional requirements.

C. Frequency Coding of Motor Unit Force

Because of their longer CT and 1/2 RT, the force generated by type S units summates at lower frequencies of activation than type F units (Fig. 9). Maximum tetanic forces are reached at lower rates of stimulation in type S units, and the ratio of twitch to maximum tetanic forces is higher in type S units than in type F units. Thus, the range of frequency coding in type S units is narrower than in type F units.

In the adult cat, we recorded the spontaneous discharge of diaphragm motor units during different sleep and waking states (Sieck et al., 1984). We found that

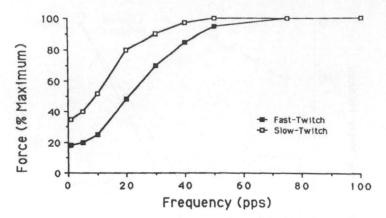

Figure 9   Force–frequency relation of fast- and slow-twitch units in the cat diaphragm.

those diaphragm motor units recruited early during inspiration (presumably type S units) have modal discharge rates ranging from 8 to 12 Hz. Motor units recruited later during inspiration (presumably type FR units) have modal discharge rates ranging from 13 to 16 Hz. Occasionally, diaphragm motor units are recruited very late during inspiration (presumably type FInt units), with modal discharge rates of 20–25 Hz. If it is assumed that the motor units consistently recruited during inspiration are type S or FR, the forces generated at these rates of activation would be approximately 50–75% of maximum tetanic force. Importantly, these discharge rates are on the steep portion of the force–frequency curves for type S and FR units (see Fig. 9). If the late and infrequently recruited units (i.e., those with discharge rates of 20–25 pps) are type FInt units, the forces generated at these discharge rates would also be approximately 50–75% of maximum. Again, these discharge rates are on the steep portion of the force–frequency curves of fast-twitch units (see Fig. 9). Thus, the spontaneous discharge rates of diaphragm motor units permit optimal frequency coding of force generation.

V. Central Versus Peripheral Fatigue of Muscle Units

Muscle fatigue has been defined as an inability of the muscle to maintain an expected or required level of force (Edwards, 1981). Fatigue may occur at any one of several potential sites, which have been generally grouped as of either central or of peripheral origin (Bigland-Ritchie, 1981). If motoneurons fail to generate action potentials, central fatigue of motor units results (Kernell and Monster, 1982b). This could be due to reduced synaptic drive, or to an accommodation of motoneuronal discharge (Kernell and Monster, 1982a,b). Peripheral fatigue results from a failure at any one of several potential sites, including axonal propagation, neuromuscular transmission, excitation–contraction coupling, sarcoplasmic reticulum release of calcium, muscle fiber contractile mechanisms, or energy production within muscle fibers. Central fatigue is bypassed by stimulating the motor axon; however, discrimination among the various potential sites of peripheral fatigue is more difficult.

A. Neuromuscular Transmission Failure

The relative contribution of neuromuscular transmission failure to diaphragm fatigue can be assessed by comparing force loss during nerve stimulation with that occurring with direct muscle stimulation; namely, bypassing the neuromuscular junction (Aldrich et al., 1986; Kelsen and Nochomovitz, 1982; Kuei et al., 1990; Pagala et al., 1984; Fig. 10). In a study of the adult rat, we compared the forces generated by these two modes of stimulation and estimated the relative contribution of neuromuscular transmission failure to diaphragmatic fatigue at various rates of stimulation (Kuei et al., 1990). At a stimulation rate of 20 Hz, we estimated that neuromuscular transmission failure contributes approximately 16% to diaphragm fatigue after 2 min of repetitive stimulation. At 40 Hz, neuromuscular transmission failure contributes approximately 35%, and at 75 Hz, approximately 42%. Thus, in the adult rat diaphragm, most of the peripheral fatigue appears to be of muscular origin.

In a study of the neonatal rat diaphragm, we found that forces generated by

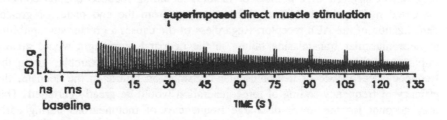

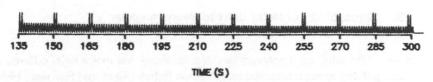

Figure 10 Neuromuscular transmission failure in the rat diaphragm muscle was estimated by comparing forces generated by superimposed direct muscle stimulation with those generated by phrenic nerve stimulation. (From Kuei et al., 1990.)

tetanic phrenic nerve stimulation (greater than 10 Hz) are significantly less than those produced by direct muscle stimulation (Fournier et al., 1991). The difference in forces generated by these two modes of stimulation increases markedly as stimulation frequency is increased. We estimated that, in the neonate, neuromuscular transmission failure contributes approximately 85% of the fatigue induced by 40-Hz stimulation. By the third postnatal week (i.e., at the time of weaning), the contribution of neuromuscular transmission failure to diaphragm fatigue approximates that found in the adult muscle.

The greater susceptibility of the neonatal rat diaphragm to neuromuscular transmission failure could be related to an inability of phrenic axons to follow higher rates of activation (e.g., axonal branch point failure of action potential propagation), or to a failure at the neuromuscular junction. To examine these possibilities, we recorded evoked end-plate potentials (EPP) during repetitive activation. The failure to generate an EPP was taken as evidence of axonal propagation failure, whereas a decrease in EPP amplitude was taken as evidence of diminished efficacy of neuromuscular transmission by either reduced release of acetylcholine (ACh) or desensitization of the postsynaptic ACh receptor. With repetitive stimulation, in the neonatal diaphragm there is both an increased incidence of action potential propagation failure and a diminished efficacy of neuromuscular transmission, compared with the 3-week-old or adult animal (Table 4). The increased incidence of action potential propagation failure may relate to the presence of polyneuronal innervation in the neonate and, hence, the expanded motor unit size at this age. The diminished efficacy of neuromuscular transmission in the neonatal diaphragm may reflect any one of a number of factors, including reduced quantal content, increased hydrolysis of ACh or diffusion away from the end plate, or greater densitization of the ACh receptor. Regardless of the cause, a greater susceptibility to neuromuscular transmission failure in the neonatal diaphragm would greatly impinge on the neuromotor control of the diaphragm. For example, given the frequency dependence of neuromuscular transmission failure in the neonate, the efficacy of frequency coding of force generation would be greatly curtailed. This may account for the lower discharge frequencies of motoneurons during early postnatal development (Navarrette and Vrbova, 1983), which is due to the intrinsic electrophysiological properties of motoneurons (Fulton and Walton, 1986; Walton and Fulton, 1986).

B. Susceptibility of Motor Units to Neuromuscular Transmission Failure

In a study of the adult cat diaphragm, we demonstrated that motor units differed in their susceptibility to neuromuscular transmission failure (Sieck and Fournier, 1990; Fig. 11 and 12). Neuromuscular transmission failure was assessed by changes in evoked muscle unit action potentials (MUAP). These electromyographic (EMG) signals were analyzed in different ways, including waveform shape and amplitude,

Table 4 Summary of the Incidence in Axonal Propagation Failure and Extent of Decrement in EPP Amplitude During Repetitive Stimulation at Different Ages[a]

| | Propagation failure rate (%) | | | | % Decrement in EPP amplitude | | | |
| | Stimulation rate (Hz) | | | | Stimulation rate (Hz) | | | |
Age	10	20	40	75	10	20	40	75
1st wk	4.4 ± 1.7*	14.5 ± 3.5*	40.5 ± 3.8*	65.6 ± 2.2	52.2 ± 10.8	70.0 ± 8.2	87.2 ± 7.7*	91.3 ± 4.4*
3rd wk	0 ± 0	2.0 ± 1.0	16.7 ± 4.2**	37.5 ± 4.8**	63.7 ± 9.7	61.2 ± 5.2	78.5 ± 3.1	77.4 ± 2.8
Adults	0 ± 0	2.5 ± 0.5	4.0 ± 2.4	26.0 ± 5.1	61.3 ± 7.8	62.8 ± 6.2	73.2 ± 2.7	75.1 ± 1.3

[a]Propagation failure rate calculated as the proportion of absent evoked EPPs in the first 10 pulses of each train.
Values are means ± S.D.
*Significantly different from older animals ($p < 0.01$).
**Significantly different from adults ($p < 0.05$).
Source: Fournier et al. (1991).

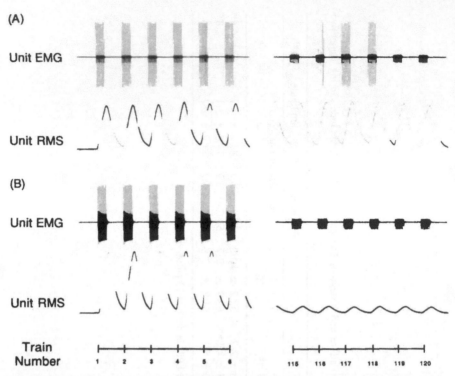

Figure 11   Motor unit action potentials (unit EMG) for two fast-twitch units from the cat diaphragm (A and B) were recorded during a 2-min fatigue test (40 Hz, 330-ms duration, one train per second). The unit EMG and calculated root-mean-square (RMS) values for the first six stimulus trains are compared with the final six stimulus trains. Note that very little change in unit EMG occurred for the unit displayed in A, but a substantial decrement in unit EMG RMS values was observed for the unit shown in B. (From Sieck and Fournier, 1990.)

and calculation of root mean square (RMS), a form of integration of the MUAP. Fatigue-resistant units (i.e., type S and FR) showed little change in evoked MUAP during the fatigue test. In contrast, some FF and FInt units showed marked changes in evoked MUAP. These changes included a prolongation of MUAP duration, a decrease in peak MUAP amplitude, and a decrease in the integrated (RMS) MUAP waveform. It should be noted that, in most cases, these changes in MUAP did not correlate with motor unit force loss during the fatigue test. Some units showed very abrupt changes in MUAP waveform, a result that was also observed by Sandercock et al. (1985) in motor units of the cat medial gastrocnemius muscle. These authors reported that the abrupt changes in MUAP waveform correlated with a failure in the generation of action potentials in some muscle unit fibers (i.e., direct evidence for neuromuscular transmission failure). In such cases, a concomitant decrease in motor unit force would also be expected. As for the muscle as a whole, the

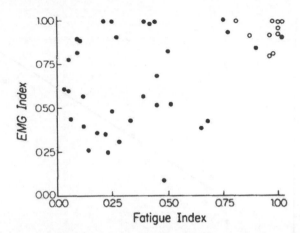

Figure 12 Scatter plot relating the changes in unit EMG (unit EMG RMS after 2-min stimulation to the initial RMS value; see Fig. 11) to the changes in motor unit force (fatigue index). Solid circles are fast-twitch units in the cat diaphragm and open circles are slow-twitch units. Note that fatigue-resistant units (fatigue index > 0.75) displayed little changes in unit EMG (EMG index > 0.75), whereas among fast-twitch units, the changes in force and unit EMG varied. However, note that the relative change in force generally exceeded the relative change in unit EMG. (From Sieck and Fournier, 1990.)

susceptibility of motor units to neuromuscular transmission failure depends on the rate of stimulation (Clamann and Robinson, 1985; Sandercock et al. 1985). Thus, in these units, frequency coding of force, especially at higher rates of activation, would be less effective.

C. Fatigue Resistance and Muscle Oxidative Capacity

By using the technique of glycogen depletion to identify muscle unit fibers (Edström and Kugelberg, 1968), we examined the correlation between diaphragmatic motor unit contractile and fatigue properties and the metabolic properties of muscle unit fibers (Enad et al., 1989). In this study, we used a microphotometric procedure, whereby the activity of the oxidative enzyme succinate dehydrogenase (SDH) could be quantified in individual muscle fibers (Blanco et al., 1988; Sieck et al., 1986, 1987). With this procedure, we found a significant correlation between diaphragm motor unit fatigue resistance and the mean SDH activity of muscle unit fibers (Fig. 13). In a more recent study, Martin et al. (1988) used a similar quantitative histochemical procedure and reported comparable results for motor units in the cat tibialis anterior muscle. With a microbiochemical procedure, oxidative enzyme activities have also been measured in dissected muscle unit fibers of the rat extensor digitorum longus (Nemeth et al., 1981) and cat tibialis posterior muscles (Hamm et al., 1988; Nemeth et al., 1986). These studies also reported that motor unit fatigue resistance

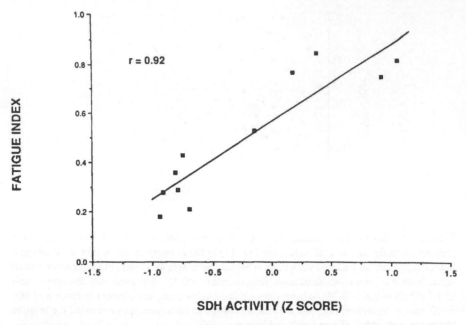

Figure 13 The fatigue resistance (fatigue index) of motor units in the cat diaphragm correlated significantly with the mean SDH activity of muscle unit fibers (SDH activity normalized across animals by calculating Z-scores). (From Enad et al., 1989.)

and oxidative capacity were correlated in these muscles. Several other studies have suggested a correlation between muscle unit fatigue resistance and oxidative capacity, based on a subjective assessment of oxidative enzyme-staining intensities (Burke, 1981; Burke et al., 1973; Edström and Kugelberg, 1968). These subjective studies have suggested that adult muscle units are composed of fibers with homogeneous histochemical properties. Indeed, these studies have provided the functional basis justifying the histochemical classification of different muscle fiber types.

If neurogenic factors exert a predominant influence on the enzymatic activities of muscle fibers, it might be expected that muscle unit fibers would have homogeneous enzymatic properties. In the cat diaphragm, the variability of SDH activity among diaphragm muscle unit fibers was significantly less than that noted for the muscle as a whole, and similar to that observed along the length of muscle fibers (Fournier and Sieck, 1986; Sieck, 1988). This indicated that, in the adult diaphragm, innervation exerts an important influence on the enzymatic properties of muscle fibers. The microbiochemical studies of Nemeth and co-workers (Hamm et al., 1988; Nemeth et al., 1981, 1986) also found that oxidative enzyme activities among muscle unit fibers were more homogeneous than in the muscle as a whole. However, in another quantitative histochemical study, Martin et al. (1988) reported that, in the cat tibialis anterior muscle, the variability of SDH among muscle unit fibers was greater than that found along the length of muscle fibers. These authors concluded that the metabolic enzyme activities of muscle fibers are not under the complete control of neurogenic factors.

D. Fatigue Resistance and Muscle Unit Capillary Density

We have examined the distribution of capillaries surrounding muscle unit fibers in the cat diaphragm (Enad et al., 1989). Muscle unit fibers were identified by glycogen depletion, and capillaries were identified in sections stained for ATPase after preincubation at pH 4.2. We found correlations between the fatigue resistance of diaphragm motor units and both the mean number of capillaries and the mean capillary density (i.e., number of capillaries per fiber cross-sectional area) of muscle unit fibers (Fig. 14). In addition, we noted a correlation between capillary density and fiber SDH activity. These results suggested that, in the adult cat diaphragm, motor unit fatigue resistance is at least partly related to the delivery and utilization of oxygen for energy production.

E. Fatigue Resistance and Muscle Fiber Cross-Sectional Area

In studies of the adult cat diaphragm, we measured the cross-sectional area of identified muscle unit fibers, using an image-processing system calibrated for

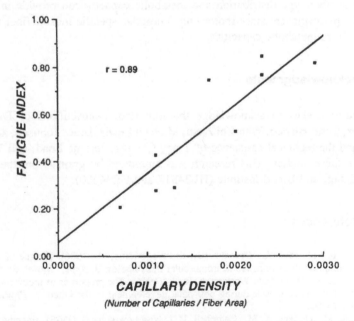

Figure 14 The fatigue resistance (fatigue index) of motor units in the cat diaphragm correlated significantly with the mean capillary density of muscle unit fibers. (From Enad et al., 1989.)

morphometry (Enad et al., 1989). The more fatigable diaphragm motor units (i.e., FF and FInt) were composed of fibers with larger cross-sectional areas and lower SDH activities. In contrast, fatigue-resistant units (i.e., S and FR) were composed of smaller fibers with higher SDH activities (see Table 2). The average fiber size of muscle units is correlated with both the maximum tetanic tensions produced by these units and their fatigability (see Table 2). These results suggest that motor unit fatigue resistance may be correlated with the distance for diffusion of oxygen and energy substrates into muscle fibers.

VI. Summary

Classification of different motor unit and muscle fiber types in the diaphragm muscle provides an invaluable framework to assess muscle contractile and fatigue properties. From our studies, it is clear that not all motor units are recruited to accomplish ventilatory behaviors of the diaphragm muscle. The fractional recruitment of motor units varies from species to species, but certainly the selective recruitment of fatigue resistant (S and FR) units in redundant ventilatory behaviors is requisite. Alterations in ventilatory demands with exercise or disease undoubtedly affects the recruitment of motor units and may lead to adaptations in motor unit composition. Assessment of muscle fiber type distribution and metabolic capacity can provide insight into muscular performance, since motor units comprise specific muscle fiber types that have uniform metabolic capacities.

Acknowledgments

The author wishes to acknowledge the important contributions of Drs. Mario Fournier, Cesar Blanco, Wen-Zhi Zhan, Michael Lewis, Bruce Johnson, and Joseph Kuei, and the technical assistance of Tracy Cheung, Jerome Enad, and Weizheng Wang in these studies. This research was supported by grants from the National Heart, Lung, and Blood Institute (HL34817 and HL34680).

References

Aldrich, T. K., Shander, A., Chaudhry, I., and Nagashima, H. (1986). Fatigue of isolated rat diaphragm: role of impaired neuromuscular transmission. *J. Appl. Physiol.* 61: 1077–1083
Bagust, J., Lewis, D. M., and Westerman, R. A. (1974). The properties of motor units in a fast and slow twitch muscle during post-natal development in the kitten. *J. Physiol. (Lond.)* 237: 75–90.
Baldwin, K. M., Hooker, A. M., Campbell, P. J., and Lewis, R. E. (1978). Enzyme changes in neonatal skeletal muscle: Effect of thyroid deficiency. *Am. J. Physiol.* 50: 197–218.
Bar, A., and Pette, D. (1988). Three fast myosin heavy chains in adult rat skeletal muscle. *FEBS Lett.* 235: 153–155.

Barany, M. (1967). ATPase activity of myosin correlated with speed of muscle shortening. *J. Gen. Physiol.* 235: C97–C102.

Belcastro, A. N. (1987). Myofibril and sarcoplasmic reticulum changes during muscle development: Activity vs inactivity. *Int. J. Biochem.* 19: 945–948.

Berger, A. J. (1979). Phrenic motoneurons in the cat: Subpopulations and nature of respiratory drive potentials. *J. Neurophysiol.* 42: 76–90.

Bigland-Ritchie, B. (1981). EMG and fatigue of human voluntary and stimulated contractions. In *Human Muscle Fatigue: Physiological Mechanisms.* Ciba Foundation Symposium 82. Edited by R. Porter and J. Whelan. London, Pitman Medical, pp. 130–148.

Blanco, C. E., and Sieck, G. C. (1992). Quantitative determination of calcium-activated myosin adenosine triphosphatase activity in rat skeletal muscle fibres. *Histochem. J.* 24: 431–444.

Blanco, C. E., Sieck, G. C., and Edgerton, V. R. (1988). Quantitative histochemical determination of succinic dehydrogenase activity in skeletal muscle fibres. *Histochem. J.* 20:230–243.

Blanco, C. E., Fournier, M., and Sieck, G. C. (1991). Metabolic variability within individual muscle fibres of the cat tibialis posterior and diaphragm muscles. *Histochem. J.* 23: 366–374.

Bodine, S. C., Roy, R. R., Eldred, E., and Edgerton, V. R. (1987). Maximal force as a function of anatomical features of motor units in the cat tibialis anterior. *J. Neurophysiol.* 57: 1730–1745.

Botterman, B. R., Iwamoto, G. A., and Gonyea, W. J. (1986). Gradation of isometric tension by different activation rates in motor units of cat flexor carpi radialis muscle. *J. Neurophysiol.* 56:494–506.

Bottinelli, R., Schiaffino, S., and Reggiani, C. (1991). Force–velocity relations and myosin heavy chain isoform compositions of skinned fibres from rat skeletal muscle. *J. Physiol.* 437: 655–672.

Brooke, M. H., and Kaiser, K. K. (1970). Muscle fiber types: How many and what kind? *Arch. Neurol.* 23: 369–379.

Brooke, M. H., Williamson, E., and Kaiser, K. K. (1971). The behavior of four fiber types in developing and reinnervated muscle. *Arch. Neurol.* 25: 360–366, 1971.

Buller, A., Eccles, J., and Eccles, R. (1960). Differentiation of fast and slow muscles in the cat hind limb. *J. Physiol. (Lond.)* 150:399–416.

Burke, R. E. (1981). Motor units: Anatomy, physiology and functional organization. In *Handbook of Physiology*, Section I, The Nervous System, Vol. III, Part 1. Edited by J. M. Brookhart and V. B. Mountcastle. Bethesda, MD, American Physiological Society, pp. 345–422.

Burke, R. E., Levine, D. N., Zajac, F. E. III, Tsairis, P., and Engel, W. K. (1971). Mammalian motor units: Physiological–histochemical correlation in three types in cat gastrocnemius. *Science* 174: 709–712.

Burke, R. E., Levine, D. N., Tsairis, P., and Zajac, F. E. (1973). Physiological types and histochemical profiles of motor units of cat gastrocnemius. *J. Physiol. (Lond.)* 234: 723–748.

Butler-Browne, G. S., Bugaisky, L. B., Cuenoud, S., Schwartz, K., and Whalen, R. G. (1982). Denervation of newborn rat muscles does not block the appearance of adult fast myosin heavy chain. *Nature* 299: 830–833.

Butler-Browne, G. S., Herlicoviez, D., and Whalen, R. G. (1984). Effects of hypothyroidism on myosin isozyme transitions in developing rat muscle. *FEBS Lett.* 166: 71–75.

Butler-Browne, G. S., Barbet, J. P., and Thornell, L.-E. (1990). Myosin heavy and light chain expression during human skeletal muscle development and precocious muscle maturation induced by thyroid hormone. *Anat. Embryol.* 181: 513–522.

Caiozzo, V. J., Herrick, R. E., and Baldwin, K. M. (1991). Influence of hyperthyroidism on maximal shortening velocity and myosin isoform distribution in skeletal muscles. *Am. J. Physiol.* 261: C285–C295.

Carraro, U., Morale, D., Mussini, I., Lucke, S., Cantini, M., Betto, R., Catani, C., Dalla Libera, L., Danieli Betto, D., and Noventa, D. (1985). Chronic denervation of rat hemidiaphragm: Maintenance of fiber heterogeneity with associated increasing uniformity of myosin isoforms. *J. Cell Biol.* 100: 161–174.

Chamberlain, S., and Lewis, D. M. (1989). Contractile characteristics and innervation ratio of rat soleus motor units. *J. Physiol. (Lond.)* 412: 1–21.

Clamman, H. P., and Henneman, E. (1976). Electrical measurement of axon diameter and its use in relating motoneuron size to critical firing level. *J. Neurophysiol.* 39: 844–851, 1976.

Clamann, H. P., and Robinson, A. J. (1985). A comparison of electromyographic and mechanical fatigue properties in motor units of the cat hindlimb. *Brain Res.* 327: 203–219.

Crow, M. T., and Kushmerick, M. J. (1982). Chemical energies of slow- and fast-twitch muscles of the mouse. *J. Gen. Physiol.* 79: 147–162.

d'Albis, A., Chanoine, C., Janmot, C., Mira, J.-C., and Couteaux, R. (1990). Muscle-specific response to thyroid hormone of myosin isoform transitions during rat postnatal development. *Eur. J. Biochem.* 193: 155–161.

Dhoot, G. K., and Perry, S. V. (1983). Effect of denervation at birth on the development of skeletal muscle cell types in the rat. *Exp. Neurol.* 82: 131–142.

Dick, T. E., Kong, F. J., and Berger, A. J. (1987a). Correlation of recruitment order with axonal conduction velocity for supraspinally driven motor units. *J. Neurophysiol.* 57: 245–259.

Dick, T. E., Kong, F. J., and Berger, A. J. (1987b). Recruitment order of diaphragmatic motor units obeys Henneman's size principle. In: *Respiratory Muscles and Their Neuromotor Control.* Edited by G. C. Sieck, S. C. Gandevia, and W. E. Cameron. New York, Alan R. Liss, pp. 249–261.

Diffee, G. M., Haddad, F., Herrick, R. E., and Baldwin, K. M. (1991). Control of myosin heavy chain expression: Interaction of hypothyroidism and hindlimb suspension. *Am. J. Physiol.* 261: C1099–C1106.

Donnelly, D. F., Cohen, M. I., Sica, A. L., and Zhang, H. (1985). Responses of early and late onset phrenic motoneurons to lung inflation. *Respir. Physiol.* 61: 69–83.

Dubowitz, V. (1967). Cross-innervated mammalian skeletal muscle: Histochemical, physiological, and biochemical observations. *J. Physiol. (Lond.)* 193: 481–496.

Dum, R. P., O'Donovan, M. J., Toop, J., Tsairis, P., Pinter, M. J., and Burke, R. E. (1985). Cross-reinnervated motor units in cat muscle. II. Soleus muscle reinnervated by flexor digitorum longus motoneurons. *J. Neurophysiol.* 54: 837–851.

Edström, L., and Kugelberg, E. (1968). Histochemical composition, distribution of fibers and fatiguability of single motor units. *J. Neurol. Neurosurg. Psychiatry* 31: 424–433.

Edwards, R. H. T. (1981). Human muscle function and fatigue. In: *Human Muscle Fatigue: Physiological Mechanisms.* Ciba Foundation Symposium 82. Edited by R. Porter and J. Whelan. London, Pitman Medical, pp. 1–18.

Enad, J. G., Fournier, M., and Sieck, G. C. (1989). Oxidative capacity and capillary density of diaphragm motor units. *J. Appl. Physiol.* 67: 620–627.

Fitzsimmons, D. P., Herrick, R. E., and Baldwin, K. M. (1990). Isomyosin distributions in rodent muscles: Effects of altered thyroid state. *J. Appl. Physiol.* 69: 321–327.

Fleshman, J. W., Munson, J. B., Sypert, G. W., and Friedman, W. A. (1981). Rheobase, input resistance, and motor unit type in medial gastrocnemius motoneurons in the cat. *J. Neurophysiol.* 46: 1326–1338.

Fournier, M., and Sieck, G. C. (1986). Variability in SDH activity among diaphragm muscle unit fibers. *Soc. Neurosci. Abstr.* 12: 1082.

Fournier, M., and Sieck, G. C. (1987). Topographical projections of phrenic motoneurons and motor unit territories in the cat diaphragm. In: *Respiratory Muscles and Their Neuromotor Control.* Edited by G. C. Sieck, S. C. Gandevia, and W. E. Cameron. New York, Alan R. Liss, pp. 215–226.

Fournier, M., and Sieck, G. C. (1988a). Somatotopy in the segmental innervation of the cat diaphragm. *J. Appl. Physiol.* 64: 291–298.

Fournier, M., and Sieck, G. C. (1988b). Mechanical properties of muscle units in the cat diaphragm. *J. Neurophysiol.* 59: 1055–1066.

Fournier, M., Alula, M., and Sieck, G. C. (1991). Neuromuscular transmission failure during postnatal development. *Neurosci. Lett.* 125: 34–36.

Fulton, B. P., and Walton, K. (1986). Electrophysiologic properties of neonatal rat motoneurones studied in vitro. *J. Physiol. (Lond.)* 370: 651–678.

Gambke, B., Lyons, G. E., Haselgrove, J., Kelly, A. M., and Rubinstein, N. A. (1983). Thyroidal and neural control of myosin transitions during development of rat fast and slow muscles. *FEBS Lett.* 156: 335–339.

Gauthier, G. F., Lowey, S., and Hobbs, A. W. (1978). Fast and slow myosin in developing muscle fibers. *Nature* 274: 25–29.

Gorza, L. (1990). Identification of a novel type 2 fiber population in mammalian skeletal muscle by combined use of histochemical myosin ATPase and anti-myosin monoclonal antibodies. *J. Histochem. Cytochem.* 38: 257–265.

Green, H. J., Reichman, H., and Pette, D. (1984). Inter- and intraspecies comparisons of fiber type distribution and of succinate dehydrogenase activity in type I, IIA, and IIB fibers of mammalian diaphragm. *Histochemistry* 81: 67–73.

Hamm, T. M., Nemeth, P. M. Solanki, L., Gordon, D. A., Reinking, R. M., and Stuart, D. G. (1988). Association between biochemical and physiological properties in single motor units. *Muscle Nerve* 11: 245–254.

Henneman, E. (1957). Relation between size of neurons and their susceptibility to discharge. *Science* 126: 1345–1346.

Henneman, E., and Mendell, L. M. (1981). Functional organizational of motoneuron pool and its inputs. In: *Handbook of Physiology*, Section 1. The Nervous System, Vol. III, Part 1. Edited by J. M. Brookhart and V. B. Mountcastle. Bethesda, MD, American Physiological Society, pp. 423–507.

Henneman, E., Somjen, G., and Carpenter, D. O. (1965). Functional significance of cell size in spinal motoneurons. *J. Neurophysiol.* 28: 560–580.

Hilaire, G., Gauthier, P., and Monteau, R. (1983). Central respiratory drive and recruitment order of phrenic and inspiratory laryngeal motoneurones. *Respir. Physiol.* 51: 341–359.

Hilaire, G., Monteau, R., and Khatib, M. (1987). Determination of recruitment order of phrenic motoneurons. In: *Respiratory Muscles and Their Neuromotor Control*. Edited by G. C. Sieck, S. C. Gandevia, and W. E. Cameron. New York, Alan R. Liss, pp. 249–261.

Hoh, J. F., Hughes, S., Hale, P. T., and Fitzsimmons, R. B. (1988). Immunocytochemical and electrophoretic analyses of changes in myosin gene expression in cat limb fast and slow muscles during postnatal development. *J. Muscle Res. Cell Motil.* 9: 30–47.

Ianuzzo, D., Chen, V., O'Brien, P., and Keens, T. G. (1984). Effect of experimental dysthyroidism on the enzymatic character of the diaphragm. *J. Appl. Physiol.* 56: 117–121.

Ianuzzo, D., Patel, P., Chen, V., O'Brien, P., and Williams, C. (1977). Thyroidal trophic influence on skeletal muscle myosin. *Nature* 270: 74–76.

Iscoe, S., Dankoff, J., Migicovsky, R., and Polosa, C. (1976). Recruitment and discharge frequency of phrenic motneurons during inspiration. *Respir. Physiol.* 26: 113–128.

Jodkowski, J. S., Viana, F., Dick, T. E., and Berger, A. J. (1987). Electrical properties of phrenic motoneurons in the cat: Correlation with inspiratory drive. *J. Neurophysiol.* 58: 105–124.

Johnson, B. D., and Sieck, G. C. (1993). Differential susceptibility of diaphragm muscle fibers to neurotransmission failure. *J. Appl. Physiol.* (in press).

Johnson, B. D., Watchko, J. F., Daood, M. J., Wilson, L. E., Prakash, Y. S., and Sieck, G. C. (1993a). Maximum shortening velocity of developing diaphragm correlates with myosin heavy chain phenotype. *FASEB J.* 7: A232.

Johnson, B. D., Wilson, L. E., and Sieck, G. C. (1993b). Denervation alters myosin heavy chain phenotype and maximum shortening velocity in developing diaphragm. *Am. Rev. Respir. Dis.* 147: A690.

Johnson, M. A., Olmo, J. L., and Mastaglia, F. L. (1983). Changes in histochemical profile of rat respiratory muscles in hypo- and hyperthyroidism. *Q. J. Exp. Physiol.* 68: 1–13.

Kelly, A. M. (1983). Emergence of muscle specialization. In: *Handbook of Physiology*, Section 10. Skeletal Muscle. Edited by L. D. Peachey and R. H. Adrian. Bethesda, MD, American Physiological Society, pp. 507–537.

Kelly, A. M., and Rubinstein, N. A. (1980). Why are fetal muscles-slow? *Nature* 288: 266–269.

Kelly, A. M., Rosser, B. W. C., Hoffman, R., Panettieri, R. A., Schiaffino, S., Rubenstein, N. A., and Nemeth, P. M. (1991). Metabolic and contractile protein expression in developing rat diaphragm muscle. *J. Neurosci.* 11: 1231–1242.

Kelsen, S. G., and Nochomovitz, M. L. (1982). Fatigue of the mammalian diaphragm in vitro. *J. Appl. Physiol.* 53: 440–447.

Kernell, D., and Monster, A. W. (1982a). Time course and properties of late adaptation in spinal motoneurons of the cat. *Exp. Brain Res.* 46: 191–196.

Kernell, D., and Monster, A. W. (1982b). Motoneuron properties and motor fatigue. An intracellular study of gastrocnemius motoneurones of the cat. *Exp. Brain Res.* 46: 197–204.

Krnjevic, K., and Miledi, R. (1958). Failure of neuromuscular propagation in rats. *J. Physiol. (Lond.)* 140: 440–461.

Krnjevic, K., and Miledi, R. (1959). Presynaptic failure of neuromuscular propagation in rats. *J. Physiol. (Lond.)* 149: 1–22.

Kuei, J. H., Shadmehr, R., and Sieck, G. C. (1990). Relative contribution of neurotransmission failure to diaphragm fatigue. *J. Appl. Physiol.* 68: 174–180.

Laskowski, M. B., and Sanes, J. R. (1987). Topographic mapping of motor pools onto skeletal muscles. *J. Neurosci.* 7: 252–260.

Liddell, E. G. T., and Sherrington, C. S. (1925). Recruitment and some other factors of reflex inhibition. *Proc. R. Soc. Lond. (Biol.)* 97: 488–518.

Mahdavi, V., Strehler, E. E., Periasamy, D., Wieizouk, S., Izumo, S., Gunds, S., Strehler, M. A., and Nadal-Ginard, B. (1986). Sarcomeric myosin heavy chain gene family: Organization and pattern of expression. In: *Molecular Biology of Muscle Development*. Edited by C. Emerson, D. Fischman, B. Nadal-Ginard, and M. A. Q. Siddiqui. New York, Alan R. Liss, pp. 345–362.

Martin, T. P., Bodine-Fowler, S., Roy, R. R., Eldred, E., and Edgerton, V. R. (1988). Metabolic and fiber size properties of cat tibialis anterior motor units. *Am. J. Physiol.* 255: C43–C50.

Maxwell, L. C., McCarter, J. M., Keuhl, T. J., and Robotham, J. L. (1983). Development of histochemical and functional properties of baboon respiratory muscles. *J. Appl. Physiol.* 54: 551–561.

Mier, A., Brophy, C., Wass, J. A. H., Besser, G. M., and Green, M. (1989). Reversible respiratory muscle weakness in hyperthyroidism. *Am. Rev. Respir. Dis.* 139: 529–533.

Miyashita, A., Suzuki, S., Suzuki, M., Numata, H., Suzuki, J., Akahori, T., and Okubo, T. (1992). Effect of thyroid hormone on in vivo contractility of the canine diaphragm. *Am. Rev. Respir. Dis.* 145: 1456–1462.

Monteau, R., Khatib, M., and Hilaire, G. (1985). Central determination of recruitment order: Intracellular study of phrenic motoneurons. *Neurosci. Lett.* 56: 341–346.

Narusawa, M., Fitzsimmons, R. B., Izumo, S., Nadal-Ginard, B., Rubinstein, N. A., and Kelly, A. M. (1987). Slow myosin in developing rat skeletal muscle. *J. Cell Biol.* 104: 447–459.

Navarrete, R., and Vrbova, G. (1983). Changes of activity patterns in slow and fast muscles during postnatal development. *Dev. Brain Res.* 8: 11–19.

Nemeth, P., and Pette, D. (1981). Succinate dehydrogenase activity in fibers classified by myosin ATPase in three hind limb muscles of rat. *J. Physiol. (Lond.).* 320: 73–80.

Nemeth, P., Pette, D., and Vrbova, G. (1981). Comparison of enzyme activities among single muscle fibers within defined motor units. *J. Physiol. (Lond.)* 311: 489–495.

Nemeth, P. M., Solanki, L., Gordon, D. A., Hamm, T. M., Reinking, R. M., and Stuart, D. G. (1986). Uniformity of metabolic enzymes within individual motor units. *J. Neurosci.* 6: 892–898.

Nguyen, H. T., Gubits, R. M., Wydro, R. M., and Nadal-Girard, B. (1982). Sarcomeric myosin heavy chain is coded by a highly conserved multigene family. *Proc. Natl. Acad. Sci. USA* 79: 5230–5234.

Pagala, M. K. D., Namba, T., and Grob, D. (1984). Failure of neuromuscular transmission and contractility during muscle fatigue. *Muscle Nerve* 7: 454–464.

Periasamy, M., Gregory, P., Martin, B. J., and Stirewalt, W. S. (1989). Regulation of myosin heavy-chain gene expression during skeletal muscle hypertrophy. *Biochem. J.* 257: 691–698.

Peter, J. B., Barnard, R. J., Edgerton, V. R., Gillespie, C. A., and Stempel, K. E. (1972). Metabolic profiles of three fiber types of skeletal muscle in guinea pigs and rabbits. *Biochemistry* 11: 2627–2634.

Petrof, B. J., Kelly, A. M., Rubinstein, N. A., and Pack, A. I. (1992). Effect of hypothyroidism on myosin heavy chain expression in rat pharyngeal dilator muscles. *J. Appl. Physiol.* 73: 179–187.

Pette, D., and Vrbova, G. (1985). Invited review: Neural control of phenotypic expression in mammalian muscle fibers. *Muscle Nerve* 8: 676–689.

Pierobon-Bormioli, S., Sartore, S., Dalla Libera, L., Vitadello, M., and Schiaffino, S. (1988). "Fast" isomyosins and fiber types in mammalian skeletal muscle. *J. Histochem. Cytochem.* 29: 1179–1188.

Reichmann, H., and Pette, D. (1982). A comparative microphotometric study of succinate dehydrogenase activity levels in type I, IIA, and IIB fibers of mammalian and human muscles. *Histochemistry* 74: 27–41.

Reiser, P. J., Moss, R. L., Giulian, G. G., and Greaser, M. L. (1985). Shortening velocity and myosin heavy chains of developing rabbit muscle fibers. *J. Biol. Chem.* 260: 14403–14405.

Reiser, P. J., Greaser, M. L., and Moss, R. L. (1988a). Myosin heavy chain composition of single cells from avian slow skeletal muscle is strongly correlated with velocity of shortening during development. *Dev. Biol.* 129: 400–407.

Reiser, P. J., Kasper, C. E., Greaser, M. L., and Moss, R. L. (1988b). Functional significance of myosin transitions in single fibers of developing soleus muscle. *Am. J. Physiol.* 254: C605–C613.

Russell, S. D., Cambon, N., Nadal-Ginard, B., and Whalen, R. G. (1988). Thyroid hormone induces a nerve-independent precocious expression of fast myosin heavy chain mRNA in rat hindlimb skeletal muscle. *J. Biol. Chem.* 263: 6370–6374.

Sandercock, T. G., Faulkner, J. A., Albers, J. W., and Abbrecht, P. H. (1985). Single motor unit and fiber action potentials during fatigue. *J. Appl. Physiol.* 58: 1073–1079.

Schiaffino, S., Ausoni, S., Gorza, L., Saggin, L., Gundersen, K., and Lømo, T. (1988a). Myosin heavy chain isoforms and velocity of shortening of type 2 skeletal muscle fibers. *Acta Physiol. Scand.* 134: 575–576.

Schiaffino, S., Gorza, L., Pitton, G., Saggin, L., Ausoni, S., Sartore, S., and Lømo, T. (1988b). Embryonic and neonatal myosin heavy chain in denervated and paralyzed rat skeletal muscle. *Dev. Biol.* 127: 1–11.

Sherrington, C. S. (1929). Ferrier lecture: Some functional problems attaching to convergence. *Proc. R. Soc. Lond. (Biol.)* 105: 332–362.

Sieck, G. C. (1988). Diaphragm muscle: Structural and functional organization. In: *Respiratory Muscle: Function in Health and Disease.* Clinics in Chest Medicine, Vol. 9. Edited by M. J. Belman. Philadelphia, W. B. Saunders, pp. 195–210.

Sieck, G. C. (1991a). Diaphragm motor units and their response to altered use. *Sem. Respir. Med. Respir. Failure* 12: 258–269.

Sieck, G. C. (1991b). Neural control of the inspiratory pump. *NIPS* 6: 260–264.

Sieck, G. C., and Blanco, C. E. (1991). Postnatal changes in the distribution of succinate dehydrogenase activities among diaphragm muscle fibers. *Pediatr. Res.* 29: 586–593.

Sieck, G. C., and Fournier, M. (1989). Diaphragm motor unit recruitment during ventilatory and nonventilatory behaviors. *J. Appl. Physiol.* 66: 2539–2545.

Sieck, G. C., and Fournier, M. (1990). Changes in diaphragm motor unit EMG during fatigue. *J. Appl. Physiol.* 68: 1917–1926.

Sieck, G. C., and Fournier, M. (1991). Developmental aspects of diaphragm muscle cells: Structural and functional organization. In: *Developmental Neurobiology of Breathing.* Edited by G. G. Haddad and J. P. Farber. New York, Marcel Dekker, pp. 375–428.

Sieck, G. C., Trelease, R. B., and Harper, R. M. (1984). Sleep influences on diaphragmatic motor unit discharge. *Exp. Neurol.* 85: 316–335.

Sieck, G. C., Sacks, R. D., Blanco, C. E., and Edgerton, V. R. (1986). SDH activity and cross-sectional area of muscle fibers in cat diaphragm. *J. Appl. Physiol.* 60: 1284–1292.

Sieck, G. C., Sacks, R. D., and Blanco, C. E. (1987). Absence of regional differences in the size and oxidative capacity of diaphragm muscle fibers. *J. Appl. Physiol.* 63: 1076–1082.

Sieck, G. C., Fournier, M., and Enad, J. G. (1989a). Fiber type composition of muscle units in the cat diaphragm. *Neurosci. Lett.* 97: 29–34.

Sieck, G. C., Zhan, W.-Z., and Fournier, M. (1989b). Adaptations of diaphragm muscle to altered use. *Nature J. (China)* 12: 656–663.

Sieck, G. C., Cheung, T. S., and Blanco, C. E. (1991a). Diaphragm capillarity and oxidative capacity during postnatal development. *J. Appl. Physiol.* 70: 103–111.

Sieck, G. C., Fournier, M., and Blanco, C. E. (1991b). Diaphragm muscle fatigue resistance during postnatal development. *J. Appl. Physiol.* 71: 458–464.

Sieck, G. C., Watchko, J., Zhan, W. Z., and Prakash, Y. S. (1992). Classification of muscle fiber types: Relation to SDH activity and cross-sectional area. *Am. Rev. Respir. Dis.* 145: A141.

Sieck, G. C., Zhan, W. Z., Wilson, L. E., Gosselin, L. E., and Megirian, D. (1993). Hypothyroidism alters myosin heavy chain phenotype and contractility of developing rat diaphragm. *FASEB J.* 7: A232.

Smith, D., Green, H., Thomson, J., and Sharratt, M. (1988). Oxidative potential in developing rat diaphragm, EDL, and soleus muscle fibers. *Am. J. Physiol.* 254: C661–C668.

Staron, R. S., and Pette, D. (1987). The multiplicity of combination of myosin light chains and heavy chains in histochemically typed single fibres. *Biochem. J.* 243: 695–699.

Stockdale, F. E., and Miller, J. B. (1987). The cellular basis of myosin heavy chain isoform expression during development of avian skeletal muscle. *Dev. Biol.* 123: 1–9.

Swynghedauw, B. (1986). Developmental and functional adaptation of contractile proteins in cardiac and skeletal muscles. *Physiol. Rev.* 66: 710–771.

Sypert, G. W., and Munson, J. B. (1981). Basis of segmental motor control: Motoneuron size or motor unit type? *Neurosurgery* 8: 608–621.

Wagner, P. D. (1981). Formation and characterization of myosin hybrids containing essential light chains and heavy chains from different muscle myosin. *J. Biol. Chem.* 256: 2493–2498.

Walmsley, B., Hodgson, J. A., and Burke, R. E. (1978). Forces produced by medial gastrocnemius and soleus muscles during locomotion in freely moving cats. *J. Neurophysiol.* 41: 1203–1216.

Walton, K., and Fulton, B. P. (1986). Ionic mechanisms underlying the firing properties of rat neonatal motoneurons studied in vitro. *Neuroscience* 19: 669–683.

Watchko, J. F., and Sieck, G. C. Respiratory muscle fatigue resistance relates to SDH activity and myosin phenotype during development. *J. Appl. Physiol.* (in press).

Watchko, J. F., Brozanski, B. S., O'Day, T. L., Guthrie, R. D., and Sieck, G. C. (1992). Contractile properties of the rat external abdominal oblique and diaphragm muscles during development. *J. Appl. Physiol.* 72: 1432–1436.

Webber, C. L., Jr., and Pleschka, K. (1976). Structural and functional characteristics of individual phrenic motoneurons. *Pflugers Arch.* 364: 113–121.

Whalen, R. G., Sell, S. M., Butler-Browne, G. S., Schwartz, K., Bouveret, P., and Pinset-Härström, I. (1981). Three myosin heavy chain isozymes appear sequentially in rat muscle development. *Nature* 292: 805–809.

Wilson, L. E., Johnson, B. D., Gosselin, L. E., and Sieck, G. C. (1993). Hypothyroidism alters myosin phenotype and unloaded shortening velocity of developing rat diaphragm. *Am. Rev. Respir. Dis.* 147: A959.

Woolson, R. F. (1987). *Statistical Methods for Analysis of Biomedical Data*. New York, John Wiley & Sons, pp. 59–64.

Zajac, F. E., and Faden, J. S. (1985). Relationship among recruitment order, axonal conduction velocity, and muscle-unit properties of type-identified motor units in cat plantaris muscle. *J. Neurophysiol.* 53: 1303–1322.

Zengel, J. E., Reid, S. A., Sypert, G. W., and Munson, J. B. (1985). Membrane electrical properties and prediction of motor-unit type of medial gastrocnemius motoneurons in the cat. *J. Neurophysiol.* 53: 1323–1344.

Zhan, W.-Z., and Sieck, G. C. (1992). Adaptations of diaphragm and medial gastrocnemius muscles to inactivity. *J. Appl. Physiol.* 72: 1445–1453.

Zhan, W. Z., Megirian, D., and Sieck, G. C. (1993). Effect of denervation on diaphragm MHC phenotype transitions and contractility during postnatal development. *FASEB J.* 7: A232.

28

Reflex Influences Acting on the Respiratory Muscles of the Chest Wall

ANN M. LEEVERS

Queen's University
Kingston, Ontario, Canada

JEREMY DAVID ROAD

University of British Columbia
Vancouver, British Columbia, Canada

I. Introduction

The respiratory muscles of the chest wall may be divided into the diaphragm and the muscles of the rib cage. The contraction of these muscles during quiet breathing follows the pattern of neural input from respiratory motoneurons. In early inspiration, some respiratory motoneurons reach their firing threshold, and then, additional motoneurons are recruited in response to activity from descending inspiratory bulbospinal neurons (Iscoe et al., 1976). Respiratory muscle contraction and the resultant muscle shortening then follow an augmenting pattern (Fig. 1). Respiratory muscle shortening moves the chest wall, which subsequently expands the lung. Lung expansion creates a pressure gradient between the upper airway and the lung; hence, air flows into the lung. Although the muscles of the chest wall are involved in many other functions, they are required to contract continually in this manner to support breathing.

Afferent nerves from a variety of sources can reflexly influence the depolarization and firing of respiratory motoneurons and, thereby, effectuate chest wall muscular contraction. These afferents can project to the spinal cord and produce an effect: spinal reflexes. For example, intercostal spindle afferents can facilitate the depolarization of spinal respiratory motoneurons and bring them to their firing threshold. Or, afferent nerves can project beyond the spinal cord to the brain stem

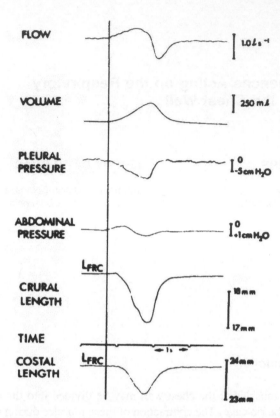

Figure 1 Example of typical strip-chart recording during spontaneous breathing. Resting length at functional residual capacity (L_FRC) is shown for crural and costal parts. Thin vertical line, onset of inspiration. (Reprinted with permission from Newman et al., 1984.)

respiratory neurons. These afferents then can influence respiratory timing [duration of inspiration (TI) and expiration (TE)], as well as the quantity of respiratory motoneuron output per breath. The afferent nerves that produce a change in brain stem respiratory neurons are traditionally termed part of a supraspinal reflex pathway. Thus, afferent nerves from peripheral structures can influence breathing reflexly at the spinal or supraspinal level. The peripheral structures that contain the nerve receptors include, for example, the chest wall muscles themselves, the lung, the abdominal viscera, the upper airway, and peripheral chemoreceptors, among others.

   The type of muscle contraction can be altered by these reflex influences on respiratory motoneuron discharge. Muscle contraction can be altered in a variety of ways. The mechanics of muscle contraction dictate that rapid muscle shortening results in force loss owing to the force–velocity relationship. At rest, the diaphragm shortens slowly (Newman et al., 1984); however, when respiratory motoneuron input to the muscle increases, the velocity of shortening increases (Road et al., 1986a), and this may lead to force loss owing to the force–velocity relationship. Alternatively, peripheral inputs can alter the configuration of the chest wall and change the respiratory muscles' initial length. As a result, the force–length relationship of muscle can influence the subsequent muscular contraction. For example, reflex contraction of the abdominal muscles in expiration can lengthen the diaphragm. The subsequent inspiration may be produced by a greater diaphragmatic force of contraction for a given respiratory motoneuronal input. The greater force is produced because the muscle's length is closer to its optimal length (Farkas and Rochester, 1988; Kim et al., 1976; Road et al., 1986b). Respiratory motoneuron activity can also determine muscle fiber type recruitment (as discussed in Chap. 27).

The balance of respiratory motoneuron output to the chest wall muscles is of considerable relevance, because it controls the coordination of chest wall muscle activity. For example, activation of the inspiratory intercostal muscles, without a corresponding activation of the diaphragm, can lead to lengthening of the diaphragm during inspiration. Therefore, some intercostal muscle shortening that could have produced airflow is lost on distortion of the diaphragm. Activation of supraspinal and spinal reflex pathways by visceral afferents (Kostreva et al., 1978; Albano and Garnier, 1983) produces a similar pattern of chest wall muscular activation favoring the rib cage muscles. The upper airway muscles are also an important part of this coordinated respiratory motoneuronal output. These muscles are normally activated before the chest wall muscles (Strohl et al., 1980), reducing upper airway resistance. Without such a coordinated activation, upper airway resistance during inspiration would impose a considerable load on the chest wall muscles.

Chest wall muscular activation occurs in a coordinated manner during sneezing, coughing, and vomiting. In this instance, an afferent neural pathway initiates a complex pattern of chest wall muscular contraction. The pattern of chest wall activation may be a result of a central neural circuit activated by the appropriate afferent nerves and results in a distinctive sequence of chest wall muscular activation.

Reflexes acting on the chest wall muscles have been studied in a variety of species and under a variety of conditions, including anesthesia, sleep, and wakefulness. The effects of reflexes in one situation may not be generally applicable. For example, results from the anesthetized cat may not be applied to humans. However, proving that a reflex present in one preparation is present or not in humans is not always easy, partly because of the effect consciousness has on reflex responses. Nevertheless, some differences have been identified among species. Recruitment of the expiratory muscles in response to lung inflation is a strong, readily reproducible reflex from the vagus nerve in anesthetized or awake quadrupeds; whereas in humans the reflex has proved difficult to detect (Wakai et al., 1992). In this chapter, the effects of spinal and supraspinal reflexes on the chest wall muscles in a variety of conditions and from a variety of peripheral structures will be discussed.

II. Reflex Influences from the Lower Airways

There are three types of receptors in the lower airways, the activity of which exerts reflex effects on the respiratory muscles of the chest wall. Activity from slowly adapting receptors (SARs) and rapidly adapting receptors (RARs), or from pulmonary stretch receptors and "irritant" receptors, is carried by myelinated nerve fibers, primarily within the vagus nerves (Paintal, 1973; Coleridge and Coleridge, 1986; Sant'Ambrogio, 1982). Activity from the third type of receptor, J-receptors (Paintal, 1973), is mediated by nonmyelinated vagal afferents, called pulmonary C-fibers.

Detailed descriptions concerning identification, location, general properties, and activation of these three types of receptors are given in several extensive review articles (Widdicombe, 1981; Coleridge and Coleridge, 1984, 1986; Sant'Ambrogio, 1982, 1987). Briefly, SARs and RARs can be distinguished on the basis of their discharge pattern and respiratory modulation (Paintal, 1973; Coleridge and Coleridge, 1986; Sant'Ambrogio, 1982). Afferent nerves from slowly adapting receptors tend to be larger in diameter and have a corresponding higher conduction velocity than rapidly adapting receptors (e.g., 32.3 m/s versus 23.3 m/s in the dog; Sampson and Vidruk, 1975), although there is considerable overlap (Paintal, 1973; Coleridge and Coleridge, 1986). In general, SARs exhibit a regular pattern of discharge that increases during inspiration and adapts slowly to maintained lung inflation (Adrian, 1933; Sant'Ambrogio, 1982; Coleridge and Coleridge, 1986). In contrast, rapidly adapting receptors show an irregular rate of discharge and respond to lung inflation (at a higher volume threshold) with a short-lasting, rapidly adapting increase in discharge (Coleridge and Coleridge, 1986; Sant'Ambrogio, 1982). Unlike most SARs, RARs are stimulated by forced lung deflation (Armstrong and Luck, 1974) and, in some cases, by chemical and mechanical stimuli (Sampson and Vidruk, 1975); hence, the term irritant receptors. Augmentation of RAR activity during lung inflation also appears to be influenced by the rate of inflation (Pack and DeLaney, 1983). There is some evidence that SARs may also act as rate receptors, especially at higher inflation volumes (Pack et al., 1986). Pulmonary C-fiber afferents have a slow conduction velocity, in keeping with their nonmyelinated nature (Armstrong and Luck, 1974; Coleridge and Coleridge, 1984). The J-receptors respond to large, maintained lung volumes and mechanical and chemical stimuli (Coleridge and Coleridge, 1984, 1986). C-fibers are by far the predominant afferents in the vagus nerve.

Vagal afferent feedback from the lower airways affects the timing and magnitude of motor output to the respiratory muscles and includes both inhibitory and excitatory influences. The net result of vagal afferent feedback on respiratory motor output depends on the relative contribution from each receptor (SAR, RAR, and J-receptor), which will be determined by a complex combination of factors and conditions. The quality and magnitude of reflex effects vary with state of consciousness: awake versus asleep (Sullivan et al., 1978; Bouverot et al., 1970; Hamilton et al., 1988); unanesthetized versus anesthetized (Sant'Ambrogio and

Widdicombe, 1965; Richardson and Widdicombe, 1969; Bjurstedt, 1953; Phillipson et al., 1971); among different species (Gautier, 1976; Gautier et al., 1981; D'Angelo and Agostoni, 1975; Coleridge and Coleridge, 1986; Trenchard, 1977); and with degree of interaction with other central and peripheral reflex influences (Cohen et al., 1986; Younes et al., 1974; Xi et al., 1993; Arita and Bishop, 1983). The functional significance of these reflexes may be to help coordinate the activity and relative contribution of the different respiratory muscles and, thereby, stabilize the breathing pattern and minimize the work of breathing (Milsom, 1990; von Euler, 1991; Agostoni et al., 1970).

Are vagal afferent reflexes operating during resting breathing? On the basis of studies from several different animal species, before and after vagotomy or vagal blockade, it would appear that these reflexes are involved in the coordination of respiratory muscle activity, even during spontaneous breathing (Smith et al., 1990; Younes et al., 1978; Gautier et al., 1981; Sant'Ambrogio and Widdicombe, 1965; Brice et al., 1991; Ainsworth et al., 1992; van Lunteren et al., 1988a). Despite many claims that vagal reflexes play no role in resting breathing in humans, there is as yet no definitive answer. Until recently, it was difficult to assess the function of vagal afferents in humans, since vagal blockade is impractical. However, with the development of successful lung transplantation techniques, there is a growing population of individuals with vagally denervated lungs. These individuals provide a unique model in which to explore the role of pulmonary vagal afferents in resting breathing and under a variety of different conditions.

It is difficult to distinguish specific receptor effects from studies in which vagotomy or complete vagal blockade were used, since all reflex effects would be eliminated. However, selective blockade or differential stimulation of vagal afferents has provided some information about the relative contribution of individual receptors under different conditions. The effects produced by each type of receptor can be separated and examined on the basis of inspiratory and expiratory consequences.

A. Reflex Effects from Slowly Adapting Receptors

Slowly adapting receptor reflex effects have been, by far, the most extensively studied of the pulmonary vagal reflexes. Of these, the Hering–Breuer inflation reflex, an inspiratory inhibitory–expiratory facilitatory reflex, has been the most completely examined (Adrian, 1933; Clark and von Euler, 1972; Bradley et al., 1976; D'Angelo and Agostoni, 1975; Coleridge and Coleridge, 1986). A variety of neurophysiological investigations have confirmed that it is afferent input from SARs that is indeed responsible for the Hering–Breuer inflation reflex (Zuperku et al., 1982; Trenchard, 1977; Russell and Bishop, 1976; Iscoe et al., 1979; Bartoli et al., 1975).

This discussion will be limited primarily to those studies that have been concerned specifically with the effects on respiratory motor output and have recorded activity directly from inspiratory or expiratory neurons, motor nerves, or muscles (i.e., diaphragm, intercostal, or abdominal muscle electromyography; EMG).

Effects on Inspiratory Muscles

The most common effect of SAR afferent input on inspiratory motor output is the Hering–Breuer inspiratory-inhibiting, lung inflation reflex (Adrian, 1933). The discharge of pulmonary SARs activated by lung inflation exerts a graded, volume-related inhibition of inspiration when lung volume exceeds a time-dependent threshold (Younes et al., 1978; Younes and Remmers, 1981; Baker et al., 1979b). As inhibition progresses, it subsequently induces an inspiratory termination (Cross et al., 1980; Clark and von Euler, 1972; Younes and Remmers, 1981). The inhibition from both tonic and phasic volume influences can be demonstrated either by lung inflation above FRC or by withholding inflation, thereby removing inhibitory influences.

Moderate, maintained lung inflation (i.e., increased end-expiratory lung volume; EELV), results in inhibition of inspiratory neurons (Koepchen et al., 1973), inspiratory motoneurons (phrenic and intercostal) (Cross et al., 1980; Davies et al., 1978; Sant'Ambrogio and Widdicombe, 1965; Baker et al., 1979b; Bartoli et al., 1975), and diaphragm and inspiratory intercostal motor activity (Arita and Bishop, 1983; Davies et al., 1980; Smith et al., 1990; Ainsworth et al., 1992; Yasuma et al., 1993) in a number of different animal species. An example of the integrated phrenic motoneuronal response to maintained lung inflation of anesthetized rabbits is shown in Figure 2. This particular example demonstrates that the inhibitory response is dependent on SARs, since it is absent when the SARs are blocked. In the rabbit, selective blockade of SARs is accomplished by inhalation of sulfur dioxide (Davies et al., 1978). Another example of inspiratory motor response to maintained lung inflation is shown in Figure 3. In this example, also from an anesthetized rabbit, the diaphragm and external oblique (EMGs) are activated by positive-pressure breathing and head-up tilting, both of which increase EELV (i.e., tonic vagal influences). When the response after selectively blocking SAR activity, by inhalation of sulfur dioxide, is compared with the response following cervical vagotomy, it is clear that SARs provide inhibitory, volume-related feedback to the inspiratory muscles (Davies et al., 1980).

Prevention of or withholding lung inflation by airway occlusion or by halting the ventilator in paralyzed animals, respectively, results in prolongation of inspiratory motoneuron (Cross et al., 1980; Sant'Ambrogio and Widdicombe, 1965; St. John and Zhou, 1990) or motor output (Smith et al., 1990; Younes et al., 1978; Gautier et al., 1981; Brice et al., 1991; Ainsworth et al., 1992; van Lunteren et al., 1988a) in cats, dogs, rabbits, and ponies, thereby demonstrating that afferent input from SARs is operative during resting breathing in these species. Although this is true for either anesthetized (Cross et al., 1980; Sant'Ambrogio and Widdicombe, 1965; Brice et al., 1991) or awake (Sant'Ambrogio and Widdicombe, 1965; Ainsworth et al., 1992;

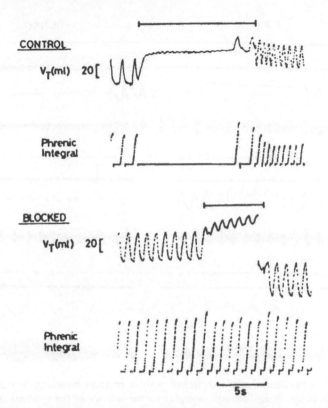

Figure 2 Phrenic motoneuron responses to lung inflation before and after selective blockade of SARs by 10-min exposure to 200 ppm SO_2, in an anesthetized rabbit. The traces are tidal volume and integrated phrenic discharge. The lungs were inflated by a positive pressure of 10 cm H_2O (horizontal bars). The shift in the baseline in the lower volume trace was due to resetting the airflow integrator. *Note* the absence of the Hering–Breuer reflex after exposure to SO_2. (Reprinted with permission from Davies et al., 1978.)

Brice et al., 1991) dogs, rabbits, and ponies, Gautier (1976) suggested that it is not evident in awake cats. However, the observation that subsequent to bilateral, cervical vagotomy, awake cats exhibit an increase in VT and a decrease in breathing frequency would support the presence of a functioning Hering–Breuer reflex during eupnea (Gautier, 1976). An example of the effects of withholding phasic lung inflation on inspiratory motor activity in anesthetized cats is shown in Figure 4 (St. John and Zhou, 1990). In this example, the activity of phrenic nerve and nerves innervating the thyroarytenoid muscle (an upper airway expiratory muscle) are increased, by virtue of a prolongation of TI, when lung inflation is withheld.

The presence of the Hering–Breuer lung inflation reflex has been demonstrated in humans, although not in the conscious state. Lung inflation to 40% of inspiratory

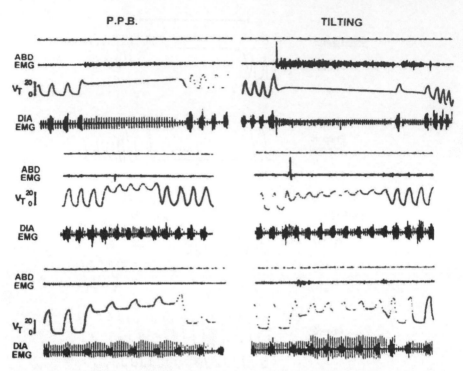

Figure 3 Anesthetized rabbit. Effect of positive-pressure breathing (P.P.B.; tracings on left) and head-up tilting (tracings on right) on the activity of the external oblique muscle (ABD, EMG), the diaphragm (DIA, EMG) and tidal volume (VT) in control condition (top tracings), after SO_2 inhalation (middle tracings) and postvagotomy (bottom tracings). Positive pressure breathing and tilting both increase EELV. Note inhibition of diaphragm and excitation of EO activity by increasing EELV during control and lack of effect after block of SARs. Time marker = 1 s. (Reprinted with permission from Davies et al., 1980.)

capacity in sleeping human subjects resulted in termination of inspiration (Hamilton et al., 1988) and inhibition of diaphragm EMG activity (Iber et al., 1991), which was absent in vagally denervated lung transplant patients (Iber et al., 1991). In anesthetized human subjects, a significant inhibitory effect of lung inflation on diaphragm activity was also found in the normal tidal volume range (Polachek et al., 1980). Furthermore, anesthetized (Polachek et al., 1980) and sleeping (Iatridis and Iber, 1992) humans exhibit TI prolongation with airway occlusion. Figure 5 demonstrates the inhibitory effects of lung inflation on inspiratory motor output in humans. The duration of diaphragm EMG activity is increased with occlusion at end-expiration and is decreased with augmentation of inspiratory flow (inflation) (Polachek et al., 1980).

In addition to inspiratory inhibitory consequences, evidence is accumulating that suggests that phasic lung inflation also exerts an excitatory influence on

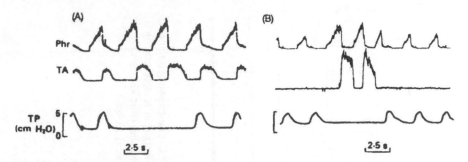

Figure 4 Alterations of inspiratory and expiratory neural activities upon withholding phasic lung inflation in two paralyzed, decerebrate cats (A and B). Note that the peak thyroarytenoid (TA) activity during the early portion of neural expiration rose during noninflation cycles. Peak integrated phrenic activity (Phr) increased during the noninflation cycles, and its postinspiratory activity declined. TP, tracheal pressure. Noninflation is indicated by the absence of changes of tracheal pressure during periods of phrenic activity. (Reprinted with permission from St. John and Zhou, 1990.)

inspiratory motor output before inspiratory off-switch (Cross et al., 1980; Pack et al., 1981; Dimarco et al., 1981; Cohen et al., 1986; Baker et al., 1979b; Bartoli et al., 1975; Hwang et al., 1987). Positive-feedback facilitation, probably from pulmonary SARs (Dimarco et al., 1981), occurs as the lungs are inflated. Inspiratory facilitation appears to have a low-volume threshold, since it can be elicited by small changes in volume, well within eupneic V_T range (Cross et al., 1980; Dimarco et al., 1981; Cohen et al., 1986). It is manifest as an increase in the slope of the phrenic or intercostal neurogram (i.e., increase in rate of rise of activity with lung inflation; Cross et al., 1980; Dimarco et al., 1981; Pack et al., 1981; Cohen et al., 1986; Baker et al., 1979b). Figure 6 shows an example of positive-feedback facilitation of phrenic and external intercostal motoneuron activity (Dimarco et al., 1981). The slopes of motoneuron discharge are increased during lung inflation, compared with withholding inflation.

How can both inspiratory facilitatory and inspiratory inhibitory feedback from SARs occur concurrently? It is likely that these opposing affects do not occur simultaneously, since these reflexes are graded; that is, inhibition from the inhibitory reflex would not occur until the threshold for the inspiratory off-switch was reached (Younes and Remmers, 1981), by which time inspiratory facilitation would be declining (Dimarco et al., 1981). Furthermore, these reflexes are most likely not expressed equally on all the motoneurons. For example, the facilitatory effect of phasic lung inflation appears to be stronger on the external intercostal motoneuron than on the phrenic (Dimarco et al., 1981).

Effects on Expiratory Muscles

In contrast with the inspiratory inhibitory effects of the Hering–Breuer inflation reflex, the general consensus in the current literature is that moderate lung inflation

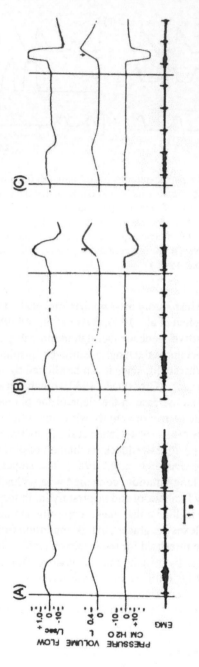

Figure 5 Representative tracings in one subject, illustrating response (A) to airway occlusion and (B,C) to augmenting inspiratory flow. In C, bag was squeezed harder than in B (note tracheal pressure tracing). EMG burst was prolonged in A, shortened in B, and markedly shortened in C. Arrows in B and C indicate volumes at termination of inspiration. Note that latter volumes are not substantially higher than spontaneous tidal volumes. (Reprinted with permission from Polachek et al., 1980.)

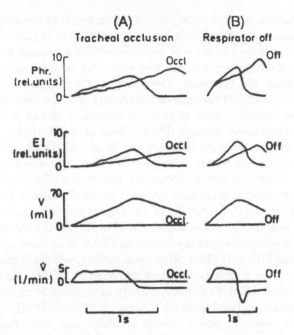

Figure 6 Inspiratory-facilitating and "off-switch" effects of volume-related feedback (A) in a spontaneously breathing cat and (B) in a paralyzed animal ventilated by "servorespirator." Superimposed records with and without volume changes. In A volume changes were prevented by tracheal occlusions (Occl) and, in B, by switching off the servorespirator (Off). From above: Phrenic activity (Phr), external intercostal activity (EI), volume (V), and airflow ($\dot{V}$). Computer-averaged records ($n = 5$). In the presence of lung movements, inspiratory activity is facilitated and inspiratory duration is shortened. Note different time scales in A and B. (Reprinted with permission from Dimarco et al., 1981.)

has a facilitatory effect on chest wall, expiratory motor output. The conclusion that lung inflation excites expiratory motor output is based on studies of expiratory neuron (Cohen et al., 1985; Baker et al., 1979a; Koepchen et al., 1973; Bajic et al., 1992), expiratory (intercostal and abdominal) motoneuron (Cohen et al., 1985; St. John and Zhou, 1990; Bajic et al., 1992), or muscle (Bishop and Bachofen, 1972; Bishop, 1964; Russell and Bishop, 1976; De Troyer et al., 1989; Farkas et al., 1988; Arita and Bishop, 1983; Farber 1982; Davies et al., 1980; Leevers and Road, 1993; Farkas and Schroeder, 1990; Brice et al., 1991; Begle and Skatrud, 1990; Yasuma et al., 1993) responses to tonic and phasic volume feedback. Tonic vagal feedback related to the end-expiratory volume is present at functional residual capacity (FRC) and increases linearly with increments in FRC. Increases in EELV almost invariably leads to recruitment of expiratory muscles, which are silent at FRC during resting breathing (Farber, 1982; Arita and Bishop, 1983; Bishop and Bachofen, 1972; Bishop, 1964; Russell and Bishop, 1976) or increased activation of expiratory muscles in which resting activity is present (Leevers and Road, 1989, 1993, 1995; Brice et al., 1991; Bellemare et al., 1991), in vagally intact animals. Expiratory muscle resting activity or recruitment and activation by increases in EELV is eliminated or greatly attenuated by vagotomy or vagal blockade (Yasuma et al., 1993; Farkas and Schroeder, 1990; Farber, 1982; Bellemare et al., 1991; Ainsworth et al., 1992). Experimental maneuvers that increase EELV include positive-pressure breathing, such as continuous positive airway pressure (CPAP) and positive end-expiratory pressure (PEEP) (Road et al., 1991a,b), and changing posture from supine to upright (Leevers and Road, 1991). Recruitment of the expiratory muscles in response to an increase in EELV is an important mechanism to defend tidal volume or load-compensating mechanism (Cherniack and Altose, 1981). Expiratory muscle recruitment mediated by vagal feedback is important for optimization of the work of breathing of the diaphragm (Road et al., 1991a) and coordination of respiratory muscle activity (Road et al., 1991b). An example of the response of an abdominal expiratory muscle to CPAP in an anesthetized opossum is shown in Figure 7 (Farber, 1982). After vagal cooling, which eliminated primarily SARs, the abdominal muscle is no longer activated by CPAP. Studies in awake animals have shown that this expiratory activity in response to increased EELV is not solely dependent on vagal afferents (Leevers and Road, 1994).

Until quite recently, phasic volume feedback was also considered to be excitatory to expiratory motor output. However, a few investigators have reported that, in anesthetized cats and dogs, lung inflation has both excitatory and inhibitory effects on expiratory neurons and motoneurons that are mediated by afferent input

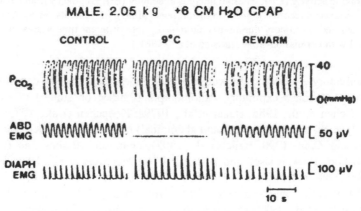

Figure 7 Bilateral vagal cooling and complete inhibition of expiratory muscle output during CPAP in adult opossum. Polygraph records show breath-by-breath EMG activity (integrated to give moving average values) from the abdominal muscles (middle traces) and diaphragm (bottom traces), along with end-tidal P_{CO_2} (top traces), after cooling the vagi to 9°C. Control patterns before cooling and after rewarming the vagi are also illustrated. (Reprinted with permission from Farber, 1982.)

from pulmonary SARs (Cohen et al., 1985; Fregosi et al., 1990; Koepchen et al., 1973; Bajic et al., 1992; Bianchi and Barillot, 1975). In general, expiratory inhibitory effects appear to be confined primarily to upper airway muscles (St. John and Zhou, 1990; Bianchi and Barillot, 1975). However, there are reports of rib cage expiratory muscle (triangularis sterni and internal intercostal) inhibition by lung inflation (Cohen et al., 1985; Ainsworth et al., 1992; Bajic et al., 1992).

Like their biphasic reflex effects on the inspiratory muscles, the SAR reflexes appear to act on the expiratory muscles in a graded fashion, and the effects are linearly related to tracheal pressure (Baker et al., 1979a; Koepchen et al., 1973; Bajic et al., 1992). It is likely that these opposing facilitatory and inhibitory effects play a role in the control of expiratory airflow (Bajic et al., 1992).

B. Reflex Effects from Rapidly Adapting Receptors

Similar to the slowly adapting receptors, feedback from rapidly adapting receptors (RARs) has both excitatory and inhibitory effects on the respiratory muscles of the chest wall. The RARs appear to be activated by lung inflation (at the peak of inspiration), particularly at higher lung volumes, and their activity is augmented by increased rates of inflation (Pack and DeLaney, 1983). Other mechanisms of activation include forced lung deflation (Green and Kaufman, 1990); decreases in lung compliance (Pisarri et al., 1990), resulting, for example, from restrictive lung diseases and pulmonary edema (Hargreaves et al., 1991; Ravi and Kappagoda, 1992); and decreased TI and TE with increased minute ventilation, for example, during acute respiratory failure (Coleridge and Coleridge, 1986).

Effects on Inspiratory Muscles

Activation of RARs during lung inflation is considered to be the primary mechanism mediating the inspiratory facilitation that leads to an "augmented breath" (Bartlett, 1971; Glogowska et al., 1972; Cherniack et al., 1981; Pisarri et al., 1990; Green and Kaufman, 1990; Pack and DeLaney, 1983). Augmented breaths occur spontaneously in several animal species, including humans, under conditions of wakefulness, sleep, and anesthesia (Shea et al., 1988; Barlett, 1971; Bendixen et al., 1964; Reynolds and Flom, 1968). A spontaneous augmented breath may serve to prevent atelectasis (Reynolds and Flom, 1968) and is thought to be stimulated by a decrease in lung compliance (Reynolds and Flom, 1968; Glogowska et al., 1972). Augmented breaths have a characteristic pattern in which inspiration has two phases, of which the first phase is essentially a normal spontaneous inspiration, and the second phase begins at or near the peak of a normal inspiration. The net result is a breath that has a larger inspiratory volume and a longer TI than the preceding tidal breaths (Glogowska et al., 1972; Cherniack et al., 1981). An example of a spontaneous augmented breath in an anesthetized cat is shown in Figure 8 (Cherniack et al., 1981).

In addition to their role in augmented breaths, it has been suggested that

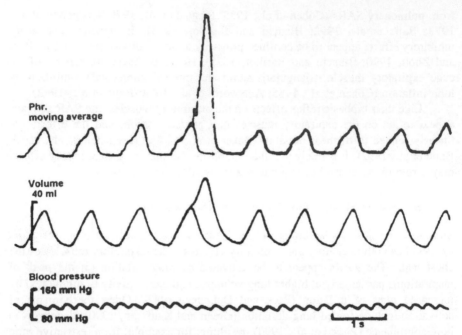

Figure 8 Characteristics of a spontaneous-augmented breath in records of tidal phrenic activity (upper trace) and tidal volume (middle trace). The "control" breath preceding the augmented breath has been retraced and superimposed on the records of the augmented breath to show the similarity between control breath and the basal portion (i.e., phase I) of the augmented breath. (Reprinted with permission from Cherniack et al., 1981.)

activation of RARs during lung inflation, even during resting tidal breathing, may play a role in the initiation of inspiration (Davies et al., 1981). The functional significance of RARs in the onset of inspiration would be to contribute to the termination of expiration in concert with the decreasing central inhibition.

Effects on Expiratory Muscles

In contrast to the facilitation of inspiratory muscle activity by RARs during spontaneous augmented breaths, an inhibition of expiratory motor output was suggested in earlier studies, showing a transient reduction in VT and TE following the augmented breath (Cherniack et al., 1981; Reynolds and Flom, 1968; van Lunteren et al., 1988b). A more recent study confirmed that expiratory muscle activity (triangularis sterni) was inhibited during augmented breaths (van Lunteren et al., 1988b). It was suggested that the reduction of expiratory muscle activity during an augmented breath may contribute to the increase in EELV that occurs (van Lunteren et al., 1988b).

C. Reflex Effects from C-Fiber Afferents

Effects on Inspiratory Muscles

To determine the reflex effects of C-fiber or nonmyelinated afferents, various techniques have been used to eliminate the activity of the myelinated afferents. For example, electrical stimulation and anodal hyperpolarization can eliminate myelinated afferents. An alternative method is to use nerve cooling. Jonzon et al. (1988) have shown that cooling the vagus nerve progressively blocks activity in myelinated and, subsequently, in nonmyelinated afferents. They found that cooling the vagus nerve below 7°C reduced neural traffic to a much larger degree in the myelinated fibers and left the conduction in nonmyelinated fibers relatively intact. The effects of nonmyelinated afferents on inspiration can then be explored.

Russell and associates (1984) used hyperpolarizing block of the myelinated afferents and explored the ventilatory response to hypercapnia. When activity in the vagus nerve was eliminated completely by vagotomy, there was no increase in breathing frequency during hypercapnia. However, when conduction in nonmyelinated afferents was left intact, breathing frequency did increase in response to hypercapnic breathing. Therefore, one effect of nonmyelinated afferents is on respiratory timing. A similar effect on respiratory timing was observed by Holmes and Remmers (1989). They used cold block of the vagus nerve to explore the effects of artificially induced nonmyelinated afferent activity. In this setting a tachypnea resulted. In addition to the tachypnea, the effects of activation of these thin-fiber afferents was to break expiration; that is, there was prolongation of postinspiratory activity of the diaphragm and increased phasic activity in the thyroarytenoid muscle.

Another reflex effect of afferents in the vagus nerve has been attributed to nonmyelinated and thin myelinated afferents. This reflex consists of a tonic inspiratory activity in response to lung deflation. Badier et al. (1989) showed this tonic activity in the muscles of the chest wall (i.e., the diaphragm and intercostals). Tonic activity could be induced by lung deflation or by injections of carbachol, histamine, or phenyl diguanide. In that study, selective block with procaine eliminated, or reduced, the reflex, which suggested to these authors that thin myelinated and nonmyelinated afferents were responsible for the tonic inspiratory activity that was observed in the diaphragm and intercostal muscles.

Effects on Expiratory Muscles

The effects of nonmyelinated afferents on the expiratory muscles have been studied in a similar manner. Haxhiu et al. (1988) found that injection of capsaicin and subsequent activation of nonmyelinated afferents led to apnea. This apnea was blocked by vagotomy and, during the apnea, there was tonic expiratory activity in the expiratory muscles of the rib cage (i.e., the internal intercostal muscles and the triangularis sterni muscles). However, activity in one abdominal muscle, the transversus abdominis, was not tonically activated by this pathway. Hollstien et al.

(1991) used cold block to study the differential effects of myelinated and nonmyelinated afferents on expiratory abdominal muscle activity. Blockade of myelinated afferents in this manner led to a 40% reduction in activity of the external oblique muscle; however, with further cooling, and a reduction in nonmyelinated activity, expiratory abdominal activity returned back toward the control level. Thus, nonmyelinated afferents from the lung would appear to have an inhibitory effect on abdominal expiratory muscle activity and can increase tonic activity in the rib cage expiratory muscles.

III. Reflex Effects from the Upper Airway

The muscles of the chest wall are frequently subjected to additional loads produced by relaxation of the upper airway dilator muscles. The patency of the upper airway depends on a balance of forces between the force of contraction of the inspiratory chest wall muscles, which tend to collapse the upper airway by reducing upper airway intraluminal pressure, and the upper airway dilator muscles. Sleep frequently shifts this balance in favor of the chest wall muscles (Remmers et al., 1978; Brouillette and Thach, 1979). The subsequent narrowing of the upper airway leads to strong contraction of the inspiratory and expiratory muscles in response to the developing hypercapnia and hypoxia (Wilcox et al., 1988).

Mathew et al. (1982a) have shown a reflex mechanism that tends to prevent upper airway collapse and hence reduce the load on the muscles of the chest wall. The first occluded breath (anesthetized rabbits) was observed to be associated with an immediate increase in activity in a major upper airway dilating muscle, the genioglossus (Fig. 9). Increasing negative pressure in the upper airways (mimicking the effect of stronger chest wall muscle contraction) led to increased activation of the genioglossus muscle. The afferent pathway of this reflex involved the superior laryngeal branch of the vagus nerve (Mathew et al., 1982b). Sant'Ambrogio et al. (1983) recorded from afferent nerves during upper airway occlusion and confirmed that afferent nerves, particularly in the internal branch of the superior laryngeal nerve were activated. Mathew and co-workers (1982b) divided the upper airway into two compartments. Negative pressure applied to the compartment between the larynx and lower pharynx activated a reflex that included the superior laryngeal nerve the afferent pathway. A similar reflex arising from the nasopharyngeal compartment was shown probably to involve mucosal receptors in the airway, since topical anesthesia completely abolished the response. Thus, there are reflexes that tend to maintain upper airway patency and hence reduce the required force of contraction of the chest wall muscles needed to maintain tidal volume.

This reflex that maintains upper airway patency also had a supraspinal pathway as respiratory timing was altered by its activation. Respiratory frequency decreased, and TI was prolonged (Mathew et al., 1982c).

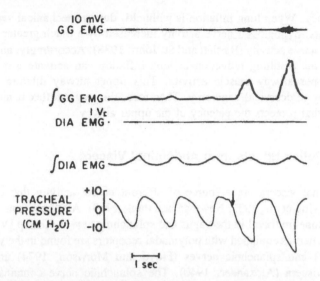

Figure 9 Effect of a respiratory-loading maneuver (nasal occlusion) in a vagotomized animal. Traces are (from top) genioglossus (GG) muscle EMG, integrated GG EMG, diaphragm (DIA) EMG, integrated DIA EMG, and tracheal pressure. Animal is breathing through its nose. Arrow indicates onset of nasal occlusion at end expiration. Note decrease in tracheal pressure and coinciding marked increase in-phase inspiratory activity of GG during first occluded breath. No such increase is seen in DIA EMG. (Reprinted with permission from Mathew et al., 1982.)

Augmentation of two additional upper airway muscles—the posterior crico-arytenoid and the alae nasi—also has been observed during upper airway obstruction (van Lunteren, 1984). Negative upper airway pressure also tended to increase the phase lag between onset of activity in the upper airway muscles and activation of the chest wall inspiratory muscles. The increase in the phase lag also preserves upper airway patency by increasing the level of activation of upper airway dilating muscles, before chest wall muscle activation occurs (Kurtz et al., 1978; Strohl et al., 1980). Selective reflex activation of upper airway dilating muscles (the genioglossus) also has been shown to occur in awake humans (Leiter and Daubenspeck, 1990). It has also been shown that high-frequency oscillations in the upper airway can activate the genioglossus muscle of sleeping dogs (Plowman et al., 1990). The oscillations were in the range of those produced by snoring and this reflex activation of the upper airway muscles may be an important mechanism maintaining upper airway patency during sleep.

The reflex increase in upper airway muscle activity during upper airway obstruction has been associated with a reduction in diaphragmatic activation (Hwang et al., 1984). This is another mechanism tending to maintain upper airway patency. Interestingly, the vagus nerve also appears to mediate a reflex, preserving upper airway patency. When lung inflation is withheld, during mechanical ventilation in paralyzed cats, hypoglossal nerve activity increased by a much greater proportion than phrenic nerve activity (Bartlett and St. John, 1988). Accordingly, an obstructed breath with the resulting reduction in lung inflation can activate a reflex which increases upper airway muscle activity. This upper airway dilating effect was eliminated by midcervical vagotomy. Therefore, this vagal reflex is an additional mechanism that protects the patency of the upper airway.

IV. Reflex Effects from Abdominal Viscera

The abdominal viscera are a source of afferent neural activity that can modify breathing (Irving et al., 1937; Newman and Paul, 1969). Afferents from the viscera and the peritoneum travel in the vagus and splanchnic nerves. Group IV unmyelinated afferent nerves equipped with polymodal receptors are found in the vagus nerve (Iggo, 1957) and splanchnic nerves (Floyd and Morrison, 1974) arising from abdominal viscera (Alexander, 1940). The splanchnic nerve contains group III myelinated afferents as well (Floyd and Morrison, 1974), which also have polymodal receptors. Polymodal receptors respond to a multiplicity of stimuli: thermal, mechanical or chemical, with slow or rapid adaptation (Iggo, 1959; Morrison, 1973). Compression or distension of the gallbladder, for example, activates tonic discharges in these afferent nerves, and receptors responding to these stimuli have been found within most of the abdominal viscera (Morrison, 1973).

That visceral afferents may modify breathing was suggested by Reeve and coauthors (1950). They noted inhibition of breathing, in humans, during stimulation of upper abdominal viscera at the time of surgery. Downman (1955) recognized inhibitory effects on phrenic nerve activity following stimulation of splanchnic afferents in decerebrate cats, and Kostreva et al. (1978) noted a similar inhibition during sympathetic afferent nerve stimulation in anesthetized dogs and primates. Therefore, the major effect on breathing with electrical stimulation of visceral afferents, at least splanchnic visceral afferents, is an inhibition of breathing.

Interestingly, however, the inhibition of breathing is greater in the diaphragm than the inspiratory intercostals. Prabhakar and colleagues (1985) showed that, although the diaphragm was inhibited by visceral afferent stimulation, the intercostal muscles were not. The result was a shift in the type of breathing favoring rib cage expansion, with little abdominal displacement. Kostreva et al. (1978) found similar results during electrical stimulation of splanchnic afferents. Reflex inhibition of the diaphragm can also be produced by distension of the esophagus. De Troyer and Rosso (1982) found this inhibition occurred preponderantly in the crural part of the diaphragm (periesophageal), with some inhibition of the costal part of the diaphragm and sparing of the major rib cage inspiratory muscle, parasternal intercostal, activity (Fig. 10). Vagotomy eliminated this inhibition. Therefore, predominant diaphragmatic inhibition, as opposed to rib cage inspiratory muscle inhibition is seen

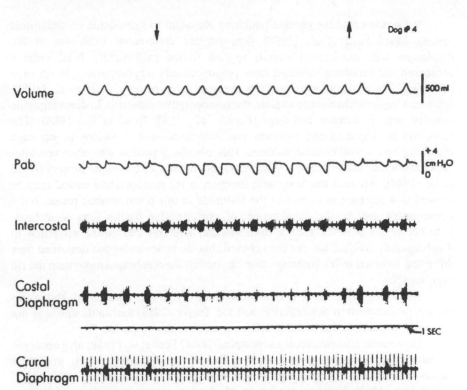

Figure 10 Effects of esophageal distension on the spontaneous electrical activity of the parasternal intercostals and of the costal and crural parts of the diaphragm in an anesthetized dog: Pab, abdominal pressure. Inflation of a balloon situated in the middle third of the esophagus with 150 ml of air (left arrow) causes immediate diaphragmatic inhibition; at the same time, the intercostal electrical activity increases. With deflation of the balloon (right arrow), all electrical activities return to control levels. (Reprinted with permission from DeTroyer and Rosso, 1982.)

following stimulation of vagal afferents from the esophagus as well as following stimulation of abdominal splanchnic afferents.

What are the functional correlates of the phrenic inhibition? Esophageal distension presumably signals the passage of ingested material and the need for relaxation of the grastroesophageal sphincter. This sphincter is partly formed by the crural diaphragm (Altschuler et al., 1985). Monges and associates (1978) recognized inhibition of periesophageal (crural) diaphragmatic muscle activity during vomiting as well as during esophageal distension in anesthetized dogs. Thus, diaphragmatic inhibition, particularly, periesophageal, may be viewed as an important reflex function allowing movement of material up or down the esophagus without impeding ventilation.

What role could the phrenic inhibition attendant to stimulation of abdominal viscera have? Ford et al. (1988) demonstrated preferential inhibition of the diaphragm with mechanical stimuli applied to the gallbladder. Tidal volume decreased and breathing switched from preponderantly diaphragmatic, to rib cage breathing. These effects were partially reversed by vagotomy. Ford et al. (1988) were seeking a mechanism to explain the postoperative reduction in diaphragmatic function seen in humans and dogs (Ford et al., 1983; Road et al., 1984). The reduction in diaphragmatic function was associated with a switch to rib cage breathing and a smaller tidal volume. This breathing pattern was observed after upper abdominal surgery (cholecystectomy), but not lower abdominal surgery (Road et al., 1984). Reduced diaphragmatic function in the postoperative period may be viewed as a mechanism to protect the abdomen in this posttraumatic phase, but a consequence may be the development of postoperative basilar lung atelectasis. Whether or not a reflex arising from visceral afferents causes the reduction in diaphragmatic function has not been proved, but the reflex pathways described here do reveal potential reflex pathways that can inhibit the diaphragm more than the rib cage muscles.

A midline laparotomy reduces EMG activity in the transversus abdominis muscle in anesthetized dogs (Farkas and De Troyer, 1989) and, although it is not known, it is possible that visceral afferents mediate this response.

Do visceral afferents act at a supraspinal level? Ford et al. (1988) also observed a change in respiratory timing with gallbladder stimulation, which implies a supraspinal affect. They noted a prolongation of TE and a reduction of TI. Schondorf and Polosa (1980) found an inhibition of phrenic and recurrent laryngeal nerve activity, with a prolongation of TE following stimulation of urinary bladder afferents. Albano and Garnier (1983) indeed observed that stimulation of splanchnic afferents arising from the pancreaticoduodenal area produced an inhibition of inspiratory bulbospinal neurons in the VRG and an excitation of expiratory bulbospinals. Interestingly, the phrenic inhibition was observed in spinalized cats (C1–C2), suggesting that this inhibition may occur at the spinal as well as the supraspinal level (Albano and Garnier, 1983). Therefore, visceral afferents may act at spinal and supraspinal levels.

Activation of visceral afferents has excitatory effects. Electrical stimulation of the vagus nerve below the diaphragm elicited an increase in minute ventilation (Mei, 1976). Waldrop et al. (1984) specifically activated thin-fiber afferents by applying capsaicin or bradykinin to the serosal surface of the stomach or gallbladder. They elicited an increase in the ventilatory output and an increase in blood pressure. Splanchnic nerve section, but not vagotomy, eliminated the response. Thus, chemical activation of thin-fiber splanchnic afferents had an excitatory effect and, since timing was altered, a supraspinal effect. This result contrasts with the effects of mechanical or electrical stimulation of visceral afferents, which produced an inhibition. The different types of stimulation may have activated nerve fibers to a different degree, for example, electrical stimulation could have activated different thin fibers. Therefore, the effects on breathing of these afferents probably depends on the type of nerve fiber activated and, accordingly, the stimulus.

V. Reflex Effects of Chemoreceptor Stimulation

Many studies have lent support to the concept that the breathing pattern and activation of the chest wall muscles differs between hypoxic and hypercapnic stimulation of breathing. These differences have been demonstrated in humans (Gautier, 1969) and in awake and anesthetized animals (Fitzgerald, 1973; Garcia and Cherniack, 1967; Gautier, 1976; Smith et al., 1989a,b). Brain stem respiratory-related neurons also respond differently to hypoxia than hypercapnia (St. John and Wang, 1977; St. John, 1981). However, the possibility remains that phrenic or other inspiratory motoneurons differ in their integration of descending inputs in response to differing chemical stimulation (Mitchell and Berger, 1975).

In general, the respiratory response to hypoxia reveals a greater reduction in T_I and T_E, compared with the respiratory response to hypercapnia at equivalent levels of ventilatory drive: that is, a relative tachypnea. Ledlie et al. (1981) confirmed these observations and demonstrated that, for any tidal volume, a greater increase in phrenic output was required with hypoxia than with hypercapnia. A similar difference in timing was observed between hypoxia and hypercapnia (Road et al., 1986a); in addition, however, the consequence of this breathing pattern on diaphragmatic shortening was measured. Hypoxia led to a faster velocity of diaphragmatic shortening for any given tidal volume, which could lead to some pressure loss owing to force–velocity considerations. Furthermore, diaphragmatic initial length decreased with hypoxia owing to an increase in FRC. Crural diaphragmatic initial length decreased by about 5% and, since the crural diaphragm's optimal pressure-generating length is 5% longer than the supine length (Road et al., 1986b), its pressure-generating capacity may well have been reduced. Thus, from the chest wall muscle aspect, hypoxia may invoke both force–velocity and force–length properties of muscular contraction. These properties may then reduce the efficiency of such contractions.

What is the mechanism of the increase in FRC during hypoxia? Bouverot and Fitzgerald (1969) attributed it to a decrease in tonic activity of the expiratory, internal intercostal muscles, as measured in anesthetized dogs. An increase in end-expiratory esophageal pressure was observed during the FRC increases in a similar preparation (Road et al., 1986a). The more positive pressure suggested that gas trapping may be occurring during hypoxia. Smith et al. (1989a,b), however, noted no increase in esophageal pressure in awake dogs, but did observe an increase in FRC. They speculated that there was a vagally mediated bronchodilation in the awake dog that prevented gas trapping and that possibly the increased postinspiratory inspiratory activity (PIIA) in hypocapnic hypoxia led to the increase in FRC. Increased FRC has also been observed during hypoxic gas breathing in humans (Gautier et al., 1976; Saunders et al., 1977).

Hypoxic stimulation of breathing also has a different effect on expiratory muscle recruitment compared with hypercapnia (St. John, 1981; Sears et al., 1982). Indeed, during hypocapnic hypoxia, expiratory muscle activity is not apparent until ventilation increases to three to five times above eupneic levels in awake dogs (Smith et al., 1989b). In comparison, hypercapnia and isocapnic hypoxia resulted in a prompt increase in expiratory muscle activity, and there was an attendant reduction in FRC. Therefore, during hypercapnia, each inspiration was begun at a lung volume below FRC, because at end expiration, the expiratory muscles reduced lung volume below FRC. As a result, therefore, early inspiration may be passive owing to chest wall recoil. However, the rate of relaxation of expiratory muscle contraction and the subsequent chest wall recoil is slow (Smith et al., 1989a; Road and Leevers, 1990). The reduction in expiratory muscle activity during hypocapnic hypoxia may be related to the hypocapnia per se, rather than hypoxia, as carotid body stimulation alone without hypocapnia led to expiratory muscle recruitment similar to that of hypercapnia (Saupe et al., 1992). This result suggests that it is not the hypoxia that reduces expiratory muscle activation, but rather, the attendant hypocapnia. These observations support the conceptual framework of shifts in expiratory and inspiratory activity, dependent on the underlying chemical drive proposed by Sears (1990).

Smith et al. (1989b) also found that the rib cage and abdominal expiratory muscles may contract independently in awake dogs during stimulated breathing. Loss of expiratory activity in either the rib cage or abdominal expiratory muscles may distort the chest wall. For example, isolated contraction of the rib cage expiratory muscles leads to distortion of the chest wall so that, for any given lung volume, diaphragmatic length is reduced (Road et al., 1991b); hence, the diaphragm is less effective as a pressure generator.

In sum, the type of chemoreceptor activation can significantly influence the relative amount of activity of the inspiratory and expiratory muscles, end-expiratory lung volume, and the chest wall configuration. The optimization of gas exchange during hypoxia produced by an increase in FRC must be weighed against the potential impairment of inspiratory muscle function produced by the increase in FRC and increased velocity of contraction.

VI. Reflex Effects from Muscles of the Limbs and Chest Wall

A. Spinal Somatic Reflexes

Spinal effects of afferents from chest wall proprioceptors can inhibit or facilitate respiratory motoneurons, but do not alter respiratory timing. As mentioned in the introduction, if respiratory timing is altered, the reflex effect is termed supraspinal. In this section, spinal somatic reflexes will be described.

Proprioceptors within the chest wall, capable of affecting the muscles of the chest wall include the muscle spindles and golgi tendon organs. Both types of receptors are found within the rib cage muscles and the diaphragm. Muscle spindles respond to muscle stretch, and the tendon organ to muscle tension.

The reflex effects of chest wall afferent nerves have largely been determined by electrical stimulation. Electrical stimulation can activate many of the different nerve fiber groups. Selective activation of Group IA fibers—afferents from the primary endings—in the intercostal nerve produces a monosynaptic excitation of both inspiratory and expiratory thoracic motoneurons at the same spinal segment and adjacent segments (Downman, 1955; Eccles et al., 1962; Sears, 1964a,b; Kirkwood and Sears, 1982). No inhibition of antagonistic muscles (e.g., expiratory intercostal inhibition) following inspiratory muscle (external intercostal) nerve excitation at IA strength has been recorded. The intercostal muscle afferents are, thus, different from many limb muscle afferents where antagonistic muscles are reciprocally inhibited (Baldissera et al., 1981).

Muscle spindle afferents are active in the intercostal nerves during the breathing cycle. The mean amplitude of the single-fiber excitatory postsynaptic potential (EPSP) from all primary spindle afferents was measured at 171 μV (Kirkwood and Sears, 1982). It has been suggested that the combined input of single-fiber EPSPs (15 mV) to the thoracic motoneurons is not adequate to raise them to their firing threshold. It would therefore appear that the contribution of this excitatory input has to be combined with other inputs.

Reflex effects of tendon organ afferents (group IB fibers) have been difficult to study, as electrical stimulation of these higher threshold fibers inevitably activates IA fibers. However, electrical activation of nerve fibers with a threshold higher than IA fibers produced inhibition in expiratory motoneurons at the same spinal segment (Sears, 1964a,b). Cutaneous nerve afferents in the internal intercostal nerve with similar threshold may also have been activated.

The limited excitatory potential produced by muscle spindle afferents mentioned above should be contrasted with the recorded effects of thoracic dorsal root section on the response to inspiratory loading (Corda et al., 1965; Shannon and Zechman, 1972). These studies show that an increase in inspiratory intercostal muscle activity on the first loaded breath of anesthetized cats was eliminated by cutting the dorsal roots. Thus, when combined with other inputs to the motoneuron, intercostal afferents can raise thoracic motoneurons above their firing threshold. During eupnea, the results of dorsal root section have been conflicting; hence, a strong role for these afferents during eupnea is not established (Shannon, 1977; Speck and Webber, 1979). Interestingly, the diaphragm did not show a similar immediate load compensation in response to inspiratory loading (Corda et al., 1965). The factors that do bring respiratory motoneurons to their firing threshold include descending inputs from the dorsal and ventral respiratory groups (DRG and VRG), Bötzinger complex, central nonrespiratory-related areas, and inputs from spinal networks (including neighboring motoneurons and spinal interneurons), and spinal afferents (see Monteau and Hilaire (1991) for review). These additional inputs can thus combine or compete with the reflex effects of peripheral afferents.

A mechanism for gating peripheral inputs is important, because of potentially conflicting effects of activation of muscle spindle afferents from inspiratory and expiratory muscles during different breathing maneuvers or during postural change. One such gating mechanism is the slow potentials recorded from thoracic motoneurons. These potentials are both inspiratory and expiratory and are slow rhythmic changes in membrane potential that have been termed *central respiratory drive potentials* (CRDPs) (Sears, 1964b; Eccles et al., 1962). These potentials arise from a supraspinal source and during inspiration produce a depolarization of inspiratory motoneurons and a hyperpolarization of expiratory motoneurons (see Fig. 11). By this mechanism, expiratory excitation, for example, during inspiration, can be reduced.

How can these thoracic reflex pathways influence breathing in humans? Since the results from studies in the cat had shown that intercostal afferents can influence breathing during loading, studies have been performed during inspiratory loading

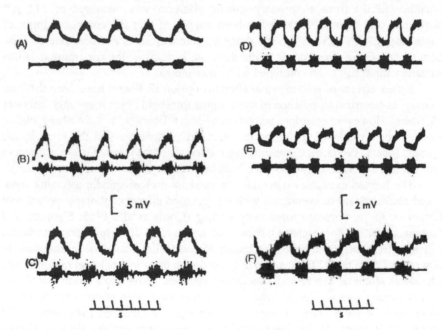

Figure 11   Central respiratory drive potentials (CRDPs) of inspiratory and expiratory motoneurons, identified by antidromic invasion from the external and internal intercostal nerve respectively. Upper traces, intracellular d.c. recordings from inspiratory and expiratory motoneurons; lower traces, electromyogram of the diaphragm. (A,B,C) inspiratory motoneurons; (D,E,F) expiratory motoneurons. Note the difference in amplification from the records from the two types of motoneuron. (Reprinted with permission from Sears, 1964b.)

in humans (Newsom Davis and Sears, 1970). In conscious humans intercostal EMG activity revealed an immediate inhibition (latency 22 ms) followed by an excitatory response (latency 50–60 ms) in response to a brief inspiratory load. In view of the relatively long latencies of the facilitatory effect, the only possible spinal effect was inhibitory and not consistent with a load-compensating reflex. No early facilitation was observed as has been commonly recorded in limb muscles.

In addition to the spinal segmental reflexes mentioned, a facilitatory intercostal-to-phrenic reflex has been described. This reflex does have supraspinal components. Group IB and II afferent nerve fibers in the internal intercostal nerve (T9–T13) and group II fibers in the external intercostal nerve appear to be involved (Downman, 1955; Decima et al., 1969; Remmers, 1973; Shannon, 1980).

Proprioception in the diaphragm is mainly due to the activity of Golgi tendon organs. No facilitation or segmental excitation from spindle afferents has been recorded in the diaphragm (Glebovskii, 1962; Sant'Ambrogio et al., 1962; Corda, Eklund and von Euler, 1965), and this is due to the paucity of muscle spindles in the diaphragm (Duron et al., 1978). Reflex effects at the spinal level are inhibitory on phrenic motoneuron activity (phrenic-to-phrenic reflex) (Gill and Kuno, 1963; Jammes et al., 1986; Rijlant, 1942; Speck and Revelette, 1987). Large diameter myelinated afferent nerves possibly tendon organs mediate the ipsilateral inhibition (Speck and Revelette, 1987). The contralateral inhibition of phrenic motoneuron activity, however, is mediated by Group III fibers, based on nerve conduction studies (Speck and Revelette, 1987).

Both phrenic and intercostal afferent nerves have central projections that can influence respiratory timing; supraspinal effects. These reflex pathways, as well as the spinal effects, will be discussed in more detail in the following chapters.

B. Reflex Effects from Contracting Muscles

The chest wall muscles are vigorously recruited during the hyperpnea of exercise; however, the stimulus for the hyperpnea has been a subject of some debate. Cross-circulation experiments showed that the return of blood from contracting muscle was not necessary for initiation of the hyperpnea (Kao and Ray, 1954). A neural reflex was postulated to produce the hyperpnea (Comroe and Schmidt, 1943; Asmussen et al., 1943). Subsequently, group III and group IV thin-fiber afferent nerves from contracting skeletal muscles were shown to form the afferent limb of a reflex pathway that stimulated breathing (Johansson, 1962; Kalia et al., 1972; Kaufman et al., 1983). The reflex hyperpnea occurred whether exercising muscles contract and shorten (Tibes, 1977), or contract isometrically. The ventilatory response, specifically the breathing pattern, could be altered, depending on how the reflex was activated. Rhythmic contractions produced a tachypnea with reduced T_E, whereas continuous isometric contractions produced an increase in tidal volume, rather than a change in timing (Tallarida et al., 1983). The reflex stimulation of ventilation produced by contracting muscle was associated with an increase in heart rate and mean arterial pressure and has been termed the exercise pressor reflex (McCloskey and Mitchell, 1972).

What factors activate thin-fiber afferents in contracting muscle? The afferents arise from polymodal receptors, free nerve endings on the surface of, and within, muscle (Stacey, 1969; Kumazawa and Mizumura, 1977). These receptors respond to a variety of stimuli: mechanical, chemical, and thermal (Kumazawa and Mizumura, 1976, 1977). Some of the receptors respond more to muscle contraction and were mainly innervated by group III fibers, whereas ischemic contractions activated receptors innervated by preponderantly group IV fibers (Mense and Stahnke, 1983). Recent observations (Duranti et al., 1991), have shown that activation of these afferents by ischemic muscle in awake humans produces a similar augmentation of ventilation.

Nerve afferents from contracting muscles have both spinal and supraspinal effects. These afferent nerves are distributed to multiple CNS locations (Iwamoto et al., 1985), and the effects on respiratory timing by activation of these afferents clearly indicates a supraspinal reflex. However, spinal phrenic motoneurons can be inhibited directly by activation of limb muscle afferents in cats (Eldridge et al., 1981). A reduction in phrenic motoneuron output has also been observed in the poststimulus period (i.e., after activation of thin-fiber limb muscle afferents; Waldrop et al., 1982). This reduction was attenuated by prior administration of naloxone (Waldrop et al., 1983), suggesting endogenous opioides, released in the CNS following stimulation, may have caused the poststimulus decrease in breathing. Endogenous opioides are known to depress ventilation (Shook et al., 1990).

The phrenic nerve, which also arises from a contracting muscle, the diaphragm, produces effects similar to activation of limb muscle afferents; namely, an excitatory effect on ventilation and a pressor effect (Fig. 12; Kohrman et al., 1947; Road et al., 1987; Revelette et al., 1988). Marlot and associates (1987) have also described an excitatory effect on ventilation after stimulation of myelinated thin-fiber afferents, but they also observed a short-term inhibition. Also, a poststimulus decrease in phrenic motoneuron output occurs after activation of these thin-fiber afferents from the diaphragm (Road et al., 1993). Therefore, activation of thin-fiber afferents in the phrenic nerve can produce a reflex excitation or inhibition of breathing. Since ventilatory timing is altered in the excitatory response, a supraspinal component is implied (Road et al., 1987). The role of these thin-fiber afferents and myelinated afferents is described in more detail in the forthcoming sections.

C. Reflex Effects in Response to Decreased Inspiratory Muscle Length

An increase in end-expiratory lung volume (EELV) is associated with a reduction in inspiratory muscle length. Lung volume increases following a change in posture from supine to upright, in a variety of obstructive lung diseases and following application of respiratory devices such as continuous positive airway pressure

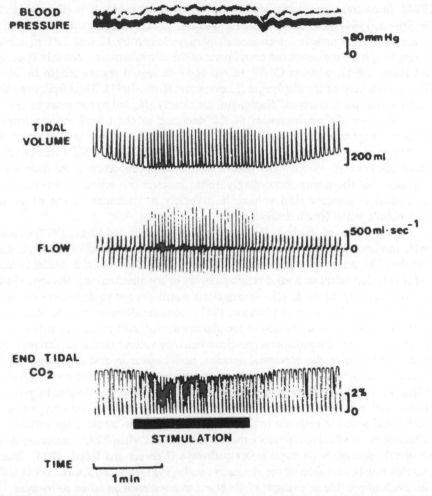

Figure 12 Example of stimulation of phrenic nerve, showing the maximum response in airflow, tidal volume, and blood pressure in one dog. With onset of stimulation (frequency 50 Hz, duration 1 ms, and voltage 60 times twitch threshold), these parameters increase over two to three breaths and at cessation of stimulation, subsequently decrease over two to three breaths. There was an associated reduction in end-tidal CO_2. (Reprinted with permission from Road et al., 1987.)

(CPAP). How are the muscles of the chest wall affected by an increase in EELV? It has been observed that the diaphragm shortens more than the major rib cage inspiratory muscles—the parasternal intercostal muscles—during lung inflation in dogs. Indeed the diaphragm length decreases by 30–40% of its resting length when lung volume increases from residual volume to total lung capacity (Newman et al.,

1984). In contrast, parasternal intercostal length decreases by 10% (Decramer and De Troyer, 1984). A shift in posture from supine to near upright, without activation of the abdominal muscles, decreased diaphragm length by 10 and 22% of supine resting length for the costal and crural parts of the diaphragm, respectively (Leevers and Road, 1991), whereas CPAP 18 cm H_2O decreased resting length by about 20% in both parts of the diaphragm (Leevers and Road, 1991). Therefore, the chest wall muscles, particularly the diaphragm, are clearly affected by increases in EELV.

What are the consequences of the decrease in chest wall muscle length? Reduced diaphragmatic length leads to a prompt reduction in diaphragmatic shortening at a time when activation of the muscle (ENG and EMG) was constant (Road and Leevers, 1988). Tidal volume decreased in proportion to the decrease in diaphragmatic shortening. Accordingly, reflex mechanisms acting on the chest wall are critical to preserve tidal volume in a variety of situations during which the diaphragm's initial length decreases.

In anesthetized (Bishop, 1964) and awake (Leevers and Road, 1993) quadrupeds, increases in EELV are associated with strong recruitment of the expiratory muscles. This recruitment preserves the diaphragm's initial length and tidal volume and is very dependent on a vagal reflex pathway in anesthetized cats (Bishop, 1964). The rib cage expiratory muscle—triangularis sterni—is not so dependent on vagal reflex pathways (DeTroyer and Ninane, 1987). Somatic afferents from the abdominal muscles, activated by distension of the abdomen, may also make a contribution to reflex activation of the abdominal muscles when lung volume increases (Davies et al., 1980). Furthermore, the intercostal muscles, both inspiratory and expiratory, can be tonically activated by reflex mechanisms arising from the labyrinth and cerebellum (Massion, 1976). All of the foregoing mechanisms can also be activated by postural change and will tend to maintain the length of the chest wall muscles and their mechanical action in response to the increase in EELV. In awake dogs without the influence of anesthesia, expiratory muscle recruitment when EELV increases is not absolutely dependent on vagal reflex pathways (Leevers and Road, 1995). These muscles may be recruited by the alternative pathways mentioned above. These latter observations provide an example of the effect of anesthesia on reflex pathways.

An alternative reflex mechanism preserving diaphragmatic shortening when its initial length decreases is an immediate reflex increase in diaphragmatic EMG activity (Banzett et al., 1981). Such a reflex has been termed an "operating-length" compensating reflex. In anesthetized dogs or cats this reflex has not been apparent (Iscoe, 1989; Road and Leevers, 1988), as increases in EELV are not associated with an immediate increase in diaphragmatic activation (Fig. 13), and there is no preservation of tidal volume. However, T_I has been prolonged following increased EELV in vagotomized, spinalized cats, suggesting that a supraspinal reflex through phrenic afferents can have some effect on tidal volume (Fryman and Frazier, 1987). This reflex affects inspiration by an increase in T_I, not in increase in the rate of rise of phrenic activity.

What mechanisms preserve tidal volume in humans following an increase in

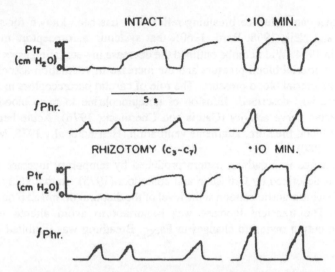

Figure 13 First-breath and steady-state responses to application of an expiratory threshold load of 10 cm H$_2$O in a cat with intact cervical dorsal roots (top) and after section of dorsal roots C3–C7 (bottom). Onset of load is indicated by upward deflection of tracheal pressure (Ptr). ʃPhr, integrated phrenic activity. (Reprinted with permission from Iscoe, 1989.)

EELV? One mechanism that could defend tidal volume at increased end-expiratory lung volume is activation of the expiratory muscles, as occurs in quadrupeds. In awake and sleeping humans, however, there is no activation of the expiratory muscles in response to increased EELV, unless the individual hyperventilates (Wakai et al., 1992). Tonic activation of abdominal muscles does occur in humans with postural change (Floyd and Silver, 1950; DeTroyer et al., 1983), but has not been demonstrated after an increase in end-expiratory lung volume alone. Increased activation of the inspiratory muscles, evidenced by a progressive increase in tidal volume in response to increased EELV, can occur over time in sleeping subjects, probably in response to increased Pa$_{CO_2}$ (Hamilton et al., 1990). Thus, a gradual increase in activation of inspiratory muscles in response to increased chemical drive appears to be the main mechanism compensating for increased lung volume in humans. Immediate increases in inspiratory EMG have not been been definitively documented, possibly because of problems encountered with reliably recording EMG of the diaphragm when lung volume increases (Gandevia and McKenzie, 1986).

VII. Reflex Effects from Cardiovascular Afferents

The interaction between the heart and lungs is described elsewhere in this text. There are, however, well-recognized reflexes arising from the heart or vascular structures that can influence breathing reflexly. It has been known for some time (Heymans and Neil, 1958; Bard, 1960), that systemic baroreceptors may inhibit breathing. In 1964, Widdicombe outlined the decrease in ventilation associated with elevations in arterial blood pressure and the increase in ventilation associated with reductions in arterial blood pressure. The role of carotid baroreceptors in mediating this response was described. Infusion of norepinephrine to raise blood pressure inhibits phrenic nerve activity (Garcia and Cherniack, 1976). Acute hemorrhage, with loss of blood pressure, augments ventilation (Heistad et al., 1975; Miserocchi and Quinn, 1980).

The change in breathing pattern produced by temporary increase in arterial pressure was described by Grunstein and coauthors (1975). In that study, transient inflation of an intra-aortic balloon at the level of the diaphragm, raised blood pressure transiently. The transient increase was important to avoid altered respiratory motoneuron output owing to changes in Pa_{CO_2}. Breathing was inhibited (Fig. 14).

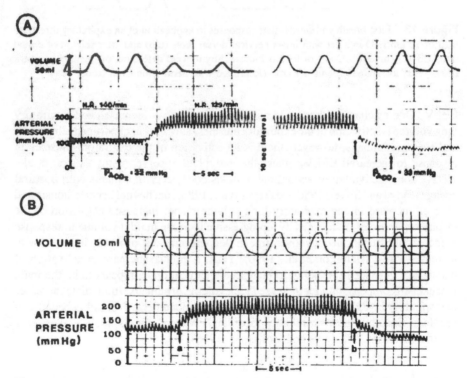

Figure 14   (A) Record of lung volume and brachial artery pressure in a cat breathing 100% O_2. Point b, inflation of aortic balloon catheter. Point c, deflation of aortic balloon catheter. Note 10-s gap in record during aortic obstruction. (B) Same cat as in A following bilateral sinus nerve section. Arrows at a and b represent point of aortic balloon inflation and deflation, respectively. (Reprinted with permission from Grunstein et al.)

Transient hypertension produced a decrease in tidal volume and an increase in T_I and T_E. Concomitant activation of the expiratory muscles was recorded, and this activation was removed by section of the carotid sinus nerves. The changes in breathing pattern were attributed to baroreceptor stimulation. Indeed Bishop (1974) showed that bilateral occlusion of the common carotid artery and a concomitant increase in baroreceptor firing rate resulted in an increase in diaphragmatic and abdominal expiratory activity, whereas saline distension of the carotid sinus produced a reduction in diaphragmatic and abdominal EMG activity. Therefore, although these authors agreed on the effects of baroreceptor activity on inspiratory activity, the effects on expiratory activity were opposite. In the latter experiments, however, expiratory muscle activity was stimulated by positive-pressure breathing at baseline, and this may have influenced the results.

The abdominal muscles may have an important role to play during hypotension. Occlusion of the ascending aorta before the carotid arteries produces an immediate reduction in expiratory muscle activity (Youmans et al., 1963). This reduction was then followed by a gradual increase in expiratory muscle activity. Indeed, Youmans et al. (1963) showed that occlusion of the inferior vena cava produced an immediate augmentation of expiratory activity. They concluded that reduced intravascular pressure between the postcaval vein and the ascending aorta led to activation of expiratory muscles. This activation of expiratory muscles, the so-called abdominal compression reflex, may be an important mechanism to attempt to restore right-sided cardiac-filling pressures during hypotension. These results may also explain why expiratory muscle activity increased in the study of Grunstein et al. (1975), because venous return would eventually have been markedly impaired by aortic occlusion and Youmans et al. (1963) demonstrated that, although expiratory muscle activity was initially inhibited by aortic occlusion, it slowly increased above control with time.

Most of the foregoing studies have explored the effects of transient increases or decreases in arterial pressure. The response to sustained increases or decreases in arterial pressure has recently been studied by Grundy and co-workers (1986). They controlled Pa_{CO_2} and observed a 28% reduction in phrenic nerve activity when mean arterial pressure showed a substantial increase from 114 to 167 mm Hg, and a 22% increase in phrenic nerve activity when mean arterial pressure decreased from 128 to 82 mm Hg (Figs. 15 and 16). Thus, these reflex responses are maintained over time. Because of the changes in breathing pattern, a supraspinal effect is implied. It is well known that the brain stem areas for cardiovascular and respiratory control are in close proximity in the brain stem (Jordan and Spyer, 1986), and these observations may be a manifestation of this proximity.

Intracardiac sensory receptors have been described of several types (Coleridge et al., 1964). Stimulation of thin-fiber afferents—sympathetic afferents—from the heart produce tachypnea (Uchida, 1976). Kostreva et al. (1979) reported that left atrial distension or stretch produced tachypnea. Subsequent studies by Lloyd (1986, 1990) have demonstrated that increased left atrial pressure elicits tachypnea in dogs.

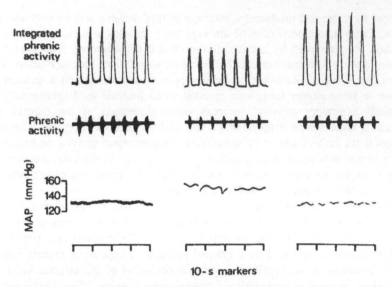

Figure 15   The changes induced by an infusion of angiotensin II 150 μg kg^{-1} min^{-1} on mean arterial pressure and phrenic nerve activity; each recording during a steady state. (Reprinted with permission from Grundy et al., 1986.)

The tachypnea was mediated by myelinated afferents in this isolated heart model. The increase in left atrial pressure required to produce this reflex was about 20 cm H_2O and, therefore, this reflex may be activated in left ventricular failure or mitral stenosis, for example. Distension of the left ventricle alone produced a depression of ventilation (Kostreva et al., 1979).

VIII.   Chest Wall Muscle Activation During Vomiting

The pattern of activation of chest wall muscles during vomiting is characteristic and reproducible. Activation occurs in a coordinated manner. In both the retching and expulsive phase, the diaphragm, external intercostal, and abdominal muscles contract. A series of bursts of EMG activity is seen in these muscles. The internal intercostals are activated out of phase with these bursts of EMG activity during the retching phase and are not activated in expulsion. As a result, during retching, the rib cage expiratory muscles are activated out of phase with the abdominal expiratory muscles (McCarthy and Borison, 1974). In the expulsive phase, expiratory activity in the internal intercostal nerve is absent, but expiratory activity in the abdominal muscles strengthens. Therefore, the expiratory muscles of the rib cage and abdomen are dissociated, which mechanically should aid vomiting. Although the diaphragm remains active in the expulsive phase, it is displaced into the chest (McCarthy et al.,

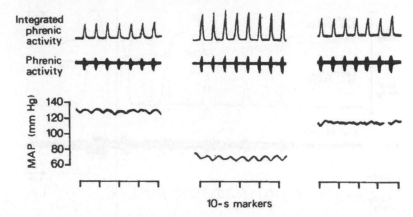

Figure 16 The changes induced by an infusion of sodium nitroprusside 200 μg kg^{-1} min^{-1} on mean arterial pressure and phrenic nerve activity; each recording during a steady state. (Reprinted with permission from Grundy et al., 1986.)

1974) and intra-abdominal and intrathoracic pressure become extremely positive, up to 300 cm H_2O (Fig. 17). As mentioned previously, the crural part of the diaphragm becomes inactive during the expulsive phase of vomiting (Monges et al., 1978).

Recordings from expiratory bulbospinals in the brain stem during fictive vomiting reveal some cells active in-phase with the diaphragm and some out of phase (Miller et al., 1987). The out-of-phase cells represent the rib cage expiratory muscles (internal intercostal nerve; Fig. 18), which contract out of phase with the other expiratory muscles (the abdominal muscles).

Vomiting is usually produced by stimulation of the subdiaphragmatic vagus nerve or by chemical stimulation of the emetic center. In either event, activation of this reflex produces a coordinated pattern of chest wall muscle activation. The pattern generator in the CNS which produces this behavior is thought to consist of a network of inspiratory and expiratory respiratory neurons (Miller and Ezure, 1991). Some of these neurons are also active during other respiratory-related behavior such as coughing (Jakus et al., 1985) and sneezing (Batsel and Lines, 1978). Furthermore, during vomiting the phrenic motoneurons activated are similar to those active during breathing (Milano et al., 1992). The difference is that their discharge rates increase considerably.

IX. Chest Wall Muscle Activity During Coughing and Sneezing

Coughing and sneezing are two important airway defense mechanisms that incorporate the chest wall muscles in a coordinated act. The afferent pathways initiating coughing will be described elsewhere in this text. Sneezing can be induced by a

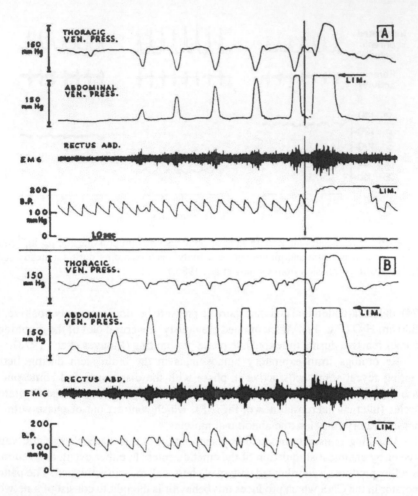

Figure 17 Effect of tracheostomy on thoracic and abdominal pressure changes during retching and expulsion: (A) tracheostomy closed; (B) tracheostomy open. Circumventing glottis markedly reduced negative thoracic pressure pulses and increased positive abdominal pressure pulses during retching, but had little effect on thoracic pressure wave during expulsion. LIM marks the channel-recording limit. (Reprinted with permission from McCarthy et al., 1974.)

wide range of stimuli (Korpas and Tomori, 1980). Stimuli applied to the nasal mucosa appear most effective (Brubaker, 1919; Malcolmson, 1959). Electrical stimulation of the ethmoidal and nasal branches of the trigeminal nerve can produce sneezing (Batsel and Lines, 1975; Wallois et al., 1991).

Much like vomiting, the act of sneezing or coughing is thought to involve a CNS pattern generator involving inspiratory and expiratory respiratory neurons

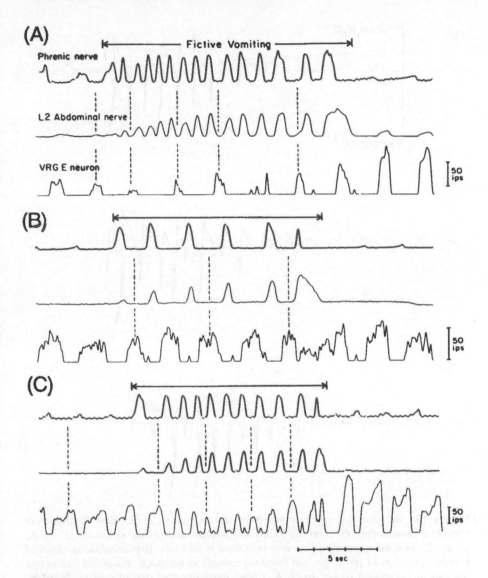

Figure 18 Examples of three ventral respiratory group (VRG) expiratory (E) neurons that, during fictive vomiting, were most active between bursts of abdominal and phrenic nerve coactivation (INT neurons). All three of these neurons were classified as having a step–ramp-augmenting firing pattern. The VRG expiratory neurons fired out of phase with the abdominal nerve and represented expiratory neurons believed to be innervating the internal intercostal muscles. (Reprinted with permission from Miller et al., 1987.)

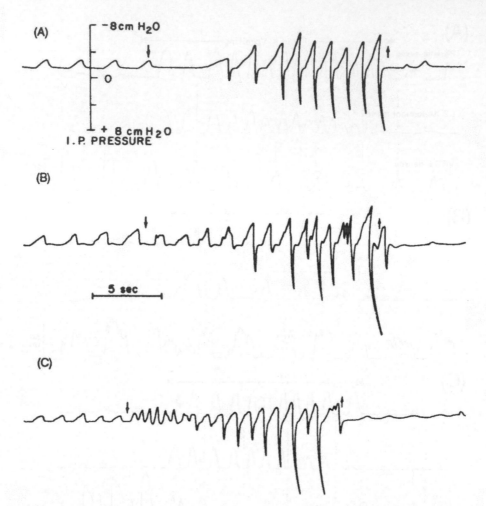

Figure 19 Intrapleural pressure recordings of sneezes induced by electrical stimulation of ethmoidal nerve in three different cats. Time and pressure calibrations were same in cats A, B, and C. Inspiration (negative pressure) is upward in all cases. Repetitive stimulations of ethmoidal nerve at 17 Hz, 10 μs, and threshold strength was begun at downward arrows and discontinued at upward arrows. In cat A, a brief apnea preceded start of sneezes. In cat B, diminished inspiratory excursions preceded sneezes. In cat C, a rapid series of inspirations preceded start of sneezing. In all of these cases, intensity of active expiration was incrementing as stimulation was continued. (Reprinted with permission from Miller and Ezure, 1991.)

(Miller and Ezure, 1991). A sequence of chest wall activation occurs with coughing and sneezing. Coughing and sneezing are preceded by a deep inspiration that lengthens the expiratory muscles, allowing greater expiratory pressure generation (Fig. 19). Glottic closure occurs, and this is followed by intense expiratory muscle activity—a compressive phase—followed by opening of the glottis and the rapid exhalation of air—expulsive phase. In humans, intrathoracic pressures during compression are usually 80–120 cm H_2O, but can reach 250 cm H_2O. The deep inspiration preceding the cough or sneeze appears to be accentuated by a vagal inflation reflex, activated by the deep inspiration (Bucher, 1958). Bucher (1958) thought that the vagal inflation reflex enhanced the subsequent expiration during cough. However, Widdicomb (1964) pointed out that additional mechanisms were needed to explain this effect, including stretch reflexes from the chest wall muscles and the mechanical advantage given to the expiratory muscles by the preceding deep inspiration. Inspiratory activity in the diaphragm during vomiting was accomplished by increased firing frequency of units that were already active during breathing. Similarly, during coughing, the phrenic motoneurons that were already active are recruited more vigorously (Milano et al., 1992).

The expiratory act during sneezing differs slightly, compared with coughing. The pharynx is constricted during exhalation with the sneeze and the expiratory airflow, therefore, is directed through the nose as well as the mouth (Brubaker, 1919; Birch, 1959).

References

Adrian, E. D. (1933). Afferent impulses in the vagus and their effect on respiration. *J. Physiol. (Lond.)* 79: 332–358.

Agostoni, E., Campbell, E. J. M., and Freedman, S. (1970). Energetics. In: *The Respiratory Muscles*, Edited by E. J. M. Campbell, E. Agostoni, and J. Newsom-Davis. London, Lloyd-Luke, pp. 115–137.

Ainsworth, D. M., Smith, C. A., Johnson, B. D., Eicker, S. W., Henderson, K. S., and Dempsey, J. A. (1992). Vagal contributions to respiratory muscle activity during eupnea in the awake dog. *J. Appl. Physiol.* 72: 1355–1361.

Albano, J. P., and Garnier, L. (1983). Bulbo-spinal respiratory effects originating from the splanchnic afferents. *Respir. Physiol.* 51: 229–239.

Alexander, W. F. (1940). The innervation of the biliary system. *J. Comp. Neurol.* 72: 357–370.

Altschuler, S. M., Boyle, J. T., Nixon, T. E., Pack, A. I., and Cohen, S. (1985). Simultaneous reflex inhibition of lower esophageal sphincter and crural diaphragm in cats. *Am. J. Physiol.* 249: C586–C591.

Arita, H., and Bishop, B. (1983). Responses of cat's internal intercostal motor units to hypercapnia and lung inflation. *J. Appl. Physiol.* 54: 375–386.

Armstrong, D. J., and Luck, J. C. (1974). A comparative study of irritant and type J receptors in the cat. *Respir. Physiol.* 21: 47–60.

Asmussen, E., Nielsen, M., and Wieth-Pederson, G. (1943). On the regulation of circulation during muscular work. *Acta Physiol. Scand.* 6: 353–358.

Badier, M., Jammes, Y., Romero-Colomer, P., and Lemerre, C. (1989). Tonic activity in inspiratory muscles and phrenic motoneurons by stimulation of vagal afferents. *J. Appl. Physiol.* 66: 1613–1619.

Bajic, J., Zuperku, E. J., Tonkovic-Capin, M., and Hopp, F. A. (1992). Expiratory bulbospinal neurons of dogs. I. Control of discharge patterns of pulmonary stretch receptors. *Am. J. Physiol.* 262: R1075–R1086.

Baker, J. P., Jr., Frazier, D. T., Hanley, M., and Zechman, F. W. (1979a). Behavior of expiratory neurons in response to mechanical and chemical loading. *Respir. Physiol.* 36: 337–351.

Baker, J. P., Remmers, J. E., and Younes, M. K. (1979b). Graded inspiratory inhibition: Specific effects of flow rate. *J. Appl. Physiol.* 46: 669–674.

Baldissera, F., Hultborn, H., and Illert, M. (1981). Integration in spinal neuronal systems. In: *Handbook of Physiology*, Section 1. Motor Control, Vol. II, Part 1. Edited by J. M. Brookhart, and V. B. Mountcastle. Bethesda, MD, American Physiological Society, pp. 509–595.

Banzett, R. B., Inbar, G. F., Brown, R., Goldman, M., Rossier, A., and Mead, J. (1981). Diaphragm electrical activity during negative lower torso pressure in quadriplegic men. *J. Appl. Physiol.* 51: 660–664.

Bard, P. (1960). Anatomical organization of the central nervous system in relation to the control of the heart and blood vessels. *Physiol. Rev.* 35: 247–300.

Bartlett, D., Jr. (1971). Origin and regulation of spontaneous deep breaths. *Respir. Physiol.* 12: 230–238.

Bartlett, D., Jr., and St. John, W. M. (1988). Influence of lung volume on phrenic, hypoglossal and mylohyoid nerve activities. *Respir. Physiol.* 73: 97–110.

Bartoli, A., Cross, B. A., Guz, A., Huszczuk, A., and Jefferies, R. (1975). The effect of varying tidal volume on the associated phrenic motoneurone output: Studies of vagal and chemical feedback. *Respir. Physiol.* 25: 135–155.

Batsel, H. L., and Lines, A. J. (1975). Neural mechanisms of sneeze. *Am. J. Physiol.* 229: 770–776.

Batsel, H. L., and Lines, A. J. (1978). Discharge of respiratory neurons in sneezes resulting from ethmoidal nerve stimulation. *Exp. Neurol.* 58: 410–424.

Begle, R. L., and Skatrud, J. B. (1990). Hyperinflation and expiratory muscle recruitment during NREM sleep in humans. *Respir. Physiol.* 82: 47–64.

Bellemare, F., Bono, D., and D'Angelo, E. (1991). Electrical and mechanical output of the expiratory muscles in anesthetized dogs. *Respir. Physiol.* 84: 171–183.

Bendixen, H. H., Smith, G. M., and Mead, J. (1964). Pattern of ventilation in young adults. *J. Appl. Physiol.* 19: 195–198.

Bianchi, A. L., and Barillot, J. C. (1975). Activity of medullary respiratory neurones during reflexes from the lungs in cats. *Respir. Physiol.* 25: 335–352.

Birch, A. C. (1959). Sneezing. *Practitioner* 182: 122–124.

Bishop, B. (1964). Reflex control of abdominal muscles during positive pressure breathing. *J. Appl. Physiol.* 19: 224–232.

Bishop, B. (1974). Carotid baroreceptor modulation of diaphragm and abdominal muscle activity in the cat. *J. Appl. Physiol.* 36: 12–19.

Bishop, B., and Bachofen, H. (1972). Vagal control of ventilation and respiratory muscles during elevated pressures in the cat. *J. Appl. Physiol.* 32: 103–112.

Bjurstedt, H. (1953). Influence of the abdominal muscle tone on the circulatory response to positive pressure breathing in anesthetized dogs. *Acta Physiol. Scand.* 29: 145–162.

Bouverot, P., and Fitzgerald, R. S. (1969). Role of arterial chemoreceptors in controlling lung volume in the dog. *Respir. Physiol.* 7: 203–215.

Bouverot, P., Crance, J. P., and Dejours, P. (1970). Factors influencing the intensity of the Breuer–Hering inspiration-inhibiting reflex. *Respir. Physiol.* 8: 376–384.

Bradley, G. W., Noble, M. I. M., and Trenchard, D. (1976). The direct effect of pulmonary stretch receptor discharge produced by changing lung carbon dioxide concentration in dogs on cardiopulmonary bypass and its action on breathing. *J. Physiol. (Lond.)* 261: 359–373.

Brice, A. G., Forster, H. V., Pan, L. G., Lowry, T. F., Murphy, C. L., and Mead, J. (1991). Effects of increased end-expiratory lung volume on breathing in awake ponies. *J. Appl. Physiol.* 70: 715–725.

Brouillette, R. T., and Thach, B. T. (1979). A neuromuscular mechanism maintaining extrathoracic airway patency. *J. Appl. Physiol.* 46: 772–779.

Brubaker, A. (1919). The physiology of sneezing. *JAMA* 73: 585–587.

Bucher, K. (1958). Pathophysiology and pharmacology of cough. *Pharmacol. Rev.* 10: 43–58.

Cherniack, N. S., and Altose, M. D. (1981). Respiratory responses to ventilatory loading. In: *The Regulation of Breathing*. New York, Marcel Dekker, pp. 905–964.

Cherniack, N. S., von Euler, C., Glogowska, M., and Homma, I. (1981). Characteristics and rate of occurrence of spontaneous and provoked augmented breaths. *Acta Physiol. Scand.* 111: 349–360.

Clark, F. J., and von Euler, C. (1972). On the regulation of depth and rate of breathing. *J. Physiol. (Lond.)* 222: 267–295.

Clifford, P. S., Litzow, J. T., and Coon, R. L. (1987). Pulmonary depressor reflex elicited by capsaicin in conscious intact and lung-denervated dogs. *Am. J. Physiol.* 252: R394–R397.

Cohen, M. I., Feldman, J. L., and Sommer, D. (1985). Caudal medullary expiratory neuron and internal intercostal nerve discharges in the cat: Effects of lung inflation. *J. Physiol. (Lond.)* 368: 147–178.

Cohen, M. I., See, W. R., Sica, A. L., and Moss, I. R. (1986). Influence of central nervous system state on inspiratory facilitation by pulmonary afferents. In: *Neurobiology of the Control of Breathing*. Edited by C. von Euler and H. Lagercrantz. New York, Raven Press, pp. 251–256.

Coleridge, J. C. G., and Coleridge, H. M. (1984). Afferent vagal C-fibre innervation of the lungs and airways and its functional significance. *Rev. Physiol. Biochem. Pharmacol.* 99: 1–110.

Coleridge, H. M., and Coleridge, J. C. G. (1986). Reflexes evoked from tracheobronchial tree and lungs. In *Handbook of Physiology*. Section 3. The Respiratory System, Vol. II. Edited by A. P. Fishman. Baltimore, MD, Williams & Wilkins, pp. 395–429.

Coleridge, H. M., Coleridge, J. C. G., and Kidd, C. (1964). Cardiac receptors in the dog, with particular reference to two types of afferent ending in the ventricular wall. *J. Physiol. (Lond.)* 174: 323–339.

Comroe, J. H., Jr., and Schmidt, C. F. (1943). Reflexes from limbs as a factor in the hyperpnea of muscular exercise. *Am. J. Physiol.* 138: 536–547.

Corda, M., Eklund, G., and von Euler, C. (1965). External intercostal and phrenic α motor responses to changes in respiratory load. *Acta Physiol. Scand.* 63: 391–400.

Cross, B. A., Jones, P. W., and Guz, A. (1980). The role of vagal afferent information during inspiration in determining phrenic motorneuron output. *Respir. Physiol.* 39: 149–167.

D'Angelo, E., and Agostoni, E. (1975). Tonic vagal influences on inspiratory duration. *Respir. Physiol.* 24: 287–302.

Davies, A., Sant'Ambrogio, F. B., and Sant'Ambrogio, G. (1981). Onset of inspiration in rabbits during artificial ventilation. *J. Physiol. (Lond.)* 318: 17–23.

Davies, A., Dixon, M., Callanan, D., Huszczuk, A., Widdicombe, J. G., and Wise, J. C. M. (1978). Lung reflexes in rabbits during pulmonary stretch receptor block by sulphur dioxide. *Respir. Physiol.* 34: 83–101.

Davies, A., Sant'Ambrogio, F. B., and Sant'Ambrogio, G. (1980). Control of postural changes of end expiratory volume (FRC) by airways slowly adapting mechanoreceptors. *Respir. Physiol.* 41: 211–216.

De Troyer, A., and Ninane, U. (1987). Effect of posture on expiratory muscle use during breathing in the dog. *Respir. Physiol.* 67: 311–322.

De Troyer, A., and Rosso, J. (1982). Reflex inhibition of the diaphragm by esophageal afferents. *Neurosci. Lett.* 30: 43–46.

De Troyer, A., Sampson, M., Sigrist, S., and Kelly, S. (1983). How the abdominal muscles act on the rib cage. *J. Appl. Physiol.* 54: 465–469.

De Troyer, A., Gilmartin, J. J., and Ninane, V. (1989). Abdominal muscle use during breathing in unanesthetized dogs. *J. Appl. Physiol.* 66: 20–27.

Decima, E., von Euler, C., and Thoden, C. (1969). Intercostal-to-phrenic reflexes in the spinal cat. *Acta Physiol. Scand.* 75: 568–579.

Decramer, M., and De Troyer, A. (1984). Respiratory changes in parasternal intercostal length. *J. Appl. Physiol.* 57: 1254–1260.

Dimarco, A. F., von Euler, C., Romaniuk, J. R., and Yamamoto, Y. (1981). Positive feedback facilitation of external intercostal and phrenic inspiratory activity by pulmonary stretch receptors. *Acta Physiol. Scand.* 113: 375–386.

Downman, C. B. B. (1955). Skeletal muscle reflexes of splanchnic and intercostal nerve origin in acute spinal and decerebrate cats. *J. Neurophysiol.* 18: 217–235.

Duranti, R., Pantaleo, T., Bellini, F., Bongianni, F., Scano, G. (1991). Respiratory responses induced by activation of somatic nociceptive afferents in humans. *J. Appl. Physiol.* 71: 2440–2448.

Duron, B., Jung-Caillol, M. C., and Marlot, D. (1978). Myelinated nerve supply and muscle spindles in the respiratory muscles of cat: Quantitative study. *Anat. Embryol.* 152: 171–192.

Eccles, R. M., Sears, T. A., and Shealy, C. N. (1962). Intracellular recording from respiratory motoneurons of the thoracic spinal cord of the cat. *Nature* 193: 844–846.

Eldridge, F. L., Gil-Kumar, P., Millhorn, D. E., and Waldrop, T. G. (1981). Spinal inhibition of phrenic motoneurons by stimulation of afferents from peripheral muscles. *J. Physiol. (Lond.)* 311: 67–79.

Farber, J. P. (1982). Pulmonary receptor discharge and expiratory muscle activity. *Respir. Physiol.* 47: 219–229.

Farkas, G. A., and De Troyer, A. (1989). Effects of midline laparotomy on expiratory muscle activation in anesthetized dogs. *J. Appl. Physiol.* 67: 599–605.

Farkas, G. A., and Rochester, D. F. (1988). Functional characteristics of canine costal and crural diaphragm. *J. Appl. Physiol.* 65: 2253–2260.

Farkas, G. A., and Schroeder, M. A. (1990). Mechanical role of expiratory muscles during breathing in prone anesthetized dogs. *J. Appl. Physiol.* 69: 2137–2142.

Farkas, G. A., Baer, R. E., Estenne, M., and De Troyer, A. (1988). Mechanical role of expiratory muscles during breathing in upright dogs. *J. Appl. Physiol.* 64: 1060–1067.

Fitzgerald, R. S. (1973). Relationships between tidal volume and phrenic nerve activity during hypercapnic and hypoxia. *Acta Neurobiol. Exp.* 33: 419–425.

Floyd, K, and Morrison, J. F. B. (1974). Splanchnic mechanoreceptors in the dog. *Q. J. Exp. Physiol.* 59: 361–366.

Floyd, W. F., and Silver, P. H. S. (1950). Electromyographic study of patterns of activity of the anterior abdominal wall muscles in man. *J. Anat.* 84: 132–145.

Ford, G. T., Whitelaw, W. A., Rosenal, T. W., Cruse, P. J., and Guenter, C. A. (1983). Diaphragm function after upper abdominal surgery in humans. *Am. Rev. Respir. Dis.* 127: 431–436.

Ford, G. T., Grant, D. A., Rideout, K. S., Davison, J. S., and Whitelaw, W. A. (1988). Inhibition of breathing associated with gallbladder stimulation in dogs. *J. Appl. Physiol.* 65: 72–79.

Fregosi, R. F., Bartlett, D., Jr., and St. John, W. M. (1990). Influence of phasic volume feedback on abdominal expiratory nerve activity. *Respir. Physiol.* 82: 189–200.

Fryman, D. L., and Frazier, D. T. (1987). Diaphragm afferent modulation of phrenic motor drive. *J. Appl. Physiol.* 62: 2436–2441.

Gandevia, S. C., and McKenzie, D. K. (1986). Human diaphragmatic EMG: Changes with lung volume and posture during supramaximal phrenic stimulation. *J. Appl. Physiol.* 60: 1420–1428.

Garcia, A., and Cherniack, N. S. (1976). Integrated phrenic activity in hypercapnia and hypoxia. *Anesthesiology* 28: 1029–1035.

Gautier, H. (1969). Effets comparés de stimulations respiratories spécifiques et de l'activité mentale sur la forme due spirogramme de l'homme. *J. Physiol. (Paris)* 61: 31–44.

Gautier, H. (1976). Pattern of breathing during hypoxia or hypercapnia of the awake or anesthetized cat. *Respir. Physiol.* 27: 193–206.

Gautier, H., Remmers, J. E., Bartlet, D., Jr. (1973). Control of the duration of expiration. *Respir. Physiol.* 18: 205–221.

Gautier, H., Bonora, M., and Gaudy, J. H. (1981). Breuer–Hering inflation reflex and breathing pattern in anesthetized humans and cats. *J. Appl. Physiol.* 51: 1162–1168.

Gill, P. K., and Kuno, M. (1963). Excitatory and inhibitory actions on phrenic motoneurons. *J. Physiol.* 168: 274–289.

Glebovskii, V. D. (1962). Stretch receptors of the diaphragm. *Fiziol. Zhur. SSSR* 48: 545 [Trans. in *Fed. Proc.* (1963). 22(2): T405–T410.]

Glogowska, M., Richardson, P. S., Widdicombe, J. G., and Winning, A. J. (1972). The role of the vagus nerves, peripheral chemoreceptors and other afferent pathways in the genesis of augmented breaths in cats and rabbits. *Respir. Physiol.* 16: 179–196.

Green, J. F., and Kaufman, M. P. (1990). Pulmonary afferent control of breathing as end-expiratory lung volume decreases. *J. Appl. Physiol.* 68: 2186–2194.

Grundy, E. M., Chakrabarti, M. K., and Whitwam, J. G. (1986). Effect of phrenic nerve activity during induced changes in arterial pressure. *Br. J. Anaesth.* 58: 1414–1421.

Grunstein, M. M., Derenne, J. P., and Milic-Emili, J. (1975). Control of depth and frequency of breathing during baroreceptor stimulation in cats. *J. Appl. Physiol.* 39: 395–404.

Hamilton, R. D., Winning, A. J., Horner, R. L., and Guz, A. (1988). The effect of lung inflation on breathing in man during wakefulness and sleep. *Respir. Physiol.* 73: 145–154.

Hamilton, R. D., Horner, R. L., Winning, A. J., and Guz, A. (1990). Effect on breathing of raised end-expiratory lung volume in sleeping laryngectomized man. *Respir. Physiol.* 81: 87–98.

Hargreaves, M., Ravi, K., and Kappagoda, C. T. (1991). Responses of slowly and rapidly adapting receptors in the airways of rabbits to changes in the Starling forces. *J. Physiol. (Lond.)* 432: 81–97.

Haxhiu, M. A., van Lunteren, E., Deal, E. C., and Cherniack, N. S. (1988). Effect of stimulation of pulmonary C-fiber receptors on canine respiratory muscles. *J. Appl. Physiol.* 65: 1087–1092.

Heistad, D. D., Abboud, F. M., Mark, A. L., and Schnied, P. G. (1975). Effect of baroreceptor activity on ventilatory response to chemoreceptor stimulation. *J. Appl. Physiol.* 39: 411–416.

Heymans, C., and Neil, E. (1958). *Reflexogenic Areas of the Cardiovascular System.* London, J. A. Churchill, p. 95.

Hollstien, S. B., Carl, M. L., Schelegle, E. S., and Green, J. F. (1991). Role of vagal afferents in the control of abdominal expiratory muscle activity in the dog. *J. Appl. Physiol.* 71: 1795–1800.

Holmes, H. R., and Remmers, J. E. (1989). Stimulation of vagal C-fibers alters timing and distribution of respiratory motor output in cats. *J. Appl. Physiol.* 67: 2249–2256.

Hwang, J.-C., St. John, W. M., and Bartlett, D., Jr. (1984). Afferent pathways for hypoglossal and phrenic responses to changes in upper airway pressure. *Respir. Physiol.* 55: 341–354.

Hwang, J., St. John, W. M., and Bartlett, D., Jr. (1987). Influence of pulmonary inflations on discharge patterns of phrenic motoneurons. *J. Appl. Physiol.* 63: 1421–1427.

Iatridis, A., and Iber, C. (1992). The role of neural reflex mechanisms in response to inspiratory resistive loads during sleep. [abstract]. *Am. Rev. Respir. Dis.* 145: A405.

Iber, C., Simon, P. M., Skatrud, J. B., and Dempsey, J. A. (1991). Pulmonary afferents mediate the lung inflation reflex in humans [abstract]. *Am. Rev. Respir. Dis.* 143: 191.

Iggo, A. (1957). Gastro-intestinal tension receptors with unmyelinated afferent fibres in the vagus of the cat. *Q. J. Exp. Physiol.* 42: 130–143.

Iggo, A. (1959). Cutaneous heat and cold receptors with slow conducting C afferent fibers. *Q. J. Exp. Physiol.* 44: 362–370.

Irving, J. T., McSwiney, B. A., and Suffold, S. F. (1937). Afferent fibers from the stomach and small intestines. *J. Physiol. (Lond.)* 89: 407–420.

Iscoe, S. (1989). Phrenic afferents and ventilatory control at increased end-expiratory lung volumes in cats. *J. Appl. Physiol.* 66: 1297–1303.

Iscoe, S., Dankoff, J., Migicowsky, and Polosa, C. (1976). Recruitment and discharge of phrenic motoneurons during inspiration. *Respir. Physiol.* 26: 113–128.

Iscoe, S., Feldman, J. L., and Cohen, M. I. (1979). Properties of inspiratory termination by superior laryngeal and vagal stimulation. *Respir. Physiol.* 36: 353–366.

Iwamoto, G. A., Waldrop, T. G., Kaufman, M. P., Botterman, B. R., Rybicki, K. J., and

Mitchell, J. H. (1985). Pressor reflex evoked by muscle contraction: Contribution by neuraxis levels. *J. Appl. Physiol.* 59: 459–467.

Jakus, J., Tomori, Z., and Stránsky, A. (1985). Activity of bulbar expiratory neurons during cough and other respiratory tract reflexes in cats. *Physiol. Bohemoslov.* 34: 127–136.

Jammes, Y., Buchler, B., Delpierre, S., Rasidakis, A., Grimaud, C., and Roussos, C. (1986). Phrenic afferents and their role in inspiratory control. *J. Appl. Physiol.* 60: 854–860.

Johansson, B. (1962). Circulatory responses to stimulation of somatic afferents with special reference to the depressor effects from muscle nerves. *Acta Physiol. Scand. [Suppl.]* 198.

Jonzon, A., Pisarri, T. E., Roberts, A. M., Coleridge, J. C. G., and Coleridge, H. M. (1988). Attenuation of pulmonary afferent input by vagal cooling in dogs. *Respir. Physiol.* 72: 19–34.

Jordan, D., and Spyer, K. M. (1986). Brainstem integration of cardiovascular and pulmonary afferent activity. *Progr. Brain Res.* 67: 295–314.

Kalia, M., Senapati, J. M., Parida, B., and Panda, A. (1972). Reflex increase in ventilation by muscle receptors with nonmedullated fibers (C fibers). *J. Appl. Physiol.* 32: 189–193.

Kao, F. F., and Ray, L. H. (1954). Regulation of cardiac output in anesthetized dogs during induced muscular work. *Am. J. Physiol.* 179: 255–260.

Kaufman, M. P., Longhurst, J. C., Rybicki, K. J., Wallach, J. H., and Mitchell, J. H. (1983). Effects of static muscular contraction on impulse activity of group III and IV afferents in cats. *J. Appl. Physiol.* 55: 105–112.

Kim, M. J., Druz, W. J., Danon, J., Machnach, W., and Sharp, J. T. (1976). Mechanics of the canine diaphragm. *J. Appl. Physiol.* 41: 369–382.

Kirkwood, P. A., and Sears, T. A. (1982). Excitatory post-synaptic potentials from single muscle spindle afferents in external intercostal motoneurons of the cat. *J. Physiol.* 322: 287–314.

Koepchen, H. P., Klussendorf, D., and Philipp, U. (1973). Mechanisms of central transmission of respiratory reflexes. *Acta Neurobiol. Exp.* 33: 287–299.

Kohrman, R. M., Nolasco, J. B., and Wiggers, C. J. (1947). Types of afferents in the phrenic nerve. *Am. J. Physiol.* 151: 547–553.

Korpas, J., and Tomori, Z. (1980). Cough and other respiratory reflexes. *Progr. Respir. Res.* 12: 23–40, 219–223, 356.

Kostreva, D. R., Hopp, F. A., Zuperku, E. J., Igler, F. O., Coon, R. L., and Kampine, J. P. (1978). Respiratory inhibition with sympathetic afferent stimulation in canine and primate. *J. Appl. Physiol.* 44: 718–724.

Kostreva, D. R., Hopp, F. A., Zuperku, E. J., and Kampine, J. P. (1979). Apnea, tachypnea and hypotension elicited by cardiac vagal afferents. *J. Appl. Physiol.* 47: 312–318.

Kumazawa, T., and Mizumura, K. (1976). The polymodal C-fiber receptor in the muscle of the dog. *Brain Res.* 101: 589–593.

Kumazawa, T., and Mizumura, K. (1977). Thin-fiber receptors responding to mechanical, chemical and thermal stimulation in the skeletal muscles of the dog. *J. Physiol. (Lond.)* 273: 179–194.

Kurtz, D., Krieger, J., and Stierle, J. C. (1978). EMG activity of cricothyroid and chin muscles during wakefulness and sleeping in the sleep apnea syndrome. *Electroencephalogr. Clin. Neurophysiol.* 45: 777–784.

Ledlie, J. F., Kelsen, S. G., Cherniack, N. S., and Fishman, A. P. (1981). Effects of hypercapnia and hypoxia on phrenic nerve activity and respiratory timing. *J. Appl. Physiol.* 51: 732–738.

Leevers, A. M., and Road, J. D. (1989). Mechanical response to hyperinflation of the two abdominal muscle layers. *J. Appl. Physiol.* 66: 2189–2195.

Leevers, A. M., and Road, J. D. (1991). Effect of lung inflation and upright posture on diaphragmatic shortening in dogs. *Respir. Physiol.* 85: 29–40.

Leevers, A. M., and Road, J. D. (1993). Abdominal muscle activation by expiratory threshold loading in awake dogs. *Respir. Physiol.* 93:289–303.

Leevers, A. M., and Road, J. D. (1995). Effect of vagal blockade on abdominal muscle activation in awake dogs. *J. Physiol. (London)* (in press).

Leiter, J. C., and Daubenspeck, J. A. (1990). Selective reflex activation of the genioglossus in humans. *J. Appl. Physiol.* 68: 2581–2587.

Lloyd, T. C., Jr. (1986). Control of breathing in anesthetized dogs by a left-heart baroreflex. *J. Appl. Physiol.* 61: 2095–3001.

Lloyd, T. C., Jr. (1990). Effect of increased left atrial pressure on breathing frequency in anesthetized dog. *J. Appl. Physiol.* 69: 1973–1980.

Malcolmson, K. G. (1959). The vasomotor activities of the vagal mucous membrane. *J. Laryngol. Otol.* 73: 73–98.

Marlot, D., Macron, J.-M., and Duron, B. (1987). Inhibitory and excitatory effects on respiration by phrenic nerve afferent stimulation in cats. *Respir. Physiol.* 69: 321–333.

Massion, J. (1976). Postural function of the respiratory muscles. In: *Respiratory Centres and Afferent Systems.* Edited by B. Duron. Paris, INSERM, pp. 178–181.

Mathew, O. P., Abu-Osba, Y. K., and Thach, B. T. (1982a). Influence of upper airway pressure changes on genioglossus muscle respiratory activity. *J. Appl Physiol.* 52: 438–444.

Mathew, O. P., Abu-Osba, Y. K., and Thach, B. T. (1982b). Genioglossus muscle responses to upper airway pressure changes: Afferent pathways. *J. Appl. Physiol.* 52: 445–450.

Mathew, O. P., Abu-Osba, Y. K., and Thach, B. T. (1982c). Influence of upper airway pressure changes on respiratory frequency. *Respir. Physiol.* 49: 223–233.

McCarthy, L. E., and Borison, H. L. (1974). Respiratory mechanics of vomiting in decerebrate cats. *Am. J. Physiol.* 226: 738–743.

McCarthy, L. E., Borison, H. L., Spiegel, P. K., and Friedlander, R. M. (1974). Vomiting: Radiographic and oscillographic correlates in the decerebrate cat. *Gastroenterology* 67: 1126–1130.

McCloskey, D. I., and Mitchell, J. H. (1972). Reflex cardiovascular and respiratory responses originating in exercising muscle. *J. Physiol. Lond.* 224: 173–186.

Mei, N. (1976). Respiratory effects produced by vagal afferents originating from the gastro-intestinal tract. In: *Respiratory Centres and Afferent Systems.* Edited by B. Duron. Paris, INSERM, pp. 225–229.

Mense, S., and Stahnke, M. (1983). Responses in muscle afferent fibers of slow conduction velocity to contractions and ischaemia in the cat. *J. Physiol. (Lond.).* 342: 383–397.

Milano, S., Grélot, L., Bianchi, A. L., and Iscoe, S. (1992). Discharge patterns of phrenic motoneurons during fictive coughing and vomiting in decerebrate cats. *J. Appl. Physiol.* 73: 1626–1636.

Miller, A. D., and Ezure, K. (1991). Behaviour of inhibitory and excitatory propriobulbar respiratory neurons during fictive vomiting. *Brain Res.* 578: 168–176.

Miller, A. D., Tan, L. K., and Suzuki, I. (1987). Control of abdominal and expiratory intercostal muscle activity during vomiting: Role of ventral respiratory group expiratory neurons. *J. Neurophysiol.* 57: 1854–1866.

Milsom, W. K. (1990). Mechanoreceptor modulation of endogenous respiratory rhythms in vertebrates. *Am. J. Physiol.* 259: R898–R910.

Miserocchi, G., and Quinn, B. (1980). Control of breathing during acute haemorrhage in anesthetized cats. *Respir. Physiol.* 41: 289–295.

Mitchell, R. A., and Berger, A. J. (1975). Neural regulation of respiration. *Am. Rev. Respir. Dis.* 111: 206–224.

Monges, H., Salducci, J., and Naudy, B. (1978). Dissociation between the electrical activity of the diaphragmatic dome and crura muscle fibers during esophageal distension, vomiting and eructation. An electromyographic study in the dog. *J. Physiol. (Paris)* 74: 541–554.

Monteau, R., and Hilaire, G. (1991). Spinal respiratory motoneurons. *Progr. Neurobiol.* 37: 83–144.

Morrison, J. F. B. (1973). Splanchnic slowly adapting mechanoreceptors with punctate receptive fields in the mesentery and gastrointestinal tract of the cat. *J. Physiol. (Lond.)* 233: 349–361.

Newman, P. P., and Paul, D. H. (1969). The projection of splanchnic afferents on the cerebellum of the cat. *J. Physiol. (Lond.)* 202: 223–237.

Newman, S. L., Road, J., Bellemare, F., Clozel, J. P., Lavigne, C. M., and Grassino, A. (1984). Respiratory muscle length measured by sonomicrometry. *J. Appl. Physiol.* 56: 753–763.

Newsom Davis, J., and Sears, T. A. (1970). The proprioceptive reflex control of the intercostal muscles during their voluntary activation. *J. Physiol.* 209: 711–738.

Pack, A. I., and DeLaney, R. G. (1983). Response of pulmonary rapidly adapting receptors during lung inflation. *J. Appl. Physiol.* 55: 955–963.

Pack, A. I., DeLaney, R. G., and Fishman, A. P. (1981). Augmentation of phrenic neural activity by increased rates of lung inflation. *J. Appl. Physiol.* 50: 149–161.

Pack, A. I., Ogilvie, M. D., Davies, R. O., and Galante, R. J. (1986). Responses of pulmonary stretch receptors during ramp inflations of the lung. *J. Appl. Physiol.* 61: 344–352.

Paintal, A. S. (1973). Vagal sensory receptors and their reflex effects. *Physiol. Rev.* 53: 159–221.

Phillipson, E. A., Hickey, R. F., Graf, P. D., and Nadel, J. A. (1971). Hering–Breuer inflation reflex and regulation of breathing in conscious dogs. *J. Appl. Physiol.* 31: 746–750.

Pisarri, T. E., Jonzon, A., Coleridge, J. C. G., and Coleridge, H. M. (1990). Rapidly adapting receptors monitor lung compliance in spontaneously breathing dogs. *J. Appl. Physiol.* 68: 1997–2005.

Plowman, L., Lauf, D. C., Berthon-Jones, M., and Sullivan, C. E. (1990). Waking and genioglossus muscle responses to upper airway oscillation in sleeping dogs. *J. Appl. Physiol.* 68: 2564–2573.

Polachek, J., Strong, R., Arens, J., Davies, C., Metcalf, I., and Younes, M. (1980). Phasic vagal influences on inspiratory motor activity in anesthetized humans. *J. Appl. Physiol.* 49: 609–619.

Prabhakar, N. R., Marek, W., Loeschcke, H. H. (1985). Altered breathing pattern elicited by stimulation of abdominal visceral afferents. *J. Appl. Physiol.* 58: 1755–1760.

Ravi, K., and Kappagoda, C. T. (1992). Responses of pulmonary C-fibre and rapidly adapting receptor afferents to pulmonary congestion and edema in dogs. *Can. J. Physiol. Pharmacol.* 70: 68–76.

Reeve, E. B., Nanson, E. M., and Rundle, F. F. (1950). Observations on inhibitory respiratory reflexes during abdominal surgery. *Clin. Sci. (Lond.)* 10: 65–87.

Remmers, J. E. (1973). Extra-segmental reflexes derived from intercostal afferents: Phrenic and laryngeal responses. *J. Physiol.* 233: 45–62.

Remmers, J. E., DeGroot, W. J., Sauerland, E. K., and Anch, A. M. (1978). Pathogenesis of upper airway occlusion during sleep. *J. Appl. Physiol.* 44: 931–938.

Revelette, W. R., Jewell, L. A., and Frazier, D. T. (1988). Effect of small-fiber afferent stimulation on ventilation in dogs. *J. Appl. Physiol.* 65: 2097–2106.

Reynolds, L. B., Jr., and Flom, M. H. (1968). Changes in vagal neurogram with spontaneous deep breath in anesthetized cats. *J. Appl. Physiol.* 25: 238–243.

Richardson, P. S., and Widdicombe, J. G. (1969). The role of the vagus nerves in the ventilatory responses to hypercapnia and hypoxia in anaesthetized and unanaesthetized rabbits. *Respir. Physiol.* 7: 122–135.

Rijlant, P. (1942). Contribution a l'etude du control reflex de la respiration. *Bull. Acad. Med. Belg.* 7: 58–107.

Road, J. D., and Leevers, A. M. (1988). Effect of lung inflation on diaphragmatic shortening. *J. Appl. Physiol.* 65: 2383–2389.

Road, J. D., and Leevers, A. (1990). Inspiratory and expiratory muscle function during continuous positive airway pressure in dogs. *J. Appl. Physiol.* 68: 1092–1100.

Road, J. D., Burgess, K. R., Whitelaw, W. A., and Ford, G. T. (1984). Diaphragm function and respiratory response after upper abdominal surgery in dogs. *J. Appl. Physiol.* 57: 576–582.

Road, J. D., Newman, S. L., and Grassino, A. (1986a). Diaphragm length and breathing pattern changes during hypoxia and hypercapnia. *Resp. Physiol.* 65: 39–53.

Road, J. D., Newman, S. L., Derenne, J. P., and Grassino, A. (1986b). The in vivo length–force relationship of the canine diaphragm. *J. Appl. Physiol.* 60: 63–70.

Road, J. D., West, N. H., and Van Vliet, B. N. (1987). Ventilatory effects of stimulation of phrenic afferents. *J. Appl. Physiol.* 63: 1063–1069.

Road, J. D., Leevers, A. M., and Grassino, A. E. (1991a). The effect of continuous positive airway versus positive end expiratory pressure on the diaphragm. *J. Crit. Care* 6: 136–142.

Road, J. D., Leevers, A. M., Goldman, E., and Grassino, A. E. (1991b). Respiratory muscle coordination during expiratory threshold loading. *J. Appl. Physiol.* 70: 1554–1562.

Road, J. D., Osborne, S., and Wakai, Y. (1993). Delayed poststimulus decrease of phrenic motoneuron output produced by phrenic nerve afferent stimulation. *J. Appl. Physiol.* 74: 68–72.

Russell, J. A., and Bishop, B. (1976). Vagal afferents essential for abdominal muscle activity during lung inflation in cats. *J. Appl. Physiol.* 41: 310–315.

Russell, N. J. W., Raybould, H. E., and Trenchard, D. (1984). Role of vagal C-fiber afferents in respiratory response to hypercapnia. *J. Appl. Physiol.* 56: 1550–1558.

Sampson, S. R., and Vidruk, E. H. (1975). Properties of "irritant" receptors in canine lung. *Respir. Physiol.* 25: 9–22.

Sant'Ambrogio, G. (1982). Information arising from the tracheobronchial tree of mammals. *Physiol. Rev.* 62: 531–569.

Sant'Ambrogio, G. (1987). Nervous receptors of the tracheobronchial tree. *Annu. Rev. Physiol.* 49: 611–627.

Sant'Ambrogio, G., and Widdicombe, J. G. (1965). Respiratory reflexes acting on the diaphragm and inspiratory intercostal muscles of the rabbit. *J. Physiol. (Lond.)* 180: 766–779.

Sant'Ambrogio, G., Wilson, M. F., and Frazier, D. T. (1962). Somatic afferent activity in reflex regulation of diaphragmatic function in the cat. *J. Appl. Physiol.* 17: 829–832.

Sant'Ambrogio, G., Mathew, O. P., Fisher, J. T., and Sant'Ambrogio, F. B. (1983). Laryngeal receptors responding to transmural pressure, airflow and local muscle activity. *Respir. Physiol.* 54: 317–330.

Saunders, N. A., Betts, M. F., Pengelly, L. D., and Rebuck, A. S. (1977). Changes in lung mechanics induced by acute isocapnic hypoxia. *J. Appl. Physiol.* 42: 413–419.

Saupe, K. W., Smith, C. A., Henderson, K. S., and Dempsey, J. A. (1992). Respiratory muscle recruitment during selective central and peripheral chemoreceptor stimulation in awake dogs. *J. Physiol. (Lond.)* 448: 613–631.

Schondorf, R., and Polosa, C. (1980). Effects of urinary bladder afferents on respiration. *J. Appl. Physiol.* 48: 826–832.

Sears, T. A. (1964a). Some properties and reflex connections of respiratory motoneurons of the cat's thoracic spinal cord. *J. Physiol.* 175: 386–403.

Sears, T. A. (1964b). The slow potentials of thoracic respiratory motoneurons and their relation to breathing. *J. Physiol.* 175: 404–424.

Sears, T. A. (1990). Central rhythm generation and spinal integration. *Chest* 97: 45S–51S.

Sears, T. A., Berger, A. J., and Phillipson, E. A. (1982). Reciprocal tonic activation of inspiratory and expiratory motoneurons by chemical drives. *Nature* 299: 728–730.

Shannon, R. (1977). Effects of thoracic dorsal rhizotomies on the respiratory pattern in anesthetized cats. *J. Appl. Physiol.* 43: 20–26.

Shannon, R. (1980). Intercostal and abdominal muscle afferent influence on medullary dorsal respiratory group neurons. *Respir. Physiol.* 39: 73–94.

Shannon, R., and Zechman, F. W. (1972). The reflex and mechanical response of the inspiratory muscles to an increased airflow resistance. *Respir. Physiol.* 16: 51–69.

Shea, S. A., Horner, R. L., Banner, N. R., McKenzie, E., Heaton, R., Yacoub, M. H., and Guz, A. (1988). The effect of human heart–lung transplantation upon breathing at rest and during sleep. *Respir. Physiol.* 72: 131–150.

Shook, J. E., Watkins, W. D., and Camporesi, E. M. (1990). Differential rates of opioid receptors in respiration, respiratory disease and opiate-induced respiratory depression. *Am. Rev. Respir. Dis.* 142: 895–909.

Smith, C. A., Ainsworth, D. M., Henderson, K. S., and Dempsey, J. A. (1989a). Differential timing of respiratory muscles in response to chemical stimuli in awake dogs. *J. Appl. Physiol.* 66: 392–399.

Smith, C. A., Ainsworth, D. M., Henderson, K. S., and Dempsey, J. A. (1989b). Differential responses of expiratory muscles to chemical stimuli in awake dogs. *J. Appl. Physiol.* 66: 384–391.

Smith, C. A., Ainsworth, D. M., Henderson, K. S., and Dempsey, J. A. (1990). The influence of carotid body chemoreceptors on expiratory muscle activity. *Respir. Physiol.* 82: 123–136.

Speck, D. F., and Revelette, W. R. (1987). Attenuation of phrenic motor discharge by phrenic nerve afferents. *J. Appl. Physiol.* 62: 941–945.

Speck, D. F., and Webber, C. L., Jr. (1979). Thoracic dorsal rhizotomy in the anesthetized cat: Maintenance of eupnic breathing. *Respir. Physiol.* 38: 347–357.

St. John, W. M. (1981). Respiratory neuron responses to hypercapnia and carotid chemoreceptor stimulation. *J. Appl. Physiol.* 51: 816–822.

St. John, W. M., and Wang, S. C. (1977). Response of medullary respiratory neurons to hypercapnia and isocapnic hypoxia. *J. Appl. Physiol.* 43: 812–821.

St. John, W. M., and Zhou, D. (1990). Discharge of vagal pulmonary receptors differentially alters neural activities during various stages of expiration in the cat. *J. Physiol. (Lond.)* 424: 1–12.

Stacey, M. J. (1969). Free nerve endings in skeletal muscle of the cat. *J. Anat.* 105: 231–254.

Strohl, K. P., Hensley, M. H., Hallett, M., Saunders, N. A., and Ingram, R. H., Jr. (1980). Activation of upper airway muscles before onset of inspiration in normal humans. *J. Appl. Physiol.* 49: 638–642.

Sullivan, C. E., Kozar, L. F., Murphy, E., and Phillipson, E. A. (1978). Primary role of respiratory afferents in sustaining breathing rhythm. *J. Appl. Physiol.* 45: 11–17.

Tallarida, G., Baldoni, F., Peruzzi, G., Raimondi, G., Massaro, M., Abate, A., and Sangiorgi, M. (1983). Different patterns of respiratory reflexes originating in exercising muscle. *J. Appl. Physiol.* 55: 84–91.

Tibes, U. (1977). Reflex inputs to the cardiovascular and respiratory centers from dynamically working canine muscles. Some evidence for involvement of group III or IV nerve fibers. *Circ. Res.* 41: 332–341.

Trenchard, D. (1977). Role of pulmonary stretch receptors during breathing in rabbits, cats and dogs. *Respir. Physiol.* 29: 231–246.

Uchida, Y. (1976). Tachypnea after stimulation of afferent cardiac sympathetic nerve fibers. *Am. J. Physiol.* 230: 1003–1007.

van Lunteren, Van de Graaff, W. B., Parker, D. M., Mitra, J., Haxhiu, M. A., Strohl, K. P., Cherniack, N. S. (1984). Nasal and laryngeal reflex responses to negative upper airway pressure. *J. Appl. Physiol.* 56: 746–752, 1984.

van Lunteren, E., Arnold, J. S., and Cherniack, N. S. (1988a). Vagal influences on parasternal intercostal muscle inspiratory shortening during hypercapnia and airway occlusion. *Respir. Physiol.* 71: 201–212.

van Lunteren, E., Prabhakar, N. R., Cherniack, N. S., Haxhiu, M. A., and Dick, T. E. (1988b). Inhibition of expiratory muscle EMG and motor unit activity during augmented breaths in cats. *Respir. Physiol.* 72: 303–314.

von Euler, C. (1991). Neural organization and rhythm generation. In: *The Lung: Scientific Foundations.* Edited by R. G. Crystal and J. B. West. New York, Raven Press, pp. 1307–1318.

Wakai, Y., Welsh, M. M., Leevers, A. M., and Road, J. D. (1992). Expiratory muscle activity in the awake and sleeping human during lung inflation and hypercapnia. *J. Appl. Physiol.* 72: 881–887.

Waldrop, T. G., Rybicki, K. J., Kaufman, M. P., and Ordway, G. A. (1984). Activation of visceral thin-fibre afferents increases respiratory output in cats. *Respir. Physiol.* 58: 187–196.

Waldrop, T. G., Eldridge, F. L., and Millhorn, D. E. (1982). Prolonged post-stimulus inhibition of breathing following stimulation of afferents from muscle. *Respir. Physiol.* 50:239–254.

Waldrop, T. G., Eldridge, F. L., and Millhorn, D. E. (1983). Inhibition of breathing after stimulation of muscle is mediated by endogenous opiates and GABA. *Respir. Physiol.* 54:211–222.

Wallois, F., Macron, J. M., Journieaux, U., and Duron, B. (1991). Trigeminal afferences implied in the triggering or inhibition of sneezing in cats. *Neurosci. Lett.* 122: 145–147.

Widdicombe, J. G. (1964). Respiratory reflexes. In: *Handbook of Physiology.* Section 3. Respiration, Volume 1. Edited by W. O. Fenn and H. Rahn. Washington, DC, American Physiological Society, pp. 585–630.

Widdicombe, J. G. (1981). Nervous receptors in the respiratory tract and lungs. In: *Regulation of Breathing*. Edited by T. F. Hornbein, New York, Marcel Dekker, pp. 429–472.

Wilcox, P., Road, J. D., Paré, P. D., and Fleetham, J. A. (1988). Inspiratory muscle function during obstructive sleep apnea. *Am. Rev. Respir. Dis.* 137: 74–80.

Xi, L., Smith, C. A., Saupe, K. W., and Dempsey, J. A. (1993). Effects of memory from vagal feedback on short-term potential of ventilation in conscious dogs. *J. Physiol. (Lond.)* 462: 547–561.

Yasuma, F., Kimoff, R. J., Kozar, L. F., England, S. J., Bradley, T. D., and Phillipson, E. A. (1993). Abdominal muscle activation by respiratory stimuli in conscious dogs. *J. Appl. Physiol.* 74: 16–23.

Youmans, W. B., Murphy, Q. R., Turner, J. K., Davis, L. D., Briggs, D. I., and Hoye, A. S. (1963). Activity of abdominal muscles elicited from the circulatory system. *Am. J. Phys. Med.* 42: 1–70.

Younes, M. K., and Remmers, J. E. (1981). Control of tidal volume and respiratory frequency. In: *The Regulation of Breathing*. New York, Marcel Dekker, pp. 621–671.

Younes, M., Vaillancourt, P., and Milic-Emili, J. (1974). Interaction between chemical factors and duration of apnea following lung inflation. *J. Appl. Physiol.* 36: 190–201.

Younes, M. K., Remmers, J. E., and Baker, J. P. (1978). Characteristics of inspiratory inhibition by phasic volume feedback in cats. *J. Appl. Physiol.* 45: 80–86.

Zuperku, E. J., Hopp, F. A., and Kampine, J. P. (1982). Central integration of pulmonary stretch receptor input in the control of expiration. *J. Appl. Physiol.* 52: 1296–1315.

29

The Role of Small-Fiber Phrenic Afferents in the Control of Breathing

SABAH N. A. HUSSAIN

McGill University
Montreal, Quebec, Canada

CHARIS ROUSSOS

National and Kapodistrian University
of Athens Medical School
Athens, Greece
McGill University
Montreal, Quebec, Canada

I. Introduction

Phrenic motoneuron activity is controlled by efferent drive emanating from pontine and medullary respiratory controllers. The activity of these controllers is influenced by inputs from higher centers, as well as by afferent inputs from various peripheral effectors. These peripheral afferent inputs provide the respiratory controllers with essential feedback concerning the functional status of these effectors to aid the respiratory controllers in modulating their output in accordance with the mechanical activity and metabolic needs of the peripheral organs. Although several of these afferent inputs, such as vagal and skeletal muscle afferent sources, had received considerable attention in the past, the functional significance of afferent inputs originating from the respiratory muscles, particularly the diaphragm, in the modulation of central respiratory output, received much less attention. Moreover, the available data on physiological properties of phrenic afferents have been a source of considerable debate.

Several investigators have advocated the notion that phrenic afferent inputs have a negligible role in the modulation of phrenic motoneuron activity (Sant'Ambrogio and Widdicombe, 1965). These authors investigated the role of phrenic afferents in anesthetized rabbits and noticed that, after sectioning the cervical vagi, phrenic motor activity was not affected by lung inflation or deflation. Phrenic motor discharge also remained unchanged in response to airway occlusion. Corda and co-workers (1965), in a subsequent study, showed that phrenic motor activity was not augmented when phrenic afferents were activated by airway occlusion. In accordance with these findings, morphological studies documenting the paucity of proprioceptors in the cat diaphragm have been published (Duron et al., 1978).

Data from the clinical settings, on the other hand, revealed, as early as 1800, that the diaphragm is equipped with a significant sensory innervation. Stimulation of the central part of the diaphragm has long been known to elicit referred pain in the shoulder. Moreover, the distribution of sensory phrenic fibers to diaphragmatic pleura has also been described by Capps (1911). In 1960, Nathan and Sears described the development of diaphragmatic paresis in patients who had undergone therapeutic section of the cervical dorsal roots. These findings are in favor of an important role for phrenic afferents in the regulation of eupneic breathing in normal subjects. Green and co-workers (1978) have also concluded that activation of phrenic afferents may mediate the decline in diaphragmatic activation in response to positive-pressure breathing in humans. In addition, there is increasing evidence that phrenic afferents are involved in respiratory load compensation. For instance, Banzett et al. (1981) showed, in awake paraplegic patients, that negative pressure applied to the lower body was associated with augmentation of diaphragmatic activation. These authors postulated that fast-conducting phrenic afferent fibers might be involved in this reflex. In a similar study on cats, Fryman and Frazier (1987) pointed out that the ventilatory response to lower-body negative-pressure application was eliminated by sectioning the cervical dorsal roots. Although these findings indicate a role for large-fiber (fast-conducting myelinated) phrenic afferents during eupneic breathing, the functional importance of the more abundant afferent fibers in the phrenic nerve (small-diameter myelinated and unmyelinated) remains unclear.

The existence of thin-fiber afferents in the phrenic nerves of various mammalian species has been previously documented by several authors. However, despite their abundance, little attention was paid to the possible involvement of these fibers in the control of breathing. In the last several years, there has been emerging evidence that activation of these fibers elicits profound changes in the respiratory and cardiovascular systems. Our main objective in this review is to elaborate on the current understanding concerning the morphological and functional characteristics of thin-fiber phrenic afferents. The subject of large-fiber intercostal afferents and their role in the control of breathing has been previously summarized by Shannon (1992).

II. Fiber Type Composition

Afferent fibers supplying the striated mammalian muscles can be classified according to either the conduction velocity or diameter. Four main types of afferents have been identified in striated muscle nerves.

Group I fibers are myelinated, with diameters ranging between 12 and 20 μm and conduction velocities between 79 and 114 m/s (Rexed, 1944). These fibers supply muscle spindles (primary endings or group IA) and Golgi tendon organs (group IB fibers). The neurophysiological characteristics of groups IA and IB fibers are very similar. *Group II* fibers are also myelinated, but are thinner (diameters ranging between 2 and 16 μm) and slower (conduction velocities of 30–65 m/s) than group I fibers. In addition, these fibers provide an additional afferent supply to muscle spindles (secondary afferent fibers). They may also supply extrafusal muscle fibers (Barker, 1974). *Group III* fibers have a thin myelin sheath and diameters ranging between 1 and 6 μm and conduction velocities of 3.6–15 m/s. The majority of these fibers terminate as free nerve endings; however, a few fibers also innervate muscle spindles and paciniform corpuscles (Stacey, 1969). *Group IV* fibers are similar in characteristics to group III (both fibers are often grouped as **thin-fiber afferents**); however, they have no myelin sheath and have diameters and conduction velocities of less than 2 μm and 2 m/s, respectively. Most group IV fibers terminate as free nerve endings. The distribution of free nerve endings within striated muscles and the pattern of branching of these fibers is not very well known. Stacey (1969) revealed that the endings of a great proportion of thin-fiber afferents terminate in various locations in the muscle, including connective tissues, arterioles, venules, the capsules of Golgi tendon organs, tendon tissues, and the interstitium between intrafusal and extrafusal muscle fibers.

The majority of the nerves supplying limb muscles are composite nerves (i.e., contain motor as well as sensory fibers). In most previous studies, one can find a detailed analysis of the myelinated fiber composition of various peripheral nerves, with little information about the number and distribution of unmyelinated nerve fibers. This is because of the difficulty in identifying these fibers with light microscopy. With the introduction of electron microscopy, it is now generally agreed that the number of unmyelinated fibers is almost twofold higher than large myelinated fibers in the peripheral nerves.

A. Diaphragm Innervation

Innervation of the diaphragm has been a subject of interest since the last decades of the 19th century. In his landmark article, Ferguson (1891) noticed that cat phrenic nerve contains sensory as well as motor fibers. He proposed that the sensory fibers may also be present in human phrenic nerve. Subsequent studies on the composition of the phrenic nerve focused on the distribution of myelinated fibers, with little attention paid to unmyelinated fibers. These studies revealed that the phrenic nerve in cats, dogs, and rats contains two populations of myelinated fibers (bimodal distribution) (Duron and Condamin, 1970; Gasser and Grundfest, 1939; Landau et al., 1962; Langford and Schmidt, 1983; Lubinska and Waryszewskia, 1974). In humans, Duron (1981) studied fiber type composition of the phrenic nerve in two accident victims and reported a similar bimodal distribution to that found in the cat.

Yasargil and Koller (1964; Yasargil, 1967), on the other hand, have indicated that fiber distribution in rabbit phrenic nerve is unimodal with most myelinated fibers having diameters ranging between 6 and 10 μm.

The size of small myelinated fiber population in the phrenic nerve varies among different species. At least 16% of myelinated fibers of the cat phrenic nerve have diameters of less than 6 μm (Duron et al., 1978; Duron and Condamin, 1969). Similar findings have been reported in the human phrenic nerve (Duron, 1981). In the phrenic nerve of dogs, Landau and co-workers (1962) found that 80–85% of myelinated fibers have diameters ranging from 9 to 12 μm, whereas only 8–10% of myelinated fibers have diameters ranging between 2 and 4 μm. Similarly, about 54% of myelinated fibers in the rat phrenic nerve have diameters ranging between 5 and 8 μm (Lubinska and Waryszewskia, 1974). Only 18% of these fibers have a diameter of less than 4 μm.

The number of fibers in the phrenic nerve may also vary according to the location along the nerve. At a given location, the number of myelinated fibers in right and left phrenic nerves appears to be similar; however, it was reported that the superior portion of the thoracic phrenic nerves has 40 or so more fibers than the inferior portion (Duron et al. 1978; Duron and Condamin, 1970; Duron, 1981). This increase in the number of myelinated fibers in the upper thoracic portion of the phrenic nerve is probably because a few of the fibers in the superior portion may also supply the pericardium.

Unlike myelinated fibers, the distribution of unmyelinated fibers in the phrenic nerve has not been assessed extensively because of the difficulties in identifying these fibers. Duron and Condamin (1970) used electron microscopy and reported unusually large number of unmyelinated fibers in cat phrenic nerve. In several nerve samples studied, these investigators counted more than 70% of total nerve fibers to be unmyelinated, with most having diameters ranging between 0.1 and 2.7 μm. It remains to be seen whether these unmyelinated fibers are sensory or motor. In a subsequent study, Duron and Marlot (1980) reported that unmyelinated fibers represent 70–80% of the total number of fibers in cat phrenic and external intercostal nerves, compared with 82% of fibers in a cutaneous nerve (Table 1). The bulk of unmyelinated fibers appears to have very small diameters (less than 1 μm). It was also proposed that unmyelinated fibers with diameters larger than 2 μm may provide sensory supply to the peritoneum and pleural surfaces. In a similar study, Langford and Schmidt (1983) counted 700 axons in rat phrenic nerve, 43% of which were unmyelinated.

B. Phrenic Afferent Population

Although the phrenic nerve is generally considered a motor nerve, the primary function of which is to provide the motor innervation to the diaphragm, investigators using deafferentation procedures, such as removing dorsal root ganglia or sectioning of the cervical dorsal roots, have documented the existence of afferent fibers. The

Table 1 Minimal Values of Myelinated and Nonmyelinated Nerve Fibers Counted From Phrenic, Intercostal, and Cutaneous Nerve Samples in Cats

	Number of nonmyelinated fibers	Number of myelinated fibers	Total
Phrenic nerve	1970	791	2751
4th external intercostal nerve	402	106	508
4th internal intercostal nerve	4539	698	5237
9th internal intercostal nerve	4272	484	4756
4th collateral cutaneous nerve	6570	1195	7765

Source: Duron and Marlot (1980).

proportion of phrenic afferents appears to vary considerably between different species. Most studies of phrenic afferents focused on the distribution of myelinated fibers. The number of unmyelinated fibers (group IV), therefore, have been grossly underestimated.

The existence of sensory fibers in the phrenic nerve of cats was assessed by Ferguson in 1891. He reported that one-third of myelinated fibers in the phrenic nerve had undergone degeneration after the removal of cervical dorsal root ganglia. More recently, Duron (1981) excised the 3rd, 4th, 5th, and 6th cervical ganglia of cats and examined phrenic nerves 35–40 days later. He found that 25% of myelinated fibers were degenerated and the degeneration was more evident in small fibers (diameters between 2 and 6 μm). Accordingly, between 20 and 30% of total myelinated fibers in cat phrenic nerve appear to be sensory, and less than 2% of these fibers supply muscle spindles. In contrast with these findings, much lower estimates of afferent fibers have been reported by Hinsey and colleagues (Hinsey et al., 1939). These authors claimed that the sensory component of cat phrenic nerve amounts to about 10% of total myelinated fibers.

In rats, Langford and Schmidt (1983) performed dorsal root ganglionectomy, ventral rhizotomy, and sympathectomy to quantitate the axonal characteristic of the phrenic nerve. They reported that 59% of afferent fibers traveling through the dorsal roots are small unmyelinated fibers, whereas only 31% of afferents are large myelinated fibers. In addition, few unmyelinated fibers appear to travel through the sympathetic chain. These fibers may have been a preganglionic efferent supply to diaphragmatic vessels.

Landau and colleagues (1962) reported that only 55–65% of the total number of phrenic axons in dogs are efferent. They also suggested that a portion of afferent axons may be connected to Golgi tendon organs or to free nerve endings inside the diaphragm, as well as in the peritoneal and pleural surfaces.

Besides species differences, some of the reasons behind the contradictory results on the size of the sensory component of phrenic nerve can be attributed to methodological difficulties in the surgical procedures to remove dorsal root ganglia or sectioning of the dorsal roots without inflicting major damage on the ventral roots. More selective techniques have been implemented recently for the assessment of the size and distribution of phrenic afferent fibers. Rose and co-workers (Rose et al., 1990) have used retrograde labeling of dorsal root ganglia with horseradish peroxidase to assess the afferent fiber component of cat phrenic nerve. They estimated that 67% of phrenic afferents are small unmyelinated fibers, compared with 33% representing large myelinated fibers. These results clearly indicate that a relatively large proportion of cat phrenic afferent fibers are small unmyelinated (group IV) fibers.

Similarly to limb muscle, phrenic afferent axons are connected to a variety of muscle receptors. These receptors include *muscle spindle*, which averages 5–6 mm in length and consists of a bundle of muscle fibers ensheathed by a lamellated capsule with a dilated central region. Two types of myelinated afferent fibers supply each muscle spindle. Primary (group IA) afferent endings give rise to annulospiral terminals that surround the central region of the intrafusal fibers. Secondary afferent endings (group II) are connected mainly to the nuclear chain fibers.

The motor supply of muscle spindle is provided by myelinated gamma-fibers (2–6 μm in diameter). Another source of motor supply to the spindles is provided by beta-motor fibers, which may also provide motor control to the extrafusal muscle fibers. Muscle spindles have been detected in various respiratory muscles in most mammalian species. Most investigators, however, agree that the number of muscle spindles in the diaphragm is unusually low when compared with other skeletal or respiratory muscles. Hinsey and colleagues (1939), for example, could not detect any muscle spindle in the cat diaphragm. Duron and colleagues (1978) counted only seven to nine muscle spindles that were exclusively located in the crural portion of the cat diaphragm. Furthermore, these investigators estimated that each phrenic nerve contains about five group IA and eight group II afferent fibers (12% of total afferent fibers).

Phrenic afferents are also attached to another type of receptors; namely, the *Golgi tendon organ* that consists of a fascia of tendinous fibers attached at one end to a large number of muscle fibers. Tendon organ receptors are located at the junction of the muscle and its tendon and measure 1600×122 μm in humans. The afferent supply of these receptors is myelinated fibers of group IB, which usually divide into numerous endings on the tendinous fibers. The electrophysiological characteristics of group IB fibers are very similar to those of group IA fibers. Golgi tendon organs have a relatively higher threshold of activation when compared with muscle spindles and, when activated, they elicit a powerful inhibition of the alpha-motor fibers of the corresponding muscle. The presence of Golgi tendon organs and muscle spindles in the human diaphragm had been reported by Winkler and Delaloye (1957). The number of these receptors, however, has not been clearly identified.

The third type of muscle receptors are *pacinian and paciniform corpuscles*, which are rapidly adapting mechanoreceptors and consist basically of a nerve ending surrounded by a lamellated capsule. The paciniform corpuscle, 177×21 μm in dimension, is located adjacently to the Golgi tendon organs and has about eight laminae surrounding the nerve ending. The pacinian corpuscles, in comparison, are larger, less frequent, and have 20–60 laminae, as compared with the paciniform corpuscles. The afferent supply of both of these receptors consists of myelinated nerve fibers, ranging in diameter between 2.8 and 11.2 μm. Rapidly adapting receptors, such as the pacinian corpuscles, are evenly distributed throughout the diaphragm (Corda et al., 1965). Moreover, Goshgarian and Roubal (1986) suggested, based on the distribution of axonal branching of phrenic afferents in the dorsal spinal columns, that a few afferent axons arise from pacinian corpuscles inside the diaphragm. The diaphragm also contains special receptors with characteristic terminal arborization, which has been described by Dogiel (1902). The functional importance of these receptors has not yet been identified.

Most unmyelinated and small myelinated afferent fibers generally end as *free nerve endings* in striated mammalian muscles. In limb muscles, Stacey (1969) estimated that 66% of group IV and at least 30% of group III fibers arise from free nerve endings. Accordingly, the number of afferent fibers with free nerve ending receptors is about 75% of the total afferent population. The receptive fields and modalities of activation of group III and IV afferent endings have been comprehensively studied in limb muscles. Both types of thin-fiber afferents can be activated by a variety of mechanical, chemical, and thermal stimuli. From their sensitivity to different stimuli, these fibers have been generally classified into two major categories: low-threshold units *(ergoreceptors)* that are activated by nonnoxious touch, pressure, and routine muscle contraction; and high-threshold units *(nociceptors)* that are sensitive to chemical stimuli, noxious agents, and ischemia. Nociceptors are also known as polymodal fibers (Kao, 1963).

Detailed studies on cat gastrocnemius–soleus muscle provided evidence that even polymodal receptors of groups III and IV fibers are not a homogeneous group. Indeed, the response of these receptors to touch, pressure, contraction, and ischemia revealed a significant heterogeneity. When local touch or pressure is applied to limb muscles of dogs and cats, about 40% of group IV fibers become strongly activated, whereas more than 50% of group III fibers are activated by these stimuli (Kniffki et al., 1978). In addition, about 70% of group IV fibers become active in response to strong noxious pressure (Kniffki et al., 1978). In contrast, there is a small proportion of group III and IV fibers that are insensitive to even strong noxious pressure.

Limb muscle thin-fiber afferents, particularly those of group III, are also sensitive to muscle stretching. Kniffi and co-workers (Kniffki et al., 1978) noticed that roughly 50% of group III fibers of gastrocnemius–soleus muscle responded to stretching of muscle tendon, compared with only 17% of group IV fibers. In addition to stretching, active muscle contraction provides another stimulus for thin-fiber afferents in limb muscles. Sustained muscle contractions are usually associated with activation of about one-third of group III and 40% of group IV fibers in hindlimb muscles (Kniffki et al., 1978). However, the degree of, and the time course of, activation of these afferents in relation to muscle contraction vary considerably among different types of fibers. For instance, most contraction-sensitive group III fibers are responsive to muscle tension, ranging between 20 and 100% of maximum, whereas high levels of tension are usually required to activate group IV fibers. Mense (1978) also classified contraction-sensitive thin-fiber afferents into two major categories: (1) afferent fibers with firing characteristics that are related to the time course and magnitude of muscle tension; the ratio of group III to IV fibers that belong to this category in cat limb muscles is 3:1; and (2) afferent fibers with irregular and delayed-firing characteristics that do not follow the time course of muscle contraction. These fibers are also sensitive to thermal and chemical stimuli. Both group III and IV fibers contribute equally to this category. Mense (1978) also described a subgroup of group III fibers that is active only when muscle contraction is accompanied by ischemia (ischemia-sensitive fibers). In a subsequent study, Kaufman et al. (1983) assessed the effect of static contraction, induced by electrical stimulation of the ventral roots, of cat gastrocnemius muscle on the firing rate of groups III and IV afferents. Stimulation of the ventral roots at 20–40 Hz for 30–45 s significantly increased the firing rates of 63% of group III afferents, with an average latency of 224 ms after the onset of stimulation. In most group III fibers, the activity declined to baseline level within 20 s of the contraction period. Moreover, the initial increase in firing rate of group III fibers appears to be related to the level of muscle tension. Strong muscle contraction also elicited a significant increase in the firing rate of 68% of group IV muscle afferents, with activity increasing 3.8 s after the onset of contraction. The augmentation of activity of these fibers was either maintained throughout the contraction period or declined after reaching an initial peak.

Muscle thin-fiber afferents are also sensitive to exogenous and endogenous pain-producing substances (noxious), such as bradykinin, serotonin, and K^+, that may be released during severe muscle contraction. These substances, however, are not particularly selective in activating only nociceptors. Studies by Mense and Schmidt (1974) indicated that a considerable portion of low-threshold and temperature-sensitive afferents are activated by these substances. In addition, the sensitivity of afferents to these endogenous substances is influenced by the presence of other endogenous metabolites. For example, the sensitivity of group IV fibers to bradykinin is enhanced significantly in the presence of serotonin or prostaglandins (Mense, 1981). Thin-fiber afferents are also sensitive to exogenous noxious substances, such as capsaicin, an extract from the plant *Capsicum*. Capsaicin is known to stimulate unmyelinated afferent fibers in various tissues. Kaufman and colleagues (1982) investigated the effect of capsaicin injection on thin-fiber afferent activation in dog hindlimb muscles. Intra-arterial injections of capsaicin elicited a strong activation in 24 of 34 group IV afferent fibers, whereas only 17 of 33 group III fibers became active in response to capsaicin injection. By contrast, capsaicin has no effect on the activity of group I and II afferent fibers.

The effect of muscle ischemia on thin-fiber afferent activity was assessed by Kaufman and colleagues (1984), who recorded the impulse activity of 24 group III and 30 group IV afferents with endings in the triceps surae, while statically contracting this muscle group both when the abdominal aorta was occluded and when it was patent. Ischemia increased the responses to static contraction of 46% of group IV fibers, compared with only 12% of group III fibers. In addition, ischemic contraction was associated with two patterns of afferent activation, an increase in firing rate of afferent fibers that were active during nonischemic contraction and activation of fibers that were not stimulated by nonischemic contraction.

III. Characteristics, Neurotransmitters, and Projections of Phrenic Afferents

The existence of a nociceptive afferent pathway originating from the diaphragm has long been known. Referred pain in the shoulder region elicited by stimulation of the central part of the diaphragm in humans was described by Felix in 1992. Hinsey and Phillips (1937) also observed a nociceptive response on central stimulation of phrenic nerves in cats. They also noticed that these responses persisted even after removal of cervical sympathetic chain, transection of spinal cord at T-4, or sectioning of vagosympathetic trunks, suggesting that thoracolumbar and vagal pathways are not essential for nociceptive transmission from the central portion of the diaphragm. These observations apparently refute the suggestion of Pollock and Davis (1935) that viscerocutaneous pathways are implicated in the transmission of nociception from diaphragmatic surfaces. In another experiment, Green (1935) found that stimulation of phrenic nerve afferents elicited a significant dilation of coronary vessels. Little and MacSwiney (1938) have also proposed that afferent fibers in the phrenic nerves may transmit pain impulses. These investigators used pupillodilatory reflex as an index of nociceptive reflex activity. In accordance with this proposal, Gernandt (1946) recorded action potential from the peripheral end of cut phrenic nerve and noticed that phrenic afferent activity increased significantly in response to noxious stimuli, such as pinching or the injection of acetic acid. Morphological evidence of nociceptive phrenic afferents were also documented by Goshgarian and Roubal (1986). These investigators found that phrenic afferent collaterals terminate in laminae I and II in the spinal cord. Given these findings, Goshgarian and Roubal concluded that phrenic afferents may be involved in mediating nociceptive transmission.

With the introduction of more sensitive-recording techniques, several investigators have characterized the response of phrenic afferents to a variety of noxious or mechanical stimuli. Our group (Jammes et al., 1986) recorded, for example, 44 group IV afferent fibers from the cervical branches of phrenic nerves in cats. These fibers were strongly activated in response to intra-arterial injections of lactic acid, hypertonic saline, or phenyl diguanide (PDG; Fig. 1). In a similar experiment, Graham et al.

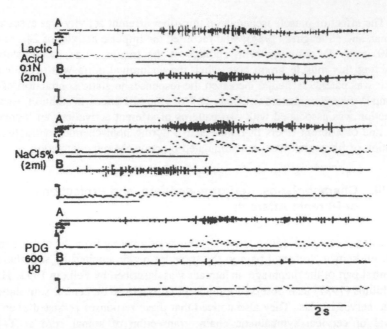

Figure 1 Effects of injecting lactic acid (0.1 N, top), NaCl (15%, middle panel), and phenyl diguanide (PDG) into the general circulation on phrenic sensory activity. Conduction velocities of these fibers are in the range of small unmyelinated fibers. A, unblocked phrenic nerve; B, conduction in the phrenic nerve blocked by local application of procaine. The first line of each tracing is the raw signal and the second line is the impulse frequency of one selected afferent unit. Horizontal black bars beneath each recording represent period of drug injection. With conduction intact (A), strong afferent activity is elicited by all three drugs. During conduction block with procaine (B), previous activity elicited by drug activation is severely depressed. (From Jammes et al., 1986.)

(1986) recorded spontaneous phrenic afferent activities from 50 fibers in the phrenic nerves of cats. Half of these units were thin-fibers with slow and tonic activity. A significant increase in the activity of these fibers was evident when lactic acid and hypertonic saline were injected intra-arterially. Thin-fiber phrenic afferent activity also increased in response to a severe reduction of diaphragmatic blood flow, induced by aortic occlusion. Experiments in our laboratory have also confirmed that thin-fiber afferents that are sensitive to capsaicin and bradykinin exist in the phrenic nerve of dogs (Hussain et al., 1990; Wilson et al., 1991). Revelette et al. (1988) also used capsaicin to demonstrate the existence of nociceptive phrenic afferents.

A. Neurotransmitters

The neurotransmitters involved in the synaptic activity of phrenic afferents have not been extensively investigated. Holtman (1989) used retrograde tracing with fluorescent dye and immunohistochemistry to localize the putative neurotransmitter substance in phrenic afferents. A total of 11% of phrenic afferent neurons contained substance P, a possible neurotransmitter of primary afferent neurons that are involved in processing nociceptive information. Several investigators have also reported that the percentage of dorsal root ganglia and axons labeled with substance P in other areas of the spinal cord ranged between 8 and 33% (Dalsgaard et al., 1982; Gibbons et al., 1987; Hokfelt et al., 1976). Other peptides, such as calcitonin gene-related peptide, somatostatin, and bombesin, all have been demonstrated immunocytochemically in subpopulations of dorsal root ganglion cells of the lumbar region in the rat (McNeill et al., 1989). Although not yet proved, these peptides are believed to be functioning as neurotransmitters in the unmyelinated afferent fibers.

B. Projections

To comprehend the influence of thin-fiber phrenic afferent activation on the respiratory and cardiovascular systems, it is vital to establish the extent of afferent projections at various levels in the central nervous system (CNS). Several authors have attempted to localize the central pathways of phrenic afferents. In most of the published studies, however, the type of phrenic afferent fibers studied has not been clearly identified. Nevertheless, there is evidence indicating that thin-fiber phrenic afferents travel through separate pathways and project to different supraspinal structures than those of large-fiber (groups I and II) phrenic afferents.

As in limb muscles, thin-fiber phrenic afferents enter the spinal cord through the dorsal roots. In addition to the dorsal roots, Langford and Schmidt (1983) have indicated that few unmyelinated phrenic fibers enter the spinal cord through the ventral roots. It was unclear in that study whether these fibers were sensory or motor. More recently, Revelette and co-workers (1988) used capsaicin to selectively activate thin-fiber phrenic afferents in dogs. These authors concluded that the ventral roots may be the pathway of spinal cord entry for a few thin-fiber phrenic afferents. Whether these fibers that enter through the ventral roots are functionally distinct from those of the dorsal roots remains unclear.

At the spinal level, the central processes of phrenic afferents in cats descend and ascend in the dorsal column, before terminating in the laminae I to IV of the dorsal horns of C-4 and C-5 (Goshgarian and Roubal, 1986). At this level, phrenic afferents appear to exert an important influence on the ipsilateral and contralateral phrenic motoneuron discharge. Early suggestion of a segmental reflex initiated by phrenic afferents was advocated by Goshgarian (1981). In rats exposed to spinal cord hemisection at C-2, Goshgarian noticed that the ipsilateral diaphragm became paralyzed. When the dorsal roots of contralateral C6–C8 were then sectioned, the paralyzed diaphragm recovered partially, indicating that phrenic afferents exert an inhibitory effect on the contralateral phrenic motoneurons. It was not obvious in that study whether supraspinal structures are also involved in this reflex. In a subsequent morphological study, Goshgarian and Roubal (1986) doubted the existence of a segmental phrenic-to-phrenic inhibitory reflex when they failed to localize any projection from phrenic afferents to the contralateral phrenic motor nuclei. These doubts were laid to rest subsequently by the physiological recordings of Gill and Kuno (1963) and Rijlant (1942). Both groups have documented segmental phrenic motoneuron inhibition by electrical stimulation of phrenic nerve afferents. More recently, Speck and Revelette (1987a) characterized the distinctive reflex effect of phrenic group III afferents on the motor discharge of phrenic neurons. They described a short-latency inhibition of ipsilateral motor discharge, combined with a relatively long-latency inhibition of contralateral phrenic motoneurons, in response to electrical stimulation of upper cervical roots of the phrenic nerve in cats (Fig. 2). Another important finding in that study is the persistence of inhibitory reflex after decerebration and decerebellation, implying that supraspinal structures are of negligible importance in the expression of this reflex. The existence of segmental spinal inhibitory reflex has also been confirmed by Marlot et al. (1988). These authors recorded phrenic motor activity in response to ipsilateral and contralateral phrenic nerve stimulation. Both stimulations inhibited phrenic motor activity; however, the duration of inhibition was shorter in response to contralateral afferent stimulation, compared with ipsilateral stimulation.

Phrenic afferents traveling through the dorsal spinal column also project to various supraspinal structures, such as external cuneate nucleus (Larnicol et al., 1985) and lateral reticular nucleus, which receives projections mainly from

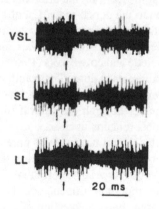

Figure 2   Neurograms demonstrating three types of phrenic motor response observed with various stimulation and recording paradigms. Top: very short latency (VSL) attenuation of right cervical phrenic nerve (CPN) elicited by stimulation of ipsilateral thoracic phrenic nerve (TPN). Middle: short latency (SL) attenuation of CPN discharge resulting from stimulation of a cervical phrenic rootlet. Bottom: long latency (LL) attenuation of CPN discharge in response to contralateral stimulation of TPN. Each trace contains ten superimposed sweeps. Stimulus pulses are indicated by arrows. (From Speck and Revelette, 1987a.)

large-fiber phrenic afferents (Macron et al., 1985). More recent experiments in our laboratory suggest indirectly that thin-fiber phrenic afferents may indeed project to the neurons of the reticular formation (Ward et al., 1992a). In addition to these sites, phrenic afferent projections to dorsal and ventral respiratory neurons have been identified by several groups (Macron et al., 1986; Speck and Revelette, 1987b). However, the types of afferent fibers involved in these projections were not clearly identified. From the latencies of dorsal and ventral neuron activation in response to electrical stimulation of the phrenic nerve, it was proposed that group III afferents are involved in these projections, including those on the lateral reticular nucleus. In addition, the apparent similarity in the latency periods of reticular formation activation elicited by phrenic and cardiac afferent stimulation suggests that these phrenic afferent fibers may be involved in mediating pain sensation from the diaphragm.

After a short latency period (10 ms) activation of phrenic afferents in cats also elicits evoked potentials in the sensorimotor cortex, in an area located medial to forelimb and lateral to hindlimb afferent projections (Davenport et al., 1985). These results suggest that the afferent representation of the diaphragm in the sensorimotor cortex is related to its position in the body and, to a lesser extent, on the spinal segments through which its afferents enter. In addition to the cerebral cortex. Marlot and colleagues (1984) reported that phrenic afferent activation elicits evoked potentials on the cerebellar cortex. The significance of these cerebral and cerebellar projections remains unclear.

IV. Spontaneous Activity

Spontaneous phrenic afferent activities during eupneic breathing have been recorded and classified according to their relation to the ventilatory rhythm. Most of these activities appear to originate from proprioceptors, with very little data available on the activity of thin-fiber afferents.

Afferent impulses in phase with respiration can be expiratory, inspiratory, or mixed. In supine cats, Glebovskii (1962), Corda et al. (1965), and Duron and Caillol (1973) recorded phasic phrenic afferent activities during the expiratory phase of the breathing cycle, with a mean firing frequency of 50 Hz. These activities may have been related to diaphragmatic muscle spindles. This conclusion is supported by the observation that, when fusimotor fiber activation was blocked with lidocaine (lignocaine), spontaneous afferent activity during expiration declined significantly. In a few animals, tonic expiratory proprioceptive activities were also recorded. In addition, about 18–25% of diaphragmatic muscle spindles are active during the inspiratory phase of the breathing cycle, with a mean firing frequency of 100 Hz. A small portion of phrenic spindles exhibit a mixed activation pattern (both inspiratory and expiratory), suggesting that spindles may be activated by active muscle contraction and passive muscle stretching.

Despite the recording of spontaneous afferent activities during eupneic breathing in several animal species, morphological studies indicate that the diaphragm contains very few muscle spindles. These findings, therefore, cast some doubt on the importance of spindle activity for normal diaphragmatic recruitment. The decline in diaphragmatic activation in response to airway occlusion, on the other hand, seems to suggest that Golgi tendon activity may have a more important influence on phrenic motoneurons than on muscle spindles (Jammes et al., 1986). Experiments by Graham and colleagues (1986) confirm this proposal. These investigators recorded phasic and tonic inspiratory afferent activities from the cervical roots of cat phrenic nerves. Revelette and colleagues (1992) have also recorded spontaneous tendon organ afferent activities from the dorsal root ganglia of anesthetized cats. They noticed that the frequency of firing of these afferents during spontaneous eupneic breathing averaged 47 Hz. Firing frequencies rose to 61 Hz when active diaphragmatic tension was increased by abdominal compression. Increased activity of these afferents could explain the reflex inhibition of phrenic motor discharge in response to abdominal compression (Cheeseman and Revelette, 1990).

Unlike proprioceptor activity, very few investigators were successful in recording spontaneous thin-fiber phrenic afferent activity during eupneic breathing. This may be due to either relatively low levels of afferent activation, or to the difficulty in recording afferent action potentials. The first report documenting spontaneous thin-fiber phrenic afferents activity during eupneic breathing was published by Gernandt (1946). He recorded phrenic action potentials from the cervical branches of cats and dogs and noticed a tonic discharge of slowly conducting small spike potentials that he attributed to group IV afferents. The activities of these fibers were augmented in response to pinching of the diaphragm or the local application of acetic acid. In more recent experiments, Jammes and co-workers (1986) recorded spontaneous activity from 44 units, with conduction velocities of 0.8–1.3 m/s. The spontaneous activity of these fibers was irregular and slow; however, it increased substantially in response to the injection of hypertonic saline or phenyl diguanide (see Fig. 1). Furthermore, Graham et al. (1986) attempted to characterize the spontaneous tonic activity of thin-fiber phrenic afferents by recording from cervical root filaments in cats. These authors noticed slow-firing afferent activity, with an average firing frequency of 14 Hz. This activity increased moderately when lactic acid was injected intra-arterially. Despite these recordings of spontaneous afferent activity during eupneic breathing, the functional significance of this activity for normal phrenic motor discharge is still questionable. Jammes and co-workers (1986) have demonstrated, on one hand, that phrenic motor discharge remained unchanged when thin-fiber activity was blocked by procaine application, suggesting a negligible role for these fibers during eupneic phrenic motor drive. On the other hand, the same authors proposed that spontaneous thin-fiber phrenic afferent activity may provide a weak tonic sensory background, with an effect on the phrenic motor discharge that may become evident with strong diaphragmatic contractions or when blood flow to the diaphragm becomes severely curtailed. Clearly, more studies are needed to elucidate the importance of spontaneous firing of thin-fiber phrenic afferents.

V. Stimulated Activity

Our current understanding of the functional significance of thin-fiber afferents has been primarily derived from animal experiments in which these fibers are activated either electrically or chemically. It is now generally accepted that activation of these fibers is associated with significant alterations in the cardiovascular and respiratory systems. In most studies, thin-fiber phrenic afferent activation elicits qualitatively similar, but quantitatively smaller, changes in the ventilatory motor drive and blood flow distribution, compared with those elicited by limb muscle afferents. This is consistent with the presence of fewer thin-fiber afferents in the phrenic nerve than in the limb muscles.

A. Effects on the Cardiovascular System

It has long been established that electrical stimulation of afferent fibers emanating from limb muscle is associated with profound changes in arterial pressure and blood flow distribution (Fell, 1968; Gordon, 1943; Johansson, 1962). It has also been recognized that the pattern and the magnitude of these vascular changes are highly dependent on the stimulus characteristics. A few investigators have described a significant decline in arterial pressure and heart rate when the central end of cut muscle nerves was stimulated at low intensities and at frequencies of 5–20 Hz (Johansson, 1962; Katz et al., 1965). Evidence published by Johansson (1962) suggests that this response is mediated through supraspinal and segmental projections of group III afferent fibers. Stimulation at frequencies ranging from 40 and 100 Hz and high intensities, on the other hand, evoked a substantial increase in arterial pressure and heart rate. Group IV afferent fibers were implicated in this response (Fell, 1968; Johansson, 1962). It remains unclear whether this rise in arterial pressure is associated with an increase in cardiac output, or with peripheral vascular resistance. Fell (1968) described a moderate increase in cardiac output in response to limb muscle afferent activation. This finding is in disagreement with those of Kumada and colleagues (1975), who reported an increase in total peripheral vascular resistance, along with a slight decline in the cardiac output.

In addition to the changes in arterial pressure and heart rate, electrical stimulation of limb muscle thin-fiber afferents elicits a distinctive redistribution of blood flow to various organs. Similar to arterial pressure and heart rate, the direction and the magnitude of blood flow redistribution appear to depend on stimulation parameters. Stimulation of limb muscle afferents at low intensities and low frequencies has been associated with a moderate vasodilation in the renal, intestinal, and limb muscle vascular beds (Fell, 1968; Johansson, 1962). Severe renal and intestinal vasoconstriction and a moderate decline in limb muscle blood flow, on the other hand, were observed, along with a significant increase in arterial pressure, when high-intensity stimulation was applied to muscle nerves. The reason behind the development of two different patterns of vascular alterations in response to electrical stimulation of limb muscle afferents is generally believed to be the activation of different types of afferent fibers. It was speculated that the hypotensive response might have been mediated by the activation of groups I, II, and few of group III fibers. Activation of mainly group III and IV fibers, on the other hand, has been implicated in the pressor response. The most definitive evidence supporting this notion has been provided by experiments in which capsaicin injection was used to selectively stimulate group III and IV fibers. Many authors reported that injection of capsaicin into an isolated limb muscle vasculature is consistently followed by a substantial increase in arterial pressure and heart rate (Crayton et al., 1981; Webb-Peploe et al., 1972). Capsaicin injections also evoke a moderate renal vasoconstriction, with no change in blood flow to the brain, heart, and limb muscles.

In the respiratory system, electrical stimulation of phrenic afferent fibers has long been known to evoke profound vascular responses. Kowaleski and Adamuk (1947) reported that electrical stimulation of the phrenic nerve elicited an increase in arterial pressure. Shortly thereafter, the same author confirmed this observation in another experiment. Dingle and co-workers (1940) also reported that electrical stimulation of phrenic afferents in dogs was followed by an increase in mean arterial pressure, ranging from 22 to 38 mm Hg. The vascular responses to phrenic afferent stimulation, however, are not always predictable. For instance, Mussgnug reported in 1930 (Mussgnug, 1947) that blood pressure rose in two dogs and a hypotension response was observed in a third dog when electrical current was applied to the phrenic nerve. In addition, it has been established that the vascular responses evoked by phrenic afferent stimulation are highly dependent on the intensity and frequency of stimulation. This has been clearly demonstrated by Khorman and colleagues (1947). These authors noticed that stimulation of the central end of phrenic nerves decreased arterial pressure in a few dogs, with no changes in heart rate. In another group of animals, a significant decline in heart rate was observed when stimulation frequency was reduced to less than 25 Hz. In yet a third group of dogs, a pressor response was noticed, provided that the intensity of stimulation was sufficiently high, with frequencies ranging from 1 to 100 Hz.

Early investigators have also attempted to correlate the changes in arterial pressure evoked by phrenic afferent activation with redistribution of cardiac output and changes in total peripheral vascular resistance. Until recently, the data on how phrenic afferents affect cardiac output and peripheral vascular resistance were scanty. Dingle and colleagues (1940) reported that peripheral vascular resistance rose by 10–30%, along with a significant increase in arterial pressure. In addition, a moderate augmentation of coronary blood flow has been observed in response to phrenic nerve stimulation (Green, 1935). In contrast, a decline in renal blood volume was reported when the central cut end of the phrenic nerve in dogs was stimulated at high intensities (Kohrman et al., 1947). In none of these reports, however, was the type of phrenic afferents responsible for the cardiovascular alterations identified.

More definite correlation between the type of phrenic afferent and the vascular changes they elicit has been established (McCallister et al., 1986). These authors demonstrated no change in arterial pressure when groups I and II and a few of group III phrenic afferent fibers were electrically stimulated. Only when group IV fibers were activated by increasing the intensity of stimulation did these investigators observe an increase in arterial pressure (Fig. 3). These findings are in favor of an important facilitatory influence of group IV phrenic afferent fibers on the cardiovascular system. This conclusion is also supported by Road and co-workers (1987).

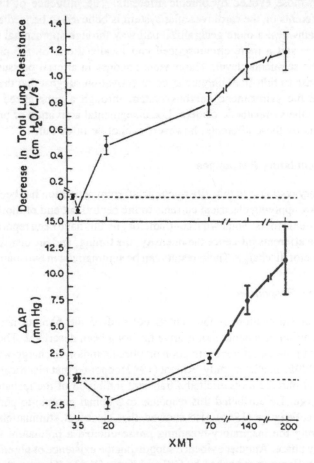

Figure 3 Changes in total lung resistance (top) and mean arterial pressure (bottom) evoked by phrenic nerve stimulation at 3, 5, 20, 70, 140, and 200 times motor threshold. (From McCallister et al., 1986.)

These investigators observed only a small attenuation in the pressor response evoked by high-intensity stimulation of phrenic afferents when conduction in large-fiber (groups I and II) was blocked. In a more recent study, we (Hussain et al., 1991a) used capsaicin injections to selectively activate group III and IV phrenic afferents in anesthetized dogs. Capsaicin injection into the phrenic artery was associated with roughly 15 and 7% increase in mean arterial pressure and heart rate, respectively. We also found that along with the increase in heart rate and blood pressure, capsaicin injection into the phrenic artery elicited approximately 16 and 10% decline in renal and superior mesenteric arterial flow and approximately 13% increase in carotid arterial flow. Injection of capsaicin into the arterial supply of the isolated gastrocnemius muscle produced qualitatively similar, but stronger, vascular responses than those evoked by phrenic afferents. The influence of limb muscles thin-fiber afferents on the cardiovascular system is believed to be mediated through two major pathways: a more generalized pathway through supraspinal sympathetic reflex centers, and a more circumscribed and localized one on the preganglionic neurons at the segmental level. The notable changes in arterial pressure and heart rate in response to thin-fiber phrenic afferent activation suggest that these afferents may activate the sympathetic nervous system through a generalized supraspinal projection on the sympathetic centers. Local segmental activation of preganglionic efferent fibers by these afferents, however, cannot be ruled out.

B. Ventilatory Responses

The ventilatory response to thin-fiber phrenic afferent activation has been characterized mainly by applying electrical currents to the central cut end of thoracic phrenic or cervical phrenic roots. Somewhat contradictory results have been reported concerning how these afferents influence the intensity, the timing, and the distribution of the ventilatory motor discharge. These results can be summarized in two main categories:

Inhibitory Responses

That electrical stimulation of the central cut end of the phrenic nerve elicits a transient inhibition of phrenic motor drive has long been described. The first report of the effect of phrenic afferent activation on phrenic motor discharge was published by Porter in 1895. In a later study, Rijlant (1942) reported that electrical stimulation of the cervical phrenic roots elicited a transient inhibition of the ipsilateral phrenic motor discharge. He attributed this response to a spinal phrenic-to-phrenic reflex. Fleisch and colleagues (1946) also showed that electrical stimulation of phrenic afferents during the inspiratory-breathing phase elicited a premature transition to the expiratory phase. Another evidence supporting the existence of phrenic-to-phrenic inhibitory reflex was published by Gill and Kuno (1963). These authors recorded intracellular phrenic motoneuron potentials in spinalized cats in which the dorsal and ventral roots of the phrenic nerve were left intact. They noticed that low-intensity stimulation of the central cut phrenic nerve evoked hyperpolarization (inhibition) of the contralateral motoneurons that lasted between 15 and 20 ms. This reflex was abolished, however, when the cervical roots were severed. The intensity of phrenic nerve stimulation used in Gill and Kuno's study suggests that the afferent fibers involved in this reflex are groups I and II. Duron et al. (1976) have also described an ipsilateral inhibition of phrenic motoneurons in response to phrenic afferent activation. More recently, Jammes et al. (1986) selectively stimulated group IV phrenic afferents in vagotomized cats and noticed a moderate inhibition of contralateral phrenic motor discharge. In addition, group IV fiber activation was associated with about 17% reduction in the inspiratory time (Table 2). Whereas Jammes et al. (1986) noticed a sustained inhibition of phrenic motor discharge, a transient phrenic-to-phrenic inhibitory response was described by Speck and Revelette (1987a). These authors demonstrated that stimulation of group III phrenic afferents evoked a contralateral and ipsilateral inhibition of phrenic motoneurons (see Fig. 2). This reflex was attenuated after sectioning of the cervical dorsal roots. The contribution of supraspinal structure to the inhibitory phrenic-to-phrenic reflex is still debatable. The changes in respiratory timing demonstrated by Jammes and colleagues (see Table 2) is in favor of an important supraspinal component. Duron and co-workers (1976) have demonstrated that the transient inhibition of phrenic motoneuron by phrenic afferent activation was eliminated by decerebration. Contradicting these findings of Duron et al. is the observation of Speck and Revelette (1987a), who showed that the short-latency inhibition of phrenic motor discharge by group III phrenic afferent activation was not influenced by decerebration. From these results, one can postulate the existence of two different pathways for ipsilateral and contralateral phrenic-to-phrenic inhibitory reflex. Evidence supporting this hypothesis stems from the differences in the latency periods between ipsilateral and contralateral inhibition demonstrated by Speck and Revelette. In addition, Speck (1987), in a later study, showed that the short-latency ipsilateral inhibition is indeed mediated by segmental circuits, whereas the long-latency contralateral inhibition of

Table 2 Changes in Motor Phrenic Discharge Induced by Contralateral Phrenic Nerve Stimulation at 40 V, 80 Hz, 1-ms Pulse Duration

	f impulse/s	Tphr	T_T	Tphr/T_T
Control	177 ± 9	2.66 ± 0.04	4.94 ± 0.06	0.55 ± 0.01
Stimulation	127 ± 8*	2.20 ± 0.05*	4.55 ± 0.09*	0.50 ± 0.01+
%	(−28%)	(−17%)	(−8%)	(−9%)

Values are means ± SE. Changes in motor phrenic discharge (right nerve cut) were induced by central stimulation of the left phrenic nerve. f, Peak impulse frequency measured on 100-ms period of the whole phrenic motor discharge; Tphr, phrenic motor discharge time; T_T, total breathing cycle duration; *, + $p < 0.05$ and 0.01, respectively.

Source: Jammes et al. (1986).

phrenic motor discharge requires the presence of intact supraspinal pathways. He did not, however, indicate which brain stem structures are involved in these reflexes.

Excitatory Responses

A substantial number of investigators have reported that stimulation of phrenic afferents in intact animals elicits a significant augmentation of the ventilatory motor drive. Khorman et al. (1947), for instance, stimulated the central end of the cut phrenic nerve in anesthetized dogs and noticed a substantial increase in tidal volume and breathing frequency, lasting throughout the period of stimulation. These authors concluded that phrenic afferent fibers mediate this reflex through projections to the respiratory and vasomotor centers. Macron and colleagues (1985, 1986) have demonstrated in a subsequent study that, indeed, electrical stimulation of groups III and IV phrenic afferents elicited a significant activation of lateral reticular formation neurons that are responsible for the integration of cardiovascular and somatic afferents. In addition, Road and co-workers (1987) have recently applied electrical stimulation to the cut central end of phrenic nerve in dogs and showed that minute ventilation and arterial pressure rose substantially in response to high-intensity and high-frequency stimulation of phrenic afferents (Fig. 4). Since the increase in ventilation required stimulation intensities greater than 20 times twitch threshold, and since sectioning C5–C7 dorsal roots abolished the response, whereas cold blockade of group I and II fibers did not, Road et al. concluded that the facilitatory ventilatory response was mediated by groups III and IV afferents. In a similar fashion, breathing frequency and tidal volume increased significantly in response to prolonged repetitive stimulation of group III phrenic afferents in vagotomized cats (Marlot et al., 1987).

The major pitfall in the use of electrical stimulation procedures to activate thin-fiber afferents has been the poor selectivity in differentiating various types of afferents. For example, investigators used high intensities to activate high-threshold thin-fiber afferents. However, since large-fiber afferents are also activated at these intensities, one could argue that the ventilatory and vascular responses observed in response to electrical stimulation of phrenic nerve may be partly attributed to the activation of large-fiber afferents. Although Road and colleagues (1987) and McCallister and co-workers (1986) reported no changes in arterial pressure or minute ventilation at intensities low enough to activate large-fiber only, the contribution of these fibers to changes evoked by high intensities of electrical stimulation of phrenic nerve is difficult to assess. The poor selectivity of electrical stimulation was clearly demonstrated by Marlot and colleagues (1987). These investigators showed that augmentation of minute ventilation following electrical stimulation of the phrenic nerve became evident when action potentials of groups I, II, and III phrenic afferents were recorded from the cervical roots.

To avoid the activation of large-fiber afferents, investigators have recently used selective chemical probes to stimulate thin-fiber afferents. Revelette and

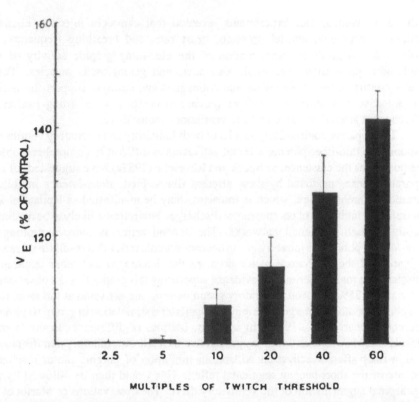

Figure 4 Results obtained during electrical stimulation of the central end of phrenic nerve. Minute ventilation (VE) is shown in relation to increasing stimulation intensities (multiple of twitch threshold). No change in ventilation was observed at low intensities. At all intensities ≥20 times twitch threshold a significant increase in ventilation was noticed. Bars, ± SE.

co-workers (1988) injected capsaicin into the phrenic artery of vagotomized dogs to stimulate thin-fiber afferents. They observed a short period of apneusis during which tonic activity of the diaphragm and hypoglossal muscles increased significantly. This was followed by an increase in the phasic activity of these two muscles, combined with an increase in breathing frequency. When capsaicin was reinjected after spinal cord section at C-7, only an increase in tonic diaphragmatic activity was observed. Revelette and co-workers concluded that thin-fiber phrenic afferents have a stimulatory effect on the inspiratory motor drive. Moreover, we have assessed the effect of thin-fiber phrenic afferent activation on the inspiratory motor drive by injecting capsaicin into the arterial supply of an in situ diaphragm preparation (Hussain et al., 1990). This preparation enabled us to completely separate diaphragmatic circulation from the systemic circulation so that contamination of systemic circulation with capsaicin, which may stimulate afferents in other vascular beds, was avoided. Our experiments revealed that capsaicin injection elicits a moderate increase in arterial pressure, heart rate, and breathing frequency, in addition to a significant augmentation of the electromyographic activity of the diaphragm, parasternal intercostal, alae nasi, and genioglossus muscles. These results confirm those of Revelette and colleagues and strongly support the notion that selective activation of thin-fiber phrenic afferents have a strong excitatory influence on arterial pressure and the ventilatory motor drive.

The apparent contradictory results of both inhibitory and excitatory ventilatory responses to thin-fiber phrenic afferent activation is difficult to comprehend unless one postulates the existence, as Speck and Revelette (1987a) have suggested, of two separate reflexes mediated by these afferent fibers: First, *short-latency* inhibitory phrenic-to-phrenic reflex, which is transient, may be manifested as ispilateral and contralateral inhibition of phrenic motor discharge. This reflex is likely to be mediated mainly through segmental networks. The second reflex is more a prolonged, *long-latency* phrenic–respiratory group neuron–phrenic reflex that results in increased activation of the inspiratory motor drive to the diaphragm and other respiratory muscles. The main experimental evidence supporting this proposal is the observation that roughly 25% of dorsal respiratory group neurons are activated at the same time that phrenic motor discharge is inhibited by ipsilateral stimulation of group III phrenic afferents (Scharf et al., 1986). In addition, because of differences in the latency periods of the two reflexes, one may predict that the earliest ventilatory manifestations of thin-fiber afferent activation will be an inhibition of phrenic motor discharge because of the short-latency segmental reflex. This would then be followed by the supraspinal augmentation of the ventilatory drive. The observations of Marlot et al. (1987) showed that a biphasic ventilatory response (a short inhibition, followed by prolonged excitation) was observed when phrenic afferents are activated in vagotomized cats. Interestingly, a biphasic ventilatory response also occurs in response to limb muscle afferent stimulation (Eldridge et al., 1981). In addition, Eldridge and co-workers showed that stimulation of calf muscle afferents in intact cats elicited a significant increase in breathing frequency and phrenic motor discharge. When afferent stimulation was repeated in high spinal animals, there was a transient inhibition of spontaneous phrenic motor discharge. These findings favor an existence of two simultaneous reflexes initiated by thin-fiber afferent. The inhibitory segmental reflex demonstrated by Eldridge and colleagues appears to dominate only when the supraspinal connections of muscle afferents are severed. Clearly, more elaborate studies are needed to elucidate the extent of segmental versus supraspinal reflexogenic components elicited by phrenic afferent activation.

Until recently, the effects of diaphragmatic fatigue on the discharge pattern of phrenic thin-fiber afferents have never been studied. In a recently published study, Jammes and Balzamo (1992) assessed the changes in the discharge frequency of large-fiber and thin-fiber phrenic afferents in response to diaphragmatic fatigue induced by direct high-frequency stimulation of the diaphragm in cats. Under control condition, large-fiber afferent activity was manifested as high-frequency (100–150

Hz) discharge that coincided with diaphragmatic contraction. By comparison, spontaneous thin-fiber afferent discharge was tonic and of low frequency (firing rate of 2.2 Hz). Diaphragmatic mechanical failure elicited a progressive increase in tonic activity of thin-fiber afferents, with the firing rate increasing to 15–20 Hz and a progressive decline in phasic large-fiber afferent discharge. Along with these changes in phrenic afferent activation, diaphragmatic mechanical failure was associated with significant prolongation of the inspiratory time and total breathing duration. No changes in respiratory timing were observed when diaphragmatic fatigue was induced after sectioning both phrenic nerves. These results demonstrate the influence of phrenic afferents on the respiratory control during diaphragmatic fatigue. This effect appears to be mediated through alterations in the activation of both large-fibers (groups I and II) and thin-fiber (groups III and IV) phrenic afferents. Changes in phrenic sensory activity during diaphragmatic fatigue may also alter the transmission of phrenic action potentials to the cortex and also the spontaneous electroencephalographic (EEG) activity. Indeed, the increase in tonic thin-fiber activity and the decline in phasic large-fiber afferent activity during diaphragmatic electrical stimulation was associated with progressive lengthening in onset and peak latencies of cortical phrenic-evoked potentials (Balzamo et al., 1992). The EEG changes were manifested as an initial increase in energy in the delta-frequency band followed by decreased energy in the theta-frequency band.

C. Pattern of Muscle Recruitment

In recent years, it became evident that afferent inputs from peripheral skeletal muscles affect the ventilatory motor discharge in an inhomogeneous fashion, resulting in different patterns of chest wall muscle recruitment. Our recent studies (Ward et al., 1992a) have confirmed that this is true of thin-fiber phrenic afferents. When electrically activated in vagotomized dogs, thin-fiber afferents in the left phrenic nerve elicited a 66% increase in minute ventilation, with a similar increase in right diaphragmatic, parasternal, and alae nasi muscle activities, whereas the activities of genioglossus and transverse abdominis muscles rose by more than 6- and 12-fold, respectively (Fig. 5). Interestingly, stimulation of thin-fiber afferents of gastrocnemius muscle at the same intensities and frequencies evokes changes in the pattern of respiratory muscle recruitment that are stronger than, but qualitatively similar to, those elicited by phrenic afferents (Hussain et al., 1991b).

The interpretation of these specific recruitment patterns initiated by muscle afferents remains speculative. We related these patterns of muscle recruitment to changes in diaphragmatic contractile performance. For example, strong recruitment of abdominal muscles through phrenic afferent activation may be interpreted to indicate facilitation of high expiratory flow rate and reduction of diaphragmatic shortening, such that the diaphragm will be placed at a better mechanical advantage relative to its force–length and force–velocity characteristics. The out of proportion increases in genioglossus muscle activity by electrical stimulation of thin-fiber phrenic afferents

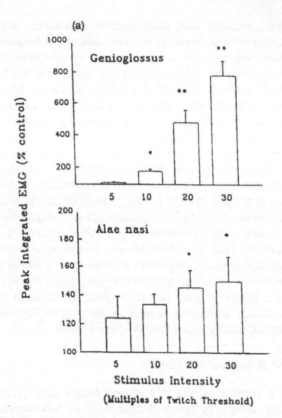

Figure 5 Percentage increase from control values of peak integrated inspiratory activity of (a) genioglossus, alae nasi, (b) right diaphragm, and parasternal intercostal muscles in response to electrical stimulation of cut central end of left phrenic nerve at 40-Hz, 1-ms stimulus duration and stimulation intensities of 5, 10, 20, and 30 times twitch-threshold. (From Ward et al., 1992.)

have also been observed following selective chemical activation of these fibers by capsaicin (Hussain et al., 1990) or bradykinin (Wilson et al., 1991). These findings are consistent with a significant convergence of phrenic afferent collaterals on the brain stem reticular-activating system that controls the hypoglossal nerve activity. It is possible that the genioglossal response to phrenic afferents may aid in reducing upper airway resistance, especially in the face of increased airflow, as during exercise.

D. Ventilatory Interaction

Many conditions exist during which simultaneous stimulation of phrenic and limb muscle afferents may occur. For example, shock state is accompanied by accumulation of lactic acid in both limb and respiratory muscles. Similarly, in exercise, an increase in the intensity of contraction develops in the diaphragm and other skeletal

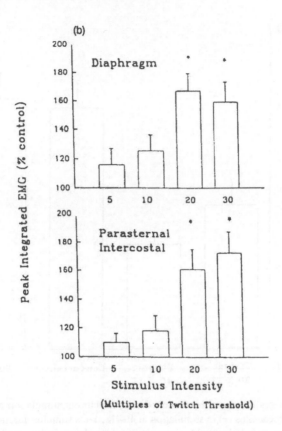

muscles. Under such conditions, the magnitude and the pattern of respiratory muscle recruitment will be modified by simultaneous afferent inputs from different muscular sources. Little is known about the nature of interaction between phrenic afferents and other respiratory-related afferent inputs. We studied the ventilatory interaction between phrenic and limb muscle thin-fiber afferents by stimulating the central cut ends of phrenic and gastrocnemius nerves, both separately and simultaneously, in vagotomized dogs (Ward et al., 1992b). Gastrocnemius nerve stimulation at 40 times motor threshold elicited a 90% increase in ventilation, whereas stimulation of phrenic nerve alone evoked about a 66% increase in ventilation. When both nerves were stimulated simultaneously, minute ventilation rose by 150%, suggesting that the ventilatory interaction between phrenic and gastrocnemius afferents is additive (Fig. 6). A similar degree of summation was found for respiratory muscle recruitment pattern. Because of the widespread projections of limb muscle and phrenic afferents on supraspinal structures, it is difficult to identify the level of afferent interaction of these muscles. However, it is likely that summation may occur at various sites, such as the reticular-activating system that modulates activity

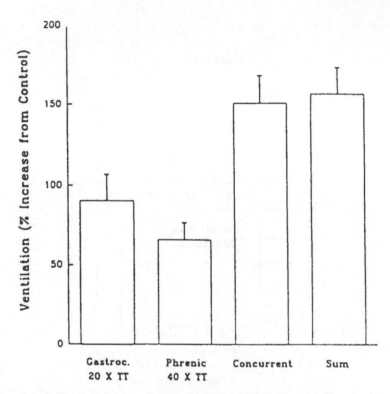

Figure 6 Changes in minute ventilation during concurrent stimulation of central ends of phrenic and gastrocnemius nerve stimulation at 40-Hz, 1-ms stimulus duration and intensities of 40 and 20 times twitch threshold, respectively. Also shown is the ventilatory response to individual gastrocnemius stimulation at 20 times twitch-threshold. Notice that the change in ventilation during concurrent nerve stimulation is similar to that obtained by algebric summation of individual phrenic and gastrocnemius stimulation.

of the genioglossus muscle. Enhancement of activity in this region may be by the summed inputs from afferents arising from the diaphragm and gastrocnemius muscle, in conjunction with less specific influences on the ventilatory site. Another site that may mediate afferent summation is the dorsal and ventilatory respiratory medullary neurons on which both gastrocnemius and phrenic afferents are known to project. The nature of a possible interaction between thin-fiber phrenic afferents and other inputs from vagal, baroreceptor, chemoreceptor, and thin-fibers afferents emanating from other respiratory muscles remains to be investigated.

E.   Poststimulus Inhibition

In addition to the immediate stimulatory effect on the ventilatory motor drive, stimulation of limb muscle thin-fiber afferents in intact animals is followed by a prolonged period of poststimulus inhibition of phrenic motor discharge (Kumazawa et al., 1983; Waldrop et al., 1982). This poststimulation inhibition of the respiratory drive is usually attenuated by naloxone or bicuculline, suggesting that this response may be mediated by the release of endogenous opoids or γ-aminobutyric acid (Waldrop et al., 1983). Recently, Road et al. (1990) studied the nature of poststimulus inhibition of phrenic motor discharge by electrically stimulating contralateral thin-fiber phrenic afferents in paralyzed anesthetized dogs. These authors reported that phrenic motor discharge increased substantially during 60-s periods of phrenic afferent stimulation. On cessation of stimulation, phrenic motor discharge then declined significantly for a period of about 30 min. These findings imply that strong activation of thin-fiber phrenic afferents and, possibly, afferents from other respiratory muscles may activate certain central mechanisms that inhibit ventilatory motor drive. It remains to be seen how these observations relate to the control of ventilatory motor drive.

F. Effects on Airway Resistance

In addition to alterations in the ventilatory motor drive, electrical stimulation of thin-fiber limb muscle afferents exert a substantial influence on bronchomotor tone and airway resistance. Rybicki and Kaufman (1985) found that stimulation of the gastrocnemius nerve at high intensities produced a significant decline in total pulmonary resistance. In a later study, Kaufman and colleagues (1985) observed the same response during tetanic and repetitive contraction of hindlimb muscles. These authors attributed the decline in transpulmonary resistance to the activation of contraction-sensitive groups III and IV fibers. Along with the decline in total pulmonary resistance, activation of contraction-sensitive limb muscle afferents evokes a moderate degree of trachealis muscle relaxation (Kaufman and Rybicki, 1984). In a similar fashion, activation of thin-fiber phrenic afferents strongly influences the bronchomotor tone. Thornton (1932) was the first to notice, during the course of setting up isolated bronchial preparations, that traction on the phrenic nerve caused a sharp dilation of the isolated bronchus. In a later study, the same author stimulated the phrenic nerve electrically and concluded that phrenic afferent activation evoked a bronchodilator response that was independent from the pressor response (Thornton, 1937). The type of fiber activated in that study, however, was not identified. More recently, McCallister et al. (1986) assessed the influence of phrenic afferent activation on total pulmonary resistance in paralyzed dogs. Electrical stimulation of group I and II fibers elicited no change in total pulmonary resistance. By contrast, when stimulation intensity was increased to activate groups III and IV fibers, total pulmonary resistance declined from a mean value of 5.4 to 4.2 cm H_2O L^{-1} s^{-1} (see Fig. 3). This response was not influenced by propranolol or phentolamine, but was abolished by atropine, suggesting that, as in limb muscles, thin-fiber phrenic afferents reflexly decreased total pulmonary resistance by withdrawing cholinergic tone to airway smooth muscles. Thin-fiber phrenic afferents also influence the tone of large airways. This was evident in our recent experiments in which we measured the changes in trachealis muscle tension in response to the activation of thin-fiber phrenic and gastrocnemius muscles in paralyzed dogs. In most animals, trachealis muscle tension declined moderately in response to either phrenic or gastrocnemius afferent stimulation. These results lend further credence to the notion that the ventilatory effects of thin-fiber phrenic afferent stimulation is qualitatively similar to those of limb muscle afferents.

G. Response to Ischemia

Our understanding of the physiological role of thin-fiber phrenic afferents has been derived primarily from experiments in which nonphysiological stimuli, such as electrical stimulation or capsaicin injections, were used to produce sudden and simultaneous activation of these afferents. Until very recently, no attempts were made to use physiological stimuli, such as muscle ischemia, to activate thin-fiber phrenic afferents. The presence of phrenic afferent fibers that are sensitive to ischemia have been documented by Graham and colleagues (1986). However, it was unknown, until very recently, whether activation of thin-fiber phrenic afferents by ischemia exerts any influence on the ventilatory control, because of the difficulty in inducing diaphragmatic ischemia without interfering with the blood flow of other organs. With the development of in situ, isolated innervated diaphragmatic preparation, we were recently able to assess the effect of diaphragmatic ischemia on the inspiratory motor drive (Teitelbaum et al., 1992a). The blood flow to the isolated left diaphragm was selectively reduced by occluding the phrenic arterial flow for a period of 20 min, during which chemical ventilatory drive was maintained constant. Diaphragmatic ischemia elicited a significant and progressive increase in the inspiratory motor drive to the ischemic diaphragm, nonischemic right diaphragm, and parasternal and alae nasi muscles. In addition, diaphragmatic ischemia was associated with a significant increase in breathing frequency. To investigate the type of afferent fibers responsible for the ventilatory response to diaphragmatic ischemia, we injected capsaicin repeatedly into the phrenic artery to desensitize phrenic nociceptors. When ischemia was induced after the last injection of capsaicin, no changes were observed in the inspiratory motor drive (Teitelbaum et al., 1992b). These results confirm that the facilitatory effect of diaphragmatic ischemia on the inspiratory motor drive is mediated through the activation of thin-fiber phrenic afferents. In addition, the changes in respiratory timing and the increase in alae nasi muscle activity during diaphragmatic ischemia suggest that thin-fiber phrenic afferents exert their influence on the ventilatory motor drive through supraspinal pathways.

VI. Summary

The phrenic nerves, similar to other muscular nerves, contain a variety of afferent fibers, a significant proportion of which have thin diameters and slow-conduction velocities and are either thinly myelinated or unmyelinated. Most of these fibers terminate in the diaphragm as free nerve endings and have been classified as either ergoceptors (sensitive to touch and contraction) or nociceptors (sensitive to chemical stimuli, noxious substances, and ischemia). Thin-fiber phrenic afferents enter the spinal cord mainly through the dorsal roots and project to various supraspinal structures, such as the reticular formation and dorsal and ventral medullary respiratory neurons. The spontaneous activity of thin-fiber phrenic afferents during eupneic breathing appears to be irregular and slow. When artificially stimulated by electrical or chemical means, thin-fiber phrenic afferents elicit substantial changes in the cardiovascular system, such as a rise in arterial pressure, in heart rate, and in redistribution of blood flow to various organs. In the respiratory system, inhibitory, excitatory, or biphasic changes in the ventilatory drive have been reported in response to artifical stimulation of thin-fiber phrenic afferents. In spite of these findings, the functional significance of thin-fiber phrenic afferents in the control of respiratory neural drive is far from clear, because very few investigators employ physiological stimuli to activate these afferents. More recent studies from our group suggest that increased phrenic thin-fiber afferent activity was associated with significant changes in the inspiratory motor drive during diaphragmatic ischemia or mechanical failure of the diaphragm. It is apparent that more extensive studies are needed to assess whether thin-fiber phrenic afferents play a significant modulatory influence on phrenic motor discharge during various physiological or pathological stimuli.

References

Balzamo, E., Lagier-Tessonnier, F., and Jammes, Y. (1992). Fatigue-induced changes in diaphragmatic afferents and cortical activity in the cat. *Respir. Physiol.* 90: 213–226.

Banzett, R. B., Inbar, G. F., Brown, R., Goldman, M., Rossier, R., and Mead, J. (1981). Diaphragm electrical activity during negative lower torso pressure in quadriplegic men. *J. Appl. Physiol.* 51: 654–659.

Barker, D. (1974). The morphology of muscle receptors. In: *Handbook of Sensory Physiology. Muscle Receptors.* Edited by C. C. Hunt. New York: Springer-Verlag, pp. 1–90.

Capps, J. A. (1911). An experimental study of the pain sense in the pleural membranes. *Arch. Intern. Med.* 6: 718–733.

Cheeseman, M., and Revelette, W. R. (1990). Phrenic afferent contribution to reflexes elicited by changes in diaphragm length. *J. Appl. Physiol.* 69: 640–647.

Corda, M., von Euler, C., and Lennerstrand, G. (1965). Proprioceptive innervation of the diaphragm. *J. Physiol. (Lond.)* 178: 161–177.

Crayton, S. C., Mitchell, J. H., and Payne, F. C. (1981). Reflex cardiovascular response during injection of capsaicin into skeletal muscle. *Am. J. Physiol.* 240: H315–H319.

Dalsgaard, C. J., Vincent, S. R., Hokfelt, T., et al. (1982). Coexistence of cholecystokinin- and substance P-like peptides in neurons of the dorsal root ganglia of the rat. *Neurosci. Lett.* 33: 159.

Davenport, P. W., Thompson, F. J., Reep, R. L., and Freed, A. N. (1985). Projection of phrenic nerve afferents to the cat sensorimotor cortex. *Brain Res.* 328: 150–153.

Dingle, J. T., Kent, G. T., Williams, L. L., and Wiggers, C. J. (1940). A study of alleged quantitative criteria of vasomotor action. *Am. J. Physiol.* 130: 63–68.

Dogiel, A. S. (1902). Die Nervenendigungen in Bauchfell, in den Sehnen, den Muskelspindeln und dem Centrum tendineum des Diaphragma beim Menschen und bei Saugethieren. *Arch. Mikrosk. Anat. Entwicklungsmech.* 59: 1–31.

Duron, B. (1981). Intercostal and diaphragmatic muscle endings and afferents. In: *Regulation of Breathing.* Edited by T. F. Hornbein. New York: Marcel Dekker, pp. 473–541.

Duron, B., and Caillol, M. C. (1973). Investigation of afferent activity in the intact phrenic nerve with bipolar electrodes. *Acta Neurobiol. Exp.* 33: 427–432.

Duron, B., and Condamin, M. (1969). L'innervation intercosta le accessoire du diaphragme chez le chat. *C. R. Soc. Biol.* 163: 1859–1864.

Duron, B., and Condamin, M. (1970). Etude au microscope electronique de la composition amyelinique du nerf phrenique du chat. *C. R. Soc. Biol.* 164: 577–583.

Duron, B., and Marlot, D. (1980). The non-myelinated fibers of the phrenic and the intercostal nerves in the cat. *Z. Mikrosk. Anat. Forsch. (Leipz.)* 2: 257–268.

Duron, B., Jung-Caillol, M. C., and Marlot, D. (1976). Reflexe inhibiteur phrenico-phrenique. In: *Respiratory Centres and Afferent Systems.* Edited by B. Duron. Paris, INSERM, pp. 193–197.

Duron, B., Jung-Caillol, M. C., and Marlot, D. (1978). Myelinated nerve fiber supply and muscle spindles in the respiratory muscles of cat: Quantitative study. *Anat. Embryol.* 152: 171–192.

Eldridge, F. L., Gill-Kumar, P., Millhorn, D. E., and Waldrop, T. G. (1981). Spinal inhibition of phrenic motoneurons by stimulation of afferents from peripheral muscles. *J. Physiol.* 311: 67–79.

Felix, W. (1922). *Dtsch. Z. Chir.* 171: 283.

Fell, C. (1968). Changes in blood flow distribution produced by central sciatic nerve stimulation. *Am. J. Physiol.* 214: 561–565.

Ferguson, J. (1891). The phrenic nerve. *Brain* 14: 282–283.

Fleisch, A., Grandjean, E., and Crusaz, R. (1946). Contribution a l'etude de la fonction des fibres affereentes du phrenique. *Physiol. Pharmacol. Acta* 4: 127–134.

Fryman, D. L., and Frazier, D. T. (1987). Diaphragm afferent modulation of phrenic motor drive. *J. Appl. Physiol.* 62: 2436–2441.

Gasser, H. S., and Grundfest, H. (1939). Axon diameters in relation to the spike dimensions and the conduction velocity in mammalian fibers. *Am. J. Physiol.* 127: 393–414.

Gernandt, B. (1946). Pain conduction in the phrenic nerve. *Acta Physiol. Scand.* 12: 255–260.

Gibbons, H., Furness, J. B., and Costa, M. (1987). Pathway-specific patterns of the coexistence of substance P and dynorphin in neurons of the dorsal root ganglia of the guinea-pig. *Cell Tissue Res.* 248: 417.

Gill, P. K., and Kuno, M. (1963). Excitatory and inhibitory actions on phrenic motoneurons. *J. Physiol. (Lond.)* 168: 274–289.

Glebovskii, V. D. (1962). Stretch receptors of the diaphragm. *Fiziol. Z. SSSR Im. I. M. Sechenova* 48: T405–T410.

Gordon, G. (1943). The mechanism of the vasomotor reflexes produced by stimulating mammalian sensory nerves. *J. Physiol. (Lond.)* 102: 95–107.

Goshgarian, H. G. (1981). The role of cervical afferent nerve fiber inhibition of the crossed phrenic phenomenon. *Exp. Neurol.* 72: 211–225.

Goshgarian, H. G., and Roubal, P. J. (1986). Origin and distribution of phrenic primary afferent nerve fibers in the spinal cord of the adult rat. *Exp. Neurol.* 92: 624–638.

Graham, R., Jammes, Y., Delpierre, S., Grimaud, C., and Roussos, C. (1986). The effects of ischemia, lactic acid and hypertonic sodium chloride on phrenic afferent discharge during spontaneous diaphragmatic contraction. *Neurosci. Lett.* 67: 257–262.

Green, C. W. (1935). *Am. J. Physiol.* 113: 390.

Green, M., Mead, J., and Sears, T. A. (1978). Muscle activity during chest wall restriction and positive pressure breathing in man. *Respir. Physiol.* 35: 283–300.

Hinsey, J. C., and Phillips, R. A. (1937). Studies on diaphragmatic sensation. *Am. J. Physiol.* 119: 336.

Hinsey, J. C., Hare, K., and Phillips, R. A. (1939). Sensory components of the phrenic nerve of the cat. *Proc. Soc. Exp. Biol. Med.* 41: 411–414.

Hokfelt, I., Elde, R., Johansson, O., Luft, R., Nilsson, G., and Arimura, A. (1976). Immunohistochemical evidence for separate populations of somatostatin-containing and substance P-containing primary afferent neurons in the rat. *Neuroscience* 1: 131.

Holtman, J. R., Jr. (1989). Localization of substance P immunoreactivity in phrenic primary afferent neurons. *Peptides* 10: 53–56.

Hussain, S. N. A., Magder, S., Chatillon, A., and Roussos, C. (1990). Chemical activation of thin-fiber phrenic afferents: Respiratory responses. *J. Appl. Physiol.* 69: 1002–1011.

Hussain, S. N. A., Chatillon, A., Comtois, A., Roussos, C., and Magder, S. (1991a). Chemical activation of thin-fiber phrenic afferents 2. Cardiovascular responses. *J. Appl. Physiol.* 70: 77–86.

Hussain, S. N. A., Ward, M. E., Gatensby, A. G., Roussos, C., and Deschamps, A. (1991b). Respiratory muscle activation by limb muscle afferent stimulation in anesthetized dogs. *Respir. Physiol.* 84: 185–198.

Jammes, Y., and Balzamo, E. (1992). Changes in afferent and efferent phrenic activities with electrically induced diaphragmatic fatigue. *J. Appl. Physiol.* 73: 894–902.

Jammes, Y., Buchler, B., and Delpierre, S. (1986). Phrenic afferents and their role in inspiratory control. *J. Appl. Physiol.* 60: 854–860.

Johansson, B. (1962). Circulatory responses to stimulation of somatic afferent (with special reference to depressor effects from muscle nerves). *Acta Physiol. Scand.* 198: 1–95.

Kao, F. F. (1963). An experimental study of the pathway involved in exercise hyperpnea employing cross-circulation technique. In: *The Regulation of Human Respiration.* Edited by D. J. C. Cunningham and B. B. Lloyd. Oxford, Blackwell, pp. 461–502.

Katz, S., and Perryman, J. H. (1965). Respiratory and blood pressure responses to stimulation of peripheral afferent nerves. *Am. J. Physiol.* 208: 993–999.

Kaufman, M. P., and Rybicki, K. J. (1984). Muscular contraction reflexly relaxes tracheal smooth muscle in dogs. *Respir. Physiol.* 56: 61–72.

Kaufman, M. P., Iwamoto, G. A., Longhurst, J. C., and Mitchell, J. H. (1982). Effects of capsaicin and bradykinin on afferent fibers with endings in skeletal muscle. *Circ. Res.* 50: 133–139.

Kaufman, M. P., Longhurst, J. C., Rybicki, K. J., Wallach, J. H., and Mitchell, J. H. (1983). Effects of static muscular contraction on impulse activity groups III and IV afferents in cats [abstract]. *J. Appl. Physiol. Respir. Environ. Exerc. Physiol.* 55: 105–112.

Kaufman, M. P., Rybicki, J., Waldrop, T. G., and Ordway, G. A. (1984). Effect of ischemia on responses of group III and IV afferent to contraction. *J. Appl. Physiol. Respir. Environ. Exerc. Physiol.* 57: 644–650.

Kaufman, M. P., Rybicki, K. J., and Mitchell, J. H. (1985). Hindlimb muscular contraction reflexly decreases total pulmonary resistance in dogs [abstract]. *J. Appl. Physiol.* 59: 1521–1526.

Kniffki, K. D., Mense, S., and Schmidt, R. F. (1978). Responses of group IV afferent units from skeletal muscle to stretch, contraction and chemical stimulation. *Exp. Brain Res.* 31: 511–522.

Kohrman, R. M., Nolasco, J. B., and Wiggers, C. J. (1947). Types of afferent fibers in the phrenic nerve. *Am. J. Physiol.* 151: 547–557.

Kowaleski, N., and Adamuk, E. (1947). Cited in: Types of afferent fibers in the phrenic nerve. *Am. J. Physiol.* 151: 547–557.

Kumada, M., Nogami, K., and Sagawa, K. (1975). Modulation of carotid baroreceptor reflex by sciatic nerve stimulation. *Am. J. Physiol.* 228: 1535–1541.

Kumazawa, T., Tadaki, E., Mizumura, K., and Kim, K. (1983). Post-stimulus facilitatory and inhibitory effects on respiration induced by chemical and electrical stimulation of thin-fiber muscular afferents in dogs. *Neurosci. Lett.* 35: 283–287.

Landau, B. E., Akert, K., and Roberts, T. S. (1962). Studies on the innervation of the diaphragm. *J. Comp. Neurol.* 119: 1–10.

Langford, L. A., and Schmidt, R. F. (1983). An electron microscopic analysis of the left phrenic nerve in the rat. *Anat. Rec.* 205: 207–213.

Larnicol, N., Rose, D., and Duron, B. (1985). Identification of phrenic afferents to the external cuneate nucleus: A fluorescent double-labeling study in the cat. *Neurosci. Lett.* 62: 163–167.

Little, M. G. A., and McSwiney, B. A. (1938). Afferent fibers from the diaphragm. *J. Physiol.* 94: 2–3.

Lubinska, L., and Waryszewskia, J. (1974). Fiber population of the phrenic nerve of rat: Changes of myelinated fiber dimensions along the nerve and characteristics of axonal branchings. *Acta Neurobiol. Exp.* 34: 525–541.

Macron, J. M., and Marlot, D. (1986). Effects of stimulation of phrenic afferent fibers on medullary respiratory neurons in cat. *Neurosci. Lett.* 63: 231–236.

Marlot, D., Macron, J. M., and Duron, B. (1984). Projections of phrenic afferents to the cat cerebellar cortex. *Neurosci. Lett.* 44: 95–98.

Macron, J. M., Marlot, D., and Duron, B. (1985). Phrenic afferent input to the lateral medullary reticular formation of the cat. *Respir. Physiol.* 59: 155–167.

Marlot, D., Macron, J. M., and Duron, B. (1987). Inhibitory and excitatory effects on respiration by phrenic nerve afferent stimulation in cats. *Respir. Physiol.* 69: 321–333.

Marlot, D., Macron, J. M., and Duron, B. (1988). Effects of ipsilateral and contralateral cervical phrenic afferent stimulation on phrenic motor unit activity in the cat. *Brain Res.* 450: 373–377.

McCallister, L. W., McCoy, K. W., and Connelly, J. C. (1986). Stimulation of groups III and IV phrenic afferents reflexly decreases total lung resistance in dogs. *J. Appl. Physiol.* 61: 1346–1351.

McNeill, D. L., Westlund, K. N., and Coggeshall, R. E. (1989). Peptide immunoreactivity of unmyelinated primary afferent axons in rat lumbar dorsal roots. *J. Histochem. Cytochem.* 37: 1047–1052.

Mense, S. (1978). Muskelreceptoren mit dunnen markhaltigen und marklosen afferenten Fasern: Receptive Eigenschaften und mogliche Funktion. *Kiel, Federal Republic of Germany*: *Christian-Albrechts-Universitat (Habilitationsschiift)*.

Mense, S. (1981). Sensitization of group IV muscle receptors to bradykinin by 5-hydroxytryptamine and prostaglandin E_2. *Brain Res.* 225: 95–105.

Mense, S., and Schmidt, R. F. (1974). Activation of group IV afferent units from muscle by algesic agents. *Brain Res.* 72: 305–310.

Mussgnug, H. (1947). Cite in: Type of afferent fibers in the phrenic nerve. *Am. J. Physiol.* 151: 547–557.

Nathan, P. W., and Sears, T. A. (1960). Effects of posterior root section on the activity of some muscles in man. *J. Neurol. Neurosurg. Psychiatry* 23: 10–22.

Pollock, L. J., and Davis, L. (1935). Visceral and referred pain. *Arch. Neurol. Psychiatry* 34: 1041–1054.

Porter, W. T. (1895). The path of the respiratory impulse from the bulb to the phrenic nuclei. *J. Physiol. (Lond.)* 17: 455–485.

Revelette, W. R., Jewell, L. A., and Frazier, D. T. (1988). Effect of diaphragm small-fiber afferent stimulation on ventilation in dogs. *J. Appl. Physiol.* 65: 2097–2106.

Revelette, R., Reynolds, S., Brown, D., and Taylor, R. (1992). Effect of abdominal compression on diaphragmatic tendon organ activity. *J. Appl. Physiol.* 72: 288–292.

Rexed, B. (1944). Contributions to the knowledge of the postnatal development of the peripheral nervous system in man. *Acta Psychiat. Neurol. [Suppl.]* 33:

Rijlant, P. (1942). Contribution a l'etude du controle reflexe de la respiration. *Bull. Acad. Med. Belg.* 7: 58–107.

Road, J. D., West, N. H., and Van Vliet, B. N. (1987). Ventilatory effects of stimulation of phrenic afferents. *J. Appl. Physiol.* 63: 1063–1069.

Road, J. D., Osborne, S., and Wakai, Y. (1990). Delayed inhibition of ventilation produced by phrenic afferent stimulation in dogs. *FASEB J.* 4: A540.

Rose, D., Larnicol, N., and Duron, B. (1990). The cat cervical dorsal root ganglia: Generalized cell-size characteristics and comparative study of neck muscle, neck cutaneous and phrenic afferents. *Neurosci. Res.* 7: 341–357.

Rybicki, K. J., and Kaufman, M. P. (1985). Stimulation of group III and IV muscle afferents reflexly decreases total pulmonary resistance in dogs. *Respir. Physiol.* 59: 185–195.

Sant'Ambrogio, G., and Widdicombe, J. G. (1965). Respiratory reflexes acting on the diaphragm and inspiratory intercostal muscles of the rabbit. *J. Physiol. (Lond.)* 180: 766–779.

Scharf, S. M., Bark, H., Einhorn, S., and Tarasiuk, A. (1986). Blood flow to the canine diaphragm during hemorrhagic shock. *Am. Rev. Respir. Dis.* 133: 205–211.

Shannon, R. (1992). Reflexes from respiratory muscles and costovertebral joints. In: *Handbook of Physiology—The Respiratory System.* Bethesda, MD, American Physiological Society, pp. 431–447.

Speck, D. F. (1987). Supraspinal involvement in the phrenic-to-phrenic inhibitory reflex. *Brain Res.* 414: 169–172.

Speck, D. F., and Revelette, W. R. (1987a). Attenuation of phrenic motor discharge by phrenic nerve afferents. *J. Appl. Physiol.* 62: 941–945.

Speck, D. F., and Revelette, W. R. (1987b). Excitation of dorsal and ventral respiratory group neurons by phrenic nerve afferents. *J. Appl. Physiol.* 62: 946–951.

Stacey, M. J. (1969). Free nerve endings in skeletal muscle of the cat. *J. Anat.* 105: 231–254.

Teitelbaum, J. S., Magder, S., Roussos, C., and Hussain, S. N. A. (1991a). Effects of diaphragmatic ischemia on the inspiratory motor drive. *J. Appl. Physiol.* 72: 447–454.

Teitelbaum, J. S., Vanelli, G., and Hussain, S. N. A. (1992b). Effects of diaphragmatic ischemia on the inspiratory motor drive: The role of groups III and IV afferent fibers. *Am. Rev. Respir. Dis.* (in press).

Thornton, J. W. (1932). Reactions of isolated bronchi. *Q. J. Exp. Physiol.* 21: 305–314.

Thornton, J. W. (1937). Bronchodilatation by stimulation of the phrenic nerve. *J. Physiol.* 90: 85P–87P.

Waldrop, T. G., Eldridge, F. L., and Milhorn, D. E. (1982). Prolonged post-stimulus inhibition of breathing following stimulation of afferents from muscle. *Respir. Physiol.* 50: 239–254.

Waldrop, T. G., Eldridge, F. L., and Millhorn, D. E. (1983). Inhibition of breathing after stimulation of muscle is mediated by endogenous opiates and GABA. *Respir. Physiol.* 54: 211–222.

Ward, M. E., Deschamps, A., Roussos, C., and Hussain, S. N. A. (1992a). Effect of phrenic afferent stimulation on pattern of respiratory muscle activation. *J. Appl. Physiol.* 73: 563–570.

Ward, M. E., Vanelli, G., Hashefi, M., and Hussain, S. N. A. (1992b). Ventilatory effects of the interaction between phrenic and limb muscle afferents. *Respir. Physiol.* 88: 63–71.

Webb-Peploe, M. M., Brender, D., and Shepherd, J. T. (1972). Vascular responses to stimulation of receptors in muscle by capsaicin. *Am. J. Physiol.* 222: 189–195.

Wilson, C. R., Vanelli, G., Magder, S., and Hussain, S. N. A. (1991). The effect of phrenic afferent stimulation by bradykinin on the distribution of ventilatory drive [abstract]. *Clin. Invest. Med.* 145: 11.

Winckler, G., and Delaloye, B. (1957). A propos de la presence de fuseaux neuromusculaires dans le diaphragme humain. *Acta Anat.* 29: 114–116.

Yasargil, G. M. (1967). Systematische Untersuchung der motorischen Innervation des Zwerchfells beim Kaninchen. *Helv. Physiol. Pharmacol. Acta [Suppl.]* 18: 1–63.

Yasargil, G. M., and Koller, E. A. (1964). Uber die motorische Innervation des Zwerchfells beim Kaninchen. *Helv. Physiol. Acta* 22: 137–147.

30

The Role of Myelinated Afferents from the Intercostal Muscles and Diaphragm

W. ROBERT REVELETTE

University of Kentucky
Lexington, Kentucky

PAUL W. DAVENPORT

University of Florida
Gainesville, Florida

I. Introduction

The functional significance of proprioceptors in the intercostal muscles and diaphragm has been a topic of intense research and debate for more than 40 years. Much is known concerning the distribution, projection pathways, transduction properties, and reflexes associated with intercostal muscle afferents. Compared with intercostal afferents, relatively little is known about proprioceptors in the diaphragm. Review articles concerning the innervation of chest wall muscles reflect this lack of information on the role of diaphragmatic proprioceptors in the control of breathing (Sant'Ambrogio and Remmers, 1985; Shannon, 1986). Only within the past few years has it been recognized that chest wall proprioceptors may provide sensations important in adjusting respiratory motor drive in the face of added loads to breathing. Evidence is also emerging that inspiratory muscle afferents are activiated by inspiratory loads and reach the somatosensory cortex in conscious human subjects (Road, 1991; Frazier and Revelette, 1991).

The aim of this chapter is to focus on the role of intercostal and diaphragmatic proprioceptors in the control of breathing. The location and numbers of end organs in the respiratory muscles will be reviewed. Emphasis is placed on the transduction properties of the afferents and the reflexes associated with their activation. Projection pathways and the potential contribution that chest wall proprioceptors make in the perception of added loads to breathing are also considered.

II. Intercostal Muscle Afferents

A. Distribution

Huber (1902) was the first to describe the population of muscle spindle fibers in the intercostal muscles of the cat. His results suggested that the absolute number of muscle spindles per rib space decreased as one moved in a cephalocaudal direction along the rib cage. The work of Huber was extended by Duron et al. (1978), who performed quantitative analysis of the myelinated nerve supply to the intercostal muscles of the cat. In addition, these authors counted the number of muscle spindle organs present in the intercostal muscles at selected rib spaces. In the external intercostal muscles, the fraction of myelinated axons that are sensory ranges from 25 to 30%. This includes axons carrying information from muscle spindle primary (group IA) and secondary (group II) endings, as well as Golgi tendon organs (group IB). The density of muscle spindles in the intercostal muscles, determined by dividing the number of spindles by the dry weight of the muscle, was highest for the rostral spaces and decreased in the more caudal spaces (Table 1).

The distribution of sensory innervation in the internal intercostal muscles is similar to that of the external intercostal muscles. The proportion of myelinated axons that are sensory ranges from 24% for the intercostal nerve supplying the third space, to 18% for the nerve supplying the seventh space. The density of muscle

Table 1 Distribution of Muscle Spindle Endings in the Intercostal, Intercartilaginous, and Diaphragm Muscles

Muscles	Density[a]	Total per muscle	Total number of myelinated fibers
Intercostals			
External 3rd space	110	18	100
Internal 3rd space	61	30	300
External 4th space	130	26	100
Internal 4th space	50	25	350
External 8th space	60	18	140
Internal 8th space	30	24	550
Intercartilaginous			
2nd space	22	8	150
3rd space	16	6	110
4th space	13	5	
Diaphragm			
Crural	3.4	4.5	780 (phrenic)
Costal	0	0	

[a]Density is represented by the number of spindles per gram of dry weight of muscle.
Source: Duron et al. (1978).

spindles in the internal intercostal muslces is lower than that of the external intercostal muscles, but follows a similar pattern, decreasing density in the cephalocaudal direction. Although the density of muscle spindles varies, depending on the intercostal space examined, the absolute number of muscle spindles in each muscle is relatively constant. For exmaple, there is but one more muscle spindle (25) in the internal intercostal muscle of the fourth space compared with the eighth (24). Results of samples from the second, third, and fourth intercartilaginous intercostal muscles revealed comparatively fewer muscle spindles compared with data from the interosseous intercostal muscles, as just reported.

Duron et al. (1978) estimated that most of the myelinated afferents in the intercosal muscles were of muscle spindle origin. They speculated that 60 of the 72 sensory fibers in the third internal intercostal nerve were either group Iᴀ or group II afferents. These data suggest that muscle spindles are more abundant than Golgi tendon organs in the intercostal muscles. This conclusion is consistent with neurophysiological studies by Critchlow and von Euler (1964) and Sears (1964b), who reported in their sample that muscle spindles outnumbered Golgi tendon organs by nearly 6.5:1.

B. Projections of Intercostal Muscle Proprioceptors

Projection pathways of intercostal muscle proprioceptors are similar to those of other skeletal muscles and involve the thalamus, cerebellum, and cerebral cortex. However, the intercostal afferents are unique in that additional pathways involve the connections with spinal cord and brain stem structures affecting the activation and coordination of respiratory muscles.

The spinal circuits of the intercostal muscle proprioceptors are remarkable in their complexity. Connections between these afferents and the alpha motoneurons of the homonymous intercostal muscles produce the "intercostal-to-intercostal" reflex. Another pathway connects the intercostal afferents with the phrenic moto-neuron pool and is responsible for the "intercostal-to-phrenic" reflex. The significance of these reflexes will be discussed later in the chapter.

Projections from intercostal afferents to brain stem respiratory-related neurons was first suggested by Downman (1955). He found that stimulation of intercostal nerve afferents in the decerebrate cat produced inhibition of phrenic efferent drive. However, these afferents produced excitation of the phrenic nerve following high cervical spinal cord transection. Shannon (1980a) was the first to record the response of neurons in the dorsal respiratory group (DRG) to intercostal afferent stimulation. Stimulation of cranial or caudal intercostal nerve roots produced inhibition of activity in 51 of 53 inspiratory cells. Termination of DRG activity associated with intercostal afferent stimulation was accompained by simultaneous inhibition of phrenic efferent activity.

Rosen (1969b) and Rosen and Sjolund (1973a,b) have shown that group I and II intercostal afferents project to the cuneate and external cuneate nuclei. This projection pathway is typical of large myelinated afferents entering the spinal cord above the midthoracic roots. Recent experiments have demonstrated that stimulation of intercostal muscle mechanoreceptors produces activation of neurons in the ventroposteriolateral (VPL) nucleus of the ventrobasal complex in the thalamus in the cat (P. W. Davenport, unpublished results). The VPL represents an integration center for skeletal muscle proprioceptors (Rosen, 1969a).

Coffey et al. (1971) mapped the cerebellar projections of the intercostal nerves in the anesthetized cat. With low-intensity stimulation, in an effort to isolate responses to large myelinated afferents alone, activation of the intercostal afferents produced low-amplitude, surface-positive potentials over the ipsilateral intermediate cortex and the lateral margin of the vermis of the cerebellum. Stimulation of individual intercostal nerves produced a localized response on the surface of the cerebellum. There was a slight preponderance of lower thoracic (T6–T10) projections to the rostral intermediate cortex and upper thoracic (T2–T5) projections to the caudal intermediate cortex. The rostral region also receives input from hindlimb afferents, whereas the caudal region receives projections from forelimb afferents. The onset latency for the evoked potentials of less than 7 ms was consistent with the activation of large-diameter afferents. Section of the dorsal columns plus the dorsal and ventral spinocerebellar tracts abolished the response to nerve stimulation.

Baker et al. (1990) have recently shown that the response of cerebellar neurons to stimulation of intercostal nerve afferents is dependent on the ventilatory cycle. They found that the amplitude of the response was lowest during the inspiratory phase. These investigators concluded that inputs from these afferents are gated by brain stem respiratory neurons.

The cerebral cortex also receives projections from intercostal muscle afferents. Electrical stimulation of the muscular branch of the intercostal nerve elicits evoked potentials in area 3a of the somatosensory cortex in the cat (Davenport et al., 1985). Area 3a represents a strip of neurons in the somatosensory cortex that receives projections from proprioceptors. Low-amplitude stretch of the intercostal muscles, a maneuver intended to activate muscle spindles, also produces evoked potentials in the cerebral cortex. The amplitude of the response is proportional to the degree of stretch, suggesting that the information coded by the muscle spindles is relayed to the somatosensory cortex (Davenport et al., 1987).

Gandevia and Macefield (1989) used microelectrodes to stimulate either the second parasternal or fifth lateral intercostal muscles in conscious human subjects. Scalp electrodes were used to record the evoked potentials associated with intercostal muscle contraction. Stimulation of the second parasternal intercostal muscle produced a short-onset (latency 19.2 ms), negative potential that was similar in amplitude to those elicited by limb nerve stimulation. Consistent with the longer conduction distance, the onset latency was slightly longer for the evoked potentials associated with activation of the fifth intercostal muscle. The recordings from the vertex produced the evoked potentials with the greatest amplitudes, suggesting that these afferents project to sites in or near the trunk area on the somatosensory cortex.

These authors concluded that group I or II afferents, or both, from the intercostal muscles project to the somatosensory cortex in humans.

C. Reflexes Elicited by Intercostal Proprioceptors

The Intercostal-to-Intercostal Reflex

Although deafferentation of intercostal muscles produces minimal (Shannon, 1972) or no alteration (Stella, 1938; Speck and Weber, 1979) in the pattern of respiratory muscle activation, several studies have demonstrated that activation of proprioceptors in these muscles by inspiratory loads or rib cage distortion elicits reflexes affecting respiratory motor drive. Our current understanding of the importance of intercostal muscle proprioceptors in the regulation of respiratory muscle activation is based on the elegant studies by Eccles et al. (1962), Sears (1964a,c,d), Critchlow and von Euler (1963), and Eklund et al. (1964). Collectively, these experiments established that mono- and polysynaptic reflexes exist between intercostal muscle proprioceptors and intercostal motoneurons. In addition, these studies showed that intercostal proprioceptors are active during spontaneous breathing in the anesthetized cat, and indicated that many of the intrafusal fibers in the intercostal muscle spindles receive phasic activation from gamma motoneurons. These experiments also revealed that the activity of muscle spindles is enhanced by maneuvers, such as tracheal occlusion, during inspiration or expansion of the chest wall.

Sears (1958) provided early evidence that spinal pathways were involved in the reflexes produced by the distortion of the chest wall. He described a reflex that was initiated by lung inflation and produced excitation of internal (expiratory) intercostal and abdominal muscles. This reflex was not dependent on the vagus nerve and was reduced or eliminated by section of the thoracic dorsal roots ipsilateral to the recording site. These data argued strongly for the existence of spinal reflexes mediated by intercostal muscle proprioceptors.

Eccles et al. (1962) made intracellular recordings from alpha motoneurons in the thoracic spinal cord (T8–T10) in the spontaneously breathing, anesthetized cat. These investigators found that cells active during the inspiratory phase supplied the external intercostal muscles, whereas those active during expiration supplied the internal intercostal muscles. Stimulation of the intercostal nerve with threshold pulses evoked monosynaptic and polysynaptic excitatory potentials in the neurons supplying the external intercostals. Stronger stimuli elicited inhibitory synaptic potentials of magnitudes great enough to block the excitatory inputs to the motoneuron.

More detailed examination of the intercostal-to-intercostal reflex by Sears (1964a) revealed that most of the intercostal motoneurons at all thoracic segments receive monosynaptic exictatory synaptic input from the ipsilateral intercostal nerves from the same and adjacent spinal nerves. Glebovskii (1966) described what he termed the "intercostal stretch reflex," in the anesthetized cat. Activation of the intercostal muscles occurred when the muscles were stretched, suggesting that it represented a spinal reflex, mediated by muscle spindle afferents. Thus, the early studies provided evidence of a monosynaptic, excitatory pathway from large-diameter–myelinated afferents in the inspiratory muscles to alpha motoneurons supplying those muscles.

Subsequent studies focused on the activity of proprioceptors during breathing in an effort to describe their transduction properties and to understand how their activity was affected by chest wall distortion. Activation of gamma motoneurons produces contraction of muscle spindle intrafusal fibers and leads to distortion and activation of the group IA afferent nerve ending. Knowing that coactivation of alpha and gamma motoneurons occurred during contraction of other skeletal muscles, Critchlow and Euler (1963) set out to determine whether gamma efferents were involved in the control of intercostal muscle spindles. Single-fiber recordings were made from thoracic dorsal root filaments to quantitate the activity of 168 muscle spindles in 41 cats. Most of the muscle spindles exhibited phasic activity, being most active during contraction of the muscle in which it was located. A follow-up study by von Euler and Peretti (1966) showed that approximately three-quarters of the IA and II intercostal afferents were phasically active. Figure 1A, shows the activity of one such muscle spindle located in the external (inspiratory) intercostal muscle. The phasic nature of the activity is this recording is clearly evident, and the peak activity occurs near the end of the inspiratory phase. To determine the extent to which gamma motor drive influenced the activity of this fiber, a 0.25% lidocaine solution was applied to the nerve to selectively block conduction of the

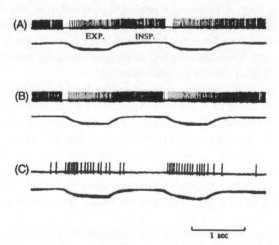

Figure 1 Relationship between intercostal muscle spindle activity and lung volume in the anesthetized cat. Muscle spindle activity is shown on the top trace in each panel, while spirometer traces are shown in the lower portion of each panel. Refer to text for explanation. (From Critchlow and von Euler, 1963.)

gamma fibers. Figure 1B is a recording taken $2^1 2$ min after lidocaine application, before significant effects on gamma fiber conduction. One minute later (see Fig. 1C), gamma fiber conduction block appears complete, and the activity of the fiber has changed phases and is now active during expiration. Without activation of the intrafusal fibers by the gamma motoneuron, the spindle functions as a passive stretch receptor; falling silent during intercostal muscle contraction and being activated during passive relaxation of the muscle.

The results from the study by Critchlow and von Euler (1963) were confirmed and extended in later investigations involving direct recording from gamma motoneurons. The alpha and gamma motoneurons supplying the same intercostal muscle received similar inputs from brain stem premotor neurons. Coactivation of alpha and gamma fibers was confirmed during eupneic breathing and during changes in the chemical drive to breathing (Eklund et al., 1964; Sears, 1964c). Similar to the alpha motoneurons, the gamma motoneurons also receive excitatory synaptic input from muscle spindle afferents (Eklund et al., 1964).

The Intercostal-to-Phrenic Reflex

The effects of stimulating intercostal muscle afferents on phrenic nerve efferent drive varies with the origin of the afferent fibers along the rib cage. Stimulation of intercostal nerves in the cranial rib cage produces inhibition of phrenic motoneurons. The reflexes elicited by activation of caudal intercostal nerves are facilitatory. Adding to the complexity of these reflexes is that they involve both spinal and supraspinal neural circuits.

Studies of the spinal component of the intercostal-to-phrenic reflex were performed by Decima et al. (1967) in cats and rabbits after decerebration or high spinal transection. Single shocks or brief, high-frequency stimuli applied to the internal or external intercostal nerves from T-9 to T-11 produced a short latency (10 to 16-ms) excitatory response of the phrenic nerve. The greatest response was elicited by stimulation of the most caudal intercostal nerves. Decima et al. (1967) also studied the reflexes associated with mechanical stimulation of proprioceptors in intercostal muscles. Tetanic stimulation of the peripheral cut ends of the phrenic nerve was used to produce contraction of the diaphragm and distortion of the lower rib cage and abdomen. The authors postulated that rib cage distortion activates proprioceptors in the intercostal and abdominal muscles. Rib cage distortion produced a transient burst in phrenic efferent discharge recorded from the proximal end of the cut phrenic nerve.

In follow-up experiments, Decima et al. (1969) and Decima and von Euler (1969) extended their previous findings and showed that the excitatory phrenic nerve response could be produced only by stimulation of the intercostal nerves of the caudal rib cage. Stimulation of the cranial intercostal nerves produced no such excitation. They also observed that this reflex did not require a circuit that passed through the brain stem, since it could be elicited following transection of the spinal cord at C-1.

A long-latancy inhibitory response to intercostal nerve stimulation was also described. The late inhibitory response could occur in the absence of the earlier excitation, suggesting that the depression in phrenic activity was due to synaptic inhibition, rather than to postexcitatory depression. Others later showed that muscle spindle afferents (group IA and II) from the external intercostal muscles make excitatory monosynaptic connections with the alpha motoneurons supplying homonymous muscles of the same and adjacent spinal segments (Kirkwood and Sears, 1974, 1982; Sears, 1964d). Golgi tendon organs, acting through an interneuron, have an inhibitory input on homonymous external intercostal muscles of the same segment (Sears, 1964d).

Decima et al. (1969) also noted that stimulation of the ipsilateral lobule IV of the anterior cerebellum produces inhibition of brain stem inspiratory output, leading them to postulate that the inhibitory circuit passed through the cerebellum. However, Speck and Weber (1982) later studied the influence of the cerebellum on the inhibitory response to intercostal nerve stimulation and discovered that, although stimulation of the cerebellum can produce similar inhibitory effects, the cerebellar connection was not required for the intercostal-to-phrenic inhibitory reflex.

Remmers (1973) and Remmers and Tsiaras (1973) performed a series of experiments designed to systematically examine the extrasegmental component of the intercostal-to-phrenic reflex. In an earlier study, Remmers (1970) noted that intercostal nerve stimulation not only inhibited efferent activity, but also produced changes in respiratory timing. This suggested that the primary target in this reflex was the pool of inspiratory neurons in the brain stem, rather than the phrenic motoneurons in the spinal cord. To separate the spinal and supraspinal components of the reflex, Remmers (1973) recorded the phrenic and recurrent laryngeal nerve responses to intercostal nerve stimulation. Intercostal nerve stimulation that produced a reduction in phrenic efferent activity was associated with a concomitant increase in recurrent laryngeal nerve activity. Results from this study suggested that the primary effect of intercostal afferent input at the brain stem level was to suppress the activity of neurons synapsing on inspiratory muscles and to facilitate those neurons directing expiratory muscle activity.

Homma et al. (1978) examined the role of intercostal muscle afferents in the control of breathing in conscious human subjects. These authors used vibration in an attempt to activate intercostal muscle proprioceptors. Vibration of the upper or lower rib cage was done while recording the electromyographic (EMG) activity of the underlying intercostal muscles and the diaphragm. Vibration always produced activation of the underlying intercostal muscles. Stimulation of the upper rib cage had little effect on the diaphragm EMG, whereas vibration of the lower rib cage produced a reduction in the amplitude of the diaphragm EMG. Later studies (Homma, 1980) showed that vibration of the lower, anterior rib cage produced reductions in the peak amplitude of the integrated diaphragm EMG, a fall in tidal volume, and decreases in both inspiratory and expiratory duration. Homma (1980) suggested that intercostal muscle afferents might play a role in influencing the phase-switching mechanism in the brain stem.

Remmers and Tsiaras (1973) suggested that the nerve tracts carrying intercostal muscle afferent impulses ascended in the lateral spinal cord, which includes the spinocerebellar tract ipsilateral to the stimulation site. Lesions of these tracts eliminated the inhibitory effects of intercostal nerve stimulation. In decerebrate cats, bilateral lesions of these pathways also produced changes in the pattern of respiration. These authors concluded that phasic activity from intercostal muscle proprioceptors may be important in producing normal respiratory motor outflow from brain stem neurons.

In his review, Shannon (1986) cautions that the inhibitory effects of intercostal muscle afferents should be considered as a global reflex, affecting outflow from brain stem inspiratory neurons, rather than one that is specific for the phrenic efferent drive alone. Shannon (1980a) found phrenic nerve inhibition with stimulation of either the internal or external intercostal nerves caudal to T-3. He also confirmed the early-onset, excitatory response with stimulation of intercostal nerves from T-9 to T-11. Recordings from inspiratory neurons of the dorsal respiratory group and the phrenic nerve revealed simultaneous inhibition with intercostal nerve stimulation. Shannon (1980a) concluded that the inhibitory intercostal-to-phrenic reflex was mediated through inhibition of inspiratory neurons of the brain stem that drive phrenic motoneurons. Bolser and Remmers (1989) used intracellular recordings to determine that the suppression in inspiratory neuronal activity associated with intercostal nerve stimulation was the result of a chloride-dependent inhibitory postsynaptic mechanism. They also suggested that the increased activity of expiratory neurons was produced by a direct, excitatory synaptic mechanism rather than disfacilitation.

Distortion of the lower rib cage by compression, rib cage expansion, or stimulation of the peripheral cut ends of the phrenic nerve affects phrenic efferent drive (Decima et al., 1969; Remmers, 1973). However, the specific type(s) of afferents responsible for these reflexes were unknown. Remmers (1970) attempted to preferentially stimulate muscle spindles and tendon organs by rib vibration, intercostal muscle stretch, or rib cage compression in the anesthetized dog and cat: Each maneuver produced an inhibitory inspiratory reflex. The effects of selective stimulation of intercostal muscle spindles or tendon organs on the activity of inspiratory (Bolser et al., 1987) and expiratory (Shannon et al., 1987) brain stem neurons was performed later in decerebrate cats. Bolser et al. (1987) isolated the T-6 intercostal muscle and nerve. A dorsal laminectomy was performed to expose the T-6 dorsal roots, the ventral root was cut and placed on stimulating electrodes. Stimulation of the ventral root produced contraction of the intercostal muscle. Recordings from dorsal root fibers were made to document the response of muscle afferents. The activity of inspiratory neurons in the dorsal and ventral respiratory groups was recorded with tungsten microlectrodes. Phrenic efferent activity was also recorded. These authors found that impeded contractions of the external or internal T-6 intercostal muscle was associated with preferential activation of tendon organs and reductions in the activity of inspiratory neuron and phrenic nerve activity.

Data from one experiment are shown in Figure 2. Vibration applied to the muscle excited muscle spindles, but produced no significant effects on inspiratory neuron or phrenic nerve activity. Bolser et al. (1987) concluded that intercostal tendon organs have an inhibitory effect on inspiration, whereas muscle spindles do not produce significant effects on the activity of medullary inspiratory neurons.

Shannon et al. (1987) employed the same technique to study the effects of stimulating intercostal muscle spindles or tendon organs on the activity of medullary expiratory neurons. Augmentation of medullary expiratory laryngeal motoneuron activity was associated with intercostal tendon organ stimulation only; muscle spindle activation had no significant effect. The bulbospinal expiratory neurons supplying the intercostal and abdominal muscles showed no change in activity to either tendon organ

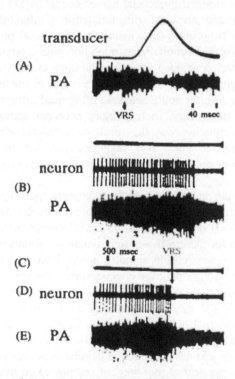

Figure 2 Responses of an inspiratory neuron in the dorsal respiratory group and phrenic nerve efferent activity (PA) to impeded contraction of the intercostal muscles. (A) A transient reduction in PA associated with T-6 ventral root stimulation (VRS): The tracing from the force transducer indicates that VRS was associated with an increase in muscle tension. (B) Control activity of the neuron and the PA. (C) Premature termination of inspiration occurred with VRS. Cycle triggered histograms of the neuron (D) and the PA (E) are shown for control (dotted line) and VRS (solid lines). Each represents the average of 22 trials and shows neuron and PA termination with VRS. (From Bolser et al., 1987.)

or muscle spindle stimulation. The current working hypothesis is that tendon organs represent the primary source of proprioceptive input from intercostal muscles to the inspiratory neurons of the dorsal and ventral respiratory groups and to the expiratory laryngeal motoneurons. Muscle spindles appear to have no significant role in the regulation of respiratory motor activity at the spinal or brain stem level.

One curious result from the study by Shannon et al. (1987) was that vibration of the ribs with high-amplitude displacements produced inhibition of brain stem inspiratory activity. This effect was not attributed to muscle spindles, because they are maximally activated with low-amplitude vibration. Nor were tendon organs implicated, since they were not adequately stimulated by rib vibration. From previous work (Shannon, 1980b) which showed that costovertebral joint receptor stimulation inhibited phrenic efferent drive, these authors postulated these same receptors were responsible for inspiratory inhibition during high-amplitude rib vibration. To study this, vibration of the T-6 intercostal muscle at amplitudes sufficient to activate tendon organs was performed while recording phrenic efferent activity. Vibration at amplitudes greater than 1200 μm reduced phrenic activity (Fig. 3). Denervation of the T-6 intercostal muscle eliminated the response in most animals, but only attenuated it in others. In those animals in which the response was attenuated, denervation of the T-6 costovertebral joint receptors eliminated the effects of vibration. Thus, these authors proposed that, in addition to intercostal muscle tendon organs, costovertebral joint receptors have an inhibitory effect on brain stem inspiratory neurons.

D. Functional Considerations: The Intercostal Muscle Proprioceptors

The information that chest wall distortion affects the activity of inspiratory muscles by an intercostal afferent mechanism (Remmers and Tsairas, 1973; Shannon, 1979),

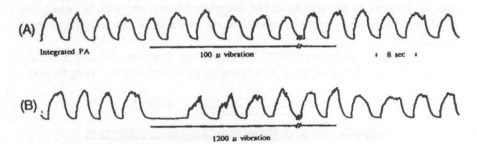

Figure 3 Effect of vibration of the T-6 intercostal muscle on the integrated phrenic nerve efferent activity (PA). (A) Vibration at 200 Hz and amplitudes of 100 or 400 μm (not shown) were sufficient to stimulate up to 98% of all intercostal muscle spindle endings, but produced no significant change in PA. (B) Increasing the vibration amplitude to 1200 μm activated intercostal muscle tendon organs and was associated with a significant reduction in PA amplitude. This response was reduced or eliminated by T-6 intercostal nerve transection. (From Bolser et al., 1988.)

and that intercostal proprioceptors áre phasically active in the spontaneously breathing animal (Critchlow and von Euler, 1963; Eklund et al., 1964; Sears, 1964c), suggests that intercostal muscle proprioceptors could be involved in respiratory load compensation. Given the knowledge that external intercostal alpha and gamma motoneurons receive simultaneous excitatory synaptic input during inspiration, Sears (1964c) proposed that reflexes involving muscle spindle afferents were important in the control of breathing. He suggested that forces that opposed the contraction of the inspiratory intercostal muscles, such as tracheal occlusion, would reduce the rate of shortening of the extrafusal, but not the intrafusal, fibers. Such misalignment in the rates of shortening would increase the activity of the muscle spindle afferent discharge and produce, through the spinal circuit, mono-synaptic excitation of the alpha motoneuron. This reflex would act to automatically assist the extrafusal fibers in overcoming the load. Sears (1964c) proposed a similar mechanism for the expiratory intercostal muscles. Although studies involving electrical stimulation of intercostal nerves had established the existence of these pathways, the functional significance had not been demonstrated. At issue was whether added loads to breathing did indeed lead to increased activity in the intercostal muscle spindle fibers.

Results from an earlier study by Critchlow and von Euler (1963) suggested that the discharge frequency of inspiratory intercostal muscle spindle afferents increases during tracheal occlusion. Corda et al. (1965a) recorded the activity of external intercostal muscle spindle in the spontaneously breathing cat and noted a substantial augmentation in spindle discharge produced by tracheal occlusion. Figure 4 shows the tidal volume trace and the afferent discharge of an inspiratory intercostal muscle spindle. During the unoccluded breaths, the afferent activity was maximal early in inspiration. Tracheal occlusion (indicated by the bracket beneath the volume trace) produced a profound increase in afferent activity. This was also associated with an increase in the activity of the inspiratory intercostal muscle, which was eliminated by cutting the dorsal root filaments of the same and adjacent thoracic spinal segments.

Shannon and Zechman (1972) showed that the load-compensating reflex also operated during stepped increases in inspiratory airflow resistance. They found, as

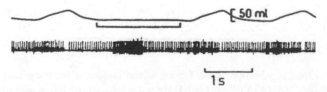

Figure 4   Recording of intercostal muscle spindle during unimpeded and occluded inspi-rations in the anesthetized cat. The top trace represents the spirogram and the lower trace is the recording from an external intercostal muscle spindle. Tracheal occlusion (bracket) was associated with a marked increase in the activity of the muscle spindle. (From Corda et al., 1965a.)

did Corda et al. (1965a), that the excitatory reflex associated with inspiratory loading was eliminated by thoracic dorsal root section in the anesthetized, vagotomized cat.

Studies of the potential role of this reflex in conscious human subjects were conducted by Sears and Newson Davis (1968), who recorded the activity of inspiratory and expiratory intercostal muscles during respiratory loading. They observed that, when loads that opposed the contraction of the intercostal muscle were applied at the mouth, the activity of the muscle increased. The response latency ranged from 33 to 80 ms and was much less than the minimal voluntary reaction time of 140 ms. Sears and Newsom Davis (1968) hypothesized that the reflexes they observed in human subjects operated through the excitatory muscle spindle-to-intercostal pathway, previously demonstrated in animals.

The effects of elastic and resistive loading on changes in brain stem inspiratory neuron activity were studied by Shannon et al. (1972). The objective of their study was to determine whether intercostal proprioceptors excited by inspiratory loading could alter the activity of brain stem inspiratory neurons. Tracheal occlusion and elastic loads were associated with a reduction in the rate of activity (3 of 14 cells, and 4 of 12 cells, respectively) in some inspiratory neurons in the vicinity of the nucleus ambiguous. However, there was no appreciable alteration in the duration of inspiration, and these authors suggested that the load-compensation reflex, at least as far as it affected brain stem control of breathing, was probably not very important. Given the results of more recent studies (Bolser et al., 1987, 1988; Shannon et al., 1987), tendon organs in the external intercostal muscles were the probable source of input onto these brain stem neurons.

III. Diaphragmatic Afferents

During eupneic breathing, the diaphragm is the principal ventilatory muscle, and the contribution of other chest wall muscles (the intercostals) and the abdomen to ventilation is minimal. The level of activation of the diaphragm is altered to compensate for changes in the impedance of the chest wall and abdomen, often within the first one or two breaths following changes in load. The behavior of the diaphragm when presented with changes in mechanical demands suggests that proprioceptors, located in the diaphragm, modulate alterations in respiratory muscle activation. This topic has been a matter of intense debate. This section will review evidence from several laboratories that supports and refutes the hypothesis that diaphragmatic proprioceptors are capable of modifying respiratory motor output at the spinal, brain stem, and higher levels of the nervous system.

A. Distribution

When compared with nerves supplying other skeletal muscles, the phrenic nerve is unique in having relatively few myelinated sensory fibers. Hinsey et al. (1939)

counted the number of myelinated sensory fibers in the phrenic nerves of the cat. They estimated that of the 1000 or so myelinated axons in the right phrenic nerve, only 100 were sensory. When contrasted with the femoral nerve, which has 30–40% of the myelinated population representing sensory fibers, it appears that there is a significant underrepresentation of proprioceptors in the phrenic nerve. Their data also indicate that there are only 20 large myelinated sensory axons consistent with group I fibers in the phrenic nerve. Data from Landau et al. (1962) suggest that very few large-diameter–myelinated afferents exist in the phrenic nerve of the dog. However, Langford and Schmidt (1983) found that 31% of the myelinated axons of the left phrenic nerve of the rat were sensory. A detailed analysis of the fiber diameters was not performed by these authors, so it is not possible to determine how many large-diameter afferent fibers are in the nerve.

Another approach in enumerating the proprioceptors in the diaphragm is to employ neurophysiological techniques. Yasargil (1962) recorded from, and attempted to classify, group I afferents in the phrenic nerve. His data suggested that relatively few muscle spindles exist in the diaphragm. Corda et al. (1965b) performed an extensive survey of the proprioceptive innervation of the diaphragm by recording afferent activity from the cut dorsal root filaments of the cervical spinal cord in cats. Results from their study confirmed the earlier work of Yasargil (1962) in showing that very muscle spindles and tendon organs exist in the diaphragm. Their data do not permit estimates of the average numbers of each afferent type per animal, but these authors did find, in contrast with limb skeletal muscle, that tendon organs outnumbered muscle spindles.

Histological examination of the diaphragm of the cat (Duron et al., 1978) reveals that no more than ten muscle spindles can be found (see Table 1). These data are in agreement with the small numbers of fibers in the gamma efferent and group II afferent categories from studies of phrenic nerve axon diameter (Landau et al., 1962). Duron et al. (1978) also found that all muscle spindles were confined to the crural region, with none found in the costal diaphragm. Diaphragmatic muscle spindles have also been identified in humans (Winkler and Delaloye, 1957) and other mammals (Cuneod, 1961; Dogiel, 1902; Hudson, 1966).

The number of large-diameter afferents in the phrenic nerve is at least 20 and appears to be several hundred in some studies. If muscle spindles and tendon organs are so few, what end organs do the remaining fibers supply? An answer has been suggested by Goshgarian and Roubal (1986), who proposed that most of the large-diameter afferent axons arise from pacinian corpuscles in the diaphragm. There have been no studies aimed at determining the role of these afferents in the control of breathing.

B. Projections of Diaphragmatic Afferents

Compared with intercostal afferents, little is known about the projection pathways for phrenic nerve proprioceptors. The spinal distribution and termination patterns of phrenic nerve afferents were studied by Goshgarian and Roubal (1981). They examined the spinal distribution of phrenic nerve afferent fibers of the rat, using horseradish peroxidase (HRP). Although they observed phrenic afferent axon branches ascending in the fasciculus cuneatus, there were no observable terminations in lamninae VI, VII, and IX. This implies that if connections between diaphragmatic proprioceptors and phrenic motoneurons occur, they must do so by way of interneurons. Attempts to obtain transganglionic transport of HRP in the phrenic nerve of other species have been largely unsuccessful. Larnicol et al. (1984, 1985) used a fluorescent double-labeling technique in the cat and showed that a small population of phyrenic nerve afferents traveled in the dorsal columns of the spinal cord. Some phrenic nerve afferents also ascend the spinal cord in the spinothalamic tract. By using electrophysiological techniques, Bolser et al. (1991) have presented evidence in the monkey that some group II and III phrenic fibers also ascend by the spinothalamic tract.

Afferents from the diaphragm project to respiratory-related neurons in the dorsal (Macron and Marlot, 1986) and ventral (Macron et al., 1985) respiratory group of the medulla. Speck and Revelette (1987b) measured the response of neurons in the dorsal (DRG) and ventral (VRG) respiratory neurons to phrenic nerve stimulation in the anesthetized cat. Approximately 25% of the inspiratory-modulated neurons in the DRG were excited by stimulation of the ipsilateral phrenic nerve. A very weak projection from phrenic nerve afferents to neurons of the VRG was found, whereas only 3 of 28 neurons were activated by nerve stimulation. Estimates of the conduction velocity of afferents responsible for these effects were consistent with group III fibers. The response was not dependent on pathways ascending in the dorsal columns of the spinal cord, nor on connections through the cerebellum or the cerebral cortex.

Consistent with the presence of afferent axon collaterals in the fasciculus cuneatus (Goshgarian and Roubal, 1986), phrenic afferents project to the external cuneate nucleus (Marlot et al., 1985a,b; Larnicol et al., 1985) and ipsilateral intermediate and posterior part of the anterior lobe of the cerebellum (Marlot et al., 1984). The projection sites on the cerebellum show overlap with forelimb afferents. Marlot et al. (1985a) stimulated the cervical phrenic nerve and recorded evoked potentials from the cerebellum of the anesthetized cat. The response had a mean onset latency of 9.5 ms and a duration of 19.5 ms. The projection site for phrenic nerve afferents was centered in the ipsilateral intermediate cortex (lobule V) and a large portion of the vermis. Lobule V also receives inputs from forelimb afferents.

Projection of phrenic nerve afferents to the cerebral cortex has also been demonstrated (Frankstein et al., 1979; Davenport et al., 1985). A detailed mapping study of phrenic afferent projection sites was performed by Davenport et al. (1985). Electrical stimulation of myelinated phrenic nerve afferents produced evoked potentials in the somatosensory region of the cerebral cortex in the anesthetized cat. These authors reported that the majority of phrenic afferents project to areas 3a and 3b of the contralateral somatosensory cortex. Projection sites for these afferents were restricted to areas 3a and 3b of the trunk region on the rostral medial edge of the postcruciate dimple. In a subsequent study (Davenport et al., 1987), focal localization of the phrenic afferent projection to cortical neurons showed activation at a depth of 400–1500 μm (lamina III). Sallach et al. (1990) later confirmed previous electrophysiological studies with fluorescent labeling of neurons projecting from the VPL to the sensorimotor cortex. The projection pathway for diaphragmatic proprioceptors is similar to that for proprioceptors located in other skeletal muscles. Collaterals of group I afferent fibers from forelimb muscles ascend within the dorsal columns of the spinal cord and synapse in the cuneate nucleus (Rosen, 1969b). Second-order neurons cross the midline at the medial lemniscus, and terminate on neurons in the VPL of the thalamus (Landgren et al., 1967; Oscarsson and Rosen, 1963; Rosen, 1969a). Neurons from the VPL then project to area 3a of the somatosensory cortex. Various studies have shown that group I afferents from the forelimb and hindlimb muscles also project to area 3a (Amassian and Berlin, 1958; Hore et al., 1976; Landgren and Silfvenuis, 1969; Oscarsson et al., 1966; Phillips et al., 1971). These studies indicate that diaphragmatic proprioceptors have projection pathways to the somatosensory cortex that are consistent with pathways established for proprioceptors in other skeletal muscles. Small myelinated afferents (group III) from the diaphragm have recently been shown to project by the spinothalamic tract to the area 4 of the motor cortex (Bolser et al., 1991).

Phillips et al. (1969) have suggested that area 3a, acting as an integration center for information derived from group I skeletal muscle afferents, participates in a cortical load-compensation mechanism. Through a transcortical servoloop, information arriving at the somatosensory cortex helps to shape the output of the motor cortex. This loop might be particularly important in controlling the activation of inspiratory muscles, since the spinal reflexes appear to be inhibitory.

C. The Phrenic-to-Phrenic and Crossed Phrenic Phenomena

Electrical stimulation of the phrenic nerve activates both segmental and supraseg-mental reflex pathways. Gill and Kuno (1963) made intracellular recordings from phrenic motoneurons in the cat to study ascending and segmental synaptic connections. Electrical stimulation of the contralateral phrenic nerve produced short-latency (5.8- to 9.1-ms) hyperpolarization of 40% of the motoneurons tested. The hyperpolarization usually lasted for 15–20 ms. The authors confirmed that this reflex had a segmantal component, since high spinal transection did not alter the response. Given the short latency of the response, Gill and Kuno concluded that the contralateral inhibitory reflex was mediated by large-diameter afferents. Speck and Revelette (1987a) studied the phrenic-to-phrenic inhibitory reflex in the anesthetized cat. They found that the short latency inhibitory response to ipsilateral phrenic nerve stimulation was mediated by afferents with conduction velocities of approximately 50 m/s.

Porter (1895) was the first to propose that contralateral phrenic nerve afferents provide inhibitory input to the phrenic motoneuron pool. In what he termed the "crossed-phrenic phenomenon," Porter was able to show that the activity of a hemidiaphragm, paralyzed by hemisection of the spinal cord, could be restored by cutting the contralateral phrenic nerve. He used these observations to postulate that descending drive from the medulla crosses to innervate the contralateral phrenic motoneuron pool. This drive is apparently inhibited by input from the contralateral phrenic nerve afferents. Goshgarian (1981) performed follow-up studies in the rat and showed that similar recovery of function in the parazlyzed diaphragm could be accomplished by contralateral dorsal rhizotomy, or by interrupting transmission along the contralateral phrenic nerve by anesthesia or crush injury. These data suggest that input from phrenic nerve afferent fibers produces inhibition of contralateral phrenic motoneurons. The neural circuit responsible for this phenomenon could be restricted to the spinal cord (Gill and Kuno, 1963; Speck and Revelette, 1987a), or travel through supraspinal structures (Macron and Marlot, 1986; Speck and Revelette, 1987a,b). A combination of the two is also possible.

D. Activity and Loading Response of Diaphragmatic Proprioceptors

Corda et al. (1965b) recorded the spontaneous discharge pattern of muscle spindle fibers in the anesthetized cat. Of the 38 different spindles in their study, only 7 exhibited maximal activity during the inspiratory phase. These 7 were shown to be driven by gamma motor fibers. The remaining 31 muscle spindles were maximally active during expiration. These authors concluded that most muscle spindles in the diaphragm function as passive length receptors.

Jammes et al. (1986) made multifiber recordings of phrenic nerve afferents in the anesthetized cat. Many afferent fibers exhibited phasic activity with respiration. The maximum frequency occurred during inspiration for most of the fibers. Tracheal occlusion during inspiration was associated with an increase in the activity of the phasically active fibers. These authors also examined the effects of large, myelinated afferents on phrenic nerve efferent drive. Cold block, a technique designed to interrupt transmission through large, myelinated axons, but not smaller fibers, was performed on the phrenic nerve in ventilated animals. This caused an increase in inspiratory duration. Consistent with these results, Jammes et al. (1986) also showed that electrical stimulation of the phrenic nerve at intensities sufficient to preferentially activate large-diameter afferents results in a reduction in inspiratory duration. Selective block of small-diameter afferents with procaine injection into the phrenic nerve failed to produce significant effects in respiratory timing.

Holt et al. (1991) recorded mechanoreceptor activity from the rat diaphragm in vitro. They found muscle spindles and tendon organs in both the costal and crural regions of the diaphragm. Pressure-sensitive receptors were also localized in the central tendon. These three types of end organs were supplied by axons with conduction velocities ranging from 30 to 65 m/s. Muscle spindles were sensitive to length changes of 4–8 mm, which is within the range of length changes associated with eupneic breathing in the intact animal.

Jammes et al. (1986) studied the effects of tracheal occlusion during the inspiratory phase on large-diameter afferent activity and on phrenic efferent drive. Data from their paper (Fig. 5) show that occlusion is associated with an increase in afferent activity, but a reduction in the efferent drive to the diaphragm. These authors concluded that large-diameter phrenic nerve afferents are sensitive to changes in diaphragm muscle length or tension, and have an inhibitory effect on inspiratory duration and efferent drive to the diaphragm. These authors also noted that interruption of input from large, myelinated phrenic nerve afferents, by cold block, was associated with a prolongation in the neural inspiratory duration. Given these data, diaphragmatic tendon organs might also play a role in modulating inspiratory duration.

Various studies have suggested that phrenic nerve afferents have no effect on the response of anesthetized animals to added loads to breathing. Arita and Bishop (1972) measured response of single motor units in the diaphragm to inspiratory occlusion in the cat. Their data showed that deafferentation of the diaphragm (by sectioning the dorsal roots of the cervical spinal cord) has no significant effect on the single motor unit response to loading. Similar conclusions were reached by others using resistive (Breslav et al., 1980) or elastic loading (Bradley, 1972) in the anesthetized animal. Since more recent studies have shown that phrenic nerve afferents can modulate inspiratory motor drive, the discrepancies in results are likely due to different methods.

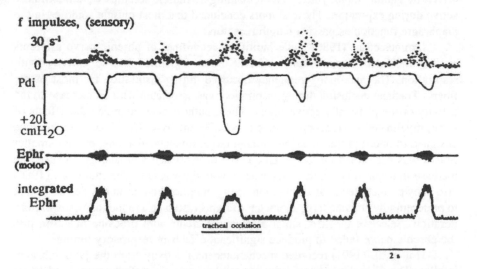

Figure 5   Effect of inspiratory occlusion on the activity of large, myelinated phrenic afferent fibers in the anesthetized cat. Tracheal occlusion was associated with a reduction in phrenic efferent drive (third and fourth traces), and an increase in the impulse frequency of phrenic nerve afferents. (From Jammes et al., 1986.)

The ability of a skeletal muscle to generate tension varies as a function of its length: within limits the greater the length, the greater the tension; the diaphragm is no exception. Its length–tension relation is similar to that observed for other skeletal muscles (Kim et al., 1976; Road et al., 1986). Green et al. (1978) had demonstrated that chest wall restriction and positive-pressure breathing elicited adjustments in respiratory muscle activation in conscious human subjects. These authors produced increases in the functional residual capacity (FRC) of their subjects by using positive airway pressure. Increasing FRC acts to shorten the operating length of the diaphragm, which reduces its force-generating ability for a given level of efferent drive. When subjected to positive pressures, their subjects increased the level of activation of the inspiratory muscles. Such increases acted to minimize changes in ventilation. Green et al. (1978) suggested that respiratory muscle afferents might mediate the response to positive-pressure breathing. Mead (1979) later suggested that an operational length-compensation reflex existed for the diaphragm, and that afferents residing within the diaphragm itself might be involved in the response.

Follow-up studies with quadriplegic human subjects were performed by Banzett et al. (1981). The subjects were fitted with a cuirass that covered the chest and abdomen. The activity of the diaphragm was recorded with surface electrodes over the lower margin of the rib cage. Evacuation of the cuirass was done to increase FRC. When FRC was suddenly increased, the authors noted that the amplitude of the diaphragm EMG rose as well. Banzett et al. (1981) discussed the mechanisms responsible for the alterations in diaphragmatic activation. Since the subjects had complete lower cervical spinal lesions, afferent activity from intercostal and abdominal muscles and costovertebral joint receptors could not influence phrenic motoneuron activity. Although the vagus nerves were intact in their subjects, lung inflation would be expected to reduce, rather than augment, phrenic efferent drive. The authors suggested the remaining possibility, and speculated that phrenic nerve afferents were sensitive to changes in the length–tension relation of the diaphragm and acted by a reflex arc to modify phrenic motoneuron activity.

Fryman and Frazier (1987) showed that lower body negative pressure, which reduced the length of the diaphragm, was associated with a prolongation in inspiratory duration in the anesthetized cat. They showed that this reflex response was partly due to phrenic nerve afferents. In contrast, Iscoe (1989) suggested that phrenic nerve afferents have little, if any, influence on respiratory muscle activation. It is difficult to reconcile such differences in conclusions, other than to note that different methods were used to increase FRC. Fryman and Frazier (1987) used lower body negative pressure, whereas Iscoe (1989) used positive airway pressure to increase FRC. The latter would be expected to elicit a more vigorous response from airway receptors. Iscoe (1989) did find that when the vagus nerves were intact and the cervical dorsal roots were cut, no change in timing or peak integrated phenic efferent activity occurred with increases in end-expiratory lung volume. It should be noted that neither study assessed whether the operating length of the diaphragm was altered by the experimental interventions. It is possible that more significant changes in the operating length of the diaphragm occurred in the study by Fryman and Frazier (1987).

If the phrenic efferent drive is increased when the operating length of the diaphragm is reduced, then it is logical to assume the opposite would hold true; that is, when the operating length is increased and the diaphragm is placed at a greater mechanical advantage, the phrenic efferent drive will fall appropriately. Reid et al. (1985) tested this hypothesis by measuring the effects of abdominal compression on the diaphragm EMG in conscious human subjects. Their subjects were seated and submerged to the hips in a tank of warm water. Immersion of the subjects were seated and submerged to the hips in a tank of warm water. Immersion of the subjects to the level of the xiphoid process increased abdominal pressure, a maneuver that should have also increased the operating length of the diaphragm. In the breaths following immersion, the amplitude of the diaphragm EMG was noted to be reduced. Reid et al. (1985) suggested that afferents in the diaphragm might mediate this response.

Cheeseman and Revelette (1990) addressed this issue in anesthetized cats. The effects of increasing abdominal pressure on the diaphragm EMG was studied in C-7 cordotomized, vagotomized animals. Inflation of a cuff around the abdomen was used to increase abdominal pressure. Changes in the operating length of the crural diaphragm were measured by sonomicrometry. Cuff inflation during the expiratory phase was associated with an increase in the operating length of the diaphragm and a significant reduction in the peak integrated EMG in the breath that immediately followed. Bilateral cervical rhizotomy, performed to interrupt phrenic afferent transmission, abolished the response. These investigators concluded that diaphragmatic afferents sensitive to increases in operating length or to active tension were responsible for the reduction in phrenic efferent drive.

Tendon organs typically show the highest activity during the inspiratory phase (Corda et al., 1965a; Revelette et al., 1992). This is consistent with the transduction properties of tendon organs, which are stimulated by increases in the active tension of the muscle in which they reside. Revelette et al. (1992) showed that elevations in abdominal pressure produced significant increases in the peak phasic activity of diaphragmatic tendon organs (Fig. 6). These results, along with studies in human (Green et al., 1978; Reid et al., 1985) and animal (Cheeseman and Revelette, 1990) subjects showing that abdominal compression is associated with an immediate decrease in phrenic efferent drive, suggest that diaphragmatic tendon organs sense increases in the active tension generated by the diaphragm and reduce phrenic nerve efferent outflow. In this manner, phrenic efferent drive might be appropriately matched with the mechanical efficiency of the diaphragm.

Recent studies by Revelette et al. (submitted) have attempted to determine whether preferential activation of muscle spindle afferents in the diaphragm produces significant alterations in respiratory muscle activation. Experiments were performed on anesthetized, vagotomized, C-7 cordotomized cats. The tendinous attachments

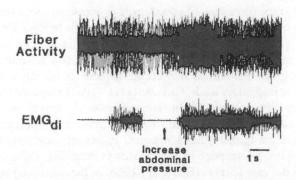

Figure 6 Response of a diaphragmatic tendon organ to abdominal compression in the neurologically intact, anesthetized cat. The upper trace shows dorsal root fiber activity and the lower is the electromyogram from the diaphragm. Inflation of a cuff around the abdomen was used to increase intra-abdominal pressure. (From Frazier and Revelette, 1991.)

of the right crural diaphragm to the vertebral bodies were isolated through an abdominal incision, ligated, and cut. The ligature was passed through a tube in the dorsal abdomen and connected to a vibrator. Vibration of the crural tendon at amplitudes and frequencies known to excite muscle spindle afferents in other skeletal muscle systems (Bolser et al., 1987) was performed to activate diaphragmatic muscle spindles. Spinal cord dorsum-evoked potentials were used to confirm that afferent activation occurred with crural tendon vibration. Results of this study indicated that crural tendon vibration had no significant effect on the rate of rise, peak, or duration of the integrated diaphragm EMG. Revelette et al. (submitted) concluded that reflexes mediated by diaphragmatic muscle spindles are weak or absent.

Emergent in the studies performed to date are two working hypotheses. The first is that changes in the operating length of the diaphragm are accompanied by adjustments in the phrenic motoneuron activity that are independent of feedback from chemoreceptors, from afferent fibers in the vagus nerve, and from afferents in the intercostal and abdominal muscles. The second is that diaphragmatic tendon organs respond to changes in the active tension generated by the diaphragm. These afferents probably mediate the reflexes observed in previous studies (Green et al., 1978; Reid et al., 1985; Jammes et al., 1987; Cheeseman and Revelette, 1990). It is clear that maneuvers that act to increase the active tension of the diaphragm are associated with reduction in the efferent drive to the diaphragm, whereas those that reduce the active tension are accompanied by increases in the efferent drive.

E. Evoked Potentials and Loading

As detailed earler in this chapter, both intercostal and diaphragmatic proprioceptors project to the somatosensory cortex. There is evidence to suggest that these afferents may contribute to the perception of added loads to breathing. An extensive review of the literature on perception of added loads in humans is beyond the scope of this chapter and is covered by Killian and Campbell in Chapter 56; however, it is appropriate to mention the potential role of diaphragmatic afferents here. From previous observations that human subjects are capable of reliably detecting either resistive or elastic inspiratory loads, Campbell et al. (1961) proposed that inspiratory muscle afferents detect subtle modifications in muscle length and tension and contribute to one's perception. Their "length–tension inappropriateness" model formed the basis for further studies designed to identify the source of afferent information supplying perception of added loads to breathing. Others later showed that afferents in the vagus nerves (Guz et al., 1966) or the intercostal and abdominal muscles (Chaudhary and Burki, 1978) could be eliminated, with no significant effects on perception of added loads. Zechman (1967) also showed that detection thresholds for resistive loads were within normal ranges in two subjects with lower cervical spinal cord lesions. Perception of added inspiratory loads in normal human subjects is unaffected by chest cage restriction (Zechman and Wiley, 1977), suggesting that intercostal muscle and joint receptors are not required. Zechman et al. (1985) also showed that the detection time for inspiratory resistive and elastic loads was correlated with load-induced changes in transdiaphragmatic pressure. These authors suggested that activation of proprioceptors in the diaphragm contributed to the sensation of added loads to breathing. These studies, along with numerous others, suggest that afferents within the inspiratory muscles are involved in the sensations elicited by added inspiratory loads and contribute to the perception of added loads to breathing.

Recent studies from several laboratories indicate that application of inspiratory loads is associated with evoked potentials that can be recorded over the somatosensory cortex in human subjects. Davenport et al. (1986) was the first to describe cerebral evoked potentials produced by occluding inspiratory airflow in six conscious adult subjects. Gold cup electrodes placed on the scalp over the left cerebral hemisphere (C_z–C_3) recorded cortical activity. The signals were filtered and amplified, then digitized and averaged by computer. Subjects reclined in a chair and breathed through a mouthpiece connected to a two-way nonrebreathing valve. Occlusion of the inspiratory inlet was performed randomnly every two to five breaths. Averaged data from the occluded breaths were compared with data from control (unoccluded) breaths. Results from their study are shown in Figure 7.

Inspiratory occlusion consistently produced evoked potentials with four identifiable peaks. A positive potential (P_1) with a mean peak latency of 60 ms, was followed by an N_1 at 117 ms, a P_2 at 170 ms, and an N_2 at 212 ms. No such activity was recorded during the unoccluded breaths. These authors concluded that inspiratory occlusion excites afferents associated with the airway or inspiratory muscles, or both, and produces activation of cerebral structures.

Davenport et al. (1986) speculated that the afferent system(s) responsible for

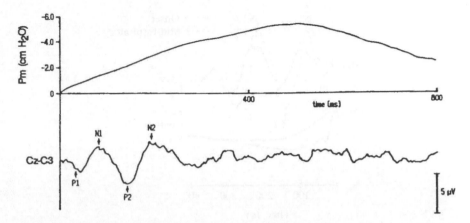

Figure 7 Averaged mouth pressure (Pm) and electroencephalographic recording from C_z–C_3 in one subject. Data represent the average response from 256 inspiratory occlusions over the initial 800 ms of inspiration. Reproducible peaks are indicated by their polarity (P = positive, N = negative) and order of occurrence on the recording. (From Davenport et al., 1986.)

the evoked potentials related to inspiratory occlusion were sensitive to sudden decreases in airway pressure or to abrupt increases in tension on the inspiratory muscles. To determine the relation between the magnitude of the drop in airway pressure and the peak latency and amplitude of the evoked potentials, Revelette and Davenport (1990) compared evoked potentials elicited by occlusion from the onset of inspiration with those produced by midinspiratory occlusion. Interruption of airflow during the early part of inspiration produced a steeper drop in mouth pressure. The evoked potenials associated with midinspiratory occlusion had significantly greater amplitudes and shorter peak latencies (Fig. 8). Midinspiratory occlusion was also associated with a significantly faster reaction time for detection by the subjects. These results supported the hypothesis that the afferents responsible for producing the evoked potentials coded for changes in airway pressure or in muscle tension, or both.

If the evoked potentials recorded with inspiratory occlusion represent the arrival of afferent input from airway or inspiratory muscle afferents, then the peak amplitude and latency of the potentials should also vary with the magnitude of the load. Recently, Bloch et al. (1991) approached this problem by measuring the evoked potentials associated with inspiratory resistive loads. Resistive loads of 3.6 and 9.4 cm H_2O L^{-1} s^{-1} were presented in random order 50 times each to awake, adult human subjects. These authors found that the evoked potential peak latency was greater and amplitude less with the lower load. These data show that neural activity that correlates with the magnitude of the load can be recorded in human subjects.

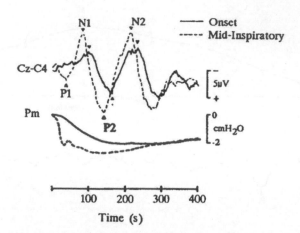

Figure 8 Comparison of evoked potentials recorded from C_z–C_4 electrode pair and mouth pressure (Pm) in one subject. Solid lines represent the average of 64 occlusions from the onset of inspiration. Dashed lines are the average of 64 midinspiratory occlusions. (From Revelette and Davenport, 1990.)

IV. Conclusions

Given the evidence from studies summarized in this chapter, there is little question that proprioceptors in the intercostal muscles and diaphragm are capable of modulating inspiratory muscle activation. Many intercostal muscle spindles receive gamma motor drive and are activated by inspiratory loads. Excitation of intercostal muscle spindles elicits an excitatory reflex involving motoneurons of the external intercostal muscles. The excitatory reflex mediated by these afferents functions to stiffen the rib cage, thereby stabilizing it against the collapsing effects of exaggerated intrathoracic pressures associated with loading. Although functional reflexes at the spinal cord level have been demonstrated, there is no evidence to suggest the existence of supraspinal reflexes mediated by intercostal muscle spindle fibers. Stimulation of muscle spindles in the intercostal muscles or the diaphragm has no influence on the amplitude or timing of the output from inspiratory neurons in the brain stem.

Tendon organs of the inspiratory muscles play a more important role in the control of breathing. High-amplitude inspiratory loads or distortion of the chest wall and abdomen are associated with tendon organ activation in the intercostal muscles and diaphragm. Through spinal and supraspinal pathways, inspiratory motor drive is attenuated and inspiratory duration is shortened. Thus, it appears that loading produces two effects on inspiratory motoneuron output. With low loads, external intercostal muscles are excited and the rib cage stiffens by muscle spindle reflexes. With greater loads, activation of tendon organs inhibits inspiratory motor drive and limits collapse of the rib cage.

The role of inspiratory muscle proprioceptors in the control of breathing at the supramedullary level is more obscure. Although the projection pathways through the midbrain to the cerebellum and sensory cortex of the cerebrum are similar to those of other skeletal muscle afferents, the importance of these pathways in the control of breathing is poorly understood. It is possible that activation of these afferents by inspiratory loading provides information on the magnitude of the added load and helps modify the output of the motor cortex.

The evidence supporting a role for inspiratory muscle afferents in the control of breathing is strong. These afferents may help modulate inspiratory muscle activity during eupneic breathing and substantially affect activation during inspiratory loading. They also may provide sensations contributing to the perception of added loads to breathing. Many questions remain.

References

Amassian, V. E., and Berlin, L. (1958). Early cortical projection of group I afferents in the forelimb muscle nerves of cat. *J. Physiol. (Lond.)* 143: 61.

Arita, H., and Bishop, B. (1983). Firing profile of diaphragm single motor units during hypercapnia and airway occlusion. *J. Appl. Physiol.* 55: 1203–1210.

Baker, S. C., Seers, C. P., and Sears, T. A. (1990). Respiratory modulation of afferent transmission to the cerebellum [abstract]. In *Modulation of Respiratory Pattern: Peripheral and Central Mechanisms*, International Conference, Oct. 1990, Lexington, KY, p. 24.

Banzett, R. B., Inbar, G. F., Brown, R., Goldman, M., Rosier, A., and Mead, J. (1981). Diaphragm electrical activity during negative lower torso pressure in quadriplegic men. *J. Appl. Physiol.* 51: 654–659.

Bloch, E., Harver, A., and Squires, N. K. (1990). Differential effects of inspiratory resistance loading and unloading on respiratory-related cortical potentials [abstract]. In: *Modulation of Respiratory Pattern: Peripheral and Central Mechanisms*, International Conference, Oct. 1990, Lexington, KY. p. 110.

Bloch, E., Harver, A., and Squires, N. K. (1990). Differential effects of inspiratory resistance loading and unloading on respiratory-related cortical potentials [abstract]. In: *Modulation of Respiratory Pattern: Peripheral and Central Mechanisms*, International Conference, Oct. 1990, Lexington, KY. p. 110.

Bolser, D. C., and Remmers, J. E. (1989). Synaptic effects of intercostal tendon organs on membrane potentials of medullary respiratory neurons. *J. Neurophysiol.* 61: 918–926.

Bolser, D. C., Lindsey, B. G., and Shannon, R. (1987). Medullary inspiratory activity: Influence of intercostal tendon organs and muscle spindle endings. *J. Appl. Physiol.* 62: 1046.

Bolser, D. C., Lindsey, B. G., and Shannon, R. (1988). Respiratory pattern changes produced by intercostal muscle/rib vibration. *J. Appl. Physiol.* 64: 2458–2462.

Bolser, D. C., Hobbs, S. F., Chandler, M. J., Ammons, S., Brennan, T. J., and Foreman, R. D. (1991). Convergence of phrenic and cardiopulmonary spinal afferent information of cervical and thoracic spinothalamic tract neurons in the monkey: Implications for referred pain from the diaphragm and heart. *J. Neurophysiol.* 65: 1042–1054.

Bradley, G. W. (1972). The response of the respiratory system to elastic loading in cats. *Respir. Physiol.* 16: 142–160.

Breslav, I. A., Klyueva, O., and Konza, E. A. (1980). Mechanisms of regulation of respiration under a resistive load. *Bull. Exp. Biol. Med.* 89: 408–411.

Campbell, E. J. M., Freedman, S., Smith, P. S., and Taylor, M. E. (1961). The ability of man to detect added elastic loads to breathing. *Clin. Sci.* 20: 223–231.

Chaudhary, B. A., and Burki, N. K. (1978). Effect of airway anesthesia on the ability to detect added inspiratory resistive loads. *Med. Sci. Mol. Med.* 54: 621–626.

Cheeseman, M., and Revelette, W. R. (1990). Contribution of diaphragm afferents in the crural response to an increase in the operating length of the diaphragm. *Appl. Physiol.* 69: 640–647.

Coffey, G. L., Godwin-Austen, R. B., MacGillevray, B. B., and Sears, T. A. (1971). The form and distribution of the surface evoked responses in cerebellar cortex from intercostal nerves in the cat. *J. Physiol. (Lond.)* 212: 129–145.

Corda, M., Eklund, G., and von Euler, C. (1965a). External intercostal and phrenic alpha motor responses to changes in respiratory load. *Acta Physiol. Scand.* 63: 391–400.

Corda, M., von Euler, C., and Lennerstrand, G. (1965b). Proprioceptive innervation of the diaphragm. *J. Physiol. (Lond.)* 178: 161–177.

Critchlow, V., and von Euler, C. (1963). Intercostal muscle spindle activity and its gamma motor control. *J. Physiol. (Lond.)* 168: 820–847.

Cuneod, M. (1961). Reflexes proprioceptifs du diaphragme chez le lapin. *Helv. Physiol. Acta* 19: 360–372.

Davenport, P. W., Thompson, F. J., Reep, R. L., and Freed, A. N. (1985). Projection of phrenic nerve afferents to the cat sensorimotor cortex. *Brain Res.* 328: 150–153.

Davenport, P. W., Freidman, W. A., Thompson, F. J., and Franzen, O. (1986). Respiratory related cortical evoked potentials in humans. *J. Appl. Physiol.* 60: 1843–1848.

Davenport, P. W., Mercak, A., Shannon, R., and Lindsey, B. G. (1987). Sensorimotor cortical evoked potentials (CEP) elicited by intercostal muscle vibration. *Fed. Proc.* 46: 1103.

Decima, E. E., and von Euler, C. (1969). Excitability of phrenic motoneurons to afferent input from lower intercostal nerves in the spinal cat. *Acta Physiol. Scand.* 75: 580–591.

Decima, E. E., and von Euler, C., and Thoden, U. (1967). Spinal intercostal–phrenic reflexes. *Nature* 214: 312–313.

Decima, E. E., and von Euler, C., and Thoden, U. (1969). Intercostal-to-phrenic reflexes in the spinal cat. *Acta Physiol. Scand.* 75: 568–579.

Dogiel, A. S. (1902). Die Nervenendigungen in Bauchfell, in dem Schnen, Den Musckelspindelund dem Centrum Tendineum des diaphragma beim Menschen und dei Saugenthieren. *Arch. Mikrosk. Anat. Entwicklungsmech.* 59: 1–31.

Downman, C. B. B. (1955). Skeletal muscle reflexes of splanchnic and intercostal nerve origin in acute spinal and decerebrate cats. *J. Neurophysiol.* 18: 217–235.

Duron, B., Jung-Caillol, M. C., and Marlot, D. (1978). Myelinated nerve fiber supply and muscle spindles in the respiratory muscles of cat: quantitative study. *Anat. Embryol.* 152: 171–192.

Eccles, R. M., Sears, T. A., and Shealy, C. N. (1962). Intra-cellular recording from respiratory motoneurones of the thoracic spinal cord of the cat. *Nature* 193: 844–846.

Eklund, G. von Euler, C., and Rutkowski, S. (1964). Spontaneous and reflex activity of intercostal gamma motoneurones. *J. Physiol. (Lond.)*. 171: 139–163.

Frankstein, S. I., Smolin, L. N., Sergeeva, Z. N., and Sergeeva, T. I. (1979). Cortical representation of the phrenic nerve. *Exp. Neurol.* 63: 447–449.

Frazier, D. T., and Revelette, W. R. (1991). Role of phrenic nerve afferents in the control of breathing. *J. Appl. Physiol.* 70: 491–496.

Fryman, D. L., and Frazier, D. T. (1987). Diaphragm afferent modulation of phrenic motor drive. *J. Appl. Physiol.* 62: 2436–2441.

Gandevia, S. C., and Macefield, G. (1989). Projection of low-threshold afferents from human intercostal muscles to the cerebral cortex. *Respir. Physiol.* 77: 203–214.

Gill, P. K., and Kuno, M. (1963). Excitatory and inhibitory actions on phrenic mononeurons. *J. Physiol. (Lond.)* 168: 274–289.

Glebovskii, V. D. (1966). Stretch reflexes of intercostal muscles. *Trans. Fed. Proc.* 25: T937–T942.

Goshgarian, H. G. (1981). The role of cervical afferent nerve fiber inhibition of the crossed phrenic phenomenon. *Exp. Neurol.* 72: 211–225.

Goshgarian, H. G., and Roubal, P. J. (1986). Origin and distribution of phrenic primary afferent nerve fibers in the spinal cord of the adult rat. *Exp. Neurol.* 92: 624–638.

Green, M., Mead, J., and Sears, T. A. (1978). Muscle activity during chest wall restriction and positive pressure breathing in man. *Respir. Physiol.* 35: 283–300.

Guz, A., Nobel, M. I. M., Widdecombe, J. G., Trenchard, D., Mushin, W. W., and Makey, A. R. (1966). The role of vagal and glossopharyngeal nerves in respiratory sensation, control of breathing and arterial pressure regulation in conscious man. *Clin. Sci. (Lond.)* 30: 161–170.

Hinsey, J. C., Hare, K., and Phillips, R. A. (1939). Sensory components of the phrenic nerve of the cat. *Proc. Soc. Exp. Biol. Med.* 41: 411–414.

Holt, G. A., Dalziel, D. J., and Davenport, P. W. (1991). The transduction properties of diaphragmatic mechanoreceptors. *Neurosci. Lett.* 122: 117.

Homma, I., Eklund, G., and Hagbarth, K.-D. (1978). Respiration in man affected by TVR contractions elicited in inspiratory and expiratory intercostal muscles. *Respir. Physiol.* 35: 335–348.

Homma, I. (1980). Inspiratory inhibitory reflex caused by the chest wall vibration in man. *Respir. Physiol.* 39: 345–353.

Hore, J., Preston, J. B., Durdovic, R. G., and Cheney, P. D. (1976). Responses of cortical neurons (areas 3a and 4) to ramp stretch of hindlimb muscles in the baboon. *J. Neurophysiol.* 39: 484–500.

Huber, G. C. (1902). Neuromuscular spindles in the intercostal muscles of the cat. *Proc. Assoc. Am. Anat.* 1: 520–521.

Hudson, B. V. (1966). Afferent discharge from the phrenic nerve of a rat diaphragm preparation. *J. Physiol. (Lond.)* 189: 9–10.

Iscoe, S. (1989). Phrenic afferents and ventilatory control at increased end-expiratory lung volumes in cats. *J. Appl. Physiol.* 66: 1297–1303.

Jammes, Y., Buchler, B., Delpierre, S., Rasidakis, A., Grimaud, C., and Roussos, C. (1986). Phrenic afferents and their role in inspiratory control. *J. Appl. Physiol.* 60: 854–860.

Kim, M. J., Druz, W. S., Danon, J., Machach, W., and Sharp, J. T. (1976). Mechanics of the canine diaphragm. *J. Appl. Physiol.* 41: 369–382.

Kirkwood, P. A., and Sears, T. A. (1974). Monosynaptic excitation of motoneurones from secondary endings of muscle spindles. *Nature* 252: 243–244.

Kirkwood, P. A., and Sears, T. A. (1982). Excitatory post-synaptic potentials from single muscle spindle afferents in external intercostal motoneurones of the cat. *J. Physiol. (Lond.)* 322: 287–314.

Landau, B. R., Akert, K., and Roberts, T. S. (1962). Studies on the innervation of the diaphragm. *J. Comp. Neurol.* 119: 1–10.

Landgren, S., nd Silfvenius, H. (1969). Projection to cerebral cortex of group I muscle afferents from the cat's hindlimb. *J. Physiol. (Lond.)* 200: 353–372.

Landgren, S., Silvenius, H., and Wolsk, D. (1967). Somato-sensory paths to the second cortical projection area of the group I muscle afferents. *J. Physiol. (Lond.)* 191: 543–559.

Langford, L. A., and Schmidt, R. F. (1983). An electron microscopic analysis of the left phrenic nerve in the rat. *Anat. Rec.* 205: 297–213.

Larnicol, N., Rose, D., and Duron, B. (1984). Identification of phrenic afferents in the dorsal columns: A fluorescent double-labeling study in the cat. *Neurosci. Lett.* 52: 49–53.

Larnicol, N., Rose, D., and Duron, B. (1985). Identification of phrenic afferents to the external cuneate nucleus: A fluorescent double-labelling study in the cat. *Neurosci. Lett.* 62: 163–167.

Macron, J.-M., and Marlot, D. (1986). Effects of stimulation of phrenic afferent fibers on medullary respiratory neurons in cat. *Neurosci. Lett.* 63: 231–236.

Macron, J.-M., Marlot, D., and Duron, B. (1985). Phrenic afferent input to the lateral medullary reticular formation of the cat. *Respir. Physiol.* 59: 155–167.

Marlot, D., Macron, J.-M., and Duron, B. (1984). Projections of phrenic afferents to the cat cerebellar cortex. *Neurosci. Lett.* 44: 95–98.

Marlot, D., Macron, J.-M., and Duron, B. (1985a). Projection of phrenic afferents to the external cuneate nucleus in the cat. *Brain Res.* 327: 328–330.

Marlot, D., Macron, J.-M., and Duron, B. (1985b). Central projections of phrenic afferent fibers.

In: *Neurogenesis of Central Respiratory Rhythm*. Edited by A. L. Bianchi and M. Denavit-Saubie. Lancaster, UK, MTP Press, pp. 235–242.

Mead, J. (1979). Responses to loaded breathing. *Bull. Physiol. Pathol. Respir.* 15(Suppl.): 61–71.

Oscarsson, O., and Rosen, I. (1963). Projection to cerebral cortex of large muscle spindle afferents in forelimb nerves of the cat. *J. Physiol. (Lond.)* 169: 924–945.

Oscarsson, O., and Rosen, I., and Sulg, I. (1966). Organization of neurons in the cat cerebral cortex that are influenced from group I muscle afferents. *J. Physiol. (Lond.)* 183: 189–200.

Phillips, C. G., Powell, T. P. S., and Wisendanger, M. (1969). Projection from low-threshold muscle afferents of hand and forearm area 3a of baboon's cortex. *J. Physiol. (Lond.)* 217: 419–446.

Porter, W. T. (1895). The path of the respiratory impulse from the bulb to the phrenic nuclei. *J. Physiol. (Lond.)* 17: 455–485.

Reid, M. B., Banzett, R. B., Fieldman, H. A., and Mead, J. (1985). Reflex compensation of spontaneous breathing when immersion changes diaphragm length. *J. Appl. Physiol.* 58: 1136–1142.

Remmers, J. E. (1970). Inhibition of inspiratory activity by intercostal muscle afferents. *Respir. Physiol.* 358–383.

Remmers, J. E. (1973). Extra-segmental reflexes derived from intercostal afferents: Phrenic and laryngeal responses. *J. Physiol. (Lond.)* 233: 45–62.

Remmers, J. E., and Tsiaras, W. G. (1973). Effect of lateral cervical cord lesions on the respiratory rhythm of anaesthetized, decerebrate cats after vagotomy. *J. Physiol. (Lond.)* 233: 63–74.

Revelette, W. R., and Davenport, P. W. (1990). Effects of timing of inspiratory occlusion on cerebral evoked potentials in humans. *J. Appl. Physiol.* 68: 282–288.

Revelette, W. R., Reynolds, S., Brown, A., and Taylor, R. (1992). Effect of abdominal compression on diaphragmatic tendon organ activity. *J. Appl. Physiol.* 72: 288–292.

Revelette, W. R., Taylor, R. F., Davenport, P. W., Frazier, D. T., and Reynolds, S. M. (submitted). Length–tension characteristics of the crural diaphragm.

Revelette, W. R., Taylor, R. F., Davenport, P. W., Frazier, D. T., and Reynolds, S. M. (submitted). Reflex effects of vibratory stimuli delivered to the crural diaphragm.

Road, J. (1990). Phrenic afferents and ventilatory control. *Lung* 168: 137–149.

Road, J., Newman, S., Derenne, J. P., and Grassino, A. (1986). In vivo length–force relationship of canine diaphragm. *J. Appl. Physiol.* 60: 63–70.

Rosen, I. (1969a). Excitation of group I activated thalamocortical relay neurons in the cat. *J. Physiol. (Lond.)* 205: 237–255.

Rosen, I. (1969b). Localization in caudal brain stem and cervical spinal cord of neurons activated from forelimb group I afferents in the cat. *Brain Res.* 16: 55–71.

Rosen, I., and Sjolund, B. (1973a). Organization of group I activated cells in the main and external cuneate nuclei of the cat: Identification of muscle receptors. *Exp. Brain Res.* 16: 221–237.

Rosen, I., and Sjolund, B. (1973b). Organization of group I activated cells in the main and external cuneate nuclei of the cat: Convergence patterns demonstrated by natural stimulation. *Exp. Brain. Res.* 16: 238–246.

Sant'Ambrogio, G., and Remmers, J. E. (1985). Reflex influences acting on the respiratory muscles of the chest wall. In: *The Thorax*. Edited by C. Roussos and P. T. Macklem. New York, Marcel Dekker, pp. 531–580.

Sallach, J., Reep, R. L., and Davenport, P. W. (1990). Thalamocortical connections related to respiratory muscle afferents in the cat. *Neurosci. Abstr.* 16: 226.

Sears, T. A. (1958). Electrical activity in expiratory muscles of the cat during inflation of the chest. *J. Physiol. (Lond.)* 142: 35P.

Sears, T. A. (1964a). Investigations on respiratory motoneurons of the thoracic spinal cord. *Prog. Brain Res.* 12: 259–272.

Sears, T. A. (1964b). The fibre-calibre spectra of sensory and motor fibres in the intercostal nerves of the cat. *J. Physiol. (Lond.)* 172: 150–161.

Sears, T. A. (1964c). Efferent discharges in alpha and fusimotor fibres of intercostal nerves of the cat. *J. Physiol. (Lond.)* 174: 295–315.

Sears, T. A. (1964d). Some properties and reflex connexions of respiratory motoneurons of the cat's thoracic spinal cord. *J. Physiol. (Lond.)* 175: 386–403.

Sears, T. A., and Newsom Davis, J. (1968). The control of respiratory muscles during voluntary breathing. *Ann. N. Y. Acad. Sci.* 155: 183–190.

Shannon, R. (1977). Effects of thoracic dorsal rhizotomies on the respiratory pattern in anesthetized cats. *J. Appl. Physiol.* 43: 20–26.

Shannon, R. (1980a). Intercostal and abdominal muscle afferent influence on medullary dorsal respiratory group neurons. *Respir. Physiol.* 39: 73–94.

Shannon, R. (1980b). Respiratory pattern changes during costovertebral joint movement. *J. Appl. Physiol.* 48: 862–867.

Shannon, R. (1986). Reflexes from respiratory muscles and costovertebral joints. In: *Handbook of Physiology*. Section 3. The Respiratory System. Vol. I. Edited by N. S. Cherniack and J. G. Widdicombe. Washington, DC, American Physiological Society, pp. 431–447.

Shannon, R., and Zechman, F. W. (1972). The reflex and mechanical response of the inspiratory muscles to an increased airflow resistance. *Respir. Physiol.* 16: 51–69.

Shannon, R., Frazier, D. T., and Zechman, F. W. (1972). First-breath response of medullary inspiratory neurones to the mechanical loading of inspiration. *Respir. Physiol.* 16: 70–78.

Shannon, R., Bolser, D. C., and Lindsey, B. G. (1987). Medullary expiratory activity: influence of intercostal tendon organs and muscle spindle endings. *J. Appl. Physiol.* 62: 1057–1062.

Speck, D. F., and Revelette, W. R. (1987a). Attenuation of phrenic motor discharge by phrenic nerve afferents. *J. Appl. Physiol.* 62: 941–945.

Speck, D. F., and Revelette, W. R. (1987b). Excitation of dorsal and ventral respiratory group neurons by phrenic nerve afferents. *J. Appl. Physiol.* 62: 946–951.

Speck, D. F., and Webber, C. L. (1979). Thoracic dorsal rhizotomy in the anesthetized cat: Maintenance of eupneic breathing. *Respir. Physiol.* 38: 347–357.

Speck, D. F., and Weber, C. L. (1982). Cerebellar influence on the termination of inspiration by intercostal nerve stimulation. *Respir. Physiol.* 47: 231–238.

Stella, G. (1938). On the mechanism of production and the physiological significance of "apneusis." *J. Physiol. (Lond.)* 93: 10–23.

von Euler, C., and Peretti, G. (1966). Dynamic and static contributions to the rhythmic gamma activation of primary and secondary spindle endings in external intercostal muscle. *J. Physiol. (Lond.)* 187: 501–516.

Winkler, G., and Delaloye, B. (1957). A propos de la presence de fuseaux neuro-musculaires dans le diaphragme humain. *Acta Anat.* 29: 114–116.

Yasargil, G. M. (1962). Proprioceptive afferenzen in J. phrenicus der Katze. *Helv. Physiol. Acta* 20: 39–58.

Zechman, F. W., and Wiley, R. L. (1977). Effect of chest cage restriction on perception of added airflow resistance. *Respir. Physiol.* 31: 71–79.

Zechman, F. Z., O'Neill, O., and Shannon, R. (1967). Effect of low cervical spinal cord lesions on detection increased airflow resistance in man. *Physiologist* 100: 356.

Zechman, F. Z., Muza, S. R., Davenport, P. W., Wiley, R. L., and Shelton, R. (1985). Relationship of transdiaphragmatic pressure and latencies for detecting added inspiratory loads. *J. Appl. Physiol.* 58: 236–243.

31

Functional Role of Respiratory Muscle Reflexes

YVES JAMMES

Institut Jean Roche
Marseille, France

I. Introduction

Before describing and commenting on the functional role of reflexes elicited by the activation of respiratory muscle afferents, I will present an overview of the different sensory nerve endings in these muscles and their tendons, including the physiological and nonphysiological stimuli, respective afferent fibers, central projections, and spontaneous afferent pathways.

Table 1 summarizes the literature data, all obtained in cats. Roughly, three categories of receptors are described: length-, force-, and metaboreceptors. The first two are considered to be proprioceptors and are encapsulated, complex structures represented by primary (group IA afferent fibers) and secondary (group II fibers) muscle spindles and Golgi tendon organs (group IB fibers). The third category is composed of free nerve endings that detect the changes in extracellular fluid composition (i.e., local acidosis and hyperosmolarity, caused by the outflow of intracellular potassium with fatigue) and are also activated by injection of foreign chemicals such as phenyl diguanide or capsaicin (Jammes et al., 1986a; Graham et al., 1986). They are connected to group III and, mostly, group IV fibers, which represent the larger sensory component in the phrenic nerve (Hinsey, 1939; Duron and Condamin, 1970). However, limb muscle studies by Mense (1986) and Kaufman and Rybicki (1987) have revealed that group III afferent fibers are also responsive

Table 1 Characteristics of Respiratory Muscle Receptors

	Muscle spindles	Golgi tendon organs	Muscular free nerve endings	
Origin	All respiratory muscles including the crural portion of the diaphragm[6]	All respiratory muscles	Diaphragm[4,6,7] probably the other respiratory muscles	
Afferent fibers	group IA (primary) group II (secondary)	group IB	groups III	and IV
Fiber type	Large myelinated fibers		Thin myelinated	Unmyelinated
Diameter	Peak: 13 μm [2,5]		Peak: $3-4$ μm[5]	Range: $0.3-1.4$ μm^2
Conduction velocity	50 m s$^{-1(4)}$		10 m s$^{-1(4)}$	$0.8-1.3$ m s$^{-(4)}$
% sensory component	25%[5] / <50%[2]			75%[5] >50%[2]
Stimuli	Length receptors	Force receptors	Force plus metaboreceptors	Metaboreceptors
Spontaneous activity Discharge pattern	"Active" spindles Phasically active during contraction[1,3,4,6,7] (75% of phasically-active diaphragmatic afferents) "Passive" spindles Phasically active during relaxation	Tendon organs		Tonically active
Firing rate	Mean: 37 imp s$^{-1(4,7)}$		Mean: 14 imp s$^{-1(4,7)}$	
Functional role	Postural adaptations Load-compensatory mechanisms Respiratory sensations (ventilatory motion?)		Reflex responses to muscle fatigue Respiratory sensations (dyspnea?)	

Source: From data collected in Corda et al. (1965)[1], Duron and Condamin (1970)[2], Glebovskii (1963)[3], Graham et al. (1986)[4], Hinsey (1939)[5], Jammes et al. (1986)[6], Jammes and Balzamo (1992)[7], Shannon (1986)[8].

to mechanical stimuli, such as distorsion of their receptive field and tendon stretch, whereas group IV fibers are mostly responsive to metabolic changes, such as muscular acidosis or ischemia. In addition, the specificity of the aforementioned physiological stimuli should be attenuated. Indeed, some studies in limb muscles (see a review and also the original data by Lagier-Tessonnier et al., 1992) and the diaphragm (Graham et al., 1986; Jammes and Balzamo, 1992) have demonstrated that the activation of muscular metaboreceptors by lactic acid injection, local ischemia, or hypoxemia is associated with a parallel decrease in the spontaneous or mechanically activated high-frequency discharge proprioceptors. Thus, in numerous circumstances that combine increased strength of muscle contraction plus the changes in muscle fiber metabolism, as during fatigue, the response of the motor centers may result from complex modifications in the sensory pathways from the muscle groups participating to the effort.

Afferents from the respiratory muscles project on numerous central nervous structures, including the spinal cord (Gill and Kuno, 1963; Sears, 1964; Speck, 1987), the medulla (Shannon, 1986; Speck and Revelette, 1987), the lateral reticular nuclei (Macron et al., 1985), the cerebellum (Marlot et al., 1984), and also the sensorimotor cortex (Davenport et al., 1985; Balzamo et al., 1992). However, all the aforementioned data were obtained by single or repetitive electric shocks applied to the cut central end of intercostal or phrenic nerves. Thus, very few observations indicated what group of afferent fibers was more specifically concerned in the activation (or inhibition) of central neurons. Some information exists concerning the phrenic afferents. In decerebrated or C-2 spinalized cats, Speck (1987) has demonstrated that the long-latency, contralateral inhibitory phrenic response to phrenic afferent stimulation involves supraspinal connections of group III and perhaps IV phrenic afferents, whereas the short-latency, ipsilateral inhibitory response of phrenic motoneurons is due to spinal cord circuits activated by large phrenic afferent fibers. Gill and Kuno (1963) have also recorded inhibitory postsynaptic potentials in phrenic motoneurons in response to the dorsal root stimulation with shocks of short duration that are able to activate only the largest myelinated fibers. By using a differential block of conduction in either large (cold block at 6°C) or thin phrenic fibers, including the unmyelinated ones (procaine block), we have shown that the electrical stimulation of groups III and IV phrenic afferents in cats was responsible for both the inhibition of phrenic motoneuron impulse frequency and phrenic discharge time (Jammes et al., 1986a). On the other hand, injection of capsaicin, a well-known chemical stimulus of unmyelinated fibers, into the phrenic artery induced excitatory effects on the respiratory system in dogs (Revelette et al., 1988; Hussein et al., 1990). However, the very short latency of capsaicin-induced diaphragmatic response is contradictory with the minimal 3- to 5-s delay needed for the activation of group IV diaphragmatic afferents by injection of chemicals (Jammes et al., 1986a; Graham et al., 1986; Jammes and Balzamo, 1992). All the aforementioned data concern the ventilatory response to electrical nerve stimulation or to foreign chemicals (i.e., nonphysiological test agents). A recent study in cats (Jammes and Balzamo, 1992) reveals that the changes in breathing pattern observed during the development of diaphragmatic fatigue correspond to the successive activation of mechanoreceptors and metaboreceptors. All effects are inhibitory on the inspiratory activity, but the afferent paths of metaboreceptors are primarily responsible for the decrease in breathing frequency.

II. Role in the Control of Eupneic Breathing

Data concerning the role played by the rib cage and diaphragmatic afferents during quiet breathing are often contradictory. Dorsal root sectioning from T-1 to T-12 or spinal cord section at the C-8 level elicits either a decrease in tidal volume, with inconstant increased respiratory frequency (Duron, 1973; Gautier, 1973; Shannon, 1977; Jammes et al., 1983a, 1986a), or has no effect (Stella, 1938; Speck and Webber, 1979). The discrepancies between data obtained in the different animal preparations may result because the central integration of somatic reflexes depends on the depth and type of anesthesia. Thus, the ventilatory effects of spinal cord section at the C-8 level are negligible in cats under pentobarbital sodium anesthesia, a powerful depressor of spinal reflexes, but very pronounced under chloralose-ethyl carbamate which enhances these refexes (Jammes et al., 1986b). In the latter, the recruitment of phrenic motoneurons is facilitated after low cervical spinal section, which unmasks the inhibitory influences exerted by somatic afferents on the respiratory neurons. Moreover, vagal and spinal afferents seem to interact centrally in the control of eupneic ventilation; indeed, when spinal section was performed first, a significant and marked increase in the amplitude of breath, with no change in the ventilatory timing, occurred, whereas the suppression of spinal afferents in vagotomized animals decreased the tidal breath and shortened the inspiratory period (Jammes et al., 1986b). Despite the apparent differences in the aforementioned observations, the overall conclusion drawn from the spinal cord section or the thoracic rhizotomy studies is that chest wall and, perhaps also, abdominal muscle transmission is not a major factor determining the breathing pattern in anesthetized animals. However, this does not allow one to claim that these peripheral communications cannot participate in determination of a spontaneous-breathing pattern in awake animals or in humans, primarily in an upright posture.

Few studies have been devoted to the role played by diaphragmatic afferents in the control of eupnea. In rabbits, Dolivo (1952) reported that the selective blockade of myelinated phrenic fibers, using anodal block, lengthened the inspiratory time; however, this was studied in animals breathing spontaneously, and the consequences of diaphragmatic paralysis on chest wall mechanics or on respiratory gas exchange may influence the ventilatory control. Anesthetized cats presenting spontaneous diaphragmatic contractions were studied under artificial ventilation, and the spinal cord was sectioned at the C-8 level to suppress the thoracic and abdominal afferents (Jammes et al., 1986a); then, cold block (6°C) of large phrenic fibers prolonged the phrenic discharge, whereas procaine block of thin phrenic fibers had no effect. Under the same experimental conditions tested in other individuals of the same species, section of the phrenic trunks exerted significant changes in the ventilatory timing ($\Delta T_I = +13\%$; $\Delta T_{tot} = +16\%$) and also markedly modified the recruitment strategy of phrenic motoneurons with enhanced high-frequency power toward the end of inspiration (Jammes and Balzamo, 1992; Fig. 1). Thus, phrenic sensory pathways seem to play a role in the control of the ventilatory timing and also to govern the rate-coding pattern of phrenic motoneurons under resting conditions. Data on the effects of differential block of phrenic conduction by cold or procain (Jammes et al., 1986a), added to the electrophysiological recordings of the phrenic afferent activity (Corda et al., 1965; Graham et al., 1986; Jammes et al., 1986a; Jammes and Balzamo, 1992), concur to show that the spontaneous high-frequency phasic discharge of diaphragmatic mechanoreceptors and not the low-frequency, erratic activity of groups III and IV fibers, is responsible for the eupneic ventilatory control. This suggests the existence of a phrenic-to-phrenic reflex

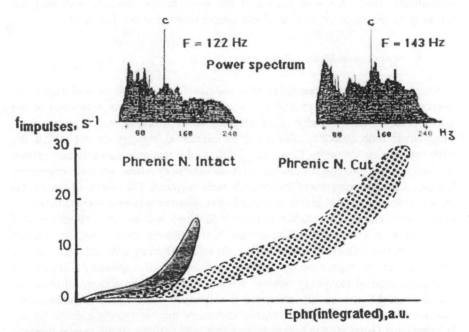

Figure 1 The spontaneous diaphragmatic contractions influence the motor phrenic discharge, even in anesthetized, vagotomized, artificially ventilated cats with the chest opened. This proprioceptive reflex loop reduces the integrated phrenic activity (Ephr) and also the impulse rate of motoneurons, as assessed from the changes in $f_{impulses}$ counted from discriminated impulses or in the centroid frequency of phrenic neurogram power spectrum). Sectioning of the phrenic nerves unmasks these inhibitory influences. (From Jammes and Balzamo, 1992.)

loop that informs the phrenic motoneurons and also the respiratory centers of the length–tension relations in the diaphragm.

III. Role in Compensation for Posture Changes

Changes in operating length of the respiratory muscles and primarily of the diaphragm occur during the transition from the supine to the upright posture. This leads to shortened muscle fiber length and, thus, a decreased pressure-generating ability of the muscle. If there were no compensatory reflex increase in neural drive, the amplitude of breath (VT) would fall. Since the first work by Fleisch (1938), numerous studies have been devoted to the description of proprioceptive reflex loops within intercostal and abdominal muscles and within the diaphragm. Most of these reflex actions have been described in the well-documented review by Shannon (1986). However, although segmental and intersegmental reflexes, as well as the supraspinal effects are well known at the level of the thoracic wall and the diaphragm, less information is available concerning the abdominal wall.

A. Intercostal Muscle Afferents

Afferents from primary muscle spindle endings from inspiratory and expiratory intercostal muscles monosynaptically excite the homonymous motoneurons of the same spinal segment and also of adjacent segments. Unlike group IA afferents of antagonistic limb muscles, afferents from intercostal muscles do not inhibit the heteronymous motoneurons (Shannon, 1986). Golgi tendon organ afferents (group IB fibers) from intercostal muscles exert an inhibitory effect on their respective homonymous motoneurons of the same thoracic segment. The effects of intercostal muscle proprioceptive afferents on medullary inspiratory and expiratory neurons are more controversial. Two studies in cats by Shannon and his team (Bolser et al., 1987; Shannon et al., 1987) demonstrate that intercostal muscle spindle endings have no direct influence on medullary neurons, whereas external and internal intercostal tendon organs exert an inhibitory effect on all inspiratory neurons and on a population of expiratory neurons driving intercostal and abdominal muscles, constituting the arm of an intercostal-to-abdominal reflex loop. Intercostal-to-phrenic reflexes also exist. Afferents of secondary muscle spindle endings (group II fibers) and Golgi tendon organs from intercostal muscles in the caudal thoracic segments (T9–T12) project to phrenic motoneurons. These proprioceptive afferents are involved in a facilitatory intercostal-to-phrenic reflex. Some studies reviewed by Shannon (1986) have also suggested the existence of an inhibitory intercostal-to-phrenic reflex, elicited by the electrical stimulation of the intercostal nerves, chest compression in vagotomized animals, or sustained high-frequency mechanical vibrations in the lower thoracic regions. However, in a more recent work, Bolser et al. (1988) have shown that costovertebral joint mechanoreceptors contribute to primarily the inspiratory inhibitory effect of intercostal muscle–rib vibration.

B. Abdominal Muscle Afferents

A facilitatory stretch reflex can be elicited in abdominal motoneurons of cats and rabbits (Bishop, 1964). Also, a tonic vibratory response (TVR) was recorded in the transversus muscle in vagotomized dogs when mechanical vibrations were applied on the linea alba (Jammes et al., 1983a; Fig. 2A). Abdominal muscle afferents also project on distal spinal segments and supraspinal structures. Indeed, the TVR of abdominal muscles is associated with a marked depression of the diaphragmatic activity and a slight tachypnea, mostly due to shortened expiratory time (see Fig. 2B). These inhibitory influences exerted by abdominal muscle afferents on the phrenic motoneurons and the respiratory centers are much more pronounced when all afferents are recruited by electrical nerve stimulation (Shannon, 1986) or direct tetanic muscle stimulation (Jammes et al., 1983a).

C. Diaphragmatic Afferents

The existence of a diaphragmatic autogenic load-compensation reflex is controversial. Sant'Ambrogio et al. (1962), Sant'Ambrogio and Widdicombe (1965), Corda et al. (1965), and von Euler (1966) reported no change in the motor phrenic activity in vagotomized animals in response to diaphragmatic distension. However, an operational length compensation, characterized by increased amplitude of breath (VT) associated with increased diaphragmatic electromyographic (EMG) activity and prolonged inspiratory duration, was observed in response to diaphragmatic distension produced by inflating an abdominal balloon (Cuenod, 1961); application of lower body negative pressure in C-7 spinalized, vagotomized cats (Fryman and Frazier, 1987); body immersion (Reid et al., 1985); or postural changes in cats (van Lunteren et al., 1985) or men (Brancatisano et al., 1989). van Lunteren et al. (1985) observed that the activity of both costal and crural portions of the diaphragm was greater in the head-up, compared with supine posture. However, increased crural activity was greater than that of costal activity as a result of changes in posture. In quadriplegic men, Banzett et al. (1981) found that application of a negative lower torso pressure within a cuirass increased VT. Also, the immediate ventilatory response to postural changes persisted after human heart–lung transplantation (i.e., permanent pulmonary denervation; Kinnear et al., 1989).

IV. Role in the Response to Ventilatory Loading or Muscle Fatigue

The role of respiratory muscle afferents during mechanical ventilatory loading includes the response to external mechanical loading, such as resistive or elastic

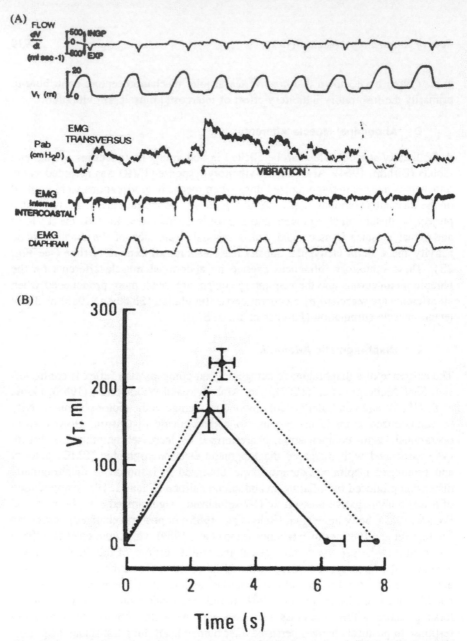

Figure 2 Proprioceptive afferents from the abdominal muscles influence the breathing pattern in dogs. (A) The tonic vibratory response (TVR) recorded in the rectus abdominis muscle is associated with a marked reduction in the amplitude of breath (V_T) and integrated diaphragmatic EMG. (B) TVR (dashed line) is associated with modifications of the mean spirogram; namely, decreased V_T and shortened expiratory duration, compared with control (solid line). (Redrawn from Jammes et al., 1983a.)

loads, chest compression, and tracheal occlusion, or to internal loading, as drug- or antigen-induced bronchospasm, high-density gas breathing, and also passive hyperinflation or deflation of the lungs. In some circumstances (external loads or passive lung volume changes), single-breath loading may be performed, avoiding the stimulation of the chemoreflex drive of breathing. The response to single-breath loads must be distinguished from that reported during multibreath (or steady-state) ventilatory loading, for which data analysis requires that the arterial blood gas levels are maintained constant. In all cases, load-induced changes in ventilatory activity must be considered in intact, rather than in vagotomized, animals, to differentiate the specific effects produced by activation of vagal afferents.

Chest compression or tracheal occlusion (TO) at end-expiration (infinite inspiratory load) decreases the thoracic gas volume. Shannon et al. (1985) have shown that, in vagotomized animals with the spinal cord intact, these loads lengthen the inspiratory activity for the first loaded breath, and this corresponds to the prolonged firing duration for 50% of medullary inspiratory neurons in the dorsal and ventral inspiratory groups. These effects disappear after cervical plus thoracic dorsal rhizotomies, but they persist with either the cervical or thoracic dorsal roots intact. In vagotomized and C-8 spinal lesioned cats, for which only the diaphragmatic afferents are intact, TO at end-expiration induced no change in the duration of phrenic nerve activity, but markedly reduced the amplitude of breath (Jammes et al., 1986b, 1988a; Fig. 3). Electrophysiological studies reveal that TO increases the discharge of both spindle endings and tendon organs in external intercostal and

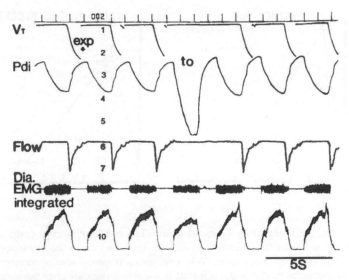

Figure 3 Tracheal occlusion (to) at end-expiration elicits a marked reduction in the integrated diaphragmatic activity in vagotomized, C-8 spinalized cats, a preparation leaving only the phrenic afferents intact. (From Jammes, 1988a.)

parasternal muscles (Shannon, 1986) and of Golgi tendon organs in the diaphragm (Jammes et al., 1986a). Thus, both the chest wall and diaphragmatic afferents seem to participate in the immediate response to an extreme mechanical loading, the latter being mainly involved in the control of the inspired volume under these circumstances. Multibreath TO at end-expiration or long-term breathing against external inspiratory loads markedly prolongs the activity of external intercostal muscles and the diaphragm, inducing a near tonic activity in these muscle groups (Shannon and Zechman, 1972; Seaman et al., 1983; Badier et al., 1989). In rabbits, bivagotomy suppresses the tonic inspiratory response (Badier et al., 1989), but this was inconstantly observed in cats (Shannon et al., 1985). Increased thoracic gas volume is produced by expiratory threshold load breathing (ETL) or positive-pressure breathing. These situations enhance the strength of diaphragmatic contractions, with lengthening of the expiratory period because of evoked expiratory activities in intercostal and abdominal muscles. This was observed in dogs under cardiopulmonary bypass, condition during which the chemoreflex drive of breathing was held constant (Jammes et al., 1983a). However, the different components of this ventilatory response need the integrity of vagal afferents to be maximal (Jammes et al., 1983a; Russel and Bishop, 1986; Fig. 4). Elastic loading increases the respiratory frequency in vagotomized dogs and cats, but this no longer occurs when the chemical drive is held constant (Shannon, 1986). Thus, respiratory muscle afferents do not participate in this response. Similarly, the ventilatory responses to

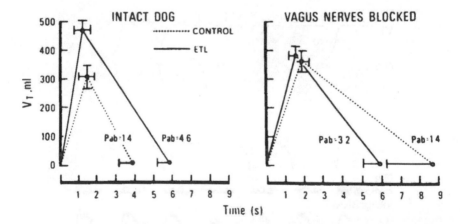

Figure 4 Prolonged expiratory threshold load (ETL) breathing in dogs under cardiopulmonary bypass increases the amplitude of breaths and slows down the respiratory rhythm owing to prolonged expiratory time. This ventilatory response results mostly from the activation of mechanosensitive vagal afferents because it disappears after the conduction in large vagal fibers is blocked by cold at 6°C. Then, reverse changes in ventilatory timing are observed in response to ETL. This confirms that the activation of expiratory muscle afferents shortens the expiratory period. (From Jammes et al., 1983a.)

an increase in the respiratory system impedance, as produced by histamine-, carbachol-, or antigen-induced bronchospasm, are very reduced or absent in vagotomized animals (for review see Badier et al., 1989). In summary, despite the existence of well-known segmental and plurisegmental spinal reflexes between the respiratory muscle groups, which may play a role in some postural adaptations, the changes in the ventilatory timing elicited by severe mechanical loading of the respiratory system involves a weak participation of respiratory muscle afferents in anesthetized animals. In conscious, quadriplegic men, ventilatory adjustments to elastic or resistive loads, including the changes in timing, are qualitatively the same as those found in healthy subjects (Kenneth, 1984). This indicates that sensory inputs from the airways and lungs and, perhaps also, from the diaphragm are sufficient to mediate normal patterns of ventilatory adjustments during loaded breathing.

Fragmentary observations concern the role of respiratory muscle afferents during muscle ischemia or fatigue. Both circumstances are able to activate the muscular metaboreceptors by the local acidosis associated with extracellular fluid hyperosmolarity caused by the outflow of intracellular potassium. In dogs, Aubier et al. (1981) reported changes in ventilatory timing during the response to breathing against a fatiguing load or in a state of reduced diaphragmatic blood flow, as in shock: initial tachypnea was followed by bradypnea. Because this response was not affected by vagotomy or cross-perfusion of the head, which eliminated the activation of arterial and central chemoreceptors, it was tempting to speculate that the activation of diaphragmatic metaboreceptors may play a role in the observed delayed bradypnea. More recently, opposite observations were reported by Supinski et al. (1989), who have shown, in the same species, that fatigue of in situ muscle strips from the left diaphragm elicited a slight increase in respiratory frequency. However, in all the foregoing studies, there were never simultaneous recordings made of the changes in the ventilatory pattern and phrenic sensory pathways during a fatigue run. This was performed in artificially ventilated cats, in which diaphragmatic fatigue was produced by the direct electrical stimulation of the two cupolae with trains of pulses (Jammes and Balzamo, 1992). When muscle failure occurred after 10–15 min of stimulation the firing rate of diaphragmatic metaboreceptors markedly increased (Fig. 5). This was associated with a progressive lengthening in inspiratory and total breath durations, whereas the leftward shift in the power spectrum of a motor phrenic neurogram (reduced impulse rate of motoneurons) began early during the fatigue trial (i.e., before muscle failure could be assessed). Section of the phrenic nerves abolished the changes in the motor phrenic activity as well as the ventilatory timing during fatigue. This suggests that the activation of the different categories of diaphragmatic receptors (proprioceptors and groups III and mostly IV phrenic afferents) exerts specific influences on the phrenic motoneurons and also the supraspinal structures that govern the respiratory frequency; the latter being mostly influenced by the peripheral inputs from the metaboreceptors. In addition, recent studies in the diaphragm (Jammes and Balzamo, 1992) and limb muscles of cats (Lagier-Tessonnier et al., 1992) have

Phrenic N. Intact

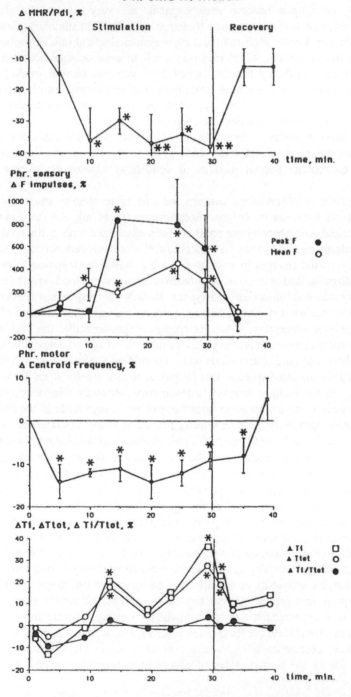

demonstrated that enhanced anaerobic metabolic paths produced by muscle fatigue or hypoxia not only activated the muscular metaboreceptors, but also depressed the discharge of mechanoreceptors. Thus, the aforementioned reflex changes in ventilatory pattern associated with the occurrence of diaphragmatic fatigue may result from both enhanced sensory pathways from metaboreceptors and depressed afferent phasic discharge of mechanoreceptors.

V. Role in the Control of the Autonomic Nervous System

It has been firmly established that static exercise of limb muscles increases heart rate and arterial pressure. The activation of groups III and IV muscle afferents plays a major role in this "pressor" reflex (Kaufman et al., 1984 and 1988; Rotto et al., 1989). This vasomotor response is associated with decreased total pulmonary resistance, a bronchomotor effect caused by the withdrawal of the tonic cholinergic vagal input to the airways. Both vasomotor and bronchomotor effects—combined to increased cardiac output and minute ventilation—are supposed to enhance the oxygen blood supply to the working muscles.

Some observations suggest that the activation of groups III and IV phrenic afferents exert the same influences on the control of the vasomotor and bronchomotor tone. In dogs, Hussain et al. (1990) demonstrated that the chemical activation of unmyelinated phrenic afferents by capsaicin, injected into the phrenic artery of an in situ isolated and innervated hemidiaphragm, elicits an increase in arterial pressure and heart rate associated with a decline in phrenic blood flow, measured with an electromagnetic flow probe. As with the stimulation of limb muscle afferents (Rybicki and Kaufman, 1985), high-voltage electrical stimulation of all phrenic afferents, including group IV fibers, evokes a decrease in lung resistance, a bronchomotor effect abolished by atropine (McCallister et al., 1986). Low-voltage stimulation of the phrenic nerve, which can activate only the largest afferent fibers, has no effect on the bronchomotor tone.

Thus, as is well known for vagal afferents from the lungs and airways (Jammes, 1988b), the sensory pathways from the respiratory muscles influence the neural networks involved in both the control of ventilation and bronchomotor tone.

Figure 5 Electrically induced diaphragmatic fatigue in anesthetized cats under artificial ventilation occurs after 10 min of intermittent muscle stimulation, as assessed from decreased maximum relaxation rate of twitches (MRR/Pdi). Muscle failure is associated with a marked activation of the tonic phrenic afferent discharge of metaboreceptors and also the progressive lengthening of both inspiratory and total breath durations. However, the changes in impulse rate of phrenic motoneurons (reduced centroid frequency of motor phrenic power spectrum) begin before diaphragmatic failure and the activation of metaboreceptors. (Redrawn from Jammes and Balzamo, 1992.)

VI. Role in Respiratory Sensations and Integrated Central Mechanisms

Projection of phrenic afferents to the cat sensorimotor cortex have been described (Davenport et al., 1985; Balzamo et al., 1992). Also, the existence of intercostal afferent projections to the cortex is well known (Davenport et al., 1985). The aforementioned data result from the location of cortical phrenic potentials (CPEPs) evoked by single shocks applied to one of the two phrenic nerves. These observations, in combination, demonstrate that a restricted area in the posterior sygmoid gyrus (PSG) receives primary (i.e., shortest latency) CPEPs, whereas secondary CPEPs are more spread out over the PSG (Balzamo et al., 1992). Respiratory-related potentials are also evoked on the sensorimotor cortex in humans, as evidenced by measurement of occluded mouth pressure (Davenport et al., 1986). However, complete occlusion of the inspiratory line stimulates numerous afferents, including the chest wall and the bronchopulmonary vagal receptors (Jammes et al., 1986b).

Continuous recordings with quantitative analysis of the spontaneous cortical activity throughout a diaphragmatic fatigue run in vagotomized, artificially ventilated cats reveal a marked early depression of low-frequency theta–delta EEG rhythms. Further modifications in the cortical activity occur in association with diaphragmatic fatigue, as diagnosed from twitch transdiaphragmatic pressure changes. The absence of any cortical response after diaphragmatic denervation demonstrates the role played by the phrenic sensory pathways (Balzamo et al., 1992). These observations constitute the electrophysiological basis of the cortical integration of diaphragmatic sensory pathways during ventilatory loading and respiratory muscle fatigue. However, pulmonary vagal afferents, also activated under the condition of loaded breathing, are integrated at the level of the sensorimotor cortex in cats (Balzamo et al., 1990). Thus, the sensation of breathlessness during loaded breathing must result from the additive effects of the activation of vagal, diaphragmatic, and probably, chest wall afferents.

The activation of respiratory muscle afferents during expiratory threshold-load breathing is responsible for a progressive depression of the central integration of peripheral information from the lungs and airways (namely, PSR afferents) and also the chemosensory afferents (Jammes et al., 1983b; Fig. 6). Such a negative interaction between somatic (muscle afferents) and vegetative respiratory afferents occurs after about 10 min of loaded ventilation and persisted for at least 10 min during recovery. Inhibitory effects also occur with the activation of diaphragmatic metaboreceptors. They combine ventilatory (i.e., brain stem) effects (bradypnea) and higher inhibitory events: depression of EEG rhythms plus delayed transmission of CPEPs (Jammes and Balzamo, 1992; Balzamo et al., 1992). This central inhibition developed progressively throughout the fatigue run, and part of the cortical effects persisted during the recovery of the fatigue trial. Thus, the central delivery of inhibitory neurotransmitters is probably involved. Studies by Kaufman et al.

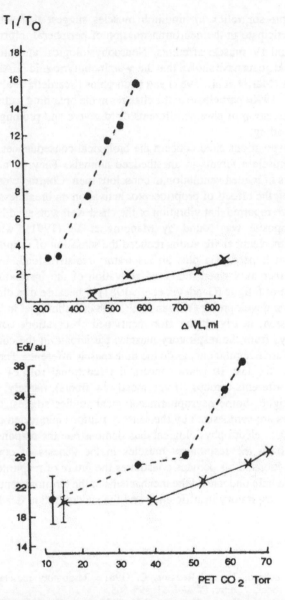

Figure 6 Prolonged ETL breathing (x) in dogs under cardiopulmonary bypass progressively and markedly reduces the inhibitory ventilatory response to the stimulation of the vagal pulmonary stretch receptors (upper diagram: Breuer–Hering reflex) and also the response to hypercapnia (lower diagram). (Redrawn from Jammes et al., 1983b.)

(1988) on the pressor reflex in hindlimb muscles suggest that substance P and somatostatin participate in the neurotransmission of peripheral information carried by groups III and IV muscle afferents. Neurophysiological and pharmacological studies in cats and goats have shown that the γ-aminobutyric acid (GABA) inhibitory neurotransmitter (Marlot et al., 1987) and endorphins (Scardella et al., 1986, 1989; Petrozzino et al., 1990) participate in the changes in the breathing pattern in response to electrical stimulation of phrenic afferents or to severe and prolonged inspiratory flow-resistive loading.

All the observations cited concern the biological consequences for activation of respiratory muscle afferents in anesthetized animals. They do not involve the cognitive aspects of loaded ventilation in conscious men. Contradictory findings are found concerning the effects of proprioceptor activation on breathlessness. Homma et al. (1984) have reported that vibration of the chest wall worsened breathlessness, whereas the opposite was found by Manning et al. (1991), who found that high-frequency mechanical vibrations reduced the sensation of dyspnea induced by a combination of hypercapnia plus an inspiratory resistive load. In humans, the sense of effort increases when increased activation of the inspiratory muscles is required because of fatigue (Gandevia et al., 1981) or because of a disadvantageous length for tension development (Killian et al., 1984; Stubbing et al., 1983).

In conclusion, nearly all the aforementioned observations confirm that the sensory pathways from the respiratory muscles participate in the control of motor output and vegetative regulations, as do the limb muscle afferents. The most striking data obtained in the last 10 years concern the functional role of diaphragmatic metaboreceptor afferents (groups III and mostly IV fibers); namely, in association with muscle fatigue. Some neuropharmacological studies suggest that inhibitory neurotransmitters are synthesized by the sensory neurons connected to the metaboreceptors and, also, electrophysiological data demonstrate the responsibility of thin afferent fibers from the respiratory muscles in the genesis of complex central inhibitory interactions. This perhaps constitutes the future of respiratory neurobiology, which could help understand the mechanisms of the terminal central ventilatory failure of severe respiratory insufficiency and the sudden infant death syndrome.

References

Aubier, M., Trippenbach, T., and Roussos, C. (1981). Respiratory muscle fatigue during cardiogenic shock. *J. Appl. Physiol.* 51: 499–508.

Badier, M., Jammes, Y., Romero-Colomer, P., and Lemerre, C. (1989). Tonic activity in inspiratory muscles and phrenic motoneurons by stimulation of vagal afferents. *J. Appl. Physiol.* 66: 1613–1619.

Balzamo, E., Gayan-Ramirez, G., and Jammes, Y. (1990). Pulmonary vagal sensory afferents and spontaneous EEG rhythms in the cat sensorimotor cortex. *J. Auton. Nerv. Syst.* 30: 149–158.

Balzamo, E., Lagier-Tessonnier, F., and Jammes, Y. (1992). Fatigue-induced changes in diaphragmatic sensory pathways and cortical activity of cats. *Respir. Physiol.* 90: 213–226.

Banzett, R. B., Ingbar, G. F., Brown, R., Goldman, M., Rossier, A., and Mead, J. (1981). Diaphragm electrical activity during negative lower torso pressure in quadriplegic men. *J. Appl. Physiol.* 51: 654–659.

Bishop, B. (1964). Reflex control of abdominal muscles during positive-pressure breathing. *J. Appl. Physiol.* 19: 224–232.

Bolser, D. C., Lindsey, B. G., and Shannon, R. (1987). Medullary inspiratory activity: Influence of intercostal tendon organs and muscle spindle endings. *J. Appl. Physiol.* 62: 1046–1056.

Bolser, D. C., Lindsey, B. G., and Shannon, R. (1988). Respiratory pattern changes produced by intercostal muscle/rib vibration. *J. Appl. Physiol.* 64: 2458–2462.

Brancatisano, A., Kelly, S. M., Tully, A., Loring, S. H., and Engel, L. A. (1989). Postural changes in spontaneous and evoked regional diaphragmatic activity in dogs. *J. Appl. Physiol.* 66: 1699–1705.

Corda, M., von Euler, C., and Lennerstrand, G. (1965). Proprioceptive innervation of the diaphragm. *J. Physiol. (Lond.)* 178: 161–178.

Cuenod, M. (1961). Reflexes proprioceptifs du diaphragme chez le Lapin. *Helv. Physiol. Acta* 19: 360–372.

Davenport, P. W., Thompson, F. J., Reep, R. L., and Freed, A. N. (1985). Projection of phrenic nerve afferents to the cat sensorimotor cortex. *Brain Res.* 328: 150–153.

Davenport, P. W., Friedman, W. A., Thompson, F. J., and Franzen, O. (1986). Respiratory-related cortical potentials evoked by inspiratory occlusions in humans. *J. Appl. Physiol.* 60: 1843–1848.

Dolivo, M. (1952). Effets de l'interruption de la conduction nerveuse dans un nerf phrénique sur la fréquence respiratoire. *Helv. Physiol. Acta* 10: 366–371.

Duron, B. (1973). Postural and ventilatory function of intercostal muscles. *Acta Neurobiol. Exp.* 33: 355–380.

Duron, B., and Condamin, M. (1970). Etude au microscope électronique de la composition amyélinique du nerf phrénique du Chat. *C. R. Soc. Biol.* 164: 577–585.

Fleisch, A., and Tripod, J. (1938). Die afferente Komponente der Atmungssteuerung. *Pfluegers Arch. Gesamte Physiol. Menschen Tiere* 240: 676–679.

Fryman, D. L., and Frazier, D. T. (1987). Diaphragm afferent modulation of phrenic motor drive. *J. Appl. Physiol.* 62: 2436–2441.

Gandevia, S. C., Killian, K. J., and Campbell, E. J. M. (1981). The effect of respiratory muscle fatigue on respiratory sensations. *Clin. Sci. (Lond.)* 60: 463–466.

Gautier, H. (1973). Respiratory responses of the anesthetized rabbit to vagotomy and thoracic dorsal rhizotomy. *Respir. Physiol.* 17: 238–247.

Gill, P. K., and Kuno, M. (1963). Excitatory and inhibitory actions on phrenic motoneurons. *J. Physiol. (Lond.)* 168: 274–289.

Glebovskii, V. D. (1963). Stretch receptors of the diaphragm. *Fed. Proc.* 22: T405–T410.

Graham, R., Jammes, Y., Delpierre, S., Grimaud, C., and Roussos, C. (1986). The effects of ischemia, lactic acid and hypertonic sodium chloride on phrenic afferent discharge during spontaneous diaphragmatic contractions. *Neurosci. Lett.* 67: 257–262.

Hinsey, J. C., Hare, K., and Philips, R. A. (1939). Sensory components of the phrenic nerve of the cat. *Proc. Soc. Exp. Biol.* 41: 411–414.

Homma, I., Obata, T., Sibuya, M., and Uchida, M. (1984). Gate mechanism in breathlessness caused by chest wall vibrations in humans. *J. Appl. Physiol.* 56: 8–11.

Hussain, S., Magder, S., Chatillon, A., and Roussos, C. (1990). Chemical activation of thin-fibre phrenic afferents: Respiratory response. *J. Appl. Physiol.* 69: 1002–1011.

Jammes, Y. (1988a). Chest wall and diaphragmatic afferents: Their role during external mechanical loading and respiratory muscle ischemia. In: *Respiratory Muscles in Chronic Obstructive Pulmonary Disease.* Edited by A. Grassino. London, Springer-Verlag, pp. 49–57.

Jammes, Y. (1988b). Tonic sensory pathways of the respiratory system (Cournand Lecture). *Eur. Respir. J.* 1: 176–183.

Jammes, Y., and Balzamo, E. (1992). Changes in afferent and efferent phrenic activities with electrically-induced diaphragm fatigue. *J. Appl. Physiol.* 73: 894–902.

Jammes, Y., Bye, P. T. P., Pardy, R. L., Katsardis, C., Esau, S., and Roussos, C. (1983a). Expiratory threshold load under extracorporeal circulation: Effects of vagal afferents. *J. Appl. Physiol.* 55: 307–315.

Jammes, Y., Bye, P. T. P., Pardy, R. L., and Roussos, C. (1983b). Vagal feedback with expiratory threshold load under extracorporeal circulation. *J. Appl. Physiol.* 55: 316–322.

Jammes, Y., Buchler, B., Delpierre, S., Rasidakis, A., Grimaud, C., and Roussos, C. (1986a). Phrenic afferents and their role in inspiratory control. *J. Appl. Physiol.* 60: 854–860.

Jammes, Y., Mathiot, M. J., Delpierre, S., and Grimaud, C. (1986b). Role of vagal and spinal sensory pathways on eupneic diaphragmatic activity. *J. Appl. Physiol.* 60: 479–485.

Kaufman, M. P., and Rybicki, K. J. (1987). Discharge properties of group III and IV muscle afferents: Their response to mechanical and metabolic stimuli. *Circ. Res.* 61: 160–165.

Kaufman, M. P., Rybicki, K. J., Waldrop, T. G., and Mitchell, J. H. (1984). Effect on arterial pressure of rhythmically contracting the hindlimb muscles of cats. *J. Appl. Physiol.* 56: 1265–1271.

Kaufman, M. P., Rotto, D. M., and Rybicki, K. J. (1988). Pressor reflex response to static muscular contraction: Its afferent arm and possible neurotransmitters. *Am. J. Cardiol.* 62: 58E–62E.

Kenneth, A. (1984). Adaptations of quadriplegic men to consecutively loaded breaths. *J. Appl. Physiol.* 56: 1099–1103.

Killian, K. J., Gandevia, S. C., Summers, E., and Campbell, E. J. M. (1984). Effect of increased lung volume on perception of breathlessness, effort and tension. *J. Appl. Physiol.* 57: 686–691.

Kinnear, W., Higenbottam, T., Shaw, D., Wallwork, J., and Estenne, M. (1989). Ventilatory compensation for changes in posture after human heart–lung transplantation. *Respir. Physiol.* 77: 75–88.

Lagier-Tessonnier, F., Balzamo, E., and Jammes, Y. (1993). Comparative effects of ischemia and acute hypoxemia on muscle afferents from tibialis anterior in cats. *Muscle Nerve* 16: 135–142.

Macron, J. M., Marlot, D., and Duron, B. (1985). Phrenic afferent input to the lateral medullary reticular formation of the cat. *Respir. Physiol.* 59: 155–167.

Manning, H. L., Basner, R., Ringler, J., Rand, C., Fenci, V., Weinberger, S. E., Weiss, J. W., and Schwartzstein, R. M. (1991). Effect of chest wall vibration on breathlessness in normal subjects. *J. Appl. Physiol.* 71: 175–181.

Marlot, D., Macron, J. M., and Duron, B. (1984). Projections of phrenic afferences to the cat cerebellar cortex. *Neurosci. Lett.* 44: 95–98.

Marlot, D., Macron, J. M., and Duron, B. (1987). Inhibitory and excitatory effects on respiration by phrenic nerve afferent stimulation in cats. *Respir. Physiol.* 69: 321–333.

McCallister, L. W., McCoy, K. W., Connelly, J. C., and Kaufman, M. P. (1986). Stimulation of group III and IV phrenic afferents reflexly decreases total lung resistance in dogs. *J. Appl. Physiol.* 61: 1346–1351.

Mense, S. (1986). Slowly conducting afferent fibres from deep tissues: Neurobiological properties and central nervous actions. In: *Progress in Sensory Physiology 6*. Edited by D. Ottoson. Berlin, Springer-Verlag, pp. 149–219.

Petrozzino, J. J., Scardella, A. T., Li, J. K. J., Krawciw, N., Edelman, N. H., and Santiago, T. V. (1990). Effects of naloxone on spectral shifts of the diaphragm EMG during inspiratory loading. *J. Appl. Physiol.* 68: 1376–1385.

Reid, M. B., Banzett, R. B., Feldman, H. A., and Mead, J. (1985). Reflex compensation of spontaneous breathing when immersion changes diaphragm length. *J. Appl. Physiol.* 58: 1136–1142.

Revelette, W. R., Jewell, L. A., and Frazier, D. T. (1988). Effect of diaphragm small-fibre afferent stimulation on ventilation in dogs. *J. Appl. Physiol.* 65: 2097–2106.

Rotto, D. M., Stebbins, C. L., and Kaufman, M. P. (1989). Reflex cardiovascular and respiratory responses to increasing H^+ activity in cat hindlimb muscle. *J. Appl. Physiol.* 67: 256–263.

Russel, J. A., and Bishop, B. (1986). Vagal afferents essential for abdominal muscle activity during lung inflation in cats. *J. Appl. Physiol.* 41: 310–315.

Rybicki, K. J., and Kaufman, M. P. (1985). Stimulation of group III and IV muscle afferents reflexly decreases total pulmonary resistance in dogs. *Respir. Physiol.* 59: 185–195.

Sant'Ambrogio, G., and Widdicombe, J. G. (1965). Respiratory reflexes acting on the diaphragm and inspiratory intercostal muscles of the rabbit. *J. Physiol. (Lond.)* 180: 766–779.

Sant'Ambrogio, G., Wilson, M. F., and Frazier, D. T. (1962). Somatic afferent activity in reflex regulation of diaphragmatic function in the cat. *J. Appl. Physiol.* 17: 829–832.

Scardella, A. T., Parisi, R. A., Phair, D. K., Santiago, T. V., and Edelman, N. H. (1986). The role of endogenous opioids in the ventilatory response to acute flow-resistive loads. *Am. Rev. Respir. Dis.* 133: 26–31.

Scardella, A. T., Santiago, T. V., and Edelman, N. H. (1989). Naloxone alters the early response to an inspiratory flow-resistive load. *J. Appl. Physiol.* 67: 1747–1753.

Seaman, R. G., Zechman, F. D., and Frazier, D. T. (1983). Response of ventral respiratory group inspiratory neurons to mechanical loading. *J. Appl. Physiol.* 54: 254–261.

Sears, T. A. (1964). Some properties and reflex connections of respiratory motoneurons of the cat's thoracic spinal cord. *J. Physiol. (Lond.)* 175: 386–403.

Shannon, R. (1977). Effects of thoracic dorsal rhizotomies on the respiratory pattern in anesthetized cats. *J. Appl. Physiol.* 43: 20–26.

Shannon, R. (1986). Reflexes from respiratory muscles and costo-vertebral joints. In: *Handbook of Physiology. The Respiratory System II*. Edited by A. P. Fishman. Bethesda, MD, American Physiological Society, pp. 431–447.

Shannon, R., and Zechman, F. W. (1972). The reflex and mechanical response of the inspiratory muscles to an increased airflow resistance. *Respir. Physiol.* 16: 51–69.

Shannon, R., Shear, W. T., Mercak, A. R., Bosler, D. C., and Lindsay, B. G. (1985). Non-vagal reflex effects on medullary inspiratory neurons during inspiratory loading. *Respir. Physiol.* 60: 193–204.

Shannon, R., Bosler, D. C., and Lindsay, B. G. (1987). Medullary expiratory activity: Influence of intercostal tendon organs and muscle spindle endings. *J. Appl. Physiol.* 62: 1057–1062.

Speck, D. F. (1987). Supraspinal involvement in the phrenic-to-phrenic inhibitory reflex. *Brain Res.* 414: 169–172.

Speck, D. F., and Revelette, W. R. (1987). Excitation of dorsal and ventral respiratory group neurons by phrenic nerve afferents. *J. Appl. Physiol.* 62: 946–951.

Speck, D. F., and Webber, C. L. (1979). Thoracic dorsal rhizotomy in the anesthetized cats: Maintenance of eupnoeic breathing. *Respir. Physiol.* 38: 347–357.

Stella, G. (1938). On the mechanism of production and the physiological significance of "apneusis." *J. Physiol. (Lond.)* 93: 10–23.

Stubbing, D. G., Ramsdale, E. H., Killian, K. J., and Campbell, E. J. M. (1983). Psychophysics of inspiratory muscle force. *J. Appl. Physiol.* 54: 1216–1221.

Supinski, G. S., Di Marco, A. F., Hussein, F., and Altose, M. D. (1989). Alterations in respiratory muscle activation in the ischemic fatigued canine diaphragm. *J. Appl. Physiol.* 67: 720–729.

van Lunteren, E., Haxhiu, M. A., Cherniack, N. S., and Goldman, M. D. (1985). Differential costal and crural diaphragm compensation for posture changes. *J. Appl. Physiol.* 58: 1895–1900.

von Euler, C. (1966). The control of respiratory movement. In: *Breathlessness*. Edited by J. B. L. Howell and E. J. M. Campbell. Oxford, Blackwell, pp. 19–32.

32

Mechanical Aspects of Loaded Breathing

J. ANDREW DAUBENSPECK

Dartmouth Medical School
Lebanon, New Hampshire

I. Introduction

Feedback control of breathing, based on control of respiratory depth and timing, serves to regulate arterial blood gas tensions within limits consistent with tissue function, respiratory energy cost, and perceived discomfort. Respiratory control in adult humans and animals involves complex interactions among humoral and neural reflex processes, and behavioral reactions acting through the respiratory muscles on the mechanics of the respiratory pump. Each of these factors is affected directly or indirectly by perturbations in the mechanical characteristics of the respiratory muscles, airways, and gas exchanger, whether the mechanics are altered by the applicaton of external loads, or by changes in mechanics intrinsic to the respiratory system. The respiratory system responds passively to load perturbations through intrinsic characteristics, and may respond actively by means of reflexes reacting to afferent nerve information.

The application of mechanical loads is a useful technique to investigate respiratory control responses in humans and animals under a wide variety of conditions. Mechanical loading has joined exercise and inhalation of hypercapnic and hypoxic gas mixtures to become an important forcing stimulus with which to evaluate respiratory control characteristics. It is not the purpose of this commentary to review the history of mechanical loading or to provide detailed analyses of loading response patterns, as this has been extensively done elsewhere (Cherniack and Altose, 1981; Cherniack and Milic-Emili, 1985; Milic-Emili and Zin, 1986). Rather, the intent of this discussion will be to review the physiological processes involved in loading responses, to establish a basis for evaluation of the diverse modes of loading, and to consider the character of breathing pattern regulation in loading relative to reflex and behavioral influences.

II. The Respiratory Pattern Regulation Diagram

The schematic diagram in Figure 1 shows the arrangement of processes involved in control of the respiratory pattern in mechanical loading. The respiratory controller at the left of the diagram activates the pool of respiratory motoneurons with a time-dependent drive signal, D(t), that combines with a voluntary (behavioral) activation signal, B(t), to determine the neural activation of respiratory muscles, N(t). Activation of specific respiratory muscles can be measured from activity in

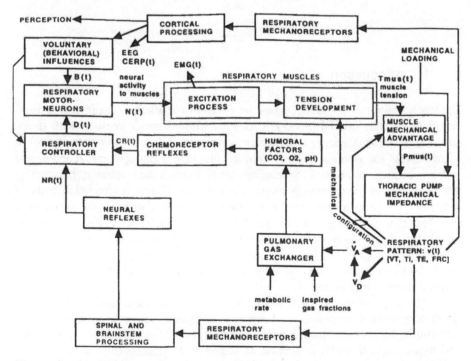

Figure 1 Block diagram of respiratory control system including controller components, mechanical aspects of muscles (including spindle reflexes) and the respiratory pump, gas exchanger, and sensory pathways providing feedback to the controller about respiratory performance. See text for explanation of individual blocks.

afferent nerves to the individual muscles, or can be monitored by measuring the electromyogram, EMG(t), associated with each muscle. The latter technique is the only approach for monitoring respiratory muscle activation in human subjects.

Consequent to this activation, the respiratory muscles generate tension, $T_{mus}(t)$, dependent on the mechanical conditions under which they operate. It has long been appreciated that respiratory muscle performance is limited by the length–tension and force–velocity relations that govern muscle performance. The mechanical configuration of the breathing muscles is another important determinant of the driving pressure, $P_{mus}(t)$, developed by muscle activation. The driving pressure that operates on the respiratory mechanical pump is a function of the developed $T_{mus}(t)$ and of the mechanical advantage available to the muscle to transform this tension into a pressure acting on the mechanical impedance of the thoracic pump. The mechanical advantage of the diaphragm, the single most important inspiratory muscle, is significantly influenced by the Laplace relationship, showing that the pressure developed within a hemispherical viscus is directly proportional to the wall tension in the shell, and inversely related to the radius of curvature of the shell. The radius of curvature of the diaphragm is related to the volume of the thoracic cavity, so that if the diaphragm were to operate by simply flattening with inspiration as $T_{mus}(t)$ increases, its mechanical advantage would decrease (Marshall, 1962). This may not accurately reflect the way in which the diaphragm operates (Whitelaw et al., 1983), as will be discussed in more detail later, but the transformation of $T_{mus}(t)$ into $P_{mus}(t)$, reflecting the mechanical advantage of the respiratory muscles, is an important issue in evaluating the direct and secondary effects of mechanical loading on the respiratory system.

To consider the action of $P_{mus}(t)$ on the thoracic pump, it is useful to apply a model of the respiratory mechanical system patterned after that of Mead and Milic-Emili (1964). Figure 2 shows such a model, demonstrating the intrinsic mechanical properties of the respiratory pump, together with the point of application of various mechanical loads. This model assumes that the respiratory mechanical impedance is dominated by viscance and elastance elements, and that the range of breathing frequencies to be considered is sufficiently low that inertial factors can be neglected. This model also neglects viscoelastic characteristics of the tissues that have been incorporated into more recent models (Similowski et al., 1989), but are omitted here in the interests of simplicity. The respiratory muscles are lumped into a single pressure source, $P_{mus}(t)$, producing a driving pressure that operates on the lumped, intrinsic mechanics of the respiratory system plus any applied external loads or pressures. The force–velocity and length–tension characteristics of the muscles are incorporated into the P_{mus} pressure source. $P_{mus}(t)$ must supply sufficient energy to provide the required ventilatory output in the face of both intrinsic and external loads. Changes in the respiratory system impedance presented to the P_{mus} generator result from alterations in internal as well as external mechanics. Loading can be produced by changes in pressure at the body surface, as well as at the airway opening (usually the mouth, although nasal loading can be applied).

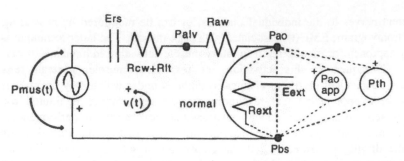

Figure 2 Electrical analog of respiratory mechanical system adapted from Mead and Milic-Emili (1964). Intrinsic elastance of lungs and chest wall are lumped into Ers, and resistance of chest wall and lung tissue into Rcw+lt. Airway resistance Raw conducts airflow (v(t)) proportional to the alveolar (Palv) pressure to airway opening (Pao) pressure difference, where Pao is normally identical with atmospheric pressure at the body surface (Pbs). Pao may differ from Pbs owing to the application of external resistance (Rext) or elastance (Eext) loads, bias pressures applied to the airway opening (Pao app), or threshold pressures (Pth). The driving pressure (Pmus) represents the net action of all the respiratory muscles acting on the mechanics, after accounting for losses internal to the muscle force generator. Omitted as negligible are inertial factors and gas compressibility.

The immediate effect of mechanical loading is to alter the usual relation between the N(t) and the mechanical output, airflow v(t). The volume and timing aspects, as well as the end-expiratory volume of the loaded breath, may be influenced by the change in impedance as the loaded breath continues. The mechanical configuration will be affected within the loaded breath, and this will alter the capability of the muscle to generate tension by changes in both intrinsic muscle characteristics and the mechanical advantage of the muscles as the breath proceeds. Thus, within-breath changes in the activation of mechanoreceptors will occur, and the resultant alteration in airflow is dependent on the passive mechanical effect of the load along with any reflex response that may develop within the breath.

Any perturbation in airflow caused by loading may affect alveolar ventilation and directly cause changes in arterial blood chemistry, which can entirely account for the progressive compensation in tidal volume subsequent to elastic loading in anesthetized cats (Younes et al., 1973). In addition, mechanical loading may induce changes in pulmonary blood volume and the distribution of ventilation relative to perfusion as intrathoracic pressure varies from normal (Milic-Emili and Zin, 1986). Loading may also induce respiratory pattern changes that influence gas exchange indirectly. For example, application of small elastic loads in normal humans decreases the occurrence of the spontaneous large breaths that may be useful in maintaining patent gas exchange areas in the lung (Daubenspeck, 1981). Thus, loading may perturb humoral factors and instigate chemoreflex responses. The relatively slow time course of humoral perturbations, however, minimizes chemo-receptor-initiated responses over the first breath or two following load application.

Rapid, within-breath responses to loading depend on a wide variety of mechanoreceptors responding to changes in the time course of airflow and lung volume or to mechanical distortion of respiratory structures. The sensory components of these responses include spindle receptors within the muscle fibers, joint and tendon receptors, and mechanoreceptors within the tracheobronchial tree, including the upper airway. The characteristics of these receptors have been extensively reviewed elsewhere (Sant'Ambrogio, 1982; Shannon, 1986; Milsom, 1990). Targets of peripheral sensory afferent information include spinal reflexes along with supraspinal actions and cortical processing networks, integral components of the conscious perception of mechanical loads. In this discussion, spinal load-compensating reflexes are incorporated into the muscle characteristics. The block titled "Neural Reflexes" in Figure 1 refers to the supraspinal, subconscious actions of peripheral afferent mechanoreceptor information on the brain stem respiratory controller. These neural reflexes, designated NR(t), combine and interact with the more slowly developing chemoreflex signal, CR(t), in the controller to determine the reflex component of respiratory drive, D(t).

Also capable of contributing to the within-breath response to mechanical loading is the behavioral component at the top of Figure 1, dependent on mechanoreceptor sensory input to the cortical perception process. Abundant evidence exists to the influence of learning in human responses to mechanical loading, and the removal of cortical involvement from loading responses by sleep or anesthesia qualitatively changes them, as will be discussed later. Thus, cortical involvement in the pattern responses to loading cannot be ignored once loading is perceived, and learning and prior experience influence this regulation.

Perception and behavioral response aspects of pattern regulation require access of mechanoreceptor afferent information to cortical processes subserving these functions. The mechanoreceptor pool providing this input may include all the receptors involved in neural reflex modulation of the pattern, but recent evidence suggests that receptors in the upper airway may play a more dominant role in perception than in pattern regulation (O'Donnell et al., 1988b; Younes et al., 1990; Puddy et al., 1992). Evaluation of mechanoreceptor stimulation of higher brain processes can be made by using cortical event-related potentials (CERPs) evoked in the electroencephalogram (EEG) by application of various mechanical stimuli. Davenport and Revelette and co-workers (Davenport et al., 1986; Revelette and Davenport, 1990) have used inspiratory occlusions in humans to demonstrate the influence of mechanoreceptor afferents on mid- and long-latency (60–300 ms) components of the CERP. Bloch et al. (1990) reported that similar CERPs could be generated by sudden imposition of flow-resistive loads in normal humans. In addition, brief pressure pulses, perceptible, but of small magnitude, evoke shorter-latency (25 to 45-ms) CERPs in normal subjects (Strobel and Daubenspeck, 1993). It is thus apparent that respiratory mechanoreceptors have rapid access to the cortex, and that cortical processes responsible for behavioral responses to loading can act nearly as rapidly as neural reflexes within the breath.

Figure 1 shows that the N(t) response to the application of a mechanical load is determined immediately by the combined influences of the neural reflex and behavioral responses NR(t) and B(t), and within a few breaths of loading by the added contribution of the chemoreflex signal, CR(t), if the load reduces alveolar ventilation relative to metabolism. The long-term response to mechanical loading involves all three of these pathways: neural and chemoreflexes and behavioral reactions. The behavioral component includes any response patterns adopted to minimize perceived discomfort, and as naive subjects experience repeated mechanical loading, these learned strategies can be applied immediately on perception of loading. Thus loading history may be a major factor in determining the immediate as well as the long-term pattern responses to mechanical loading. The individual contribution of each of these components to immediate and long-term pattern regulation needs to be determined to evaluate how these processes interact and combine to determine N(t) during loading.

III. Character of Mechanical Loads and of Pattern Responses to Loading

A. Definition of a Mechanical Load

It is appropriate to define what constitutes a mechanical load to the respiratory system. One viewpoint from which to classify mechanical loading is to distinguish between situations that result in an increased mechanical impedance of the respiratory system and those that put the respiratory muscles at a mechanical disadvantage (Milic-Emili and Zin, 1986). It is also useful to evaluate the effect of various types of mechanical loading using the change in the effective driving pressure (P_{mus}) that would be required to maintain some defined aspect of respiratory performance at the preloaded control level. Alternatively, the effect of a load could be assessed in terms of the effect on breathing if it could be ensured that neural drive was fixed.

As noted by Cherniack and Milic-Emili (1985), a *mechanical load* may be considered to be any factor perturbing adversely the operating characteristics of the respiratory muscles or the forces required of them to produce a given respiratory action. For the purposes of this discussion, that definition will be considered for neural drive requirements consequent to mechanical perturbations. A *mechanical load* is defined here to be anything that requires an increased muscle pressure, generated by tension developed in the respiratory muscles acting on mechanical structures of the respiratory musculoskeletal system, to maintain the normal (nonloaded control) ventilatory pattern. Loading can consist of changes in intrinsic mechanical properties, addition of extrinsic mechanical loads, or application of external forces perturbing the respiratory muscles from their normal mechanical operating point, as discussed in the following. Although the respiratory pattern may adapt in response to the load application, the stress of various loading conditions will be evaluated here concerning the P_{mus} resulting from the initial neural activation signal.

The use of P_{mus} as the measure of muscle performance may be questioned, since it is obvious that respiratory muscles directly produce contractile tension (T_{mus}), which determines P_{mus} through action of T_{mus} on the musculoskeletal mechanics. For biomechanical arrangements less geometrically complex than those presented by the respiratory system, it would be possible to transform tension in specific muscles into forces exerted on skeletal elements. The respiratory system, however, is sufficiently complex to make it impracticable to incorporate the wide range of primary and accessory muscles of breathing into an isomorphic T_{mus}–P_{mus} transformation. This question will be addressed in greater depth later.

B. Classification of Mechanical Loads

Because there are many ways to change the load presented to the respiratory muscles, categorization of loads requires evaluation of a variety of qualities. Mechanical loads can be separated into two categories, depending on whether the magnitude of the load varies with the activity of the respiratory muscles. The magnitudes of pure pressure-biasing and threshold loads are independent of gas flow and volume, and these can be considered to be *static loads*. The added driving pressure requirement consequent to a flow-resistive or elastic load, however, is a function of how airflow or volume change with time, and these loads can be considered to be *dynamic loads*. If the pressure demanded varies proportionally with airflow or volume, then the load is considered to be *linear*, almost exclusively a characteristic of external loads designed by physiologists. In addition, mechanical loads can be separated into *continuous* or *discontinuous* types, depending on whether they cause abrupt pressure discontinuities in P_{mus} and airway pressure. Further classification considers whether the load is applied during both inspiration and expiration, or is limited to one or the other phase of the cycle.

Static Loads

Static loads include the application of continuous, steady pressure above or below atmospheric, either to the mouth or to the body surface. Continuous positive airway pressure (CPAP) is commonly used in patients to alleviate problems of airway collapse by splinting the airway open throughout the respiratory cycle. A necessary consequence of this procedure is that end-expiratory lung volume is increased as the lungs are inflated, leaving the inspiratory muscles at a shorter initial length and at a mechanical disadvantage. Continuous negative airway pressure is used experimentally to reduce lung volume and transairway pressure, and serves to promote inspiratory, and impede expiratory, muscle performance.

Continuous positive pressure affects the end-expiratory volume (EEV) in the same way changing from the supine to the upright position in gravity produces an increased EEV. Humans accommodate to a postural increase in FRC about 0.5 L every time they stand up, and it is possible that reflex responses to this mechanical disadvantage play a role in maintaining ventilation (Green et al., 1978), although the character of this reflex is controversial (McKenzie and Gandevia, 1986). Use of CPAP also increases transmural pressure across the extrathoracic airway, changing the stretch on airway mechanoreceptors, so continuous pressure loading does not necessarily simulate postural perturbations accurately. Because the effect of pressure loading is to produce a steady-state shift in the configuration of the respiratory muscles, this is a continuous static load.

Inspiratory or expiratory threshold pressure (P_{THin}, P_{THex}) loads are applied by allowing flow only after mouth pressure exceeds a threshold level. The character of this type of load is static, in the sense that a fixed pressure is required to overcome the threshold limit, and the intensity of the load does not vary with respiratory effort, once the threshold is achieved. Threshold loads have been applied only at the mouth, and cause the demand on the muscle to increase continuously until the point at which airflow begins, after which the added load is constant. This discontinuous type of load differs importantly from the application of continuous pressures relative to the passive system response (the response without alteration of respiratory muscle activation from the control pattern). This difference occurs at the phase transitions in which the respiratory muscles are required to contract or relax isometrically to match the airway pressure conditions before flow can occur. Also, although an expiratory threshold load does produce an elevated end-expiratory lung volume, an inspiratory threshold load does not directly affect EEV. With the possible exception of overcoming a labile airway obstruction, there is no naturally occurring physiological stress that threshold loading simulates.

Dynamic Loads

Dynamic loads serve to increase the respiratory muscle tension requirements in a manner dependent on the temporal pattern of flow or volume. Flow-resistance loading varies the requirement for muscle tension in proportion to the instantaneous airflow, and elastance loading varies this demand in proportion to the change in lung volume. External dynamic loads can be applied to either inspiration or expiration separately, or to both phases of the respiratory cycle. Resistance loading of either or both phases of breathing is continuous, in the sense that the load builds and decays smoothly with airflow changes. Elastic loading of the entire respiratory cycle is also continuous, but elastic loading of either cycle alone represents a discontinuous load, since an abrupt change in airway pressure is required to connect the end of the loaded to the following, nonloaded phase. Elastic loading correlates, in some degree, to fibrotic disease effects, and viscous loading may perturb the normal mechanics similarly to asthma or bronchitis. Although these loads partially imitate changes in intrinsic viscous and elastance characteristics, mouth application may involve extrathoracic airway mechanoreceptors in ways that are not analogous to intrinsic loading. To more accurately mimic intrinsic impedance changes, loads can be applied to the body surface, using a servocontrolled pressure chamber around the thorax (Younes et al., 1990). This approach minimizes influences on the upper airway, which can be affected only indirectly through thoracic tethering to tracheal structures (Brown et al., 1985; Van de Graaff, 1988).

IV. Evaluation and Comparison of Various Types of Loading

A. Identification of Separate Effects of Loading

It is difficult to compare the respiratory stress of one type of load versus another, or to evaluate the net effect of applying multiple types of loads simultaneously. It is quite rare and takes carefully planning to apply only one type of mechanical stress in an experimental situation, and the effects of disease on the overall mechanical status of the system usually include multiple mechanical aspects. For example, the application of CPAP to relieve obstructive airway occlusion in sleep apnea patients is intended to reduce the flow-resistance of the airways that was previously elevated to the point of obstruction. This would reduce the muscle tension requirements to provide a given level of ventilation. At the same time, however, the application of CPAP to the mouth results in an elevated end-expiratory volume as the pulmonary system is inflated to a new equilibrium between the increased elastic recoil of the lung–thorax system and the elevated mouth pressure holding the lungs inflated. The driving pressure required of the inspiratory muscles to produce a given airflow pattern is assisted, and expiration is opposed by the application of CPAP. The increased elastic recoil at end expiration consequent to the elevated EEV is balanced by the CPAP, and expiration may remain passive or expiratory muscle activity may be initiated to drive expiration. If the expiratory muscles force the EEV below the relaxation equilibrium with the given level of CPAP, then the applied positive pressure will directly cause inspiratory airflow as the expiratory muscles relax at end expiration. This transfers load from the inspiratory to the expiratory muscles directly. Inspiratory muscle requirements are further reduced by the effect of CPAP to prevent increased airway resistance owing to collapse and moderately to reduce thoracic airway resistance as pulmonary volume increases (Fisher et al., 1968). However, there are important, direct effects of CPAP on the tension requirements of the inspiratory muscles because of changes in their initial length and their mechanical advantage.

The effect of increasing FRC on the mechanical advantage of the diaphragm was once thought to be clearly disadvantageous if the change in FRC was produced by lowering the diaphragmatic dome of a hemispheric thoracic model (Marshall, 1962). Whitelaw et al. (1983) have incorporated a more realistic configurational model of the diaphragm, forcing it to remain tangent to the rib cage as lung volume changes, and more closely approximating the zone of apposition between diaphragm and rib cage. This results in a decreased mean radius of curvature of the diaphragm as it descends, opposite the change in the hemispheric model. This model was used to examine the relation between transdiaphragmatic pressure, Pdi, and tension in the diaphragm in the relaxed state, and shows that the mechanical advantage of the diaphragm may not necessarily decrease with increasing volume. The question is not whether the Laplace relationship applies to the diaphragm; as a physical force balance, it must always apply. Rather, the questions concerning the mechanical advantage of the diaphragm relate to (1) the appropriate mean radius of curvature to be used in estimating muscle tension from geometry and pressure measurements; and (2) the relative influence of the mechanical advantage limitation compared with that consequent to the length–tension effect.

Given the complex geometry of the human diaphragm, shaped like a saddle between the hemispheres and, thus, having opposite radii of curvature in some portions, it is obvious that uniform tension in diaphragmatic tissue is unlikely (Whitelaw, 1987; Paiva et al., 1992). Neither is it simple to judge the effect of changes in functional reserve capacity (FRC) upon the length of specific muscles, since costal and crural components of the diaphragm may have different initial muscle lengths, compared with the length at which peak tension is developed. In the supine dog, for example, increasing FRC may actually increase costal diaphragm force capability, since its resting length is above the optimal for force generation (Road et al., 1986). Thus, the assumptions that the diaphragm operates as a simple membrane, with even tension throughout, and has uniform length–tension changes with changing lung volume are not tenable.

It is impossible to compare the combined influences of multiple mechanical perturbations without establishing a basis by which to account for loading effects. The approach proposed in the next section uses a neuromechanical model to determine the effect of an added load on respiratory mechanical output, given a neural activating signal of fixed amplitude and timing characteristics. Loads that have very different influences on the time course of volume and flow can be compared for their net mechanical effect, incorporating the intrinsic muscle characteristics, without reflex responses. The depression of VT is used as an index to assess the relative effect of each load type, as a function of load magnitude, and to compare the relative stress of each type and level of load on the respiratory muscles taken as a group.

This approach represents a simple method for estimating the demands placed on the respiratory musculature by various types of mechanical loads. It can be criticized for its simplistic assumptions, but it is intended to be no more than an indication of how one might provide a basis for evaluating the stress of various types of loads singly or in combination. Although the eventual goal of such modeling is to incorporate the activation and action of each respiratory muscle acting on an anatomically realistic thorax, this is not yet possible; therefore, the strategy adopted here is appropriate.

B. Respiratory Mechanical Modeling

The approach taken is to use the neuromechanical model of Younes and Riddle (1981) to estimate the loading effect from the change in tidal volume, without any neural driving signal adaptation. The model requires a neural activation signal, and produces a net muscle driving pressure output after accounting for losses owing to factors intrinsic to the muscles and the geometry (force–velocity, length–tension, and configuration), using empirical curves to account for observed responses as described next. The net P_{mus} is applied to a mechanical system similar to that depicted in Figure 2.

The Younes–Riddle model applies a neural activation signal [N(t)] to muscle through a first-order activation process (60-ms time constant) to generate a potential driving pressure. From this pressure, they deduct intrinsic volume and configuration losses by using analyses of experimental results from the literature for normal human subjects. Flow- and velocity-related losses intrinsic to the musculoskeletal thorax are similarly deducted as the applied force causes the thoracic pump to move from its relaxed position, and the resultant force is applied to a lumped parameter model of the respiratory system, similar to Figure 2, to determine the actual airflow and volume time courses. The temporal trajectories of volume and flow feedback are used to determine the flow- and volume-related losses intrinsic to the muscles. The implementation of their model showed that the results were not critically dependent on a particular set of assumptions (Riddle and Younes, 1981), and the model has been used to predict the time course of occlusion pressure in humans (Younes et al., 1981) and the neural component of human pattern responses to loads (Daubenspeck and Bennett, 1983; Im Hof et al., 1986b). This model incorporates the essential features for converting neural activation into airflow in humans and has been accepted as a useful tool for estimating loading effects (Daubenspeck and Bennett, 1983; Im Hof et al., 1986a,b; Poon et al., 1987; Sanii and Younes, 1988; Gallagher et al., 1989; Gallagher and Younes, 1989; Harver and Daubenspeck, 1989; Younes and Sanii, 1989).

The particular application here is to compare the loading stress (as indicated by the reduction of V_T) over various types and sizes of loads, using a fixed amplitude and timing of the neural activation signal, N(t) (see Fig. 1). N(t) is assumed to have a ramp increase from the start until the end of neural inspiration (NTI), when it achieves a maximum level, N_{peak}. N(t) then ramps down to zero activity during NTE_{decay}, and maintains quiescence throughout the rest of neural expiration ($NTE_{quiescent}$) until the start of the next inspiration. It is not implied that this is the only possible form for N(t), nor that this temporal pattern would accurately describe the waveform in response to loading. The pattern is realistic in that it is adequate to describe human resting breathing, and the essence of the approach is to evaluate the effects of loading without N(t) compensation.

The model is set up with timing and amplitude values as listed in Table 1 to achieve a respiratory frequency of 15 breaths per minute (BPM). A control $V_T =$

0.5 L was achieved by finding the appropriate value for the peak neural amplitude N_{peak}. Lumped respiratory system resistance and elastance were assumed to be normal at 3.0 cm H_2O $L^{-1}s^{-1}$ (LPS), and 10 cm H_2O/L, respectively. Table 1 lists the results of application of external flow resistive (R_{ex}) and elastic (E_{ex}) loads, and of CPAP and expiratory threshold (P_{THEX}) loading, all adjusted in size to decrease the V_T to 80% of control, without neural compensation.

At the breathing frequency selected for this comparison, the load magnitudes listed in Table 1 represent equivalent stresses to the respiratory system from the standpoint of V_T depression. It is not implied that this is the only parameter by which to judge the effect of various load types. Rather, the point is that a specific criterion can be defined (here, V_T depression) to compare load intensities using a modeling appoach. Given the assumptions of this example, two points can be made from the results. First, the effects of loads that represent changes in existing mechanical parameters are not proportionally equivalent, depending on the control-breathing pattern. For the chosen pattern, the change in R required to depress V_T by 20% is 133% (R_{ex}/R_{normal}), whereas the comparable change in E is only 40%. Second, it does not require very large levels of CPAP or P_{THEX} to depress V_T significantly without compensatory reflexes. Both these pressure loads cause an

Table 1 Model Results Using Added External Resistance (R_x), Elastance (E_x), Continuous Positive Pressure at the Airway Opening (CPAP), or Positive End-Expiratory Pressure (PEEP) Loads for a Respiratory Pattern Giving 7.5 L/mm Minute Ventilation

Load[a]	ΔLoad for V_T = 80% control[b]
R_{ex}	4.0 cm H_2O/LPS
E_{ex}	4.0 cm H_2O/L
CPAP	4.05 cm H_2O
P_{THEX}	1.05 cm H_2O

[a]R_{ex}, the external resistance; E_{ex}, the external elastance; CPAP, the level of continuous airway pressure applied; P_{THEX}, the expiratory threshold load.
[b]The normal reference pattern uses N_{peak} = 8.7 units to achieve a control V_T = 0.5 L, with neural T_I (NTI) = 1.52 s, NTE_{decay} = 0.2 s, and $NTE_{quiescent}$ = 2.28 s, to result in a cycle frequency of 15 B/M and minute ventilation of 7.5 LPM. One neural unit causes a 1 cm H_2O change in the isometric muscle pressure at FRC. See text for description of modeling process.
Source: Younes and Riddle (1981).

increase in the end-expiratory volume, and influence performance through the intrinsic muscle (length–tension) and mechanical advantage factors considered earlier. Expiratory threshold loading does not elevate EEV as much as CPAP in this iso-effect comparison, but involves a longer zero flow phase in inspiration than does CPAP. There is no inspiratory assistance provided by an external pressure source in Pᴛʜᴇx as in CPAP to balance the increased elastic recoil at the elevated EEV, so the inspiratory muscles must offset this recoil themselves. In anesthetized animals, much larger decreases in Vᴛ are seen with Pᴛʜᴇx of the same magnitude as CPAP (Bishop and Bachofen, 1972), and normal human subjects are aware of increased respiratory effort with Pᴛʜᴇx compared with CPAP (O'Donnell et al., 1988a). The level of Pᴛʜᴇx predicted to depress Vᴛ 20% is not uncommon in respiratory apparatus with a slightly sticky expiratory valve.

These results show the effects of loads on the passive system, without neural drive compensation. This is not how the intact respiratory system responds to loading. Indeed, responses of virtually every aspect of the neural driving signal N(t) can contribute to loading responses under various conditions (Younes and Riddle, 1984).

V. Responses to Loading

A. General Characteristics of Loading Responses

Responses attributable to intrinsic muscle properties and their anatomical arrangement, and to spinal load-compensating reflexes have been categorized by Mead (1979) as "nonneural." Inclusion of spinal reflexes involved in mechanical loading responses means that these nonneural responses do not represent strictly mechanical components, but do reflect the capabilities intrinsic to the muscle and its inherent load-compensating reflexes. These will be categorized as "passive" responses here, predictable from the modeling results of the previous section. Passive responses, as noted, do not include loading-induced compensation in N(t).

The respiratory control system responsible for operative reflex responses (considered by Mead to be neural and to be active responses in this chapter) has been characterized by a hierarchical structure. It regulates ventilation of the gas exchanger to accommodate to the metabolic demands of the organism at one level, and at a lower level adjusts the respiratory pattern to optimize some criterion within constraints set at the higher level (Tenenbaum, 1971; Hamalainen and Viljanen, 1978a). The idea that optimal criteria may be relevant to the control of respiratory pattern has fascinated physiologists for decades ever since Rohrer's early analysis (Rohrer, 1925).

The degree to which an observed response to loading is considered "compensatory" has also been considered for many indexes of respiratory performance, including ventilatory-, pattern-, and effort-related aspects. The interpretation of such pattern responses to applied loads has provided the basis for evaluating physiological and philosophical hypotheses concerning the usefulness of a particular response in terms of its potential benefit to the organism (Rohrer, 1925; Otis et al., 1950; Mead, 1960, 1970; Tenenbaum, 1971; Yamashiro and Grodins, 1971, 1973; Ruttiman and Yamamoto, 1972; Grodins and Yamashiro, 1973; Yamashiro et al., 1975; Hamalainen and Viljanen, 1978b; Lafortuna et al., 1984; Poon, 1986, 1987, 1988, 1991; Cha et al., 1987; Minetti et al., 1987; Luijendijk and Milic, 1988; Poon et al., 1992). This section will consider observed loading responses, without considering the optimal nature of those responses. The relation of pattern selection and respiratory effort will be considered in the last section of this discussion.

Responses to perturbations in mechanical impedance have been well reviewed elsewhere (Cherniack and Altose, 1981; Cherniack and Milic-Emili, 1985; Milic-Emili and Zin, 1986), and the reader is referred to those reviews for the classic results and viewpoints, which will be only summarized here. Previous work has established the need to consider the type and magnitude of load applied (flow-resistive, elastic, pressure-biasing), the phase of the cycle in which the perturbation is applied, the state of consciousness of the subject, and the level of concurrent ventilatory stimuli, such as exercise or hypercapnia.

Milic-Emili and Zin (1986) concluded that the "respiratory system has a remarkable capacity to maintain ventilation within relatively narrow limits despite considerable changes in mechanical loading and pressure biasing," and work since then supports that statement. The responses to loading involve all the aspects depicted in the control system diagram of Figure 1, and it is helpful to consider pattern accommodations to loading in two time frames. The immediate pattern response to loading involves combined contributions of intrinsic muscle characteristics with spinal load-compensating reflexes, together with any supraspinal load reflex responses (neural reflexes) and behavioral responses. After sufficient time has passed to allow a humoral stimulus to develop, chemoreflexes can contribute to the accommodation to loading. The number of breaths that can be considered to represent only nonhumoral responses is dependent on the control pattern characteristics and the magnitude of the applied load, but can be as short as a one or two breaths (Younes et al., 1973).

Earlier analyses of immediate V_T responses to elastic loading used a simplified model of respiratory mechanics and airflow to predict the expected V_T depression immediately after loading, for comparison with observed values. The results showed that V_T was less depressed than would have been predicted from the model used (Lynne-Davies et al., 1971). The concept that the mechanical impedance of the respiratory system was immediately augmented by loading led to the idea that rapid reflex responses acted to provide an "effective" impedance greater than the passive control value, and served to stabilize the respiratory system in the face of increased mechanical loads. The increase in effective elastance seen immediately after loading in dogs is dependent on vagal pathways during anesthesia (McClelland et al., 1972), but not during wakefulness or sleep (Phillipson et al., 1976). So this reflex response to loading probably depends on information from multiple receptor pathways.

Read et al. (1974) found that the assumptions inherent in the computation of the effective impedance (steady-state sinusoidal driving pressure and airflow) were not valid, judging from their observations in humans. It is obvious from their volume traces for resistance and elastic loading that the airflow patterns differ between these load types. Thus, to generate accurate predictions concerning intrinsic and reflex responses to loading, it is necessary to use more complex models, based on specific measurements of responses, as done by Read et al., or on more basic assumptions about neural drive (N(t)), as done by Younes and Riddle (Younes and Riddle, 1981, 1984).

It has been emphasized by others (e.g., Mead, 1979; Cherniack and Milic-Emili, 1985; Milic-Emili and Zin, 1986) that from a gas-exchange view, effective load compensation must protect alveolar ventilation. Cherniack and Milic-Emili (1985) derived an equation to separate a drive-related term from one related to respiratory timing:

$$\dot{V}_A = \left(\frac{V_T - V_D}{T_I}\right)\left(\frac{T_I}{T_{TOT}}\right) \tag{1}$$

where the factor $(V_T - V_D)/T_I$ represents mean inspiratory flow to the alveolar exchanger, considered to be alveolar ventilatory drive, and (T_I/T_{TOT}), the timing or inspiratory duty cycle factor. This equation is useful in a qualitative sense to evaluate observed pattern responses to loading relative to gas exchange, but the two factors are not necessarily independent, as they pointed out. The variation of lung volume within T_I may not follow a linear path, so the same mean inspiratory flow could reflect many different compensation strategies. In fact, Younes and Riddle (Younes and Riddle, 1984) showed that curvilinear changes in the neural activation of inspiratory muscle provide a sensitive mode for control of tidal volume that could contribute to the loading response.

The inverse relation between inspiratory time and the volume achieved at end inspiration shown by Clark and von Euler (1972), together with the direct correlation they found between T_I and the subsequent T_E, can also be applied to analyze loading responses. They proposed that the locus of inspiratory-terminating volumes versus times of inspiration defined an inspiratory off-switch mechanism, the threshold of which declined with time during inspiration. For a fixed off-switch locus, any effect of loading to alter mean inspiratory flow rate necessarily causes intersection with the inspiratory off-switch to occur at a different T_I, and this could define the respiratory frequency through the T_I–T_E correlation. Responses to loading may incorporate shifts in this inspiratory off-switch threshold. Thus, volume–timing aspects of the pattern response to loading can be examined using this model.

Younes and co-workers have more recently applied a neuromechanical model (Younes and Riddle, 1981; described earlier) to assess human-breathing pattern responses to loading in terms of the amplitude, shape, or timing parameters of the signal describing the occlusion pressure at FRC (the driving muscle pressure signal before flow- and volume-related losses), closely related to the neural signal N(t) of

Figure 1 (Im Hof et al., 1986a,b; Poon et al., 1987; Sanii and Younes, 1988; Gallagher et al., 1989; Younes and Sanii, 1989). Others have used the same model to determine the predicted pattern response in the absence of neural reflex effects on N(t) for contrast with observed responses (Daubenspeck and Bennett, 1983; Harver and Daubenspeck, 1989). This approach has the advantage that the model includes intrinsic characteristics of the muscles and their mechanical configuration, permitting assessment of the effects of loading on neural drive and allowing evaluation of pattern regulation reflexes.

These viewpoints will be applied to the reported pattern responses to flow-resistive, elastic, and pressure loads.

B. Flow-Resistive Loading

The classic, steady-state response to inspiratory resistance loading (IRL) in awake humans is a smaller augmentation of VT than of TI, such that the mean inspiratory flow (VT/TI) is decreased and respiratory frequency is reduced (McIlroy et al., 1956; Zechman et al., 1957; Altose et al., 1979; Daubenspeck, 1981; Im Hof et al., 1986b; O'Donnell et al., 1988b). Inspiratory resistance-unloading has been performed with a servocontrolled ventilatory assist device and has shown pattern responses opposite those shown for loading (Gallagher et al., 1989). It is important to stress that these findings, and those prior, primarily apply to subjects conditioned to the experimental protocol: immediate pattern responses of untrained subjects are impressively variable (Axen and Haas, 1979). This will be considered later relative to the importance of behavioral influences on pattern adaptations to loading.

Nonrapid eye movement (NREM) sleep attenuates the immediate augmentation of inspiratory electromyographic (EMG) activity to IRL found in wakeful goats, although TI prolongation was similar (~20%) in wakefulness and sleep (Hutt et al., 1991). In humans, on the other hand, the awake response to acute IRL was maintenance of the control ventilation by increasing inspiratory EMG amplitude and complete VT compensation, with little change in TI (Badr et al., 1990). During NREM sleep, the EMG response was absent and TI was only slightly prolonged. Previously, Iber et al. (1982) showed that, after five IRL breaths during wakefulness, both VT and TI increased, and breathing frequency (f) fell so that minute ventilation stabilized; NREM sleep resulted in a fall in VT, coupled with no change in TI, and an increase in f.

Anesthesia attenuates the prolongation of TI in humans caused by resistance loading, although an augmented amplitude of the calculated driving pressure (P_{mus}) followed loading in this state (Read et al., 1974). Similarly, Zin et al. (1986) showed only small timing responses to IRL during anesthesia. Thus, sleep and anesthesia share the ability to minimize the prolongation of TI seen in conscious responses to IRL.

The effect of flow-resistance loading only during the expiratory phase results in prolongation of TE in awake humans (Zechman et al., 1957; Gothe and Cherniack,

1980; Daubenspeck and Bartlett, 1983; Hill et al., 1985; Poon et al., 1987; Barnett and Rasmussen, 1988), and an increased EEV is frequently, but not always, observed. Poon et al. (1987) used an indirect approach to calculate the effect of expiratory loading alone on the driving pressure (occluded P_{mus} at FRC) waveform, and found that both the neural and mechanical phase durations lengthened with this load, and the peak amplitude increased in normal, awake subjects. They assumed that expiratory muscles were not activated by the degree of expiratory load used (8 cm H_2O/LPS), and that laryngeal resistance was unaltered in response to the applied load. They concluded that EEV did not change with this degree of loading. The effect of expiratory-resistance loading to elevate the EEV is controversial and depends on the balance among the longer expiratory time constant, tending to slow expiratory flow; the lengthening of T_E to give a longer duration for expiration to continue; and any effect of loading, to reduce expiratory braking by laryngeal actions or changes in respiratory muscle activation.

Laryngeal braking of expiratory flow occurs in humans and animals and may be an important mechanism for FRC regulation in small animals (Remmers and Bartlett, 1977). In humans, however, the laryngeal aperture response to expiratory-resistance loading of the airway is not consistent with maintaining FRC, since the expiratory aperture narrows with such loading (Daubenspeck and Bartlett, 1983; Brancatisano et al., 1985) and with bronchoconstriction (Higenbottam, 1980), further increasing the expiratory resistance. Expiratory muscle activity increases with elevation of EEV in anesthetized cats (Koehler and Bishop, 1979) and awake humans (Green et al., 1978), and this could help return EEV toward the nonloaded level.

If the resistance load is applied throughout the cycle, both phases lengthen, and respiratory frequency, consequently, decreases. The effect of R loading throughout the respiratory cycle on EEV is similar to that of expiratory loading alone (Zechman et al., 1957).

When the pattern response to flow-resistive loading is considered relative to Eq. (1), evaluating the effect on alveolar ventilation, it is apparent that all the components are affected, and that the steady-state change in pattern with resistance loading minimizes depression of alveolar ventilation. If V_T increases slightly and V_D is relatively stable (Poon et al., 1987), then an increase in T_I/T_{TOT} could balance the increase in T_I. The mean values reported by Im Hof et al. (1986b) indicate that this is indeed what happens with IRL (inspiratory duty cycle increases from 0.38 to 0.45 with loading, data from their Table 1). With ERL, Poon et al. (1987) indicate a decline in T_I/T_{TOT}, yet the mean change in P_{ETCO_2} in both these studies was much less on a relative basis than the decrease in minute ventilation. Thus, the pattern responses to loading appear to protect alveolar ventilation, although minute ventilation is depressed.

These pattern responses can be viewed considering the Clark–von Euler inspiratory off-switch curve, discussed previously. A change in the V_T-T_I pattern can result from a change in the mean inspiratory flow (V_T/T_I), a shift in the off-switch curve owing to loading, or both. Since resistance-loading produces an increase in Tᵢ that is greater than the increase in Vᴛ, this corresponds to a shallower approach to an inspiratory-terminating threshold that must move to the right for humans (breathing in the vertical "range 1" portion of the Clark–von Euler plot) or upward in animals (breathing on the hyperbolic portion of the curve relating Vᴛ to Tᵢ) to permit both pattern parameters to increase.

There are subtle effects of loading on respiratory muscle activity that have been interpreted relative to promoting the mechanical advantage of various muscles. Very large inspiratory loads in upright, but not supine, humans activate phasic activity in abdominal muscles that correlates with a reduction in abdominal volume and an enhanced mechanical advantage for the diaphragm (Martin and De Troyer, 1982). Martin et al. (1982) also showed that inspiratory loading in humans can cause a reduction in expiratory braking by inspiratory muscles, together with expiratory muscle recruitment, both of which promote expiratory flow, and they reported that EEV fell with inspiratory loading. Application of a large IRL in humans resulted in an earlier decay of diaphragmatic EMG (EMGdi) relative to the onset of mechanical expiration, such that most of the postinspiratory diaphragmatic activity promoted inspiration rather than retarded expiration, and expiratory flow increased with a variable effect upon EEV (Agostoni and Zocchi, 1987). One influence of very small resistance loads applied throughout the cycle was to reduce the tonic EMGdi (Kobylarz and Daubenspeck, 1992), similar to the effect of mass loading of the abdomen (Muller et al., 1979). Such a decrease in diaphragmatic expiratory tone favors a reduction of FRC and an increased mechanical advantage for the diaphragm.

C. Elastic Loading

Application of elastic loads to the respiratory system in humans depresses Vᴛ and increases respiratory frequency in the steady state; the steady-state level of ventilation often returns close to the control level (McIlroy et al., 1956; Freedman and Weinstein, 1965; Bland et al., 1967; Pope et al., 1968; Agostoni et al., 1978). The immediate effect of elastic loading in anesthetized or decerebrate cats is to prolong Tᵢ, dependent on vagal information (Bradley, 1972). In conscious humans, the immediate effect of elastic loading is to shorten Tᵢ (Read et al., 1974; Agostoni et al., 1978), but experienced subjects may adopt quite different strategies (Daubenspeck, 1979). Axen and Haas (1979) demonstrated that naive subjects exhibit a wide range of responses, although most subjects tend to reduce Vᴛ and Tᵢ immediately, with progressive Vᴛ compensation following in the succeeding breaths (Axen et al., 1983).

Margaria et al. (1973) showed that respiratory frequency increased immediately after application of elastic loads in conscious humans, but that this response was eliminated by anesthesia. They interpreted this to indicate the role of cortical influences on pattern regulation, a conclusion also made by Read et al.

(1974) from observations of the effect of anesthesia on resistance-loading responses. Agostoni et al. (1977) applied elastic loading, by strapping the rib cage or the abdomen in conscious and anesthetized men, and found that anesthetized subjects did not show the reduction in V_T, T_I, and T_E that characterized conscious responses to rib cage strapping. Baydur and Sassoon (1986) showed a similar absence of timing response to elastic loading in anesthetized subjects.

However, Puddy and Younes (1991) demonstrated that a slowly increasing elastic load, applied over the entire respiratory cycle and undetected in normal subjects, caused decreases in T_I, T_E, and T_{TOT}, with an increase in f. Since their subjects were unaware of the load, it is not likely that the pattern responses were due to cortical influences, suggested by previous investigators to be behavioral and related to minimization of discomfort (Freedman and Weinstein, 1965). Thus, it is possible that the effects of anesthesia on responses to mechanical loading involve both removal of conscious, behavioral responses and attenuation of reflex pathways. The influence of sleep on human pattern responses to inspiratory elastic loading is to eliminate any augmented occlusion pressure seen in wakefulness, and to abolish the reduction in T_I in wakefulness in the single subject showing that (Wilson et al., 1984). Animal experiments suggest that sleep may not affect the immediate reduction in V_T on elastic loading; timing responses were not reported (Phillipson et al., 1976; Bowes et al., 1983).

The typical awake response to elastic loading includes reductions in V_T, T_I, and T_{TOT}, such that respiratory frequency increases and minute ventilation is often maintained. O'Donnell et al. (1988b) and Puddy and Younes (1991) showed that elastic loading had no significant effect upon P_{ETCO_2}, indicating that alveolar ventilation was well defended in the face of loads of the size used in these studies (<13 cm H_2O/L). Thus, in Eq. (1), alveolar volume $V_A (=V_T-V_D)$, T_I, and T_{TOT} fall with elastic loading, apparently in equal measure.

The effect of elastic loading to reduce both V_T and T_I requires a leftward or downward shift in the Clark–von Euler inspiratory termination threshold, opposite the effect of flow-resistive loading. A curve somewhat analogous to the inspiratory off-switch threshold on the $V(t)$ versus time plot is shown in the plot of integrated diaphragmatic EMG activity against time demonstrated by Lopata and Pearle (1980). There, the inspiratory terminus shifts leftward with elastic loading.

An intriguing question is how the respiratory control system operates to produce the quite different pattern responses to resistance and elastic loading. Sanii and Younes (1988) addressed this in experiments designed to test the importance of the timing of pressure changes applied to the mouth, relative to airflow in normal humans. Mouth pressure changes that were strictly proportional to airflow were more effective in prolonging T_I than were half-sinewave pressures, indicating great sensitivity of the control system to the phase difference between the airway pressure and respiratory airflow. They confirmed this sensitivity to phase in experiments where they electronically varied the relative phase between mouth pressure and flow (Younes and Sanii, 1989). Younes et al. (1978) had previously demonstrated that the action and effectiveness of inspiratory inhibition by afferent feedback (the basic mechanism of the Clark–von Euler off-switch threshold scheme) varied with time during inspiration. Inhibition of inspiration occurs through both vagal (volume-related) and nonvagal afferent pathways, and the general scheme they envision is that the latter dominate in the regulation of timing responses to loading. They note that withdrawal of an inhibitory stimulus before inspiratory termination results in inspiratory prolongation, and this is what happens as the mouth pressure declines after midinspiration with resistance loading. Elastic loading, on the other hand, presents an ever-increasing inhib·tory stimulus to the off-switch mechanism as inspiration continues, resulting in inspiratory termination earlier than with a nonloaded breath. Supporting this hypothesis are the results of Woodall and Mathew (1986) showing that the relative timing within inspiration of brief negative-pressure pulses applied to the upper airway in anesthetized rabbits was critical in determining the effect on inspiratory duration. Negative-pressure pulses applied early in inspiration prolonged inspiration, whereas those applied in late inspiration terminated that phase.

D. Pressure-Loading Responses

Continuous positive airway pressure (CPAP) inflates the lungs and thorax above the relaxation volume and puts the inspiratory muscles at a mechanical disadvantage. As shown in Table 1, the predicted response of the passive respiratory system to such a load would be to depress VT and minute ventilation. In anesthetized animals, a consequence of lung inflation is immediate abdominal muscle activation and diaphragm inhibition (both vagally dependent), and depression of f, VT, and minute ventilation, regardless of the state of vagal afferent input (Bishop and Bachofen, 1972). D'Angelo and Agostoni (1975b) found that CPAP resulted in increased TE and a small shortening of TI, with a decrease in VT/TI in vagally intact animals, consistent with a Hering–Breuer reflex.

Conscious human responses to pressure breathing differ from those seen in anesthetized animals. The results of Flenley et al. (1971) show that VT decreases with CPAP, and that acute exposure to CPAP did not stimulate expiratory activity in abdominal or intercostal muscles, but that sustained exposure (1–4 min) was required for expiratory muscle activation and a reduction in FRC. The immediate fall in VT that they observed was coupled to an increased respiratory rate on the first loaded breath, and ventilation was nearly unaffected by the immediate pressure load. Margaria et al. (1973) showed that there was no tendency for respiratory frequency to increase in anesthetized subjects with similar CPAP, and minute ventilation fell proportionally to the increase in FRC, without the increase in frequency they observed in conscious subjects.

Green et al. (1978) applied CPAP of 10 cm H$_2$O to four normal subjects and found VT was generally reduced, with a variable tendency for f to increase. Two of their subjects were tested twice, before and after instruction about how they should respond to PPB. They reported results from these subjects with and without increased EEV. In the four situations when EEV increased, they saw an increase in f in one subject, with no change or a decrease in three. Since V_T decreased in all four situations, minute ventilation was not defended. As these investigators noted, cortical influences played an important role in the responses, particularly with the EEV. Cortical influences on the entire respiratory pattern must be considered, because subjects were either knowledgeable about the physiological aspects or trained to think about their responses.

These authors also reported that when EEV increased with positive-pressure breathing (PPB) (in four of six of the cases reported), activation of inspiratory muscles increased (diaphragm EMG up in four of four cases, inspiratory intercostal activity increased in three of three for whom data were reported). They postulated that this reflected operation of a reflex that compensated for the reduced mechanical advantage of the diaphragm with elevated EEV by increasing neural activation of the muscle. This "operational length-compensating" reflex (OLC; Mead, 1979) may assist in adaptation to postural perturbations in EEV. There is, however, evidence that a volume-related artifact in measurement of EMGs in humans may be responsible for some portion, if not all the increased EMG activity with increased EEV in PPB (McKenzie and Gandevia, 1986). Esophageal and surface electrode measurements of diaphragmatic compound muscle action potentials (CMAPs), following supramaximal electrophrenic stimulation in humans, resulted in a CMAP amplitude that varied directly with the inspiratory position of the diaphragm (Gandevia and McKenzie, 1986). When the EMG responses to PPB induced elevation of EEV were calibrated for the effect of this maneuver on the CMAP amplitude, McKenzie and Gandevia (1986) concluded that there was evidence for diaphragmatic inhibition, rather than excitation, with increased EEV. Thus, the question of the existence and extent of the OLC reflex in humans is open and subject to further investigation, using within-subject calibration of potential volume-related artifacts to correct diaphragmatic EMG responses when volume changes.

As summarized by Cherniack and Milic-Emili (1985), the immediate effects of CPAP on the factors of Eq. (1) indicate that alveolar ventilation is not well protected by the observed responses in animals or humans under anesthesia. On the other hand, conscious human responses to decrease T_{TOT}, while supporting V_T by behavioral or reflex pathways, do assist maintenance of alveolar ventilation. In the awake human, CPAP appears to depress V_T, with little effect on T_I (Green et al., 1978), yet this occurs from an elevated EEV, so that the effect on the inspiratory off-switch threshold curve reflects starting at an increased end-inspiratory lung volume and reducing the mean inspiratory flow rate. Since the responses to this type of load include important behavioral aspects, it is not possible to identify separately the reflex contributions to this shift.

Expiratory threshold loading (P_{THex}) represents a similar, yet importantly different, type of stress to the respiratory system, compared with CPAP. Similar to CPAP, P_{THex} loading serves to increase EEV in humans and animals on the first breath, without an altered frequency, and this was seen in conscious and anesthetized subjects (Campbell et al., 1961). D'Angelo and Agostoni (1975a) showed that vagal reflexes were active in the augmented end-inspiratory volume seen immediately with this type of loading in anesthetized animals. As noted earlier, P_{THEX} of equivalent expiratory pressure to CPAP causes a more marked depression in V_T in animals (Bishop and Bachofen, 1972) and a more intense sense of respiratory effort in humans (O'Donnell et al., 1988a). The results of Freedman and Weinstein (1965) demonstrate the influence of experience in inspiratory threshold loading in humans. Initial exposures to negative inspiratory threshold loads caused a substantial fall in V_T, but subsequent load application elicited immediate inspiratory compensation such that V_T often exceeded control. Respiratory frequency was unaffected by this type of load, so the experienced responder suffered no depression of ventilation once the response was learned. As with CPAP, human responses to P_{THEX} include major behavioral components, and reflex responses are not separately identifiable.

VI. Behavioral Contributions to Loading Responses

A. Minimization of Discomfort

As shown in Figure 1, besides neural and humoral reflex contributions, the respiratory controller output reflects the influence of behavioral reactions to the perception of impeded breathing. Conscious control of the respiratory pattern during loading is well demonstrated by the ability of subjects to regulate aspects of their response as directed by the experimenter (e.g., Green et al., 1978), and by possible discomfort minimization through appropriate pattern adjustment to large mechanical loads (Freedman and Weinstein, 1965; Chonan et al., 1990). Since nearly all the information related to load sensation and behavioral responses is from human experiments, the focus of this section is on pattern regulation in humans, but this does not preclude the possibility that minimization of discomfort influences loading responses in awake animals. Dogs can be trained to indicate when a mechanical load has just reached the level of detection (Davenport et al., 1991). Since these dogs can perceive loads and initiate voluntary action, there is no reason to suspect that one who preempts the most comfortable chair will not find the most comfortable breathing pattern response to an applied mechanical load.

With elevated, controlled respiratory drive (P_{ETCO_2} = 55 torr), Schwartzstein et al. (1989) reported human subjects to be quite sensitive to the match between the level of ventilation spontaneously chosen (chemically driven ventilation; CDV) and changes in that level. When asked to ventilate below the CDV level with CO_2 clamped, all subjects in their study became more dyspneic, and half of their subjects felt more dyspneic when asked to ventilate above the CDV level at the same P_{ETCO_2}. The latter subjects breathed with higher frequency at a given V_T than the subjects who did not become more dyspneic with ventilation above the CDV, although their T_I was unchanged, and thus they had a longer inspiratory duty cycle. Consequently, the matching of actual ventilatory performance to that required by chemical drive is important in determining the sensations associated with comfort. The authors note that mechanoreceptors in the lungs and chest wall are an important source for those sensations.

Chonan et al. (1990) performed a similar study with controlled chemical drive while normal subjects maintained a target ventilation equal to the spontaneous control level as they adopted different f–VT combinations. Subjects judged the difficulty of breathing with each f–VT combination, and demonstrated that the minimum sense of effort occurred with the spontaneously selected pattern. Increasing or decreasing respiratory frequency from that point resulted in an increased sensation of discomfort. Figure 3 shows the variation of perceived effort observed in one subject at a P_{ETCO_2} = 50 torr, as f varied from below 10 to above 30 BPM with ventilation maintained at a constant level.

Their results are consistent with the idea that respiratory pattern regulation may operate by minimizing the perceived discomfort as the work of breathing increases. Many previous reports have shown that indexes of respiratory effort vary with pattern parameters when the overall output is fixed (e.g., Rohrer, 1925; Otis et al., 1950; Mead, 1960; Ruttiman and Yamamoto, 1972; Yamashiro et al., 1975), much the way the sense of effort varies with respiratory frequency at a fixed

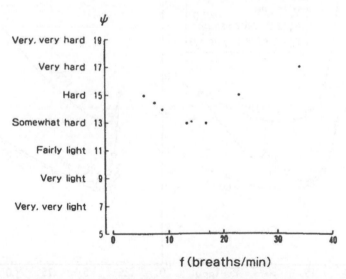

Figure 3 Variation of "sensation of difficulty in breathing (dyspnea)" (Chonan et al., 1990) with respiratory frequency as a normal subject adjusts f–VT, maintaining isoventilation during controlled P_{ETCO_2} (=50 torr). The asterisk marks the spontaneous pattern. Note the spontaneous respiratory pattern choice minimizes the relative discomfort. Compare the shape of this curve to that of Figure 4, which shows the optimal pattern related to the respiratory work rate. (From Chonan et al., 1990.)

ventilation level, as shown by Chonan et al. (1990). Figure 4 shows the predicted variation in respiratory work rate as the f–Vт pattern changes, constraining alveolar ventilation at 5 L/min, under control and mechanically loaded conditions using a total cycle work rate model (Yamashiro et al., 1975). It is apparent that applied loads move the f:Vт optimum in directions consistent with mean observed responses to the specific loading types in awake subjects.

B. Role of Conscious Perception

It would be incorrect to conclude that conscious perception of respiratory effort is necessary to regulate the breathing pattern in the face of applied loads. Even though consciousness is required to provide the timing responses to resistance and elastic loads, as discussed in the foregoing, this does not mandate effort sensation as the sole mechanism of pattern adaptation to loading. Evidence for this comes from several sources. In studies where elastic loading gradually increased over the course of many minutes, starting from an imperceptible level, Puddy and Younes (1991)

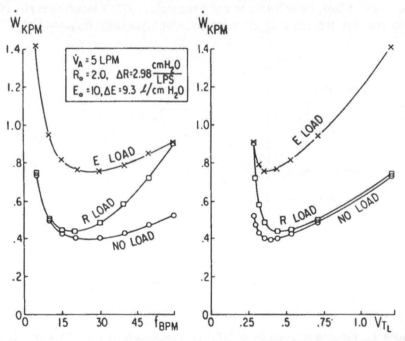

Figure 4 Variation of the calculated external work rate of breathing with respiratory pattern during control, and flow resistive (R) and elastic (E) loading at resting ventilation from the model of Yamashiro et al. (1975). Note that loading shifts the optimal frequency–Vт pattern (minimum work rate point) in opposite directions with R and E loading. (From Daubenspeck, 1981.)

showed that respiratory frequency increased and VT fell at the earliest point shown, 2 min after the start of the progressively increased loading when the elastic load was less than 1 cm H_2O/L. The increase in f, caused by decreases in both TI and TE, continued without the subjects' conscious awareness, until the load reached 6 cm H_2O/L. Thus, minimization of perceived effort could not have accounted for the observed pattern responses, since they occurred without conscious awareness.

In another approach, Daubenspeck and Bennett (1983) developed a technique for loading that applied loads according to a pseudorandom binary sequence (PRBS loading). This approach permitted determination of first-breath pattern responses to resistance and elastic loads that were near or below the perceptual threshold in normal subjects. These immediate responses are free of humoral influences, and should be uninfluenced by conscious reactions to perceptions of impeded breathing.

The three studies that have used this approach have shown consistent effects of these loads to evoke immediate mechanical volume and timing responses in normal humans (Daubenspeck and Bennett, 1983; Harver and Daubenspeck, 1989; Kobylarz and Daubenspeck, 1992). Resistance loading of 1 cm H_2O/LPS and elastic loading of 2 cm H_2O/L of the entire respiratory cycle was unreliably detected by most of the subjects, given the background impedance of the experimental apparatus, and behavioral contributions to the responses are most likely absent. The average immediate effects found for PRBS ΔR include no change in VT, an increase in mechanical TI, and a prolongation of mechanical TE, so that respiratory frequency decreased on the first loaded breath. The PRBS elastic loading produced an immediate fall in VT, little effect on mechanical TI, and a reduction in mechanical TE, so that there was an immediate increase in respiratory frequency. Predictions using the Younes and Riddle (1981) model and responses of diaphragmatic EMG to such loading indicate that the immediate mechanical TI responses to these small loads, when observed, do not indicate a change in neural TI (Daubenspeck and Bennett, 1983; Harver and Daubenspeck, 1989; Kobylarz and Daubenspeck, 1992). The effect of both loads on neural TE was consistent and significant, such that neural frequency increases with ΔE and decreases with ΔR. These responses are consistent in direction with pattern adaptation reflexes that minimize work rate (Fig. 4).

The foregoing PRBS responses should be useful to evaluate loading response reflexes by exclusion of behavioral and humoral influences, but are not representative of the spectrum of reflex possibilities, which probably include components activated only with higher levels of loading. Thus, the subthreshold approach cannot evoke the full range of pattern regulation reflexes. The responses to these small loads, however, are somewhat dependent on the background impedance on which they are applied (Harver and Daubenspeck, 1989). Imperceptible R loads applied on a background of elevated R did not induce prolongation of TI or TE to the same degree as occurred with the control background. Elevation of the background elastic load served to expose a reduction in TI with PRBS ΔE loading that was not apparent in the control condition. This subperceptual loading approach and that of Puddy and Younes are useful to explore the influences of state of consciousness, drugs, and disease on respiratory pattern control.

C. Relative Magnitude of Behavioral Contribution to Loading Response

Once the applied load is perceived, human pattern responses include reflex and humoral factors, plus a variable contribution from behavioral reaction. How large is this behavioral component? One way to estimate the relative contribution of behavioral to reflex responses is to examine the immediate pattern responses to applied loads in subjects who have not had prior exposure to external mechanical loading and, therefore, have not had an opportunity to learn how to minimize discomfort by pattern adaptation consistent with this (Chonan et al., 1990). The wide range of first-breath responses to applied resistance and elastic loads in naive humans has been amply demonstrated by Axen and associates (Axen and Haas, 1979; Axen et al., 1983, 1984). Their data show that, although the mean pattern responses seem to be consistent with the reflex predictions from the experiments of Puddy and Younes (1991) for elastic loading, and with those using the PRBS approach (see previous section), there is a wide variation in individual subjects. With the lowest elastic load (7.5 cm H_2O/L, above the threshold for conscious detection), the Axen group's data show many first-breath responses that increase VT above, or drop f below the control level. This tactic is inefficient from an energetic standpoint and ought to be less comfortable than adopting a smaller VT–higher-f pattern with elastic loading. Similarly, in response to the lowest level resistance load (10 cm H_2O/LPS, also well above the perceptual threshold), a large number of subjects immediately dropped their VT or increased frequency, or both, also inefficient relative to work and comfort. Most, but not all, subjects decreased TE immediately with the lowest E load, whereas the TI response seems distributed evenly about the control level. Their lowest R load, however, tended to prolong TI and shorten TE in most subjects, although the latter effect is less pronounced. The immediate responses to the highest loads show pattern responses more uniformly in accord with expected reflexes and comfort optimization, but their experimental protocol applied increasing loads within a load type, so the responses to higher loads include a load size effect confounded with a learning effect owing to exposure to the previous loads. Conclusions from their results are that behavioral reactions can dominate reflex responses to impeded breathing, and that when the load is sufficiently high, after previous exposure to lower loads of similar type, adaptation to minimize discomfort may govern pattern regulation.

Another way to minimize the effect of behavioral influences on pattern regulation is to examine responses to loading in the absence of perception. Conscious subjects can be tested with imperceptible loads, as described earlier (Daubenspeck and Bennett, 1983; Harver and Daubenspeck, 1989; Puddy and Younes, 1991; Kobylarz and Daubenspeck, 1992), or pattern responses determined in the absence of consciousness, during sleep or anesthesia. As described earlier, removal of consciousness minimizes human timing responses to applied loads, but interpretation of reflexes and behavioral contributions is problematic, since the responses include the obvious effect of consciousness on behavioral responses per se, confounded with unknown effects of sleep or anesthesia on pattern regulation reflexes. Experiments could be done to evaluate the effect of sleep or anesthesia on the pattern responses to imperceptible loads, to explore the effects of these conditions on the responses to perceived loads that include behavioral reactions.

D. Role of Personality in Determining Individual Responses to Loading

Since the observed first-breath responses reported by Axen's group for the lowest level of loading encompass such a wide range of pattern options, it is intriguing to question whether individual characteristics determine how subjects adjust their pattern in response to an unexpected load. As Green et al. (1978), and others, have shown, subjects can be coached in aspects of pattern responses to conform to the desires and expectations of physiologists. They note that, "the strictly rational response of the ordinary man to PPB [positive-pressure breathing] would be to come off the mouthpiece!" (Green et al., 1978). Once a subject decides to remain on the apparatus during a relatively uncomfortable loading procedure, what is it that determines how he or she adapts to the applied load? One suspects that psychological as well as physiological issues pertain here, however much we might prefer to ignore personality characteristics in interpretation of physiological responses.

Little attention has been paid to the role of personality characteristics in setting breathing pattern responses to respiratory stimuli in normal subjects. Aitken et al. (1970) reported the pattern responses to various levels of PTHex, and showed that normal subjects tended to use a lower- f–higher-VT pattern with a smaller minute ventilation than subjects categorized as neurotic. Arkinstall et al. (1974) used established personality assessment instruments to compare respiratory pattern responses to CO_2 in twins. They reported that the twin rating higher on the aggressive scale of the Jackson Personality Research Form (Jackson, 1967) also exhibited a higher frequency of breathing in response to elevated P_{ETCO_2}.

In her Ph.D. thesis of 1980, Haas used multiple personality measures to categorize the psychological makeup of 80 male and 80 female subjects (all healthy, normal volunteers, naive to the purposes of the study), who were then subjected to mechanical loading. Three levels of flow resistance and four levels of elastic loads were applied for three single breaths, with the initial load type selected randomly. Within a load type, however, the loads were applied in ascending order. Psychological profile analysis was done on the responses to the highest loads used ($\Delta R = 37$ cm H_2O/LPS; $\Delta E = 40$ cm H_2O/L), and using only data from the responders who fit into extremes of the distributions (the lowest and highest 20% bins of each aspect of the pattern responses). This permitted categorization of subjects into those whose immediate (first-breath) response was "efficient" to loads (R: slow, deep pattern; E: rapid, shallow pattern), or "inefficient" (opposite responses).

The subjects so classified into the efficient–inefficient categorization showed interesting pattern profiles, with some gender and load type differences. General contrasts resulted between "the stable, capable and confident individual vs. the cautious, easily hurt, usually passive and dependent individual" and between "those who chafe under restrictions vs. those who tolerate them particularly well" (Haas, 1980, p. 90). Table 2 shows summarizations abstracted from Haas' thesis for these two types of responders.

E. Role of Reflex Regulation of the Breathing Pattern During Loading

The evidence presented here supports the idea that behavioral factors may explain some of the puzzling loading responses seen by every experimenter who has done mechanical loading in awake humans. It is difficult to minimize the potential influence of nonreflex components to pattern regulation, given that personality may influence immediate adoption of a pattern that results in more discomfort than a more appropriate one (Axen and Haas, 1979; Chonan et al., 1990). In evaluation of reflex responses, the probability that behavioral responses can so dominate the pattern response to applied loads makes it imperative to account for this factor. The behavioral factor is ubiquitous and plastic, depending on experiences, perceptual sensitivity, and perhaps personality traits.

The possibility that perceived discomfort modulates responses to loading in conscious animals cannot be dismissed. An interesting question concerns the role of reflex contributions in awake humans and animals. It is entirely possible that the

Table 2 Psychological Characteristics Common to Male and Female "Efficient" and "Inefficient" Responders to Resistance (ΔR) and Elastic (ΔE) Loading

Load	Efficient[a]	Inefficient[b]
ΔR	*Males and females*: stable, outgoing, spontaneous, tolerant or ambiguity and disorder, risktaker, unafraid of anger, not easily offended, not bothered by restrictions, less nurturant	*Males and females*: Passive, cautious, fearful, serious, need for structure and order, dislikes restrictions, nurturant, easily offended, mistrustful
ΔE	*Males*: stable, strong, tolerant of restrictions *Females*: stable, social, tolerant of restrictions	*Males*: Passive, dislikes restrictions *Females*: Aggressive, mistrustful, cautious loners, dislikes restrictions

[a]*Efficient*: responds with slower f, larger V_T pattern to ΔR; faster f, smaller V_T pattern to ΔE.
[b]*Inefficient*: opposite efficient.
Source: Summary characteristics abstracted from Haas (1980; pp. 88–90).

main effect of neural and humoral reflex pathways is to "train" the behavioral regulation of pattern during repeated loading, by providing afferent information related to sensation and performance. It is also possible that psychological factors may determine the degree to which the behavioral response is even trainable. Interpretation of loading responses in the conscious state, therefore, must be made with consideration of these nonreflex contributions. As anesthesia and sleep depress the operation of behavioral contributions, they also may attenuate neural and humoral reflexes. It is a considerable challenge to design experimental protocols to evaluate the normal state of these subconscious somatic reflexes.

References

Agostoni, E., and Zocchi, L. (1987). Postinspiratory-ramp activity of diaphragm under inspiratory resistive load. *Respir. Physiol.* 69: 369–385.

Agostoni, E., D'Angelo, E., Torri, G., and Ravenna, L. (1977). Effects of uneven elastic loads on breathing pattern of anesthetized and conscious men. *Respir. Physiol.* 30: 153–168.

Agostoni, E., D'Angelo, E., and Piolini, M. (1978). Breathing pattern in men during inspiratory elastic loads. *Respir. Physiol.* 34: 279–393.

Aitken, R. C. B., Zealley, A. K., and Rosenthal, S. V. (1970). Some psychological and physiological considerations of breathlessness. *Breathing: Hering-Breuer Centenary Symposium*. London, Churchill.

Altose, M. D., Kelsen, S. G., and Cherniack, N. S. (1979). Respiratory responses to changes in airflow resistance in conscious man. *J. Appl. Physiol.* 36: 249–260.

Arkinstall, W., Nirmel, K., Klissouras, V., and Milic-Emili, J. (1974). Genetic differences in the ventilatory response to inhaled CO_2. *J. Appl. Physiol.* 36: 6–11.

Axen, K., and Haas, S. S. (1979). Range of first-breath ventilatory responses to added mechanical loads in naive men. *J. Appl. Physiol.* 46: 743–751.

Axen, K., Haas, S. S., Haas, F., Gaudino, D., and Haas, A. (1983). Ventilatory adjustments during sustained mechanical loading in conscious humans. *J. Appl. Physiol.* 55: 1211–1218.

Axen, K., Haas, F., Gaudino, D., and Haas, S. S. (1984). Effect of mechanical loading on breathing patterns in women. *J. Appl. Physiol.* 56: 175–181.

Badr, M. S., Skatrud, J. B., Dempsey, J. A., and Begle, R. L. (1990). Effect of mechanical loading on expiratory and inspiratory muscle activity during NREM sleep. *J. Appl. Physiol.* 68: 1195–1202.

Barnett, T. B., and Rasmussen, B. (1988). Separate resistive loading of the respiratory phases during mild hypercapnia in man. *Acta Physiol. Scand.* 133: 355–364.

Baydur, A., and Sassoon, C. S. H. (1986). Mechanisms of respiratory elastic load compensation in anesthetized humans. *J. Appl. Physiol.* 60: 613–617.

Bishop, B., and Bachofen, H. (1972). Vagal control of ventilation and respiratory muscles during elevated pressure in the cat. *J. Appl. Physiol.* 32: 103–112.

Bland, S., Lazerou, L., Dyck, G., and Cherniack, R. M. (1967). The influence of the "chest wall" on respiratory rate and depth. *Respir. Physiol.* 3: 47–54.

Bloch, E., Harver, A., and Squires, N. K. (1990). Event-related potentials elicited by resistive loads in normal subjects [abstract]. *Am. Rev. Respir. Dis.* 141: A308.

Bowes, G., Kozar, L. F., Andrey, S. M., and Phillipson, E. A. (1983). Ventilatory responses to inspiratory flow-resistive loads in awake and sleeping dogs. *J. Appl. Physiol.* 54: 1550–1557.

Bradley, G. W. (1972). The response of the respiratory system to elastic loading in cats. *Respir. Physiol.* 16: 142–160.

Brancatisano, T. P., Dodd, D. S., Collett, P. W., and Engel, L. A. (1985). Effect of expiratory loading on glottic dimensions in humans. *J. Appl. Physiol.* 58: 605–611.

Brown, I. G., McClean, P. A., Webster, P. M., Hoffstein, V., and Zamel, N. (1985). Lung volume dependence of esophageal pressure in the neck. *J. Appl. Physiol.* 59: 1849–1854.

Campbell, E. J. M., Dickinson, C. J., Dinnick, O. P., and Howell, J. B. L. (1961). The immediate effects of threshold loads on the breathing of men and dogs. *Clin. Sci.* 21: 309–320.

Cha, E. J., Sedlock, D., and Yamashiro, S. M. (1987). Changes in lung volume and breathing pattern during exercise and CO_2 inhalation in humans. *J. Appl. Physiol.* 62: 1544–1550.

Cherniack, N. S., and Altose, M. D. (1981). Respiratory responses to ventilatory loading. In: *Regulation of Breathing, Part II*. New York, Marcel Dekker.

Cherniack, N. S., and Milic-Emili, J. (1985). Mechanical aspects of loaded breathing. In: *The Thorax*. Edited by C. Roussos and P. T. Macklem. New York, Marcel Dekker.

Chonan, T., Mulholland, M. B., Altose, M. D., and Cherniack, N. S. (1990). Effects of changes in level and pattern of breathing on the sensation of dyspnea. *J. Appl. Physiol.* 69: 1290–1295.

Clark, F. J., and von Euler, C. (1972). On the regulation of depth and rate of breathing. *J. Physiol. (Lond.)* 222: 267–295.

D'Angelo, E., and Agostoni, E. (1975a). Immediate response to expiratory threshold load. *Respir. Physiol.* 25: 269–284.

D'Angelo, E., and Agostoni, E. (1975b). Tonic vagal influences in inspiratory duration. *Respir. Physiol.* 24: 287–302.

Daubenspeck, J. A. (1979). Ventilatory responses to elastic loading at constant P_{ACO_2} in hypercapnic hyperpnea. *J. Appl. Physiol.* 47: 778–786.

Daubenspeck, J. A. (1981). Influence of small mechanical loads on variability of breathing pattern. *J. Appl. Physiol.* 50: 299–306.

Daubenspeck, J. A., and Bartlett, D. J. (1983). Expiratory pattern and laryngeal responses to single-breath expiratory resistance loads. *Respir. Physiol.* 54: 307–316.

Daubenspeck, J. A., and Bennett, F. M. (1983). Immediate human breathing pattern responses to loads near the perceptual threshold. *J. Appl. Physiol.* 55: 1160–1166.

Davenport, P. W., Friedman, W. A., Thompson, F. J., and Franzen, O. (1986). Respiratory-related cortical potentials evoked by inspiratory occlusion in humans. *J. Appl. Physiol.* 60: 1843–1848.

Davenport, P. W., Dalziel, D. J., Webb, B., Bellah, J. R., and Vierck, C. J. (1991). Inspiratory resistive load detection in conscious dogs. *J. Appl. Physiol.* 70: 1284–1289.

Fisher, A. B., DuBois, A. B., and Hyde, R. W. (1968). Evaluation of the forced oscillation technique for the determination of resistance to breathing. *J. Clin. Invest.* 47: 2045–2057.

Flenley, D. C., Pengelly, L. D., and Milic-Emili, J. (1971). Immediate effects of positive-pressure breathing on the ventilatory response to CO_2. *J. Appl. Physiol.* 30: 7–11.

Freedman, S., and Weinstein, S. A. (1965). Effects of external elastic and threshold loading on breathing in man. *J. Appl. Physiol.* 20: 469–472.

Gallagher, C. G., and Younes, M. (1989). Effect of pressure assist on ventilation and respiratory mechanics in heavy exercise. *J. Appl. Physiol.* 66: 1824–1837.

Gallagher, C. G., Sanii, R., and Younes, M. (1989). Response of normal subjects to inspiratory resistive unloading. *J. Appl. Physiol.* 66: 1113–1119.

Gandevia, S. C., and McKenzie, D. K. (1986). Human diaphragmatic EMG: Changes with lung volume and posture during supramaximal phrenic stimulation. *J. Appl. Physiol.* 60: 1420–1428.

Gothe, B., and Cherniack, N. S. (1980). Effects of expiratory loading on respiration in humans. *J. Appl. Physiol.* 49: 601–608.

Green, M., Mead, J., and Sears, T. A. (1978). Muscle activity during chest wall restriction and positive pressure breathing in man. *Respir. Physiol.* 35: 283–300.

Grodins, F. S., and Yamashiro, S. M. (1973). Optimization of the mammalian gas transport system. *Annu. Rev. Biophys. Bioengr.* 2: 115–130.

Haas, S. S. (1980). *Relationships between individual differences in personality and respiratory behavior: an exploratory study*. Ph.D. Thesis, City University of New York.

Hamalainen, R. P., and Viljanen, A. A. (1978a). A hierarchical goal-seeking model of the control of breathing. Part I: Model description. *Biol. Cybern.* 29: 151–158.
Hamalainen, R. P., and Viljanen, A. A. (1978b). Modelling the respiratory airflow pattern by optimization criteria. *Biol. Cybern.* 29: 143–149.
Harver, A., and Daubenspeck, J. A. (1989). Human breathing pattern responses to loading with increased background impedance. *J. Appl. Physiol.* 66: 680–686.
Higenbottam, T. (1980). Narrowing of glottis opening in humans associated with experimentally induced bronchoconstriction. *J. Appl. Physiol.* 49: 403–407.
Hill, A. R., Kaiser, D. L., Lu, J.-Y., and Rochester, D. F. (1985). Steady-state response of conscious man to small expiratory resistance loads. *Respir. Physiol.* 61: 369–381.
Hutt, D. A., Parisi, R. A., Edelman, N. H., and Santiago, T. V. (1991). Responses of diaphragm and external oblique muscles to flow-resistive loads during sleep. *Am. Rev. Respir. Dis.* 144: 1107–1111.
Iber, C., Berssenbrugge, A., Skatrud, J. B., and Dempsey, J. A. (1982). Ventilatory adaptations to resistive loading during wakefulness and non-REM sleep. *J. Appl. Physiol.* 52: 607–614.
Im Hof, V., Dubo, H., Daniels, V., and Younes, M. (1986a). Steady-state response of quadriplegic subjects to inspiratory resistive load. *J. Appl. Physiol.* 60: 1482–1492.
Im Hof, V., West, P., and Younes, M. (1986b). Steady-state response of normal subjects to inspiratory resistive load. *J. Appl. Physiol.* 60: 1471–1481.
Jackson, D. N. (1967). *Manual for Personality Research Form.* Goshen, NY, Research Psychology Press.
Kobylarz, E. J., and Daubenspeck, J. A. (1992). Immediate diaphragmatic electromyogram responses to imperceptible mechanical loads in conscious humans. *J. Appl. Physiol.* 73: 248–259.
Koehler, R. C., and Bishop, B. (1979). Expiratory duration and abdominal muscle responses to elastic and resistive loading. *J. Appl. Physiol.* 46: 730–737.
Lafortuna, C. L., Minetti, A. E., and Mognoni, P. (1984). Inspiratory flow pattern in humans. *J. Appl. Physiol.* 57: 1111–1119.
Lopata, M., and Pearle, J. L. (1980). Diaphragmatic EMG and occlusion pressure response to elastic loading during CO_2 rebreathing in humans. *J. Appl. Physiol.* 49: 669–675.
Luijendijk, S. C., and Milic, E. J. (1988). Breathing patterns in anesthetized cats and the concept of minimum respiratory effort. *J. Appl. Physiol.* 64: 31–41.
Lynne-Davies, P., Couture, J., Pengelly, L. D., and Milic-Emili, J. (1971). Immediate ventilatory response to added elastic loads in cats. *J. Appl. Physiol.* 30: 512–516.
Margaria, C. E., Iscoe, S., Pengelly, L. D., Couture, J., Don, H., and Milic-Emili, J. (1973). Immediate ventilatory response to elastic loads and positive pressure in man. *Respir. Physiol.* 18: 347–369.
Marshall, R. (1962). Relationships between stimulus and work of breathing at different lung volumes. *J. Appl. Physiol.* 17: 917–921.
Martin, J. G., and De Troyer, A. (1982). The behavior of the abdominal muscles during inspiratory mechanical loading. *Respir. Physiol.* 50: 63–73.
Martin, J., Aubier, M., and Engel, L. A. (1982). Effects of inspiratory loading on respiratory muscle activity during expiration. *Am. Rev. Respir. Dis.* 125: 352–358.
McClelland, A. R., Benson, G. W., and Lynne-Davies, P. (1972). Effective elastance of the respiratory system in dogs. *J. Appl. Physiol.* 32: 626–631.
McIlroy, M. B., Eldridge, F. L., Thomas, J. P., and Christie, R., V. (1956). The effect of added elastic and non-elastic resistances on the pattern of breathing in normal subjects. *Clin. Sci.* 15: 337–344.
McKenzie, D. K., and Gandevia, S. C. (1986). Changes in human diaphragmatic electromyogram with positive pressure breathing. *Neurosci. Lett.* 70: 86–90.
Mead, J. (1960). Control of respiratory frequency. *J. Appl. Physiol.* 15: 325–336.
Mead, J. (1979). Responses to loaded breathing. A critique and a synthesis. *Bull. Eur. Physiopathol. Respir.* 15: 61–71.
Mead, J., and Milic-Emili, J. (1964). Theory and methodology in respiratory mechanics with

glossary of symbols. In: *Handbook of Physiology*: Section 3. Respiration Volume 1. Edited by W. O. Fenn and H. Rahn. Washington, DC, American Physiological Society.

Milic-Emili, J., and Zin, W. A. (1986). Breathing responses to imposed mechanical loads. In: *The Respiratory System. Control of Breathing, Part 2*. Bethesda, MD, American Physiological Society.

Milsom, W. K. (1990). Mechanoreceptor modulation of endogenous respiratory rhythms in vertebrates. *Am. J. Physiol.* 259: R898-R910.

Minetti, A. E., Brambilla, I., and Lafortuna, C. L. (1987). Respiratory airflow pattern in patients with chronic airway obstruction. *Clin. Physiol.* 7: 283–295.

Muller, N., Volgyesi, G., Becker, L., Bryan, M. H., and Bryan, A. C. (1979). Diaphragmatic muscle tone. *J. Appl. Physiol.* 47: 279–284.

O'Donnell, D. E., Sanii, R., Giesbrecht, G., and Younes, M. (1988a). Effect of continuous positive airway pressure on respiratory sensation in patients with chronic obstructive pulmonary disease during submaximal exercise. *Am. Rev. Respir. Dis.* 138: 1185–1191.

O'Donnell, D. E., Sanii, R., and Younes, M. (1988b). External mechanical loading in conscious humans: Role of upper airway mechanoreceptors. *J. Appl. Physiol.* 65: 541–548.

Otis, A. B., Fenn, W. O., and Rahn, H. (1950). Mechanics of breathing in man. *J. Appl. Physiol.* 2: 592–607.

Paiva, M., Verbanck, S., Estenne, M., Poncelet, B., Segebarth, C., and Macklem, P. T. (1992). Mechanical implications of in vivo human diaphragm shape. *J. Appl. Physiol.* 72: 1407–1412.

Phillipson, E. A., Kozar, L. F., and Murphy, E. (1976). Respiratory load compensation in awake and sleeping dogs. *J. Appl. Physiol.* 40: 895–902.

Poon, C. S. (1986). Estimation of response curves in closed-loop physiological control. *J. Appl. Physiol.* 61: 1481–1491.

Poon, C. S. (1987). Ventilatory control in hypercapnia and exercise: Optimization hypothesis. *J. Appl. Physiol.* 62: 2447–2459.

Poon, C. S. (1988). Comments on "Optimal respiratory controller structures." IEEE Trans. Biomed. Eng. 35: 395–7.

Poon, C. S. (1991). Optimization behavior of brainstem respiratory neurons. A cerebral neural network model. *Biol. Cybern.* 66: 9–17.

Poon, C. S., Younes, M., and Gallagher, C. G. (1987). Effects of expiratory resistive load on respiratory motor output in conscious humans. *J. Appl. Physiol.* 63: 1837–1845.

Poon, C. S., Lin, S. L., and Knudson, O. B. (1992). Optimization character of inspiratory neural drive. *J Appl. Physiol.* 72: 2005–17.

Pope, H., Holloway, R., and Campbell, E. J. M. (1968). The effects of elastic and resistive loading of inspiration on the breathing of conscious man. *Respir. Physiol.* 4: 363–372.

Puddy, A., and Younes, M. (1991). Effect of slowly increasing elastic load on breathing in conscious humans. *J. Appl. Physiol.* 70: 1277–1283.

Puddy, A., Giesbrecht, G., Sanii, R., and Younes, M. (1992). Mechanism of detection of resistive loads in conscious humans. *J. Appl. Physiol.* 72:2267–2270.

Read, D. J. C., Freedman, S., and Kafer, E. R. (1974). Pressures developed by loaded inspiratory muscles in conscious and anesthetized man. *J. Appl. Physiol.* 37: 207–218.

Remmers, J. E., and Bartlett, D. J. (1977). Reflex control of expiratory airflow and duration. *J. Appl. Physiol.* 42: 80–87.

Revelette, W. R., and Davenport, P. W. (1990). Effects of inspiratory occlusion on cerebral evoked potentials in humans. *J. Appl. Physiol.* 68: 282–288.

Riddle, W., and Younes, M. (1981). A model for the relation between respiratory neural and mechanical outputs. II. Methods. *J. Appl. Physiol.* 51: 979–989.

Road, J., Newman, S., Derenne, J. P., and Grassino, A. (1986). In vivo length–force relationship of canine diaphragm. *J. Appl. Physiol.* 60: 63–70.

Rohrer, F. (1925). Physiologie der Atembevegung. In: *Handbuch der Normalen und Pathologischen Physiologie*. Berlin, Springer.

Ruttiman, U. E., and Yamamoto, W. S. (1972). Respiratory airflow patterns that satisfy power and force criteria of optimality. *Ann. Biomed. Eng.* 1: 146–159.

Sanii, R., and Younes, M. (1988). Steady-state response of normal subjects to an inspiratory sinusoidal pressure load. *J. Appl. Physiol.* 64: 511–520.

Sant'Ambrogio, G. (1982). Information arising from the tracheobronchial tree of mammals. *Physiol. Rev.* 62: 531–569.

Schwartzstein, R. M., Simon, P., Weiss, J. W., Fencl, V., and Weinberger, S. E. (1989). Breathlessness induced by dissociation between ventilation and chemical drive. *Am. Rev. Respir. Dis.* 139: 1231–1237.

Shannon, R. (1986). Reflexes from respiratory muscles and costovertebral joints. In: *Handbook of Physiology*, Section 3. The Respiratory System. Bethesda, MD, American Physiological Society.

Similowski, T. P., Levy, P., Corbiel, C., Albala, M., Pariente, R., Derenne, J. P. Bates, J. H. T., Jonson, B., and Milic-Emili, J. (1989). Viscoelastic behavior of lung and chest wall in dogs determined by flow interruption. *J. Appl. Physiol.* 67: 2219–2229.

Strobel, R. J., and Daubenspeck, J. A. (1993). Early and late respiratory-related potentials evoked by pressure pulse stimuli applied at the mouth in humans. *J. Appl. Physiol.* (in press).

Tenenbaum, L. A. (1971). On control processes of external respiratory parameters. *Automatica* 7: 407–416.

Van de Graaff, W. B. (1988). Thoracic influence on upper airway patency. *J. Appl. Physiol.* 65: 2124–2131.

Whitelaw, W. A. (1987). Shape and size of the human diaphragm in vivo. *J. Appl. Physiol.* 62: 180–186.

Whitelaw, W. A., Hajdo, L. E., and Wallace, J. A. (1983). Relationships among pressure, tension, and shape of the diaphragm. *J. Appl. Physiol.* 55: 1899–1905.

Wilson, P. A., Skatrud, J. B., and Dempsey, J. A. (1984). Effects of slow wave sleep on ventilatory compensation to inspiratory elastic loading. *Respir. Physiol.* 55: 103–120.

Woodall, D. L., and Mathew, O. P. (1986). Effect of upper airway pressure pulses on breathing pattern. *Respir. Physiol.* 66: 71–81.

Yamashiro, S. M., and Grodins, F. S. (1971). Optimal regulation of respiratory airflow. *J. Appl. Physiol.* 30: 597–602.

Yamashiro, S. M., and Grodins, F. S. (1973). Respiratory cycle optimization in exercise. *J. Appl. Physiol.* 35: 522–525.

Yamashiro, S. M., Daubenspeck, J. A., Lauritsen, T. A., and Grodins, F. S. (1975). Total work rate of breathing optimization in CO_2 inhalation and exercise. *J. Appl. Physiol.* 38: 702–709.

Younes, M., and Riddle, W. (1981). A model for the relation between respiratory neural and mechanical outputs. I. Theory. *J. Appl. Physiol.* 51: 963–978.

Younes, M., and Riddle, W. (1984). Relation between respiratory neural output and tidal volume. *J. Appl. Physiol.* 56: 1110–1119.

Younes, M., and Sanii, R. (1989). Effect of phase shifts in pressure–flow relationship on response to inspiratory resistance. *J. Appl. Physiol.* 67: 699–706.

Younes, M., Arkinstall, W., and Milic-Emili, J. (1973). Mechanism of rapid ventilatory compensation to added elastic loads in cats. *J. Appl. Physiol.* 35: 443–453.

Younes, M. K., Remmers, J. E., and Baker, J. (1978). Characteristics of inspiratory inhibition by phasic volume feedback in cats. *J. Appl. Physiol.* 45: 80–86.

Younes, M., Riddle, W., and Polacheck, J. (1981). A model for the relation between respiratory neural and mechanical outputs. III. Validation. *J. Appl. Physiol.* 51: 990–1001.

Younes, M., Jung, D., Puddy, A., Giesbrecht, G., and Sanii, R. (1990). Role of the chest wall in detection of added elastic loads. *J. Appl. Physiol.* 68: 2241–2245.

Zechman, F., Hall, F. G., and Hull, W. E. (1957). Effects of graded resistance to airflow in man. *J. Appl. Physiol.* 10: 356–362.

Zin, W. A., Behrakis, P. K., Luijendijk, S. C. M., Higgs, B. D., Baydur, A., Böddener, A., and Milic-Emili, J. (1986). Immediate response to resistive loading in anesthetized humans. *J. Appl. Physiol.* 60: 506–512.

33

Reflex Compensation for Changes in Operational Length of Inspiratory Muscles

ROBERT B. BANZETT

Harvard School of Public Health
Harvard Medical School
Boston, Massachusetts

JERE MEAD

Harvard School of Public Health
Boston, Massachusetts

I. Introduction

Changes in posture common in everyday life exert forces that, if uncompensated, would alter the operational length and, thereby, the contractile strength of respiratory muscles. The principal inspiratory muscle, the diaphragm, does the major part of the work during quiet breathing. The diaphragm is unusual among skeletal muscles in undergoing large changes in its resting length. In the supine human, the weight of the abdominal contents stretches the diaphragm slightly, allowing it to operate in an advantageous portion of its length–tension curve. When one assumes an upright posture, the weight of abdominal contents is removed from the diaphragm, resulting in shorter sarcomere operating length. If there were no compensatory changes in neural drive, this would result in a much smaller tidal volume, because the shortened muscle generates less force at any given neural drive (Pengelly et al., 1971; Eyzaguirre and Fidone, 1975; Kim et al., 1976). Quadriplegic patients, with C-1 lesions, whose diaphragms are electrically paced by the phrenic nerve provide a unique opportunity to study the function of the diaphragm with constant neural drive. When these patients are tilted from supine to upright, the tidal volume falls 50% or more, as predicted on the basis of muscle mechanics (Danon et al., 1979; Strohl et al., 1984; Fig. 1). This fall in tidal volume does not occur in the intact human because of reflex adjustments to respiratory muscle drive that are described in this chapter.

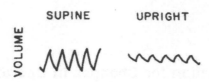

Figure 1   Fall in tidal volume resulting from upward shift in end-expiratory volume in a quadriplegic woman during bilateral phrenic pacing. (From Mead, 1981.)

The effect of the transition from supine to upright on the diaphragm has been simulated in the laboratory by application of about 10 cm H_2O continuous positive transrespiratory pressure (also termed CPAP; continuous positive airway pressure), which increases end-expiratory lung volume and shortens the operating length of the diaphragm, much like the upright posture. Although expiratory threshhold load (or PEEP; positive end-expiratory pressure) has also been used to elevate end-expiratory volume, the mechanical situation is different. Consider, for example, the situation during 10 cm H_2O PEEP: if the expiratory muscles do not come into play the inspiratory muscles must generate more than 10 cm H_2O muscle pressure before the lungs start to inflate, and about 20 cm H_2O to reach end inspiratory volume. In contrast, during 10 cm H_2O CPAP, the muscles need only generate 10 cm H_2O at end inspiration. When neural drive to the respiratory muscles is held constant, the effect of the change in operational length becomes obvious: application of 10 cm H_2O CPAP causes a 50% fall in tidal volume in phrenic nerve-paced quadriplegics (Harpin et al., 1986). When CPAP is applied in spontaneously breathing subjects, however, tidal volume does not fall as expected on the basis of inspiratory muscle mechanics (see Sec. II). Two strategies, probably reflexive, are employed separately or together to maintain tidal volume (Fig. 2). The first strategy is to increase neural drive to the diaphragm and other inspiratory muscles to restore their original force at the new, shorter length. This strategy has been termed "operational length compensation" (OLC) and is the strategy most often seen in human experiments. The second strategy is to contract abdominal and other expiratory muscles, which can restore the inspiratory muscles toward their original length, in addition to shifting some of the work of breathing to the expiratory muscles. The particular reflex strategies that are called into play in a given situation presumably depend on which of the possible reflex pathways are facilitated or suppressed by descending pathways (Stuart; summarized in Altose and Zechman, 1986). This selection of reflexes may depend on instruction given the subject, posture, respiratory task (e.g., resting breathing vs. speech), state of wakefulness, or other.

In theory, the expiratory muscles may be used in two ways. At one extreme, expiratory muscles can be tonically contracted, restoring lung volume and inspiratory muscle lengths to control values. This allows the inspiratory muscles to provide approximately the same tidal volume, at the same neural drive, as during control. At the other extreme, inspiratory muscles can be inactive, allowing phasic

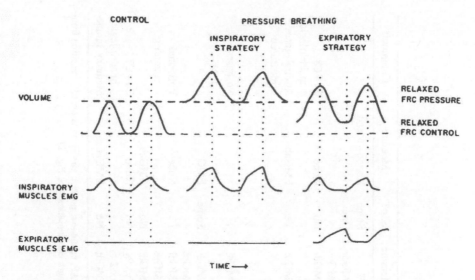

Figure 2 Diagrammatic representation of the strategies adopted to maintain tidal volume while breathing on continuous positive transrespiratory pressure sufficient to increase relaxed functional residual capacity (FRC) by 1 tidal volume equivalent.

contractions of the expiratory muscles to produce the entire tidal volume by driving lung volume down from the elevated relaxation volume during pressure. When moderate pressure, which simulates postural influence, is applied, the most common expiratory strategy is an intermediate one, in which phasic expiratory muscle contraction performs part of the work of breathing, while, at the same time, lengthening the inspiratory muscles (see Fig. 2, right-hand panel). (Newborn infants seem to use this expiratory strategy exclusively; Stark et al., 1984.) Increased abdominal muscle activity during positive pressure has been demonstrated in dogs and cats (Bishop, 1967). Pulmonary stretch receptors with fibers in the vagus nerve play the major role in this response (Bishop and Bachofen, 1972), although muscle stretch receptors may also contribute. This expiratory strategy has been well described and is not the focus of this chapter.

II. Experimental Studies in Humans

Table 1 summarizes observations in humans. In three studies (Barach et al., 1946; Grassino et al., 1973; Gillespie et al., 1979), continuous positive pressure was used to increase end-expiratory lung volume by about 1.5 L in men, thereby shortening inspiratory muscles. Although these studies were not designed to investigate this aspect of respiratory control, retrospective examination of the data revealed that tidal volume and end-tidal PCO_2 were maintained at control levels, implying that

Table 1 Summary of Reflex Experiments in Humans

Ref.	State	Intervention	OLC?	Measure	Exp?	Measure	Comments
Grassino et al. (1973)	Awake	CPAP	Sometimes	V_T	Some	Konno–Mead	
Green et al. (1978)	Awake	CPAP	Yes (¾)	EMGdi EMGps	One	None	
Banzett et al. (1981a)	Awake	Lower torso pressure	Yes	EMGdi	No	None	C5–C8 quadriplegics
Banzett et al. (1981b)	Awake	a. CPAP b. Lower torso pressure c. Tilt	Yes	EMGdi	Yes	EMGab	Arterial gases measured
Druz et al. (1981)	Awake	Posture	Yes	EMGdi			No gases measured
Reid et al. (1985)	Awake	Immersion	Yes	EMGdi EMGps	Some	EMG	
Banzett et al. (1985)	Awake	Immersion	Yes	EMGdi EMGps	?	None	Volitional breathing
Begle et al. (1987; 1990)	Sleep	CPAP	Yes	EMGdi	No	EMGab	
McCool et al. (1988)	Awake	Tilt	Yes	V_T, $P_{0.1}$ Pco_2	No	None	C4–C7 quadriplegics
Derenne et al. (1986)	Anesth	CPAP	Partial	EMGdi	No	EMGab	Methoxyflurane

EMG, electromyogram; ps, parasternal intercostal; di, diaphragm; ab, abdominal; CPAP, continuous positive airway pressure; tilt, transition from supine to upright; exp, expiratory muscle strategy; OLC, inspiratory operational length compensation (see Fig. 2).

substantial changes must have occurred in the neural drive to respiratory muscles. These changes compensated for the length–tension disadvantage of inspiratory muscles during pressure breathing, preventing the fall in tidal volume of more than 50% that is predicted on the basis of muscle mechanics. The lack of change in end-tidal Pco_2 suggested that the adjustments in drive were made in response to proprioceptive, rather than chemoreceptive, afferent information. The Konno–Mead plots of chest wall motion (see Fig. 4 of Grassino et al., 1973) hint that three of eight subjects employed the phasic expiratory muscle strategy, whereas the other five defended tidal volume by increasing inspiratory muscle activity.

The first study expressly designed to investigate operational length compensation of inspiratory muscles (Green et al., 1978) employed electromyographic (EMG) recording of diaphragm (esophageal electrodes) and intercostal muscles (implanted wire electrodes). The experimental design prevented any change in end-tidal Pco_2. When positive pressure of 10 cm H_2O was applied through a mouthpiece to seated subjects, tidal volume fell slightly, but not as much as predicted for the one tidal volume shift in end-expiratory volume. There was a rapid increase in both diaphragm and inspiratory intercostal EMG integrated amplitude when positive pressure was applied in three of four subjects, while breathing frequency did not change (Fig. 3). This was the first direct evidence of increased inspiratory neuromuscular drive when inspiratory muscles are passively shortened, although the nature of EMG recording does not provide an absolute baseline; consequently, quantitation of relative changes should be interpreted with caution. One subject chose instead to use the expiratory muscle strategy, which led the authors to conclude that instruction of the subject can affect the strategy that is employed. Indeed, when this individual was instructed to relax against the applied pressure, rather than to fight it, he showed the same increase in inspiratory activity as the other subjects. The responses were fast, occurring in the first breath following the upward shift in lung volume, which further supported the notion that the afferent limb is proprioceptive, rather than chemoreceptive.

There are a few potential questions regarding conclusions that may be drawn from the data of Green et al. (1978). The most important is that of volitional response: The subjects in this study were trained in respiratory physiology and were

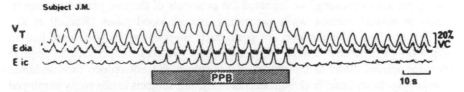

Figure 3 Representative tracings of effects of one application of positive-pressure breathing (PPB) on tidal volume and electrical activity of the diaphragm (Edi) and intercostal muscle (Eic) in one subject. Inspiration is upward. Edi and Eic are in arbitrary units. (From Green et al., 1978.)

quite aware of the pressure applied at the mouth: Were they consciously responding to the stimulus? Another question concerns the reliability of diaphragm EMG recording electrodes in an experiment that systematically alters the configuration of the diaphragm (see later discussion). The fact that an entirely different type of electrode recorded similar amplitude changes in the intercostal muscles is of some reassurance on this point. In addition, there was no direct measure of arterial Pco_2 or Po_2: Might positive pressures have increased alveolar dead space, causing end-tidal Pco_2 to underestimate arterial Pco_2 (Folkow and Pappenheimer, 1955)? What is the afferent pathway for the response? Although a chemoreceptor reflex was tentatively ruled out, several possibilities remained, including reflexes from chest wall and pulmonary mechanoreceptors or conscious response.

A study performed in supine quadriplegics having C5–C8 lesions answered several of these outstanding questions (Banzett et al., 1981a). These subjects have intact innervation of the diaphragm, but the abdominal muscles and most of the ribcage muscles are paralyzed. A cuirass extending from armpits to hips and screened from the sight of the subject was used to apply continuous positive transrespiratory pressure. With this technique, conscious perception of the stimulus was largely avoided because these subjects had no somatic sensation below the shoulders and because there was no change in upper airway pressure. Surface electrodes on the lower rib cage were used to record the diaphragm EMG. When positive transrespiratory pressure (i.e., negative pressure in the cuirass) was applied, there was an immediate increase in lung volume and a twofold increase in the amplitude of diaphragmatic EMG, which was sufficient to maintain tidal volume and P_{ETCO_2} constant. Inspiratory time did not change; thus the response was not simply a prolongation of inspiration by the Hering–Breuer reflex. (The expiratory muscles in these subjects were paralyzed, precluding use of the expiratory strategy.) Operational length changes produced by tilting quadriplegic subjects are also well compensated (McCool et al., 1988). These data confirm those of Green et al. and provide some evidence against the possibility of conscious volitional response, as the subjects were untrained, uninformed, and unaware of the respiratory nature of the experiment. Furthermore, in quadriplegic patients, possible afferent pathways were further narrowed (see Sec. IV).

To allay doubts about the correspondence of end-tidal Pco_2 to arterial Pco_2 during pressure breathing, we repeated the protocols of the two preceding experiments in normal humans while measuring arterial blood gases (Banzett et al., 1981b), and found that the levels of positive transrespiratory pressure used had no effect on the end-tidal–arterial Pco_2 difference. In these experiments, positive pressure applied either at the mouth or by cuirass did not reduce tidal volume, change inspiratory time, or change arterial Pco_2. The subjects in this study employed both strategies—changes in inspiratory muscle activation and recruitment of expiratory muscles—to cope with the positive pressure challenge; they sometimes shifted smoothly between the strategies, with no change in tidal volume (Fig. 4). Most subjects increased inspiratory drive, rather than activating expiratory muscles

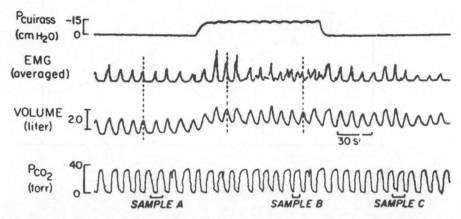

Figure 4 Negative cuirass pressure ($P_{cuirass}$) trial in one subject. Notice increase in inspiratory muscle activity as lung volume increases at the onset of pressure; then phasic expiratory muscle activity increases, allowing less inspiratory work for a given tidal volume. Expiratory muscles lower end-expiratory volume so that there is a smaller volume shift when pressure is turned off. At sample A, $Paco_2$ = 30 torr, $Petco_2$ = 33 torr; at sample B, $Paco_2$ = 28, $Petco_2$ = 33; At sample C, $Paco_2$ = 27, $Petco_2$ = 32. (From Banzett et al., 1981b.)

(perhaps a result of instruction). The transition from supine to upright was also examined; tidal volume and arterial Pco_2 were maintained, although usually the underlying changes in respiratory EMG were hard to detect among postural activity in nearby muscles. This study resolved the blood gas question, and provided more evidence for neural compensation of respiratory muscle length changes in normal, albeit aware, humans (including the first woman to be tested).

Druz and Sharp (1981) provided better EMG data showing that diaphragmatic electrical activity in the upright posture increased fourfold to maintain the same force generation in the upright posture as in the supine (Fig. 5). These recordings are of very high quality; thus the errors inherent in quantitation are likely to be small. They did not record end-tidal Pco_2 and tidal volume, so we can only surmise that the afferent mechanisms for this adjustment were the same as seen in foregoing experiments.

Immersion of the upright subject in water shifts the operating lengths of respiratory muscles in a manner more like postural change. An upright subject, immersed to the level of the xiphoid, breathes at a lung volume and chest wall configuration similar to the supine position, unimmersed. As water level falls from xiphoid to hips, the pressure on the abdomen is reduced, allowing the diaphragm to descend and shorten. This descent of the diaphragm expands the lung, lowering pleural pressure, and pulling the rib cage inward, lengthening inspiratory intercostals. In contrast, positive pressure at the mouth shortens the diaphragm, while expanding the rib cage. We studied the reflex adjustments to immersion in healthy

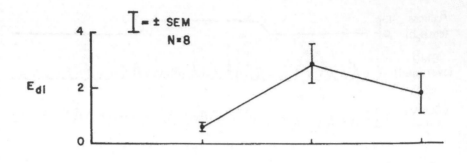

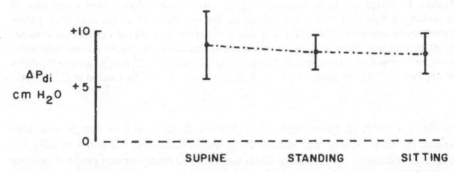

Figure 5   Diaphragmatic electrical activity (Edi) and transdiaphragmatic pressure (Pdi) data on eight normal subjects in supine, 80° head-up (standing), and erect-sitting positions. Tidal volumes were comparable, and no mouthpiece was used. (From Druz and Sharp, 1981.)

naive subjects (Reid et al., 1985). Subjects were seated in a deep tub while the water level was lowered in stages from shoulder to hips. The experience was comfortable and, unlike other methods of applying transrespiratory pressure, did not give strong clues about the respiratory nature of the experiment. Again subjects maintained constant tidal volume and end-tidal Pco_2. In the absence of compensatory changes in neural drive, tidal volume would have fallen with the lowering of water level as the diaphragm, by far the most important inspiratory muscle, was forced to operate at a shorter, less effective, length. Rather than increasing the neural drive to the diaphragm alone, these subjects increased activity of both diaphragm and inspiratory intercostals, despite the fact that the intercostals were operating at a longer, more effective, length (Fig. 6). This suggests that the compensatory reflexes are organized to globally adjust output to all muscles in the same direction, meeting the needs of the entire system (which are generally dominated by the needs of the diaphragm, because it provides the major part of tidal volume).

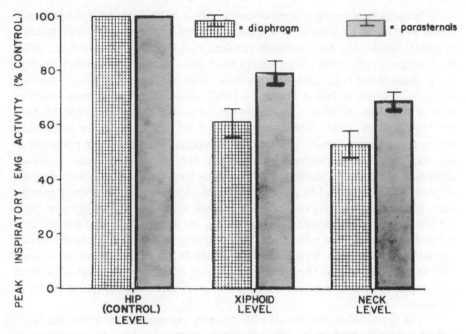

Figure 6 Changes in peak integrated inspiratory activity of diaphragm and parasternal intercostal muscles during progressive immersion of nine seated subjects. Standard errors indicated. (Data from Reid et al., 1985.)

Does operational length compensation depend on consciousness? Compensation might be a volitional response, or might require descending input associated with wakefulness to facilitate the reflex pathway. Both of these possibilities can be eliminated if unconscious humans show the response. Humans in nonrapid eye movement (NREM) sleep exposed to CPAP sufficient to shift end-expiratory volume up to 1.8 L preserved tidal volume, without increasing inspiratory time (Begle et al., 1987). This was accomplished by increased diaphragm activity (recorded with several pairs of surface electrodes) in the absence of detectable abdominal or expiratory intercostal activity (Begle et al., 1987; Begle and Skatrud, 1990). The authors concluded that sleeping humans compensate for changes in operational length very well, even though they compensate for resistive and elastic loads poorly, or not at all. Anesthetized humans, on the other hand, seem to compensate poorly for operational length change (Derenne et al., 1986). Men anesthetized with methoxyflurane increased diaphragm activity slightly, but tidal volume fell 25% when 16 cm H_2O CPAP was applied. As these subjects did not activate abdominal muscles, one would have expected tidal volume to fall 75% at this level of CPAP (Harpin et al., 1986), suggesting that operational length compensation was partially effective.

Is operational length compensation an artifact of EMG recording? Systematic artifacts have been reported in the potentials recorded from wire electrodes implanted in rabbit, human, and dog diaphragm (Banzett et al., 1977; Gandevia et al., 1986; Brancatisano et al., 1989). Other studies have failed to find these artifacts in dogs (R. B. Banzett and J. Lehr, unpublished data; Road and Leevers, 1988). Systematic artifactual changes in human diaphragm EMG amplitude have also been observed in recordings from esophageal electrodes (Gandevia and McKenzie, 1986; McKenzie and Gandevia, 1986). These authors stimulated the phrenic nerve in the neck with supramaximal intensity, and recorded compound maximal action potentials of the diaphragm, using esophageal and surface electrodes. They found *increased amplitude* of the recorded action potential when lung volume was increased or the diaphragm was shortened by positive transrespiratory pressure, isovolume maneuvers, posture, or voluntary inspiration. As this artifact acted in the sign to explain the results of studies reported in the foregoing, the authors ". . . cast doubt on the suggestion that there is a reflex increase in diaphragmatic activity when the human diaphragm is at a shorter length." The magnitude of this artifact, however, is small over the range of volume employed in most reflex experiments, and other evidence not subject to the same artifact supports the conclusion that the reflex exists, as follows:

The same studies that showed artifact in esophageal electrode recordings failed to find systematic artifacts in surface electrode recordings of diaphragm (Gandevia and McKenzie, 1986; McKenzie and Gandevia, 1986). Comparison of diaphragm EMG signals recorded by surface electrodes placed in various locations has shown that descent of the diaphragm can reduce the amplitude of surface electrodes placed high on the chest, opposite in sign to the observed reflex changes (Lansing and Savelle, 1989). These changes are consistent with changes in the proximity of diaphragm to the recording site. Electrodes placed in the usual location (seventh interspace, midaxillary line) were not much affected or were affected in a direction the sign of which is opposite that of the observed reflex changes over the range of lung volumes employed in most studies of operational length compensation. In a few experiments, the EMG response to operational length change recorded by electrodes at various sites have been compared, and similar responses have been observed (Begle et al., 1987; Begle and Skatrud, 1990; Brice et al., 1991). By and large, then, it is difficult to attribute length compensation responses recorded with surface electrodes to systematic artifact.

Even in the absence of EMG data, many experiments provide sufficient mechanical evidence to conclude that the drive to respiratory muscles is adjusted to compensate for operational length changes. Subjects who cannot, or do not, employ phasic expiratory muscle force must increase the drive to inspiratory muscles to maintain tidal volume, as observed. Unfortunately, not all studies include measurements (e.g., expiratory muscle EMG) or neural deficits (e.g., spinal lesion below the phrenic motoneurons) that exclude the expiratory strategy. In the animal experiments described in the following section, several investigators have observed

EMG changes that were later abolished by afferent section, providing further evidence against recording artifacts as a possible explanation for the observed diaphragm EMG changes.

III. Reflex Experiments in Animals

Although experiments in humans have given us some clues about afferent mechanisms, animal experiments in which afferents can be recorded or selectively interrupted, are likely to be the only source of definitive information. In the first edition of this volume we stated "Until a species is found which consistently exhibits the inspiratory muscle compensation commonly seen in humans, it will be difficult to obtain more definitive information on afferent pathways." This challenge has been taken up, and data have emerged that point the way toward the afferent path.

The principal problem in finding a suitable animal "model" of operational length compensation is that animals are generally free to employ the alternative strategy of phasic expiratory muscle recruitment—this can make it difficult to isolate and define the inspiratory strategy. Several investigators have observed variable responses in the same study, sometimes the animals showed compensatory changes in diaphragm activation, whereas at other times, they employed expiratory muscles, obviating the need to adjust inspiratory muscle drive. Not all studies include information on expiratory muscle use, making interpretation difficult. Several relevant animal experiments that have used various means to alter operational length, are summarized in Table 2. Iscoe (1989) found that phrenic nerve efferent activity increased greatly during positive pressure in some anesthetized cats, but not in others; the increases were not significant for the group as a whole. Fitting et al. (1989) showed an average 40% diaphragm EMG increase in the upright sitting position in awake dogs, but again the changes were quite variable, thus not significant; they concluded from abdominal pressure data that the expiratory strategy dominates in awake dogs. Gorini and Estenne (1991) found that the expiratory strategy alone operates on the first breath after tilting in anesthetized dogs, with no evidence for adjustments of phrenic activity, aside from those arising from altered chemical drive. Road and Leevers (1988) found no evidence of increased phrenic drive in anesthetized vagotomized dogs exposed to CPAP, even though vagotomy eliminated the expiratory strategy. In contrast with these latter data, other studies have shown more consistent operational length compensation: Anesthetized cats, tilted from supine to upright, increased activity of both costal and crural diaphragm, maintaining tidal volume and P_{ETCO_2} in the face of operational length change (van Lunteren et al., 1985). Likewise, tidal volume was maintained and diaphragm EMG increased significantly in the anesthetized dog held upright (Newman et al., 1986); the authors concluded that this was due to the operational length compensation reflex, although they did not report first-breath response, nor did they control P_{ETCO_2}. Awake ponies increased both diaphragm and transversus abdominis muscular

Table 2 Summary of Animal Reflex Experiments

Ref.	Species	State	Intervention	OLC?	Measure	Exp?	Measure	Comments
van Lunteren et al. (1985)	Cat	Anesth	Tilt	Yes	EMGdi	?	None	
Newman et al. (1986)	Dog	Anesth	Tilt	Yes	EMGdi	?	None	Lacks blood gas
Fryman et al. (1987)	Cat	Anesth	Lower body pressure	Yes[a]	EMGdi	No	None	C-7 cord section
Road et al. (1988)	Dog	Anesth	CPAP	No	EMGdi	No	P–V curve	Vagotomized
Iscoe (1989)	Cat	Anesth	PEEP	Some	Ephr	?	None	
Fitting et al. (1989)	Dog	Awake	Posture	Some	EMGdi	Yes	Pab	Dominated by expiratory strategy
Cheeseman et al. (1990)	Cat	Anesth	Abdominal compression	Yes[a]	EMGdi	?	None	Persists after C-7 cord section and vagotomy
Gorini et al. (1991)	Dog	Anesth	Tilt	No	Ephr, EMGps	Yes	EMGab	
Brice et al. (1991)	Pony	Awake	CPAP	Yes	EMGdi	Yes	EMGab	Intact
	Pony	Awake	CPAP	Yes	EMGdi	No	EMGab	Vagotomized
Teitlebaum et al. (1993)	Dog	Anesth	Paralysis	Yes[a]	EMGdi	?	None	Paralysis of one hemidiaphragm

[a]Operational length compensation response abolished by section of diaphragm afferents in these studies. Abbreviations as in Table 1.

activity in response to CPAP, preserving tidal volume and P_{ETCO_2}; carotid body denervation did not eliminate the responses (Brice et al., 1991). Other animal experiments showed compensation during less usual interventions that altered operating length: Cheeseman and Revelette (1990) lengthened the diaphragm of anesthetized cats by compressing the abdomen; this limits the animals' option to compensate with abdominal muscles. They found that diaphragm EMG was adjusted to defend tidal volume in the face of 17% length changes. (The unknown changes in mechanical impedance make it difficult to predict what tidal volume change to expect with this maneuver.) Anesthetized, vagotomized cats, with spinal section at C-7, increased diaphragm EMG by lengthening inspiratory time during lower body negative pressure (Fryman and Frazier, 1987). This technique also removes the option to employ the expiratory strategy, because the expiratory muscles are paralyzed. Although the response they observed (no change in rate of rise of diaphragm EMG, but increased TI and increased peak EMG) was different in form from the usual description of operational length compensation (increased rate of rise and peak EMG with no change in TI), the authors speculated that it was a different manifestation of the same reflex.

IV. Mechanoreceptor Afferent Pathway

What can we deduce about the afferent pathway of the response? Having determined that the compensatory changes in neural drive can occur on the first breath and without changes in $PaCO_2$, we have concluded that operational length compensation is a response to alterations in mechanoreceptor discharge. Which mechanoreceptors could account for the response? Pulmonary stretch receptors are well suited to gauge tidal volume (Adrian, 1933), and Breuer proposed, a century ago, that tidal volume was maintained breath-to-breath by volume feedback from the lung (Breuer and Hering, 1868). It is generally accepted that the reflex effect of pulmonary stretch receptors is to increase tidal volume by lengthening inspiration, different from the operational length compensation response reported by almost all observers. Furthermore, it is commonly held that this reflex does not operate during resting breathing in humans. However, we cannot entirely discount pulmonary stretch receptors on these bases. Proprioceptors in the respiratory muscles are also suited to measure the performance of the muscles. The respiratory muscles are provided with muscle spindles and Golgi tendon organs (although spindles are said to be scarce in the diaphragm), both innervated with large, myelinated fibers. The physiology of these receptors in limb muscle systems has been well studied. Spindles can signal the rate of active shortening and cause compensatory changes in drive through reflexes at segmental and supraspinal levels, thus could also theoretically initiate operational length compensation. Tendon organs can signal and regulate the developed active tension and, thus, are another possible pathway. As one might expect, large-fiber phrenic afferents alter phrenic motor output (Jammes et al., 1986; Speck and Revelette, 1987).

We begin to narrow the possibilities by examining some of the human experiments. In high quadriplegic subjects, the only proprioceptive afferents available to sense the change in respiratory mechanics are pulmonary mechanoreceptors with afferent fibers in the vagus, and diaphragm mechanoreceptors with afferent fibers in the phrenic nerves; these subjects showed complete operational length compensation, allowing us to conclude that rib cage afferents are not essential to the response (Banzett et al., 1981a). This conclusion is supported by immersion experiments in which inspiratory intercostals and diaphragm underwent opposite length changes, but altered activity in the same direction (Banzett et al., 1985; Reid et al., 1985). Although this narrows the anatomical sources, it does not speak to the type of receptor involved. Heart–lung transplant patients defended tidal volume when changing from the seated to the supine posture, suggesting that pulmonary afferents are also unnecessary for the response (Kinnear et al., 1989). Unfortunately, however, there was no measure of expiratory muscle action (EMG, or abdominal pressure swings) in this latter study, so we are unable to determine whether these subjects chose to use the expiratory strategy. Human experiments, therefore, suggest that diaphragm afferents are the key pathway, but do not rigorously eliminate alternative hypotheses.

The most clear and consistent demonstration of operational length compensation in animals is found in the studies of awake ponies (Brice et al., 1991). Like some awake humans, intact ponies showed simultaneous compensatory changes in diaphragm activity and phasic expiratory activity. Vagal denervation of the lungs did not abolish the diaphragmatic response, but did eliminate the expiratory muscle response to CPAP in these animals. Although these experiments showed that pulmonary mechanoreceptors and arterial chemoreceptors are not necessary for operational length compensation, they did not pin down the necessary pathway. For further information, we must turn to experiments in anesthetized cats, although the responses demonstrated thus far in cats are not completely like the operational length compensation responses in awake humans. Two studies showed consistent compensatory changes in diaphragm EMG with changes in operating length; in both cases, the response was eliminated by section of the phrenic dorsal roots, indicating that phrenic afferents are essential to the response (Fryman and Frazer, 1987; Cheeseman and Revelette 1990). Of these two studies, the abdominal compression study of Cheeseman and Revelette showed changes in EMG bearing the strongest resemblance to those seen in human studies. This group went on to record afferents under the same conditions as imposed in their reflex studies (Revelette et al., 1992). They found that Golgi tendon organs were active during ordinary diaphragm contractions, and that their discharge increased markedly (30%) when the abdomen was compressed (Fig. 7). As tendon organ activity is known to inhibit alpha motoneuronal discharge in other skeletal muscle, the authors suggested that tendon organs account for the alterations in diaphragm activity during abdominal compression, and speculated that this pathway could account for the operational length compensation response seen in humans.

Teitlebaum et al. (1993), using a different approach, examined the reflex response to paralysis of one hemidiaphragm in anesthetized dogs. This intervention

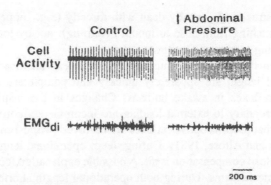

Figure 7 Response of a single diaphragm tendon organ afferent (cell activity) to increased diaphragmatic operational length, achieved by compressing the abdomen. The discharge of the tendon organ is greater, despite the reduction of neural drive to the diaphragm (EMGdi), presumably because the muscle develops more force at the longer length. (From Revelette et al., 1992.)

should abolish tendon organ firing, and it is also likely to markedly diminish spindle firing, owing to paralysis of intrafusal fibers. Paralysis of the left diaphragm doubled the activity of the right diaphragm, inspiratory intercostals, and alae nasi, with no increase in inspiratory time. The response to left diaphragm paralysis was abolished by section of the left phrenic nerve. This response did not occur if the diaphragm was held at a very short length so that it could not generate active tension. These data point strongly to a powerful diaphragm tendon organ reflex; the response to paralysis is in the sign opposite that expected from spindle reflexes. The global nature of the response was similar to the report of global activation by Reid et al. (1985) in awake humans.

It thus appears that the reflex operational length compensation observed in humans and animals is mediated by reflexes arising in Golgi tendon organs of the diaphragm and is integrated in the medulla. If this proves true, the response might better be termed "diaphragm force compensation" (DFC), and is likely to play a role in other circumstances that alter diaphragmatic force-generation capacity, such as fatigue or partial neuromuscular block. When diaphragmatic activation is altered to compensate for changes in the diaphragm's force capacity, the drive to intercostal muscles is altered in parallel, even when their local tendon organ reflexes oppose the global change. Furthermore, upper airway muscles also appear to be involved, suggesting a supraspinal level of integration. This global involvement is consistent with the diaphragm's dominant role in tidal volume production.

V. Relation of Operational Length Compensation to Load Compensation

Transient changes in inspiratory muscle operational length are common in daily life. Overall inspiratory load, however, seldom changes, aside from upper airway obstruction. Obstruction is usually dealt with directly (e.g., upper airway muscle activation or switching from nose to mouth breathing), not by load-compensating mechanisms acting to increase inspiratory drive.

Changes in the inspiratory muscles' effectiveness secondary to changes in their operational length are apparently quickly and completely compensated by proprioceptive reflexes in awake humans. Changes in the inspiratory muscles' effectiveness secondary to external loading are incompletely compensated, and it seems unlikely that proprioceptive reflexes are involved (Milic-Emili and Pengelly, 1970; Cherniack and Altose, 1981). During sleep, operational length compensation is complete, but load compensation is nil. A possible explanation for this discrepancy lies in sensory mechanisms. During both operational length shortening and during external loading, reduced motion will be sensed by pulmonary stretch receptors and muscle spindles. The two situations would, however, have opposite effects on contractile force sensed by tendon organs. When operational length is reduced, sarcomeres produce less force for a given efferent drive. On the other hand, inspiratory loading retards muscle shortening; therefore, at any time during inspiration, sarcomeres are longer and will produce greater force for a given efferent drive; termed "intrinsic load compensation" (Milic-Emili et al., 1970). Thus, force feedback is appropriate for operational length compensation, but is inappropriate for compensation of external loads. This may account for the failure of the system to compensate for external loads.

Local load-compensating mechanisms, neural or intrinsic, may have important implications for respiratory muscle coordination, however. The diaphragm and inspiratory intercostals act together to expand the lung, but they act antagonistically on one another. For instance, as the diaphragm contracts, it lowers pleural pressure, tending to collapse the rib cage. Thus, an overly strong contraction of the diaphragm will load the inspiratory intercostals, and the resulting inward deformation of the rib cage will be opposed by spindle reflex mechanisms of the inspiratory intercostals. Most breaths parallel the relaxation configuration of the rib cage, and it is possible that local load-compensation mechanisms assist this by distributing activation appropriately.

VI. Summary

The neural drive to ventilatory muscles is adjusted to compensate for changes in the muscles' effectiveness secondary to their length change. Such changes in length are brought about by altered transrespiratory pressure, immersion, and by ordinary postural changes that shift the weight of the abdominal contents. The responses seem to be organized around the effectiveness of the diaphragm, which dominates tidal volume generation and routinely undergoes greater changes in resting length than most other skeletal muscles. Two strategies are adopted: (1) increased activation of inspiratory muscles, and (2) phasic activation of expiratory muscles. The first (inspiratory) strategy is seen in adult humans and some animals; recent evidence suggests that it may be due to the reflex effects of tendon organ receptors in the diaphragm. The second (expiratory) strategy is commonly seen in humans, especially infants, and in animals; it has been attributed to pulmonary stretch receptors that sense the increase in lung volume. Recent evidence suggests that operational length compensation seen in inspiratory muscles is mediated by force feedback from Golgi tendon organs.

Acknowledgments

This work was supported by HL19170 and HL 46690.

References

Adrian, E. (1933). Afferent impulses in the vagus and their effect on respiration. *J. Physiol. (Lond.)* 79: 332–358.

Altose, M., and Zechman, F. J. (1986). Loaded breathing: Load compensation and respiratory sensation. *Fed. Proc.* 45: 114–122.

Banzett, R. B., Bruce, E., Goldman, M., and Mead, J. (1977). Artifactual changes in diaphragm EMG amplitude caused by mechanical interventions to breathing. *Physiologist* 20: 5.

Banzett, R. B., Inbar, G. F., Brown, R., Goldman, M., Rossier, A., and Mead, J. (1981a). Diaphragm electrical activity during negative lower torso pressure in quadriplegic men. *J. Appl. Physiol.* 51: 654–659.

Banzett, R., Strohl, K., Geffroy, B., and Mead, J. (1981b). Effect of transrespiratory pressure on P_{ETCO_2}–Pa_{CO_2} and ventilatory reflexes in humans. *J. Appl. Physiol.* 51: 660–664.

Banzett, R. B., Lansing, R. W., and Reid, M. B. (1985). Reflex compensation of voluntary inspiration when immersion changes diaphragm length. *J. Appl. Physiol.* 59: 611–618.

Barach, A., Eckman, M., Ginsburg, E., Rumsey, C. J., Korr, I., Eckman, I., and Besson, G. (1946). Studies of positive pressure respiration. *J. Aviat. Med.* 17: 290–320.

Begle, R. L., and Skatrud, J. B. (1990). Hyperinflation and expiratory muscle recruitment during NREM sleep in humans. *Respir. Physiol.* 82: 47–63.

Begle, R. L., Skatrud, J. B., and Dempsey, J. A. (1987). Ventilatory compensation for changes in functional residual capacity during sleep. *J. Appl. Physiol.* 62: 1299–1306.

Bishop, B. (1967). Diaphragm and abdominal muscle responses to elevated airway pressures in the cat. *J. Appl. Physiol.* 22: 959–965.

Bishop, B., and Bachofen, H. (1972). Vagal control of ventilation and respiratory muscles during elevated pressures in the cat. *J. Appl. Physiol.* 32: 103–112.

Brancatisano, A., Kelly, S. M., Tully, A., Loring, S. H., and Engel, L. A. (1989). Postural changes in spontaneous and evoked regional diaphragmatic activity in dogs. *J. Appl. Physiol.* 66: 1699–1705.

Brice, A. G., Forster, H. V., Pan, L. G., Lowry, T. F., Murphy, C. L., and Mead, J. (1991). Effects of increased end-expiratory lung volume on breathing in awake ponies. *J. Appl. Physiol.* 70: 715–725.

Cheeseman, M., and Revelette, W. R. (1990). Phrenic afferent contribution to reflexes elicited by changes in diaphragm length. *J. Appl. Physiol.* 69: 640–647.

Danon, J., Druz, W. S., Goldberg, N. B., and Sharp, J. T. (1979). Function of the isolated paced diaphragm and the cervical accessory muscles in C1 quadriplegics. *Am. Rev. Respir. Dis.* 119: 909–919.

Derenne, J. P., Whitelaw, W. A., Couture, J., and Milic, E. J. (1986). Load compensation during positive pressure breathing in anesthetized man. *Respir. Physiol.* 65: 303–314.

Druz, W. S., and Sharp, J. T. (1981). Activity of respiratory muscles in upright and recumbent humans. *J. Appl. Physiol.* 51: 1552–1561.

Fitting, J. W., Easton, P. A., Arnoux, R., Guerraty, A., and Grassino, A. (1989). Diaphragm length adjustments with body position changes in the awake dog. *J. Appl. Physiol.* 66: 870–875.

Folkow, B., and Pappenheimer, J. (1955). Components of the respiratory deadspace and their variation with pressure breathing and with bronchoactive drugs. *J. Appl. Physiol.* 8: 102–110.

Fryman, D. L., and Frazier, D. T. (1987). Diaphragm afferent modulation of phrenic motor drive. *J. Appl. Physiol.* 62: 2436–2441.

Gandevia, S. C., and McKenzie, D. K. (1986). Human diaphragmatic EMG: Changes with lung volume and posture during supramaximal phrenic stimulation. *J. Appl. Physiol.* 60: 1420–1428.

Gillespie, J. R., Bruce, E., Alexander, J., and Mead, J. (1979). Breathing responses of unanesthetized man and guinea pigs to increased transrespiratory pressure. *J. Appl. Physiol.* 47: 119–125.

Gorini, M., and Estenne, M. (1991). Effect of head-up tilt on neural inspiratory drive in the anesthetized dog. *Respir. Physiol.* 85: 83–96.

Grassino, A. E., Lewinsohn, G. E., and Tyler, J. M. (1973). Effects of hyperinflation of the thorax on the mechanics of breathing. *J. Appl. Physiol.* 35: 336–342.

Green, M., Mead, J., and Sears, T. A. (1978). Muscle activity during chest wall restriction and positive pressure breathing in man. *Respir. Physiol.* 35: 283–300.

Harpin, R. P., Gignac, S. P., Epstein, S. W., Gallacher, W. N., and Vanderlinden, R. G. (1986). Diaphragm pacing and continuous positive airway pressure. *Am. Rev. Respir. Dis.* 134: 1321–1323.

Iscoe, S. (1989). Phrenic afferents and ventilatory control at increased end-expiratory lung volumes in cats. *J. Appl. Physiol.* 66: 1297–1303.

Jammes, Y., Buchler, B., Delpierre, S., Rasidakis, A., Grimaud, C., and Roussos, C. (1986). Phrenic afferents and their role in inspiratory control. *J. Appl. Physiol.* 60: 854–860.

Kinnear, W., Higenbottam, T., Shaw, D., Wallwork, J., and Estenne, M. (1989). Ventilatory compensation for changes in posture after human heart–lung transplantation. *Respir. Physiol.* 77: 75–88.

Lansing, R. W., and Savelle, J. (1989). Chest surface recordings of diaphragm potentials in man. *Electroencephalogr. Clin. Neurophysiol.* 72: 59–68.

McCool, F. D., Brown, R., Mayewski, R. J., and Hyde, R. W. (1988). Effects of posture on stimulated ventilation in quadriplegia. *Am. Rev. Respir. Dis.* 138: 101–105.

McKenzie, D. K., and Gandevia, S. C. (1986). Changes in human diaphragmatic electromyogram with positive pressure breathing. *Neurosci. Lett.* 70: 86–90.

Mead, J. (1981). Mechanics of the chest wall. *Adv. Physiol. Sci.* 10: 3–11.

Newman, S. L., Road, J. D., and Grassino, A. (1986). In vivo length and shortening of canine diaphragm with body postural change. *J. Appl. Physiol.* 60: 661–669.

Pengelly, L. D., Alderson, A. M., and Milic, E. J. (1971). Mechanics of the diaphragm. *J. Appl. Physiol.* 30: 797–805.

Reid, M. B., Banzett, R. B., Feldman, H. A., and Mead, J. (1985). Reflex compensation of spontaneous breathing when immersion changes diaphragm length. *J. Appl. Physiol.* 58: 1136–1142.

Revelette, R., Reynolds, S., Brown, D., and Taylor, R. (1992). Effect of abdominal compression on diaphragmatic tendon organ activity. *J. Appl. Physiol.* 72: 288–292.

Road, J. D., and Leevers, A. M. (1988). Effect of lung inflation on diaphragm shortening. *J. Appl. Physiol.* 65: 2383–2389.

Speck, D. F., and Revelette, W. R. (1987). Attenuation of phrenic motor discharge by phrenic nerve afferents. *J. Appl. Physiol.* 62: 941–945.

Stark, A. R., Waggener, T. B., Frantz, I., Cohlan, B. A., Feldman, H. A., and Kosch, P. C. (1984). Effect on ventilation of change to the upright posture in newborn infants. *J. Appl. Physiol.* 56: 64–71.

Strohl, K. P., Mead, J., Banzett, R. B., Lehr, J., Loring, S. H., and O'Cain, C. F. (1984). Effect of posture on upper and lower rib cage motion and tidal volume during diaphragm pacing. *Am. Rev. Respir. Dis.* 130: 320–321.

Teitlebaum, J., Borel, C. O., Magder, S., Traystman, R. J., and Hussain, S. N. A. (1993). Effect of selective diaphragmatic paralysis on the inspiratory motor drive. *J. Appl. Physiol.* 74: 2261–2268.

van Lunteren, E., Haxhiu, M. A., Cherniack, N. S., and Goldman, M. D. (1985). Differential costal and crural diaphragm compensation for posture changes. *J. Appl. Physiol.* 58: 1895–1900.

34

The Neuropharmacology of Central Fatigue in Respiratory Control

ANTHONY T. SCARDELLA and NORMAN H. EDELMAN

University of Medicine and Dentistry of New Jersey
Robert Wood Johnson Medical School
New Brunswick, New Jersey

I. Introduction

Fatigue of the neuromuscular system has been defined as the inability of a muscle or muscle groups to sustain the required or expected force (Asmussen, 1979). This phenomenon can occur at, at least, three sites (Bigland-Ritchie and Woods, 1984): failure of the central nervous system to provide adequate motor drive for a given command; failure of transmission at the neuromuscular junction; failure of the contractile process itself. The focus of most of investigations into the causes and consequences of neuromuscular fatigue has centered on processes occurring within the muscle itself (peripheral fatigue; Porter and Whelan, 1981). It has been long recognized, however, that "central fatigue" may also play a role in the reduction in force output seen during fatiguing exercise of skeletal muscle (Merton, 1954). For purposes of this discussion *central fatigue*, as defined by Bigland-Ritchie and Woods (1984), refers to conditions under which a decline in force output can be ascribed to a level of motor drive inadequate to sufficiently activate the muscle (i.e., to achieve the effect of a given command). In addition to the demonstration of central fatigue in limb skeletal muscle, Bellemare and Bigland-Ritchie (1987) demonstrated the occurrence of central fatigue in the diaphragm. The purpose of this discussion will be to define the concept of central fatigue, examine the proposed relation between skeletal muscle metabolism and central fatigue, and explore the relation between central fatigue in unanesthetized animals and activation of endogenous opioid pathways.

II. Central Fatigue of the Neuromuscular System

A. Central Components of Diaphragm Fatigue

Bellemare and Bigland-Ritchie (1987) tested whether, following repetitive contractions of the diaphragm in normal human subjects to the limits of its endurance, the nervous system would be able to fully activate the diaphragm in response to a command for maximal voluntary effort. For this purpose they employed the method of twitch occlusion (Bellemare and Bigland-Ritchie, 1984). This method examines the transdiaphragmatic pressure (Pdi) response to bilateral phrenic nerve stimulation superimposed on graded voluntary contractions of the diaphragm. The amplitude of Pdi twitches in response to phrenic nerve stimulation decreases as the voluntary Pdi increases. During maximal voluntary contractions of the diaphragm (Pdimax), no superimposed twitches can to be detected. A stylized representation of the expected result using this method is shown in Figure 1.

Diaphragm fatigue was induced by repetitive contractions of the diaphragm, loaded by either inspiratory resistive loads at 50 and 30% of Pdimax, or by expulsive contractions against a bound abdominal wall. Resistive or expulsive contractions were continued until either the target Pdi could no longer be sustained, or for a

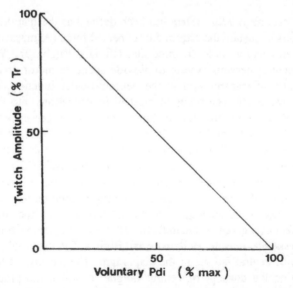

Figure 1   The relation between voluntary Pdimax and the superimposed twitch amplitude (expressed as a percentage of the twitch amplitude of the relaxed diaphragm, Tr). As voluntary Pdimax increases, the magnitude of the superimposed twitch decreases.

maximum of 30–45 min. During loading, single bilateral phrenic shocks were administered during (Ts) and between (Tr) contractions. Single shocks were also administered during voluntary Pdimax contractions. At the start of the experiment, central respiratory drive was able to fully activate the diaphragm, since no superimposed twitches could be detected during Pdimax contractions, a finding consistent with their previous study (Bellemare and Bigland-Ritchie, 1984). During the course of loaded breathing the degree to which the full muscle activation could be achieved decreased, as evidenced by the finding that superimposed twitches could be demonstrated at the limits of endurance when each contraction involved a maximal effort on the part of the subject. At the limits of diaphragm endurance, voluntary Pdimax had decreased by 50%, whereas the Pdimax estimated from the twitch occlusion had decreased by only 25%. A representation modified from the original data depicting the major finding of this study is shown in Figure 2. The

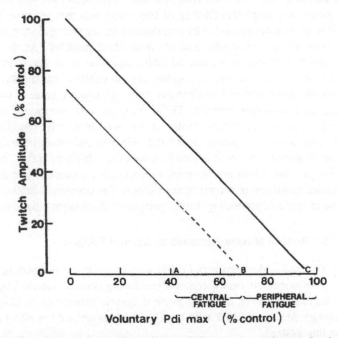

Figure 2 The relation between the voluntary Pdimax and superimposed twitch amplitude during control experiments performed before loading (upper line) and during loading after the limits of endurance had been reached (lower line). The contribution of central fatigue to the decrease in Pdimax is represented by the difference between the actual and predicted Pdimax following loading (difference between points A and B). The contribution of peripheral fatigue is represented by the difference between predicted Pdimax during loading and control voluntary Pdimax (difference between points B and C). (Adapted from the data of Bellemare and Bigland-Ritchie, 1987.)

difference between the point where the lower line (generated after the limit of endurance was reached) intersects the x-axis (predicted voluntary Pdimax if the diaphragm were fully activated, point B) and the actual maximal voluntary Pdi (point A) represents the contribution of the lack of central drive in generating Pdimax (the difference between points A and B). The difference between the point where the upper line (generated during control measurements before the fatigue experiments) intersects the x-axis, the unfatigued Pdimax (point C), and the point where the lower line intersects the x-axis (point B) represents the contribution of peripheral muscle fatigue to the generation of Pdimax (the difference between points B and C). The presence of peripheral muscle fatigue was also demonstrated by the finding that there was a significant decline in the twitch amplitude of stimulations performed while the diaphragm was relaxed (Tr). Thus, this study showed that at the limits of diaphragm endurance, even though peripheral diaphragm fatigue was present, a significant portion of the reduction in the force-generating capacity of the diaphragm was due to failure of the central nervous system to completely activate this muscle.

One potentially important finding of this study was that resistive loading in these experiments was accompanied by increases in the measured electromyographic (EMG) activity of the intercostal and sternomastoid muscles. At the limits of endurance, intercostal and sternomastoid EMG activities were approximately 300 and 500% of their control activities, respectively. In contrast, the diaphragm EMG at the limits of endurance was unchanged from its control values, which were recorded during a voluntary Pdimax. These findings were interpreted to indicate that the reduction in respiratory motor drive was relatively specific for the diaphragm. One possible explanation for the selective reduction in central motor output to the diaphragm is that it is due to a specific inhibitory reflex, originating in the diaphragm, that results in a decrease in respiratory motor drive to this muscle and not a global reduction in central motor output. The potential adaptive nature of this response in terms of preventing further peripheral diaphragm fatigue is apparent.

B.   The Role of Muscle Ischemia in Central Fatigue

A study by Garland and co-workers (1988) sought to define the peripheral signal resulting in the reduction in central motor drive during skeletal muscle fatigue. They tested the idea that low-level, indirect electrical muscle stimulation to fatigue would reduce voluntary force and EMG activity. They also examined the effect of muscle ischemia in this system.

In healthy subjects, stimulation of the ankle dorsiflexor muscles was performed to fatigue by repetitive stimulation of the peroneal nerve at 15 Hz. The muscles were kept ischemic by inflation of a blood pressure cuff to above arterial pressure. The method of twitch occlusion was used to assess the peripheral and central components of fatigue: When 15-Hz tetanic torque was reduced by 25%, the maximal voluntary torque was also significantly reduced. Unlike the findings of Bellemare and Bigland-Ritchie for the diaphragm, at this time point the maximal voluntary integrated EMG was also reduced. The reduction in EMG activity and maximal voluntary torque persisted as long as the cuff remained inflated, but recovered rapidly after release of the pressure in the cuff. This study shows that potentially fatiguing muscle contractions can result in reductions in both voluntary force and EMG activity and that this effect was potentiated by muscle ischemia.

In a similar experiment, Bigland-Ritchie and colleagues (1986) induced fatigue of the biceps brachii using sustained maximal voluntary contractions (mvc) of 20 s. To occlude biceps brachii blood flow, studies were performed with a blood pressure cuff both inflated and deflated: Motoneuron discharge rates decreased progressively during the 20-s maximal contraction. Following a 3-min rest with the blood supply, intact motoneuron discharge rates recovered to 95% of their initial value. When the blood supply was occluded between a first and second mvc, motoneuron discharge rates remained decreased. Since recovery was rapid after restoration of blood supply, the authors concluded that the reduction in EMG must be due to a peripheral reflex generated in response to changes within the muscle caused by peripheral fatigue.

C. The Role of Thin-Fiber Afferents in Reductions in Central Motor Output

Two studies have examined the reflex nature of the decrease in respiratory motor output in response to stimulation of thin-fiber muscle afferents (Jammes et al., 1986; Kumazawa and Tadaki, 1983). In anesthetized, paralyzed, vagotomized, and mechanically ventilated cats, Jammes and colleagues (1986) selectively stimulated small-fiber (group III and IV) phrenic afferents. During repetitive stimulation of these afferents, they found reduced phrenic impulse frequency and firing time of the motor phrenic discharge, which recovered to control values when stimulation was stopped. In a similar preparation, Kumazawa and Tadaki (1983) examined the respiratory response to gastrocnemius nerve stimulation. Stimulation of thin-fiber afferents resulted in an immediate suppression of phrenic nerve activity and a delayed phase of suppression that occurred several minutes after the cessation of stimulation. The ability of thin muscle fiber afferents to also respond to metabolic by-products is well known and has been reviewed elsewhere (Rotto and Kaufman, 1988).

In summary, central fatigue of the neuromuscular system can be demonstrated to occur under conditions for which peripheral fatigue is likely or is present. Central fatigue has been described in both limb skeletal muscle and diaphragm. Studies in limb skeletal muscle have shown that central fatigue may result in reductions in both voluntary force generation and EMG activity. These studies have also suggested that central fatigue may occur as a result of events related to the accumulation of by-products of metabolism generated during fatiguing contractions, as this phenomenon is potentiated by muscle ischemia and rapidly reverses after restoration of blood flow. Reductions in respiratory motor output may also occur as a consequence of electrical stimulation of group III and IV afferent nerves. Finally, in central fatigue of the diaphragm, this reflex may be relatively specific and not the result of a global inhibition, as other respiratory muscles increase their activity at a time when inhibition of the diaphragm can be demonstrated.

III. Endogenous Opioid Pathways

The respiratory depressant effects of opiate drugs, such as morphine and meperidine, have been well described (Weil et al., 1975; Santiago et al., 1980; Kryger et al., 1976). The discovery of endogenous opioid receptors and ligands in the brain stem led to the speculation that these peptides might also be involved in ventilatory control (Atweh and Kuhar, 1983). High concentrations of opiate ligands and receptors have been demonstrated in the nucleus tractus solitarius (NTS) and nucleus ambiguus (Santiago and Edelman, 1985). β-Endorphin and corticotropin (adrenocorticotropic hormone; ACTH) have been isolated from the NTS of rats and guinea pigs, with use of cation-exchange chromatography and radioimmunoassay (Dores et al., 1986). It has been further demonstrated that cell bodies in this region are the major source of proopiomelanocortin (POMC), the common precursor of these peptides (Dores et al., 1986). The effect of endogenous opioids on neurons in all brain regions is depression of spontaneous activity (Bloom, 1983). In some cases, these effects have been due to membrane hyperpolarization (Bloom, 1983; Johnson and North, 1992).

The presence of endogenous opioid receptors and ligands in areas of the brain associated with ventilatory control led to investigations of the possible role of these peptides in ventilatory control in humans. An early study by Santiago and colleagues (1981) demonstrated that the opioid antagonist naloxone could restore the flow-resistive load compensation reflex in those patients with chronic obstructive pulmonary disease (COPD) in whom it was initially absent. They postulated that, in these patients, endogenous opioids were elaborated in response to the stress of a permanently increased airway resistance, and this resulted in attenuation of the respiratory compensation for the increased airway resistance, perhaps as a mechanism by which the sense of dyspnea in these patients might be reduced. We have had the opportunity to extend these findings and hypotheses by studing the effects of endogenous opioid elaboration on central respiratory output in an unanesthetized animal model.

All the studies cited in the following were performed in permanently instrumented male goats at least 1 week following surgery. Only one loading protocol was performed on each day. An inspiratory flow-resistive load composed of fine wire mesh disks was used in each study. During all studies 25% O_2 was given to prevent hypoxemia.

A. The Effect of an Inspiratory Load on the Immediate Ventilatory Response and on Cerebrospinal Fluid Levels of β-Endorphin

We attempted to extend the observations of Santiago and co-workers (1981) on elaboration of endogenous opioids in response to increased airway resistance and, in this study, tested the hypothesis that relatively short-term, but high-intensity, flow-resistive loading would be sufficient to activate the endogenous opioid system and modify the subsequent respiratory response (Scardella et al., 1986). We exposed unanesthetized goats to 2.5 h of inspiratory flow-resistive loading at two levels (50 and 80 cm H_2O L^{-1} s^{-1}) on separate days. Endogenous opioid effects were assessed by intravenous administration of naloxone (NLX: 0.1 mg/kg) at the conclusion of the loading period. Control studies (experimental situation, but no load imposed, followed by NLX) were also performed. To directly test for endogenous opioid elaboration in this model, we measured immunoreactive β-endorphin in the cisternal cerebrospinal fluid (CSF). The effect of an 80 cm H_2O L^{-1} s^{-1} inspiratory load and NLX on tidal volume (VT) is shown in Figure 3. Tidal volume fell significantly during loading to a mean of 82.5 ± 7.5 SEM% of the baseline value at 2.5 h. Administration of NLX increased tidal volume significantly, but transiently, after its administration, whereas saline administration had no effect. The effect of inspiratory loading and NLX during the studies with the lower load were similar, but smaller in magnitude.

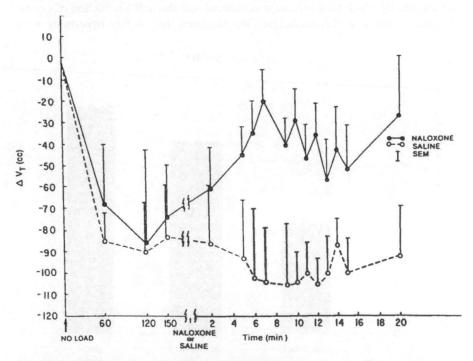

Figure 3 Tidal volume response to 2.5 h of high inspiratory flow-resistive loading before and following the administration of naloxone. The tidal volume decrease associated with loading is partially reversed by naloxone. (Note the change in time scale on the *x* axis.) Closed circles, naloxone; open circles, saline control.

The CSF β-endorphin levels in each of the unloaded and loaded experiments are shown in Figure 4. β-Endorphin immunoreactivity was higher in either of the two loading conditions than in the unloaded control. β-Endorphin levels tended to be higher with the 80 cm H_2O L^{-1} s^{-1} load than with the lower load and were linearly related to the relative minimum tidal volume after the first 30 min of loading.

These data support the hypothesis of Santiago and colleagues that an increase in airway resistance can activate the endogenous opioid system. Furthermore, the increase in tidal volume immediately following NLX during short-term, inspiratory loading suggests that these potentially fatiguing, flow-resistive loads reduce tidal volume, before the onset of overt muscle fatigue, by a mechanism that, in addition to the direct mechanical effect of the load, involves the endogenous opioid system.

B. The Effect of Endogenous Opioids on Abdominal Muscle Activity During Inspiratory Loading

From our initial finding that activation of the endogenous opioid system attenuates the tidal volume response during inspiratory loading, we postulated that the mechanism by which tidal volume was reduced was through a reduction of central respiratory output to the diaphragm. We reasoned that, if this hypothesis were

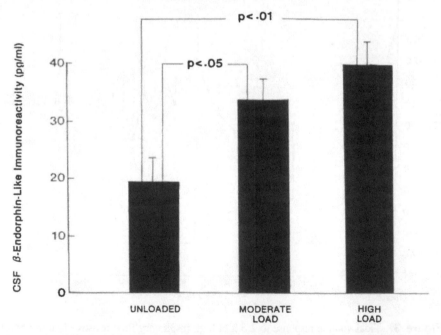

Figure 4 β-Endorphin-like immunoreactivity in cisternal CSF in control (unloaded) and under two loading conditions. β-Endorphin immunoreactivity was significantly increased with the moderate ($p < 0.05$) and high ($p < 0.01$) loads when compared with the unloaded state.

correct, a constant infusion of naloxone (NLX) during the loading period would increase ventilation, relative to loading without NLX, by increasing respiratory output to the diaphragm. In addition, we hypothesized that the increase in diaphragm activity might predispose it to fatigue (Scardella et al., 1989).

Fifteen minutes before the imposition of a 120 cm H_2O L^{-1} s^{-1} inspiratory load, NLX (0.1 mg/kg) was given intravenously and repeated every 15 min thereafter. Loading was maintained for 4 h. Figure 5 shows the mean tidal volume and frequency response to loading, with and without (saline control), a continuous NLX infusion. In the control animals, the load caused a sustained reduction in tidal volume, similar to that seen in the previous study (Scardella et al., 1986). During NLX infusion, loading was not accompanied by a reduction in tidal volume, which remained significantly above its baseline for 2 h. As expected, transdiaphragmatic pressure was significantly greater during NLX than in the saline control. However, the increase in diaphragmatic EMG (EMGdi) following loading was not different

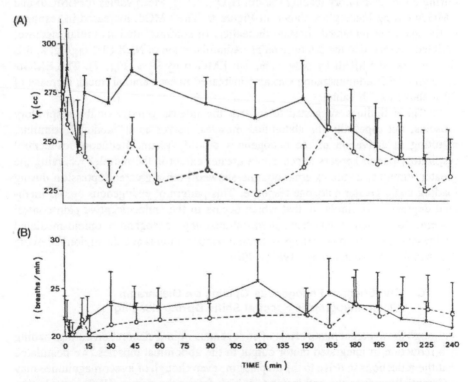

Figure 5 Tidal volume (A) and frequency (B) response during 4 h of inspiratory loading. Loading resulted in tidal volume depression in the saline group. It did not fall during NLX administration and was significantly above that of saline up to 2.5 h. (Open circles, saline; X, naloxone.)

between saline and NLX studies. No evidence of diaphragm fatigue was present, as assessed by spectral analysis of the diaphragm EMG performed by examination of the high/low ratio. We did note a greater end-expiratory gastric pressure during loading in the animals given NLX, implying increased activity of the abdominal muscles. An additional important finding of this study included the observation that, although ventilation was greater in the NLX group for the initial 2 h of loading, Pco_2 did not differ between the two groups. Thus, the greater ventilation during NLX was offset by a greater CO_2 production, again supporting the idea that endogenous opioids play an adaptive role in terms of overall energy expenditure of the respiratory muscles.

Since EMGdi did not appear to be greater during loading with a continuous NLX infusion, we investigated the possible role of activation of the endogenous opioid system in selective inhibition of the abdominal muscles (Scardella et al., 1990). The EMGdi and the EMG activity of two abdominal muscles, the external oblique EMG (EMGeo) and transversus abdominis EMG (EMGta), were monitored during 3 h of inspiratory loading (50 cm H_2O L^{-1} s^{-1}). Mean values for EMGdi and EMGeo during loading are shown in Figure 6. The EMGdi increased in response to the load, but remained constant thereafter. In contrast, after its initial increase, EMGeo decreased at the 3-h time point. Administration of NLX (0.1 mg/kg) at this time increased EMGdi by only 15%, but EMGeo by 91% (Fig. 7). The EMGta following NLX administration was also increased in each animal (mean increase of 30% above its 3-h value).

These findings suggested to us that the intense activity of the respiratory muscles, but especially the abdominal muscles, serves as a "noxious" stimulus, resulting in activation of the endogenous opioid system. Reduction of central respiratory output appears to occur to a greater extent in the muscles receiving the greater stimulus, as the external oblique showed both a greater depression during loading and a greater naloxone response. This pattern of endogenous opioid-mediated depression is similar to that which occurs in the antinociceptive pain control system, for which it has been demonstrated that endogenous opioid-mediated analgesia is specific to both the peripheral noxious stimulus and the region receiving the stimulus (Scardella et al., 1989, 1990).

C. The Effect of Endogenous Opioids on Diaphragm Electromyographic Spectral Shifts During Loading

Although the apparent major effect of endogenous opioid elaboration during loading is a reduction in integrated motor output to the abdominal muscles, we postulated that the reductions in drive to the diaphragm, even though of lesser magnitude, may differentially reduce the end-inspiratory high-frequency power (HFP) contribution to the diaphragmatic EMG (EMGdi) power spectrum (Petrozzino et al., 1990). We based this hypothesis on the finding that, during inspiration, there exists an orderly discharge pattern of phrenic motoneurons from low- to high-frequency, with the

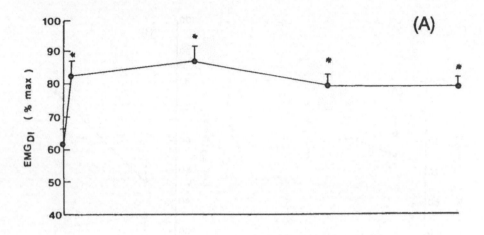

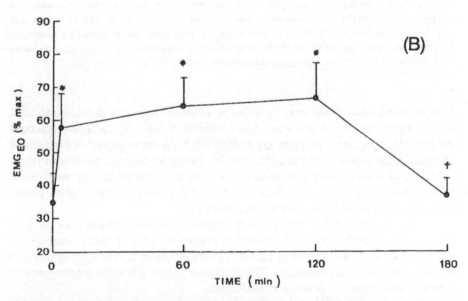

Figure 6 EMGdi (A) and EMGeo (B) during 3 h of inspiratory loading. The EMGdi increased in response to the load and was significantly above baseline for all 3 h. The EMGeo increased immediately and was significantly above baseline until 180 min, when it decreased. (*$p < 0.05$ vs. baseline; + $p < 0.05$ vs. 120 min.)

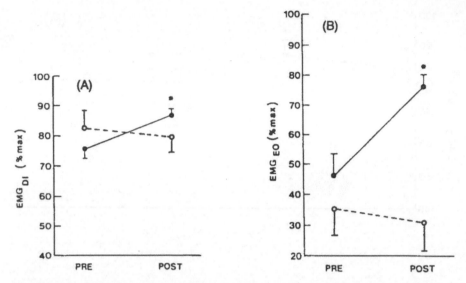

Figure 7 The EMGdi (A) and EMGeo (B) at 180 min of loading (PRE) and after 0.1 mg/kg naloxone (POST). After naloxone administration, the increase in EMGdi (15%) was significantly greater ($p < 0.05$) than after saline because each animal showed a response. Note the large increase in EMGeo (91%) after naloxone administration compared with saline ($p < 0.05$). Closed circles, naloxone; open circles, saline. (*$p < 0.05$ vs. PRE.)

later-recruited units being more sensitive to either increases or decreases in total neural input than the earlier ones. Since coherence between the power spectral content of the phrenic neurogram and EMGdi has been demonstrated, we examined changes in the power spectrum of the EMGdi during loading and postulated that a reduction of overall motor unit activation is likely to be biased toward inactivation of high-frequency units, as reflected in the HFP content of the EMGdi power spectrum, thereby reducing centroid frequency (f_c).

We recorded EMGdi during 3 h of inspiratory loading (50 cm H_2O L^{-1} s^{-1}). The effects of loading on f_c are shown in Figure 8. After an initial increase, f_c decreased throughout the loading period. The reduction in f_c was entirely due to a reduction in HFP to approximately 70% of its peak value early in the loading period, whereas low-frequency power was unaffected.

The effect of NLX (0.1 mg/kg) on f_c shown in Figure 9. As previously shown, f_c had decreased significantly by 180 min of loading. Administration of NLX completely reversed the decrease in f_c, whereas saline administration had no effect.

The findings of this study suggest that spectral shifts in EMGdi in this model arise from alterations mediated by the central nervous system (CNS). These observations raise the possibility that part of the reduction in centroid frequency

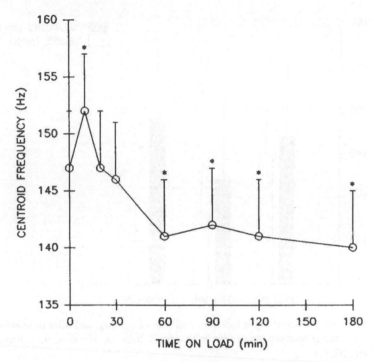

Figure 8 The change in f_c (expressed in Hz) during 180 min of loading. After an initial increase (T_{peak}), f_c decreased significantly throughout the loading period. (*$p < 0.05$ vs. baseline.)

associated with daphragmatic fatigue may result from reductions in central respiratory output associated with elaboration of endogenous opioids.

D. The Relation Between Respiratory Muscle Lactic Acidosis and Endogenous Opioid Activity During Inspiratory Loading

We next sought to define the peripheral stimulus that would activate the endogenous opioid system in a manner that was both linked to muscle activity and would result in differential reduction in respiratory output to the diaphragm and abdominal muscles. Since lactic acid is a metabolic by-product related to intense muscle activity and is a strong stimulant of afferent (group III and IV) fibers that can signal the release of endogenous opioids, we hypothesized that lactic acid is the stimulus that triggers their release during loading (Kumazawa et al., 1985; Petrozzino et al., 1992).

During 2 h of inspiratory loading (50 cm H_2O L^{-1} s^{-1}), goats were exposed to a constant infusion of either saline or dichloroacetate (DCA), a compound that enhances the activity of pyruvate dehydrogenase and, thereby, lessens the production of lactic acid (McAllister et al., 1973). Figure 10 shows the response to naloxone

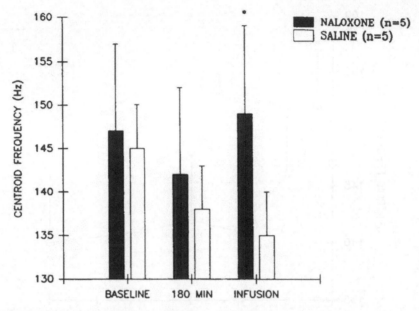

Figure 9 Centroid frequency at baseline, 180 min of loading, and after infusion of NLX or saline. Naloxone reversed the decline in f_c. (*$p < 0.05$ vs. 180 min; open bars, saline; closed bars, NLX.)

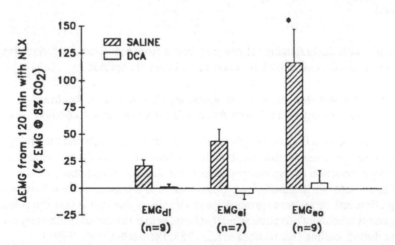

Figure 10 The EMG responses to NLX administration after 120 min of loading, with saline or DCA. With saline NLX caused an increase in all EMGs; DCA blocked the NLX response. (Open bars, DCA; hatched bars, saline; *$p < 0.05$ vs. EMGdi.)

(NLX, 0.3 mg/kg) given at the conclusion of the loading period. In the goats given saline, NLX significantly increased both EMGdi and EMGeo (as well as external intercostal EMG). Consistent with our previous findings, the greatest response was in the external oblique. Infusion of DCA completely blocked the NLX effect on respiratory activity, suggesting that lactic acid is the stimulus signaling the activation of the endogenous opioid system.

If increased respiratory muscle lactic acid is the peripheral stimulus that activates the endogenous opioid system, then a greater decrease in pH in the external oblique compared with the diaphragm may account for the differential reduction in its activity during loading. We measured interstitial pH in the external oblique (pHeo) and diaphragm (pHdi), during 2 h of inspiratory loading (50 cm H_2O L^{-1} s^{-1}) in unanesthetized goats, with flexible glass pH electrodes. Figure 11 shows the change in pHdi and pHeo from baseline during 2 h of loading. A greater decrease in pHeo compared with pHdi was noted throughout the loading period. A continuous infusion of DCA completely blocked the decrease in pHdi (Fig. 12) and significantly attenuated the decrease in pHeo (Fig. 13). From this study, we concluded that the reduction in central respiratory output secondary to increased endogenous opioid activity is linked to lactic acid accumulation (and pH fall) in the respiratory muscles.

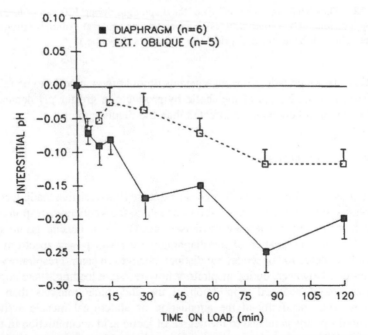

Figure 11 The change in interstitial pH of the diaphragm and external oblique during 120 min of loading. There was a greater decrease in pHeo compared with pHdi throughout loading.

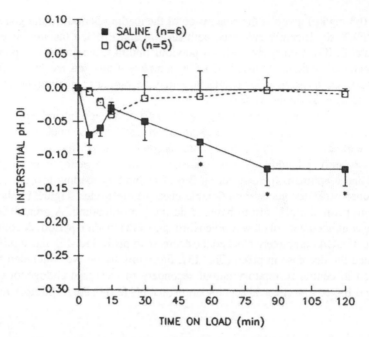

Figure 12   The change in interstitial pH of the diaphragm during 120 min of loading with a constant infusion of DCA (open squares) or saline (closed squares). Administration of DCA completely blocked the decrease in pHdi. (*$p < 0.05$ vs. baseline.)

In addition, the magnitude of the endogenous opioid effect appears to be related to the degree of accumulation of metabolic by-products (a greater pH decrease), in that the external oblique is more affected than the diaphragm.

IV.   Conclusions

In unanesthetized animals, acute, intense inspiratory flow-resistive loading activates endogenous opioid pathways that serve to attenuate the ventilatory response to the load by reducing overall respiratory muscle activity in a muscle group-specific manner. Careful examination of the diaphragmatic EMG power spectrum during loading allows detection of subtle, but distinct, changes in central respiratory output to this muscle. However, during inspiratory flow-resistive loading, there appears to be greater opioid-mediated suppression of the abdominal muscles than of the diaphragm. The specificity of the attenuation of abdominal muscle activity by endognenous opioids is related to the degree of lactic acid accumulation in the two muscles. Two lines of evidence support this concept. First, dichloroacetate blocks the naloxone-mediated increase in respiratory muscle activity during loading and,

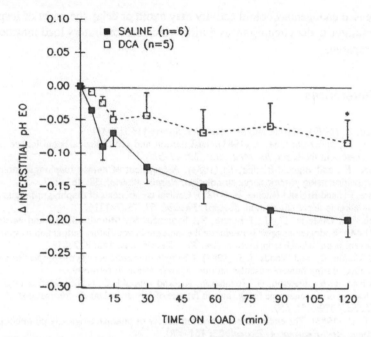

Figure 13   The change in interstitial pH of the external oblique during 120 min of loading, with a constant infusion of DCA (open squares) or saline (closed squares). Administration of DCA significantly attenuated the decrease in pHeo during loading.

second, the decrease in interstitial pH during loading is greater in the external oblique abdominal muscle than in the diaphragm. Finally, activation of the endogenous opioid system during inspiratory loading appears to be adaptive, since the increase in ventilation following naloxone administration is not accompanied by a reduction in arterial P_{CO_2}. That is, inefficient excess muscle contraction is avoided, probably delaying the onset of overt peripheral muscle fatigue. This pattern of endogenous opioid-mediated suppression is similar to the pattern that occurs in the endogenous opioid antinociceptive pain control system. In such studies, analgesia is specific for both the type of peripheral noxious stimulus and the region that receives the stimulus.

   Does this phenomenon occur in humans? One possible example of endogenous opioid activation in the face of an increased respiratory load in humans was recently described by Bellofiore and co-workers (1990). In asthmatics with methacholine-induced severe reductions in FEV_1, naloxone pretreatment resulted in an increased breathing frequency, occlusion pressure, and mean inspiratory flow rate when compared to saline pretreatment. These findings suggest that, similar to our findings in the unanesthetized goat, endogenous opioid pathways are activated in response to the acute increase in airway resistance, reducing overall ventilatory output. Our findings would suggest that reduction in respiratory muscle activity in the presence of increased endogenous opioid activity may avoid or delay the onset of respiratory muscle fatigue under circumstances during which the respiratory load may be severe or inescapable.

References

Asmussen, E. (1979). Muscle fatigue. *Med. Sci. Sports* 11: 313–321.

Atweh, S. F., and Kuhar, M. J. (1983). Distribution and physiological significance of opioid receptors in the brain. *Br. Med. Bull.* 39: 47–52.

Bellemare, F., and Bigland-Ritchie, B. (1984). Assessment of human diaphragm strength and activation using phrenic nerve stimulation. *Respir. Physiol.* 58: 263–277.

Bellemare, F., and Bigland-Ritchie, B. (1987). Central components of diaphragm fatigue assessed by phrenic nerve stimulation. *J. Appl. Physiol.* 62: 1307–1316.

Bellofiore, S., DiMaria, G. U., Privitera, S,, Sapienza, S., Milic-Emili, J., and Mistretta, A. (1990). Endogenous opioids modulate the increase in ventilatory output and dyspnea during severe acute bronchoconstriction. *Am. Rev. Respir. Dis.* 142: 812–816.

Bigland-Ritchie, B., and Woods, J. J. (1984). Changes in muscle contractile properties and neural control during human muscular fatigue. *Muscle Nerve* 7: 691–699.

Bigland-Ritchie, B., Dawson, N., Johansson, R., and Lippold, O. (1986). Reflex origin for the slowing of motoneurone firing rates in fatigue of human voluntary contractions. *J. Physiol.* (*Lond.*) 379: 451–459.

Bloom, F. E. (1983). The endorphins: A growing family of pharmacologically pertinent peptides. *Annu. Rev. Pharmacol. Toxicol.* 23: 151–170.

Dores, R. M., Jain, M., and Akil, H. (1986). Characterization of the forms of β-endorphin and α-MSH in the caudal medulla of the rat and guinea pig. *Brain Res.* 377: 251–260.

Garland, J., Garner, S., and McComas, A. (1988). Reduced voluntary electromyographic activity after fatiguing stimulation of human muscle. *J. Physiol.* (*Lond.*) 401: 547–556.

Jammes, Y., Buchler, B., Delpierre, S., Rasidakis, A., Grimmaud, C., and Roussos, C. (1986). Phrenic afferents and their role in inspiratory control. *J. Appl. Physiol.* 60: 854–860.

Johnson, S. W., and North, R. A. (1992). Opioids excite dopamine neurons by hyperpolarization of local interneurons. *J. Neurosci.* 12: 483–488.

Kryger, M. H., Yacoub, O., Dosman, J., Macklem, P. T., and Anthonisen, N. R. (1976). Effect of meperidine on occlusion pressure responses to hypercapnia and hypoxia with and without external inspiratory resistance. *Am. Rev. Respir. Dis.* 114: 333–340.

Kumazawa, T., and Tadaki, E. (1983). Two different inhibitory effects on respiration by thin-fiber muscular afferents in cats. *Brain Res.* 272: 364–367.

Kumazawa, T., Eguchi, K., and Tadaki, E. (1985). Naloxone-reversible respiratory inhibition induced by muscular thin-fiber afferents in decerebrate cats. *Neurosci. Lett.* 53: 81–85.

McAllister, A., Allison, S. P., and Randle, P. J. (1973). Effects of dichloroacetate on the metabolism of glucose, pyruvate, acetate, 3-hydroxybutyrate and palmitate in rat diaphragm and heart muscle in vitro and on extraction of glucose, lactate, pyruvate and free fatty acids by dog heart in vivo. *Biochem. J.* 134: 1067–1081.

Merton, P. (1954). Voluntary strength and fatigue. *J. Physiol.* (*Lond.*) 128: 553–564.

Petrozzino, J. J., Scardella, A. T., Li, J-K. J., Krawciw, N., Edelman, N. H., and Santiago, T. V. (1990). Effect of naloxone on spectral shifts of the diaphragm EMG during inspiratory loading. *J. Appl. Physiol.* 68: 1376–1385.

Petrozzino, J. J., Scardella, A. T., Santiago, T. V., and Edelman, N. H. (1992). Dichloroacetate blocks endogenous opioid effects during inspiratory flow-resistive loading. *J. Appl. Physiol.* 72: 590–596.

Porter, R., and Whelan, J. (eds.). Ciba Foundation Symposium 82 (1981). *Human Muscle Fatigue: Physiological Mechanisms*. London, Pitman Medical.

Rotto, D., and Kaufman, M. (1988). Effect of metabolic products of muscular contraction on discharge of group III and IV afferents. *J. Appl. Physiol.* 64: 2306–2313.

Santiago, T. V., and Edelman, N. H. (1985). Opioids and breathing. *J. Appl. Physiol.* 59: 1675–1685.

Santiago, T. V., Goldblatt, K., Winters, K., Pugliese, A., and Edelman, N. H. (1980). Respiratory consequences of methadone: The response to added resistance to breathing. *Am. Rev. Respir. Dis.* 122: 623–628.

Santiago, T. V., Remolina, C., Scoles, V., and Edelman, N. H. (1981). Endorphins and control of breathing: Ability of naloxone to restore the impaired flow-resistive load compensation in chronic obstructive pulmonary disease. *N. Engl. J. Med.* 304: 1190–1195.

Scardella, A. T., Parisi, R. A., Phair, D. K., Santiago, T. V., and Edelman, N. H. (1986). The role of endogenous opioids in the ventilatory response to acute flow-resistive loads. *Am. Rev. Respir. Dis.* 133: 26–31.

Scardella, A. T., Santiago, T. V., and Edelman, N. H. (1989). Naloxone alters the early response to an inspiratory flow-resistive load. *J. Appl. Physiol.* 67: 1747–1753.

Scardella, A. T., Petrozzino, J. J., Mandel, M., Edelman, N. H., and Santiago, T. V. (1990). Endogenous opioid effects on abdominal muscle activity during inspiratory loading. *J. Appl. Physiol.* 69: 1104–1109.

Weil, J. V., McCullough, R. E., Kline, J. S., and Sodal, I. E. (1975). Diminished ventilatory response to hypoxia and hypercapnia after morphine in normal man. *N. Engl. J. Med.* 292: 1103–1106.

T - #0227 - 101024 - C0 - 229/152/58 [60] - CB - 9780824795047 - Gloss Lamination